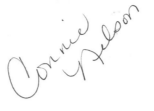

P9-CBE-319

Pharmacology:

Drug Therapy and

Nursing

Considerations

Contributors:

Zoriana Kawka Malseed, Ph.D.
Associate Professor of Anatomy and Physiology,
University of Pennsylvania School of Nursing,
Philadelphia, Pennsylvania

Freddy Grimm, M.S., Pharm.D.
Director, Outpatient Pharmacy,
Hospital of the University of Pennsylvania;
Clinical Assistant Professor,
Philadelphia College of Pharmacy and Science,
Philadelphia, Pennsylvania

Consultants:

Marie Brandt Andrews, R.N., M.S.
Nursing Lecturer, Texas Woman's University
College of Nursing at Houston,
Houston, Texas

Ruth M. Steinfurth Harboe, R.N., B.S., M.S.
Assistant Professor, University of Colorado
School of Nursing, University of Colorado
Health Sciences Center,
Denver, Colorado

Martha M. Lamberton, R.N., M.S.N.
Assistant Head Nurse, Northwest Institute of Psychiatry,
Fort Washington, Pennsylvania

Michael Reichgott, M.D., Ph.D.
Medical Director, Bronx Municipal Hospital Center;
Associate Professor of Medicine,
Albert Einstein College of Medicine,
Bronx, New York

Pharmacology

Drug Therapy and Nursing Considerations

Second Edition

Roger T. Malseed, Ph.D.

Adjunct Associate Professor of Pharmacology,
University of Pennsylvania School of Nursing and
Philadelphia College of Pharmacy and Science
Philadelphia, Pennsylvania

J. B. Lippincott Company   Philadelphia
London   Mexico City   New York
St. Louis   São Paulo   Sydney

Sponsoring Editor: David T. Miller/Joyce Mkitarian
Manuscript Editor: Virginia M. Barishek
Indexer: Ruth Low
Art Director and Designer: Tracy Baldwin
Design Coordinator: Earl Gerhart
Production Supervisor: N. Carolyn Kerr
Production Assistant: Don Wilby
Compositor: Tapsco, Inc.
Printer/Binder: The Murray Printing Company

Second Edition

6 5 4 3

Library of Congress Cataloging in Publication Data

Malseed, Roger T. (Roger Thomas)
    Pharmacology, drug therapy and nursing considerations.

    Bibliography: p.
    Includes index.
    1. Pharmacology. 2. Nursing. I. Title.
[DNLM: 1. Drug Therapy—nurses' instruction.
2. Pharmacology—nurses' instruction.   QV 4 M259p]
RM300.M183 1985   615.7'024613   84-20169
ISBN 0-397-54460-X

The author and publisher have exerted every effort to ensure
that drug selection and dosage set forth in this text are in
accord with current recommendations and practice at the
time of publication. However, in view of ongoing research,
changes in government regulations, and the constant flow
of information relating to drug therapy and drug reactions,
the reader is urged to check the package insert for each
drug for any change in indications and dosage and for added
warnings and precautions. This is particularly important when
the recommended agent is a new or infrequently employed
drug.

To my father,
  for taking so little
  and giving so much

Preface

The publication of the second edition of *Pharmacology: Drug Therapy and Nursing Considerations* only three years after the appearance of the first edition reflects the rapidly metamorphosing field of nursing pharmacology and the consequent need for a drug reference source to be current and topical. While retaining the general outline style and tabular format of the first edition, which has proven so successful in simplifying information retrieval and facilitating comparisons among similar drugs, the second edition contains many new drug entries, as well as discussions of several newer concepts of drug action, such as drug-induced changes in receptor sensitivity and differential activation of narcotic receptor sites. Newer methods for administering drugs, such as transdermal application, are given expanded consideration, and new uses, both approved and investigational, for many drugs are reviewed.

The increasing tendency toward multiple drug therapy, including over-the-counter medications, has resulted in a burgeoning of reports of heretofore unsuspected drug interactions. The increased potential of many drugs to interact with one another is noted throughout the text.

Knowledge of the pharmacokinetic profile of a drug can often be of considerable value in planning a dosage regimen and minimizing the danger of untoward reactions or treatment failures. To assist the reader in obtaining a greater understanding of the means by which many drugs are handled by the body, many new tables have been added (and others expanded) that compare the pharmacokinetic parameters of drugs such as beta-blockers, calcium-channel blockers, penicillins, cephalosporins, and antiarrhythmics.

As in the first edition, the physiology of the various organ systems is reviewed in the lead chapter in each part of the book. These physiology reviews have been further developed in certain areas to provide an even greater knowledge base for understanding the pharmacologic and toxicologic aspects of drug therapy. Likewise, the introductory section of the book, which deals with general principles of drug action, drug interactions, and pediatric and geriatric pharmacology, also has undergone some expansion.

Integral components of the book are the nursing alerts and nursing considerations. These have been expanded and thoroughly reviewed by the nurse–consultants for completeness and relevance. The consultants' contributions to the new edition are invaluable and are reflected in the comprehensive and germane nature of the nursing implications found throughout the text.

The wide acceptance of the first edition has been most gratifying to the author. Every effort has been made to present a second edition that is improved in many ways while at the same time retaining those features, such as extensive use of comparative tables, comprehensive nursing considerations, physiology reviews, listings of cancer chemotherapy regimens and anti-infective drugs of choice, that so many readers found so helpful. It is hoped that the second edition of this text will continue to evoke in its readers a genuine respect for both the potential good and the possible harm inherent in drug use. The nurse is in a unique position to ensure that drugs are properly used; and armed with sufficient knowledge, the nurse can play a vital role in safe and effective drug therapy. This book is an attempt to provide that knowledge base.

Roger T. Malseed, Ph.D.

Acknowledgments

The second edition of this book has come to fruition through the efforts of many people. I am greatly indebted to Joyce Mkitarian, who as editor was responsible for the overall development of the book. Her professionalism is evident in every aspect of her work, and the book is better for her efforts.

Mary Murphy coordinated the entire flow of events and expertly typed all the new sections of manuscript. Her efficiency is remarkable, and I am deeply appreciative of her efforts on my behalf.

Virginia Barishek, as manuscript editor, ably and efficiently coordinated the transition from manuscript to proofs to finished edition, and managed to keep the timetable on track. That alone deserves special commendation.

The entire J. B. Lippincott Company family has always been supportive of my work and their continued interest is most satisfying. In particular, David T. Miller, Vice President and Editor, Nursing Division, has consistently offered his wisdom and encouragement, and the insight he brings to publishing is invaluable.

Finally, I am deeply grateful to my wife and children for their patience, tolerance, and support.

Contents

Pharmacology:
Drug Therapy and
Nursing
Considerations

General Principles
of Pharmacology

Drugs may be administered by several different routes, largely determined by the intended site of action, the rapidity and duration of effect desired, and the chemical and physical properties of the drug itself. *Route of administration* is one of the most important factors influencing the effects of a drug. Some drugs may exert widely differing actions depending on their routes of administration. For example, diazoxide is a potent, rapidly acting antihypertensive agent when given IV, but following its oral ingestion, it inhibits the release of insulin from the pancreas with minimal effects on blood pressure. Magnesium sulfate is a laxative when taken orally, reduces swelling of joints when used as a concentrated soak, and exerts powerful anticonvulsant effects when injected IV or IM.

Although some drugs can be used both locally and systemically, the majority of agents are employed by a single route of administration. We shall examine the various methods of drug administration and discuss the dosage forms most commonly employed with each route of administration.

Methods of Drug Administration

1

I Topical Application

Most topically applied drugs are intended for their local effects. Drugs may be applied topically to the skin or mucous membranes (oral, nasal, vaginal, urethral, anal), instilled into the eye or ear, or inhaled into the lungs.

A Dermatologic Application

Medications are applied to the skin in several forms: lotions, creams, ointments, sprays, and liquids (wet dressings, baths, soaks). Systemic effectiveness is greatly limited by the keratinized structure of the skin, which prevents absorption of significant amounts of most drugs. Absorption may be enhanced when drugs are applied to damaged skin (wounds, burns). Incorporation of the drug in a fatty vehicle (such as waxes or wool fat) or use of a keratolytic agent (such as salicylic acid) to break down the keratin layer may also increase absorption.

Major uses for dermatologically applied drugs are the following:

1 Antiseptic/anti-infective (antibiotics, antifungal agents, alcohol, hexachlorophene)
2 Anti-inflammatory (corticosteroids)
3 Astringent (aluminum acetate, zinc oxide)
4 Antipruritic (local anesthetics, antihistamines)
5 Emollient (vitamins A, D, and E, glycerin, lanolin, mineral oil)
6 Keratolytic (salicylic acid, resorcinol)
7 Vasodilator (nitroglycerin)

Dermatologically applied drugs may also be used as protectives, absorbents, counterirritants, and corrosives to aid in sloughing off or removing damaged tissue. Diseases commonly treated by local application of drugs to the skin surface include acne, psoriasis, allergic dermatoses, and topical infections. In addition, certain systemic conditions, such as angina, are amenable to treatment by locally applied drugs that are well absorbed through the intact skin from specialized dosage forms (*e.g.,* transdermal patches).

B Mucous Membrane Application

Absorption of drugs from mucous membranes is generally good, primarily due to the thinness and vascularity of the membrane. Drugs may be applied to mucous membranes in all the forms used for dermatologic application, as well as in the form of suppositories (rectal, vaginal), powders (nasal), lozenges (oral), and tablets (buccal, sublingual). Because absorption is good, especially from aqueous solution, many drugs exert significant systemic actions following application to mucous membranes. Thus, the toxic effects of drugs may also be enhanced as a result of systemic absorption, and mucous membrane application must be undertaken more cautiously than dermatologic administration.

Major uses of drugs applied to various mucous membranes are the following:
1. *Local Effects*
   a. Antiseptic (oral lozenges, sprays, mouthwashes)
   b. Antibacterial and antifungal (vaginal creams, suppositories)
   c. Decongestant (nasal sprays, drops)
   d. Antihemorrhoidal (rectal astringents, local anesthetics, emollients)
   e. Contraceptive (vaginal foams, tablets, lotions)
2. *Systemic Effects*
   a. Antianginal (sublingual vasodilators)
   b. Laxative (rectal suppositories, retention enemas)

The rectal route (suppository, retention enema) may also be employed with antiemetics (prochlorperazine), bronchodilators (aminophylline), analgesics (aspirin), sedatives (phenobarbital), and many other drugs that cannot be administered orally because the patient is unconscious or uncooperative, or is vomiting. Rectal absorption is unpredictable and a small, cleansing enema prior to drug administration may improve absorption.

▶ **NURSING CONSIDERATIONS—DERMATOLOGIC AND MUCOUS MEMBRANE APPLICATION**

▷ *A Dermatologic*
▷ 1 Apply most ointments and creams (except topical burn preparations), in small amounts, that is, cover area thoroughly with a thin layer of medication, and use firm but gentle pressure.
▷ 2 Remove ointments, creams, or jellies from jar with a sterile tongue depressor or applicator stick—not fingers—to avoid contaminating remainder of jar contents.
▷ 3 If application stains clothing, advise patient to take adequate precautions, such as use of a protective covering. Use caution if applying adhesive tape near a wound or abraded skin area.

▷ 4 If the skin is broken or abraded, use aseptic techniques whenever possible and cleanse skin with an antiseptic (such as hexachlorophene) before application.
▷ 5 When using topically applied preparations, be alert for allergic hypersensitivity reactions such as rash, local edema, or hives, and stop medication immediately if any of these are observed.
▷ 6 Local corticosteroid application may result in spreading of an existing topical infection if appropriate antibiotic therapy is not employed concurrently.
▷ 7 When moist compresses are applied to denuded or oozing skin areas, aseptic technique is imperative. Sterile compresses should be wrung out before being applied. If *warm* compresses are needed, do not warm solution to more than body temperature.
▷ 8 Provide emotional support to patient and encourage him to talk about his feelings regarding the skin condition—a sense of rejection, loss of self-image, and a tendency toward isolation are often present. Avoid showing signs of aversion or rejection toward the person because of this condition.

▷ *B   Mucous Membrane*

▷ *Oral Mucosa*
▷ 1 Advise patient taking sublingual medication *not* to swallow tablets or take water with them.
▷ 2 Inform patient that effects of sublingually administered drugs should occur within 5 minutes. If no relief is obtained, advise physician, because dosage adjustment may be necessary.
▷ 3 Apply buccal tablets to gums above the upper incisors. Use caution when eating or drinking so that the tablet is not dislodged.

▷ *Nasal Mucosa*
▷ 1 Avoid use of oil-based preparations for nasal application because aspiration of oil droplets into lungs may cause severe irritation and lipid pneumonia.
▷ 2 Be sure nasal passages are clear; if nasal drops are used, position patient so that the head is tilted backward.
▷ 3 Do not allow tip of dropper to contact nasal mucosa because contamination can result or patient may be stimulated to sneeze.
▷ 4 Any solution remaining in dropper following each administration should be discarded—not returned to original bottle.
▷ 5 Instruct patient to hold head in backward position for several minutes, to allow time for drug absorption.
▷ 6 Do not use drops containing nasal decongestants (vasoconstrictors) for a period of more than 3 to 5 days. Tolerance will develop, lessening the effect of the drug and leading to a condition of "rebound congestion," characterized by hyperemia, inflammation, and edema of nasal membranes.
▷ 7 Advise patients with hypertension or other cardiovascular disorders about the danger of using nasal sprays containing vasoconstrictors, because systemic absorption of the drug can elevate blood pressure.

▷ 8 Clean nozzle of nasal spray applicator after each use to prevent contamination and possible bacterial growth. Do not allow use of same nasal spray bottle by more than one person.

▷ 9 Caution patients against excessive use of any nasal preparation, because significant systemic absorption can occur with time, especially if substantial amounts of the drug are swallowed rather than inhaled.

▷ *Vaginal Mucosa*

▷ 1 Instruct patient about the proper technique to be employed in insertion of vaginal tablets and suppositories, and assist patient with first insertion if necessary. Tell patient to remain in bed at least 15 minutes after insertion to allow medication sufficient time to contact target area.

▷ 2 Ensure that medication is taken for the entire duration prescribed, because many vaginal infections are difficult to treat and can be very resistant to medications.

▷ 3 If preparation causes stains, advise user to wear a sanitary napkin to prevent staining of clothing or bedsheets.

▷ 4 Caution against excessive use of douches. If they are used, provide instructions for mixing, and demonstrate proper placement of container and tubing so that force of flow does not become too great.

▷ 5 Counsel users of contraceptive foams and jellies about their proper timing and method of application according to package instructions. Stress the limitations of their effectiveness and advise those who are considering their use to seek professional advice on alternative methods of contraception.

▷ *Rectal Mucosa*

▷ 1 Most suppositories should be refrigerated, especially in warmer weather, because they tend to soften and become difficult to handle.

▷ 2 Insert suppository beyond the internal anal sphincter. Lubricate if necessary. Use gentle, firm pressure with the forefinger. Have patient lie on one side with knees drawn. Patient should remain on side for 15 minutes to prevent leakage.

▷ 3 If suppository is to be self-administered, be certain patient knows proper technique and depth and can reach anus easily (for example, arthritic conditions can restrict movement).

▷ 4 Urge bowel evacuation, if possible, just before insertion of suppository to aid drug absorption.

▷ 5 Caution patients that laxative suppositories generally have a rapid onset of action so toilet facilities should be nearby.

▷ 6 With retention enemas, give small volumes (less than 150 ml) slowly with a small-diameter rectal tube to prevent stimulation of peristalsis and subsequent expulsion of rectal contents.

▷ 7 Retention enemas should be given before meals and following a bowel movement to enhance absorption of medication.

▷ 8 Temperature of solution should be close to body temperature and the solution should flow slowly. Tell patient to lie flat for 30 minutes following administration.

II Ophthalmic Application

Drugs intended for use in the eye may be administered as drops, ointments, or washes. In addition, a special type of preparation intended for use in glaucoma is available in the form of sterile insertion units termed Ocuserts. All ophthalmic medications are packaged sterile; thus, aseptic technique is essential when handling these drugs.

Major indications for local administration of drugs in the eye are the following:

1 Glaucoma (miotics, decongestants)
2 Inflammation (corticosteroids)
3 Infection (antibiotics)

Ophthalmic drugs may also be employed to facilitate eye examinations. Mydriatics produce pupillary dilatation, and cycloplegics paralyze accommodation. Artificial "tears" can be used to provide lubrication.

▶ **NURSING CONSIDERATIONS—OPHTHALMIC APPLICATION**

▷ 1 Aseptic technique is important in handling ophthalmic drugs. Wash hands before administering drugs; do not allow tip of dropper or ointment tube to come in contact with eyelid; discard any unused portion of each dose.

▷ 2 Check solution suspension or ointment for expiration date and make sure solution is clear and free from discoloration.

▷ 3 Hold bottle or applicator parallel to the eye, rather than perpendicular, to prevent injury should the patient move or jerk.

▷ 4 Have patient look up during administration; place medication in the conjunctival sac, not directly on the cornea; wipe area near the eyes gently with a cotton ball; and instruct patient to lie or sit with head tilted backward.

▷ 5 When using ophthalmic ointments, place *small* ribbon of medication into inverted lower eyelid and tell patient to close eye. Body heat will cause dispersion of drug over eye surface.

▷ 6 Impress upon glaucoma patients the necessity of maintaining a regular schedule of drug administration to prevent deterioration of eyesight.

III Otic Application

Drugs intended for use in the ear are usually administered as drops, although irrigation of the external auditory canal can be performed as well. When the tympanic membrane is intact, sterile technique is not essential.

Primary conditions for which drugs are instilled into the ear are the following:

1 Infections (antibiotics)
2 Inflammation (corticosteroids)
3 Pain (local anesthetics)
4 Obstruction with wax (hydrogen peroxide)

Self-medication should be reserved for those minor conditions (*e.g.,* impacted wax) that can be treated safely. Most cases of ear disorders require professional diagnosis and treatment.

▶ **NURSING CONSIDERATIONS—OTIC APPLICATION**

▷ 1 Warm ear drops to body temperature before instilling in ear canal.

▷ 2 Place patient on side with affected ear uppermost; instruct patient to remain in that position for several minutes after drugs have been administered to allow sufficient time for medication to reach affected area.

▷ 3 *Adults:* pull external part of lower ear backward and upward and instill drops in the direction of the opening of the ear canal. *Children:* pull lower part of external ear downward before instilling drops.

▷ 4 If cotton is to be inserted into ear following drug administration, insert *loosely.* Never pack cotton tightly into ear canal.

▷ 5 For irrigation, place tip of special irrigating syringe inside meatus, pull auricle upward and backward, and direct a slow gentle stream of warmed solution toward the roof of the auditory canal. The patient may sit or lie with head tilted toward the side of the affected ear. Allow fluid to escape freely and collect it in a basin placed below the ear and against the face.

▷ 6 Following irrigation, place patient with affected ear downward and allow ear to drain. Dry ear when process is completed.

IV   Inhalation Application

Inhaled drugs are generally intended for their local effects on the respiratory system. In addition, certain drugs including general anesthetics and amyl nitrite exert profound systemic effects when inhaled into the lungs. Rapid absorption of many drugs occurs in the alveoli of the lungs because of the large surface area, extensive vascularity, and high permeability of the alveolar epithelium. Thus, although a drug may be given for its local effects in the lungs, systemic absorption can result in undesirable side-effects such as cardiac stimulation, and this possibility must be kept in mind. *Particle size* of the delivered drug is the most important factor determining depth of penetration into the bronchial tree, and hence extent of systemic absorption.

Major indications for inhaled drugs are the following:

1 Anesthesia (general anesthetics)
2 Acute angina (amyl nitrite)
3 Obstructive pulmonary diseases, such as asthma and emphysema (corticosteroids, bronchodilators, mucolytics, antibiotics)
4 Respiratory aid (oxygen)

Inhalation of drugs is most easily accomplished by use of a hand nebulizer or atomizer, often available in prepackaged form, although patients require careful instruction for effective use of a nebulizer. Alternately, an intermittent positive pressure breathing (IPPB) apparatus can be used, an apparatus commonly used in a hospital setting. The method provides greater depth and more extensive distribution of the drug in the bronchial tree.

▶ **NURSING CONSIDERATIONS—**
INHALATION ADMINISTRATION

▷ 1 Check directions for administering inhaled medications because many must be diluted before use.

▷ 2 Instruct patient in correct procedure for using atomizer or nebulizer. Directions are usually provided with containers.

▷ 3 Make sure nebulizer or atomizer is carefully cleaned after each usage to prevent obstruction and contamination. Discard unused medication left in nebulizer.

▷ 4 Carefully explain to patient the proper use of IPPB machine before drug administration. Place him in upright position, and tell him to close lips tightly around mouthpiece and breathe *only* through mouth at normal resting rate.

▷ 5 Observe patient carefully for signs of dizziness, nausea, or anxiety. Reassure patients who have difficulty mastering the technique.

▷ 6 Instruct patients that inhalation equipment (*e.g.,* nebulizers) used at home should be soaked for 30 minutes once every 2 weeks in a solution one half water and one half white vinegar to prevent pseudomonal contamination.

V   Oral Administration

The oral route of drug administration is the simplest, most convenient, and generally the safest and most economical means of administering medications. Commonly employed oral dosage forms are tablets, capsules, and liquids. Most drugs are well absorbed from the gastrointestinal (GI) tract, and absorption is usually enhanced if the drug is in liquid form or is administered with water. Some drugs, such as anti-inflammatory drugs, may irritate the GI mucosa and are best given with food, whereas other agents (*e.g.,* penicillins), may be inactivated by the presence of food-induced digestive enzymes and are best given between meals.

It should be recognized that following oral administration of a drug, onset of action is slower and the duration of effect is more prolonged than after sublingual and most forms of parenteral administration. This is of little consequence in most cases; however, it becomes significant in emergencies (*e.g.,* acute pain, cardiac arrest, acute asthmatic attacks).

Other important disadvantages of the oral route of administration are the following:

1 Some drugs are rapidly inactivated in the GI tract (*e.g.,* insulin) or are not absorbed (*e.g.,* tubocurarine).
2 Some drugs undergo extensive first-pass hepatic metabolism (*i.e.,* they are largely inactivated in the liver soon after absorption into the portal circulation). Thus, a large fraction of the dose never reaches the systemic circulation. Differences in the rate and extent of hepatic metabolism among patients can result in significant variations in steady state plasma levels, and hence widely differing dosage requirements. Sublingual drug administration avoids first-pass hepatic metabolism and generally results in higher plasma levels for those drugs extensively metabolized in the liver.
3 Some drugs have an objectionable odor or taste (*e.g.,* liquid potassium).
4 Some drugs (such as large doses of aspirin) may produce local stomach irritation and cause nausea and vomiting. Drugs that may irritate the stomach can be given in the form of enteric-coated tablets, which dissolve only in the intestine where the environment is more alkaline.
5 Some drugs (such as liquid iron or gastric acids) may stain or destroy the tooth enamel.

In addition, unconscious, uncooperative, or vomiting patients or those without a gag reflex should not be given drugs by the oral route.

▶ **NURSING CONSIDERATIONS—
ORAL ADMINISTRATION**

▷ 1 Know the properties of the drug being administered so that it may be given at the proper time (*e.g.,* at meals or bedtime).
▷ 2 Be aware of the intended purpose of the drug as well as the expected side-effects, and observe the response of the patient carefully.
▷ 3 Mix a disagreeable liquid preparation with juice or another palatable substance to facilitate administration.
▷ 4 Do not attempt to break unscored tablets or divide capsules, because dosage inaccuracies can result.
▷ 5 Determine the patient's ability to swallow a solid dosage form. If swallowing problems exist, consider use of a liquid preparation or parenteral administration.
▷ 6 Make sure suspensions and emulsions are well mixed before administration.
▷ 7 Instruct patient to swallow coated tablets whole and not to chew them, because breaks in the coating will alter dissolution characteristics.
▷ 8 Note expiration date on liquid preparations (*e.g.,* antibiotics), and do not use if too old. Potency may be affected.
▷ 9 Keep preparations requiring refrigeration cold, and discard unused content at end of period stated on the label.

▷ 10 Do not mix liquids together unless so instructed. Incompatibilities may result, affecting the action of the drugs.
▷ 11 Do not use liquids that are discolored, exhibit precipitation, or have an unusual odor without consulting physician or pharmacist.
▷ 12 Advise patients to avoid indiscriminate use of over-the-counter (OTC) drugs when taking prescribed oral medications, because many OTC products (such as antacids, laxatives, and cough syrups) can interfere with the other drugs' actions.
▷ 13 Instruct patients to take oral medications with a full glass of water to facilitate absorption and to ensure sufficient fluid intake.

VI Administration of Parenteral Medications

Although the term *parenteral* literally means any route other than enteral (by way of the GI tract), it is usually used to refer to the various methods of *injection* of drugs. Parenteral administration requires aseptically prepared drugs and sterile techniques, critical regulation of dosage, careful selection of site and rate of injection, and a certain degree of technical skill not necessary with most other forms of drug usage.

Parenteral administration encompasses several routes that may vary according to the route selected in onset of drug action, extent of drug effects (local vs. systemic), dosage of drug required, skill in administration, and potential hazards. We shall examine in more detail several of the more important routes of parenteral administration.

A Intravenous (IV)

Intravenous administration is accomplished by either direct injection (bolus) or slow infusion. Direct (bolus) IV injection is employed primarily in emergency situations because it provides an extremely rapid onset of action. Also, some drugs (*e.g.,* diazoxide) require bolus injection to achieve their desired effect. However, because the drug is injected directly into the bloodstream, bolus IV injection is one of the most hazardous methods as well, and great care must be taken to ensure that the proper preparation and accurate dose have been selected, and to provide prompt antidotal therapy should an overdose occur. Bolus IV injection is most commonly done into the median cubital (antecubital) or basilic vein near the bend of the elbow (Fig. 1-1), although in an emergency any accessible vein may be used.

Irritating substances that cannot be given by other parenteral routes of injection because of the production of tissue damage can sometimes be administered by slow IV injection diluted in 100 ml to 200 ml of suitable liquid (*e.g.,* Sterile Water for Injection). The lining of the blood vessels is quite

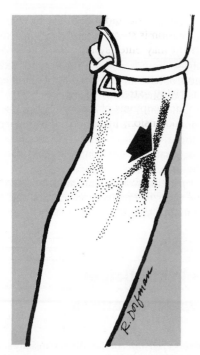

Figure 1–1 The most common bolus IV injection site is into the median cubital (antecubital) or basilic vein near the bend of the elbow (*arrow*).

resistant to the irritative effects of many drugs, and the buffering capacity of the blood may reduce local necrosis. This procedure requires selection of a large vein and assurance that the injection is properly placed into the flowing bloodstream.

Slow IV infusions are most commonly employed to replace depleted blood volume, to supply nutrients and electrolytes, to prevent or relieve tissue dehydration, and to administer drugs. The veins of the dorsal venous plexus or the cephalic vein (Fig. 1-2) are commonly used for these purposes. Very large volumes of fluids can be given by IV infusion, although care must be taken to avoid overloading the patient's circulatory capacity. A controlled rate of flow is maintained and may vary depending upon the nature of the drug and the patient's age, weight, and condition. Drugs are either contained in the infusion system itself or added to the flowing infusion.

Major advantages of the IV route of administration are the following:

1 Immediate effect—dose can be quickly adjusted to response.

2 Fairly constant blood levels can be maintained by a proper rate of infusion.

3 Irritating drugs (such as antineoplastic agents) can often be given with minimal trauma because of the buffering capacity of the blood.

4 Administration can be performed easily in the patient who is unconscious or unable to swallow.

Several disadvantages to IV administration also exist:

1 Rapid action prevents easy antagonism of undesirable drug effects—especially critical in cases of overdosage. Drug is essentially irretrievable once it has been injected.

2 Toxic effects may develop quickly and may be exacerbated by too-rapid injection.

3 Many incompatibilities exist among drugs and IV solutions, because of such variables as *p*H, temperature of solution, and salt content.

4 IV administration is technically more difficult than most other methods, often causes pain, and may result in infection.

▶ **NURSING CONSIDERATIONS—IV ADMINISTRATION**

▷ 1 Cleanse skin over injection site with alcohol swab; following needle insertion, withdraw plunger slightly. Backflow of blood indicates proper needle placement. Inject solution slowly (*e.g.,* 0.5 mg/min) and steadily, carefully observing patient at the same time.

▷ 2 Before beginning IV infusion, check that tubing is unoccluded, all connections are tight, proper drug is being given, and area of needle insertion has been disinfected.

▷ 3 Check drug and dosage *carefully* before administering any agent IV.

▷ 4 Perform IV injection slowly (1 min–2 min for most drugs) unless otherwise indicated (drugs such as diazoxide must be given very rapidly). If problems arise during injection (such as with blood pressure, respiratory, or cardiac irregularities), stop injection at once.

▷ 5 Observe area immediately around injection or infusion site for any swelling or coldness, which are indications that fluid is leaking from injected vein. If they are present, stop injection immediately.

▷ 6 Do not inject insoluble materials IV (*e.g.,* suspensions of drugs), because this may result in embolisms.

▷ 7 Check flow rate continually (*e.g.,* every 10 min initially, then at least every 1 hr or whenever the room is entered for any reason). Be alert for disruption in flow if patient is restless.

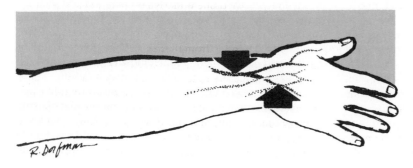

Figure 1–2 The veins of the dorsal venous plexus or the cephalic vein can be used for IV infusions.

▷ 12 Do not allow bottle and tubing to empty completely before infusion is stopped or IV bottles are changed, because air may enter system. Prevent development of negative pressure in the tubing by keeping part of tubing below the level of the extremity being infused and by placing extremity below level of heart.

▷ 13 Be alert for symptoms of embolism (cyanosis, tachycardia, hypotension, loss of consciousness) and be prepared to administer oxygen and other necessary drugs.

▷ 14 When terminating IV infusion, clamp tubing, remove dressing around needle or catheter, withdraw needle, and apply firm pressure over site until bleeding ceases. Apply a Band–Aid tightly to provide continued pressure at needle site.

B   Intra-arterial (IA)

Injection of a drug directly into an artery is an infrequently used method of administration, the purpose of which is to perfuse a specific area or organ of the body to achieve a high local concentration of the drug.

Types of drugs most frequently given by this route are the following:

1 Diagnostic agents (x-ray contrast media)
2 Antineoplastic drugs
3 Vasodilators

▶ **NURSING CONSIDERATIONS—IA ADMINISTRATION**

▷ 1 This is a very hazardous procedure requiring skilled injection techniques and should be performed only by someone specially trained in its application.

▷ 2 Even though the initial drug distribution is local, systemic spread eventually occurs. Be alert for development of toxic signs.

▷ 3 Explain the diagnostic procedure in detail to the patient before beginning injection and carefully outline any instructions the patient must follow.

▷ 4 Be especially careful to note the recommended dilution and rate of administration.

C   Subcutaneous (SC)

Subcutaneous injections are given beneath the skin into the fat and connective tissue underlying the dermis. Most common sites of SC injections are the upper lateral aspect of the arm, the anterior portion of the thigh, and the abdomen (Fig. 1-3). Absorption from these sites through the capillary network is generally rapid (although slower than with IM injection) but can be reduced by local cooling of the area or by the addition of vasoconstrictors to the injection solution. The maximum volume that can comfortably be given by this route is about 2 ml, and the drugs used must be highly soluble and nonirritating to tissues.

A special form of SC injection is termed *hypodermoclysis,*

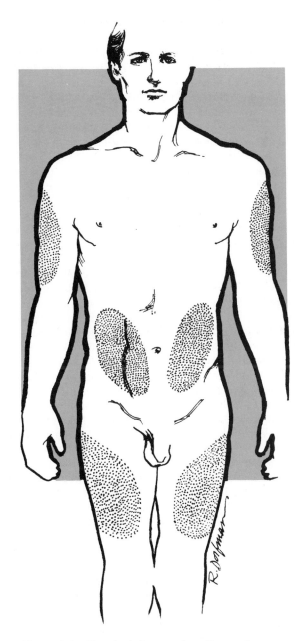

Figure 1-3   The shaded areas show the most common sites for SC injections.

▷ 8 Correct needle placement on IV infusion may be checked by lowering bottle below level of vein. If blood flows back into needle, vein has been correctly punctured.

▷ 9 Be alert for symptoms of extravasation (leakage). These include reduction in flow rate, edema, pain, and coldness at area of infusion. Stop infiltration at once if these signs are evident.

▷ 10 Note symptoms of developing venous phlebitis (pain, tenderness, erythema), and discontinue infusion if observed.

▷ 11 Do not attempt to flush a clogged IV system, because dislodgement of embolus into circulation may result.

in which large volumes of fluid are given *very slowly* into the loose connective tissue on the upper surface of the thigh or the outer side of the upper body surface. This procedure can be employed with an isotonic sodium chloride solution, glucose, or other parenteral fluids that cannot be given IV for some reason. Hyaluronidase, an enzyme that breaks down the connective tissue matrix, is sometimes added to the mixture to facilitate the spread and absorption of the large volume of injection. It may also reduce the discomfort associated with the injection of such a large volume (500 ml–1000 ml) of fluid.

Compressed pellets can be implanted subcutaneously to provide a "depot" form of a drug, which is continuously and evenly absorbed over a long time. This procedure requires a small incision, and sterility is essential. Absorption from SC sites can also be prolonged by suspending the drug in a protein colloid or gelatin solution.

▶ **NURSING CONSIDERATIONS—SC ADMINISTRATION**

▷ 1 Use a fine (25–26 gauge), short (⅜ in–⅝ in) needle and a small barrel syringe (2 cc). Sterile technique is required.

▷ 2 If repeated injections are necessary, vary site of administration to minimize irritation and possible tissue necrosis. Record location of each injection.

▷ 3 Grasp and lift skin over injection site, cleanse, and insert needle with a quick thrust. A 90° angle can be used with shorter needle (⅜ in–½ in) when giving insulin or possibly heparin but a 45° angle is used with most other SC injections.

▷ 4 Before injecting drug, slightly withdraw plunger to aspirate fluid, making sure needle is not in a blood vessel.

▷ 5 Inject drug slowly and continuously. When completed, withdraw needle quickly and apply pressure to injection site to retard bleeding.

▷ 6 Observe patient for later development of pain at injection site, which may indicate formation of a sterile abscess. Should this pain occur, advise physician.

▷ 7 Check for appearance of a blister or wheal at injection site, which indicates some drug was given intradermally. Injection may need to be repeated.

D Intramuscular (IM)

Drug injections can be made into several of the larger muscle masses. Sites most commonly employed are the deltoid muscle (Fig. 1-4A), the gluteal muscles (dorsogluteal and ventrogluteal sites) (Fig. 1-4B), and the vastus lateralis (especially in infants) (Fig. 1-4C). Injections are usually made with a longer, heavier needle than that used in SC injections, and larger volumes can be given IM (up to 5 cc at one site) than SC. Absorption is very rapid because of the vascularity of muscle and the large absorbing surface. The deltoid has perhaps the greatest blood flow of any muscle routinely used for IM injection.

The danger of inadvertent IV administration is increased with an IM injection because of the large number of blood vessels in muscle. Therefore, aspiration of the syringe for blood prior to injecting is essential to ensure proper needle placement. There is also an increased likelihood of nerve damage if the injection is performed incorrectly.

Drugs may be given IM as solutions or suspensions in either water or oil. Aqueous solutions are rapidly absorbed, whereas suspensions or solutions of various drugs (*e.g.,* hormones) in oil provide a depot form, which is slowly absorbed and provides a long-lasting effect. Caution must be exercised when injecting oil-based preparations; some patients may develop allergic reactions to the oil, and in some cases the oil may not be absorbed, requiring excision and drainage.

Depth of needle insertion is very important and depends mainly on the site and volume of injection and on the condition of the patient (*e.g.,* age, weight, extent of body fat).

In small children IM injections have special difficulties associated with them, primarily because of the limited muscle mass. Generally, the vastus lateralis (see Fig. 1-4C) on the anterolateral aspect of the thigh is used. Needle lengths should be shorter than with adults, and the child should be restrained to minimize the risk of sudden movement during needle insertion and injection.

There are three basic techniques that may be employed when giving an IM injection: stretching, pinching, and the "Z" method. In the first, the skin is pressed down and stretched between the thumb and fingers. This method is often used for obese patients to reduce the thickness of subcutaneous fat that must be pierced to reach the muscle. Pinching is accomplished by gathering the tissue between the thumb and fingers. This tends to raise the underlying muscle tissue and is helpful with emaciated adults and infants. Finally, the "Z" method is used with medications that might discolor the skin (*e.g.,* iron preparations) or cause subcutaneous irritation should they leak from the underlying muscle. It involves pulling the overlying skin to one side of the injection site, inserting the needle at a right angle to the skin, injecting, and withdrawing the needle quickly while releasing the pulled-back skin at the same time, which "seals off" the puncture tract.

▶ **NURSING CONSIDERATIONS—IM ADMINISTRATION**

▷ 1 Select appropriate needle size and length depending on site of injection, dosage form of medication, and condition of the patient (age, weight, body fat, scar tissue from repeated injections).

▷ 2 Decide on method of injection to be used (stretch, pinch, "Z") and palpate intended site.

▷ 3 Place patient in proper position and explain procedure to be followed. For gluteal injections, use location of bony prominences (*e.g.,* greater trochanter, anterior and posterior superior iliac spine) to identify proper site. Keep patient prone and instruct patient to turn toes inward to relax gluteal muscle.

▷ 4 When drawing medication into syringe, pull about 0.2 cc air into syringe as well. Air bubble at rear of syringe will ensure expulsion of entire contents and prevent

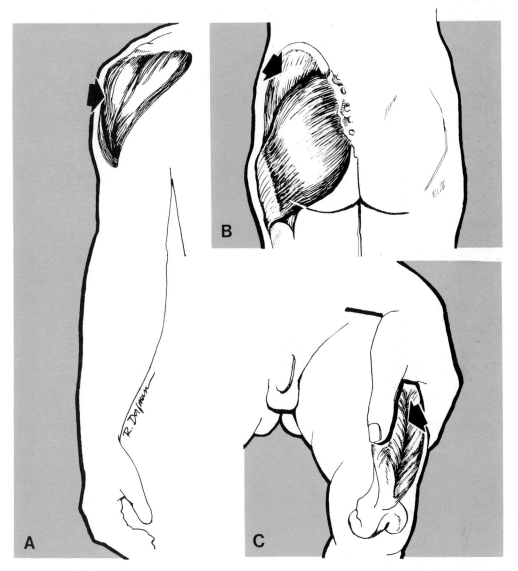

Figure 1–4 Sites most commonly employed for drug injections into the larger muscle masses are (*A*) the deltoid muscle, (*B*) the gluteal muscles, and (*C*) the vastus lateralis, especially in infants. With gluteal injections *always* use bony prominences to identify correct injection site (see Nursing Considerations—IM Administration).

drug from entering subcutaneous tissue as needle is withdrawn.

▷ 5 After cleansing area, insert needle using selected technique. Aspirate small amount of fluid into syringe to ensure needle is not in a blood vessel. If blood returns in the syringe, withdraw needle, discard medication, draw up a new dose in a fresh syringe, and inject at a different site.

▷ 6 Inject slowly and continuously. Withdraw needle at same angle as insertion and apply pressure. Massage injected site to promote distribution and absorption of drug unless a depot form of drug is used.

▷ 7 Do not administer drugs IM when blood supply to the area may be inadequate (as in shock or a paralyzed extremity), because absorption will be impaired and drug effects will be reduced and unpredictable in onset and duration.

E Other Parenteral Routes

1 Intradermal (ID)

Drugs may be injected superficially into the outer layers of the skin in very small amounts. Local anesthetics can be given this way to facilitate deeper injections, but this method is employed primarily for diagnostic purposes, as in "skin" testing for allergies, or in tuberculin testing. The injection sites commonly employed are the medial forearm area and the surface of the back. Injections are best performed with a small needle (26 gauge) and syringe, and the injection volume is usually 0.5 cc or less. Systemic absorption of intradermally injected agents is very limited, so the method is applicable only to those drugs used locally.

2   Intra-articular

This method of injection, directly into a joint, is used primarily for administration of corticosteroids in the treatment of acute local inflammatory conditions. The major advantage is attainment of high local concentrations of steroid in the affected area with minimal systemic absorption, thus reducing toxicity. The procedure requires skill and is painful to the patient.

3   Intrathecal

Injections of drugs into the spinal subarachnoid space are most often employed with local anesthetics, antibiotics, and x-ray contrast media. This technically difficult procedure is usually performed by a physician. It is frequently used for production of localized anesthesia during labor and delivery, although epidural administration of local anesthetics (*outside* the subarachnoid space) is often preferred because of a lower frequency of toxic reactions and less danger of postanesthetic complications.

▶ **NURSING CONSIDERATIONS—OTHER PARENTERAL ROUTES**
▷ 1   After ID administration, observe patient for signs of local reaction (swelling, erythema, pain).

▷ 2   Following an intra-articular injection, advise patient not to overuse the affected joint when pain is relieved, because further deterioration of the joint may occur.
▷ 3   Caution patient that pain may intensify for several hours after an intra-articular injection before relief is obtained.
▷ 4   Warn patient that severe headache may follow intrathecal injection but that it will disappear shortly.

Several other methods of parenteral administration of drugs are available, but are used only infrequently. These are briefly summarized below.

1   *Intraperitoneal.* Injection of drugs directly into the peritoneal cavity of the abdomen; widely used in animal experimentation (rapid absorption), but direct injection is not employed in humans because of danger of infection and adhesions. Peritoneal dialysis is performed in cases of renal failure, intractable edema, hepatic coma, azotemia, and uremia and in therapy for peritonitis.
2   *Intracardiac.* Direct injection into the heart; occasionally used with epinephrine and isoproterenol for emergency treatment of cardiac arrest.
3   *Intrapleural.* Administration of drugs between the lungs and chest wall (pleural cavity). Occasionally antibiotics are given this way.
4   *Intra-amniotic.* Instillation of drugs into the amniotic sac surrounding the fetus; employed with prostaglandin E_2 for second trimester abortion.

In order for a systemically administered drug to exert its desired effects, it must reach its intended site of action. Many factors control the rate and extent to which a drug attains sufficient levels at its site of action. The most important of these factors are the following:

1 *Absorption.* The processes involved in transferance of drug from its site of administration to the bloodstream, across one or more membranes.

2 *Distribution.* The means by which drugs are transported by body fluids to their intended sites of action.

3 *Biotransformation.* The metabolic processes by which a drug molecule is usually converted to a less active and more readily excreted form.

4 *Excretion.* The mechanisms whereby a drug or its metabolites are removed from the body.

Each of these processes is dependent on many variables and can be modified in several ways. We will discuss the important aspects of each of these processes and examine how each can be influenced. An outline of the major factors that influence the concentration of a drug at its site of action is shown in Figure 2-1.

In order for a drug to travel from its site of administration to its intended site of action, it usually must pass across several body membranes. Because membranes are largely lipid (fatty) in nature, the lipid-soluble form of a drug most readily crosses these membranes by means of passive diffusion. Thus, an understanding of the lipid membrane concept and how it relates to the various processes involved in the handling of a drug by the body is essential. Most drugs are either weak acids or weak bases, depending on their chemical structure. In solution, they may exist in both the ionized forms (*e.g.,* Na^+ and Cl^-) and the un-ionized forms (*e.g.,* NaCl), as with sodium chloride. Ionization results in the "splitting apart" of a drug molecule into positively and negatively charged components, and in the *ionized* state, the charged particles are incapable of diffusing across lipid membranes. On the other hand, the *un-ionized* (intact) form of a drug is the lipid-soluble form, and because membranes are primarily lipid in nature, this form most easily diffuses across these membranes. Thus, processes such as absorption, distribution, and excretion, which depend upon a drug's ability to diffuse easily through body membranes, are greatly impaired by ionization of the drug molecules.

The form in which a drug is found—ionized or un-ionized—is dependent on the *p*H of the environment (*e.g.,* gastric juice, urine) in which it exists. Thus, drugs that are acidic in nature (such as barbiturates and salicylates) are present largely in the *un-ionized* state in an acid environment, for example, gastric juice, with a *p*H of 1.2. Basic drugs, such as morphine, ephedrine, and theophylline, are *ionized* in these regions of low *p*H. Conversely, in areas of higher *p*H (*e.g.,* the intestine with *p*H of 5.5), the reverse is true, and acidic drugs are more completely ionized than basic drugs. It is evident, then, that acidic drugs, being largely un-ionized in areas of low *p*H (such as the stomach and urine), are well absorbed from the gastric mucosa and renal tubules; however, basic drugs exist predominantly in ionized form in these regions, and do not readily diffuse across the mucosal barriers. The most important factors, then, which

Interaction of Drugs with Body Tissues

2

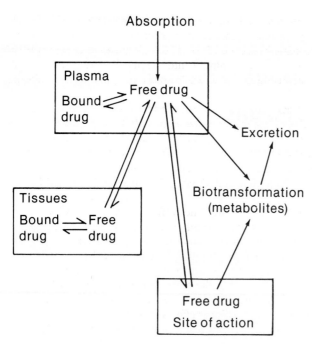

Figure 2-1 Factors influencing concentration of a drug at its site of action.

control the onset and duration of a drug's effects, are the chemical characteristics of the compound, such as the degree of ionization and the lipid solubility of the un-ionized form. These properties determine the drug's ability to readily traverse body membranes and therefore play a significant role in the movement of drug molecules throughout the body. In general, *un-ionized* drugs are better absorbed, more widely distributed, and less readily excreted than *ionized* drugs.

I   Absorption

The site and mechanisms involved in the absorption of a drug depend to a large extent on the means of administration.

1   Absorption From the GI Tract

Drugs may be absorbed from several regions of the GI tract, although most absorption occurs throughout the upper region of the small intestine. The main reasons for this are the presence of many small folds or *villi,* which greatly increase the absorbing surface area, and the highly permeable nature of the intestinal epithelium. Other factors that make the small intestine the major site for most drug absorption are the presence of special transport systems for absorption of sugars, amino acids, nutrients, and other substances; the fairly rapid gastric emptying of many drugs, which delivers

a greater fraction of unabsorbed drug to the upper intestine; and the extensive capillary network of the intestinal villi.

In general, absorption of most drugs from the GI tract is best explained by simple diffusion of the lipid-soluble form of the drug across the mucosal barrier. Some absorption, especially of low molecular weight drugs, also occurs by way of diffusion through aqueous pores in the membrane. Active (energy-requiring) transport mechanisms utilizing a carrier that can move a drug molecule *against* a concentration gradient are also involved in absorption of some drugs. Likewise, facilitated diffusion is a carrier-mediated process, but unlike active transport, it does not require energy and moves *down* the concentration gradient. It is utilized to move less lipid soluble drugs across the membrane.

Absorption of drugs from the GI tract is influenced by several factors:

A   Nature of the Drug

1 Lipid solubility of the un-ionized form, because it is this form that is capable of crossing GI membranes
2 Stability of the drug in GI fluid
3 Molecular weight and configuration of the drug, which may influence its passage through the membrane pores. Smaller molecules have a better chance of "squeezing" through the pores

B   Nature of the Dosage Form

1 Concentration of the drug if administered in solution
2 Dissolution rate of a solid dosage form of the drug
3 Presence of special (enteric) coatings on the drug molecules that resist breakdown and hence prevent absorption in the stomach

C   Nature of the Absorbing Barrier (Membrane)

1 Permeability of the mucosal epithelium
2 Blood flow in the absorbing area
3 *p*H of the region, which determines the ratio of the un-ionized to ionized form of the drug present
4 Amount of absorbing surface exposed, which is a function of the total surface area present (the length of the absorbing segment, and the presence of surface modifications such as villi)

D   Other Factors

1 Length of time the drug is in contact with the absorbing surface. This may depend on peristaltic activity, gastric emptying time, or the presence of inactivating enzymes in the GI tract

2 Presence of food, which reduces rate of absorption of many drugs, but can increase bioavailability of other drugs, presumably by slowing first-pass hepatic metabolism

3 Presence of other drugs or substances that can retard absorption by binding free drug molecules or altering GI function (*e.g.,* laxatives, anticholinergics). "Bound" drugs usually cannot be efficiently absorbed.

2 Absorption From Parenteral Sites

In general, most parenteral sites provide for a more rapid and predictable rate of absorption than the intestinal tract, all other factors being equal. Absorption following subcutaneous or intramuscular injection depends primarily on two factors:

1 Solubility of the drug
2 Blood supply to the area of injection

Drugs in aqueous solution are absorbed more rapidly than drugs in suspension. Often, however, drugs are suspended in certain vehicles to retard their rate of absorption and to provide a prolonged action. Examples of this are various penicillins (benzathine and procaine penicillin G) and long-acting hormones and steroidal agents. Certain types of insulin are combined with proteins or zinc to delay their rate of absorption.

Absorption of drugs from IM sites is usually more rapid than from SC areas because of the more extensive vascular supply per unit area of muscle compared with fatty subcutaneous tissue. The decreased peripheral blood flow present during circulatory failure (as in cases of shock) may significantly reduce the rate of absorption of injected drugs and greatly alter their efficacy. Blood flow to a superficial area can be increased and absorption enhanced by application of heat, local vasodilators, or massage; conversely, decreased blood flow and delayed absorption can result from use of cold packs, a tourniquet, or vasoconstrictors. All these factors can exert a profound influence on the onset, as well as the extent, of a drug's action.

IV administration, of course, provides the most rapid drug action because the drug enters the bloodstream directly without crossing any membranes. The advantages as well as the hazards of this method have been discussed previously.

3 Absorption From Skin
and Mucous Membranes

Absorption of most drugs through the intact skin is very poor, primarily because of the keratinized structure of the epidermis. The underlying dermis, however, is quite permeable and significant drug absorption can occur if the overlying skin is abraded or denuded. In general, drug absorption occurs to a greater extent through mucous membranes, which present a much thinner and more permeable absorbing surface than the skin. Enhanced absorption of topically applied drugs can be obtained by dissolving the drug in an oily base, vigorously massaging it into the applied area, or by simultaneously applying a keratin-softening agent (such as salicylic acid).

Increasingly, drugs intended for systemic action are being formulated in specialized topical dosage forms, such as transdermal patches, to take advantage of their ability to be consistently absorbed through the skin. Examples of such drugs are nitroglycerin and scopolamine.

Sublingually administered drugs are very rapidly absorbed, owing to the extremely thin epithelial membrane and extensive capillary network in the area of administration.

Absorption of inhaled medication depends to a large extent on the particle size of the drug, which determines the extent of penetration into the alveoli of the lungs. This is the primary site of systemic absorption of inhaled medications, because of the close proximity of capillaries to the alveolar membrane. Although most inhaled drugs are intended for their local effects, systemic absorption may be appreciable and can result in unwanted adverse effects.

II Distribution

After a drug is absorbed, it is distributed throughout the body by the circulatory system and must reach adequate levels in tissues on which it exerts its principal actions to produce a significant pharmacologic effect. Because the distribution pattern of a drug is ultimately dependent on its ability to cross body membranes, the principles governing membrane transport of a drug, discussed earlier in the chapter, apply here as well. In general, the initial distribution of a drug is dependent on cardiac output and local tissue blood flow. In addition, several other factors, addressed below, can also determine the amount of active drug that ultimately reaches the intended site of action.

1 Binding of the Drug

Drugs may bind either to constituents of plasma (*e.g.,* albumin) or to cells (*e.g.,* nucleoproteins). Binding to plasma proteins slows the disappearance of the drug from the plasma, limits the rate of accumulation in tissues, and prolongs the time that the drug remains in the body. A protein-bound drug is usually inactive, because it is only the free drug that is capable of diffusing across membranes to reach its site of action in the tissues. However, a dynamic equilibrium usually exists between the bound and free forms of a drug (Fig. 2-1) and some drug will be present in either state. Plasma protein binding may provide a reservoir of drug which gradually dissociates from the binding sites to replace the free drug which has been inactivated.

It is important to keep in mind that the binding capacity of plasma proteins is limited, and saturation can occur, although the amount of drug capable of being bound by plasma proteins is variable and difficult to determine. However, once protein-binding sites are completely occupied, further administration of the drug may result in increased effects or toxic reactions because of the presence of large amounts of non-protein-bound drug. Similarly, many different kinds of drugs are protein-bound, and *simultaneous* administration of two or more of these drugs can result in competition for the binding proteins, displacement of active drug, and subsequently enhanced drug effects. This type of drug interaction is discussed more fully in Chapter 7.

2 Lipid Solubility of the Drug

Because most membranes are lipid in nature, drug distribution across these membranes, and ultimately to the site of action, depends to an extent on the lipid solubility of the drug. Moreover, highly lipid soluble drugs tend to localize in adipose tissue where they may be stored for extended periods of time. Slow release of active drug from these storage sites can result in prolonged subtherapeutic effects with certain drugs, such as continued drowsiness following use of a highly lipid soluble central nervous system (CNS) depressant.

3 Blood–Brain Barrier

It is well established that some drugs enter the CNS with relative ease, while others do not enter this system at all. These observations have led to the concept of the existence of a blood–brain barrier. The capillaries in the CNS exhibit very tightly joined endothelial cells that lack pores and are enveloped by poorly permeable cells, termed *glial* cells, which impede the access of many water-soluble drugs to the CNS while permitting some highly lipid soluble drugs to pass. It must be remembered that this is not an absolute barrier but describes a *measurable* difference in the permeability of CNS capillaries to various drugs. In order for a drug to more easily pass the blood–brain barrier, it should possess the following properties:

1 Low ionization at plasma pH
2 High lipid solubility of the un-ionized form of the drug
3 Minimal plasma protein binding

4 Placental Barrier

Although some form of a "barrier" probably exists between the bloodstream and the placenta, it is very nonselective. Most drugs (except for strongly charged and high molecular weight molecules) are capable of readily entering the placental circulation. During the first trimester of pregnancy, many drugs have a potentially damaging effect on the developing fetus, even though they may not be harmful to the mother. Other drugs, (*e.g.,* alcohol, barbiturates, nicotine, and narcotics) may have untoward effects on both the mother and the fetus. No drug should be taken during pregnancy without consulting the physician, and drugs should be used during pregnancy only when the advantages greatly outweigh the potential risks.

III Biotransformation

Although some drugs (such as certain antibiotics and general anesthetics) are excreted from the body largely unchanged, most compounds undergo one or more metabolic transformations. These metabolic changes usually occur in the liver by way of hepatic microsomal enzyme systems. These consist of a group of enzymes located on the smooth endoplasmic reticulum of liver cells. The endoplasmic reticulum resembles a series of canals that are continuous with the cell membrane and the membrane of the nucleus. Microsomal enzymes catalyze most oxidative drug metabolism. Metabolites as well as unchanged drugs are then conjugated, for example, with glucuronic acid, which results in the formation of less active, more water-soluble, and hence more easily excreted compounds. Other enzyme systems capable of biotransforming drugs are found in the lungs, plasma, intestine, and kidneys.

Biotransformation does not always result in formation of *less active* compounds. The metabolic changes occurring with some drugs result in formation of equally active (*e.g.,* imipramine, ephedrine) or more active (*e.g.,* chloral hydrate) products. Similarly, metabolism may bring about formation of a product *more* toxic than the administered agent; an example is ethanol metabolized to acetaldehyde.

Some drugs are administered in the form of an inactive *prodrug,* which is then converted to an active metabolite. An example of such a drug is dipivefrin, an eye drop that is converted to epinephrine, the active component, in the eye. Dipivefrin is better absorbed than epinephrine, hence less drug is required.

Many types of chemical reactions are involved in biotransformation processes and will be reviewed only briefly. The most common are the following:

1 *Oxidation*—for example, side chain oxidation, dealkylation, oxidative deamination, desulfuration
2 *Reduction*—for example, azo dye reduction, nitro-reduction
3 *Hydrolysis*—for example, protease, peptidase, and phosphatase enzyme reactions (hydrolysis of amides and esters)
4 *Conjugation*—for example, glucuronide, glycine and sulfate formation, methylation, acetylation (production of soluble, inactive complexes that are readily excreted)

There is often considerable variation in the rate at which different individuals metabolize drugs. Several factors are important in determining the capacity of an individual to inactivate a drug:

1 Diseases that alter liver function
2 Age (immature liver functioning in the infant, and impaired liver functioning in the geriatric patient)
3 Presence of other drugs (such as barbiturates, phenytoin, pesticides, and dyes) that may increase liver enzyme function and enhance metabolism (this is termed *enzyme induction,* and is discussed in Chap. 7).
4 Genetically determined differences in metabolic activity (which may explain hypersensitive, drug-resistant, or drug-tolerant persons)

A significant factor in determining the efficacy of many orally administered drugs is *hepatic first-pass metabolism.* Following their absorption from the GI tract, drugs enter the portal circulation and are immediately transported to the liver, where they may be taken up by hepatic cells and metabolized. In some cases, the metabolism of the drug is virtually complete upon first-pass, and drugs such as morphine and lidocaine, which undergo extensive first-pass metabolism, cannot be used orally. Other drugs, such as propranolol, also undergo extensive first-pass metabolism but are converted in part to an active intermediate. Other drugs cleared to a considerable extent by first-pass inactivation include chenodeoxycholic acid, desipramine, hydralazine, oxyphenbutazone, propranolol, reserpine, and verapamil.

IV Excretion

Elimination of a drug or its metabolites from the body is accomplished by several routes including the kidney, lungs, intestine, and, to a lesser extent, the sweat, salivary, and mammary glands. Of these, the most important for the majority of drugs is the kidney.

1 Kidney

Renal excretion can occur by either passive glomerular filtration or active tubular secretion.

A Glomerular Filtration

This is the process whereby drug molecules diffuse out of the blood perfusing the glomeruli of the nephron, and pass into the tubules of the kidney. The drug may then either be reabsorbed into the bloodstream at various segments of the tubule or excreted in the urine. Several factors can influence renal excretion by glomerular filtration.

1 *Molecular size.* The amount of drug filtered by the glomerulus depends on its molecular size; smaller molecules are more easily filtered.
2 *Plasma protein binding.* Since only free drug can be filtered by the kidney, binding to plasma proteins will decrease renal excretion.
3 *Blood level of the drug.* The greater the drug concentration in the plasma, the more readily the drug can be filtered and ultimately excreted.
4 *Ionization of drug at urinary* p*H.* Because only unionized molecules are reabsorbed in the kidney, drugs that are largely in the ionized state in the acidic urine will be more readily excreted.

Altering the *p*H of the urine can markedly affect excretion of a drug. Weak acids, such as salicylates, barbiturates, and sulfonamides, are excreted more readily as the *p*H of tubular fluid increases, because weak acids ionize more as the urine is made more basic. Conversely, weak bases like amphetamines, ephedrine, and meperidine are best excreted in an acidic urine, because they are largely ionized at low *p*H. Acidification or alkalinization of the urine with drugs such as ascorbic acid and sodium bicarbonate, respectively, are techniques that can be employed to hasten excretion of certain drugs taken in overdosage. For example, phenobarbital intoxication may be managed in part by administration of sodium bicarbonate to raise the urinary *p*H, thus promoting ionization of the drug molecules in the tubular fluid.

B Tubular Secretion

The proximal renal tubule can actively secrete certain drugs, transporting them from the bloodstream directly into the tubular fluid. This process is not significantly affected by protein binding as long as the binding is reversible. Many drugs that are secreted are also filtered by the glomeruli and thus have a very short period of action. An example is penicillin. The tubular secretion process for one drug can be inhibited by another drug. For example, probenecid is often given with penicillin to inhibit its active tubular secretion by competing for a saturable transport system. The duration of action of penicillin in the body is therefore prolonged.

2 Intestine

Drugs that are unabsorbed from the GI tract or secreted into the GI tract by the bile, salivary glands, and digestive glands can be excreted in the feces. Because many drugs are metabolized in the liver, their metabolites are often secreted into the bile, which passes to the intestine. The metabolite may then be excreted in the feces, but most often is reabsorbed from the intestine into the bloodstream and ultimately excreted in the urine. Thus, biliary and fecal excretion is important mainly for those drugs (such as penicillin or colchicine) that cannot be reabsorbed from the intestine because of their ionization at the intestinal pH.

3   Lungs

This relatively minor route of excretion is important primarily in the case of the gaseous and volatile liquid general anesthetics, which can be excreted from the bloodstream across the alveolar membrane into the expired air. Many other volatile substances (including alcohols, paraldehyde, and oils) can appear in the expired air in limited amounts, but are mainly broken down in the liver and excreted by the kidneys. Enough alcohol can be eliminated unchanged by the lungs to be detected and measured, and this procedure (breathometer) is often used to determine the degree of intoxication.

4   Mammary Glands

Many drugs can be excreted by the mammary glands, although the amounts present are generally minimal. However, some drugs, such as anticoagulants, barbiturates, corticosteroids, penicillins, and sulfonamides, may be transferred to the infant in breast milk in significant amounts; thus, use of such drugs during lactation should be restricted as much as possible. Specific mention of drugs that are likely to appear in milk is made throughout the text.

In order for a drug to exert its desired pharmacologic effect, it must either act on abnormal parasites or growths (*e.g,* microorganisms, neoplasms) or modify existing physiologic processes. The actions of a drug in the body must be viewed as the consequence of a complex series of physical and chemical interactions with certain cellular constituents of the living organism. Although much remains to be learned about the molecular basis of a drug's effects, sufficient information exists to establish a fairly detailed picture of the sites at which drugs act and the biochemical mechanisms involved in their actions.

Virtually all body tissues are exposed to systemically administered drugs, but certain tissues appear to be affected much more than others. Most drugs exert their *primary* actions at specific sites in the body, although they may affect several tissues or organs depending upon their distribution. In order to explain a drug's pattern of action, the "receptor theory" of drug action was proposed.

Drugs are believed to produce their effects by combining with cell constituents, thus altering the functioning of the target cell and ultimately the target tissue. This drug–cell constituent combination is believed to be in the form of a chemical bond with reactive sites on the cell constituent. The reactive sites that have an affinity for the drug are termed *receptors.* Although the precise structure of most receptors is still uncertain, several concepts relating to drug–receptor interactions can be stated:

1 Drugs exert a quantitative, not a qualitative, effect at receptor sites; that is, drugs alter the *rate* of ongoing physiologic processes, but cannot create new functions.

2 Receptors have specific molecular conformations, corresponding to certain kinds of drugs ("lock and key" theory).

3 Forces must be present to attract and hold a drug in contact with a receptor so that the drug may exert its effect.

4 Drugs "fitting" the receptor may either activate it (*agonists*) or inhibit it (*antagonists*), depending upon many factors.

5 Not all receptors on a particular cell need to be occupied for a drug effect to occur; potent drugs may be effective at very low concentrations, occupying only a fraction of the receptors.

In considering drug–receptor interactions, it is important to have an understanding of several basic concepts:

1. *Affinity*—the tendency for a drug to bind or attach to its receptor site

2. *Intrinsic activity*—the ability of a drug to produce an effect when bound to the receptor

3. *Intensity of effect*—the magnitude of the response to a drug-receptor interaction. The intensity of a drug effect may be explained by two theories:

   a. *Receptor occupation theory*—the intensity is proportional to the fraction of receptors occupied; this probably only holds true to a certain extent.

   b. *Rate theory*—the intensity is proportional to the rate at which the drug-receptor combinations occur.

Basic Sites and Mechanisms of Drug Action

3

A drug that combines with receptors and initiates an effect possesses both affinity and intrinsic activity, and this drug is termed an *agonist.* A drug that combines with a receptor, fails to produce an effect itself, but prevents an agonist from eliciting a response at the same receptor site is termed an *antagonist.* For example, acetylcholine functions as a cholinergic agonist, but its effects are inhibited by atropine, a cholinergic antagonist capable of occupying the same receptor sites but possessing no intrinsic cholinergic activity of its own.

Potency Versus Efficacy

Two terms relating to drug action that are often confused are *potency* and *efficacy.* A drug is said to be *potent* when it possesses high intrinsic activity at low unit weight doses. Potencies are compared based on doses that elicit the same intensity of effect, rather than based on magnitudes of effects elicited by the same dose. Knowledge of a drug's potency is important for approximating the appropriate dosage level to be administered but is relatively unimportant in deciding which of two drugs exhibiting the same maximal effect should be used. It makes little difference if the dose of a drug is 5 mg or 500 mg as long as the dosage is convenient to administer. There is no rationale for believing the more potent drug is the clinically preferred drug, as is sometimes implied in drug advertising.

Efficacy, on the other hand, refers to the maximal effect produced by a drug, and it is an important determinant in the drug selection process. For example, oral administration of 4 mg of hydromorphone (Dilaudid) results in much greater pain relief than 65 mg of propoxyphene (Darvon). Therefore, hydromorphone is more effective as well as more potent than propoxyphene.

Therapeutic Index

The therapeutic index (TI) for a given drug is a measure of its safety margin and is defined as the TD_{50}/ED_{50}, where the TD_{50} is the dose producing a certain toxic reaction in 50% of an experimental population and the ED_{50} is the dose eliciting the *desired* effect in 50% of an experimental population. The greater the TI, the wider is the safe dosage range for the drug. It is important to recognize, however, that the TI is simply one measure of a drug's safety and has no bearing on the efficacy. Further, the TI must be viewed in general terms, because certain patients display extreme sensitivity to certain drugs, and thus have a very low TI for that particular drug. As an example, aspirin is a very safe drug in normal doses in the majority of individuals; however, severe hypersensitivity reactions to small doses of aspirin have occurred in some patients. Therefore, while the TI for aspirin is quite high in the general population, it is very low in those few allergic individuals.

Factors Modifying Drug Effects

In determining the proper drug and dosage to employ, it is important to recognize that many factors can alter an individual's response to a drug. The important factors are the following:

A   Body Weight

Drug dosages should be adjusted in proportion to the body weight, because the greater the body weight, the more the drug can become diluted in the body. This factor becomes especially critical in infants and small children and will be explored in more detail in Chapter 4. Similarly, the reduced body weight frequently noted in elderly or debilitated persons can increase the effects of drugs.

B   Age

In general, the pediatric and geriatric populations are very sensitive to the effects of many drugs, principally because of altered metabolic activity, reduced body mass, and decreased excretory capacity.

C   Sex

Females are thought to be more susceptible to the actions of some drugs, exhibiting either a more intense or a more prolonged effect. This may be due to their smaller body weight and greater proportion of body fat, wherein many drugs are metabolized much more slowly, and possibly also to the influence of hormonal factors.

D   Route and Time of Administration

Absorption is greatly affected by the route of administration (as discussed in Chap. 2) as well as the time of administration; for instance, greater absorption of most orally administered drugs occurs when the stomach is empty.

E   Pathologic Conditions

Rates of absorption, metabolism, and excretion can be markedly altered by changes in the normal physiologic state of the individual. Examples include nutritional disorders, thyroid dysfunction (increased sensitivity toward epinephrine), hepatic or renal disease (delayed metabolism and clearance of drugs), cardiovascular impairment and presence of pain (paradoxical excitatory effect with barbiturates), fever, anxiety (decreased analgesic efficacy), or infection.

F   Drug Idiosyncrasies

These may take the form of an abnormal drug response or an allergic drug reaction. Many appear to be genetically determined enzyme deficiencies that may interfere with the normal metabolism of drugs or increase the vulnerability of certain cells to the adverse effects of drugs.

G   Repeated Dosage

Variations in the response to an individual drug over time may take several forms:

1   *Cumulative effect*—a progressively increasing response to repeated doses that occurs if the rate of dosing exceeds the rate of excretion

2   *Tolerance*—decreased response to a drug resulting from its repeated administration. Although the mechanism is not entirely understood, it may result from increased rates of drug metabolism or cellular adaptation to a drug's local action. It is frequently observed with prolonged use of hypnotics and sedatives. *Rapid* development of tolerance, such that the response becomes progressively less with subsequent doses of drug, is known as *tachyphylaxis*.

3   *Resistance*—impaired response to a dose that normally is effective. It is a type of tolerance usually seen in connection with anti-infective drugs, where the microorganism becomes resistant to the bactericidal effects of the antibiotic. The phenomenon of resistance is considered in greater detail in Chapter 58.

H   Combined Effects of Drugs

Effects of one drug may be modified in several ways by the presence of a second drug.

1. *Synergism*—an enhanced pharmacologic response resulting from the simultaneous use of two drugs
   a. *Additive effect*—the net response is equal to the algebraic sum of the individual drug responses; that is, if the dose of each were reduced by half, the resultant effect would *equal* that observed with full dosage of either drug alone (*e.g.,* alcohol and barbiturates).
   b. *Potentiation*—the net response is greater than the algebraic sum of the individual drug responses. It is usually seen when two drugs exert the same clinical effect by different mechanisms (*e.g.,* propranolol and hydrochlorothiazide for hypertension).
2. *Antagonism*—a reduced or abolished drug effect due to the presence of a second drug

   a. *Competitive*—competition for the same receptor sites (*e.g.,* acetylcholine and atropine)
   b. *Chemical*—inactivation of a drug by formation of a chemical complex (*e.g.,* chelating agents in metal poisoning)
   c. *Physiologic*—use of two drugs having opposing biological effects (*e.g.,* amphetamine and barbiturates)

I   Psychological Factors

The attitude and expectations of the person taking the drug can greatly determine its effectiveness. A perfect example of this kind of response is the "placebo effect." This is the appearance of a clinical effect to a dose of a pharmacologically inactive substance (*e.g.,* dextrose) given to a patient who believes he is receiving an active drug. The importance of patient reassurance and encouragement in enhancing clinical effectiveness of drugs cannot be overemphasized in this respect.

Mechanisms of Drug Action

Although the *clinical* effects of a drug can be described in terms of alterations in physiologic function, the underlying biochemical and biophysical mechanisms of drug action are less well understood. As discussed earlier in the chapter, the interaction of a drug molecule with a receptor site is the initial event by which the majority of drugs evoke a biological response. This drug–receptor interaction subsequently initiates a chain of biochemical or physiologic events that determine the ultimate therapeutic response to the drug. Several theories have been advanced to help explain how the chemical complexation between a drug molecule and a reactive site in the body can lead to the enormous range of clinical manifestations that constitute the response to drug therapy.

A   Enzyme Inhibition

Many drugs have been shown to interfere with enzymes necessary for the normal functioning of the organism, such as dopa decarboxylase inhibitors, or cholinesterase inhibitors. Because practically all biological reactions are catalyzed by enzymes, inhibition of these compounds can result in a wide range of pharmacologic responses.

B   Enzyme Stimulation

Activation of synthesizing enzymes (*e.g.,* adenyl cyclase) may increase the effects of many drugs and body hormones such as cyclic AMP. Conversely, stimulation of the activity of hepatic metabolizing enzymes by one drug can inactivate other drugs, and this situation, known as enzyme induction, is discussed further in Chapter 7.

C   Alterations in Membrane Permeability

Drugs such as local anesthetics, insulin, or antibiotics may either increase or decrease permeability of cellular membranes, alter active transport processes, or redistribute the concentration of ions on either side of the cellular membrane, thereby changing its resting potential. As discussed previously, passage of drugs across body membranes is essential for most of the interactions between a drug and body tissues.

D   Interaction with Neurohormones

Most physiologic processes are regulated by neurohormonal activity (*e.g.*, catecholamines, acetylcholine). Drugs may modify the actions of these neurohormones in several ways:

1   Altering their rate of synthesis (*e.g.*, carbidopa)
2   Interfering with their binding and storage (*e.g.*, reserpine)
3   Varying their rates of release (*e.g.*, guanethidine, amphetamine)
4   Interfering with their receptor interaction (*e.g.*, propranolol, atropine)
5   Modifying their rate of inactivation (*e.g.*, imipramine, physostigmine)

In addition to the general types of drug mechanisms discussed above, a variety of other mechanisms are responsible for the clinical effects of many drugs. Chemical neutralization of gastric acid, a detergent action on bronchiolar mucus, physical debridement of dead tissue, adsorption of toxins onto the surface of drug particles, and osmotic swelling of muciloids to provide a laxative action are just a few examples of mechanisms of action for other drugs.

The net results of a drug's action on a biochemical level is an alteration in the normal physiologic functioning of the organism. If this alteration occurs in an abnormal parasite or growth on the body such as bacteria, virus, or neoplastic tissue, the drug is termed a *chemotherapeutic agent* (*e.g.*, antibiotics, antineoplastics). If a change in the normal physiologic function of the body occurs in response to a drug (*e.g.*, reduction in blood pressure, slowing of the heart rate, or increased urine output), the drug is termed a *pharmacodynamic* agent. Most drugs, of course, fall into the latter category. It should be apparent that the effect of a pharmacodynamic agent is strictly quantitative; that is, these drugs are capable of modifying *existing* physiologic functions but are unable to induce a system to perform an action other than a preexisting physiologic one.

An infant or small child should not be considered a "little adult" for the purpose of administering drugs. Unique and potentially serious problems exist in the use of pharmacologic agents in the pediatric population, and perhaps nowhere is the choice of the proper dose and route of administration so important as with the small child. Yet critically defined guidelines for safe and efficient use of pediatric drugs do not always exist. Thus, much drug therapy in small children is undertaken simply by scaling down the recommended adult dose, largely based upon differences in body weight. However, a small child has many immature physiologic processes that greatly alter the handling of drugs by the body. Especially important are the lesser metabolic and excretory capacities of the infant compared to the adult, which severely impair the infant's ability to detoxify and eliminate many drugs safely.

Although it is difficult to arbitrarily divide the pediatric population according to age and developmental characteristics, certain stages in a child's growth are important in relation to drug handling. These may be described as follows:

1 *Neonatal period* (0 mo–1 mo)—period of marked physiological immaturity and rapid change; a dangerous time for drug administration.

2 *Infancy* (1 mo–12 mo)—period of gradually improving capacity of the body to efficiently handle drugs.

3 *Toddler period* (1 yr–3 yr)—fairly well-developed metabolic excretory processes; child resists many medications when they are presented; however, may ingest toxic substances on his own.

4 *Preschool age and adolescence* (3 yr and up)—few anatomical problems but occasional behavioral problems associated with drug administration; probably the most important consideration for safe drug therapy is body weight.

Pediatric Pharmacology

4

Factors that Affect

Therapeutic Response

Many factors determine the drug dosage and therapeutic response in infants and children. In one respect, children and adults are similar because each individual has a peculiar biochemical system that handles a drug in its own way. Thus, individual differences in drug responses are as apparent in children as in adults. However, the pediatric population must contend with many more variables in drug handling than the adult population. Such variables include immaturity of enzymatic processes, incomplete development of metabolic and excretory functions, increased tissue responsiveness to many drugs, and acceptance and ease of drug administration.

During the neonatal period, there is rapid physical growth and continual changes in organ functioning that persist through the early years of life, although at a somewhat reduced rate. This period of rapid growth and development represents the most critical time with regard to potential hazards of drug usage. Persons administering drugs to infants and children should recognize the complex nature of the many variables affecting drug activity and attempt to understand as clearly as possible the major determinants of drug responsiveness in the pediatric population.

A   Absorption

In general, absorption of *orally* administered drugs in infants is somewhat reduced compared to the adult, because children exhibit slowed GI motility, prolonged gastric emptying time, increased gastric acidity, decreased absorptive capacity of the various segments, and differences in the composition of intestinal flora. Also, transport mechanisms that carry drug molecules across the intestinal membranes into the bloodstream may be underdeveloped in small infants. Thus, a drug like riboflavin is absorbed much more slowly in infants (16 hr) than in adults (3 hr–4 hr).

Conversely, absorption of *topically* applied drugs is often greatly enhanced in small children compared to adults, largely because of a child's reduced keratin layer and thinner epithelium. This can be particularly significant with the prolonged use of topically applied corticosteroids for conditions such as diaper rash and eczema, where significant absorption through the skin can lead to many untoward systemic reactions.

Absorption of drugs from IM injection sites (*e.g.,* vastus lateralis muscles) may be more erratic in small infants than in older children, partly because of the small muscle mass. Drugs used to treat serious illnesses in hospitalized infants are often most effectively given by the IV route, frequently through the frontal or superficial scalp veins in very young infants.

B   Distribution

Differences in drug distribution among various pediatric age groups may depend on circulatory dynamics, extent of body water, binding of the drug in the plasma, membrane permeability, and the specificity of the drug for tissue receptor sites.

1   Circulatory Dynamics

Therapeutic agents generally penetrate highly perfused organs (*e.g.,* liver, kidney, brain) to a greater extent than organs receiving less blood flow (bone and muscle). As the growth of these organs progresses at different rates, the amount of drug distributed to each will change with development of the child. Young infants may have poor peripheral circulation, resulting in slowed absorption of intramuscularly or subcutaneously administered drugs.

2   Body Water

The newborn has a much higher percentage of total body water and extracellular fluid volume (80%–85%) than the older child or adult (60%–65%). Fat content, on the other hand, is markedly reduced in the neonate compared with the older child. Thus, water-soluble drugs diffuse to a greater extent in the very young, often resulting in reduced plasma concentrations compared with older children. An important consideration in this regard is that in states of dehydration, "normal" doses of a drug in the infant can result in very high plasma levels, because the overall extracellular fluid volume may be markedly reduced. Further, because of the reduced fat content of the neonate, lipid-soluble drugs will not exhibit the same distribution pattern as in the older child, and may not be stored to the same extent because there is less total adipose tissue.

3   Binding

Binding of most drugs to plasma proteins such as albumin and globulins is significantly less in the newborn compared with adults. This may be due to the following causes:

   a. Lower concentrations of plasma proteins in the neonate

   b. Altered binding characteristics of neonatal proteins

   c. Presence of endogenous substances (*e.g.,* bilirubin, steroids, hormones, fatty acids) that compete for plasma protein binding sites during the early days of life

Because reduced protein binding increases the amount of pharmacologically active drug in the plasma, this effect may predispose the child to a greater likelihood of toxic reactions, especially when multiple drug therapy is undertaken. Among the more important drugs that may exhibit reduced binding in the newborn are salicylates, barbiturates, penicillins, sulfonamides, and phenytoin.

4   Membrane Permeability

The incomplete development of the infant's body membranes, especially the blood–brain barrier, results in increased distribution of drugs to certain areas of the body, notably the brain. Lipid-soluble drugs (*e.g.,* anesthetics, sedatives, analgesics, antibiotics) readily enter the brain of the neonate and in many cases can cause serious harm (respiratory depression or brain damage). However, factors other than lipid solubility are involved in the penetration of many drugs into the brain. Blood chemistry changes (acidosis, hypoxia, hyperglycemia), body temperature fluctuations, and structural alterations in the blood–brain barrier itself (*e.g.,* reduced myelination) can all affect drug passage into the neonatal brain.

5 Drug Receptor Specificity

Differences in the responsiveness of infants and adults to certain drugs suggest that the sensitivity of some receptor sites is not equal. For example, therapeutic doses of atropine and epinephrine are proportionately greater on a mg/kg basis in the infant than in the adult, presumably because of reduced receptor responsiveness in the infant.

C Metabolism

Hepatic drug-metabolizing activity is substantially reduced in early neonatal life, and drug metabolizing enzymes in the liver mature at different rates. Liver function, therefore, changes very rapidly after birth, and major problems relating to reduced hepatic catabolism of drugs occur primarily in the first few weeks following delivery. The major consequence of the decreased hepatic drug-metabolizing capacity in the infant is that many drugs have a more prolonged duration of action, and this may predispose the child toward a cumulative toxic reaction.

On the other hand, drug metabolism in the neonate can be enhanced by administration of certain drugs—the barbiturates for example—that function as hepatic enzyme inducers. That is, certain pharmacologic agents are capable of enhancing the action of liver microsomal enzymes involved in the metabolism of other drugs (see Chap. 7). This effect becomes important when multiple drug therapy is undertaken in the infant, because addition of a second drug can markedly shorten the duration of action of the first drug, greatly reducing its efficacy. In this regard, repeated administration of certain drugs (*e.g.,* barbiturates) to the mother throughout pregnancy may lead to enzyme induction in the neonate. Infants born to such mothers often are capable of metabolizing many drugs at an accelerated rate from the time of birth. Thus, the efficacy and duration of action of drugs that may be required in the newborn can be dangerously reduced.

Reduced neonatal hepatic functioning also results in decreased synthesis of plasma proteins, allowing larger amounts of a drug to circulate unbound in the body, possibly leading to increased side-effects.

D Excretion

As with liver metabolic function, the renal excretory capacity is immature at birth and shows gradual maturation with advancing age. For example, shortly after birth the neonate's renal function is approximately 30% to 40% of that of an adult; however, a substantial increase in renal function occurs in the first week, and by the fifth day, renal filtration rates and blood flow have reached 60% to 70% of adult capacity. Glomerular filtration rates of newborns are approximately one half that of adults, but attain comparable levels by 6 months of age. Tubular secretion in infants likewise is about one third less than in adults. By nine months of age, however, renal function in the child is approximately equivalent to that of the young adult.

The significance of reduced renal elimination in the infant with respect to a particular drug depends on whether that drug is excreted largely by the kidney. Many important drugs used in pediatric pharmacology are eliminated predominantly by renal excretory processes (*e.g.,* most antibiotics, salicylates, acetaminophen, aminophylline, digoxin, thiazide diuretics) and thus may exhibit prolonged durations of action in the very young. This is an important factor to consider, especially when determining the frequency of dosage.

Drug Dosage and Administration

The pediatric population presents unique problems with regard to drug dosage and administration. As we have seen, a number of factors other than age and size can affect drug response. Thus, no one rule can be applied to the entire pediatric group with regard to dose and route of drug administration. Nevertheless, most therapy is undertaken on a milligram of drug per kilogram of body weight (mg/kg) basis. This method, of course, only considers one factor (weight) in determining a pediatric dosage, but it is probably the most applicable method for the majority of drugs prescribed for children.

Dosage

Many "rules" for pediatric dosing have been described, most of them based on a fraction of the adult dose as determined by some factor (*e.g.,* age, weight, or surface area). The most commonly used of these rules are:

a. *Young's rule* (2 yr and up)

$$\frac{\text{Age (yr)}}{\text{Age (yr)} + 12} \times \text{adult dose}$$

b. *Clark's rule* (infants and young children)

$$\frac{\text{Weight (lb)}}{150 \text{ lb}} \times \text{adult dose}$$

(150 lb = weight of "average" adult)

c. *Fried's rule* (infant under 1 year)

$$\frac{\text{Age (mo)}}{150} \times \text{adult dose}$$

d. *Surface area method* (all children except newborns)

$$\frac{\text{Surface area child (sq m)}}{1.7} \times \text{adult dose}$$

(1.7 = average sq m surface area of adult)

The surface area of the child is determined from its height and weight using standard nomograms found in many pharmacology and pediatric texts.

It is apparent that no single rule is satisfactory by itself, because the "average" dose is not necessarily the correct dose. Dosage must be individualized for the patient, the drug, and the disease, whether the patient is an adult or child. For example, doses calculated on age alone cannot compensate for the variations in body weight observed among children, especially in the proportion of body fat. Body surface area probably provides a more consistent dose schedule for older children but is not suitable for neonates, because a high percentage of their weight is water. Moreover, this method requires computation and use of nomograms. On the other hand, rules based on weight *assume* an average adult weight of 150 lb and with many drugs, infants would receive an *underdosage* if given mg/kg doses calculated by this method. Because adult doses should be individualized, it is erroneous to base a child's dose on an "average" adult weight.

Although pediatric dosage rules can provide guidelines for the use of drugs in children, they cannot guarantee safety or adequacy of dosage, especially in the newborn. Further, no rule is able to anticipate all the variables associated with pediatric therapy, especially those caused by individual differences in drug response. Thus, drug dosage in children must be critically adjusted to each patient, and careful observation must be made of the child during therapy to maximize efficacy and to minimize toxicity.

Administration

The preferred route of drug administration in children is determined by many factors, and may change quickly with the developing child. Several important routes are outlined briefly below:

A Oral

- Generally the preferred route.
- Liquid medications, especially if flavored, may facilitate administration, but should also be kept out of the child's reach to prevent self-administration and potential overdosage.
- In infants, medication may be placed along the side of the tongue by dropper or syringe.
- Tablets or capsules can be crushed and mixed with honey, syrup, jam, or fruit if the child is unable or unwilling to swallow them whole, although the parents should consult a pharmacist for the proper procedure.

B Rectal

- Can be used when oral route is contraindicated or difficult (*e.g.,* cleft palate, nausea or vomiting)
- Many drugs are erratically absorbed rectally.
- Diarrhea or constipation often makes rectal administration impractical.

C Intramuscular

- Often used for single dose administration (*e.g.,* vaccines, antibiotics).
- Buttocks and the deltoid muscle should not be used in infants and small children (under 2 yr) due to danger of nerve damage and lack of sufficient muscle mass.
- With repeated injections, sites should be alternated.
- Absorption is generally good and fairly rapid.
- Always use bony prominences to identify injection site.

D Intravenous

- Should be used in young children only where other routes have failed or are inappropriate.
- Infants and small children should be restrained so needle is not dislodged once inserted.
- Drug must be properly diluted and smallest dose given at slowest possible rate (*e.g.,* 0.5 ml/min–2 ml/min), because overdosage is most dangerous with IV route, and adverse reactions can develop quickly.
- Circulatory overload can occur more rapidly in children than in adults. As a general rule never give more than 250 ml fluid to a child under 5 yr, or 500 ml to an older child, unless special conditions warrant (*e.g.,* rapid or severe dehydration, renal impairment).

E Topical and Local (Eye, Ear, Nose)

- Possibility of significant percutaneous absorption of topically applied drugs must be considered in children, especially with repeated application.
- Eye and ear drops may be warmed before instillation.
- Oil-based preparations should not be used in the nose, because aspiration may cause lipid pneumonia.
- In infants, if nose drops are indicated, they should be instilled briefly, then aspirated with a bulb syringe.

Whatever method of drug administration is used in children, perhaps the most important single factor in successful pediatric drug usage is the relationship between the child and the practitioner. Successful and simple drug administration depends to a great extent on the cooperation between the child and the person giving the drug. Establishment of a secure, positive relationship between the drug giver and the drug receiver can overcome many obstacles to successful therapy. Each child has an individual personality that must be used to maximum advantage in administering medications. Honest explanations are essential, and medications should never be portrayed as candy, rewards, or anything less serious or important than they really are. If children are old enough, they should be told why medications are being used and the importance of proper dosage schedules in a manner appropriate to the child's age and level of understanding. A child's fears should be understood and allayed if possible. Pediatric drug administration can be exceedingly difficult and trying at times, and requires not only skill but patience, understanding, and recognition of the child's concerns and feelings.

▶ NURSING CONSIDERATIONS—PEDIATRIC PHARMACOLOGY

▷ 1 Consider the age and developmental stage of the child carefully before choosing a route of administration.

▷ 2 Be honest with the child and explain as clearly as possible what is happening. Do not lie (*e.g.,* this shot won't hurt); rather, give truthful information and provide comfort and support.

▷ 3 Stress the importance of compliance with the prescribed drug regimen.

▷ 4 Use the most convenient drug regimen, both in terms of route of administration and frequency of dosage, that is appropriate for the particular child and condition being treated.

▷ 5 Disguise disagreeable oral medications whenever feasible. Do not force any drug orally, because pulmonary aspiration can result. Try to gain the child's cooperation, but if this fails, advise physician so that an alternate drug or route of administration can be attempted.

▷ 6 Be cautious about mixing disagreeable drugs with foods in the child's normal diet (*e.g.,* milk, cereal, or juice) because the child may associate the drug with the food and an eating problem may develop.

▷ 7 Do not offer "rewards" in the form of candy, ice cream, or other sweets for drug taking, because the child will associate taking medication with something bad or unpleasant that should be rewarded if carried out. Try to develop a *positive* outlook on the part of the child that drug therapy is a beneficial and necessary function.

▷ 8 Avoid mixing a dose of medication in too large a volume of fluid or food, because the child will often not consume the entire amount and thus will not receive sufficient medication. Follow with fluid if possible.

▷ 9 Use a positive, authoritative statement to *tell* the child it is time for his medicine, rather than *asking* him if he wants to take it.

▷ 10 With very small children, dosing may be facilitated by crushing tablets or emptying capsule contents and mixing with appropriate vehicles, such as juice, formula, or milk. Obtain proper directions for mixing before attempting to do this, especially because the properties of the vehicle may alter bioavailability of some drugs.

▷ 11 When giving liquid medication to an infant, direct flow from dropper toward inside of the cheek to prevent gagging and stimulation of the cough reflex. Raise the infant's head to prevent aspiration.

▷ 12 Older children sometimes respond best to recognition of their maturity. Let the child drink unassisted, let him choose which medication he'll take first if more than one must be given, or let him pour from the bottle himself. Always check that correct dose is being used and all medication is taken.

▷ 13 Instruct parents in how to correctly measure liquid doses. Make sure they use calibrated measuring devices and not household spoons, which can vary significantly in volume.

▷ 14 If child is totally uncooperative in taking oral medication, consider rectal or parenteral administration and discuss with physician.

▷ 15 Be cautious about cutting suppository crosswise, because medication may be contained mainly at the tip or toward the distal end of the suppository. Place suppository high in rectum, and instruct child to lie prone until sufficient absorption can occur (usually 15 min to 30 min).

▷ 16 When giving parenteral medication to children, say truthfully that injection will hurt briefly and proceed promptly and smoothly with the procedure.

▷ 17 Enlist the aid of one or more individuals to restrain the child, if necessary, to prevent tissue trauma and possible needle breakage.

▷ 18 In children under 2 yr, give IM injections in vastus lateralis or rectus femoris muscle (see Chap. 1). Gluteal injections in the very young risk sciatic nerve injury, while the deltoid provides insufficient muscle mass.

▷ 19 Recognize child's fears and attempt to deal with them. Use of diversionary tactics, such as talking or singing, may work but usually is unsuccessful.

▷ 20 Do not shame the child for uncooperative behavior. Compliment him for his cooperation during the procedure and display empathy for the trauma undergone.

▷ 21 If child will not hold eye open for instillation of drug, place proper number of drops on inner corner of eye and wait for child to open eye. Drug will then be dispersed over cornea.

▷ 22 With child under 3 yr, pinna of ear is pulled down and back for administration of ear drops. With older child, pinna is pulled up and back. Gently massage outer area of ear to facilitate entry of drug.

▷ 23 With small children, nose drops should be instilled 30 minutes before feeding to facilitate suckling.

▷ 24 Check for clarity of solution where possible. Cloudy fluids may indicate contamination.

5 Geriatric Pharmacology

The aging process is associated with certain recognizable physical changes in the individual, among them decreased body weight, loss of hair, and alterations in posture and in contour of external features. Perhaps more important in terms of drug therapy are the less obvious changes occurring in the internal body organs and physiologic functions. With advancing age, there are decreases in the number of cells in most body tissues; changes in the activity of the remaining cells (e.g., metabolic function, permeability, respiration); increased proliferation of connective tissue and fat; impaired adaptation to stress; and decreases in muscle strength, circulation, oxygen utilization, and sensory perception. These deteriorations in organ and tissue functioning can result in altered responsiveness to many drugs; therefore, effects of drug therapy in the aged are often unpredictable, and untoward reactions are quite common and frequently serious.

Complicating the picture is the multiplicity of drugs that may comprise an elderly individual's therapeutic regimen. A progressively increasing life span has resulted in a greater proportion of the population reaching advanced age, with a corresponding increase in the use of drugs for treating chronic disease conditions such as congestive heart failure, hypertension, cerebrovascular disease, and carcinomas. It has been estimated that in the U.S., the elderly account for almost one third of all drug taking. They often take several drugs at one time, and close to 90% experience one or more episodes of adverse reactions to these drugs, not to mention the high likelihood of drug interactions with such a multiple drug regimen. Therefore, constant attention to the drug therapy of the aged individual is essential if maximum benefit is to be derived with minimal adverse effects.

Variables that Affect Response to Drugs

The frequent presence of multiple disease states in the elderly, as well as the wide variability in the development of organ and tissue pathology, can make determination of the proper drug and dosage a difficult matter. The safe and effective use of drugs in the aged depends on individualized therapy and requires constant reevaluation. There are a number of variables that influence the response to drugs in the geriatric as well as the pediatric population. In general, drugs tend to be absorbed, distributed, metabolized, and excreted much less efficiently in elderly patients compared with younger adults. Thus, the danger of untoward reactions as well as drug interactions is magnified. A brief examination of the changes that can occur in the handling of a drug in the elderly will highlight some of the problems that can be expected.

A Absorption

Many changes can occur in the GI tract that impair absorptive capacity. There may be a reduction in the number of absorbing cells, decreased GI motility, impaired gastric secretory cell function, reduced intestinal mucosal blood flow, and an elevated gastric pH. Such alterations can retard both active and passive absorption. In general, drugs are absorbed at a slower rate and less consistently in the aged; however, the *extent* to which drugs are absorbed is probably not significantly different from that in younger patients.

B   Distribution

Drug distribution in the elderly can be markedly curtailed simply because of reduced cardiac output and decreased perfusion of body organs. Other factors that may alter distribution in the geriatric population are smaller body size and lowered proportion of body water, decreased plasma protein binding (lower plasma albumin levels), and increased stores of body fat, leading to the possibility of accumulation of highly lipid-soluble agents (*e.g.,* barbiturates).

C   Metabolism

Significant changes in liver function generally do not occur until rather late in life (after age 70), partly because of the tremendous reserve capacity of the organ. However, decreases in hepatic function at an earlier age can often develop secondary to the presence of chronic disease states, and the decreases are frequently responsible for the toxic effects of drugs used to treat these states. Reduced metabolism of many drugs in the elderly may often be a consequence of progressive loss of liver cells as well as impaired enzyme function but is more commonly due to decreased perfusion of the liver secondary to diminished cardiac output. The important implication here is that doses of many drugs need to be reduced in the elderly, because the retarded rate of metabolism can result in a prolonged duration of action and danger of accumulation. Of course, patients with liver disease (cirrhosis, hepatitis, fatty infiltration) or decreased hepatic blood flow (congestive heart failure, pulmonary hypertension, arteriosclerosis) are extremely sensitive to those drugs that are primarily detoxified by the hepatic enzyme systems.

D   Excretion

Kidney function diminishes by approximately one third by age 65, largely due to reduced renal blood flow and loss of functioning nephrons. Glomerular filtration, tubular reabsorption, and active tubular secretion are all somewhat compromised in the elderly. The maximum amount of a drug that can be removed from the blood by the kidney depends largely on the volume of blood presented to the glomeruli—a function of renal blood flow. It is estimated that the blood flow to the kidney is reduced about one half by age 70. This decreased renal perfusion greatly limits the amount of drug that is filtered and excreted at any one time. Because the majority of drugs are eliminated primarily by the kidney through glomerular filtration, doses of these drugs should be reduced to avoid cumulation and subsequent toxicity.

E   Other Factors

Many other factors contribute to altered drug responsiveness in the geriatric population. Some of the more important of these are:

1 *Altered tissue sensitivity*—Certain drugs (*e.g.,* barbiturates) can produce greatly enhanced effects in a percentage of the elderly population. Although decreased metabolism may account for part of this effect, it appears that altered receptor sensitivity occurs to certain pharmacologic agents as the patient ages.

2 *Presence of chronic disease states*—As mentioned earlier, many elderly patients exhibit one or more chronic pathologic conditions, such as hypertension, diabetes, angina, congestive heart failure, or peripheral vascular disease. These can often markedly affect the responsiveness to a particular drug. Altered drug responses may result from interference with one or more of the basic functions discussed above (*e.g.,* absorption) or may be due to reduced compensatory reactions caused by impaired homeostatic mechanisms. For example, orthostatic hypotension is common in the elderly patient, resulting from blunted cardiovascular reflex responses normally operative in maintaining blood pressure. This condition may be exacerbated by a number of drugs, including some antihypertensives, vasodilators, and antipsychotics. Obviously, chronic liver or kidney disease can significantly prolong the effects of drugs by reducing their rate of metabolism or excretion.

3 *Hormonal changes*—Many drugs act through hormonal mechanisms and thus may elicit altered responses because of reduced endocrine secretion as the aging process continues. Decreases are often observed in thyroid function, glucose tolerance, adrenal cortical activity, and gonadal hormone release in the geriatric population. Replacement drug therapy is frequently indicated in these instances but can result in greatly enhanced effects early in therapy due to hypersensitivity of the receptor sites. Atrophic changes in certain structures (bones and genital organs) due to lack of hormonal action may likewise greatly modify a drug's effect or increase its toxicity. For example, use of steroids in the aged can result in marked glucose intolerance, osteoporosis, and susceptibility to infection.

4 *Behavioral changes*—Often overlooked, but critically important as a major determinant of drug responses in the aged, is the mental condition of the patient. Cerebral arteriosclerosis can result in confusion, loss of memory, and even dementia. These behavioral abnormalities may adversely affect normal physiologic

functioning. Also, impaired memory and disorientation frequently are responsible for poor dosage compliance, accidental overdosage, and ingestion of the wrong drug.

Drug Administration in the Elderly

Drug therapy in the geriatric population is at best difficult and in many instances quite hazardous. A thorough understanding of the altered physiology of this age group is essential for proper drug prescribing. An awareness of the potential adverse reactions that are likely to occur in this population is very important. In addition, several other considerations should be borne in mind when using drugs in the aged.

A   Necessity of Therapy

Many afflictions in the elderly do not always require drug treatment, and others should be treated only on a short-term basis. Frequent review of a patient's drug regimen as his condition changes is essential. Generally, drugs having a profile of potential adverse reactions that are worse than the symptoms described by the patient should be avoided. The benefit–risk ratio assumes critical importance in the geriatric population because of the greater likelihood that these patients will experience untoward reactions.

B   Adequacy of Therapy

Overprescribing of medications is as deleterious as inadequate therapy. The presence of multiple diseases in many geriatric patients occasionally leads to a "shot-gun" approach to prescribing that greatly increases the danger of drug toxicity and especially drug interactions. In addition, the reduced mental capacity of many older people makes it very difficult for them to manage multiple drug therapy. Thus, the fewest number of drugs that are adequate to serve the patient's needs should be prescribed.

C   Method of Administration

The dosage form and method of administration should be chosen to elicit the greatest possible degree of compliance. Because older patients may have difficulty swallowing large tablets or capsules, liquid preparations are often utilized. Parenteral self-administration generally should not be attempted by the geriatric patient. Dose regimens should be made as simple as possible, directions should be clearly indicated on the container, and labels on bottles should be easy to read. Large quantities of medications should be kept out of reach of senile or unstable patients. Close supervision of drug-taking habits in the elderly can eliminate many complications and adverse reactions.

D   Dosage Level

For many of the reasons outlined earlier in the chapter, the elderly patient generally requires smaller doses of most medications than does the younger adult. Complex dosage schedules should be avoided if at all possible, because many geriatric patients find it difficult to adhere to such schedules; single daily dosage is usually preferred. Drug therapy should be initiated with small doses, and the dose gradually increased until an optimal effect is observed. Abrupt alterations in dosage should be avoided. Whenever additional drugs are added to the regimen, the current dosage schedule should be reviewed and appropriate modifications made.

▶ **NURSING CONSIDERATIONS—GERIATRIC PHARMACOLOGY**

▷ 1 Decide whether the patient's complaint requires drug therapy. The psychological aspect of "taking a pill" is often as important as the actual medication in relieving many symptoms.

▷ 2 Use only those drugs that are absolutely necessary. Keep the dose as small as possible and the drug regimen as simple as is feasible.

▷ 3 When possible, package drugs intended for geriatric use in easily opened containers. Labels should be in large print. Keep only a minimal quantity of each drug within easy access of the patient, especially at night.

▷ 4 Closely supervise drug therapy in the elderly patient. Impress upon the patient the importance of rigid adherence to the prescribed dosage schedule, which is often necessary to maintain stable, effective blood levels and minimize adverse reactions.

▷ 5 Assist the patient to establish a daily dosing schedule for all medications being used. Suggest ways to ensure that each drug is taken when prescribed, such as setting an alarm, keeping a daily "log-book," posting reminder notes, and so forth.

▷ 6 Counsel the patient to seek advice before taking any nonprescribed drug. Warn the individual of the potential danger of serious interactions and toxic effects caused by combining medications, even over-the-counter preparations.

▷ 7 Do not leave bottles of medications, especially sedatives and hypnotics, within the patient's reach at night. Drowsiness often causes forgetfulness on the part of the patient, who may then consume additional doses, leading to possible overdosage.

▷ 8 Label all medications clearly, and if two or more drugs have a similar appearance, two green liquids, for example, place them in different types of containers to avoid confusion.

▷ 9 Give the patient a drink of water before having him take large tablets or capsules to facilitate swallowing.

▷ 10 Caution geriatric patients taking drugs that may produce orthostatic hypotension (antipsychotics, antidepressants, antihypertensives, sedatives) against changing position too rapidly or arising too quickly from bed.

▷ 11 Use of opiates for pain may induce severe respiratory depression in the elderly. Use the smallest effective dose and terminate therapy if respiratory rate falls below 10 per minute.

▷ 12 Be cautious in using CNS stimulants to combat depression in the aged; these drugs may exaggerate confusion and lead to disordered behavior in some individuals.

▷ 13 Begin digitalis or related therapy at very low doses because many geriatric patients are extremely sensitive to cardiotonic drugs. Careful observation of symptoms and critical dosage adjustment are necessary for maximum therapeutic benefit. Regular (*i.e.,* 6 mo–12 mo) evaluations of blood levels should be done to prevent excessive dosing.

▷ 14 Treatment with anticholinergic drugs may lead to confusion, delirium, and extreme dryness of the mouth. Use these drugs cautiously, avoid self-medication with proprietary products containing anticholinergics, and give liberal fluids to overcome dryness of mucous membranes.

▷ 15 Diuretic usage, coupled with inappropriate dietary and fluid intake and use of laxatives, may produce severe dehydration and electrolyte imbalances. Provide potassium supplementation and volume replacement if needed.

▷ 16 Reduce doses of oral anticoagulants in the elderly because of impaired renal and hepatic function and decreased plasma protein binding. Use extreme caution with these agents because of increased risk of hemorrhagic complications. Monitor clotting time at frequent intervals (*e.g.,* every 3 mo).

▷ 17 Give patients taking several drugs concurrently a list of those to be carried with them at all times. This information may be important in an emergency to determine proper treatment and avoid drug interaction problems.

▷ 18 Recognize that many side-effects associated with drugs used in the elderly mimic the behavior that is normally present in some older people (*e.g.,* weakness, forgetfulness, confusion, or anxiety). Careful observation of the patient is essential.

6 Pharmacologic Basis of Adverse Drug Effects

Adverse reactions to drug therapy include any unwanted, undesirable, or potentially injurious consequence of drug administration. Not all adverse reactions, however, are unexpected or unpredictable; some represent a logical extension of a drug's normal pharmacologic spectrum of action. Others can often be predicted on the basis of the patient's condition, route of drug administration, and presence of other drugs. Although the distinction is arbitrary and quite flexible, those expected and usually unavoidable untoward drug reactions are termed *side-effects,* and while frequently troublesome and annoying, they are rarely serious. Examples are drowsiness, dry mouth, and nausea. On the other hand, unpredictable, unusual, unexpected, or potentially serious reactions are generally referred to as *adverse effects (e.g.,* gastric ulceration, ocular damage, respiratory depression, blood dyscrasias). Changing the dose, dosage form, route of administration, or diet can often reduce or abolish many minor side-effects. Major adverse reactions, however, are frequently dose- and dosage-form independent, and their occurrence is more difficult to control. The propensity for a particular drug to cause reactions, the type of reactions produced, and the frequency of occurrence will determine the utility of the drug for a particular disease state. That is, the possibility of serious toxicity resulting from drug usage is generally acceptable only if the condition being treated is serious enough to warrant the risk. Conversely, drugs causing a high degree of adverse effects should never be used to treat trivial or psychosomatic illnesses. For example, chloramphenicol, a highly toxic antibacterial agent, is acceptable in the treatment of certain salmonella or meningeal infections in which other agents have failed or are inappropriate, but the drug should never be used to treat uncomplicated respiratory tract infections. Potent corticosteroids are invaluable in many types of inflammatory conditions but should not be routinely prescribed for such relatively minor ailments as poison ivy or urticaria.

Classification of Adverse Drug Reactions

Classification of adverse drug reactions is difficult because a wide range of diverse manifestations can occur. No single classification is adequate to categorize the multiplicity of adverse effects that can follow drug treatment. To discuss adverse reactions in a logical format, however, we will classify them in the following manner:

I. Pharmacologic
  A. Extension of therapeutic effect
  B. Nontherapeutic effects ("side-effects")
II. Nonpharmacologic
  A. Hypersensitivity
  B. Idiosyncrasy
  C. Photosensitivity
III. Disease-related
IV. Multiple drug reactions

V. Miscellaneous
   A. Carcinogenicity
   B. Teratogenicity
   C. Drug dependence

A brief review of these various types of adverse drug reactions will aid in their proper identification.

I   Pharmacologic Adverse Effects

Many adverse drug effects are the result of a greater than desired intensity of action or elicitation of one or more *secondary* drug effects in addition to the *primary* or intended drug effect.

A   Primary Actions (Extension of Therapeutic Effect)

Overdosage with a therapeutic agent will usually elicit, among other effects, an excessive reaction to the *primary* effect of the drug. For example, tranquilizers used as daytime sedatives in excessive amounts will generally produce drowsiness and possibly hypnosis. In this case, the adverse reaction usually can be overcome by either reducing the dosage or decreasing the frequency of administration. Other common examples of untoward reactions induced by drug overdosage are superficial hemorrhaging with anticoagulants, or excessive electrolyte and water depletion secondary to diuretic therapy.

B   Secondary Actions (Nontherapeutic— "Side-effects")

In many instances, the adverse effects caused by drug administration are the result of manifestation of one or more *secondary* actions produced by a drug molecule. In some cases, these secondary drug effects can be largely eliminated by adjusting the dose carefully in each individual. Many times, however, these adverse reactions are an inescapable consequence of normal therapeutic doses of a drug. For example, normal doses of many antihistamines are associated with a certain degree of drowsiness, a potentially dangerous occurrence. Even in small, therapeutic doses, anticholinergics used for relief of GI spasm and hypermotility usually produce xerostomia (dry mouth), blurring of vision, and some degree of urinary retention and constipation. Other examples of drug-induced secondary reactions include constipation with narcotic analgesics, potassium loss (hypokalemia) with diuretics, and orthostatic hypotension with antipsychotics.

Although these secondary effects of a drug usually cannot be controlled by dosage adjustment, because minimal therapeutic doses are already being used, the effects often can be reduced by substituting or adding other drugs to the regimen. For example, the drowsiness seen with many antihistamines can be minimized by using a mild central stimulant such as caffeine, or by switching to an antihistamine possessing minimal CNS depressant actions, such as tripelennamine.

Secondary adverse reactions may be quite serious, requiring careful patient monitoring and perhaps changes in the drug regimen. Potentially dangerous secondary effects of drugs include the possibility of thrombotic complications with oral contraceptives, arrhythmias with improper digitalis usage, and GI bleeding and ulceration with aspirin and related drugs.

Most pharmacologic adverse reactions have been extensively documented. Thus, in assessing the suitability of a particular therapeutic regimen, the disadvantages of a drug's known predictable toxicity should be weighed against its potential beneficial effects.

II   Nonpharmacologic Adverse Effects

Another group of adverse drug effects have little relationship to the pharmacologic effects of a drug. Rather, they occur as a result of an abnormal sensitivity or reactivity on the part of the drug recipient to a chemical substance. This aberrant reaction may be termed a *hypersensitivity* (or allergic) *reaction* or an *idiosyncratic reaction.* A principal hazard of this type of nonpharmacologic adverse reaction is that it is *not* predictable based upon the profile of drug action, but only occurs in a fraction of patients receiving the drug.

A   Hypersensitivity

Hypersensitivity or allergic reactions are perhaps the largest single group of untoward drug effects. Allergic reactions are usually *not* dose related and are largely independent of the pharmacologic properties of the drug molecule. These hypersensitivity reactions are associated with an altered reactivity or sensitization of the patient resulting from prior exposure to a drug or chemical that behaves like an allergen. The drug (or metabolite) interacts with a tissue or plasma protein, activating the reticuloendothelial system, resulting in production of antibodies to the drug molecule. A subsequent exposure to the same drug (or in some cases a similar one) elicits an antigen–antibody reaction that produces the symptoms of the allergic response (*e.g.,* itching, edema, congestion, wheezing).

Allergic drug reactions may be classified as either immediate (*e.g.*, anaphylaxis, urticaria) or delayed (*e.g.*, serum sickness).

1   Immediate

An immediate allergic drug reaction develops within minutes of drug exposure. The drug–antibody reaction probably releases several vasoactive substances, such as histamine and bradykinin, from their tissue stores. These substances can react with the smooth muscle of many body tissues (blood vessels, bronchioles, GI tract) to produce characteristic signs of the allergic reaction, such as bronchoconstriction or vasodilation. The symptoms may be very mild (rash, itching, urticaria) or serious enough (respiratory distress, circulatory collapse) to require immediate attention and swift medical treatment to prevent death. In general, the severity of the reaction is independent of the drug itself but probably depends to a large extent on a patient's sensitivity. It has been documented that even very small doses of common drugs, such as aspirin and penicillin, can produce violent hypersensitivity reactions in susceptible patients. The grave concern about these kinds of reactions is that often they are totally unpredictable, and quick recognition and proper treatment are essential to minimize serious consequences, such as respiratory distress, hypotension, and cardiovascular collapse.

2   Delayed

A delayed allergic drug reaction develops slowly following drug challenge. The clinical picture of delayed hypersensitivity often includes a diffuse rash, fever, and swelling and stiffness of the joints. This syndrome is frequently referred to as *serum sickness*. This name derives from the fact that the allergic response results from damage produced by *circulating* immune complexes that may lodge in small vessels and cause the characteristic symptoms. Sometimes the liver, kidney, and bone marrow may become damaged, although the factors that determine specific organ involvement are largely unknown.

B   Idiosyncrasy

Idiosyncrasy refers to a peculiarity in bodily function that causes an individual to react to a drug in an abnormal manner. Idiosyncratic reactions may manifest themselves as either a quantitative (*i.e.*, over- or under-responsiveness) or a qualitative (*e.g.*, paradoxical excitation) change from the norm.

These reactions are probably not caused by formation of an antigen–antibody complex but result from a genetically determined defect in the patient's ability to handle a particular drug. The manifestations of idiosyncratic reactions

can assume various forms; they may range from the rather mild (erythema, rash, photosensitivity) to the very serious (blood dyscrasias, exfoliative dermatitis, systemic lupus-like reaction, hemolytic anemia, malignant hyperpyrexia). A general description of some of the more important idiosyncratic drug reactions appears at the end of this chapter. A specialized field of study termed *pharmacogenetics* deals with these altered drug responses that are under hereditary control; great strides have been made in determining some of the genetic flaws that predispose certain individuals to toxic drug effects.

C   Photosensitivity

A unique type of dermatological hypersensitivity reaction following use of many drugs is observed upon exposure to sunlight, and is termed *photosensitization*. Two principal types of reactions can occur in people whose skin has been sensitized by either topical or internal use of photosensitizing drugs. A *photoallergic* reaction presents itself as a papular eruption on sun-exposed areas similar to that resulting from contact dermatitis. It is probably due to the photosensitizing drug forming an antigen by absorption of sunlight and subsequent combination with a skin protein. The resultant antibody formation sensitizes the patient to further synthesis of antigen by continued sun exposure.

A *phototoxic* reaction, on the other hand, is characterized by a severe sunburn, and as such is not always viewed as a hypersensitivity reaction. Nevertheless, it is probably the result of a photosensitizing chemical that absorbs ultraviolet radiation energy to such an extent that it becomes toxic to epidermal cells.

III   Disease-Related Adverse Effects

The pathophysiologic state of a patient is a major determinant of the potential for a drug to cause adverse effects. Underlying disease states, often unrecognized, can greatly increase the possibility of drug toxicity. The more common abnormalities are outlined briefly below.

A   Hepatic Disease

Because the liver plays a major role in the metabolism and inactivation of many drug molecules, impaired liver function can result in abnormally high plasma levels of a drug for extended periods of time. If normal dosing schedules are followed, accumulation of drug in the body can occur, resulting in symptoms of drug overdosage. Because of the tremendous reserve capacity of the liver, however, near-normal metabolic function usually is present except in the most severe forms of hepatic disease.

B Renal Disease

The presence of kidney disease can lead to many adverse reactions with those drugs that are eliminated largely through renal excretory processes. In the presence of renal disease, doses of drugs excreted by the kidney, such as the potentially toxic aminoglycoside antibiotics, need to be reduced, to avoid accumulation and subsequent toxicity. In progressive renal failure, plasma albumin stores may also be decreased, which can reduce the serum protein binding of many drugs, resulting in potentiation of their effects.

C Emotional Disorders

The mentally unstable individual should not be allowed to monitor his own drug therapy. Too often, emotionally unsound patients do not comply with proper dosing requirements, and this leads to overdosage with many dangerous drugs (*e.g.,* hypnotics, antipsychotics) or use of improper drugs. A major problem exists with misuse of, or overmedication with, the psychotherapeutic group of drugs. Because most individuals taking these drugs are emotionally unstable to some extent, these drug users represent an extremely high-risk group for potential adverse reactions.

D Other Disease States

The presence of many other pathologic conditions makes it unsafe to administer certain drugs. Specific contraindications for the various groups of drugs will be given throughout the text. Accurate assessment of a patient's overall health status before administration of any medication is perhaps the most important way to ensure the safest and most effective use of a drug.

IV Multiple Drug Reactions

The presence of a second drug may greatly modify the actions of a concurrently administered drug. In many instances, drugs are used together to achieve a better clinical response than either drug could achieve alone. This is an example of a positive clinical interaction. On the other hand, indiscriminate multiple drug therapy can be quite hazardous; the chance of untoward reactions increases dramatically as additional drugs are added to a therapeutic regimen. This problem becomes especially acute in the elderly or the seriously ill patient, for whom several different drugs may be prescribed simultaneously. Adverse effects due to multiple drug therapy can be manifested in several ways; this aspect of pharmacotherapy is examined in Chapter 7.

V Miscellaneous Adverse Reactions

A number of other adverse drug effects that do not fall within one of the above groups have been reported with certain drugs, and some of the more important of these are the following:
   a. *Carcinogenicity*—the ability of a drug or chemical to elicit malignant changes in cells
   b. *Teratogenicity*—the ability of a drug or chemical to produce structural defects in the developing fetus
   c. *Drug Dependence*—the ability of a drug or chemical to induce a state of psychological or physical need for itself (see Chap. 81)

▶ **NURSING CONSIDERATIONS—ADVERSE DRUG EFFECTS**

▷ 1 Recognize that any drug can be potentially toxic, and administer all drugs with caution.

▷ 2 When adverse reactions are expected, warn patient of their probable occurrence and provide necessary instructions for properly dealing with them.

▷ 3 Obtain a careful drug history, including any previous drug allergies, from each patient before administering any prescribed medication. This measure reduces the possibility of hypersensitivity reactions.

▷ 4 Advise the patient to carefully follow the prescribed drug regimen, avoid "extra" doses, and observe prescribing directions—before meals, with food, morning and night only, and so on.

▷ 5 Counsel patient to avoid any dietary constituents, over-the-counter drugs, and any other prescription medication that could result in increased toxic effects of the prescribed drug.

▷ 6 Ensure that the patient will report any untoward effects immediately, even if they seem insignificant (*e.g.,* sore throat, mild fever, itching) because these are often early signs of more severe adverse effects.

▷ 7 Impress upon the patient the importance of obtaining appropriate laboratory evaluations such as blood counts, or prothrombin time, to ensure that the optimal dose of the medication is being used.

▷ 8 Caution patients about trying to "treat" side-effects of drugs on their own (with aspirin for fever or antacids for gastric pain) because this may delay recognition until serious consequences have developed.

▷ 9 Carefully assess the seriousness of the condition being treated before using highly toxic medications. The potential benefit should outweigh the apparent risk, and other less toxic agents should be tried first if at all possible.

▷ 10 Always check that the dose being given is within acceptable limits for the condition and patient being treated.

▷ 11 Attempt to administer drugs to maximize the intended effects and to minimize their untoward reactions. For example, give diuretics in the morning to reduce need to void at night, and give antihistamines at night to prevent daytime drowsiness.

Adverse Drug Reactions—A Glossary

1. *Alopecia*—loss of hair sometimes accompanied by extreme drying of the scalp. Alopecia is a frequent side-effect of many antineoplastic agents.
2. *Anaphylactic reaction*—a severe systemic allergic reaction that develops suddenly, progresses rapidly, and is frequently fatal if not treated. Symptoms range from itching, hives, nasal congestion, abdominal cramping, and diarrhea to dyspnea, hypotension, fainting, choking sensation, cardiovascular collapse, and possibly death. An anaphylactic reaction can theoretically occur with any drug, but it is most commonly observed with those drugs frequently associated with drug allergies, such as penicillins, sulfonamides, and salicylates.
3. *Blood dyscrasias*—an abnormal condition of the formed elements or other clotting constituents of the blood. Several types are commonly observed:
   a. *Agranulocytosis*—an acute febrile disease characterized by an absence of granulocytes and often a corresponding reduction in monocytes and lymphocytes. Clinical symptoms include chills, fever, and extreme weakness. Because of the lack of white blood cells, the body's defense mechanism is impaired, and severe infection can result. Early warning signs are mucous membrane ulceration, sore throat, skin rash, and fever. Recovery normally occurs within 1 week to 2 weeks after drug is removed. Any existing infection should be vigorously treated. This is the most common drug-induced blood dyscrasia.
   b. *Anemia*—a reduction in the number of red blood cells, hemoglobin concentration, and volume of packed red cells. The result is a sharp curtailment in the oxygen-carrying capacity of the blood.
      Aplastic—results from drug-induced damage to the bone marrow and is marked by a deficiency of red cells, hemoglobin, and granular cells, and a predominance of lymphocytes. Clinical signs include fatigue, tachycardia, bleeding, fever, and increased susceptibility to infection. Aplastic anemia is often fatal due to hemorrhage and overwhelming infection.
      Hemolytic—characterized by a short life span of the red cell. Circulating erythrocytes are destroyed due to increased hemolytic activity induced by certain drugs or poisons. Especially common in individuals with a glucose-6-phosphate dehydrogenase deficiency. Withdrawal of offending agent usually corrects the condition.
   c. *Thrombocytopenia*—a decreased blood platelet count, resulting from either platelet destruction or depression of the platelet-forming mechanism in the bone marrow. Onset may be sudden, and symptoms include purpura (petechiae; epistaxis; oral, vaginal, or GI bleeding) and easy bruising. The platelet count returns to normal within a few weeks after cessation of drug therapy, but the count may again rise briefly immediately following stoppage of the drug. Most severe complications can result from excessive cerebral hemorrhage.
4. *Erythema multiforme*—an acute inflammatory skin disease characterized by lesions consisting of concentric circles of erythema, usually appearing on the neck, face, and legs. Occasionally blisters are observed. Often accompanied by fever, malaise, arthralgia, and gastric distress. The most severe variant, *Stevens-Johnson syndrome,* is characterized by high fever, headache, and inflammatory lesions of the mouth, eyes, and genitalia. Death can occur because of renal impairment.
5. *Exfoliative dermatitis*—erythema and scaling of the skin over large parts of the body. Symptoms include itching, weakness, malaise, fever, and weight loss. Exfoliation may include loss of hair and nails as well as skin, and mucosal sloughing can occur. The reaction is generally unpredictable in its duration and recurrence. Relapses are frequent, and secondary infections can be serious. Exfoliative dermatitis may occur secondary to pre-existing dermatoses or to contact dermatitis resulting from an underlying carcinoma, or can be caused by drug usage.
6. *Hepatotoxicity*—liver damage resulting from either infections or drug hypersensitivity. The most frequently observed drug-induced manifestation is *jaundice,* characterized by hyperbilirubinemia and deposition of bile pigments in the mucous membranes and skin, which impart the typical yellow appearance. At least three main types of jaundice are recognized:
   a. *Cholestatic*—due to interference with the normal secretion of bile by an obstruction of the biliary passages. It may result from gallstones, tumors, or drug-induced inflammation of the bile channels.
   b. *Hepatocellular*—due to impairment of the function of liver cells. It is also termed *necrotic jaundice* and closely resembles severe viral hepatitis.
   c. *Hemolytic*—due to a drug hypersensitivity or a direct toxic effect of the drug on erythrocytes, possibly interference with normal glucose metabolism in the red cells.
7. *Lupus Erythematosus* (LE)—an autoimmune inflammatory disorder that can occur in two forms,

one affecting only the skin (discoid LE) and the other, more serious, affecting multiple body organs (systemic LE). The etiology of the naturally occurring disease is unknown, but both forms occur predominantly in young women. Several drugs can also cause a lupus-like reaction. Among the many symptoms are diffuse rash; fever; malaise; alopecia; joint symptoms including stiffness, swelling, and synovitis; conjunctivitis; photophobia; pneumonitis; pleurisy; myocarditis; arrhythmias; lymphadenopathy; splenomegaly; and hemolytic anemia. Renal and neurologic features are absent in drug-induced lupus but are seen in the spontaneously occurring form of the disease. Clinical features generally revert slowly toward normal when the offending drug is withdrawn, but altered laboratory values (*e.g.,* elevated antinuclear antibody titer, leukopenia, thrombocytopenia) indicative of the disease may persist for many months.

8. *Nephrotoxicity*—damage to the functional units of the kidney, such as the glomerular filtration apparatus, blood vessels, or renal tubular cells, or a dysfunction of the components (*e.g.,* enzymes, transport carriers) involved in the tubular secretory and reabsorptive processes.

9. *Neurotoxicity*—damage to various nervous system structures.
   a. *Myasthenia-like reacton*—extreme muscle weakness due to an impairment in the transmission of impulses at the neuromuscular junction.
   b. *Extrapyramidal reactions*—disturbances of the extrapyramidal motor regulating system in the CNS, resulting in abnormal motor function. Common manifestations include immobility (akinesia); fixed positioning of the limbs (rigidity); sudden violent movement of the arms and head (dystonias); restlessness (akathisia); and rhythmic, clonic muscular activity (tremor). Extrapyramidal reactions are frequently associated with use of antipsychotic drugs.
   c. *Ototoxicity*—progressive hearing loss and tinnitus caused by damage to the eighth cranial nerve. Often accompanied by vertigo and nystagmus if the vestibular branch of the nerve is affected. It is common with the aminoglycoside antibiotics and certain diuretics.
   d. *Ocular toxicity*—disturbances in the functioning of the eye. The most common manifestation is *blurred vision,* which can occur following use of many drugs, especially those with an anticholinergic action. Other drug-induced ocular disorders include myopia, scotomata, amblyopia, optic neuritis, pigmentary retinopathy, and cataracts.

10. *Photosensitivity*—an altered responsiveness to light, usually eczematous in nature. Common manifestations are itching, scaling, urticaria, and in severe cases multiform lesions.

11. *Purpura*—localized hemorrhaging, occurring in the skin, mucous membranes, or serous membranes. The lesions may be petechiae (small blood spots) or ecchymoses (larger areas of bleeding). Purpura is commonly seen in patients with thrombocytopenia due to increased platelet destruction.

7 Drug Interactions

A drug interaction refers to the process whereby the expected therapeutic effect of a drug is modified by the presence of another factor, usually a drug or other chemical agent that may be dietary, environmental, or endogenous. When two drugs are administered in close sequence to each other, they may interact either to enhance or to diminish the intended effect of one or both drugs, or they may produce an unintended and potentially harmful reaction.

Thus, drug interactions may also be viewed as either *beneficial* or *adverse.* The means by which the presence of a second drug can augment or reduce the effects of the initial drug were briefly reviewed in Chapter 3 under "Combined Effects of Drugs." This chapter offers a more detailed look at why drug interactions occur and the mechanisms that may be involved.

The clinical significance of drug interactions, especially the adverse type, is greatly understated in many cases. When a patient on multiple drug therapy develops an unusual or disturbing symptom, it is often very difficult to determine if the reaction is caused by an alteration in the disease state being treated, by the presence of a certain drug, by the interaction of two concurrently used drugs, or by some other change in the individual's physiology. What may be a significant drug interaction might simply be viewed as a deterioration in the patient's status or the appearance of a new disease entity. It is apparent, then, that many drug reactions can go completely unheeded or fail to be recognized immediately, especially if the reaction is mild. The clinician must therefore make a careful assessment of *any* change in a patient's condition and possess sufficient knowledge of potential drug interactions to be able to recognize the possibility of a developing drug interaction problem.

The practice of multiple drug therapy is becoming increasingly prevalent as the median age of the population increases, with an attendant increase in the presence of chronic disease conditions requiring drug treatment. It stands to reason that as the number of drugs used concurrently increases, the *potential* for drug interactions increases to an even greater degree. Thus, the benefit-to-risk ratio assumes critical importance in decisions about the number and kinds of drugs to be employed in the therapy of chronic diseases. Occasional episodes of dizziness or tachycardia may be acceptable consequences of drug combinations used to control severe hypertension. On the other hand, use of aspirin is totally unwarranted in coumarin anticoagulant users when other equally effective analgesics are readily available that do not interfere with the action of the anticoagulants. Knowledge of the etiology of drug interactions and the ability to predict possible problems based upon drug mechanisms can greatly minimize the toxicity resulting from concurrent drug usage. Of themselves, most drug interactions are usually not serious or life-threatening, but ignorance of them, through either lack of knowledge or careful observation, can be annoying to the patient and frequently dangerous.

There are numerous reasons why drug interactions occur, yet many interactions can be eliminated or at least minimized by recognizing the probable causative factors and by undertaking appropriate preventive action. Some of the more common reasons are the following:

1 *Insufficient knowledge*—Safe and effective combination drug therapy requires adequate understanding of the mechanisms of action and potential complications of each type of drug employed.

2 *Dietary factors*—Many constituents of an individual's diet can interact with certain drugs. In cases in which such interactions are documented, it is important that the patient be advised to avoid the offending dietary agents. Caffeine, licorice (produces hypokalemia), calcium in dairy products, and tyramine in a variety of different foods are some common examples of food substances that can interact with other drugs.

3 *Physiologic state of the individual*—The effect of factors such as age, sex, weight, and genetic abnormalities can greatly influence the occurrence of drug interactions.

4 *Presence of disease states*—The likelihood of a drug interaction is increased in those persons whose pathologic condition (such as liver disease, kidney damage, or altered enzyme systems) may affect the handling of one or more drugs used as part of a therapeutic regimen. The fairly common practice of seeing more than one physician at a time can increase the risk of a drug interaction if each prescriber is not fully aware of all the drugs being taken by the patient. Self-medication is likewise responsible for a large number of drug interactions that could easily be avoided by proper counseling.

5 *Environmental factors*—Often overlooked as a contributory factor in drug interactions is the possibility of exposure to pollutants—industrial, agricultural, and other types of chemical agents that are pharmacologically active. Although little direct reliable information exists concerning interactions with these substances, even small amounts of insecticides, fungicides, or industrial wastes can markedly alter the effects of certain therapeutic agents. For example, chlorinated insecticides may stimulate drug metabolism by liver enzymes, whereas pesticides containing cholinesterase inhibitors can cause respiratory distress, muscle weakness, and convulsions.

6 *Dosage form factors*—Incompatibility of different dosage forms or improper preparation of a drug may result in drug interactions on either a physical or a chemical level. Generally, the major concern in this regard is one of bioavailability—that is, what fraction of the dose is available through absorption to the fluids of distribution. *In vitro* chemical interactions, *in vivo* alterations in rate, or extent of absorption resulting from the presence of a second drug can markedly influence the response to the initially administered agent. Opponents of generic equivalency (*i.e.,* similar efficacy and safety for the same drug manufactured by different companies) often cite the demonstrated differences in absorption rates, dissolution characteristics, and peak blood levels as evidence that not all forms of the same drug are therapeutically or toxicologically equal. Further, the maintenance of constant plasma levels of a drug for extended periods of time through use of a sustained-release dosage form can be upset by the presence of another drug that alters GI motility and intestinal transit time; thus, the sustained-release dosage form is eliminated too quickly.

Drug Interactions—Classification and Mechanisms

Interactions between drugs may occur *in vitro* or *in vivo*. An understanding of the basic mechanisms by which drug reactions develop can enable the practitioner either to prevent many interactions from occurring or at least to recognize potential interaction problems before they develop into serious complications. Although any classification of drug interactions represents an oversimplification, the following outline will serve as an aid to categorizing many of the important types of drug interactions according to their mechanisms of action.

A   In Vitro

The term *incompatibility* is often used to designate *in vitro* drug reactions and may refer to either a physical or chemical interaction.

1 *Physical*—occurs if the physical state of either drug is altered when the chemicals are mixed. For example, amphotericin will precipitate if mixed with Normal Saline instead of 5% Dextrose. Likewise, the anticoagulant effect of heparin, a negatively charged acid, is antagonized by protamine, a positively charged base.

2 *Chemical*—occurs when the components of a drug mixture interact to form chemically altered products. For example, chemical incompatibilities in solution exist between methicillin and kanamycin, aminophylline and chlorpromazine, and dopamine and sodium bicarbonate.

In most cases, physical and chemical incompatibilities are manifested by a visible change such as precipitate formation or color change. Occasionally, however, *in vitro* interactions can occur without any observable signs, possibly resulting in undetected loss of potency. Thus, the compatibility of two drugs should always be ascertained by reference to an appropriate source prior to mixing.

B   In Vivo

Most drug interactions occurring in the body can be categorized into one of several classes, depending on the mechanisms responsible for the interaction. It should be repeated that drug interactions can be desirable and expected and often purposely caused, or they may be unwanted and unexpected. The interaction may enhance, retard, or abolish the actions of one or both drugs. Several important mechanisms of *in vivo* drug interactions are discussed, and pertinent examples are given. While an understanding of the mechanisms of drug interactions can help the practitioner to recognize many potential problems when two or more drugs are combined, it is important that the sections of the book on each individual drug be consulted to obtain a listing of the most likely drug interactions for each agent used. The following classification is intended to serve only as an overview of this tremendously complex field.

I   Alterations in Drug Effects

Several types of interactions result from alterations in the normal pharmacologic effects of one drug due to the presence of a second drug with similar or different pharmacologic effects.

A   Similar Pharmacologic Effects

Each of two drugs possessing similar pharmacologic actions will generally enhance the pharmacologic and toxicologic effects of the other. This synergistic interaction can result in either an additive effect or potentiation (see Chap. 3). Examples of this type of reaction are the combined use of alcohol and a barbiturate (CNS depressants having an additive effect) or anticholinergics and tricyclic antidepressants (which have significant anticholinergic action) resulting in enhanced side-effects such as dry mouth, blurred vision, and urinary retention.

B   Different Pharmacologic Effects

Administration of two drugs with opposing actions usually results in a significant reduction or total abolition of the pharmacologic effects of each. This type of interaction is generally easy to predict if the mechanisms of action of the two drugs are known. Examples might be the simultaneous use of a barbiturate (depressant) and an amphetamine (stimulant) or the administration of epinephrine (a vasoconstrictor) and histamine (a vasodilator).

C   Competitive Receptor Antagonism

This form of drug interaction is similar to the above because the effects of one drug can be cancelled by the concomitant use of a second drug that blocks the access of the first drug to its receptor site of action. Again, this type of interaction can usually be avoided by an awareness of the mechanisms of action of the two agents. For example, anticholinergic drugs should not be used in patients with glaucoma because they would block the receptor actions of the cholinergic drugs (such as pilocarpine) used to treat this eye disorder. Propranolol, a beta-adrenergic blocking drug, would interfere with the bronchodilatory action of isoproterenol in the treatment of chronic obstructive pulmonary disease.

D   Blockade of Neuronal Uptake or Release

Drugs interfering with the uptake or release of other agents by the nerve endings can result in significant interactions that usually decrease the effects of one or both drugs. Phenothiazines and tricyclic antidepressants exert an inhibitory effect on uptake of drugs by the nerve endings. These agents will nullify the antihypertensive effect of guanethidine, which must be taken up by the nerve endings to produce its intended effect. Because many important endogenous pressor amines, such as tyramine and norepinephrine, are partially inactivated by neuronal uptake, these endogenous substances will be potentiated in the presence of neuronal uptake blockers such as the phenothiazines and the tricyclics. This potentiation can lead to serious consequences, such as severe hypertension or arrhythmias.

E   Altered Receptor Sensitivity

The sensitivity of a receptor for a particular drug action can be modified by the presence of a second drug. For example, thyroxine may increase the sensitivity of receptors to the anticoagulant effect of the coumarins, so that a dosage adjustment is needed. Long-term use of antipsychotic drugs can lead to a hypersensitivity of central dopamine receptors. This dopamine supersensitivity is thought to be responsible for the appearance of a series of chronic orofacial involuntary movements, known as tardive dyskinesias, that occur with prolonged antipsychotic drug use, because the endogenous dopamine is interacting with hypersensitive receptor sites. As a general rule, receptor sensitivity decreases with prolonged stimulation and increases with chronic blockade or disuse. This phenomenon helps to explain the action of many drugs that alter receptor sensitivity, and the terms *down-regulation* and *up-regulation* can be applied to drug-induced decreases or increases in receptor sensitivity, respectively. This concept is explained more fully for those drugs acting in this manner throughout the book under Mechanism of Action.

II   Alterations in Drug Metabolism

Many drug interactions occur as a result of alterations in the metabolism of one drug that are caused by the presence of other drugs. These interactions may reflect changes in the absorption, distribution, biotransformation, or excretion of one drug that result from the actions of a second pharmacologic agent.

A Absorption

Any substance capable of altering the normal physiologic processes of the GI tract can markedly impair drug absorption. Alterations in gastric absorption may be caused by the following:

1 Changes in Gastric *p*H

Drugs (*e.g.,* sodium bicarbonate or antacids) that can raise the *p*H of the GI fluid may decrease the absorption of weakly acidic drugs and may increase the absorption of weakly basic drugs. This is based on the concept that un-ionized drug molecules are lipid-soluble and thus cross the absorptive membranes easily. Acidic drugs, such as the salicylates, barbiturates, and oral anticoagulants, are largely ionized at high *p*H and therefore are poorly absorbed. Conversely, basic drugs, such as amphetamines and ephedrine, are essentially un-ionized at a high *p*H and thus are well absorbed (see Chap. 2).

2 Changes in Intestinal Motility and Function

Drugs that slow GI motility (*e.g.,* anticholinergics) prolong gastric emptying time and thus may allow for more complete gastric absorption of many orally administered agents. Substances inducing diarrhea hasten the removal of drugs from the GI tract, thereby reducing their gastric absorption. Conversely, antidiarrheal products or constipating agents, such as loperamide, diphenoxylate with atropine sulfate, and powdered opium tincture, slow passage through the gastric region and allow for more extensive absorption.

3 Chemical Binding of Drugs

Several classes of agents have the capability of forming complexes with many orally administered drugs, thereby impairing their GI absorption. The absorption of tetracyclines is inhibited by the presence of drugs (*e.g.,* antacids) or foods (*e.g.,* milk, cheese) containing calcium, magnesium, or aluminum, substances capable of chemically chelating the tetracycline molecule. Many antacids, as well as cholestyramine (an ionic-exchange resin), may interfere with the absorption of drugs such as warfarin, digitoxin, and phenylbutazone by forming a chemical complex.

4 Sequestration

Fat-soluble drugs, including vitamins A, D, and K, will be sequestered in the presence of a fatty vehicle like mineral oil, and absorption may be retarded.

5 Alteration of Intestinal Flora

Alterations in the microbial population of the GI tract can occur with many antibiotics, thereby lowering the levels of vitamin K and increasing the anticoagulant action of the coumarins. Drug-induced diarrhea can occur in response to changes in intestinal flora, affecting drug absorption as well.

6 Competition for Absorption Mechanisms

Active transport mechanisms function in the absorption of many drugs and can be inhibited by pharmacologic agents that compete for these active absorptive mechanisms. Phenytoin, for example, impedes absorption of folic acid, leading to megaloblastic anemia in many instances. Certain amino acids compete for the same transport mechanisms involved in methyldopa and levodopa absorption.

7 Miscellaneous Factors

Other factors that can result in altered absorption of one drug due to the presence of a second drug include (1) decreased mucosal blood flow, (2) altered volume and content of GI secretions, (3) direct damage to the mucosal surface, and (4) osmotic pressure changes within the intestinal lumen.

B Distribution

The distribution of drugs within the body can be significantly altered by the presence of other drugs. Among the more important mechanisms of drug interactions related to drug distribution are the following:

1 Competition for Plasma Protein Binding

Drugs bound to plasma proteins are inactive, even though present in the body. Upon release from the protein-bound stores, the free drug becomes active and is capable of exerting a pharmacologic effect. Many classes of drugs display significant protein-binding capacity, and when two highly protein-bound drugs are employed concurrently, a drug interaction is likely to occur. This interaction results from competition for the fixed number of available protein binding sites in the plasma, which quickly become saturated, leaving a significant fraction of either drug unbound, and therefore active. Highly protein-bound drugs capable of interacting with one another are salicylates, barbiturates, oral anticoagulants, oral hypoglycemics, sulfonamides, hydantoins, nonsteroidal anti-inflammatory drugs, calcium channel blockers, cyclophosphamide, clofibrate, diazoxide, chloral hydrate, and methotrexate.

2   Displacement from Storage Depots

Many endogenous substances, including neurotransmitters and hormones, are stored by various means in the body. Many drugs exert their effects by either liberating these substances from their storage sites or by preventing their release. A drug interaction can occur when two drugs affecting storage mechanisms are given concurrently. For example, due to its releasing action on stored catecholamines, amphetamine may interfere with the antihypertensive action of guanethidine but can enhance the stimulatory action of ephedrine.

3   Blood Flow Alterations

Pharmacologic agents capable of modifying blood flow to various body organs can greatly influence the distribution and handling of other drugs. For example, epinephrine is often combined with local anesthetics to restrict the spread of the anesthetic by reducing local blood flow. Some cardiovascular drugs can alter blood volume and blood pressure by producing vasoconstriction, thereby restricting the access of other drugs to certain body organs. Decreases in hepatic blood flow by vasoconstrictors likewise can significantly reduce the rate and extent of drug metabolism.

C   Biotransformation

The process of converting drugs to their respective metabolites is termed *biotransformation,* and it usually occurs in the liver. These reactions are generally mediated by enzymes, so that any drug capable of altering the enzymatic processes involved in the metabolism of other drugs can produce a drug interaction.

1   Enzyme Inhibition

There are many examples of compounds that interfere with the activity of inactivating enzymes, thereby potentiating other drugs. Monoamine oxidase (MAO) inhibitors, compounds that inhibit the normal functioning of the endogenous enzyme monoamine oxidase, elevate levels of biogenic amines and may produce severe hypertensive reactions in the presence of pressor amines. Xanthine oxidase inhibitors such as allopurinol increase plasma levels of mercaptopurine by blocking its breakdown. Cholinesterase inhibitors such as physostigmine and neostigmine block degradation of choline esters and can enhance the effects of acetylcholine, succinylcholine, and other cholinergic drugs. Carbidopa competitively inhibits the enzyme dopa decarboxylase in the plasma. This enzyme normally inactivates l–DOPA before it reaches its site of action in the CNS. Thus, dopa decarboxylase inhibition elevates the brain level of l–DOPA and increases the synthesis of dopamine in the motor regulating centers of the CNS.

2   Enzyme Acceleration

Liver microsomal enzymes involved in the metabolic breakdown of many classes of drugs can be stimulated by certain pharmacologic agents, including barbiturates, hydantoins, meprobamate, griseofulvin, and chlorinated hydrocarbon insecticides. This is termed *enzyme induction* and results in a decreased therapeutic response to those drugs metabolized by the microsomal enzymes, because the drugs are being metabolized more rapidly. There are literally hundreds of drugs and chemicals that can stimulate hepatic enzymes, and the range of potential drug interactions along these lines is enormous. For example, coumarin anticoagulants are metabolized at a much faster rate in the presence of a barbiturate, and an appropriate dosage adjustment must be made. Phenytoin reduces the effects of dexamethasone by inducing the microsomal enzymes responsible for its metabolism. Enzyme induction may be responsible for development of tolerance to certain drugs because some drugs may stimulate their own liver metabolism. Examples of such drugs are barbiturates, meprobamate, and glutethimide.

D   Excretion

Drug interactions occurring with the excretion of drugs may involve any of the renal excretory processes (glomerular filtration, tubular reabsorption, active tubular secretion). Most clinically important drug interactions occur as a result of either changes in urinary pH, altering the fraction of reabsorbed drug, or through competition for active tubular secretory mechanisms.

1   Changes in Urinary pH

Acidification of the urine with agents such as ammonium chloride can result in potentially reduced effects of basic drugs (*e.g.,* amphetamine and quinidine) because they will be largely ionized at the acidic pH and readily excreted. On the other hand, renal excretion of acidic drugs, such as salicylates, barbiturates, and anticoagulants, will be accelerated by alkalinization of urine with sodium bicarbonate, acetazolamide, or potassium citrate. Alkalinization of urinary pH is often an effective technique in treating drug overdosage with certain acidic drugs, such as phenobarbital or salicylates.

2 Competition for Tubular Mechanisms

Many drugs and metabolites are actively secreted from the renal capillary network into the tubules of the kidney and are subsequently eliminated. Drug interactions may occur when any two actively secreted drugs are used together because of competition for the active secretory mechanisms. Drugs that may interact by this means, resulting in prolonged therapeutic effects, are salicylates, sulfonamides, penicillins, thiazide diuretics, pyrazolones, dicumarol, indomethacin, probenecid, oral hypoglycemics, acetazolamide, diazoxide, and methotrexate. Small doses of aspirin may impair the uricosuric (uric acid-excreting) action of probenecid by interfering with the active secretion of uric acid into the renal tubules, and can also inhibit the excretion of methotrexate. Competition for active tubular secretion can be used to therapeutic advantage as well. For example, the use of probenecid with penicillin to delay the normally rapid excretion of the penicillin molecule significantly prolongs the effective duration of penicillin in the body.

3 Alterations in Fluid and Electrolyte Balance

Changes in fluid and electrolyte levels induced by certain drugs can markedly affect the therapeutic effectiveness and toxicity of other drugs, particularly those acting on the heart, kidney, and skeletal muscles. Hypokalemia (low serum potassium levels) produced by many diuretic agents and corticosteroids increases the likelihood of digitalis toxicity, and can antagonize the antiarrhythmic effects of quinidine, lidocaine, procainamide, and phenytoin. Potassium loss may also result in prolonged paralysis following use of antidepolarizing skeletal muscle relaxants.

Another interaction of potential clinical significance is the use of drugs that induce sodium and water retention (*e.g.,* pyrazolones or corticosteroids) with antihypertensive or diuretic drugs. These fluid-retaining drugs can negate the action of antihypertensive agents in lowering blood pressure.

III Miscellaneous Drug Interactions

A Alterations in the Immune Response

Antibody production can be altered by the presence of certain drugs. Vaccines and toxoids stimulate antibody production, whereas glucocorticoids such as hydrocortisone can markedly inhibit the immune response and should not be used with vaccines.

Although antibiotics are frequently given in combination, drug interactions can occur if both bacteriostatic and bactericidal drugs are given together. For example, penicillins are bactericidal because they interfere with cell wall synthesis in dividing bacteria. They are less effective, however, when used with tetracyclines—drugs that prevent cell division and bacterial growth. This mutual antagonism can cause serious complications when combination therapy is used to treat severe infections.

B Residual Drug Effects

A potential source of drug interactions is the prolonged period of therapeutic effectiveness that is often observed even after a drug is discontinued. Drugs with prolonged actions have the potential to interact with newly introduced drugs even though the first drugs are no longer being administered. For example, when MAO inhibitors are given within 2 weeks of tricyclic antidepressants, severe hypertension can occur due to the residual effects of the MAO inhibitors combined with the effects of the tricyclic antidepressants.

It is difficult to simply state the overall clinical importance of drug interactions. Some are beneficial, others represent mild and essentially benign reactions, requiring merely an adjustment in the dosage of one or more drugs, while others are potentially life-threatening interactions requiring immediate action. Although most drug interactions result in unwanted effects of one or more drugs, some are clinically beneficial and are often deliberately induced. Clinically significant adverse drug interactions can be minimized by an understanding of the various mechanisms involved in their production, awareness of the presence of predisposing factors, and avoidance, where possible, of multiple drug usage.

Drugs Acting on
the Nervous System

The human nervous system is an immensely complex structure, encompassing more than 12 billion nerve cells or neurons. Along with the endocrine system, it regulates and coordinates the functioning of the various organs of the body. The endocrine system provides a slowly developing but long-lasting control, whereas the nervous system evokes rapid changes in body function and therefore provides "moment-to-moment" control.

The nervous system can be categorized in the following manner:
1. Peripheral nervous system
   a. Somatic system
   b. Autonomic system
      (1) Sympathetic division
      (2) Parasympathetic division
2. Central nervous system
   a. Brain
   b. Spinal cord

While an in-depth discussion of the various divisions of the nervous system is beyond the scope of this text, a brief review of the important aspects and concepts related to the functioning of the nervous system will be presented in order to provide sufficient background to a better understanding of the subsequent chapters dealing with those classes of drugs affecting neuronal functioning.

Neurophysiology —A Review

8

I Peripheral Nervous System

The peripheral nervous system is divided into the somatic and autonomic branches, and several important differences exist between these two systems, as outlined in Table 8-1. The somatic system is mainly concerned with conveying to the CNS sensory information relative to the external environment, such as light, heat, and pressure, and mediating those skeletal muscle responses that represent one's reaction to the environment. Thus, the somatic system is viewed as a voluntary system—one over which a person exerts conscious control.

In contrast, the autonomic system includes those sensory and motor nerves that primarily innervate organs (smooth muscle, heart, glands) that usually function independently of our volition. This system is classified as an involuntary system. While responses of the somatic system, such as contraction of skeletal muscle, are almost always excitatory, those of the autonomic system can be either excitatory (*e.g.,* vasoconstriction) or inhibitory (*e.g.,* bradycardia, bronchodilation), depending on the organ and neurohormone involved.

The autonomic system is further subclassified into sympathetic and parasympathetic divisions, and the characteristics of each division are listed in Table 8-2.

The parasympathetic division is often referred to as a cholinergic system because the neurotransmitter at its postganglionic nerve endings is acetylcholine, whereas the sympathetic system is frequently considered adrenergic because its postganglionic neurotransmitter in most cases is nor-

Table 8-1. Difference Between the Somatic and Autonomic Nervous Systems

Parameter	Somatic	Autonomic
Nature of the response	Voluntary	Involuntary
Centers of neuronal origin in the CNS	Cerebrum, cerebellum, midbrain, basal ganglia, spinal cord	Midbrain, hypothalamus, pons, medulla, spinal cord
Structures innervated by efferent nerve fibers	Skeletal muscles, sensory organs	Smooth muscle, cardiac muscle, exocrine and endocrine glands
Efferent nerve pathways	Single neuron with cell body in CNS and axon terminal at effector structure (*e.g.,* skeletal muscle fiber)	Two-neuron chain, with cell body of *pre*ganglionic neuron in CNS and axon terminal in a peripheral ganglia. *Post*ganglionic neuron has cell body in ganglia (synapses with *pre*ganglionic nerve ending) and axon terminal at effector structure (*e.g.,* heart, GI tract, bronchioles, glands)
Effect of nerve impulse on innervated structures	Excitation (*e.g.,* skeletal muscle contraction)	Excitation (*e.g.,* vasoconstriction, salivation) or inhibition (*e.g.,* bradycardia, bronchodilation)

epinephrine. Most effector structures are innervated by *both* divisions of the autonomic system, and in dually innervated structures the pharmacologic effects of the two divisions are *opposite.* That is, if sympathetic activation causes excitation, parasympathetic activation causes inhibition. However, it is important to recognize that the two divisions do not exert *equal* control over all dually innervated structures. For example, the sympthetic division controls blood vessel tone, and hence blood pressure, to a much greater degree than the parasympathetic system, whereas the reverse is true in the functioning of the GI tract.

A few structures, however, are singly innervated, including the adrenal medulla, sweat glands, certain blood vessels, intrinsic eye muscles, and pilomotor muscles of the skin. The response of these structures is always *excitatory,* irrespective of their innervation. The effects of sympathetic versus parasympathetic stimulation on various structures of the body are outlined in Table 8-3, in which the opposing nature of most responses and the excitatory nature of singly innervated structures is clearly indicated. It should be noted that although the adrenal medulla and most sweat glands are innervated by sympathetic fibers, the neurotransmitter released at the nerve ending is acetylcholine, not norepinephrine. Thus, peripheral nerves are probably best classified

chemically—that is, on the basis of the principal neurohormone released from their nerve endings. Nerves releasing acetylcholine are thus termed *cholinergic,* and those releasing norepinephrine are called *adrenergic.* The various mechanisms by which these neurohormones function at nerve endings are reviewed below.

A   Neurohormonal Function

The functional unit of the nervous system is the neuron, a specialized cell capable of generating and transmitting electrical impulses. The passage of an impulse *along* a neuron, termed *conduction,* is an *electrical* process involving changes in the potential difference across the neuronal membrane caused by alterations in the flow of ions through the membrane. Drugs such as local anesthetics are capable of interrupting conduction of nerve impulses along a neuron by interfering with ionic flow across the membrane.

On the other hand, the transmission of an impulse *between* adjacent neurons is a *chemical* process mediated by substances termed *neurohormones* or *neurotransmitters* (*e.g.,* acetylcholine, norepinephrine) that are stored within

Table 8-2. Comparison of the Parasympathetic and Sympathetic Division of the Autonomic Nervous System

Parameter	Parasympathetic Division	Sympathetic Division
Outflow from CNS	Craniosacral	Thoracolumbar
	Cranial nerves (3, 7, 9, 10; *i.e.,* oculomotor, facial, glossopharyngeal, and vagus) and sacral (S2 to S4) segments of the spinal cord	Thoracic (T1 to T12) and lumbar (L1 to L3) segments of the spinal cord
Ganglia	Near or within structure innervated	Close to spinal cord
Preganglionic fiber	Long and myelinated	Short and myelinated
Postganglionic fiber	Short and nonmyelinated	Long and nonmyelinated
Response to stimulation	Localized to a restricted area	Generalized and widespread
Neurotransmitter at all ganglia	Acetylcholine	Acetylcholine
Neurotransmitter at postganglionic nerve ending	Acetylcholine	Norepinephrine

Table 8-3. Responses of Effector Structures to Autonomic Nervous System Activation

Effector	Parasympathetic (Cholinergic) Nerve Impulses	Sympathetic (Adrenergic) Nerve Impulses
Heart		
Rate	Decreased	Increased
Contractility		Increased
Blood Vessels		
Coronary		Dilated
Skeletal muscle		Dilated
Skin and mucosa		Constricted
Cerebral, pulmonary, abdominal viscera	Dilated	Constricted
Stomach and Intestine		
Motility and tone	Increased	Decreased
Sphincters	Relaxed	Contracted
Glandular secretion	Increased	
Urinary Bladder		
Detrusor muscle	Contracted	Relaxed
Trigone and sphincter	Relaxed	Contracted
Other Smooth Muscle		
Bronchial muscle, ureters, gallbladder and ducts	Contracted	Relaxed
Salivary Glands	Stimulated (profuse, watery secretion)	Stimulated (sparse, thick, mucinous secretion)
Eye		
Radial muscle of iris		Contracted (mydriasis)
Sphincter muscle of iris	Contracted (miosis)	
Ciliary muscle	Contracted (accommodated for near vision)	Relaxed
Spleen Capsule		Contracted
Liver		Glycogenolysis
Kidney		Renin secreted
Skin		
Sweat glands		Stimulated*
Pilomotor muscles		Contracted
Adrenal Medulla		Secretion of epinephrine and norepinephrine

* Neurotransmitter at nerve ending is acetylcholine rather than norepinephrine

the nerve ending and diffuse from one neuron to another across the interneuronal space or synaptic junction. It should be remembered that the *post*synaptic structure can be either a second neuron or some other type of organ or tissue, such as a muscle fiber or gland. The transmission of nerve impulses is an essential step in the functioning of the nervous system, and because it is a chemically (neurohormonally) mediated process, it is readily affected by many different classes of drugs, resulting in a wide range of pharmacologic effects.

In order to understand how drugs can affect nerve impulse transmission, it is necessary to first review the sequence of events that occur during the transmission of impulses between neurons.

1. *Biosynthesis of neurotransmitter*—Chemical substances that mediate transmission are formed from precursor substances within the nerve ending. Acetylcholine is synthesized from choline and acetyl coenzyme A by the action of the enzyme choline acetyltransferase. Norepinephrine is formed from the amino acid phenylalanine through a series of enzymatic conversions. In the adrenal medulla, as well as in certain brain areas, norepinephrine is further converted to epinephrine.

2. *Storage of neurotransmitter*—Upon formation, the neurotransmitter is taken up into specialized sites (such as vesicles) within the nerve ending and

stored. This allows the neuron to "build up" a surplus of the transmitter in anticipation of its need. Thousands of molecules of acetylcholine are stored in each vesicle. These vesicles are thought to be membranous sacs derived from the neuronal membrane. Some norepinephrine is stored in granules bound to ATP, the so-called reserve pool, whereas other norepinephrine exists in the cytoplasm and is not contained within vesicles. This latter fraction is known as the *mobile pool,* and is *not* released by a nerve action potential (see below), but can be expelled by various drugs.

3. *Release of neurotransmitter*—With the arrival of a nerve action potential at the nerve ending, depolarization of the *presynaptic* membrane occurs, resulting in release of the neurotransmitter from its storage site into the synaptic junction. Release of the neurohormones probably is due to influx of calcium ions into the nerve ending, resulting in destabilization of the storage vesicles, subsequent fusion with the terminal plasma membrane, and extrusion of the neurotransmitter into the synaptic cleft.

The release of presynaptic stores of norepinephrine can be regulated by a negative feedback mechanism that is mediated by alpha-2 receptor sites (see Table 8-4) on the presynaptic nerve ending. When the level of norepinephrine released from the nerve ending becomes excessive, some of the molecules begin to interact with the prejunctional alpha-2 receptor sites on the terminal nerve ending, thereby attenuating further release of norepinephrine. In this way, the neurotransmitter can regulate its own rate of release through a negative feedback mechanism. A number of other clinically useful drugs also influence the release of norepinephrine by either activating (*e.g.,* clonidine) or blocking (*e.g.,* imipramine) presynaptic alpha-2 receptor sites. Conversely, activation of presynaptic beta receptor sites has been postulated to facilitate neurohormonal release.

Prejunctional regulation of neurotransmitter release is not limited to norepinephrine. Evidence suggests that most substances that function as neurotransmitters (*e.g.,* serotonin, histamine, polypeptides) can regulate their own release through a negative feedback mechanism.

4. *Interaction with postsynaptic membrane*—The released neurohormone diffuses across the synaptic junction and interacts (complexes) with specific reactive areas (receptor sites) on the postsynaptic membrane. This interaction can result in either depolarization (activation) or hyperpolarization (inhibition) of the neuron or effector structure and subsequent facilitation or blockade of nerve impulse transmission.

5. *Inactivation of neurotransmitter*—Neurohormonal action can be terminated in several ways:
   a. Diffusion of the released neurotransmitter away from the synaptic area; probably important in removing excess or "overflow," but of little consequence for terminating the effects of physiologically released amounts of neurohormones.

Table 8-4. Characteristics of Peripheral Receptor Sites

Type	Location	Activators	Blockers
Cholinergic			
Muscarinic (M)	Sites innervated by postganglionic parasympathetic fibers	Acetylcholine Pilocarpine	Atropine
Nicotinic I (NI)	All autonomic ganglia	Acetylcholine Nicotine	Trimethaphan Mecamylamine
Nicotinic II (NII)	Skeletal neuromuscular junction	Acetylcholine Nicotine	d-tubocurare Gallamine Pancuronium
Adrenergic			
Alpha-1	Most blood vessels, GI tract, pancreas, eye, skin, salivary glands	Norepinephrine Epinephrine Phenylephrine	Phentolamine Prazosin
Alpha-2	*Presynaptic* terminal endings of adrenergic nerve fibers, platelets, fat cells	Norepinephrine Epinephrine Clonidine	Imipramine
Beta-1	Heart, GI tract, adipose tissue	Epinephrine Isoproterenol Dobutamine	Propranolol Metoprolol
Beta-2	Bronchioles, uterus, urinary bladder, liver, kidney, skeletal muscle vasculature	Epinephrine Isoproterenol Albuterol	Propranolol Nadolol
Dopaminergic	Renal, visceral, and coronary blood vessels	Dopamine	Haloperidol

b. Enzymatic breakdown of neurohormone; plays a greater role for acetylcholine than for norepinephrine. Acetylcholinesterase cleaves the neurotransmitter into choline and acetate, thus terminating its action. Two enzymes, MAO (intracellular) and COMT (extracellular), function to inactivate norepinephrine, but these are of little significance in *initially* terminating the action of the endogenously released hormone.

c. Uptake of released neurotransmitter, either into the presynaptic nerve terminal from where it was released (uptake I) or into surrounding non-neural glial or smooth muscle cells (uptake II). Uptake I represents the *principal means* by which norepinephrine is inactivated following its extrusion from the prejunctional nerve ending.

6. *Repolarization of postsynaptic membrane*— Following termination of neurotransmitter action, the postsynaptic receptor area membrane is repolarized—that is, returned to its original ionic polarity and responsiveness.

Drugs acting on the nervous system may affect the transmission of impulses at one or more of the preceding steps. Types of drug action at each step are listed below, along with examples of drugs described in the text that have the particular type of action specified.

1 Inhibition of biosynthesis (*e.g.,* carbidopa, metyrosine)
2 Interference with intraneuronal binding or storage (*e.g.,* reserpine)
3 Interference with transmitter release (*e.g.,* guanethidine, bretylium, clonidine)
4 Enhancement of transmitter release (*e.g.,* amphetamine, amantadine, imipramine)
5 Activation of postsynaptic receptor sites (*e.g.,* pilocarpine, isoproterenol, bromocriptine)
6 Blockade of postsynaptic receptor sites (*e.g.,* atropine, propranolol, tubocurarine)
7 Interference with neurotransmitter inactivation (*e.g.,* physostigmine, imipramine, tranylcypromine)
8 Prevention of postsynaptic membrane repolarization (*e.g.,* succinylcholine)

B Receptor Concept

A receptor site may be viewed as a chemically reactive area on the surface of a cell membrane that is capable of complexing with specific neurohormones. This interaction initiates a sequence of events that alters the ionic permeability of the membrane, eliciting biochemical changes in the postsynaptic structure that result in either stimulation or inhibition of the functional activity of the effector structure, such as a muscle fiber, gland, or neuron. A more extensive discussion of drug–receptor interactions can be found in Chapter 3.

Receptors may be classified on the basis of their location, their selective responsiveness to various activators or blockers, and their differences in effector structure responses.

Table 8-4 lists several criteria that can be utilized to distinguish the various kinds of cholinergic and adrenergic receptor sites found in the peripheral nervous system. Cholinergic receptors are differentiated primarily on the basis of their anatomical location into muscarinic (M) sites, found on effector structures innervated by postganglionic parasympathetic fibers and two types of nicotinic (N) sites, one type located at all autonomic ganglia, the N–I receptors, and the other type found at the skeletal neuromuscular junction, the N–II receptors.

Adrenergic receptors, on the other hand, may be grouped into alpha and beta receptor sites according to their location, their differential activation and/or blockade by various drugs, and the types of responses they mediate. Each receptor type is then further subdivided to reflect differences in location and function. Alpha-1 receptors are found postsynaptically in vascular smooth muscle, GI and urinary sphincter muscles, and in the eye, skin, pancreas, and salivary glands. Alpha-2 receptors occur on presynaptic nerve endings (where they control the release of norepinephrine) as well as in platelets, fat cells, and possibly also in vascular smooth muscle. Beta-1 receptors occur primarily in the heart and adipose tissue, while beta-2 sites are present in the bronchioles, skeletal muscle vasculature, liver, kidney, and urinary bladder. A review of the various responses elicited by activation of the various adrenergic receptors is presented in Table 11-1.

In addition to the receptor sites for the cholinergic and adrenergic neurohormones outlined above, other specialized types of receptors exist in peripheral and central structures. For example, two types of histamine receptors (H_1 and H_2 sites) are present in various body tissues, and these receptors selectively mediate the diverse actions of endogenous histamine on different body organs. A further discussion of histamine receptor sites is found in Chapter 14, which deals with antihistamine drugs. Serotonin, another endogenous neurohormone, interacts with at least two kinds of specific reactive sites to elicit its pharmacologic effects, and these effects can be abolished by agents that are capable of selectively blocking the different serotonin receptor sites. Antiserotonin drugs are also discussed in Chapter 14. Many other putative neurotransmitters, including glycine, glutamic acid, GABA, and bradykinin, are also believed to exert their effects by chemically combining with a corresponding receptor site.

As mentioned briefly in Chapter 7, receptor sensitivity can be significantly altered depending on the degree of activity at a particular receptor site. Persistent activation of a receptor results in a gradual loss of sensitivity; thus, when the agonist is removed, the receptor is less reactive to additional agonists for some time. The term *down-regulation* has been coined to describe this phenomenon and helps to explain the action of several drugs, such as the tricyclic antidepressants (for a further description of the mechanisms involved in down-regulation of receptor sites, see Chap. 24). Similarly, persistent receptor antagonism can result in a state of receptor supersensitivity, leading to exaggerated responses once the antagonist is removed. For example, prolonged dopamine blockade by antipsychotic drugs results in hypersensitivity of central dopamine receptors. This dopamine supersensitivity, or *up-regulation* of dopamine receptor sites, is believed to be responsible for the appearance of orofacial involuntary movements with long-term antipsychotic drug usage. Presumably, endogenous dopamine acts on hypersensitive receptor sites to elicit altered muscle activity in the facial region.

II Central Nervous System

The central nervous system (CNS) is composed of the brain and the spinal cord; together they serve to integrate and regulate a tremendous range of sensory, motor, and emotional activities. Thus, drugs that affect central neuronal function have the potential to markedly alter the behavior of an individual. The mechanisms of action of centrally acting drugs are similar to those of peripherally acting drugs, and in fact many drugs exert simultaneous effects on both the central and peripheral nervous systems (*e.g.,* sedation, hypotension). Moreover, because of the complex neuronal interconnections among various CNS areas, drugs acting at a specific central locus may exert widespread pharmacologic effects throughout the body and simultaneously alter the functioning of several physiologic systems.

The diversity of functions regulated by the CNS can best be illlustrated by outlining the major subdivisions of the brain and the principal physiologic functions controlled by each area.

A. Forebrain
  1. Telencephalon
    a. *Cerebral Cortex*
      (1) Analysis of sensory input—reception, integration, organization, facilitation of appropriate action (primary sensory areas)
      (2) Memory development (temporal lobe)
      (3) Storage of short-term information and elaboration of thought (temporal and frontal lobe)
      (4) Analysis and control of muscular coordination (superior temporal gyrus and frontal lobe)
      (5) Speech (temporal lobe)
      (6) Hearing (superior temporal lobe)
      (7) Vision (occipital lobe)
    b. *Corpus Striatum* (caudate, putamen, globus pallidus)
      (1) Planning, programming, and modulation of motor movement
      (2) Control of muscle tone
    c. *Corpus Callosum*
      (1) Connects two hemispheres of the cerebral cortex, permitting functional integration
  2. Diencephalon
    a. *Thalamus*
      (1) Relay center for discrimination of incoming sensory signals (*e.g.,* pain, temperature, touch)
      (2) Modulation of motor impulses from cerebral cortex
      (3) Integration of emotional behavior
    b. *Hypothalamus*
      (1) Regulation of cardiovascular function
      (2) Regulation of body water
      (3) Regulation of temperature
      (4) Regulation of food intake and satiety
      (5) Control of endocrine functioning
      (6) Control of sleep–wake mechanisms
      (7) Modification of behavior
B. Midbrain
  1. Mesencephalon
    a. *Corpora quadrigemina* (superior and inferior colliculus)
      (1) Relay centers for visual and hearing reflexes
    b. *Cerebral peduncles*
      (1) Control of motor coordination and postural reflexes
    c. *Red nucleus*
      (1) Regulation of motor functioning
    d. *Substantia nigra*
      (1) Regulation of motor functioning
C. Hindbrain
  1. Metencephalon
    a. *Cerebellum*
      (1) Coordination of muscle activity (synergia)
      (2) Maintenance of equilibrium and posture
    b. *Pons*
      (1) Relay center for impulses from the medulla to higher cortical centers
      (2) Regulation of respiration
  2. Myelencephalon
    a. *Medulla oblongata*
      (1) Control of respiration and cardiovascular function (heart and blood vessels)
      (2) Regulation of certain reflex activity (swallowing, salivation, vomiting)
      (3) Modulation of GI function

In addition to the specific areas outlined above, mention should be made of several groups of CNS structures that function as integrated systems to control certain aspects of behavior. The *reticular formation* is a diffuse network of cells and nuclei scattered throughout the brainstem and extending upward into the midbrain. Impulses from spinal-cord ascending pathways (by way of collateral neurons) and the cerebellum impinge on the reticular formation, which in turn makes diffuse connections with the cerebral cortex by way of relay nuclei in many subcortical areas. The reticular formation functions as part of the so-called extrapyramidal system and is capable of modifying motor activity, but the principal role of the reticular formation is the maintenance of a state of alertness or arousal in the organism. The functioning of the reticular formation and in fact of the the entire reticular activating system (RAS) can be markedly impaired by many classes of drugs, including barbiturates, anesthetics, and antipsychotics, resulting in varying degrees of CNS depression and eventually leading to unconsciousness.

The principal group of structures controlling emotional

behavior is collectively termed the *limbic system,* which is composed of several subcortical areas (thalamus, hypothalamus, hippocampus, amygdala, septum, preoptic area, and portions of the basal ganglia) and a surrounding ring of cortical tissue on the medial and ventral surfaces of each cerebral hemisphere. The limbic system functions to regulate many aspects of behavior, such as feelings of pleasure, anger, rage, and fear. It also functions in regulating biological rhythms, sexual activity, feeding, and learning. Many portions of the limbic circuit transmit their impulses through the hypothalamus, so their output is frequently expressed in the form of autonomic manifestations, such as changes in blood pressure or respiration, hormonal changes, and expressions of pain, anger, and pleasure. Drugs used in the treatment of emotional disorders, such as antipsychotics, antidepressants, and lithium, exert at least a part of their action on the structures of the limbic system.

The *basal ganglia* are composed of three areas in the forebrain—the caudate nucleus, putamen, and globus pallidus—as well as several areas in the midbrain, such as the substantia nigra, red nucleus, and subthalamic nucleus. These structures are important for the integration and regulation of locomotor activity and postural reflexes. Pathologic changes in these ganglia result in the appearance of many types of movement disorders, the most common of which is parkinsonism.

9 Cholinergic Drugs

Cholinergic drugs are substances capable of evoking biological responses similar to those elicited by the neuro-hormone acetylcholine (ACh). The effects produced by these drugs mimic those evoked by stimulation of cholinergic nerves; thus, these drugs are termed *cholinomimetic agents*.

On the basis of their principal mechanisms of action, the cholinergic drugs can be divided into two major groups, the direct acting and the indirect acting.

I. *Direct Acting*

These drugs produce their cholinomimetic effects by directly activating cholinergic receptor sites on postjunctional membranes. Drugs in this group can be categorized as one of two types:

A. Synthetic esters of choline (*e.g.,* bethanechol)
B. Cholinomimetic alkaloids (*e.g.,* pilocarpine)

II. *Indirect Acting*

These compounds exert their effects by elevating the endogenous levels of ACh in the region of the cholinergic receptors. This is accomplished by interfering with the functioning of the cholinesterase enzymes responsible for the inactivation of choline esters such as ACh. These indirect-acting drugs can be categorized further, depending on whether the enzyme inhibition is transient (hours) or prolonged (weeks).

Thus, indirect-acting cholinergic drugs are classified as either:

A. *Reversible cholinesterase inhibitors* (*e.g.,* physostigmine). Competitive, short-lived receptor blockade; enzymatic function is quickly restored
B. *Irreversible cholinesterase inhibitors* (*e.g.,* echothiophate). Extremely stable complexation with enzyme; restoration of enzymatic function depends on synthesis of new enzyme, requiring several weeks

Acetylcholine itself is of little clinical usefulness because it is rapidly hydrolyzed by esterase enzymes and therefore has a very short duration of action. Moreover, it is nonspecific in its effects, exerting an action at all cholinergic receptor sites in the body and producing a tremendous range of pharmacologic effects. The therapeutically useful synthetic cholinergic agents are much more resistant to enzymatic hydrolysis and therefore possess a much longer duration of action. In addition, their structural modifications confer a greater degree of selectivity with regard to which type of cholinergic receptors will be activated by the different synthetic compounds.

I Direct-Acting Cholinomimetic Drugs

A Choline Esters

These drugs are all direct-acting cholinergic receptor activators. They are primarily used for their local effects in the eye, although bethanechol can be administered systemically and has selective effects on the GI and urinary tract.

1 Choline Esters for Topical Administration

▶ acetylcholine
Miochol

Uses
1 During ocular surgery (*e.g.,* cataracts, iridectomy, penetrating keratoplasty) for production of rapid, complete miosis

Dosage
0.5 ml to 2 ml of 1% solution administered by instillation into the anterior chamber of the eye, before or after securing one or more sutures

Fate
Rapidly hydrolyzed (10 min–20 min), so that solution need not be removed from the eye by flushing with saline

▶ NURSING CONSIDERATIONS
▷ 1 Prepare solution immediately before use because aqueous solutions of ACh are extremely unstable.
▷ 2 Immerse whole vial (two chambers) in sterilizing solution (*e.g.,* 70% ethanol) half-hour prior to use, then mix contents and shake.
▷ 3 Instill mixed solution gently, parallel to the face of the iris.
▷ 4 In cataract surgery, use only after delivery of the lens.
▷ 5 Discard any unused solution.
▷ 6 To *maintain* miosis, pilocarpine can be applied topically.

▶ carbachol
Carbacel, Isopto Carbachol, Miostat

Uses
1 Pupillary miosis during surgery (Miostat)
2 Chronic treatment of open-angle glaucoma (especially in cases resistant to pilocarpine)

Dosage
Miostat—0.5 ml into anterior chamber of the eye
Other products—1 to 2 drops 2 to 3 times daily into lower conjunctival sac

Fate
Most potent of the direct-acting cholinergic drugs; very slowly hydrolyzed

Common Side-Effects
Headache, hyperemia of conjunctival vessels, ciliary spasm with temporarily decreased vision

Significant Adverse Reactions
Systemic absorption may cause flushing, sweating, cramping, urinary urgency, and severe headache; usually not present following ophthalmic use in small doses

Contraindications
Corneal abrasions, acute iritis

Interactions
1 Miotic effects are reversed by local atropine or other anticholinergics.

▶ NURSING ALERTS
▷ 1 Use Miostat cautiously in the presence of asthma, peptic ulcer, GI or urinary distress, hyperthyroidism, cardiac failure, and parkinsonism because systemic absorption can occur.
▷ 2 Never give carbachol orally or parenterally, only topically.

▶ NURSING CONSIDERATIONS
▷ 1 Individualize dosage to minimize headache and visual disturbances.
▷ 2 Instill Miostat *gently* into anterior chamber using sterile syringe before or after securing sutures.

2 Choline Esters for Systemic Application

▶ bethanechol
Duvoid, Myotonachol, Urecholine, Vesicholine

Uses
1 Treatment of acute, nonobstructive urinary retention and neurogenic atony of the urinary bladder
2 Relief of postoperative abdominal distention and paralytic ileus (essentially obsolete)
3 Treatment of reflux esophagitis (investigational use only)

Dosage
Should be individualized depending on type and severity of condition
Adults: PO—10 mg to 50 mg 2 to 4 times/day; SC—2.5 mg to 5 mg 3 to 4 times/day
Children: 0.6 mg/kg/day in divided doses

Fate
Effects appear within 30 minutes to 90 minutes after oral dose, and persist for up to 6 hours; SC administration is effective within 15 minutes.

Common Side-Effects
Sweating, flushing, salivation, abdominal discomfort

Significant Adverse Reactions
Diarrhea, GI pain and cramping, headache, nausea, hypotension, and asthma-like attacks

Contraindications
Hyperthyroidism, hypertension, hypotension, peptic ulcer, bronchial asthma, coronary artery disease, AV conduction

defects, pronounced bradycardia, urinary obstruction, gastrointestinal anastomosis, epilepsy, parkinsonism, pregnancy

Interactions

1 Significant drop in blood pressure can occur if used with ganglionic blocking agents.
2 Quinidine and procainamide may antagonize the action of bethanechol.

▶ **NURSING ALERTS**

▷ 1 Never give injectable form IM or IV, only SC, because severe cholinergic overstimulation (hypotension, diarrhea, abdominal cramps, shock, cardiac arrest) can occur.
▷ 2 Keep a syringe containing 0.6 mg atropine on hand to treat symptoms of toxicity. Administer SC if required.
▷ 3 Use with extreme caution following urinary bladder surgery, GI resection, and in the presence of spastic GI disturbances, acute inflammatory lesions of the GI tract, marked vagotonia, and peritonitis.

▶ **NURSING CONSIDERATIONS**

▷ 1 Administer when stomach is empty. If given after meals, nausea and vomiting can occur.

B   Cholinomimetic Alkaloids

Cholinomimetic alkaloids produce effects similar to cholinergic nerve stimulation. The only drug of clinical importance in this group is pilocarpine, which is almost exclusively used topically in the eye because systemic administration evokes profuse salivation and sweating.

Pilocarpine (Adsorbocarpine, Almocarpine, Akarpine, Isopto Carpine, Pilocar, Pilocel, Pilomiotin, P.V. Carpine)

Mechanism

Direct cholinergic receptor activation results in contraction of the ciliary muscle and ciliary body; miosis occurs and the outflow of aqueous humor from the anterior chamber is facilitated. Systemic effects include stimulation of sweat, lacrimal and nasopharyngeal secretion, decreased heart rate, vasodilation, bronchoconstriction, and increased GI motility.

Uses

1 Open-angle glaucoma
2 Narrow-angle glaucoma prior to surgery (with other cholinergics or carbonic anhydrase inhibitors)
3 Reverse effects of cycloplegics and mydriatics following surgery or eye examinations
4 Stimulate salivation (systemically only)

Dosage

1 to 2 drops of 1% to 2% solution up to 6 times/day; concentrations greater than 4% are rarely used, although solutions up to 10% are available.

Narrow angle: 1 to 2 drops every 5 minutes to 10 minutes until relief is obtained
To stimulate salivation: 5 mg PO or SC

Fate

Onset within 10 minutes to 20 minutes. Duration of miotic effect 4 hours to 8 hours, though residual effects can last for 24 hours; excreted in urine as conjugates.

Common Side-Effects

Ciliary spasm, headache, difficulty in focusing, local irritation

Significant Adverse Reactions

Allergic sensitivity, provocation of acute asthmatic attacks

Contraindications

Acute iritis and inflammatory conditions of the anterior chamber

Interactions

1 Effects may be decreased by anticholinergics, adrenergics, corticosteroids, and phenothiazines

▶ **NURSING ALERTS**

▷ 1 Use cautiously in patients with bronchial asthma, especially systemically, because bronchoconstriction can occur.
▷ 2 Advise patients to report symptoms of sweating, salivation, cramping, and nausea immediately because they may signify onset of systemic toxicity.

▶ **NURSING CONSIDERATIONS**

▷ 1 Protect solutions from light because they are unstable.
▷ 2 Do not touch eyelids with dropper tip because contamination can occur.

Pilocarpine Ocular Therapeutic System (Ocusert Pilo)

A continuous release form of pilocarpine (20 mcg or 40 mcg/hour) placed into the lower conjunctival cul-de-sac. Used primarily for continuous therapy of open-angle glaucoma. A system unit is inserted into the conjunctival sac once a week. Release rate of pilocarpine is not affected by presence of other locally acting drugs (*e.g.,* epinephrine, carbonic anhydrase inhibitors). Myopia can occur for several hours following insertion of the system but is usually mild. System can be moved to upper conjunctival sac before sleep to aid in retention during the night.

Use cautiously in presence of infectious conjunctivitis or keratitis. Safety for use in presence of retinal detachments has not been established. Signs of conjunctival irritation, erythema, and increased secretions may occur when first used but tend to lessen after the first week or two. The system is poorly tolerated, however, by many patients, and its usefulness is somewhat limited.

II Indirect-Acting Cholinomimetic Drugs

A Reversible Cholinesterase Inhibitors

Drugs in this group are generally short-acting cholinergic drugs used both topically and systemically. They are capable of increasing the amounts of functional ACh at the postsynaptic receptor site, and are primarily indicated for their local effects in the eye and for the diagnosis and treatment of myasthenia gravis. These drugs may also effectively antidote curariform and atropine-like drugs, relieve postoperative urinary bladder atony, and suppress paroxysmal atrial tachycardia.

1 Topical and Systemic Use

▶ physostigmine
Eserine, Isopto-Eserine, Antilirium

Mechanism
Competitive inhibition of cholinesterase enzymes, allowing buildup of endogenous levels of ACh, both peripherally and in the CNS. It is the only cholinesterase inhibitor that gains ready access to the CNS.

Uses
Topical (Eye)
1 Treatment of open-angle glaucoma
2 Reverses cycloplegia and mydriasis due to atropine-like agents

Systemic (Antilirium Only)
1 Antidote to toxic neurologic effects caused by drugs (*e.g.*, scopolamine, tricyclic antidepressants) having central anticholinergic activity

Dosage
Eserine—2 drops (0.25%–0.5% solution) 3 to 4 times/day (ophthalmic ointment also available)
Antilirium—0.5 mg to 2 mg IM or IV; repeat 1 mg to 4 mg as necessary (Children: 0.5 mg over 1 min by slow IV injection; repeat in 5 min–10 min if needed)

Fate
Following topical application, peak miotic effect occurs in 1 hour to 2 hours, lasting 12 to 24 hours. Systemic doses rapidly metabolized by cholinesterases. IV effects seen in 5 minutes; duration of 1 hour to 4 hours. Drug readily enters the CNS. Hydrolyzed and inactivated by cholinesterase enzyme.

Common Side-Effects
Ophthalmic—decreased visual acuity, eyelid twitching, increased tearing, mild headache
Systemic—sweating, nausea, urinary urgency, cramping, salivation

Significant Adverse Reactions
Ophthalmic—altered pigmentation of the iris, conjunctival irritation, allergic dermatitis
Systemic—vomiting, diarrhea, muscle weakness, hypotension, bradycardia, bronchospasm, convulsions, respiratory paralysis

Contraindications
Ophthalmic—inflammation of the iris or ciliary body, narrow-angle glaucoma
Systemic—asthma, gangrene, cardiovascular disease, diabetes, obstruction of intestine or bladder

Interactions
1 Systemic effects may be potentiated by depolarizing neuromuscular blocking agents (*e.g.*, succinylcholine) and choline esters.

▶ NURSING ALERTS
▷ 1 Following systemic administration, discontinue drug if extreme salivation, vomiting, urination, or defecation develops. Reduce dosage if excessive nausea or sweating occurs.
▷ 2 Have atropine sulfate injection on hand when giving drug systemically, in case of allergic reaction or accidental overdose.
▷ 3 Use cautiously in patients with epilepsy, parkinsonism, or bradycardia.

▶ NURSING CONSIDERATIONS
▷ 1 Use only clear, colorless ophthalmic solutions of the drug. Avoid exposure to light or excessive heat.
▷ 2 Apply ointment in a thin ribbon onto lower conjunctival surface. Instruct patient to close eye *gently* and massage area lightly.
▷ 3 In cases of severe anticholinergic poisoning, supportive measures (*e.g.*, oxygen or respiratory aids) should be undertaken in addition to use of physostigmine.
▷ 4 Caution patient that vision may be impaired temporarily or localized twitching may occur following instillation of the drops.

2 Topical Use Only

▶ demecarium bromide
Humorsol

Mechanism
Anticholinesterase agent with a duration of action significantly longer than that of other reversible inhibitors; powerful miotic

Uses
1 Treatment of glaucoma
2 Treatment of convergent strabismus

Dosage

Glaucoma—1 to 2 drops in conjunctival sac once or twice a day

Strabismus—1 drop daily; reduce gradually to 1 drop twice a week as condition warrants. Dosage must be titrated and individualized.

Fate

Quickly absorbed topically; miosis develops within minutes; effects are prolonged (up to 1 wk after single administration).

Common Side-Effects

Blurred vision, twitching of eyelid, brow pain, lacrimation

Significant Adverse Reactions

Photophobia, elevated intraocular pressure, cysts on iris, conjunctival thickening, lens opacities, retinal detachment (rare). Systemic absorption may produce symptoms of cholinergic overdose.

Contraindications

Narrow-angle glaucoma, inflammatory conditions of the eye

Interactions

1 May potentiate succinylcholine and systemic anticholinesterase drugs used in the treatment of myasthenia gravis.

▶ NURSING ALERTS

▷ 1 Use cautiously in individuals with asthma, ulcers and other GI disorders, bradycardia, hypotension, epilepsy, parkinsonism, and recent coronary occlusion.

▷ 2 Discontinue if signs of cholinergic overdosage appear (*e.g.,* salivation, sweating, diarrhea, or muscle weakness).

▷ 3 Warn patient of danger of added systemic cholinergic effects if exposed to organophosphorus insecticides or pesticides (*e.g.,* Malathion or Diazinon) when taking this drug.

▶ NURSING CONSIDERATIONS

▷ 1 Use precise dosage and carefully observe patient during initial 24 hours. Frequent tonometer readings are necessary to determine optimal dosage.

▷ 2 Caution patient that headache and dimness of vision may persist for up to 1 week following initiation of therapy.

▷ 3 Compress lacrimal sac immediately after instillation to minimize drainage into nasal chamber and systemic absorption.

▷ 4 Discontinue before ophthalmic surgery to reduce danger of bleeding.

---

3   Systemic Use Only

▶ neostigmine
Prostigmin

Mechanism

Unique among cholinesterase inhibitors, neostigmine inhibits the cholinesterase enzyme and has a direct ACh-like agonistic action at cholinergic receptors, especially at the neuromuscular junction. It may also increase the release of ACh from presynaptic nerve endings.

Uses

1 Diagnosis and treatment of myasthenia gravis
2 Relief of postoperative abdominal distention and urinary retention (infrequent use)
3 Antidote to curare-like muscle relaxants (parenteral use)

Dosage

Myasthenia—oral:15 mg 3 times/day up to 375 mg/day; SC, IM: 0.5 mg; repeat as required every 3 hours

Urinary retention and abdominal distention—
Treatment—0.5 mg SC or IM; repeat every 3 hours as required
Prevention—0.25 mg SC or IM before and after operation; repeat every 4 hours to 6 hours for 3 days

Curare antidote—0.5 mg to 2 mg by slow IV injection; repeat as required, not to exceed 5 mg

Fate

Unevenly absorbed following oral dose; largely inactivated in GI tract; does not enter CNS. Onset within 2 hours to 3 hours orally and 15 minutes to 30 minutes parenterally. Duration of action 3 hours to 6 hours; metabolized in liver and excreted in urine

Common Side-Effects

Nausea, diarrhea, cramping, salivation, urinary urgency, sweating, muscle twitching

Significant Adverse Reactions

CNS—dysphagia, dysphonia, irritability, restlessness

Respiratory—increased bronchial secretions, laryngospasm, bronchiolar constriction, respiratory paralysis

Ocular—miosis, cycloplegia, diplopia, lacrimation

Cardiovascular—arrhythmias, hypotension

Other—vomiting, increased peristaltic activity, weakness, muscle cramping, skin rash

Overdosage may lead to a cholinergic crisis characterized by nausea, diarrhea, sweating, increased bronchial and salivary secretions, bradycardia, and increasing muscle weakness. Death can occur due to bronchial airway obstruction and respiratory paralysis.

Contraindications

Intestinal or urinary obstruction, megacolon, peritonitis, acute peptic ulcer, hyperthyroidism

Interactions

1 Anticholinergic drugs and other drugs with nondepolarizing blocking actions (*e.g.,* aminoglycoside antibiotics, local and general anesthetics, antiarrhythmics) may interfere with action of neostigmine.

2 Neostigmine may prolong the action of succinylcholine.

▶ **NURSING ALERTS**

▷ 1 Dosage regulation is difficult, especially oral dosage. Observe patient closely for any untoward reaction indicating overdose. Monitor blood pressure, respiration, and pulse during periods of dosage adjustment.

▷ 2 Stress rigid dosage compliance for the myasthenic patient; carefully note signs of improvement (raising of eyelids or ease of swallowing). Be prepared to assist patient when symptoms prevent him from helping himself (*e.g.,* extreme muscle weakness or difficulty in breathing).

▷ 3 Have emergency measures readily available (*e.g.,* atropine, oxygen with respirator, suction apparatus) in case of a breathing crisis.

▷ 4 Be aware of the possibility of excessive cholinergic stimulation resulting from neostigmine, leading to extreme muscle weakness (cholinergic crisis). Because the symptoms of cholinergic crisis closely resemble those of a myasthenic crisis, determine if weakness is caused by patient's condition or drug overdosage by using IV test dose of edrophonium supervised by physician. Have atropine on hand as an antidote to the cholinesterase inhibitor.

▶ **NURSING CONSIDERATIONS**

▷ 1 Give drug before meals if patient experiences dysphagia when eating.

▷ 2 When drug is used as a curare antidote, be prepared to assist respiration and have atropine available.

▷ 3 Keep careful records of patient's daily condition, noting changes in muscle strength, respiration, and blood pressure, to assist in developing an optimal therapeutic regimen.

▷ 4 Tailor dose intervals and amounts to correspond to normal periods of stress and fatigue. Give largest portion of total dose before time of expected greatest muscle demands (*e.g.,* eating, shopping).

▶ **ambenonium**

Mytelase

Mechanism

Reversible inhibition of cholinesterase enzyme, thus prolonging and enhancing the action of ACh at the neuromuscular junction, improving muscle strength

Uses

1 Treatment of myasthenia gravis

Dosage

Adults: 5 mg to 25 mg 3 to 4 times/day orally. Begin at low level and gradually increase to optimally effective dose.
Children: 1.5 mg/kg/day in divided doses

Fate

Erratically absorbed from GI tract; onset occurs in 20 minutes to 30 minutes; fairly long duration of action (4 hr to 8 hr)

Common Side-Effects

See Neostigmine
Somewhat lower incidence of GI side-effects

Significant Adverse Reactions

See Neostigmine
Slightly lower incidence of bronchial secretions but may produce nervousness, dizziness, and confusion

Contraindications

Patients receiving atropine or mecamylamine

▶ **NURSING ALERT**

▷ 1 Observe patient very carefully for signs of cholinergic intoxication if dosage exceeds 150 mg to 200 mg daily. Warning of overdosage is minimal and there is a narrow margin between first appearance of side-effects and serious toxic manifestations. If signs of overdosage occur, discontinue all cholinergic medication and administer atropine (0.5 mg–1 mg IV).

▶ **NURSING CONSIDERATIONS**

See Neostigmine. In addition:

▷ 1 Note signs of CNS toxicity (jitteriness, confusion, dizziness) and make proper dosage adjustment.

▷ 2 Because duration of action is prolonged, give dose at bedtime to carry patient through the night.

▶ **edrophonium**

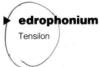
Tensilon

Mechanism

Short-acting, reversible cholinesterase inhibitor and direct cholinergic receptor activator, especially at neuromuscular junctions

Uses

1 Differential diagnosis of myasthenia gravis from cholinergic crisis

2 Antidote for poisoning with curare-like muscle relaxants

Dosage

Diagnosis of myasthenia—Adults: 2 mg IV. If there is no improvement in muscle strength as measured by several indices (*e.g.,* ptosis, diplopia, dysarthria, limb strength) in 1 minute, give 8 mg IV. Alternately, give 10 mg IM as single dose. Pediatric: IV 1 mg to 2 mg, titrated up to 5 mg; IM 2 mg to 5 mg

Curare Antagonist—10 mg IV. May be repeated to a maximum of 40 mg

Fate

Rapidly hydrolyzed; onset of action within 30 seconds to 60 seconds; duration 5 minutes to 10 minutes.

Common Side-Effects

See Neostigmine

Significant Adverse Reactions

See Neostigmine. In addition, cardiac dysrhythmias

Interactions

See Neostigmine. In addition:

1 Edrophonium may potentiate depolarizing neuromuscular blockers (*e.g.,* succinylcholine).

▶ **NURSING CONSIDERATIONS**

See Neostigmine. In addition:

▷ 1 Check patient's pulse frequently during administration.

▷ 2 When employed as curare antidote, use with oxygen and artificial respiration.

▶ **pyridostigmine**

Mestinon, Regonol

Mechanism

Reversible cholinesterase inhibitor that elevates ACh levels at the neuromuscular junction

Uses

1 Treatment of myasthenia gravis

2 Antagonist to curare-like drugs

Dosage

(Must be individualized)

Oral—average 600 mg/day in divided doses (10 tablets or tsp) up to 1500 mg/day; alternately, 1 to 3 sustained-action tablets (180 mg each) every 6 hours

IM or IV—1/30 of the oral dose; for curare antagonism 10 mg to 20 mg IV.

Fate

Poorly absorbed; onset is 30 minutes to 45 minutes orally, 15 minutes IM, and 2 minutes to 5 minutes IV. Duration of action is 3 hours to 6 hours orally and 2 hours to 4 hours IM and IV.

Common Side-Effects

See Neostigmine. In addition:

Rash

Lower incidence of GI effects than with other similar agents

Significant Adverse Reactions

See Neostigmine

Contraindications

GI and urinary obstruction, bronchial asthma

▶ **NURSING ALERTS**

▷ 1 Caution patient taking sustained-action tablets not to exceed 1 tablet every 6 hours.

▷ 2 Advise patient to report early signs of muscle weakness because this may indicate impending cholinergic crisis. See Nursing Alerts under Neostigmine.

B Irreversible Cholinesterase Inhibitors

The "irreversible" cholinesterase inhibitors are organophosphorus compounds that cause phosphorylation of the cholinesterase enzyme. This permanently inactivates the enzyme, and enzymatic activity remains impaired until a new enzyme can be synthesized, often requiring weeks or even months for full restoration. These compounds were originally developed as chemical warfare agents but are now extensively used as pesticides and insecticides. The major application of the one clinically available compound, echothiophate, is in the eye, for the production of prolonged miosis and treatment of glaucoma.

▶ **echothiophate**

Phospholine Iodide

Uses

1 Treatment of glaucoma

2 Diagnosis and treatment of accommodative convergent strabismus (often with epinephrine or carbonic anhydrase inhibitors)

Dosage

Glaucoma—1 drop (0.03%–0.125%) 1 to 2 times/day, individualized to condition

Strabismus—1 drop 0.06%/day or 0.125% every other day (maximum 0.125%/day)

Fate

Fairly rapid onset (10 min); effects may persist for several weeks. It is water soluble and does not induce excessive lacrimation.

Common Side-Effects

Stinging and burning in the eye, temporary blurred vision, lid twitching, hyperemia, browache

Significant Adverse Reactions

Iris cysts, conjunctival thickening, lens opacities, iritis, retinal detachment (rare); systemic absorption may produce symptoms of cholinergic crises.

Contraindications

Narrow-angle glaucoma (most cases), inflammatory conditions of the eye

Interactions

1 May enhance systemic effects of succinylcholine and cholinesterase inhibitors

2 Effects in eye are readily reversed by atropine.

▶ **NURSING ALERTS**

▷ 1 Discontinue drug if early signs of cholinergic overdosage appear (*e.g.,* salivation, diarrhea, sweating, or muscle weakness).

▷ 2 Use cautiously in individuals with asthma, ulcers, hypotension, epilepsy, parkinsonism, cardiovascular damage, and vagotonia.

▶ **NURSING CONSIDERATIONS**

▷ 1 Solutions are stable for approximately 1 month. Check for discoloration or cloudiness of old solution before administration.

▷ 2 Following instillation, compress inner canthus for 1 minute to 2 minutes to minimize drainage into nose and throat and to minimize danger of systemic absorption. Remove excess solution around eye following usage.

▷ 3 Use lowest concentration that will control condition. Do not exceed twice-a-day dosing. A single daily dose can be instilled at bedtime to minimize inconvenience of miosis and blurred vision during the day.

▷ 4 Tolerance may occur with prolonged use. Use drug-free periods or alternate miotics when possible to eliminate rapid development of tolerance.

▷ 5 Adhere strictly to recommended dosage. Long action of the drug increases danger of cumulative systemic toxicity.

C   Miscellaneous

▶ **guanidine**

Guanidine

Guanidine is a unique cholinergic agent that prolongs the action potential in nerve terminals. It improves the muscle weakness seen in myasthenia; however, due to its relatively high toxicity its use is generally restricted to the myasthenic syndrome of Eaton–Lambert (carcinomatous myopathy), in which muscle weakness accompanies a malignant disease, particularly bronchogenic carcinoma.

Mechanism

Enhances the release of acetylcholine following a nerve impulse; may also slow the rates of depolarization and repolarization of muscle cell membranes

Uses

1 Alleviation of the symptoms (muscle weakness, fatigability) of the myasthenic syndrome of Eaton–Lambert

2 Treatment of severe myasthenia gravis (investigational use only)

Dosage

Initially, 10 mg/kg/day to 15 mg/kg/day in 3 or 4 divided doses. Increase dosage gradually up to a maximum of 35 mg/kg/day.

Common Side-Effects

Gastric irritation, nausea, anorexia, flushing, sweating

Significant Adverse Reactions

GI—diarrhea, abdominal cramping, vomiting

Neurologic—paresthesias, lightheadedness, irritability, nervousness, trembling, ataxia, tremor, confusion, mood changes, hallucinations

Dermatologic—rash, petechiae, purpura, ecchymoses, skin eruptions, scaling of skin

Hematologic—bone marrow depression, anemia, leukopenia, thrombocytopenia

Renal—elevation of creatinine, renal tubular necrosis, interstitial nephritis

Cardiovascular—palpitations, tachycardia, hypotension, atrial fibrillation

Other—sore throat, fever

▶ **NURSING ALERTS**

▷ 1 Perform baseline and routine follow-up complete blood cell (CBC) counts and differential counts. Discontinue drug at first indication of bone marrow suppression.

▷ 2 Advise patients to note the development of sore throat, skin rash, fever or mucosal ulceration (possible early signs of a developing blood dyscrasia), and notify physician immediately if any of these occur.

▷ 3 Be aware that appearance of GI disorders (*e.g.,* anorexia, diarrhea) are often an indication that the dosage is excessive, and a dosage reduction should be considered.

▷ 4 Be prepared to treat cases of overdosage with IV atropine (for GI symptoms) and IV calcium gluconate (for neuromuscular and convulsive symptoms).

▷ 5 Monitor renal function on a regular basis, because renal abnormalities have occurred with guanidine.

▶ **NURSING CONSIDERATIONS**

▷ 1 Carefully titrate the dose in each patient, because individual tolerance may be highly variable.

▷ 2 Perform periodic serum creatinine determinations, because drug-induced elevations have been noted.

▷ 3 Alert patients to the fact that paresthesias may occur shortly following a dose of guanidine, but these are not an indication that dosage is excessive.

III   Cholinesterase Inhibitor Antidote

A specific antidote, pralidoxime chloride (PAM), is available primarily for treating overdosage with organophosphorus cholinesterase inhibitors, which usually occurs as a result of insecticide poisoning. It is also capable of antagonizing the effects of the reversible cholinesterase inhibitors (*e.g.,* neostigmine) used in the treatment of myasthenia gravis, although its effectiveness is much less with these compounds. Treatment with PAM should be initiated as soon as possible following poisoning because the enzyme-inhibitor complex which has formed undergoes a fairly rapid process of "aging." Thus, within hours, the complex becomes extremely stable and largely resistant to the action of the reactivator PAM.

▶ pralidoxime chloride

Protopam, PAM

Mechanism

Disrupts the bond between the phosphorus group of the enzyme inhibitor and the esteratic site of the cholinesterase enzyme, thus reactivating the intact enzyme.

Uses

1 Poisoning with pesticides and insecticides of the organophosphate class
2 Antidote to overdosage by anticholinesterase drugs used in treatment of myasthenia gravis

Dosage

Insecticide poisoning—Adults: 1 g to 2 g as IV infusion in 100 ml saline over 15 minutes to 30 minutes, often with atropine (2 mg–4 mg IV) PO 1 g to 3 g every 5 hours. Children: 20 mg/kg to 40 mg/kg IV infusion with 0.5 mg to 1 mg atropine. (Most effective if given within a few hours after exposure to poison; usually ineffective if 48 hr have elapsed)

Anticholinesterase overdosage—initially, 1 g to 2 g IV injection; increments of 250 mg every 5 minutes until symptoms subside.

Fate

Slowly absorbed orally; very short acting; not bound to plasma protein; metabolized in the liver and readily excreted in urine, partly as unchanged drug

Common Side-Effects

Dizziness, blurred vision, headache, drowsiness, nausea

Significant Adverse Reactions

Tachycardia, hyperventilation, laryngospasm, muscle weakness. Excitement and hypomania may occur following recovery of consciousness.

Interactions

1 Certain drugs should not be used concurrently with PAM in organophosphate poisoning (morphine, theophylline, succinylcholine, reserpine, and phenothiazines) because enzyme reactivator exerts a depolarizing effect at the neuromuscular junction.
2 Barbiturates may be potentiated by cholinesterase inhibitors.

▶ NURSING ALERTS

▷ 1 Perform IV infusion slowly because tachycardia, muscle rigidity, and laryngospasm can occur with too rapid infusion rates.

▷ 2 Use cautiously in presence of myasthenia gravis because PAM may precipitate a myasthenic crisis. Have edrophonium (Tensilon), a rapid-acting cholinesterase inhibitor, on hand.

▷ 3 When drug is used with atropine, be alert for signs of atropine toxicity (xerostomia, blurred vision, flushing, excitement) and terminate atropine administration at that point.

▶ NURSING CONSIDERATIONS

▷ 1 Observe patient closely for 72 hours following poisoning. Perform red blood cell and plasma cholinesterase determinations to determine patient's progress.

▷ 2 Thoroughly wash skin with alcohol if that is the route of contamination, or perform gastric lavage following oral ingestion of the poison.

▷ 3 Determine what insecticide is involved in the poisoning. Pralidoxime chloride is ineffective in cases of carbamate (Sevin) pesticide poisoning.

▷ 4 Do not use in cases of poisoning due to organophosphates not having anticholinesterase activity.

Summary. Cholinergic Drugs

Drug	Preparations	Usual Dosage Range
Direct Acting		
Acetylcholine (Miochol)	2-ml dual chamber vial containing 20 mg ACh, 100 mg mannitol, and sterile water—yields 1% solution when reconstituted	0.5 ml to 2 ml of 1% solution
Carbachol (Carbacel, Isopto Carbachol, Miostat)	Miostat—1.5 ml vials of 0.01% solution Others (Ophthalmic drops)—0.75%, 1.5%, 2.25% and 3.0%	Miostat—0.5 ml in a single dose Others—1 to 2 drops 2 to 3 times/day
Bethanechol (Duvoid, Myotonachol, Urecholine, Vesicholine)	Tablets—5 mg, 10 mg, 25 mg, 50 mg Injection—5 mg/ml	PO—10 mg to 50 mg 2 to 4 times/day SC—2.5 mg to 5 mg 3 to 4 times/day
Pilocarpine (Various manufacturers)	Ophthalmic drops—0.25%, 0.5%, 1%, 2%, 3%, 4%, 5%, 6%, 8%, and 10%	1 to 2 drops of 1% to 4% solution 3 to 4 times/day
Pilocarpine Ocular Therapeutic System (Ocusert)	Packets of 8 sterile systems releasing 20 mcg or 40 mcg of pilocarpine per hr	One system placed into conjunctival sac per wk, according to package directions

(continued)

Summary. Cholinergic Drugs *(continued)*

Drug	Preparations	Usual Dosage Range
Indirect Acting		
Physostigmine (Antilirium, Eserine, Isopto Eserine)	Antilirium—Injection 1 mg/ml Others Ophthalmic drops—0.25%, 0.5% Ophthalmic ointment—0.25%	Antilirium—IM, IV—0.5 mg to 2 mg by slow injection; repeat 1 mg to 4 mg as needed. (Children—0.5 mg by slow IV injection) Others Drops—2 drops 3 times/day Ointment—small ribbon in lower eyelid
Demecarium (Humorsol)	Ophthalmic drops—0.125% and 0.25%	1 to 2 drops once or twice a day to twice a wk, depending on condition
Neostigmine (Prostigmin and various manufacturers)	Tablets—15 mg Injection—1:1000, 1:2000, and 1:4000	PO—15 mg 3 times/day to 375 mg a day SC, IM—0.5 mg every 3 hr as required
Ambenonium (Mytelase)	Tablets—10 mg	5 mg to 25 mg 3 to 4 times/day
Edrophonium (Tensilon)	Injection—10 mg/ml	Myasthenia diagnosis—2 mg IV or 10 mg IM (Children: 1 mg to 2 mg IV or 2 mg to 5 mg IM) Curare poisoning: 10 mg to 40 mg IV as needed
Pyridostigmine (Mestinon, Regonol)	Tablets—60 mg Sustained-release tablets—180 mg Syrup—60 mg/5 ml Injection—5 mg/ml	PO—600 mg daily in divided doses (maximum 1500 mg/day) IM or IV—1/30 oral dose Curare antagonism—10 mg to 20 mg IV
Echothiophate Iodide (Phospholine Iodide)	Powder—1.5 mg, 3 mg, 6.25 mg, and 12.5 mg with 5 ml diluent for ophthalmic use	0.03% to 0.06% (1 to 2 drops) 1 to 2 times/day
Guanidine (Guanidine)	Tablets—125 mg	Initially, 10 mg/kg/day to 15 mg/kg/day in 3 or 4 divided doses; may increase gradually up to 35 mg/kg/day
Antagonist		
Pralidoxime (Protopam)	Tablets—500 mg Injection—1 g/20 ml or 1 g powder with one 20-ml vial of diluent	Insecticide poisoning Adults: 1 g to 2 g IV in 100 ml saline over 15 min to 30 min Children: 20 mg to 40 mg/kg IV Anticholinesterase overdosage: 1 g to 2 g IV initially; repeat with 250 mg every 5 min

10 Anticholinergic Drugs

The anticholinergic drugs inhibit the actions of acetylcholine and other cholinergic agents on effector structures innervated by postganglionic cholinergic nerves. These drugs are often referred to as antimuscarinics, because their predominant blocking action is exerted at the postganglionic parasympathetic muscarinic (M) sites. However, their site specificity is dose dependent. That is, they can also interfere with cholinergic neurotransmission at the nicotinic (N) sites (*i.e.,* autonomic ganglia, neuromuscular junction) in sufficiently high doses. Because the distribution of parasympathetic cholinergic nerves is vast, these drugs exert a wide range of pharmacologic effects. Major organs affected by the anticholinergic group of drugs include the eye, respiratory tract, heart, GI tract, urinary bladder, most nonvascular smooth muscle, exocrine glands, and, to varying degrees, the CNS. The principal pharmacologic actions of the anticholinergic group of drugs are listed in Table 10-1.

There is a diverse group of drugs classified as anticholinergics. Some of these drugs are derived from natural sources, such as atropine and scopolamine, but the majority are compounds synthesized in attempts to increase receptor site selectivity, thereby reducing the extent of disturbing side-effects associated with the nonselective, naturally occurring products. These attempts have met with only limited success, however, and most anticholinergic drugs exhibit a similar pattern of side-effects.

In light of the overall similarity of uses, side-effects, and clinical implications among the many anticholinergic drugs, the pharmacology of the group is discussed as a whole. Dosage forms, indications, and specific characteristics for each drug are then listed in Table 10-2.

Anticholinergics

Anisotropine	Hyoscyamine
Atropine	Isopropamide
Belladonna	Mepenzolate
Benztropine	Methantheline
Biperiden	Methscopolamine
Chlorphenoxamine	Orphenadrine
Clidinium	Oxybutynin
Cyclopentolate	Oxyphencyclimine
Cycrimine	Oxyphenonium
Dicyclomine	Procyclidine
Diphemanil	Propantheline
Ethopropazine	Scopolamine
Glycopyrrolate	Thiphenamil
Hexocyclium	Trihexyphenidyl
Homatropine	Tropicamide

Mechanism

Competitive antagonism of acetylcholine (or other direct-acting cholinergic drugs) at postsynaptic muscarinic cholinergic receptor sites. Large doses may block cholinergic transmission at the ganglia and neuromuscular junction. Certain drugs (*e.g.,* antiparkinsonian agents) may also decrease uptake of dopamine into presynaptic nerve endings.

Table 10-1. Pharmacologic Actions: Anticholinergics

Effects	Clinical Consequences
Cardiovascular	
Decreased heart rate in small doses (central vagal stimulation)	
Increased heart rate in large doses (peripheral vagal blockade)	
Vasodilation	
Gastrointestinal Tract	
Decreased motility	Delayed gastric emptying
Decreased smooth muscle tone	
Decreased secretions	
Urinary Tract	
Relaxation of detrusor muscle	Urinary retention
Contraction of sphincter muscle	
Eye	
Mydriasis (decreased response of sphincter muscle)	Blurring of vision
Cycloplegia (decreased response of ciliary muscle)	
Smooth Muscle	
Slight relaxation of nonvascular smooth muscle (e.g., biliary, bronchiolar, intestinal, uterine)	Relief of biliary or intestinal colic
Exocrine Glands	
Decreased sweat gland secretion	Anhidrosis, xerostomia, hyperthermia
Decreased salivation	
Decreased mucous gland secretion (nasopharynx and bronchioles)	
CNS	
Drowsiness, disorientation, hallucinations (large doses)	—
Decreased tremor and rigidity of parkinsonism	

Uses

Refer to tabular listing of individual drugs for specific uses of each agent.

1 Production of mydriasis and cycloplegia as an aid to ophthalmic examinations
2 Preoperative medication to reduce excess salivation and prevent bradycardia (scopolamine additionally produces a tranquilizing effect)
3 Decrease GI motility and secretions in cases of peptic ulcer, GI spasms, irritable bowel syndrome, or other GI disorders
4 Minimize muscarinic side-effects associated with cholinesterase inhibitor treatment of myasthenia
5 Relief of nasopharyngeal and bronchial secretions accompanying upper respiratory and allergic disorders
6 Prevention and relief of motion sickness
7 Treatment of enuresis in children
8 Treatment of sinus bradycardia and conduction block due to excessive vagal tone
9 Production of sedation and amnesia ("twilight sleep") in obstetrics
10 Relief of dysmenorrhea
11 Antidote to overdosage with cholinergic agents (anticholinesterases, organophosphate insecticides and pesticides)
12 Relief of symptoms of parkinsonism (especially tremor and rigidity), and control of extrapyramidal disorders resulting from antipsychosis treatment

Dosage
See Table 10-2

Fate
Oral absorption varies from good to poor depending on chemical configuration (*see* Table 10-2). Distribution depends largely on lipid solubility of individual drugs, more lipid soluble drugs (*e.g.,* scopolamine) readily entering the CNS. Duration of action dependent on dose, method of administration, and type of action produced (*i.e.,* local or systemic). Generally readily excreted by the kidney (80%–90% in 24 hr) both as intact drug and metabolites.

Common Side-Effects
Dry mouth, blurred vision, urinary hesitancy, constipation, palpitations, flushing

Significant Adverse Reactions
Any significant adverse reactions generally result from excessive dosage or individual hypersensitivity.

Increased intraocular pressure, vomiting, elevated body temperature, rash, muscular incoordination and ataxia, CNS excitation, photophobia, restlessness, confusion, insomnia, delirium, hallucinations, respiratory difficulties, hypertension, tachycardia, impotence, dysphagia, allergic reactions, and suppression of lactation.

Contraindications
Narrow-angle glaucoma, asthma, urinary or GI obstruction, intestinal atony, paralytic ileus, myasthenia gravis, ulcerative colitis, hiatal hernia, serious hepatic or renal disease

Interactions
1 The following drugs may increase the side-effects of anticholinergics: antihistamines, tricyclic antidepressants, antipsychotics, antiarrhythmics, antianxiety drugs, meperidine, nitrites and nitrates, methylphenidate, orphenadrine, primidone, MAO inhibitors, and amantadine.
2 Guanethidine, histamine, and reserpine can antagonize the inhibitory effects of anticholinergics on gastric acid secretion.
3 Anticholinergics may enhance the actions of bronchodilators (*e.g.,* adrenergics), isoniazid, and methotrimeprazine.
4 Antacids may impair the GI absorption of anticholinergics.

(*Text continues on p. 70.*)

Table 10-2. Anticholinergics

Drug	Preparations	Usual Dosage Range	Major Uses	Remarks
Anisotropine (Valpin 50)	Tablets—50 mg	Adults—50 mg 3 times/day	GI spasms	Oral absorption is erratic. Also available as Valpin 50-PB with 15 mg phenobarbital
Atropine (various manufacturers)	Tablets—0.4 mg Hypodermic tablets—0.3 mg, 0.4 mg, 0.6 mg Ophthalmic drops— 0.5%, 1.0%, 2.0%, 3.0% Ophthalmic ointment— 0.5%, 1% Injection—0.1, 0.3, 0.4, 0.5, 0.6, 1.0, and 1.2 mg/ml	Systemic: Adults—0.4 mg to 0.6 mg every 4 hr to 6 hr Children—0.01 mg/kg to 0.02 mg/kg to a maximum of 0.4 mg Ophthalmic: Adults—1 drop 1% 3 times/day Children—1 drop 0.5%– 1% 1 to 3 times/day For refraction: 1 drop 1 hr before examination	See general discussion of anticholinergics	Atropine flush due to peripheral vasodilation is a normal effect of the drug. When used in the eye, prevent systemic absorption by compressing lacrimal sac following instillation. Do not use in children under 6 years of age. Ophthalmic drops available with prednisolone
Belladonna alkaloids (Bellafoline)	Tablets—0.25 mg Injection—0.5 mg/ml	Adults: Tablets—0.25 mg to 0.5 mg 3 times/day Injection—0.25 ml to 1 ml SC 1 to 2 times/day Children: Tablets—0.125 mg to 0.25 mg 3 times/day	Preoperative medication, GI hypermotility, dysmenorrhea, respiratory hypersecretion	Tincture belladonna is also available for GI disturbances (spasms, hypermotility) 0.6 ml 3 times/day; often used in combination with phenobarbital and antacids
Belladonna extract	Tablets—15 mg Liquid—30 mg/100 ml	Tablets—15 mg 3 to 4 times/day Liquid—0.6 ml to 1.0 ml 3 to 4 times/day	GI hypermotility	Available in combination with phenobarbital (Chardonna-2, Belap) butabarbital (Butibel) or amobarbital (Amobell)
Benztropine (Cogentin)	Tablets—0.5 mg, 1 mg, 2 mg Injection—1 mg/ml	Parkinsonism—1 mg to 2 mg daily to a maximum of 6 mg Extrapyramidal reactions—1 mg to 4 mg 1 to 2 times/day	Parkinsonism, extrapyramidal reactions	If used with l-DOPA, adjust dose of each medication accordingly. Start with low dose and gradually increase. Sedative effect can occur. Withdraw gradually. See Chapter 26.
Biperiden (Akineton)	Tablets—2 mg Injection—5 mg/ml	Parkinsonism—1 mg to 2 mg 3 to 4 times/day with meals; 2 mg IM or IV; repeated every half hour to a maximum of 4 doses Extrapyramidal reactions—2 mg 1 to 3 times/day	Parkinsonism, extrapyramidal reactions	Most effective on akinesia and rigidity. May elevate mood. Can produce incoordination following IV or IM use. See Chapter 26.
Chlorphenoxamine (Phenoxene)	Tablets—50 mg	Initially 50 mg 3 times/day to a maximum of 100 mg 4 times/day with meals or milk	Parkinsonism	Possesses significant antihistamine activity. May produce drowsiness. See Chapter 26.
Clidinium (Quarzan)	Capsules—2.5 mg and 5 mg	2.5 mg to 5 mg 3 to 4 times/day	GI hypermotility and hypersecretion	Reduce dosage in geriatric or debilitated patients. Oral absorption is erratic. Combined with chlordiazepoxide as Librax.

Table 10-2. Anticholinergics *(continued)*

Drug	Preparations	Usual Dosage Range	Major Uses	Remarks
Cyclopentolate (Ak-Pentolate, Cyclogyl)	Ophthalmic drops— 0.5%, 1%, 2%	Refraction: Adults—1 to 2 drops 0.5% to 1% solution. Children—1 to 2 drops 0.5% solution	Ophthalmic refraction	Can produce behavioral disturbances in children (ataxia, disorientation, restlessness, incoherent speech) if absorbed systemically; ophthalmic drops available with phenylephrine (Cyclomydril) for increased mydriatic effect
Cycrimine (Pagitane)	Tablets—1.25 mg, 2.5 mg	Initially 1.25 mg 3 times/ day with meals to a maximum of 20 mg daily	Parkinsonism	Many side-effects; subside with continued therapy (*e.g.,* GI distress, blurred vision, urinary retention). May produce vertigo and weakness. See Chapter 26.
Dicyclomine (Bentyl and various other manufacturers)	Tablets—20 mg Capsules—10 mg, 20 mg Liquid—10 mg/5 ml Injection—10 mg/ml	Adults: Oral—10 mg to 20 mg 3 to 4 times/day IM—20 mg every 4 to 6 hours Children: 5 mg to 10 mg 3 to 4 times/day orally	GI spasm and hyperirritability, ulcerative colitis	Possibly effective in infant colic; usually administered with antacids in GI disorders, because it does not reduce gastric secretions; well-absorbed orally. Common side-effects are dizziness, abdominal fullness, and slight euphoria
Diphemanil (Prantal)	Tablets—100 mg	Adults—Initially 100 mg to 200 mg every 4 to 6 hours; may reduce to 50 mg to 100 mg every 4 to 6 hours for maintenance	GI hypermotility, excessive sweating	Not recommended for children. Administer before meals because oral absorption is erratic.
Ethopropazine (Parsidol)	Tablets—10 mg, 50 mg, 100 mg	Initially 50 mg 1 to 2 times/day to a maximum of 600 mg/ day	Parkinsonism, extrapyramidal reactions	Does not potentiate CNS depressants: high incidence of dose-related side-effects including drowsiness, hypotension, confusion, and GI distress. See Chapter 26.
Glycopyrrolate (Glycobarb, Robinul)	Tablets—1 mg, 2 mg Injection—0.2 mg/ml	Oral—1 mg to 2 mg 3 times/day. Parenteral (IM, IV)—0.1 mg to 0.2 mg as single dose. For overdosage—0.2 mg for every 1 mg neostigmine or equivalent received.	GI disorders, preoperative medication, cholinergic overdosage, allergic conditions (for drying effect)	Not indicated for children. May cause burning at site of injection. Do not mix with solutions of sodium chloride or bicarbonate. Oral absorption is erratic.
Hexocyclium (Tral)	Tablets—25 mg Tablets—(timed-release) 50 mg	25 mg 4 times/day; alternately, 50 mg twice a day.	GI hypermotility, hypersecretion	Do not chew tablets. Absorption is very erratic. Do not use in children
Homatropine (Isopto Homatropine, Homatrocel)	Ophthalmic drops—1%, 2%, 5%	Refraction—1 to 2 drops 2% every 10 minutes to 15 minutes to 5 doses. Other ophthalmic—1 to 2 drops 2% to 5% 2 to 3 times/day	Acidity, refraction, iritis, relief of ciliary spasm, preoperative cycloplegic and mydriatic	Cycloplegia may be prolonged and caution in driving is recommended.

(continued)

Table 10-2. Anticholinergics (continued)

Drug	Preparations	Usual Dosage Range	Major Uses	Remarks
Hyoscyamine (Anaspaz, Cystospaz, Cystospaz-M, Levamine, Levsin, Levsinex)	Tablets—0.125 mg, 0.15 mg Timed-release capsules—0.375 mg Elixir—0.125 mg/5 ml Oral drops—0.125 mg/ml Injection—0.25 mg/ml, 0.5 mg/ml	Oral Adults—0.125 mg to 0.25 mg 3 to 4 times/day Children—2 to 10 yr: ½ adult dose less than 2 yr: ¼ adult dose Parenteral—SC, IM, or IV 0.25 mg to 0.5 mg	GI spasm and hypersecretion, cholinergic poisoning, dysmenorrhea, urinary spasm, acute rhinitis	Well absorbed orally; tablets, elixir and drops are also available with phenobarbital; may be used in controlling diarrhea
Isopropamide (Darbid)	Tablets—5 mg	5 mg to 10 mg twice a day (every 12 hr)	GI spasm and hypersecretion, diarrhea, urinary spasm	Not for use in children under 12; erratically absorbed orally; iodine skin rash may occur; may alter PBI and I^{131} tests, because drug is an iodide salt; combined with prochlorperazine as Combid.
Mepenzolate (Cantil)	Tablets—25 mg	25 mg to 50 mg 4 times/day	GI hypermotility, diarrhea, ulcerative colitis	Urinary hesitancy and constipation can occur, especially at larger doses; erratically absorbed orally
Methantheline (Banthine)	Tablets—50 mg	Adults—50 mg to 100 mg 4 times/day Children—less than 1 year: 12 mg to 25 mg 4 times/day over 1 year: 25 mg to 50 mg 4 times/day	Preoperative medication, GI spasm, uretral spasm, urinary frequency, excessive sweating	Less effective than many other similar agents; tablets are very bitter, oral absorption is poor.
Methscopolamine (Pamine)	Tablets—2.5 mg	2.5 mg 3 times/day and 5 mg at bedtime	GI hypermotility, hyperhidrosis, excess salivation	Take drug one half hour before meals; may exert curare-like effect on smooth muscle
Orphenadrine (Banflex, Disipal, Flexoject, Flexon, K-Flex, Marflex, Myolin, Norflex, O'Flex, X-Otag)	Tablets—50 mg Tablets (sustained release)—100 mg Injection—30 mg/ml	Parkinsonism—50 mg orally 3 times/day up to 250 mg daily Muscle spasms—100 mg orally twice a day or 60 mg IV or IM every 12 hr	Parkinsonism, extrapyramidal reactions, skeletal muscle spasms	HCl salt (Disipal) is used in parkinsonism, whereas citrate salt (all others) is used as a skeletal muscle relaxant; major effect is on rigidity of parkinsonism. May produce dizziness and lightheadedness in addition to normal anticholinergic side effects in large doses See Chapter 26.
Oxybutynin (Ditropan)	Tablets—5 mg Syrup—5 mg/5 ml	Adults—5 mg 2 to 3 times/day Children—5 mg twice a day	Urinary incontinence (reflex neurogenic bladder)	Exerts additional direct antispasmodic effect on smooth muscle; delays desire to void; may lead to heat prostration in high temperatures; drowsiness and blurred vision can occur; do not use in children under 5 or in patients with paralytic ileus, intestinal atony, megacolon, colitis, GI obstruction, or myasthenia.

Table 10-2. Anticholinergics (continued)

Drug	Preparations	Usual Dosage Range	Major Uses	Remarks
Oxyphencyclimine (Daricon)	Tablets—10 mg	5 mg to 10 mg 2 to 3 times/day	GI, urinary, or biliary spasms	Oral absorption is generally good; may induce CNS stimulation; do not use in children under 12.
Oxyphenonium (Antrenyl)	Tablets—5 mg	10 mg 4 times/day	GI hyperacidity and hypermotility, preoperative medication	Erratically absorbed; high incidence of common anticholinergic side-effects; not for use in children
Procyclidine (Kemadrin)	Tablets—2 mg, 5 mg	Parkinsonism—2 mg to 5 mg 3 times/day Extrapyramidal reactions—2.5 mg to 5 mg 3 to 4 times/day	Parkinsonism, extrapyramidal reactions	Most effective against rigidity; may temporarily worsen tremor; in elderly, may induce confusion and psychotic reactions; note urinary output and reduce dose if necessary. See Chap. 26.
Propantheline (Pro-Banthine, Norpanth, SK-Propantheline)	Tablets—7.5 mg, 15 mg Injection—30 mg/vial	Oral—7.5 mg to 15 mg 3 times/day and 30 mg at bedtime Parenteral—30 mg every 6 hours IM or IV	GI spasm and hypersecretion, diarrhea, irritable colon, urinary spasm, chronic pancreatitis	Safety in children is not established; increased fluid intake may minimize fecal impaction and urinary hesitancy; blurring of vision and dizziness can occur.
Scopolamine (Isopto Hyoscine and various manufacturers)	Hypodermic tablets—0.4 mg, 0.6 mg Capsules—0.25 mg Injection—0.3, 0.4, 0.5, 0.6, 1.0 mg/ml Ophthalmic drops—0.2%, 0.25% Ophthalmic ointment—0.2%	Systemic: Adults—(Oral) 0.4 mg to 0.8 mg (SC, IM) 0.3 mg to 0.6 mg Prophylaxis of motion sickness—0.25 mg capsule 1 hour before travel Children—(SC, IM) 0.1 mg to 0.3 mg Ophthalmic: 1 to 2 drops. Adjust dosage to requirements	Pre-anesthetic medication, motion sickness, spastic states, obstetrical analgesia (with narcotics), ophthalmic mydriatic and cycloplegic, hyperhidrosis, excess salivation and secretions	CNS depression can occur with systemic use, overdosage results in excitement, confusion, and delirium; produces amnesia when given with narcotics; may produce delirium if used alone in severe pain; effects generally persist 4 hours to 6 hours. Neostigmine or physostigmine is an effective antidote. 0.25-mg capsule (Triptone) is available over-the-counter for prophylaxis of motion sickness.
Scopolamine Transdermal Therapeutic System (Transderm-Scop)	Adhesive patch containing 1.5 mg scopolamine and delivering 0.5 mg over 3 days at a constant rate	Apply 1 system to the postauricular skin once every 3 days, several hours before exposure	Prevention of motion sickness	A circular adhesive patch that delivers steady state blood levels of scopolamine over 3 days from a drug reservoir within the patch. An initial priming dose is released from the adhesive layer, and quickly brings the plasma level to the desired steady state level, which is maintained by continuous release of drug from the reservoir through the rate-controlling membrane. Bathing and swimming do not affect drug response as long as

(continued)

Table 10-2. Anticholinergics *(continued)*

Drug	Preparations	Usual Dosage Range	Major Uses	Remarks
				patch remains intact. The most common side-effects are dry mouth, blurred vision, and drowsiness; use with caution in presence of glaucoma, urinary or GI obstruction, impaired liver or kidney function, and in the elderly. Safe use in children has not been established.
Thiphenamil (Trocinate)	Tablets—100 mg, 400 mg	Adults—400 mg every 4 hr as required	GI hypermotility and spasm	Causes somewhat lower incidence of atropine-like side-effects; more costly than most other similar drugs; not recommended for children
Tropicamide (Mydriacyl)	Ophthalmic drops— 0.5%, 1%	Refraction—1 to 2 drops of 1%, repeat in 5 min, and every 20 min to 30 min as needed to maintain mydriasis Examination—1 to 2 drops 0.5% 20 to 30 minutes prior to examination	Ophthalmic examinations	Effects occur in 20 minutes to 30 minutes; minimize systemic absorption by compressing lacrimal sac after instillation.
Trihexyphenidyl (Artane, Tremin, THP, Trihexane)	Tablets—2 mg, 5 mg Elixir—2 mg/5 ml Capsules (sustained release)—5 mg	Parkinsonism—1 mg initially, increased by 2-mg increments every 3 to 5 days to a total dose of 6 mg to 10 mg a day; usual maintenance dose is 6 mg to 12 mg daily in divided doses. Extrapyramidal Reactions—5 mg to 15 mg in divided doses	Parkinsonism, extrapyramidal reactions	When used with l-DOPA, reduce dose of each drug proportionately; major effect is on rigidity, with minimal effects on tremor. May produce CNS stimulation and excessive drying of the mouth; often given before meals. See Chapter 26.

5 Anticholinergics may decrease the effects of cholinergics (*e.g.,* pilocarpine or physostigmine) used locally in the eye. Concurrent use of anticholinergics with haloperidol or corticosteroids may elevate intraocular pressure.

▶ **NURSING ALERTS**

▷ 1 Caution patient against driving or operating machinery if blurred vision, dizziness, or drowsiness occurs.

▷ 2 Observe patients, especially geriatrics, for signs of excitement, agitation, and delirium. Reduce dose or consider alternative medication. Caution elderly patients to take special care during physical activity because drugs may impair coordination.

▷ 3 Use cautiously in peptic ulcer patients, because drugs may delay gastric emptying time and produce abdominal distention and antral stasis.

▷ 4 Have antidotal measures (*e.g.,* cholinesterase inhibi-

tors, barbiturates, levarterenol, respiratory aids, oxygen) on hand in case of overdosage, especially when drugs are used parenterally.

▷ 5 Determine patient history before using these agents, because they may aggravate conditions such as glaucoma, asthma, duodenal ulcer, coronary heart disease, arrhythmias, hyperthyroidism, hiatal hernia, ulcerative colitis, chronic lung disease, and prostatic hypertrophy.

▶ **NURSING CONSIDERATIONS**

▷ 1 Warn patient to expect certain common side-effects with systemic use of these drugs. These effects include dry mouth, urinary hesitancy, blurred vision, tachycardia, and possibly constipation. They may be minimized by dosage reduction but often must be tolerated to obtain the beneficial effects of the drug.

▷ 2 Advise patient that dry mouth can be relieved by chewing gum or candy, if necessary.

▷ 3 Be alert for changes in pulse rate and respiration, and report any changes immediately. A dosage adjustment or another drug may be required.

▷ 4 Monitor urine output and bowel regularity. Note any significant changes and inform physician.

▷ 5 Carefully check dosages of drugs, as many are quite small (*e.g.,* atropine 0.4 mg–0.6 mg) and overdosage is easily possible.

▷ 6 Ensure that proper diet is followed, especially if medication is used for GI disorders. Administer oral medications 30 minutes before meals.

▷ 7 Inform patients using drugs for symptoms of parkinsonism that optimal effects may take several days to develop. When changing medication or adjusting the dosage, do so gradually (See Chap. 26).

▷ 8 Do not use for prolonged periods of time in the eye, because local irritation, edema, and follicular conjunctivitis may occur.

▷ 9 Discontinue ophthalmic use if rapid pulse, dizziness, dryness of the mouth, or other signs of systemic toxicity occur. Advise physician immediately.

Adrenergic Drugs

11

Adrenergic drugs are compounds, either natural or synthetic, that are capable of eliciting biological responses similar to those produced by activation of the sympathetic nervous system or resulting from adrenal medullary discharge. For this reason, these agents may also be termed *sympathomimetic drugs*—that is, drugs that mimic sympathetic nerve stimulation.

The adrenergic agents comprise a large, heterogenous group of compounds possessing a wide spectrum of pharmacologic actions. Adequate classification of these substances, therefore, is difficult. Based on their predominant mechanism of action, adrenergic drugs can be divided into three groups:

1 *Direct acting*—compounds exerting a direct activating effect at the postsynaptic adrenergic receptor site, (*e.g.,* norepinephrine, dopamine)

2 *Indirect acting*—compounds acting on the presynaptic adrenergic nerve terminals to promote the release of stored adrenergic neurohormones (*e.g.,* tyramine)

3 *Dual acting*—compounds possessing a mixture of both direct and indirect actions (*e.g.,* ephedrine, amphetamine)

Qualitative differences in the responses of effector structures to the various groups of adrenergic agents indicates the existence of different kinds of adrenergic receptor sites. A discussion of adrenergic receptors can be found in Chapter 8. It is now generally accepted that adrenergic receptor sites are of two basic types, *alpha* and *beta,* which exhibit selective differences between them. In addition, adrenergic receptors can be subdivided further into type 1 (*i.e.,* alpha 1, beta 1) and type 2 (*i.e.,* alpha 2, beta 2) sites, depending largely on their location (see Table 11-1). In addition, dopamine, one of the endogenous catecholamines, is capable of interacting not only with certain alpha and beta receptor sites but also with specific dopaminergic sites, particularly in the brain and on certain blood vessels. Table 11-1 outlines the major adrenergic receptor sites and lists the important pharmacologic effects produced by activation of each type of receptor.

The pharmacologic actions of the various adrenergic agents depend to a large extent on their affinity and specificity for the different types of adrenergic receptors, as well as their intrinsic activity at each site. An overview of the major pharmacologic effects resulting from activation of the different kinds of peripheral adrenergic receptor sites is presented in Table 11-2.

In addition to their many peripheral actions, many adrenergic compounds exert profound effects on the CNS. Alterations in catecholamine activity in various brain structures are believed to be responsible for many affective and motor disorders, and those drugs that are useful in treating these conditions function largely by modifying the availability or action of endogenous adrenergic amines. Many noncatecholamine adrenergic drugs (*e.g.,* ephedrine and amphetamine) can easily penetrate the CNS and elicit marked stimulatory effects. These agents are often abused and they are potentially dangerous drugs. They will be considered in Chapter 27 with the other CNS stimulants.

In order to discuss the adrenergic drugs in some reasonable order, the following arbitrary classification will be

Table 11-1. Adrenergic Receptor Sites

Activated by	Alpha-1 *Epinephrine Norepinephrine*	Alpha-2 *Epinephrine Norepinephrine*	Beta-1 *Epinephrine Isoproterenol*	Beta-2 *Epinephrine Isoproterenol*	Dopaminergic *Dopamine**
Major Peripheral Locations					
	Blood vessels, GI and urinary sphincters, eye (radial muscle), pancreas, spleen, skin (pilomotor muscles, sweat glands), salivary glands	Presynaptic adrenergic nerve endings, platelets, fat cells, vascular smooth muscle	Heart, GI smooth muscle, adipose tissue	Bronchioles, GI, uterine and urinary bladder smooth muscle, skeletal muscle vasculature, liver, kidney	Renal, coronary, and visceral blood vessels
Responses					
Excitatory	Vasoconstriction, contraction of GI and urinary sphincters, sweat and salivary secretions	Platelet aggregation, vasoconstriction (slow onset)	Cardiac stimulation, lipolysis	Glycogenolysis, gluconeogenesis	
Inhibitory	Decreased GI motility, impaired pancreatic secretions	Decreased release of norepinephrine from nerve ending, inhibition of lipolysis	Decreased GI motility	Bronchodilation, vasodilation in skeletal muscle, uterine relaxation, decreased GI motility, urinary bladder relaxation	Dilation of renal, coronary, and visceral blood vessels

* Dopamine also can activate cardiac beta receptors and certain vascular alpha receptors.

used with the realization that many drugs fall into more than one of the proposed categories.

I. Endogenous catecholamines (*e.g.,* epinephrine, norepinephrine, dopamine)
II. Synthetic catecholamines (*e.g.,* isoproterenol, dobutamine)
III. Vasopressor amines (*e.g.,* metaraminol)
IV. Nasal decongestants (*e.g.,* phenylephrine)
V. Ophthalmic decongestants (*e.g.,* naphazoline)
VI. Bronchodilators (*e.g.,* ephedrine, metaproterenol)
VII. Smooth muscle relaxants (*e.g.,* isoxsuprine, nylidrin, ritodrine)
VIII. CNS stimulants and anorexiants (*e.g.,* amphetamine)

I   Endogenous Catecholamines

The three major endogenous catecholamines, epinephrine, norepinephrine, and dopamine, serve to mediate the functioning of the sympathetic nervous system and are found widely throughout the body. Moreover, many other classes of pharmacologic agents exert their effects by modifying the action of one or more of these endogenous substances, so that the catecholamines participate in the action of a wide range of drugs. Catecholamines can also be prepared synthetically and are widely used in the treatment of many disease states. The therapeutic indications of the catechol-amines are primarily based on their vasoconstrictive, bronchodilatory, and cardiac stimulatory actions.

▶ **epinephrine**

Parenteral—Adrenalin, Asmolin, Sus-Phrine

Inhalation—Asthmahaler, Asthmanefrin, Bronitin Mist, Bronkaid Mist, Medihaler-Epi, Micronefrin, Primatene, Vaponefrin

Nasal—Adrenalin

Ophthalmic—Adrenalin, Epifrin, E1, E2, Epinal, Epitrate, Eppy/N, Glaucon, Mytrate

Mechanism

Direct nonspecific activation of alpha and beta adrenergic receptor sites; alpha activation elicits vasoconstriction in many vascular beds; beta-1 activation results in positive inotropic and chronotropic actions on the heart and beta-2 activation evokes bronchodilation and dilation of vessels in skeletal muscles.

Uses

1 Symptomatic relief of anaphylactic, allergic, and other hypersensitivity reactions
2 Pressor agent for acute hypotensive states
3 Nasal decongestion
4 Bronchodilation and pulmonary decongestion (relaxes bronchial smooth muscle and constricts mucosal blood vessels)

5 Restoration of normal cardiac rhythm in cases of cardiac arrest
6 Management of simple, open-angle glaucoma (decrease production and increase outflow of aqueous humor)
7 Ocular decongestion (vasoconstriction) and production of mydriasis
8 Topical hemostasis (control superficial bleeding)
9 Potentiation and prolongation of the action of local anesthetics

Dosage
1 *Parenteral*
   Cardiac arrest—5 ml to 10 ml 1:10,000 IV repeated at intervals every 5 minutes as required
   Intracardiac—3 ml to 5 ml 1:10,000
   Intraspinal—0.2 ml to 0.4 ml 1:1000 added to anesthetic solution
   Bronchospasm—0.2 ml to 1 ml 1:1000 SC or IM *or* 0.05 ml to 0.6 ml 1:400 SC or IM *or* 0.1 ml to 0.3 ml 1:200 SC (Children—0.01 mg/kg SC)
   With local anesthetic—1:20,000—1:100,000
2 *Inhalation*
   1:100 (1%) aqueous solution from metered aerosol or nebulizer. Allow 1 minute to 2 minutes between inhalations, and use least number of inhalations that are effective
3 *Topical*
   Nasal—1 to 2 drops 0.1% solution every 4 hours to 6 hours
   Hemostatic—1:1000 to 1:10,000 applied locally
4 *Ophthalmic*
   Glaucoma—1 to 2 drops 0.25% to 2% solution (individualized to patient needs)
   Ocular mydriasis and hemostasis—1 to 2 drops 0.1% solution

Fate
Readily absorbed by mucous membranes but rapidly destroyed by digestive enzymes, thus is useless orally. Aqueous solutions are very unstable, oxidize readily (amber or yellow color in solution), and should be used immediately. Effects occur quickly when given SC, IM, intraocularly, or by inhalation. Suspension forms provide more prolonged actions (6 hr–12 hr). Drug is usually rapidly inactivated by uptake into adrenergic nerve endings, or through enzymatic (MAO, COMT) hydrolysis. Circulating drug is hydrolyzed in the liver, and metabolites, chiefly vanillyl mandelic acid (VMA), are excreted in the urine.

Common Side-Effects
Systemic—nervousness, anxiety, nausea, sweating, pallor, palpitations, headache, insomnia
Ophthalmic—headache, stinging, lacrimation, rebound hyperemia
Nasal—burning, mucosal dryness, sneezing, rebound congestion

Table 11-2. Adrenergic Drug Effects

Structure	Response	Receptor Type
Cardiovascular System		
Heart	Increased rate	Beta-1
	Increased force	Beta-1
	Increased conduction velocity	Beta-1
Blood Vessels		
Skeletal	Vasoconstriction	Alpha-1, Alpha-2
	Vasodilation	Beta-2
Mucosal	Vasoconstriction	Alpha-1
Mesenteric	Vasoconstriction	Alpha-1
	Vasodilation	Dopaminergic
Coronary, renal	Vasodilation	Dopaminergic
Bronchioles	Smooth muscle relaxation	Beta-2
GI Tract		
Smooth muscle	Relaxation	Beta-2
Sphincters	Contraction	Alpha-1
Urinary Bladder		
Smooth muscle	Relaxation	Beta-2
Sphincter	Contraction	Alpha-1
Uterus	Relaxation	Beta-2
Kidney	Renin release	Beta-2
Eye		
Radial muscle	Contraction	Alpha-1
Ciliary muscle	Relaxation (weak)	Beta-1
Skin		
Pilomotor muscles	Contraction	Alpha-1
Sweat glands	Secretion (weak)	Alpha-1
Liver	Glycogenolysis	Beta-2
Adipose Tissue	Lipolysis	Beta-1
	Inhibition of lipolysis	Alpha-2
Pancreas	Decreased insulin secretion	Alpha-1

Significant Adverse Reactions
Systemic—weakness, dizziness, hypertension, anginal pain, tachycardia and arrhythmias, pulmonary edema, dyspnea, urinary retention, cerebral or subarachnoid hemorrhage, delusions, tremor, psychoses, lactic acidosis
Ophthalmic—conjunctival irritation; pigmentation of eyelids, cornea, or conjunctiva; iritis; shedding of eyelashes; scotomas

Contraindications
Severe hypertension, arrhythmias, coronary artery disease, shock, porphyria, narrow-angle glaucoma, organic brain

damage, during labor (delays second stage), and in combination with general anesthetics, especially halogenated hydrocarbons

Interactions

1 Epinephrine may be potentiated by other sympathomimetic agents (*e.g.,* phenylephrine, mephentermine), tricyclic antidepressants, MAO inhibitors, antihistamines, thyroxine, guanethidine.
2 Epinephrine may produce toxic effects when used in combination with digitalis (arrhythmias), general anesthetics (arrhythmias), isoproterenol (arrhythmias), or propranolol (bradycardia).
3 Epinephrine may produce hyperglycemia, altering the requirements for insulin or oral hypoglycemic agents.
4 Cardiac and bronchodilatory effects of epinephrine are antagonized by propranolol. Pressor effects are blocked by vasodilators such as nitrites or alpha-adrenergic blockers (*e.g.,* phentolamine), but may be intensified by beta-blockers (*e.g.,* propranolol).
5 Diuretics may increase the vascular pressor response to epinephrine.

▶ NURSING ALERTS

▷ *Systemic*

▷ 1 Do not use solutions if yellow or amber colored or if they contain a precipitate. Epinephrine is readily destroyed by alkalies, oxidizing agents, and salts of zinc, copper, and iron. Use caution in mixing solutions.
▷ 2 Do not administer simultaneously with isoproterenol, because serious cardiac arrhythmias can result.
▷ 3 Administer very cautiously to elderly patients or to those with hypertension, hyperthyroidism, diabetes, parkinsonism, cardiovascular disease, long-term bronchial asthma or emphysema, psychoneuroses, prostatic hypertrophy, or tuberculosis. Safe use in pregnancy or during lactation has not been established.
▷ 4 Carefully check solution *strength* and required dosage before administration. Use a syringe with calibrations small enough to ensure accurate dosage measurement. Serious consequences can result from slight overdosage or improper injection techniques.
▷ 5 Always aspirate syringe prior to SC or IM injection to ensure needle is not in a vein.
▷ 6 When giving drug IV, slowly inject small amount, carefully monitor blood pressure and pulse, and give repeat injections only as needed to obtain desired effect. Take blood pressure every 3 minutes to 5 minutes until patient is fully stabilized. Observe patients for signs of shock (*e.g.,* cyanosis, pallor) and be prepared with IV fluids and other measures.

▷ *Inhalation*

▷ 1 Allow 1 minute to 2 minutes between inhalations. Overdosage can produce severe systemic effects.
▷ 2 Do not give isoproterenol concurrently with epinephrine. Allow at least 4 hours between drugs.

▷ 3 If symptoms are not relieved within 15 minutes to 30 minutes, consult physician immediately.

▷ *Ophthalmic*

▷ 1 Caution patients that drug may cause blurred vision and sensitivity to light. Advise against driving or operating hazardous machinery.
▷ 2 Perform periodic tonometric evaluations during drug usage to aid in determining frequency of dosage.

▷ *Nasal*

▷ 1 Caution patient against too frequent use of epinephrine because rebound congestion and hyperemia frequently occur.
▷ 2 Use carefully in infants and the elderly because systemic absorption can produce untoward reactions (*e.g.,* tachycardia, hypertension, anxiety).

▶ NURSING CONSIDERATIONS

▷ *Systemic*

▷ 1 Do not expose solutions to heat, light, or air because deterioration rapidly ensues.
▷ 2 Massage injection site to hasten absorption, and rotate sites to prevent tissue necrosis due to localized vasoconstriction.
▷ 3 Always have antidotal drugs (*e.g.,* phentolamine, propranolol, nitrites) on hand when giving epinephrine, especially IV. Make sure patient is constantly observed following IV administration.
▷ 4 Teach patients with history of acute bronchial asthmatic attacks how to administer epinephrine SC.
▷ 5 Counsel patients to promptly report any unusual changes while taking the drug (*e.g.,* urinary hesitancy, difficulty in controlling diabetes).
▷ 6 Prolonged use may lead to "epinephrine tolerance." Instruct patients to inform physician if drug seems to be less effective over time.

▷ *Inhalation*

▷ 1 Use only the minimal number of inhalations to relieve the symptoms. Prolonged, frequent, or excessive use can produce marked adverse effects.
▷ 2 Alert patient to reduce dosage if bronchial irritation, nervousness, or insomnia is noted.
▷ 3 Tell individual to rinse mouth with water after inhalation to prevent excessive drying effects.

▷ *Ophthalmic*

▷ 1 If possible, administer drug at bedtime to minimize discomfort from mydriasis and photophobia. Caution patient that visual perception may be impaired, especially at night.
▷ 2 Advise patient to inform physician if localized symptoms (stinging, burning, headache, tearing) persist with continued use of the drug.
▷ 3 Caution users to discontinue drug and consult physician if hypersensitivity reactions develop (*e.g.,* itching, edema, watery discharge).
▷ 4 Discontinue drug prior to surgery in which certain

general anesthetics (*e.g.,* halothane, other halogenated hydrocarbons) will be used because there is danger of possible arrhythmias from systemic absorption of epinephrine.

▷ *Nasal*
▷ 1 Avoid contaminating dropper tip. Rinse dropper in hot water after each application.
▷ 2 Caution patients against prolonged use of nasal decongestants, because rebound congestion frequently occurs.
▷ 3 Give nose drops with head low or tilted back to prevent passage into throat and possible systemic absorption.
▷ 4 Tell user that instillation of nasal solution will sting, but that discomfort will be temporary.

▶ **dipivefrin**
Propine

Dipivefrin is a lipid-soluble prodrug of epinephrine; that is, it is converted to epinephrine by enzymatic hydrolysis following instillation into the eye. Due to its highly lipophilic nature, its penetration into the cornea is much greater than that of epinephrine itself. Onset of action is within 30 minutes. Dipivefrin is indicated for the control of intraocular pressure in chronic, open-angle glaucoma, and its use is associated with fewer side-effects than conventional epinephrine therapy because less drug is required due to improved absorption. Therapeutic response to twice daily administration of dipivefrin is approximately equivalent to that of 2% pilocarpine given 4 times a day, without the miosis and cycloplegia characteristic of cholinergic therapy. However, the response is somewhat inferior to that observed with 2% epinephrine. Due to its mydriatic action, dipivefrin, like epinephrine, is contraindicated in narrow-angle glaucoma.

The side-effects associated with dipivefrin therapy are similar to those noted previously for ophthalmic epinephrine administration but occur with lower frequency. Burning and stinging following instillation are the most common side-effects. In addition, systemic effects (tachycardia, increased blood pressure, arrhythmias) have been reported following ocular administration of epinephrine and can occur with use of dipivefrin as well. Dipivefrin is available as a 0.1% solution and the usual dosage is 1 drop every 12 hours.

▶ **norepinephrine (NE)**
Levarterenol, Levophed

Mechanism
Direct activation of alpha-adrenergic receptor sites on blood vessels, producing powerful vasoconstriction; also possesses slight inotropic action on cardiac beta receptors (increased force of contraction). Increases blood pressure and coronary artery blood flow, but increases work load of the heart as well; in normal doses, little effect on the CNS or on metabolic activity.

Uses
1 Management of acute hypotensive states
2 Adjunctive treatment of cardiac arrest

Dosage
Used by IV *infusion*—initially, 8 mcg/min to 12 mcg/min (2 ml/min–3 ml/min) of a 4 mcg/ml dilution (4 mg NE/1000 ml 5% dextrose); maintenance dose—2 mcg/min to 4 mcg/min (0.5 ml/min–1 ml/min)

Fate
Rapid acting; effects disappear within 2 minutes after termination of IV infusion; rapidly inactivated by uptake and enzymatic hydrolysis; excreted in the urine largely as metabolites

Common Side-Effects
Bradycardia (reflex), headache, palpitation, nervousness

Significant Adverse Reactions
Hypertension, respiratory distress, tremors, arrhythmias in the presence of certain anesthetics, tissue necrosis following extravasation; large doses can cause chest pain, photophobia, hyperglycemia, vomiting, severe hypertension, cerebral hemorrhage, and convulsions.

Contraindications
Hypovolemic shock, vascular thrombosis; extreme hypoxia or hypercapnia; pregnancy; during general anesthesia when halogenated hydrocarbons (*e.g.,* halothane) are employed.

Interactions
1 The pressor effects of norepinephrine may be potentiated in the presence of tricyclic antidepressants, MAO inhibitors, other sympathomimetic drugs, beta-blockers, antihistamines, guanethidine, and methyldopa.
2 Norepinephrine, together with oxytocic drugs, can result in severe hypertension.
3 Norepinephrine may precipitate cardiac arrhythmias in the presence of cyclopropane and the halogenated hydrocarbon general anesthetics.
4 Thiazide and high-ceiling (*e.g.,* bumetanide, furosemide) diuretics may reduce arterial responsiveness to norepinephrine.

▶ **NURSING ALERTS**
▷ 1 Take blood pressure readings every 2 minutes to 5 minutes during and following infusion. Carefully observe patient's color, skin temperature, and vital signs.
▷ 2 Check flow rate constantly, and never leave patient unattended during treatment.
▷ 3 Do not use catheter tie-in arrangement because venous stasis around tubing can occur, resulting in increased local concentration of drug.
▷ 4 Do not give infusion into veins of the leg, especially in the elderly, because occlusive vascular diseases can result.
▷ 5 Be alert for early signs of overdosage (headache, vom-

iting, blurred vision, cardiac dysrhythmias, anginal symptoms), and adjust dosage appropriately.

▷ 6 Use very cautiously in patients with hypertension, heart disease, or hyperthyroidism, and in elderly individuals.

▷ 7 Be alert to possibility of edema, hemorrhage, and organ necrosis with prolonged use of norepinephrine.

▷ 8 Should extravasation occur (blanching of skin, swelling, hardness), stop infusion and infiltrate area with 10 ml to 15 ml saline containing 5 mg to 10 mg phentolamine as soon as possible.

▷ 9 Do not use solutions that are discolored or that contain precipitated matter.

▷ 10 Do not administer whole blood or plasma with norepinephrine.

▶ NURSING CONSIDERATIONS

▷ 1 Give infusion into a large vein wherever possible, and alternate infusion sites to minimize risk of necrosis.

▷ 2 Monitor pulse for signs of bradycardia; atropine can be given if necessary.

▷ 3 Consider addition of heparin to infusion solution to prevent thromboses, especially in patients with recent infarction.

▷ 4 Determine urinary output regularly as an indicator of renal perfusion. Note decrease in output, and report immediately.

▷ 5 When using norepinephrine, maintain adequate blood volume to prevent tissue ischemia resulting from vasoconstrictive effect of the drug.

▷ 6 Continue infusion until blood pressure and tissue perfusion can be maintained on their own. Discontinue therapy by *gradually* reducing infusion rate, and continue monitoring vital signs to assure circulatory adequacy.

▷ 7 Do not infuse in saline *alone* because oxidation and loss of potency can occur rapidly. Use 5% dextrose vehicle.

▷ 8 Have atropine and propranolol on hand to treat bradycardia and arrhythmias should they develop.

▶ dopamine

Dopastat, Intropin

Mechanism

Direct activation of specific dopaminergic receptors in mesenteric and renal vasculature, resulting in vasodilation and increased renal blood flow; also stimulates myocardial beta receptors, enhancing force of contraction and increasing cardiac output with minimal cardioaccelerator action. In high doses, activates alpha receptors in other vascular beds, causing constriction. Produces less oxygen demand on the myocardium and has a lower incidence of arrhythmias than other catecholamines.

Uses

1 Correction of the hemodynamic imbalances associated with various forms of shock (*e.g.,* trauma, heart surgery, myocardial infarction, renal failure, septicemia)

Dosage

Initially—2 mcg/kg/min to 5 mcg/kg/min of diluted solution by IV infusion. May increase by 5 mcg/kg/min to 10 mcg/kg/min increments up to 20 mcg/kg/min to 50 mcg/kg/min in severely ill patients

Fate

Rapid onset (5 min) and short duration of action (5 min–10 min); largely inactivated by liver and plasma enzymes and excreted chiefly in the urine as metabolites. A portion is converted to norepinephrine in adrenergic nerve endings; does not cross the blood–brain barrier

Common Side-Effects

Nausea, vomiting, palpitations, tachycardia, slight hypotension, mild respiratory difficulty, and headache

Significant Adverse Reactions

(Usually occur with high doses) Hypertension, conduction irregularities, azotemia, decreased urinary outflow. Necrosis and tissue sloughing can occur following extravasation.

Contraindications

Ventricular arrhythmias and pheochromocytoma

Interactions

1 Pressor effects of dopamine may be potentiated by MAO inhibitors, tricyclic antidepressants, other sympathomimetics, ergot alkaloids, and furazolidone.

2 Actions of dopamine and diuretics may be mutually additive.

3 Dopamine may produce arrhythmias in the presence of cyclopropane and halogenated hydrocarbon anesthetics.

4 Severe hypertension may result from combined use of dopamine and oxytocic drugs.

5 Use of phenytoin with dopamine may lead to hypotension, bradycardia, and seizures.

▶ NURSING ALERTS

▷ 1 Always dilute solution before use. Contents of ampule are added to a sterile diluent solution (250 ml or 500 ml of Sodium Chloride, Sodium Lactate, Dextrose 5%, Lactated Ringer's), according to package instructions.

▷ 2 Do not add to alkaline IV solutions (*e.g.,* sodium bicarbonate) because dopamine will be inactivated.

▷ 3 Carefully monitor blood pressure, pulse, cardiac output, and urine flow during infusion. Rate of flow must be adjusted to maintain stable vital signs.

▷ 4 If high doses are used, check urine output continually, and reduce dosage if output begins to fall.

▷ 5 Note any changes in skin color, as well as temperature or consistency at injection site, indications of possible extravasation. To prevent necrosis, infiltrate with 10 ml to 15 ml of saline solution containing phentolamine (5 mg–10 mg).

▷ 6 Watch for symptoms of overdosage (hypertension, reduced urine flow, arrhythmias, change in color of extremities) and reduce dosage if symptoms are noted.

Antidotal measures are usually not required, because drug is very short acting.

▶ **NURSING CONSIDERATIONS**

▷ 1 Protect dopamine solutions from light and do not use if discolored.

▷ 2 Dilute just prior to administration, although solutions are stable for approximately 24 hours.

▷ 3 Check infusion system for stable flow rate, and adjust as needed to obtain desired hemodynamic and renal responses.

▷ 4 Infuse into a large vein (preferably of the antecubital fossa) to minimize danger of extravasation and tissue necrosis.

II Synthetic Catecholamines

In addition to the three catecholamines found endogenously, two synthetic derivatives, isoproterenol and dobutamine, are available. They are almost exclusively activators of *beta*-adrenergic receptor sites. Isoproterenol nonselectively activates all beta receptors, and dobutamine exerts a relatively specific activation of cardiac beta-1 receptors.

▶ isoproterenol

Oral/parenteral—Isuprel

Inhalation—Aerolone, Dispos-A-Med, Isuprel, Medihaler-Iso, Norisodrine, Vapo-Iso

Mechanism

Direct beta-adrenergic receptor activation, resulting in cardiac stimulation, vasodilation, and bronchodilation; also relaxes smooth muscle of the GI tract and uterus, releases free fatty acids, stimulates insulin secretion, and increases glycogenolysis

Uses

1 Relief of bronchospasm associated with respiratory disorders and general anesthesia

2 Adjunct in management of shock, cardiac arrest, Adams–Stokes syndrome, AV block, and carotid sinus hypersensitivity

Dosage

A. *Parenteral*

1. Bronchospasm (during anesthesia)—0.01 mg to 0.02 mg IV of a 1:50,000 solution in saline or Dextrose 5%

2. Shock—0.25 ml/min to 2.5 ml/min of 1:500,000 dilution in Dextrose 5% by IV infusion (0.5 mcg/min–5 mcg/min)

3. Cardiac arrest: IV (injection)–1 ml to 3 ml of a 1:50,000 dilution (0.02 mg–0.06 mg); IV (infusion)—1.25 ml of 1:250,000 dilution per minute (5 mcg/min); IM, SC—1 ml of 1:5000

solution undiluted (0.2 mg); Intracardiac—0.1 ml of 1:5000 solution (0.02 mg)

B. *Sublingual*

1. Bronchospasm—10 mg to 20 mg 3 to 4 times/day (children—5 mg to 10 mg 3 to 4 times/day)

2. Heart block—10 mg initially (range 5 mg–50 mg)

C. *Rectal*

5 mg initially; 5 mg to 15 mg maintenance

D. *Inhalation*

Solution—125 mcg to 250 mcg (1–2 inhalations) 4 to 6 times/day (maximum 6/hr)

Aerosol—75 mcg to 250 mcg (1–2 inhalations) 4 to 6 times/day

Powder—45 mcg to 220 mcg (1–2 inhalations) 4 to 6 times/day

Fate

Readily absorbed when given parenterally or as aerosol; oral and sublingual absorption is unreliable; duration following most forms of administration is 2 hours to 4 hours (1 hr–2 hr with inhalation); metabolites are excreted largely in the urine, within 24 hours to 48 hours following biotransformation in the GI tract, liver, lungs, and other tissues.

Common Side-Effects

Nervousness, headache, palpitations, flushing, nausea, dizziness, mild tremors, and dryness of the oropharynx

Significant Adverse Reactions

Buccal ulcerations (sublingual), bronchial irritation and edema, cardiac distress (tachycardia, dysrhythmias, anginal pain), parotid gland enlargement (rare); overdosage may result in severe bronchoconstriction, cardiac excitability, and possibly cardiac arrest.

Contraindications

Arrhythmias associated with tachycardia, concurrent administration of epinephrine; long-acting tablets should not be used in hyperexcitability states, coronary sclerosis, or hypertension.

Interactions

1 Pressor response may be potentiated by MAO inhibitors or tricyclic antidepressants.

2 Combined use with epinephrine may lead to serious arrhythmias.

3 Arrhythmias may develop if used with cyclopropane or halogenated hydrocarbon anesthetics.

4 Effects are specifically antagonized by propranolol and other beta-adrenergic blockers.

▶ **NURSING ALERTS**

▷ *Parenteral*

▷ 1 Closely observe patients in shock during infusion. If heart rate exceeds 110 beats/minute, decrease or stop infusion, due to danger of arrhythmias.

▷ 2 Carefully monitor blood pressure, heart rate and rhythm, ECG, urine volume, blood pH, and Pco_2. Adjust infusion rate to maintain stability of above parameters.

▷ 3 Never inject solutions intended for oral inhalation.

▷ *Oral/Sublingual*

▷ 1 Caution patient to swallow sustained-release tablet whole.

▷ 2 Warn patients that prolonged use of sublingual tablets can damage teeth. Instruct them to rinse mouth thoroughly after each administration.

▷ *Inhalation*

▷ 1 Discourage excessive use of inhalation products because tolerance can develop and sudden deaths have been reported.

▷ 2 Use with extreme caution in patients with cardiovascular disorders, hypertension, hyperthyroidism, or diabetes.

▷ 3 Do not use discolored or cloudy solutions.

▷ 4 When using powdered inhalation, instruct patient *not* to breathe deeply but with normal force and depth.

▷ 5 Advise patient to report immediately if usual doses are not producing the desired relief. Inform user of dangers in using too frequent doses (3–5 treatments within 6 hr–12 hr).

▶ **NURSING CONSIDERATIONS**

▷ 1 Recognize that constant ECG monitoring is essential with parenteral administration.

▷ 2 Have oxygen and other respiratory aids available when using parenteral isoproterenol.

▷ 3 Warn patients to expect mild systemic effects (*e.g.,* flushing, palpitations) with sublingual use.

▷ 4 Instruct patient to allow tablet to dissolve under tongue without sucking or swallowing saliva until drug has been absorbed.

▷ 5 Use only *sublingual* tablets rectally, if directed.

▷ 6 Carefully check dosage and method of inhalation prescribed (*e.g.,* nebulizer, aerosol, powder).

▷ 7 Instruct patients on the proper method of using the various forms of inhalation. Stress the importance of using the lowest effective dose.

▷ 8 Tell patient to rinse mouth following inhalation to minimize dryness.

▷ 9 Alert user to the fact that saliva may appear pink or red following inhalation.

▷ 10 Do not place more than a one-day supply of drug in nebulizer, and thoroughly rinse mouthpiece daily.

▷ 11 Inform user to report any untoward reactions to the drug or lack of expected relief following normal doses.

▶ **dobutamine**

Dobutrex

Mechanism

Direct activation of beta-1 adrenergic receptors on the myocardium, with minimal action at alpha or beta-2 sites; increases contractile force but produces less increase in heart rate and less decrease in peripheral vascular resistance than comparably effective doses of isoproterenol

Uses

1 Short-term treatment of acute heart failure due to depressed contractility

Dosage

2.5 mcg/kg/min to 10 mcg/kg/min IV infusion of either a 250 mcg/ml, 500 mcg/ml, or 1000 mcg/ml solution in sterile water or 5% Dextrose. Occasionally, infusion rates up to 40 mcg/kg/min are required.

Fate

Onset of action within 1 minute to 2 minutes; short duration of action; plasma half-life of 2 minutes; metabolized in the liver and excreted in urine as conjugates

Common Side-Effects

Tachycardia (5 beats/min–15 beats/min increase), palpitations, mild hypertension (10 mm Hg–20 mm Hg increase in systolic pressure)

Significant Adverse Reactions

Premature ventricular beats, anginal pain, headache, dyspnea, nausea, pronounced tachycardia, marked hypertension

Contraindications

Idiopathic hypertrophic subaortic stenosis

Interactions

1 Cyclopropane and halogenated hydrocarbons may increase the incidence of arrhythmias with dobutamine.

2 Pressor effects of dobutamine can be enhanced by MAO inhibitors, tricyclic antidepressants, other sympathomimetic amines, and oxytocic drugs.

3 Insulin requirements may be increased in the diabetic by dobutamine.

▶ **NURSING ALERTS**

▷ 1 Correct hypovolemia with volume expanders (*e.g.,* dextran) before initiating dobutamine therapy.

▷ 2 During infusion, continually monitor ECG, blood pressure, and cardiac rate and rhythm, and where possible, cardiac output and pulmonary wedge pressure.

▷ 3 Use very cautiously following myocardial infarction or in patients with atrial fibrillation (increased AV conduction may induce ventricular extrasystoles) or preexisting hypertension.

▷ 4 Administer digitalis preparation prior to dobutamine in patients with atrial fibrillation and rapid ventricular response.

▶ **NURSING CONSIDERATIONS**

▷ 1 Note that duration of action of the drug is very brief, and effects are terminated shortly after discontinuation of therapy.

▷ 2 Attempt to adjust volume of infusion by choosing appropriate solution concentration based upon the fluid requirements of the patient.

▷ 3   Do not dilute injection with alkaline solutions (*e.g.,* Sodium Bicarbonate Injection), because incompatability can occur.

▷ 4   Use dilutions for IV use within 24 hours. A color change in the solution during this period indicates slight oxidation, but there is *no* significant loss of potency during the first 24 hours.

III   Vasopressor Amines

Sympathomimetic vasopressor agents comprise a group of synthetic substances possessing both direct and indirect adrenergic activity. Their predominant pharmacologic effect is the production of generalized vasoconstriction, and they are primarily indicated for the management of acute hypotensive situations, such as those associated with cardiac arrest, circulatory shock, drug reactions, and complications of general anesthesia. They are potent drugs and must be used with extreme care.

▶ mephentermine
Wyamine

Mechanism
Direct- and indirect-acting sympathomimetic amine. Pressor effect involves both increased cardiac output (beta activation of the heart) and peripheral vasoconstriction (alpha activation of blood vessels).

Uses
1   Hypotension secondary to ganglionic blockade or spinal anesthesia
2   Maintenance of blood pressure in shock following hemorrhage while fluid replacement is accomplished

Dosage
IM, IV—30 mg to 45 mg in a single injection (30-mg supplements as needed to maintain blood pressure)
IV infusion—0.1% (1 mg/ml) in 5% Dextrose by continuous infusion at a rate of 1 mg/min; two 10-ml vials (30 mg/ml) added to 500 ml of 5% Dextrose in Water

Fate
Rapid onset following IM or IV administration; duration of pressor effect is 2 hours to 3 hours IM and 30 minutes to 60 minutes IV; readily excreted as metabolites in the urine; minimal effects on the CNS

Common Side-Effects
Occasional anxiety

Significant Adverse Reactions
(Occasionally with large doses) Tremor, arrhythmias, drowsiness, hypertension, incoherence, and convulsion

Contraindications
Patients receiving MAO inhibitors, halothane or related anesthetics or chlorpromazine

Interactions
1   Pressor effects may be potentiated by MAO inhibitors, tricyclic antidepressants, sympathomimetic amines, and oxytocic drugs.
2   Arrhythmias may result if used in combination with cyclopropane, halothane, or digitalis.
3   Pressor effects can be antagonized by guanethidine and reserpine.
4   Hypotensive effects of chlorpromazine may be potentiated by mephentermine.

▶ NURSING ALERTS
▷ 1   Monitor blood pressure, pulse, and ECG constantly during IV administration (every 2 min until stabilized, then every 5 min–15 min for duration of action).
▷ 2   Use with extreme caution in presence of hypertension, cardiovascular disease, hyperthyroidism, arteriosclerosis, or in chronically debilitated or ill patients.
▷ 3   Use cautiously in treatment of shock secondary to hemorrhage, and only until blood volume replacement is effected.

▶ NURSING CONSIDERATIONS
▷ 1   Regulate rate of infusion and duration of IV therapy according to response of the patient.
▷ 2   Be alert to possible development of tolerance with repeated injections. Do not increase dose to compensate.
▷ 3   To prevent hypotension, give IM injection 10 minutes to 20 minutes prior to spinal anesthesia.

▶ metaraminol
Aramine

Mechanism
Direct- and indirect-acting adrenergic amine; primarily stimulates alpha receptors (vasoconstriction) and can also activate beta receptors (increased force of contraction). Prolonged use depletes norepinephrine from nerve endings (displaces norepinephrine from storage sites), reducing sympathomimetic activity.

Uses
1   Acute hypotensive states associated with spinal anesthesia
2   Adjunctive management of hypotension caused by brain damage, hemorrhage, surgery, drug reactions, septicemia, or cardiogenic shock

Dosage
IM, SC—2 mg to 10 mg (prevention of hypotension)
IV injection—0.5 mg to 5 mg followed by infusion of 15 mg to 100 mg in 500 ml 5% Dextrose
IV infusion (preferred in shock)—15 mg/500 ml–100

mg/500 ml 5% Dextrose; rate adjusted to maintain desired blood pressure
(Pediatric: SC, IM—0.1 mg/kg; IV—0.01 mg/kg; IV infusion—0.4 mg/kg)

Fate
Onset 1 minute to 2 minutes with IV infusion, 10 minutes with IM and 10 minutes to 20 minutes with SC; effects persist 15 minutes to 60 minutes; partly excreted in the urine and partly taken up by adrenergic nerve endings; weak CNS stimulatory effect

Common Side-Effects
Restlessness, headache, flushing, sweating, and palpitations

Significant Adverse Reactions
(Usually in large doses) Tachycardia, anginal pain, arrhythmias, severe hypertension, convulsions, cardiac arrest, and cerebral hemorrhage. Prolonged use may perpetuate the shock state by preventing volume expansion; hypotension may occur following termination of the drug.

Contraindications
Combined use with halothane or related halogenated hydrocarbon anesthetics or MAO inhibitors, pulmonary edema, metabolic acidosis, use as the sole treatment in cases of hypovolemic shock

Interactions
1 Pressor effects may be enhanced by sympathomimetics, MAO inhibitors, tricyclic antidepressants, guanethidine, reserpine, oxytocics, and ergot alkaloids.
2 Arrhythmias may develop in combination with halogenated hydrocarbon anesthetics, digitalis, or mercurial diuretics.

▶ NURSING ALERTS
▷ 1 Closely monitor blood pressure during infusion (every 2 min–5 min). Avoid excess blood pressure response by carefully regulating rate of infusion.
▷ 2 Change flow rate cautiously because drug has a prolonged effect, and accumulation can occur if rate is too rapid.
▷ 3 Use carefully in patients with hypertension, hyperthyroidism, diabetes, or cirrhosis, and in patients taking digitalis drugs.
▷ 4 Response may be erratic in patients with coexistent shock and acidosis. Correct blood volume if possible before beginning metaraminol.
▷ 5 Avoid extravasation because tissue necrosis and sloughing can occur. Use larger veins whenever possible.
▷ 6 Withdraw drug gradually because marked hypotension often occurs following abrupt termination.

▶ NURSING CONSIDERATIONS
▷ 1 Do not use SC administration if at all possible because necrosis is likely to occur.

▷ 2 Monitor urinary output, as well as sodium and potassium loss, because changes in renal function can occur, especially in patients with cirrhosis.
▷ 3 In the case of reflex bradycardia, have atropine available for treatment.

▶ methoxamine
Vasoxyl

Mechanism
Direct alpha-adrenergic receptor stimulant, producing extensive vasoconstriction with little or no effects on the heart or the CNS; may induce reflex bradycardia, which is abolished by atropine

Uses
1 Restoration or maintenance of blood pressure during anesthesia
2 Termination of paroxysmal supraventricular tachycardia

Dosage
Hypotension
IV—3 mg to 5 mg slow injection
IM (usual route)—10 mg to 20 mg just prior to anesthesia; repeat if necessary in 15 minutes or 5 mg to 15 mg for treatment of hypotension
Paroxysmal supraventricular tachycardia
IV—10 mg slow injection
(Pediatric—IM: 0.25 mg/kg)

Fate
Onset is 10 minutes to 15 minutes following IM injection; immediately with IV use; duration 1 hour to 2 hours; not distributed to CNS

Common Side-Effects
Urinary urgency, pilomotor stimulation, bradycardia, coldness in the extremities

Significant Adverse Reactions
Sustained hypertension, severe headache, and vomiting

Contraindications
With local anesthetics to prolong their action, advanced cardiovascular disease

Interactions
See Metaraminol

▶ NURSING ALERTS
▷ 1 Use cautiously in patients with hypertension, hyperthyroidism, or myocardial damage, and following parenteral injection of the ergot alkaloids.
▷ 2 Continuously monitor blood pressure and heart rate during and for some time following administration. Have atropine available for severe bradycardia.

▶ **NURSING CONSIDERATIONS**

▷ 1 Check urinary output and report any significant changes because drug may produce urinary retention.

▷ 2 Watch for sudden changes in heart rate and blood pressure when drug therapy is terminated.

▶ **phenylephrine parenteral**

Neo-Synephrine

Mechanism

Direct, powerful activation of alpha-adrenergic receptors, resulting in marked vasoconstriction and reflex bradycardia; little direct effect on the heart or the CNS

Uses

1 Maintenance of blood pressure during spinal and inhalation anesthesia

2 Treatment of shock or drug-induced hypotension

3 Treatment of paroxysmal supraventricular tachycardia

4 Production of vasoconstriction for regional analgesia (added to local anesthetic solution)

Dosage

Hypotension

SC, IM—2 mg to 5 mg of a 1% solution

IV—0.1 mg to 0.5 mg of a 0.1% solution (may repeat in 15 min)

IV infusion—100 drops/minute to 200 drops/minute of a 1:50,000 solution until pressure is stabilized, then 40 drops/minute to 60 drops/minute for maintenance (Pediatric—0.1 mg/kg SC or IM)

Prolong spinal anesthesia

2 mg to 5 mg added to anesthetic solution

Tachycardia

0.5 mg IV injection over 20 seconds to 30 seconds; may increase by 0.1-mg increments as needed

Fate

Rapid acting following injection; duration of effects is 20 minutes to 30 minutes with IV and 45 minutes to 90 minutes with SC and IM

Common Side-Effects

Palpitations, tingling in extremities, reflex bradycardia, and lightheadedness

Significant Adverse Reactions

Tachycardia, arrhythmias, tremor, dizziness, hypertension, and weakness

Contraindications

Severe hypertension, cardiac dysrhythmias, and coronary artery disease

Interactions

See Metaraminol

▶ **NURSING ALERTS**

▷ 1 Be alert for early symptoms of overdosage (fullness in the head, tachycardia, numbness or tingling of extremities) and inform physician.

▷ 2 Use very cautiously in patients with hyperthyroidism, myocardial damage, partial heart block, arteriosclerosis, and severe hypertension, and in elderly patients.

▷ 3 Always have an alpha-adrenergic blocking agent (*e.g.,* phentolamine) on hand to treat hypertensive emergencies.

▶ **NURSING CONSIDERATIONS**

▷ 1 Check blood pressure and heart rate frequently during infusion, and avoid excessive increases by carefully controlling rate and dosage.

▷ 2 Do not use solutions that are discolored or cloudy.

IV Nasal Decongestants

Desoxyephedrine	Phenylpropanolamine
Ephedrine	Propylhexedrine
Epinephrine	Pseudoephedrine
Naphazoline	Tetrahydrozoline
Oxymetazoline	Xylometazoline
Phenylephrine	

Adrenergic drugs used for the relief of nasal congestion provide a prompt decongestant effect when applied topically to the nasal mucosa. They exert a direct vasoconstrictive action on the arterioles in the mucosa, thus reducing local blood flow, fluid exudation, and mucosal edema. Tolerance to this decongestant effect develops rapidly, however, and continued use of these drugs frequently results in the appearance of "rebound congestion," characterized by hyperemia and edema of the mucosal membrane. Most of the clinically important nasal decongestants have a reasonably long duration of action and are usually used only 2 to 3 times a day. A general discussion of adrenergic nasal decongestants is followed by more specific prescribing information concerning each individual drug in Table 11-3.

Mechanism

Direct activation of alpha-adrenergic receptor sites on smooth muscle of the nasal mucosal blood vessels; vasoconstriction reduces engorgement of mucosa and fluid exudation, thus reducing congestion.

Uses

1 Relief of nasal congestion associated with allergic reactions, colds, acute and chronic inflammatory states, and hay fever

2 Adjunctive therapy in middle ear infections (decreases congestion around eustachian tubes)

3 Relief of pressure and pain due to ear block during air travel

Table 11-3. Nasal Decongestants

Drug	Preparations	Usual Dosage Range	Remarks
Desoxyephedrine (Vicks inhaler)	Inhaler—50 mg	1 to 2 inhalations as needed	Avoid excessive use; headache can occur
Ephedrine (Efedron, Ephedsol, Vatronol)	Drops—0.5%, 1%, and 3% Jelly—0.6% Capsules—25 mg, 50 mg Syrup—11 mg/5 ml, 20 mg/5 ml	Topical—2 to 3 drops or small amount of jelly every 3 hours to 4 hours Oral—25 mg to 50 mg every 3 hr to 4 hr	Avoid swallowing nose drops because systemic effects are likely; do not use more often than recommended; other uses are discussed in Section VI, Bronchodilators, under Ephedrine.
Epinephrine (Adrenalin)	Drops—0.1%	1 to 2 drops every 4 hours to 6 hours	Do not use in children under 6; avoid prolonged or excessive use; see also epinephrine under Endogenous Catecholamines and Table 11-4
Naphazoline (Privine)	Drops—0.05% Spray—0.05%	2 drops or sprays each nostril every 4 hours to 6 hours	Insomnia is not a problem, so drug may be given at bedtime Naphazoline is incompatible with aluminum; may produce CNS depression; ophthalmic drops also available; see Table 11-4
Oxymetazoline (Afrin, Bayfrin, Dristan Long Lasting, Duramist Plus, Duration, Four Way Long Acting, Neosynephrine 12 Hour, Nostrilla, Sinex Long Lasting)	Drops—0.025%, 0.05% Spray—0.05%	Adults—2 to 3 drops or sprays of 0.05% twice a day Children under 6—2 to 3 drops of 0.025% twice a day	Long-acting preparation; do not exceed twice-a-day dosage; do not use in children under 2 years
Phenylephrine (various manufacturers)	Drops—0.125%, 0.16%, 0.2%, 0.25%, 0.5%, and 1% Spray—0.25%, 0.5% Jelly—0.5%	Adults—0.25% to 0.5% solution every 3 hours to 4 hours Children (6–12 yrs)—0.25% solution every 3 hours to 4 hours Infants—0.125% to 0.2% solution every 2 hours to 4 hours	Jelly is placed into nasal cavity and gently inhaled; do not use for prolonged periods, especially in children; avoid swallowing solution because systemic effects can occur
Phenylpropanolamine (Decongestant-P, Propagest, Rhindecon)	Tablets—25 mg, 50 mg Timed-release capsules—75 mg Syrup—12.5 mg/5 ml	Adults—25 mg every 4 hr or 50 mg every 8 hr Children—(6 yrs–12 yrs) 25 mg every 8 hours (2 yrs–6 yrs) 12.5 mg every 8 hours	Do not exceed recommended dosage, especially in children because side-effects are likely to occur; reserpine can antagonize effects of phenylpropanolamine; also available over the counter as an anorexiant of questionable efficacy, either alone or in combination with caffeine; see Summary, Section VIII
Propylhexedrine (Benzedrex)	Inhaler—250 mg	1 to 2 inhalations as needed	Do not overuse because CNS stimulation can occur; may produce headache and temporary elevation of blood pressure
Pseudoephedrine (Afrinol, Cenafed, Kodet SE, Neosynephrinol, Neofed, Novafed, Sudafed, Sudrin)	Tablets—30 mg, 60 mg Repeat-action tablets—120 mg Capsules—60 mg, 120 mg (timed release) Liquid—30 mg/5 ml	Adults—60 mg every 6 hours or 120 mg every 12 hours Children—15 mg to 30 mg every 6 hours	Fewer side-effects, less pressor action, and longer duration than ephedrine; rebound congestion is minimal; avoid taking drug near bedtime because stimulation can occur; do not use if restlessness, dizziness, tremors, or other signs of CNS excitation occur
Tetrahydrozoline (Tyzine)	Drops—0.05%, 0.1%	Adults—2 to 4 drops or 1 to 2 sprays 0.1% every 3 hours to 4 hours Children (2–6 years)—2 to 3 drops 0.05% every 3 hours to 4 hours	Large doses may produce CNS depression; not recommended in children under 2 years; ophthalmic drops also available; see Table 11-4
Xylometazoline (Chlorohist Long Acting, Corimist, NeoSynephrine II, Otrivin)	Drops—0.05%, 0.1% Spray—0.1%	Adults—2 to 3 drops or sprays every 8 hours to 10 hours Children—2 to 3 drops 0.05% every 8 hours to 10 hours	Effects persist 4 hours to 8 hours; do not use in aluminum containers; do not exceed recommended dosage because systemic effects are likely

Dosage

See Table 11-3

Fate

Topically applied drugs exert a rapid effect that persists for several hours; readily absorbed through mucous membranes; large doses may exert systemic effects

Common Side-Effects

Stinging and burning of the nasal mucosa, sneezing, dryness of mucosa, and headache

Significant Adverse Reactions

Palpitations, tachycardia, hypertension, arrhythmias, nervousness, insomnia, dizziness, blurred vision; severe overdosage and significant absorption may result in marked somnolence, sedation, hypotension, bradycardia, and coma (usually observed following systemic absorption of topically applied drug).

Contraindications

Narrow-angle glaucoma, concurrent therapy with MAO inhibitors or tricyclic antidepressants

Interactions

1 Systemic effects may be potentiated by other sympathomimetics, MAO inhibitors, tricyclic antidepressants, antihistamines, and thyroxine.

▶ **NURSING ALERTS**

▷ 1 Caution users not to exceed recommended dose and to avoid prolonged treatment with topical nasal decongestants because rebound congestion is likely to occur. If relief is not obtained within 5 days, consult physician.

▷ 2 Use cautiously in patients with hypertension, angina, hyperthyroidism, diabetes, or arteriosclerosis, and in young children and elderly patients.

▷ 3 Be alert for signs of developing systemic toxicity (sedation, bradycardia, hypotension, depressed respiration), and, if present, terminate the drug.

▶ **NURSING CONSIDERATIONS**

▷ 1 Instill drops with patient in the lateral, head-down position, to minimize possibility of swallowing solution and systemic absorption.

▷ 2 Instruct patients using spray bottles to always keep container upright to ensure that fine mist is expelled rather than a liquid stream that can result in overdosage.

▷ 3 Following nasal instillation, always rinse spray or dropper tip in hot water to prevent contamination from nasal secretions. Never use same container for more than one person.

▷ 4 Counsel user to blow nose prior to drug administration to clear nasal passages.

▷ 5 When using inhalers, advise patient to close one nostril while inhaling through open nostril.

V Ophthalmic Decongestants

Epinephrine	Phenylephrine
Hydroxyamphetamine	Tetrahydrozoline
Naphazoline	

The sympathomimetics used in ophthalmology are employed primarily to produce arteriolar vasoconstriction and pupillary dilation due to their strong alpha-adrenergic effects. Their primary advantages over the anticholinergic preparations that have many of the same actions in the eye are that ophthalmic decongestants do not produce cycloplegia (*i.e.,* paralysis of accommodation), nor do they increase intraocular pressure. They are also employed in the treatment of *open-angle* glaucoma, usually in combination with cholinergics (see Chap. 9), because they decrease the formation of aqueous humor (beta-adrenergic action) and facilitate its outflow from the anterior chamber (alpha-adrenergic action). Due to their mydriatic effect, however, they are contraindicated in *narrow-angle* glaucoma because refraction of the iris would further impair the already reduced drainage of aqueous humor resulting from occlusion of the channels by the abnormally positioned iris. A general review of this class of drugs is followed by a listing of individual drugs in Table 11-4.

Mechanism

Direct activation of alpha-adrenergic receptor sites, resulting in vasoconstriction of small blood vessels and contraction of the radial muscle, producing pupillary dilation (mydriasis)

Uses

1 Facilitate examination of the fundus of the eye
2 Reduce the incidence of synechiae formation in uveitis
3 Treatment of open-angle glaucoma (increases outflow and decreases production of aqueous humor)
4 Symptomatic relief of minor eye irritations due to colds, hay fever, dust, wind, and so forth
5 Dilation of the pupil prior to intraocular surgery

Dosage

See Table 11-4

Fate

Onset of mydriatic effect is rapid and persists for several hours.

Common Side-Effects

Stinging and burning in the eyes, headache, and blurred vision

Significant Adverse Reactions

Conjunctival irritation; pigmentation of the eyelids, cornea or conjunctiva; maculopathy with a central scotoma; systemic absorption of significant amounts may lead to palpitations, tachycardia, hypertension, anxiety, sweating, insomnia, dizziness, and pallor.

Table 11-4. Ophthalmic Decongestants

Drug	Preparations	Usual Dosage Range	Remarks
Epinephrine (various manufacturers)	Drops—0.25%, 0.5%, 1.0%, and 2%	1 to 2 drops 0.1% to 2% individualized to condition	See general discussion of epinephrine
Hydroxyamphetamine (Paredrine)	Drops—1%	1 to 2 drops as needed	Pupillary dilation persists for several hours
Naphazoline (Ak-Con, Albalon, Allerest, Clear-Eyes, Degest-2, Naphcon, VasoClear, Vasocon)	Drops—0.012%, 0.02%, and 0.1%	1 to 2 drops every 3 hours to 4 hours	Primarily used as an ocular decongestant; 0.012% and 0.02% solutions available over the counter, 0.1% by prescription only; available in combination with pheniramine (Naphcon-A) and antazoline (Albalon-A, Vasocon-A)
Phenylephrine (Ak-Dilate, Ak-Nefrin, Efricel, Eye Cool, Isopto Frin, Mydfrin, Neo-Synephrine, Optigene, Prefrin, Tear Efrin)	Drops—0.08%, 0.12%, 0.15%, 2.5%, and 10%	10%—uveitis, open-angle glaucoma, prior to intraocular surgery; 2.5%—refraction, ophthalmic exams, prior to surgery; 0.02% to 0.15%—ocular decongestion, relief of minor eye irritations	Do not use 10% solution in children; prior instillation of a local anesthetic in the eye may alleviate much of the stinging and burning caused by phenylephrine; the 2.5% solution may be used as a diagnostic test for narrow-angle glaucoma; Available over-the-counter combined with zinc sulfate (e.g., Prefrin-Z, Zincfrin), or as prescription only combined with pyrilamine (Prefrin-A) or pheniramine (Vernacel)
Tetrahydrozoline (Clear and Bright, Murine 2, Opt-Ease, Soothe Eye, Tetracon, Tetrasine, Visine)	Drops—0.05%	1 to 2 drops 2 to 3 times/day	Primarily used to relieve minor symptoms of eye irritation; available over-the-counter

Contraindications

Narrow-angle glaucoma

Interactions

1 Effects may be potentiated by MAO inhibitors, tricyclic antidepressants, or other sympathomimetic drugs.
2 Mydriatic effects can be reduced by levodopa.
3 Arrhythmias with digitalis drugs and halogenated hydrocarbon anesthetics (e.g., cyclopropane, halothane) can occur in the presence of sympathomimetics, although the incidence with ophthalmic application is rare.

▶ **NURSING ALERTS**

▷ 1 Use cautiously in the elderly, and in the presence of hypertension, heart disease, diabetes, or cerebral arteriosclerosis.
▷ 2 Do not use strong solutions of phenylephrine in infants or small children, or in the presence of arteriosclerosis or hypertension.
▷ 3 Caution patients not to exceed recommended dosage, because systemic absorption can occur.
▷ 4 Be alert to the fact that some preparations may stain contact lenses.

▶ **NURSING CONSIDERATIONS**

▷ 1 Do not contaminate dropper tip, and do not use if solution is cloudy or discolored.
▷ 2 Caution older persons that rebound miosis (e.g., blurred vision) can occur within one day following termination of phenylephrine use. Re-instillation of drug may be less effective in eliciting mydriasis.
▷ 3 Note that the stronger concentrations (2.5%–10%) are used for diagnostic eye examinations and during ocular surgery, the intermediate strengths (0.5%–2%) are indicated for treatment of glaucoma, and the weaker concentrations (0.05%–0.1%) are employed for relief of minor eye irritations.

VI Bronchodilators

Sympathomimetic agents used as bronchodilators possess prominent *beta*-adrenergic activity that elicits relaxation of the smooth muscle of the bronchioles. Some drugs in this category (epinephrine, isoproterenol) activate all beta-adrenergic receptor sites, and their use is potentially associated with a disturbing range of side-effects, particularly involving the cardiovascular system. Newer adrenergic bronchodilators (e.g., albuterol, metaproterenol, terbutaline) exhibit a greater degree of selectivity with regard to the beta-2 receptors located on bronchiolar smooth muscle, and thus produce a lower incidence of cardiac side-effects, although *complete* separation of beta-1 and beta-2 activity has still not been realized. The relative popularity of the various adrenergic bronchodilators is determined by many factors, including the type and severity of the condition being treated, physician preference, patient acceptance, and cost.

Parenteral (*i.e.*, IM, SC) injections of epinephrine are usually very effective in relieving respiratory distress during an acute asthmatic attack. Some patients who respond poorly to epinephrine, however, may be successfully treated with IV infusion of aminophylline (see Chap. 55). A second major application of the various sympathomimetic bronchodilators is for the continual symptomatic management of chronic obstructive pulmonary diseases (COPD). Those agents (*e.g.,* epinephrine, ephedrine), possessing *alpha*-adrenergic action as well as beta activity, exert a secondary vasoconstrictive effect on bronchiolar blood vessels, and the resultant mucosal decongestant action also contributes to their effectiveness in treating chronic lung diseases.

Epinephrine and isoproterenol, two widely used bronchodilators, have been discussed in detail earlier in the chapter. The remaining adrenergic drugs used in the management of respiratory diseases are outlined below.

▶ albuterol

Proventil, Ventolin

Mechanism

Relatively selective activation of beta-2 receptor sites resulting in relaxation of smooth muscle of the bronchi, uterus, and vascular smooth muscle; less cardiac stimulation than isoproterenol or epinephrine

Uses

1 Relief of bronchospasm associated with reversible obstructive airway disease

Dosage

Inhalation—1 to 2 inhalations (90 mcg–180 mcg) every 4 hours to 6 hours
Oral—Initially, 2 mg to 4 mg 3 to 4 times/day; maximum daily dose is 32 mg.

Fate

Longer acting than isoproterenol; gradually absorbed from the bronchi and GI tract; elimination half-life is approximately 4 hours; excreted primarily in the urine, most within 24 hours, as both unchanged drug and metabolites

Common Side-Effects

Nervousness, mild tremor, and headache (especially with oral use)

Significant Adverse Reactions

Palpitations, tachycardia, increased blood pressure, muscle cramps, vertigo, nausea, insomnia, dizziness, irritability, angina-like pain, unusual taste, and drying of the oropharynx with inhalation (especially with oral use)

Interactions

1 Effects of albuterol may be potentiated by other sympathomimetics, MAO inhibitors, and tricyclic antidepressants and inhibited by beta-adrenergic blocking agents.

▶ NURSING ALERTS

▷ 1 Do not exceed recommended dosage, because excessive use can result in serious complications such as acute asthmatic crisis or cardiac arrest.
▷ 2 Use cautiously in patients with cardiovascular disorders, hyperthyroidism, and diabetes and in pregnant or nursing mothers.
▷ 3 Be alert for development of paradoxical bronchospasm and discontinue drug immediately.

▶ NURSING CONSIDERATIONS

▷ 1 Do not use more frequently than every 4 hours to 6 hours unless instructed, because cumulation toxicity can occur.
▷ 2 Instruct patients in the proper use of the inhaler.
▷ 3 Caution patients against concurrent use of other inhaled medications unless prescribed by the physician.

▶ ephedrine

(See also Table 11-3)

Mechanism

Direct activation of both alpha- and beta-adrenergic receptor sites, and indirect action through release of norepinephrine from presynaptic nerve terminals; effects include tachycardia, increased blood pressure and cardiac output, mydriasis, and relaxation of bronchiolar and GI smooth muscle; bronchodilation is less intense than that produced by epinephrine but is more prolonged; central stimulatory effects are more pronounced than with epinephrine.

Uses

1 Bronchodilation in milder forms of chronic pulmonary diseases (*e.g.,* bronchial asthma, bronchitis)
2 Relief of nasal mucosal congestion
3 Maintenance of blood pressure during spinal anesthesia and control of postural hypotension (injection only)
4 Treatment of enuresis (with atropine)
5 Treatment of narcolepsy
6 Support of ventricular rate in Adams–Stokes syndrome
7 Treatment of overdosage with CNS depressants
8 Adjunctive treatment of myasthenia gravis (with cholinesterase inhibitor)

Dosage

Adults: 25 mg to 50 mg PO, SC, IM, or slow IV every 3 hours to 4 hours as necessary (not to exceed 150 mg/24 hr)
Children: 2 mg/kg/day to 3 mg/kg/day in 4 to 6 divided doses

Fate

Readily absorbed orally or parenterally; crosses blood–brain barrier and exerts a central stimulating effect; duration of effect approximately 3 hours; excreted largely unchanged in the urine

Common Side-Effects

Similar to epinephrine; in addition, nervousness, anxiety, and insomnia due to central stimulatory properties

Significant Adverse Reactions

Tachycardia, confusion, delirium, tremors (usually observed with large doses); CNS and respiratory depression can occur with overdosage.

Contraindications

Narrow-angle glaucoma, patients receiving MAO inhibitors, severe hypertension, or coronary artery disease

Interactions

1 Pressor effects may be increased by ergot alkaloids, MAO inhibitors, furazolidone, and oxytocics.
2 Ephedrine may reduce the action of guanethidine.
3 Ephedrine may be less effective in the presence of methyldopa or reserpine.
4 Arrhythmias can occur if used in combination with halothane and related anesthetics or digitalis drugs.

▶ **NURSING ALERTS**

▷ 1 Use cautiously in patients with chronic heart disease, hypertension, hyperthyroidism, and diabetes.
▷ 2 Caution patients to follow recommended dosage carefully because central stimulatory effects can lead to abuse.
▷ 3 Check blood pressure repeatedly when drug is used IV until patient is stabilized.
▷ 4 Do not use prolonged-acting forms or high doses in the elderly because they are more prone to develop hallucinations, convulsions, and CNS depression.

▶ **NURSING CONSIDERATIONS**

See Epinephrine, in addition:

▷ 1 Advise older patient to immediately report difficulty in urinating, and alert physician.
▷ 2 Tolerance can occur with prolonged use. Drug-free periods of several days may be needed to restore effectiveness.
▷ 3 If insomnia is a problem, do not administer doses at night if possible, and avoid long-acting preparations.

▶ **ethylnorepinephrine**

Bronkephrine

Mechanism

Direct activation of alpha- (weak) and beta-adrenergic receptor sites; less of an effect on blood pressure than epinephrine

Uses

1 Relief of acute bronchospasm in bronchial asthma where other agents are ineffective, or in children and diabetics

Dosage

1 mg to 2 mg (0.5 ml–1.0 ml) SC or IM
Children—0.1 ml to 0.5 ml depending on weight
Similar to isoproterenol in most respects. See isoproterenol monograph for additional information.

▶ **isoetharine**

Arm-a-Med, Beta-2, Bronkometer, Bronkosol, Dey-Lute Isoetharine, Dispos-A-Med Isoetharine

Mechanism

Preferential activation of beta-2 adrenergic sites on bronchi and arteriolar smooth muscle; minimal activity at beta-1 sites on the heart, therefore fewer side-effects than epinephrine or isoproterenol; may also inhibit histamine release

Uses

1 Acute relief of bronchial asthma and other bronchospastic states

Dosage

Solution (Beta-2, Bronkosol, Dispos-A-Med):
Undiluted—3 to 7 inhalations of 1% solution in hand nebulizer
Dilution—¼ to 1 ml of 1:3 dilution of 0.5% or 1.0% solution in saline or other diluent by oxygen aerosolization
Metered dose nebulizer (Bronkometer):
1 to 2 inhalations every 4 hours (340 mcg/metered dose)

Fate

Rapid onset and relatively long duration

Common Side-Effects

Minimal with infrequent use

Significant Adverse Reactions

(Too frequent use or excessive dosage) Tachycardia, insomnia, tremor, dizziness, palpitations, and headache

Contraindications

In combination with other sympathomimetic amines

Interactions

1 Effects can be enhanced by other adrenergic drugs

▶ **NURSING ALERTS**

▷ 1 Repeated use may lead to development of increased airway resistance. If this occurs, discontinue drug immediately because severe side-effects can develop.
▷ 2 Use with caution in presence of coronary disease, hypertension, or hyperthyroidism, and in the elderly.
▷ 3 If other sympathomimetic agents are indicated, alternate usage with isoetharine. Do not use together, because excessive tachycardia can occur.

▷ 4 Do not use more often than every 4 hours, except in severe cases because duration of action is prolonged and cumulative toxicity can result.

▶ metaproterenol
Alupent, Metaprel

Mechanism
Direct activation of beta-adrenergic receptor sites, resulting in relaxation of bronchiolar smooth muscle; exerts a more selective effect on the *beta-2* sites in the bronchioles than isoproterenol, thus is associated with a lower incidence of cardiovascular side-effects.

Uses
1 Symptomatic treatment of bronchial asthma and other bronchospastic conditions

Dosage
Oral—Adults: 20 mg orally every 6 hours to 8 hours; Children: 10 mg to 20 mg every 6 hours to 8 hours depending on weight (not recommended for children under 6 yr)

Inhalation—2 to 3 sprays of metered dose inhaler every 3 hours to 4 hours *or* 10 inhalations of 5% soluton *via* hand nebulizer.

Fate
Oral absorption is good, but a portion of the dose is quickly metabolized in the liver. Onset of action orally is about 15 minutes, and duration ranges from 2 hours to 5 hours. Onset following inhalation is about 1 minute to 2 minutes, and effect may persist up to 4 hours. Excreted in the urine in conjugated form.

Significant Adverse Reactions
Similar in most respects to isoproterenol but with a lower incidence of cardiovascular complications.

Contraindications
Arrhythmias, severe hypertension, or coronary artery disease

Interactions
1 Effects may be potentiated by other sympathomimetic agents

▶ NURSING ALERTS
▷ 1 Warn patient to adhere to prescribed dosage because excessive use can lead to severe complications, including cardiac arrest.
▷ 2 Counsel user to promptly report any diminished response to the normal dose because long-term use can result in tolerance.

▶ NURSING CONSIDERATIONS
▷ 1 Instruct patient as to proper procedure for administering aerosol dose. Allow 2 minutes between inhalations, and do not exceed 12 inhalations per day.
▷ 2 Prolonged use may result in shorter duration of action (1 hr–2 hr). Alert patients to this possibility, and instruct them to report to physician if usual dose does not provide relief for a sufficient period of time.
▷ 3 Inform user that a bad taste can occur with oral inhalation and will gradually disappear with repeated usage.

▶ terbutaline
Brethine, Bricanyl

Mechanism
Relatively selective activation of beta-2 receptor sites on bronchiolar smooth muscle, resulting in bronchodilation. Minimal effects on cardiac function at recommended doses.

Uses
1 Symptomatic treatment of bronchial asthma, bronchitis, and emphysema

Dosage
Parenteral—0.25 mg SC (repeat in 15 min–30 min, if needed)
Oral—Adults: 2.5 mg to 5 mg 3 times/day (maximum dose 15 mg/day); Children over 12: 2.5 mg 3 times/day; maximum dose 7.5 mg/day

Fate
Slowly absorbed orally and parenterally. Onset of action is 15 minutes to 30 minutes; duration is 4 hours to 8 hours orally and 2 hours to 4 hours SC. Slowly metabolized in the liver and excreted largely in the urine and partly in the feces.

Common Side-Effects
Minimal at small doses (2.5 mg); larger doses (5 mg) elicit muscle tremor in about one-third of patients.

Significant Adverse Reactions
(Usually only at high doses) Tachycardia, palpitations, dizziness, anxiety, and headache

Contraindications
See metaproterenol

Interactions
1 Effects may be enhanced by other sympathomimetics

▶ NURSING ALERTS
▷ 1 Use cautiously in the presence of diabetes, hypertension, or severe cardiovascular disease.
▷ 2 Be aware of the possibility of cardiovascular toxicity when drug is used parenterally. Specificity for beta-2 sites is observed primarily following oral dosage.

▶ **NURSING CONSIDERATIONS**
▷ 1 Do not use in children under 12 years of age.
▷ 2 Do not administer more than two SC injections 15 minutes to 30 minutes apart. If patient does not respond to second injection, other measures should be attempted.

VII Smooth Muscle Relaxants

Several adrenergic drugs have the ability to relax smooth muscle and this action has led to their use in the treatment of peripheral vascular insufficiency and premature labor.

Nylidrin and isoxsuprine are two orally effective sympathomimetics that exhibit a beta-adrenergic receptor agonistic action. Activation of beta-2 receptor sites in skeletal muscle vasculature can lead to vasodilation of normal vessels. However, the vasodilator effects of nylidrin and isoxsuprine on muscle blood flow are *not* prevented by beta-blockers. Thus, these drugs also probably exert a direct relaxant effect on vascular smooth muscle in addition to their beta-agonistic action. Despite the fact that blood flow in normal resting skeletal muscle can be increased by these drugs, there is *no* conclusive evidence that they have a beneficial effect in chronic occlusive vascular conditions such as arteriosclerosis or thromboangiitis obliterans. Because skeletal muscle and cerebral vascular beds are probably reflexly dilated by the ischemia resulting from a vascular occlusion, peripheral vasodilator drugs primarily increase blood supply to nondilated, nonischemic areas that are not in critical need of improved perfusion. Further compromising their efficacy is the fall in blood pressure that frequently accompanies their administration. Thus, their hypotensive effect may actually *reduce* cerebral blood flow and perfusion of vital organs. Therefore, use of nylidrin and isoxsuprine for treating peripheral and cerebral vascular insufficiency should be discouraged.

Isoxsuprine has also been used to delay premature labor, because it also exerts a uterine smooth muscle relaxant effect. Its effects are nonselective, however, and side-effects due to beta-receptor activation elsewhere in the body are frequent. Use of isoxsuprine as a uterine relaxant has been largely supplanted by ritodrine, another beta-agonist that exerts a somewhat more selective effect on beta-2 receptors in the uterus. These three sympathomimetic smooth muscle relaxants are discussed below.

▶ **isoxsuprine**
Vasodilan, Vasoprine

Mechanism
Activation of beta-adrenergic receptor sites on vascular smooth muscle, resulting in diminished vascular resistance and increased resting blood flow in skeletal muscles; also exerts a direct relaxant effect on vascular smooth muscle; exhibits some alpha-adrenergic blocking action, and high doses may inhibit platelet aggregation and decrease blood viscosity; elicits cardiac stimulation and uterine relaxation

Uses
(Clinical effectiveness has not been conclusively demonstrated.)
1 Symptomatic treatment of peripheral vascular insufficiency (*e.g.,* Raynaud's disease, thromboangiitis obliterans)
2 Improve circulatory function in cerebral vascular insufficiency
3 Treatment of premature labor and threatened abortion (experimental use only)

Dosage
Oral—10 mg to 20 mg 3 to 4 times/day
IM—5 mg to 10 mg 2 to 3 times/day (single dose not to exceed 10 mg)

Fate
Peak effects occur in about 1 hour and persist 2 hours to 3 hours; largely excreted in the urine

Common Side-Effects
Lightheadedness, lethargy, and flushing

Significant Adverse Reactions
Hypotension, palpitations, tachycardia (especially IM), dizziness, nausea, anxiety, abdominal distress, vomiting, and rash

Contraindications
Postpartum, arterial bleeding; IM use is contraindicated in hypotension and tachycardia.

Interactions
1 Effects may be antagonized by other sympathomimetic drugs (particularly those possessing significant alpha activity).

▶ **NURSING ALERTS**
▷ 1 Do not give IM in presence of hypotension or tachycardia.
▷ 2 Warn patient to discontinue drug at first sign of skin rash.
▷ 3 Individuals with extensive circulatory impairment may not respond to the drug. Observe patients carefully for signs of deteriorating condition (*e.g.,* numbness, coldness, paresthesias), and advise physician.
▷ 4 Use cautiously in patients with coronary artery insufficiency, thyrotoxicosis, paroxysmal tachycardia, and following an acute myocardial infarction.

▶ **NURSING CONSIDERATIONS**
▷ 1 Counsel patients with vascular insufficiency on the various adjunctive measures that can be utilized to alleviate their condition (*e.g.,* proper exercises, use of support hose and proper footwear, control of weight, cessation of smoking).

▷ 2 Monitor blood pressure and pulse of patient in standing and prone positions at frequent intervals during treatment, especially with IM use.

▷ 3 Inform patient that beneficial effects may take several weeks to appear and are usually indicated by cessation of numbness, coldness, or tingling in the extremities.

▷ 4 When drug is used for relief of premature labor (experimental use only) carefully monitor pattern of contractions, and adjust dose and rate of administration accordingly.

▶ nylidrin
Arlidin

Mechanism
Activation of vascular beta receptors, relaxing arteriolar smooth muscle and decreasing circulatory resistance; also exerts a direct relaxant effect on vascular smooth muscle; cardiac output is slightly increased.

Uses
(Clinical effectiveness has not been conclusively demonstrated.)

1 Symptomatic relief of peripheral vasospastic disorders (*e.g.,* diabetic vascular disease, acrocyanosis, Raynaud's disease, night leg cramps, ischemic ulcer, frostbite, thrombophlebitis)

2 Relief of circulatory disturbances of the inner ear (*e.g.,* cochlear cell, macular or ampullar ischemia, labyrinthine artery spasm)

Dosage
Orally—3 mg to 12 mg 3 to 4 times/day

Fate
Well absorbed orally; maximum effects appear within 30 minutes to 45 minutes and persist for 2 hours; slowly excreted in the urine

Common Side-Effects
Palpitations, nervousness, and weakness

Significant Adverse Reactions
Dizziness, vomiting, tremors, and hypotension

Contraindications
Acute myocardial infarction, paroxysmal tachycardia, severe angina, thyrotoxicosis, and uncompensated heart failure

Interactions
1 Effects can be antagonized by other sympathomimetic agents having pressor effects.

▶ NURSING ALERTS
▷ 1 Use cautiously in patients with hypertension, cardiac disorders, and peptic ulcers.

▷ 2 Urge patient to report development of palpitations. If they do not subside during continued therapy, reduce dose.

▶ NURSING CONSIDERATIONS
▷ 1 Be supportive of patient at beginning of therapy, and advise that beneficial effects may take several weeks to become manifest.

▷ 2 Provide appropriate adjunctive treatment (*e.g.,* cleansing of wounds, hygienic care of extremities) and advise patient of steps that may aid in improvement of condition (*e.g.,* exercise, cessation of smoking, proper footwear).

▶ ritodrine
Yutopar

Ritodrine is a fairly selective beta-2 adrenergic receptor agonist that can inhibit uterine contractions, and therefore is used in the management of premature labor. It is administered initially by IV infusion to arrest contractions, then orally for as long as necessary to prolong pregnancy to the desired extent. Its overall toxicity is somewhat lower than other agents employed in premature labor (alcohol, magnesium sulfate, isoxsuprine).

Mechanism
Activates beta-2 receptor sites on uterine smooth muscle, thus reducing the contractile response; also affects beta-1 receptors in higher amounts, resulting in tachycardia and blood pressure changes.

Uses
1 Management of preterm labor in suitable patients, where the gestation is greater than 20 weeks.

Dosage
Initially, 0.1 mg/min by IV infusion. May be increased by 50 mcg/min every 10 minutes to a maximum of 350 mcg/minute. Continue infusion for 12 hours after labor has ceased. Administer an oral dose of 10 mg 30 minutes before terminating infusion, then 10 mg every 2 hours for 24 hours, then 10 mg to 20 mg every 4 hours to 6 hours for as long as necessary. Maximum oral dose is 120 mg/day.

Fate
Oral bioavailability is approximately 30% of IV dose. Maximum serum levels following oral ingestion occur in 30 minutes to 60 minutes; effective half-life is 1½ hours to 2 hours; metabolized in the liver and excreted primarily in the urine, 90% within 24 hours; crosses placental barrier.

Common Side-Effects
(Especially with IV infusion) Alterations in maternal and fetal heart rates and blood pressure, transient elevations in blood glucose and insulin, hypokalemia, palpitations, nausea, tremors, headache, and erythema

Significant Adverse Reactions

(Especially with IV infusion) Vomiting, anxiety, nervousness, chest pain, arrhythmias, dyspnea, sweating, chills, weakness, diarrhea, bloating, rash, anaphylactic shock, lactic acidosis, glycosuria

Contraindications

Before the 20th week of pregnancy, any condition of mother or fetus in which continuation of pregnancy is dangerous (*e.g.,* antepartum hemorrhage, fetal death, eclampsia, cardiac disease, pulmonary hypertension), cardiac arrhythmias, severe bronchial asthma, and pheochromocytoma

Interactions

1 Combined administration of ritodrine and corticosteroids may lead to pulmonary edema.
2 Effects of other adrenergic amines may be potentiated by ritodrine.
3 Beta-blockers will reduce the effectiveness of ritodrine.
4 Ritodrine may increase the hypokalemia observed with various diuretics.

▶ NURSING ALERTS

▷ 1 Closely monitor maternal pulse rate and blood pressure as well as fetal heart rate, and observe for indications of maternal pulmonary edema (chest pain, dyspnea, sweating).
▷ 2 Do not administer earlier than the 20th week of gestation because many fetuses are abnormal when labor begins before this time.
▷ 3 Use with caution in patients with hypertension, diabetes, and cardiac impairment.

▶ NURSING CONSIDERATIONS

▷ 1 Do not administer if solution is discolored or cloudy or contains a precipitate.
▷ 2 Be prepared to initiate IV infusion if labor recurs during oral drug therapy.
▷ 3 Note that recommended dilution is 150 mg ritodrine (3 ampuls) in 500 ml either Sodium Chloride, 5%

Dextrose, 10% Dextran 40 in Sodium Chloride, or 10% Invert Sugar, yielding a final concentration of 0.3 mg ritodrine/ml infusion solution.
▷ 4 Monitor amount and rate of infusion to avoid circulatory overload.

VIII CNS Stimulants and Anorexiants

The principal adrenergic drugs used for their central stimulatory effects are the amphetamine derivatives and ephedrine. The major indications for these compounds are control of obesity, relief of depression, and treatment of the minimal brain dysfunction syndrome in children. Due to their profound central excitatory action, they are an often abused class of drugs. These compounds are discussed in Chapter 27 (CNS Stimulants), and aspects of their abuse potential will be reviewed in Chapter 81 (Drugs of Abuse—A Review).

A number of products containing phenylpropanolamine, a sympathomimetic decongestant reviewed earlier in this chapter, are promoted as nonprescription diet aids as an adjunct to caloric restriction. Many of the preparations contain caffeine as well. Their efficacy for this particular indication is subject to serious doubt by many professionals, and their use should be strictly controlled. Patients with cardiovascular disease, hypertension, diabetes, hyperthyroidism, glaucoma, or renal impairment should not use these products, and combined use of these drugs with other sympathomimetics, antihypertensives, or antidepressants should be avoided. Their administration must be discontinued at once should palpitations, dizziness, or rapid pulse occur. Recommended doses are 25 mg phenylpropanolamine 3 times a day or 50 mg to 75 mg of the long-acting preparations once daily. Continuous use for longer than three months is not recommended.

Summary. Adrenergic Drugs

Drug	Preparations	Usual Dosage Range
I. Catecholamines		
Epinephrine (various manufacturers)	Solution—1:1000, 1:10,000 Suspension—1:200, 1:400 Inhalation—1%, 2.25% Aerosol—0.16 mg/dose, 0.2 mg/dose Nasal drops—0.1% Ophthalmic drops—0.25%, 0.5%, 1%, and 2%	Parenteral: Cardiac arrest—5 ml to 10 ml 1:10,000 IV every 5 minutes as required Intracardiac—3 ml to 5 ml 1:10,000 Intraspinal—0.2 ml to 0.4 ml 1:1000 added to anesthetic solution Bronchospasm—0.2 ml to 1 ml 1:1000 SC or IM *or* 0.05 ml to 0.6 ml 1:400 SC or IM *or* 0.1 ml to 0.3 ml 1:200 SC (Children—0.01 mg/kg SC) With local anesthetic—1:20,000 to 1:100,000 Inhalation—1:100 solution (1 min to 2 min between doses) Nasal—1 to 2 drops 0.1% 4 times/day Ophthalmic—1 to 2 drops 0.25% to 2%

(continued)

Summary. Adrenergic Drugs *(continued)*

Drug	Preparations	Usual Dosage Range
Dipivefrin (Propine) (An epinephrine prodrug)	Ophthalmic drops 0.1%	1 drop every 12 hours
Norepinephrine (Levophed)	Injection—1 mg/ml	8 mcg/min to 12 mcg/min IV infusion (2 ml/min–3 ml/min) of a 4 mcg/ml dilution. Maintenance—2 to 4 mcg/min
Dopamine (Dopastat, Intropin)	Injection (for dilution)—40 mg/ml, 80 mg/ml, and 160 mg/ml Infusion solution—80 mg/100 ml, and 160 mg/100 ml	Initially 2 mcg/kg/min to 5 mcg/kg/min IV infusion of diluted solution; increase by 5 mcg/kg/min to 10 mcg/kg/min to maximum of 50 mcg/kg/min

II. Synthetic Catecholamines

Drug	Preparations	Usual Dosage Range
Isoproterenol (various manufacturers)	Injection—1:5000 (0.2 mg/ml) Sublingual tablets—10 mg, 15 mg Inhalation solution—1:100, 1:200, and 1:400 Aerosol—0.2%, 0.25% Powder—10 mg, 25 mg per cartridge	Parenteral: Bronchospasm—0.01 mg to 0.02 mg 1:50,000 solution IV injection Shock—0.25 ml/min to 2.5 ml/min 1:500,000 dilution IV infusion Cardiac arrest—1 ml to 3 ml 1:50,000 IV injection; 1.25 ml/min 1:250,000 IV infusion; 1 ml 1:5000 IM, SC; 0.1 ml 1:5000 intracardiac injection Sublingual: 10 mg to 20 mg 3 to 4 times/day (children 5 mg to 10 mg 3 to 4 times/day) Inhalation: 1 to 2 inhalations 4 to 6 times/day (dose range 45 mcg to 250 mcg)
Dobutamine (Dobutrex)	Injection—250 mg/20 ml	IV infusion—2.5 mcg/kg/min to 10 mcg/kg/min of a 250 mcg/ml to 1000 mcg/ml solution in Sterile Water or 5% Dextrose; maximum 40 mcg/kg/min

III. Vasopressors

Drug	Preparations	Usual Dosage Range
Mephentermine (Wyamine)	Injection—15 mg/ml, 30 mg/ml	IM, IV—30 mg to 45 mg single dose; 30 mg supplements as needed IV infusion—1 mg/min of a 0.1% solution in 5% dextrose
Metaraminol (Aramine)	Injection—10 mg/ml	IM, SC—2 mg to 10 mg IV injection—0.5 mg to 5 mg IV infusion—15–100 mg/500 ml 5% Dextrose (Pediatric—SC, IM: 0.1 mg/kg; IV: 0.01 mg/kg; IV infusion: 0.4 mg/kg)
Methoxamine (Vasoxyl)	Injection—20 mg/ml	IV—3 mg to 5 mg (hypotension) IV—10 mg (tachycardia) IM—10 mg to 20 mg prior to anesthesia or 5 mg to 15 mg for treatment of hypotension
Phenylephrine (Neo-Synephrine)	Injection—1% (See also Tables 11-3 and 11-4)	SC, IM—2 mg to 5 mg IV injection—0.1 mg to 0.5 mg IV infusion—100 to 200 drops/min of a 1:50,000 solution until stabilized, then 40 drops/min to 60 drops/min (Pediatric—SC, IM:0.1 mg/kg)

IV. Nasal Decongestants

See Table 11-3

V. Ophthalmic Decongestants

See Table 11-4

Summary. Adrenergic Drugs *(continued)*

Drug	Preparations	Usual Dosage Range
VI. Bronchodilators		
Albuterol (Proventil, Ventolin)	Inhaler—90 mcg/metered dose Tablets—2 mg, 4 mg	Inhalation—1 to 2 inhalations every 4 hours to 6 hours Oral—2 mg to 4 mg 3 to 4 times/day; maximum 32 mg/day
Ephedrine	Capsules—25 mg, 50 mg Syrup—11, 20 mg/5 ml Injection—25, 50 mg/ml (See also Table 11-3)	Oral and Parenteral—25 mg to 50 mg every 3 hours to 4 hours as necessary to a maximum 150 mg/24 hr (Children—6 yr–12 yr; 6.25 mg to 12.5 mg every 4 hr to 6 hr; 2 yr–6 yr; 0.3 mg/kg–0.5 mg/kg every 4 hr to 6 hr)
Ethylnorepinephrine (Bronkephrine)	Injection 2 mg/ml	SC, IM—1 mg to 2 mg (0.5 ml to 1.0 ml) (Children—0.1 ml to 0.5 ml)
Isoetharine (Arm-a-Med, Beta-2, Bronkometer, Bronkosol, Dey-Lute Isoetharine, Dispos-a-Med Isoetharine)	Solution—0.06%, 0.08%, 0.1%, 0.125%, 0.17%, 0.2%, 0.25%, 0.5%, 1% Metered-dose nebulizer—0.61% (delivers 340 mcg/metered dose)	Solution—¼ ml to 1 ml of a 1:3 dilution of 0.5% or 1% solution with saline by aerosolization or 3 to 7 inhalations of undiluted 1% solution in nebulizer. Metered dose—1 to 2 inhalations every 4 hours
Metaproterenol (Alupent, Metaprel)	Tablets—10 mg, 20 mg Syrup—10 mg/5 ml Inhaler—225 mg (0.65 mg/dose) Solution—5%, 0.6% per unit dose vial	Oral—20 mg every 6 hours to 8 hours (Children over 6—10 mg to 20 mg every 6 hr to 8 hr) Solution—10 inhalations of 5% solution in a hand nebulizer Inhalation—2 to 3 sprays every 3 hours to 4 hours to a maximum of 12/day
Terbutaline (Brethine, Bricanyl)	Tablets—2.5 mg, 5 mg Injection—1 mg/ml	Adults: Oral—2.5 mg to 5 mg 3 times/day SC—0.25 mg; repeat in 15 minutes to 30 minutes if needed (Children over 12—2.5 mg 3 times/day)
VII. Smooth Muscle Relaxants		
Isoxsuprine (Vasodilan, Vasoprine)	Tablets—10 mg, 20 mg Injection—5 mg/ml	Oral—10 mg to 20 mg 3 to 4 times/day IM—5 mg to 10 mg 2 to 3 times/day (maximum single IM dose is 10 mg)
Nylidrin (Arlidin)	Tablets—6 mg, 12 mg	Oral—3 mg to 12 mg 3 to 4 times/day
Ritodrine (Yutopar)	Tablets—10 mg Injection—10 mg/ml	Initially, 0.1 mg/min IV infusion; increase by 50 mcg/min every 10 min to maximum of 350 mcg/min; continue for 12 hr after labor has ceased; begin oral dose (10 mg) 30 min before terminating infusion, then 10 mg every 2 hr for 24 hr, then 10 mg to 20 mg every 4 hr to 6 hr for as long as needed
VIII. CNS Stimulants and Anorexiants		
Amphetamines	See Chapter 27	
Anorexiants	See Chapter 27	
Phenylpropanolamine (Dexatrim, Dietac and various other manufacturers)	Tablets—25 mg, 37.5 mg Capsules—25 mg, 37.5 mg Drops—25 mg/dose Timed-release capsules—75 mg, 150 mg Timed-release tablets—75 mg	25 mg 3 times/day or 50 mg to 75 mg timed-release once daily

Adrenergic Blocking Drugs

12

Several types of pharmacologic agents are capable of interfering with the functioning of the sympathetic nervous system as well as the actions of exogenous adrenergic drugs. Certain compounds can either deplete the catecholamine stores in adrenergic nerve endings or retard release of the catecholamine neurotransmitters (*e.g.*, norepinephrine) from the nerve ending. Many of these agents serve primarily as antihypertensive drugs and are considered in Chapter 31. Other anti-adrenergic agents antagonize the actions of sympathomimetic amines at adrenergic receptor sites in various body tissues. These drugs are termed *adrenergic receptor blockers* and are effective antagonists of either exogenously administered adrenergic compounds or endogenous catecholamines released from sympathetic nerve endings.

Reflecting the generally accepted classification of adrenergic receptor sites into *alpha* and *beta* types, the adrenergic receptor blockers are likewise separated into alpha-adrenergic and beta-adrenergic blocking agents, and the delineation is essentially complete for the currently available drugs (*i.e.*, alpha blockers do not block beta sites and *vice versa*). However, adrenergic blocking drugs have been developed that display a greater selectivity for alpha and beta receptor subtypes. Thus, while several alpha blockers are nonselective, that is, block both alpha-1 and alpha-2 receptors, some (*e.g.*, phenoxybenzamine, prazosin) are selective for the alpha-1 site. Similarly, early beta-blockers (*e.g.*, propranolol) were nonselective in their blocking action, but more recent drugs (*e.g.*, metoprolol, atenolol) are relatively selective for the beta-1 receptor. Achieving greater specificity of blockade has to some extent reduced undesirable side-effects of adrenergic receptor blockade.

Alpha-Adrenergic Blocking Agents

Compounds capable of blocking the actions of various agonists at the alpha-adrenergic receptor sites are termed *alpha-blockers* (see Table 11-2). Postsynaptic (*i.e.*, alpha-1 blocking) agents act primarily on alpha sites located on vascular smooth muscle to antagonize the pressor (vasoconstrictive) effects of epinephrine and norepinephrine. In addition, the shorter-acting drugs (see below) possess a direct relaxant effect on vascular smooth muscle that contributes to the peripheral vasodilation seen with these drugs, and a cardiac stimulant action that may result in tachycardia.

Selective alpha-2 blockers (*e.g.*, yohimbine) have become valuable laboratory tools, but their clinical significance remains to be established, and, to date, they have not become commercially available.

Among the clinically useful drugs with alpha-adrenergic blocking activity are the following:

1 *Prolonged-acting, noncompetitive antagonist (e.g., phenoxybenzamine)*—forms a stable bond between the drug and alpha receptor site; blockade can persist for days or even weeks; blocking action is limited to alpha-1 sites.

2 *Short-acting, competitive antagonists (e.g., phentol-*

amine, tolazoline)—form a reversible, competitive blockade at alpha site that persists for only a few hours; can be overcome by larger amounts of agonist (*e.g.*, norepinephrine); exerts both a presynaptic (alpha-2) and postsynaptic (alpha-1) blocking action.

3 *Ergot alkaloids* (*e.g.*, ergotamine)—possess some alpha-blocking action, but primarily exert a direct spasmogenic action on vascular smooth muscle, resulting in vasoconstriction. Used primarily for relief of vascular headaches; see Chapter 14.

In addition, prazosin is an alpha-1 selective antagonist used in the control of hypertension, and is considered in Chapter 31.

▶ phenoxybenzamine
Dibenzyline

Mechanism
Long-acting, essentially noncompetitive alpha-adrenergic blockade exerted at postsynaptic alpha-1 sites; forms stable covalent bond with receptor site, possibly inducing structural alterations; increases blood flow to skin, mucosa, and viscera; lowers blood pressure but does not increase cardiac output or perfusion of liver or kidney

Uses
1 Control hypertension and sweating associated with pheochromocytoma
2 Improve circulation in vasospastic peripheral vascular diseases (*e.g.*, Raynaud's, acrocyanosis, gangrene, frostbite) (effectiveness not conclusively determined)

Dosage
Individualized to obtain symptomatic relief with minimal side effects

Initially—10 mg orally daily. Increase by 10 mg every 4 days. Usual range 20 mg to 60 mg daily (may require several weeks to obtain optimal effect)

Fate
Oral absorption is erratic (20%–30% absorbed in active form); peak effects occur in 4 hours to 6 hours; may accumulate in adipose tissue at high doses; excreted largely through the kidney and bile, mostly within 24 hours

Common Side-Effects
Lightheadedness, nasal congestion, dryness of the mouth, flushing, tachycardia, miosis, and GI irritation (if given on empty stomach)

Significant Adverse Reactions
Dizziness, orthostatic hypotension, weakness, failure of ejaculation; overdosage can cause vomiting, CNS stimulation, and shock.

Contraindications
Congestive heart failure or other conditions when a drop in blood pressure might be dangerous (*e.g.*, angina, cerebral vascular insufficiency)

Interactions
1 May increase blood pressure lowering effects of antihypertensive agents
2 May enhance the hypotensive and cardiac stimulant effects of epinephrine

▶ NURSING ALERTS

▷ 1 Warn patient to rise from supine position slowly and to sit upright for a few moments before standing, due to danger of orthostatic hypotension. Advise patient to lie down immediately should weakness or faintness appear.
▷ 2 If severe hypotension occurs, use norepinephrine (levarterenol) infusion, *not* epinephrine, because a further drop in blood pressure can occur due to unmasking of the beta effect. Keep patient flat for 24 hours and apply leg bandages as necessary.
▷ 3 Do not increase dose sooner than 4 days following previous increase. Monitor blood pressure, heart rate and rhythm in both erect and recumbent positions during period of dosage adjustment and for at least 4 days thereafter.
▷ 4 Use with caution in presence of cerebral, coronary, or renal insufficiency.
▷ 5 Do not use in diseases involving the larger blood vessels; direct-acting vasodilators (*e.g.*, papaverine) are preferred.

▶ NURSING CONSIDERATIONS
▷ 1 Advise patient that palpitations, tachycardia, and orthostatic hypotension will disappear with continued therapy.
▷ 2 Tell patient that onset of beneficial effects may take several weeks and advise him to follow prescribed regimen closely to obtain maximal benefit.
▷ 3 Suggest taking drug with meals to minimize GI irritation.
▷ 4 Be alert to the possibility that symptoms of respiratory infections may be aggravated by the drug and that appropriate therapy must be provided.
▷ 5 Observe users closely for objective signs of clinical improvement (*e.g.*, increased skin color and temperature, less sensitivity to cold). In pheochromocytoma, watch for decreases in blood pressure and pulse rate as indications of effectiveness.

▶ phentolamine
Regitine

Mechanism
Reversible, competitive antagonism of catecholamines at presynaptic and postsynaptic alpha receptor sites and direct relaxant action on vascular smooth muscle; decreases pe-

ripheral vascular resistance and pulmonary pressure; slightly increases heart rate, cardiac output, GI motility (parasympathomimetic action), and secretion of pepsin and hydrochloric acid (histamine-like action).

Uses
Oral
1 Control of hypertension in patients with pheochromocytoma during stress periods, and prior to or during surgical excision of tumor

Parenteral
1 Prevent tissue necrosis and sloughing resulting from extravasation of norepinephrine
2 Diagnosis of pheochromocytoma (measurement of urinary catecholamines is the preferred diagnosis)
3 Treatment of hypertensive crises or rebound hypertension following withdrawal of antihypertensive drugs (investigational use only)

Dosage
Oral
Adults: 50 mg 4 to 6 times/day
Children: 25 mg 4 to 6 times/day

Parenteral
Hypertension—IV, IM—5 mg (adults), 1 mg (children)
Prevent necrosis—10 mg added to each liter IV infusion
Treat necrosis—5 mg to 10 mg in 10 ml saline infiltrated into area

Fate
Poorly absorbed orally; onset is rapid following IV or IM use; effects persist for 15 minutes with IV use and several hours following IM injection; excreted largely as metabolites

Common Side-Effects
Flushing, nasal congestion, and GI distress

Significant Adverse Reactions
(Usually following parenteral use) Tachycardia, hypotension, arrhythmias, anginal pain, myocardial infarction, shock, and cerebrovascular occlusion

Contraindications
Recent myocardial infarction, coronary insufficiency, and angina.

Interactions
See phenoxybenzamine

▶ NURSING ALERTS
▷ 1 Keep patient supine while giving drug IV, and monitor blood pressure and pulse frequently until stabilized.
▷ 2 Do not use epinephrine to treat hypotension resulting from overdosage because unmasking of beta effect may increase drop in blood pressure.
▷ 3 Use phentolamine as a diagnostic aid in pheochromocytoma only to confirm results of other tests. It is

not the procedure of choice and should be used only when relative risks have been considered.
▷ 4 Advise patient to rise slowly from bed and remain in a sitting position several minutes before standing, to avoid orthostatic hypotensive reactions.
▷ 5 Use cautiously in patients with peptic ulcer, gastritis, and coronary artery disease, or in patients using digitalis drugs.

▶ NURSING CONSIDERATIONS
▷ 1 Minimize GI irritation by giving drug with either meals or milk.
▷ 2 Carefully observe patients receiving parenteral therapy for any changes in blood pressure or heart rate. Treat overdosage vigorously and promptly.

▶ tolazoline
Priscoline

Mechanism
Reversible nonselective blockade of alpha-adrenergic receptor sites and direct relaxant effect on vascular smooth muscle; also exhibits significant beta-adrenergic activity (increased cardiac rate, force, and output), cholinergic activity (increased GI motility), and histaminergic activity (increased gastric secretions)

Uses
1 Improve blood flow in various peripheral vascular disorders associated with vasospastic conditions (effectiveness not conclusively demonstrated)
2 Dilate pulmonary vessels in infants with acutely increased pulmonary vascular resistance (investigational use only)

Dosage
Parenteral—IM, IV, SC—10 mg to 50 mg 4 times/day
Intra-arterial—25 mg initially, followed by 50 mg to 75 mg/dose 1 to 2 times a day (given only by trained personnel)

Fate
Slowly absorbed with maximal effects within 30 minutes to 60 minutes IM or SC; duration of action 3 hours to 4 hours; excreted largely unchanged by the kidney

Common Side-Effects
Flushing, tingling or loss of sensation in extremities, nausea, and tachycardia

Significant Adverse Reactions
Arrhythmias, anginal pain, orthostatic hypotension, ulcerlike pain, vomiting, epigastric distress, duodenal perforation, apprehension, rash, and edema; Intra-arterial administration may produce burning sensation at injection site, vertigo, palpitations, nervousness, and paradoxical impairment of blood flow with possible gangrene.

Table 12-1. Pharmacologic and Pharmacokinetic Properties of Beta-Blockers

Drug	Receptor Activity	Oral Absorption	Protein Binding	Elimination Half-Life	Membrane-Stabilizing Activity	Intrinsic Sympathomimetic Activity	Interpatient Variations in Plasma Levels
Atenolol (Tenormin)	B₁	50%	0%–10%	6 hr–9 hr	0	0	4-fold
Metoprolol (Lopressor)	B₁	95%–100%	10%–15%	3 hr–4 hr	+	0	10-fold
Nadolol (Corgard)	B₁, B₂	30%	30%	16 hr–24 hr	0	0	7-fold
Pindolol (Visken)	B₁, B₂	95%–100%	40%–50%	3 hr–4 hr	0	+	4-fold
Propranolol (Inderal)	B₁, B₂	90%–100%	90%–95%	3 hr–6 hr	+	0	20-fold
Timolol (Blocadren, Timoptic)	B₁, B₂	90%–95%	10%	3 hr–4 hr	0	0	7-fold

Contraindications

Coronary artery disease, cerebrovascular insufficiency

Interactions

See phenoxybenzamine

▶ **NURSING ALERTS**

See phentolamine. In addition:

▷ 1 Warn patient that ingestion of alcohol with tolazoline may result in a disulfiram-like reaction (tachycardia, sweating, dyspnea, vomiting). See Chapter 80.

▷ 2 Do not attempt intra-arterial injection unless thoroughly familiar with procedure, and perform only in a hospital or other well-equipped setting.

▶ **NURSING CONSIDERATIONS**

▷ 1 Counsel patient that most side-effects will disappear with continued therapy.

▷ 2 Tell patient to avoid overexposure to cold environments because drug effectiveness is enhanced in warm, comfortable surroundings.

▷ 3 Observe user for flushing in extremities, increased skin temperature, and piloerection, which indicate that dosage is optimal.

▷ 4 Be aware that hypotension resulting from overdosage is best treated by placing patient in head-low position, use of IV fluids, and infusion of ephedrine, not epinephrine or norepinephrine.

Beta-Adrenergic Blocking Agents

Atenolol	Pindolol
Metoprolol	Propranolol
Nadolol	Timolol

Drugs capable of exerting a reversible, competitive blocking action at beta-adrenergic receptor sites can antagonize the effects of catecholamines released from adrenergic nerve endings as well as the adrenal medulla. Beta-blocking agents effectively reduce the myocardial stimulant, vasodilator, bronchodilator, and metabolic (glycogenolytic, lipolytic) actions of the catecholamines. Although propranolol is the most widely used of these agents, it is largely nonspecific in its blocking action, and its use often is associated with a wide range of side-effects, particularly relating to the bronchopulmonary system. Newer beta blocking drugs display greater selectivity towards the beta-1 receptors in the heart, leaving the bronchiolar beta-2 sites *relatively* unblocked. To date, however, absolute dissociation of beta-1 and beta-2 blocking activity has not been attained, and all beta blockers must still be used cautiously in patients with bronchospastic disorders.

A comparison of the pharmacologic and pharmacokinetic properties of the various beta-blockers is presented in Table 12-1. Although most of the drugs exhibit a common profile of action, the recognized indications for the different compounds vary. A listing of approved and investigational uses for the individual beta blockers is found in Table 12-2.

The general pharmacology of the beta-blockers is discussed below. Unusual characteristics of individual drugs are noted where necessary. The individual beta-blockers will then be listed in Table 12-3, together with their dosage ranges and pertinent remarks. Additional information relating to their respective uses (*e.g.,* antianginal, antihypertensive, antiarrhythmic) is found in the appropriate chapter dealing with these particular classes of drugs.

Mechanism

Reversible competitive blocking action at beta-adrenergic receptor sites (see Table 12-1 for site specificity), resulting in decreased heart rate and force of contraction, slowed AV conduction, decreased plasma renin, and lowered blood pressure; a quinidine-like membrane-stabilizing action is exhibited by propranolol and to a lesser extent by metoprolol. Pindolol possesses intrinsic sympathomimetic activity (ISA), thus resting heart rate is reduced less than with other beta-blockers. Central effects of beta-blockers are exerted at the level of the vasomotor center in the brainstem to retard tonic sympathetic nerve impulse outflow. In the eye, beta-blockers decrease formation of aqueous humor without inducing miosis or hyperemia. Platelet aggregation may be impaired.

Uses
See Table 12-2

Dosage
See Table 12-3

Fate
(See Table 12-1) Oral absorption is generally good except for atenolol and nadolol. First-pass hepatic metabolism is significant for all drugs except pindolol, thus interpatient plasma levels vary widely. Food enhances the bioavailability of propranolol and metaprolol. Protein binding is minimal with the exception of propranolol. Atenolol and nadolol do not readily pass the blood–brain barrier due to low lipid solubility, and are also excreted unchanged by the kidney. The remaining beta-blockers are metabolized in the liver and are excreted as metabolites and unchanged drug by the kidney. Elimination half-lives are rather short (3 hr–6 hr), except for atenolol (6 hr–9 hr) and nadolol (16 hr–24 hr).

Common Side-Effects
(Not all effects seen with all drugs) Drowsiness, light-headedness, lethargy, nausea, cramping, and bradycardia

Significant Adverse Reactions
(Not all reactions seen with all drugs)
Cardiovascular—tachyarrhythmias, chest pain, AV block, sinoatrial block, peripheral arterial insufficiency, pulmonary edema, syncope, cerebrovascular accident, cardiac failure
CNS—dizziness, vertigo, depression, weakness, behavioral disturbances, agitation, disorientation, memory loss, emotional instability, sleep disturbances, bizarre dreams, hallucinations, catatonia
GI—diarrhea, vomiting, gastric pain, anorexia, bloating, dry mouth, ischemic colitis, hepatomegaly
Respiratory—bronchospasm, dyspnea, cough, rales, nasal congestion
Musculoskeletal—joint pain, muscle cramping
Dermatologic—rash, pruritus, skin irritation, sweating, dry skin, increased pigmentation
Other—hypoglycemia, alopecia, acute pancreatitis, agranulocytosis, thrombocytopenia, eosinophilia, urinary difficulty, fever, sore throat, psoriasis-like rash, blurred vision, elevated BUN, serum transaminase, alkaline phosphatase, lactic dehydrogenase

Table 12-2. Approved and Investigational Uses for Beta-Blockers

Indication	Drugs
Approved	
Hypertension	Atenolol, metoprolol, nadolol, pindolol, propranolol, timolol (oral)
Angina	Nadolol, propranolol
Arrhythmias	Propranolol
Migraine prophylaxis	Propranolol
Hypertrophic subaortic stenosis	Propranolol
Reduce risk of reinfarction after acute infarct	Metoprolol, propranolol, timolol (oral)
Glaucoma	Timolol (ophthalmic)
Pheochromocytoma (adjunctive therapy)	Propranolol
Hyperthyroidism	Propranolol
Investigational	
Alcohol withdrawal	
Anxiety	
Cardiogenic shock	
Digitalis intoxication	
Disseminated intravascular coagulation	
Dissecting aorta	
Essential tremor	
Hemorrhagic shock	
Hypothermia	
Insulinoma	
Lithium-induced tremor	
Mitral stenosis	
Narcolepsy	
Narcotic withdrawal	
Parkinsonism	
Phantom limb pain	
Pulmonary stenosis	
Schizophrenia	
Spastic colon	
Tetanus	
Tetralogy of Fallot	
Ureteral colic	
Urinary incontinence	

Contraindications
Sinus bradycardia, greater than first-degree heart block, right ventricular failure, severe congestive heart failure, cardiogenic shock, in combination with drugs potentiating adrenergic amines (such as MAO inhibitors or tricyclic antidepressants); in addition, nonselective beta-blockers are contraindicated in bronchial asthma.

Interactions
1 Beta-blockers can have additive cardiac depressant effects with digitalis, phenytoin, verapamil, and quinidine.

Table 12-3. Beta-Adrenergic Blocking Agents

Drug	Preparations	Usual Dosage Range	Remarks
Atenolol (Tenormin)	Tablets—50 mg, 100 mg	**Hypertension** Initially, 50 mg once a day; increase to 100 mg once a day if necessary after 1 week to 2 weeks	Long-acting, selective beta-1 antagonist; minimal protein binding; dosage may have to be reduced in patients with significant renal failure, as drug is excreted unchanged in the urine; does not pass the blood–brain barrier
Metoprolol (Lopressor)	Tablets—50 mg, 100 mg Injection—1 mg/ml	**Hypertension** Initially, 100 mg in single or divided doses; increase at weekly intervals until optimal effect is attained; usual maintenance range is 100 mg to 450 mg/day in single or divided doses **Myocardial infarction** 5 mg IV 2 minutes apart for 3 doses, then 50 mg orally every 6 hours for 48 hours, then 100 mg twice daily	Selective beta-1 blocker; well absorbed orally but undergoes significant first-pass hepatic metabolism; weakly protein bound; readily enters the CNS; if once daily administration does not provide sufficient control, may give 2- to 3 times/day in divided doses; ingestion of food enhances oral absorption
Nadolol (Corgard)	Tablets—40 mg, 80 mg, 120 mg, 160 mg	**Hypertension** Initially, 40 mg once daily; increase gradually in 40-mg to 80-mg increments; usual dosage range 80 mg to 320 mg once daily; maximum dose is 640 mg/day **Angina** Initially, 40 mg once daily; increase at 3- to 7-day intervals until desired effect; usual dosage range is 80 mg to 160 mg once daily	Long-acting, nonselective beta-blocker; does not enter the CNS; excreted essentially unchanged by the kidney, therefore dosage may need to be reduced in renal failure; presence of food does not affect rate or extent (approximately 30%) of absorption; if drug is to be discontinued, taper dosage gradually over 1 week to 2 weeks; do not administer more often than once a day
Pindolol (Visken)	Tablets—5 mg, 10 mg	**Hypertension** Initially, 10 mg twice a day or 5 mg 3 times/day; adjust dosage at 2-week to 3-week intervals in increments of 10 mg to obtain the desired reduction in pressure; maximum dose is 60 mg/day	Nonselective beta-antagonist with intrinsic sympathomimetic activity, thus exhibits slightly less slowing of heart rate than other beta-blockers; rapidly absorbed orally; peak plasma levels in 1 hour; short-acting; excreted both as unchanged drug and metabolites; no significant first-pass hepatic metabolism; use is frequently associated with weight gain
Propranolol (Inderal)	Tablets—10 mg, 20 mg, 40 mg, 60 mg, 80 mg, and 90 mg Sustained-release capsules—80 mg, 120 mg, and 160 mg Injection—1 mg/ml	**Hypertension** Initially, 40 mg twice a day or 20 mg 3 times/day; increase gradually until desired response; usual dosage range is 160 mg to 480 mg/day in 3 to 4 divided doses, or 120 mg to 160 mg of sustained-release capsules once daily **Angina** Initially, 10 mg to 20 mg 3 to 4 times/day; increase at 3-day to 7-day intervals; usual dose is 160 mg/day in a single or divided doses **Arrhythmias** 10 mg to 30 mg 3 to 4 times/day **Hypertrophic subaortic stenosis** 20 mg to 40 mg 3 to 4 times/day or 80 mg to 160 mg sustained-release capsule once daily **Myocardial infarction** 180 mg to 240 mg daily in divided doses 3 to 4 times/day	Widely used, nonselective beta blocker; also possesses a quinidine-like cardiac membrane depressant action at high doses; well absorbed orally (food enhances absorption), but undergoes extensive first-pass hepatic metabolism, and variations in plasma levels among patients are wide; highly protein bound; excreted largely as metabolites in the urine; if treatment of angina is to be discontinued, decrease dose gradually over several weeks, as severe angina or myocardial infarction can be precipitated by abrupt termination; if a satisfactory response in the treatment of migraine is not achieved within 4 to 6 weeks after reaching the maximum dose (*i.e.*, 240 mg/day), drug should be discontinued; IV injection should be undertaken with extreme caution, and central venous pressure and ECG closely monitored; transfer to oral therapy as soon as possible

(continued)

Table 12-3. Beta-Adrenergic Blocking Agents *(continued)*

Drug	Preparations	Usual Dosage Range	Remarks
		Migraine Initially, 80 mg a day in divided doses; increase as necessary; usual range is 160 mg to 240 mg/day in a single or divided doses	
		Parenteral (Emergencies only) 1 mg to 3 mg IV at a rate of 1 mg/min; a second dose may be given in 2 minutes to 3 minutes	
Timolol (Blocadren, Timoptic)	Tablets—10 mg, 20 mg Ophthalmic drops—0.25%, 0.5%	Oral Hypertension—Initially, 10 mg twice a day; usual maintenance range is 20 mg to 40 mg/day in 2 divided doses	Nonselective beta-antagonist used orally for hypertension and as prophylaxis following an acute infarction and as eye drops for the management of chronic open-angle glaucoma; oral absorption is good and protein binding is minimal; drug is short-acting and may have to be given 3 times/day if response is inadequate; effects in eye begin in 15 to 30 minutes, peak in 1 to 2 hours and persist up to 24 hours; do not give more than 1 drop 0.5% twice a day; add other antiglaucoma drugs if necessary (see Chap. 9)
		Following myocardial infarction—10 mg twice a day	
		Ophthalmic Glaucoma—1 drop of 0.25% or 0.5% solution twice a day	

2 The effects of beta-blockers can be reversed by norepinephrine, isoproterenol, dopamine, dobutamine, and other sympathomimetic drugs.

3 Plasma levels of propranolol and possibly other beta-blockers can be elevated by chlorpromazine, cimetidine, furosemide, and hydralazine.

4 Aminophylline and beta-blockers have mutually antagonistic effects.

5 The hypotensive action of beta-blockers can be increased by diuretics and other antihypertensives, and inhibited by indomethacin.

6 Barbiturates and phenytoin can reduce plasma levels of beta-blockers metabolized in the liver.

7 Beta-blockers may prolong insulin-induced hypoglycemia and mask the symptoms of lowered blood glucose.

8 Beta-adrenergic blockade may increase the incidence of the "first-dose" orthostatic hypotensive response to prazosin.

▶ **NURSING ALERTS**

▷ 1 Before beginning therapy, determine if patient has any condition (*e.g.,* asthma, allergies, congestive heart failure) that might be worsened by use of beta-blockers.

▷ 2 At first sign of impending cardiac failure (dyspnea, night cough, swelling of extremities), digitalize patient and observe carefully. If improvement is not observed, withdraw drug.

▷ 3 When drugs are administered IV, carefully monitor ECG and blood pressure. Have on hand atropine (for bradycardia), vasopressors (for hypotension), and bronchodilators for emergency use. Transfer patient to oral therapy as soon as possible.

▷ 4 Since beta-blockers may impair patient's adaptive responses to stress or exercise, weakness, fatigue, lightheadedness, and dyspnea can occur. Caution user to avoid dangerous activities (*e.g.,* driving) until reaction to the drug is established.

▷ 5 Carefully observe diabetic patient and advise him to report *any* unusual symptoms while taking a beta-blocker. Drugs may mask appearance of signs of hypoglycemia and insulin overdosage (*e.g.,* tremors, sweating, increased pulse rate).

▷ 6 In patients with confirmed or suspected angina taking a beta-blocker, withdraw drug *slowly* by gradually decreasing dosage. Abrupt cessation of therapy can markedly worsen the condition and may lead to arrhythmias or myocardial infarction.

▷ 7 Withdraw beta-blockers 48 hours before major surgery because they can impair the reflex ability of the heart to respond to stimuli.

▷ 8 Administer cautiously to patients with nonallergic bronchospasm (*e.g.,* chronic bronchitis, emphysema), peripheral vascular insufficiency, history of allergies, allergic rhinitis (especially during the pollen season), impaired renal or hepatic function, diabetes, or myasthenia gravis.

▶ **NURSING CONSIDERATIONS**

▷ 1 Make periodic determinations of hematologic, renal, and hepatic function if drugs are used for prolonged periods.

▷ 2 Carefully observe patient during initial stages of therapy because variation in response is great, and dosage must be individualized and critically titrated in each person.

▷ 3 Do not continue to use beta-blockers in angina unless there is reduced pain and increased work capacity. Routinely monitor ECG and exercise performance ability.

▷ 4 Do not administer within 2 weeks after patient has had an MAO inhibitor drug.

▷ 5 Note that propranolol and metoprolol are best given during meals, whereas the remaining drugs should be given before meals.

▷ 6 Record intake–output fluid ratio and patient's weight. Excess fluid accumulation may signify developing heart failure. Notify physician of any changes.

▷ 7 Alert patient on continual therapy that mild hypotension can occur, resulting in dizziness or lightheadedness. Advise user to rise slowly, avoid prolonged standing, and be cautious when operating machinery.

▷ 8 Warn patient that smoking may reduce effectiveness of beta-blockers, especially propranolol, and that alcohol may enhance the hypotensive and CNS depressant effects.

▷ 9 Caution individual that prolonged fasting may greatly potentiate the hypoglycemic effects produced by beta-blockers.

▷ 10 Note that nadolol and atenolol have long half-lives that permit once-daily dosing. Do not exceed recommended doses because accumulation can occur.

Summary. Adrenergic Blocking Agents

Drug	Preparations	Usual Dosage Range
Alpha-Adrenergic Blocking Agents		
Phenoxybenzamine (Dibenzyline)	Capsules–10 mg	Oral—10 mg initially; increase by 10 mg every 4 days; usual range 20 mg to 60 mg daily
Phentolamine (Regitine)	Tablets–50 mg Injection–5 mg/ml	Oral: Adults—50 mg 4 to 6 times/day; Child—25 mg 4 to 6 times/day; IV, IM: Adults—5 mg to 10 mg; Child—1 mg
Tolazoline (Priscoline)	Injection–25 mg/ml	IM, IV, SC—10 mg to 50 mg 4 times/day; Intra-arterial—25 mg initially; 50 mg to 75 mg 1 to 2 times/day as needed

Beta-Adrenergic Blocking Agents

See Table 12-3

13 Ganglionic Blocking Agents

Synaptic transmission at the ganglia of the autonomic nervous system is mediated by acetylcholine (ACh), and thus can be impeded by drugs capable of blocking the actions of the cholinergic neurotransmitter. Those specific anticholinergic compounds acting primarily at autonomic ganglia are termed *ganglionic blocking agents.* Although many experimental substances are employed to alter ganglionic function in the laboratory, there are presently only two therapeutically useful agents, and their clinical applicability is restricted to the production of hypotensive states for specialized circumstances. Because the agents are nonselective in their blocking action, transmission is reduced in both sympathetic and parasympathetic ganglia. Thus, in addition to interfering with those sympathetic impulses that constrict vascular smooth muscle, the agents likewise block impulses to many other body organs, resulting in a wide range of side-effects. Typical effects caused by parasympathetic blockade include decreased GI motility and secretions, dryness of the mouth, urinary retention, constipation, paralysis of ocular accommodation, mydriasis, and impotence. It is evident that the scope of possible untoward reactions greatly limits the clinical utility of these drugs.

Compounds impairing transmission at autonomic ganglia can be categorized by their mechanism of action as either *depolarizing* or *antidepolarizing* blocking agents. Depolarizing blockers, of which the alkaloid nicotine is an example, exert an initial stimulation of the postganglionic receptors, then block further receptor activation by persistently occupying the site and preventing repolarization of the postsynaptic membrane. Although of no therapeutic value, nicotine is of considerable toxicologic importance because it is systemically absorbed from tobacco smoke and may be accidentally inhaled from nicotine-containing insecticides. The pharmacologic effects of nicotine are quite variable and depend largely upon the amount absorbed, extent and level of exposure, and physiologic state of the individual—that is, the presence of underlying disease states such as peripheral vascular disorders, hypertension, coronary artery disease, or congestive heart failure.

The antidepolarizing group of ganglionic blocking agents, to which all the clinically useful drugs belong, function as competitive antagonists of ACh at the postganglionic receptor sites. Their predominant effect is to reduce sympathetic vascular tone, producing marked vasodilation and hypotension (primarily orthostatic), and decreasing venous return to the heart and consequently cardiac output. They are *potent* blood-pressure-lowering agents but are infrequently used today because of their extensive side-effects.

▶ **mecamylamine**
Inversine

Mechanism
Competitive antagonism of ACh at autonomic ganglia, producing prolonged (6 hr–12 hr) lowering of blood pressure predominantly of the postural type, in both normotensive and hypertensive subjects

Uses

1 Management of moderately severe to severe essential hypertension and uncomplicated malignant hypertension

Dosage

Initially 2.5 mg twice a day orally, increased by 2.5-mg increments every 2 days until optimal effect is obtained (average dose 25 mg/day in 2 to 4 divided doses)

Fate

Completely absorbed orally; onset in 30 minutes to 90 minutes; duration 6 hours to 12 hours; widely distributed and enters CNS; excreted slowly through kidneys, largely in unchanged form; excretion is enhanced in an acidic urine

Common Side-Effects

Dryness of the mouth, constipation, anorexia, weakness, fatigue, mydriasis, and blurred vision

Significant Adverse Reactions

Abdominal distention, ileus, orthostatic hypotension, dizziness, syncope, urinary retention, and impotence; tremor, confusion, convulsions, and mental aberrations are rare occurrences.

Contraindications

Coronary insufficiency, recent myocardial infarction, uremia, chronic pyelonephritis, pyloric stenosis, and glaucoma

Interactions

1 Hypotensive effect of mecamylamine can be enhanced by alcohol, other antihypertensive agents, diuretics, anesthetics, MAO inhibitors, and bethanechol.
2 Mecamylamine may potentiate sympathomimetic drugs.

▶ NURSING ALERTS

▷ 1 Be aware of development of constipation, abdominal distention, and decreased bowel sounds, because they may indicate paralytic ileus. Discontinue drug slowly as directed.

▷ 2 Withdraw drug gradually while other antihypertensives are substituted. Sudden discontinuation of drug may lead to hypertensive rebound, with possibility of cerebral vascular accident.

▷ 3 Use very cautiously in the presence of renal, cerebral, or coronary insufficiency; bladder neck or urethral obstruction; prostatic hypertrophy; elevated BUN levels.

▷ 4 Recognize that effects of mecamylamine may be enhanced by fever, infection, exercise, salt depletion (excess sweating, vomiting, diarrhea), hemorrhage, and pregnancy. See Interactions.

▶ NURSING CONSIDERATIONS

▷ 1 Dosage titration is critical to obtain optimal response. Give drug after meals to obtain smoother control. Use smaller doses in the morning and larger doses during the day because response is usually greater in early morning.

▷ 2 Consider using more than 3 daily doses if hypertension is severe. More than 4 daily doses can be used if control is difficult to sustain.

▷ 3 Determine effective maintenance doses by monitoring blood pressure in the upright position and by titrating dose to a level just below that producing signs of orthostatic hypotension (faintness, dizziness, lightheadedness).

▷ 4 Advise patient that symptoms of orthostatic hypotension can occur with rapid changes from sitting or lying to standing positions. Instruct user to rise to sitting position and pause several minutes before standing.

▷ 5 Urinary excretion is markedly affected by pH. Be aware that toxicity can be intensified by drugs that increase urinary pH (e.g., sodium bicarbonate) thus reducing excretion of mecamylamine.

▷ 6 If constipation becomes a problem, use milk of magnesia or a similar laxative. Bulk laxatives are ineffective.

▷ 7 Monitor fluid intake and output, and examine for edema. Urinary retention can occur and dosage adjustment may be required.

▶ trimethaphan
Arfonad

Mechanism

Short-lived, competitive antagonism of ACh at ganglionic receptor sites; may also exert a direct relaxant effect on vascular smooth muscle; causes pooling of blood in peripheral and splanchnic vessels; may also release histamine; blood pressure is markedly reduced and peripheral blood flow is improved.

Uses

1 Production of controlled hypotension during surgery
2 Acute control of blood pressure in hypertensive emergencies
3 Emergency treatment of pulmonary edema resulting from pulmonary hypertension
4 Management of dissecting aortic aneurysm or ischemic heart disease in cases in which other agents cannot be used (investigational use only)

Dosage

Only by IV infusion—500 mg (10 ml) diluted to 500 ml in 5% Dextrose; begin IV drip at 3 ml/min to 4 ml/min and adjust to individual needs; may range from 0.3 ml/min to 6 ml/min

Fate

Onset of action is immediate; duration approximately 10 minutes to 20 minutes; excreted partly by the kidneys

Significant Adverse Reactions

(Primarily due to overdose) Excessive hypotension, rapid pulse, cyanosis, angina-like pain, and vascular collapse

Contraindications

Conditions in which hypotension may subject the patient to undue risks such as hypovolemia, shock, asphyxia, anemia, respiratory insufficiency, impaired renal function, severe arteriosclerosis, or severe cardiac disease

Interactions

1   Hypotensive effects can be potentiated by antihypertensive agents, anesthetics, vasodilators, and diuretics.

▶ **NURSING ALERTS**

▷ 1   Monitor blood pressure, pulse, and respiratory rate continuously during infusion and frequently thereafter to ensure that response is stable.

▷ 2   Have on hand adequate amounts of oxygen, replacement fluids, respiratory aids, and vasopressor agents to treat untoward reactions. Phenylephrine and mephentermine are vasopressor drugs of choice.

▷ 3   Use cautiously if at all in patients with arteriosclerosis; cardiac, hepatic, or renal disease; Addison's disease; degenerative CNS disease; diabetes; allergies; and in the elderly, debilitated, or the very young.

▷ 4   Position patient supine to avoid cerebral anoxia. If pressure fails to drop, raise head of bed carefully to observe response.

▷ 5   Terminate infusion gradually while closely monitoring blood pressure.

▶ **NURSING CONSIDERATIONS**

▷ 1   Prepare infusion solution fresh, and discard unused portion. Do not use trimethaphan infusion as a vehicle for other drugs.

▷ 2   Monitor intake and output, because urinary retention can occur. Check for abdominal distention and report immediately.

▷ 3   Terminate infusion prior to wound closure in surgical procedures to allow pressure to return to normal. Usually occurs within 10 minutes.

▷ 4   Be aware that tolerance can develop within 48 hours. Monitor pressure closely, and report any lessening of drug effect.

Summary. Ganglionic Blocking Agents

Drug	Preparations	Usual Dosage Range
Mecamylamine (Inversine)	Tablets—2.5 mg	Initially 2.5 mg twice a day; increase by 2.5-mg increments every 2 days to optimal effect (average 25 mg/day)
Trimethaphan (Arfonad)	Injection—50 mg/ml	Dilute 500 mg (10 ml) in 500 ml 5% Dextrose; begin IV infusion at rate of 3 ml/min to 4 ml/min; adjust to individual (range 0.3 ml/min–6.0 ml/min)

I Antihistamines

Drugs that competitively block the effects of histamine at various receptor sites in the body are termed antihistamines. Histamine is present in virtually all mammalian tissues, arising from the decarboxylation of the amino acid histidine. Sites of highest histamine concentration in the body include (1) *mast cells* and *basophils,* the fixed tissue and circulating histaminocytes, respectively, where histamine is bound to heparin in an inactive form; (2) *gastric mucosal cells,* where histamine is not extensively bound; and (3) *CNS histamine-containing cells,* located primarily in the hypothalamus. Upon release from binding sites or tissue stores, histamine is capable of eliciting a tremendous range of pharmacologic effects, from mild itching to circulatory shock.

While the physiologic functions of endogenous histamine remain largely speculative (*e.g.,* neurotransmission, gastric acid secretion, tissue growth and repair), its role in several pathologic processes associated with acute and chronic allergic and hypersensitivity reactions is much more clearly established. Histamine can be released from cells by physical and chemical agents, a variety of drugs and toxins, and antigen–antibody reactions; therefore it plays a critical role in the symptomology of many allergic, anaphylactic, and hypersensitivity reactions.

The major pharmacologic actions of histamine are centered on the cardiovascular system, nonvascular smooth muscle, exocrine glands, and the adrenal medulla. The more important pharmacologic effects of histamine are the following:

1 Arteriolar and venular dilation
2 Increased capillary permeability
3 Increased heart rate
4 Contraction of nonvascular smooth muscle (*e.g.,* bronchoconstriction, GI hypermotility)
5 Stimulation of gastric hydrochloric acid secretion
6 Release of catecholamines from the adrenal medulla

These effects of histamine are mediated by an action on two distinct receptors, termed H_1 and H_2 receptor sites. H_1 receptors are those associated with the smooth muscle of the blood vessels, bronchioles, and GI tract, while H_2 receptors are found on gastric parietal cells, the myocardium, and certain blood vessels as well. Thus, it appears that the contraction of nonvascular smooth muscle is an H_1 receptor effect, the secretion of gastric acid and acceleration of the heart rate are caused by H_2 receptor activation, and vascular dilation and increased permeability result from a combined action of histamine on both H_1 and H_2 sites.

Clinical uses of histamine are essentially obsolete. Histamine itself and its structural analog betazole (Histalog) were once commonly used to test for functional achlorhydria (lack of gastric hydrochloric acid), but they have now largely been replaced by a more effective and less toxic diagnostic agent, pentagastrin (Peptavlon), which is discussed in Chapter 78. Histamine phosphate injection (0.275 mg) is occasionally used for presumptive diagnosis of pheochromocytoma (see Chap. 78), but it is a dangerous procedure and should be employed only by persons trained in its admin-

Antihistamine–Antiserotonin Agents

14

istration. The principal importance of histamine lies in its role as mediator of certain pathologic conditions, and in the therapeutic value of its antagonism by antihistamine drugs.

Antihistamines are classified as either H$_1$ or H$_2$ receptor antagonists, although the H$_1$ blockers comprise the overwhelming majority of drugs, and the term *antihistamine* has come to be associated synonymously with H$_1$ antagonists. The H$_2$ blockers exert a specific blocking effect on gastric parietal cell histamine receptor sites, markedly reducing their output of hydrochloric acid.

The antihistamines can be categorized chemically into one of several groups, each of which demonstrates slightly different pharmacologic properties.

A H$_1$ Antagonists

1 *Alkylamines*—e.g., chlorpheniramine; potent drugs that produce mild sedation; most widely used group
2 *Ethylenediamines*—e.g., tripelennamine; produce low incidence of drowsiness but significant GI upset
3 *Ethanolamines*—e.g., diphenhydramine; high incidence of drowsiness; good antiemetics
4 *Phenothiazines*—e.g., promethazine; strong sedative activity; used for motion sickness, preoperative medication, obstetrics
5 *Piperazines*—e.g., cyclizine, meclizine; primarily used for motion sickness
6 *Miscellaneous*—e.g., azatadine, diphenylpyraline; moderate sedation; also block serotonin receptors

B H$_2$ Antagonists

Examples of H$_2$ antagonists are cimetidine, ranitidine; potent inhibitors of gastric hydrochloric acid secretion.

In addition to the above classes of histamine antagonists, drugs possessing antihistaminic along with other pharmacologic actions have been used in the treatment of parkinsonism (*e.g.*, chlorphenoxamine) and pruritus (*e.g.*, cyproheptadine). These agents are discussed under their appropriate headings.

It is important to recognize that although H$_1$ antagonists can prevent effector cell responses to both exogenous and endogenous histamine, the antagonists are significantly more effective against the former; yet *endogenous* histamine is primarily responsible for most allergic reactions. Moreover, antihistamines are much more useful when given before a histamine challenge rather than after an allergic attack has begun. Finally, antihistamines are effective only to the extent that histamine is the primary causative factor in the allergic response. Therefore, H$_1$ antagonists are most effective in prevention of seasonal pollinosis and urticaria, somewhat less effective in allergic dermatoses, contact dermatitis, vasomotor rhinitis, serum sickness, and allergic transfusion reactions, and seldom useful alone in bronchial asthma, GI allergies, and systemic anaphylactic reactions.

The pharmacology of the H$_1$ receptor antagonists are discussed as a group because they are remarkably similar in most of their actions. A listing of individual drugs is given in Table 14-1.

A H$_1$ Receptor Antagonists

Azatadine	Diphenylpyraline
Brompheniramine	Doxylamine
Buclizine	Meclizine
Carbinoxamine	Methdilazine
Chlorpheniramine	Pheniramine
Clemastine	Promethazine
Cyclizine	Pyrilamine
Dexchlorpheniramine	Tripelennamine
Dimenhydrinate	Triprolidine
Diphenhydramine	

Mechanism
Competitive blockade of the actions of histamine at H$_1$ receptor sites on effector structures (*e.g.*, vascular and nonvascular smooth muscle, salivary and respiratory mucosal glands); also exert an anticholinergic (*e.g.*, drying) and sedative action

Uses
1 Relief of symptoms of various allergic disorders (*e.g.*, allergic rhinitis, vasomotor rhinitis, uncomplicated urticaria and angioedema, allergic reactions to blood or plasma)
2 Adjunctive treatment in anaphylactic reactions (with epinephrine and other measures)
3 Prevention and treatment of motion sickness
4 Temporary relief of insomnia
5 Adjunctive therapy for parkinsonism and extrapyramidal reactions due to antipsychotic drug therapy
6 Relief of coughs caused by colds, allergies, or minor throat irritations
7 Prevention and control of nausea and vomiting due to anesthesia or surgery
8 Adjunct to analgesics for obstetrics and postoperative pain, and for preoperative sedation and relief of apprehension

Dosage
See Table 14-1

Fate
Most drugs are used orally and are well absorbed; onset is normally within 10 minutes to 30 minutes; duration is 3 hours to 4 hours (sustained-action forms, 8 hr–12 hr); metabolized by liver and kidney and excreted largely in the urine, usually as metabolites; readily enter CNS and produce depression; effectiveness or dependability not significantly enhanced by parenteral administration; topical forms involve risk of sensitization

(*Text continues on p. 110.*)

Table 14-1. Antihistamines

Drug	Preparations	Usual Dosage Range	Major Uses	Remarks
Azatadine (Optimine)	Tablets—1 mg	1 mg to 2 mg twice a day	Allergic disorders	Do not use in children under 12; has antiserotonin effects as well
Brompheniramine (Bromamine, Bromphen, Dehist, Dimetane, ND-Stat, Veltane)	Tablets—4 mg Tablets (timed-release)—8 mg, 12 mg Elixir—2 mg/5 ml Injection—10 mg/ml	Oral: Adults—4 mg to 8 mg 3 to 4 times/day or 8 mg to 12 mg timed-release twice a day Children (over 6 yr)—2 mg to 4 mg 3 to 4 times/day Children (under 6 yr)—0.5 mg/kg daily in divided doses Parenteral: Adults—5 mg to 20 mg IV, IM or SC twice a day (maximum 40 mg/day) Children—0.5 mg/kg/day	Allergic disorders, cough	Keep patient lying down during IV administration; sweating, hypotension, and faintness may occur with IV use; do not use solutions with preservatives for IV use; see chlorpheniramine
Buclizine (Bucladin-S)	Tablet—50 mg	Nausea—50 mg to 150 mg/day Motion sickness—50 mg one half hour before travel, and 50 mg every 4 hours to 6 hours as needed	Nausea, vomiting, and vertigo Prevention of motion sickness	Tablets may be chewed or swallowed whole; do not use during pregnancy or in small children; may produce headache, nervousness, drowsiness, dryness of the mouth
Carbinoxamine (Clistin)	Tablets—4 mg	Adults—4 mg to 8 mg 3 to 4 times/day Children—2 mg to 6 mg 3 to 4 times/day depending on age	Allergic disorders	Low incidence of drowsiness and GI disturbances
Chlorpheniramine (Chlor-Trimeton, Teldrin, and various other manufacturers)	Chewable tablets—2 mg Tablets—4 mg Timed-release tablets—8 mg, 12 mg Timed-release capsules—8 mg, 12 mg Syrup—2 mg/5 ml Injection—10 mg/ml, 20 mg/ml, and 100 mg/ml	Oral: Adults—4 mg 3 to 6 times/day or 8 mg to 12 mg twice a day Children (6 yr–12 yr)—2 mg 3 to 6 times/day or 8 mg twice a day Children (2 yr–6 yr)—1 mg 3 to 4 times/day Parenteral: Allergy—5 mg to 20 mg IM, SC (maximum 40 mg/day) Anaphylaxis—10 mg to 20 mg IV	Allergic disorders, transfusion and drug reactions, anaphylactic reactions	May be used prophylactically for blood transfusion; when given IV (10 mg/ml solution only) or added directly to stored blood, do not use solution with preservatives; low incidence of drowsiness and other side-effects; has antiemetic, antitussive, and some local anesthetic action; do not use long-acting preparation in children under 12
Clemastine (Tavist)	Tablets—1.34 mg, 2.68 mg	Adults—1.34 mg to 2.68 mg 2 to 3 times/day (maximum 3 tablets daily)	Allergic disorders	Not recommended in children under 12
Cyclizine (Marezine)	Tablets—50 mg Injection—50 mg/ml	Oral: 50 mg one half hour before travel; repeat every 4 hours to 6 hours to a maximum of 300 mg/day Children—6 yr–10 yr—½ adult dose IM—50 mg every 4 hours to 6 hours	Prevention and treatment of motion sickness, and postoperative nausea and vomiting	Do not use in pregnancy or in children under 6; produces frequent drowsiness; for postoperative nausea and vomiting, give 20 minutes to 30 minutes before end of surgery; overdosage may produce hyperexcitability and

(continued)

Table 14-1. Antihistamines (continued)

Drug	Preparations	Usual Dosage Range	Major Uses	Remarks
				convulsions; may decrease sensitivity of labyrinthine apparatus to motion
Dexchlorpheniramine (Polaramine)	Tablets—2 mg Repeat action Tablets—4 mg, 6 mg Syrup—2 mg/5 ml	Adults—2 mg 3 to 4 times a day or 4 mg to 6 mg twice a day Children—½ adult dose Infant—¼ adult dose	Allergic disorders	Low incidence of many common side-effects; do not use repeat action tablets in children; available as an expectorant with pseudoephedrine and guaifenesin
Dimenhydrinate (Dramamine and various other manufacturers)	Tablets—50 mg Liquid—12.5 mg/4 ml Suppositories—100 mg Injection—50 mg/ml	Oral: Adults—50 mg to 100 mg every 4 hrs Children (8 yr–12 yr)—25 mg to 50 mg 3 times/day Rectal—100 mg 1 to 2 times/day IM: Adults—50 mg as needed Children—1.25 mg/kg 4 times a day up to 300 mg/day IV (adults only)—50 mg in 10 ml Sodium Chloride given over 2 minutes	Prevention and treatment of nausea, vomiting and vertigo of motion sickness, radiation sickness or anesthesia	Drowsiness is common, especially at higher doses. Caution when used in combination with aminoglycoside antibiotics because it may mask signs of ototoxicity, leading to permanent damage; tolerance develops with continued use; do not mix parenteral solutions with other drugs
Diphenhydramine (Benadryl and various other manufacturers)	Tablets—25 mg, 50 mg Capsules—25 mg, 50 mg Elixir—12.5 mg/5 ml Syrup—12.5 mg/ml, 13.3 mg/5 ml Injection—10 mg/ml, 50 mg/ml Cream—1%, 2%	Oral: Adults—25 mg to 50 mg 3 to 4 times/day Children (over 20 lbs)—5 mg/kg/day in divided doses Parenteral (IV or deep IM): Adults—10 mg to 50 mg as needed (maximum 400 mg/day) Children—5 mg/kg/day in 4 divided doses	Allergic disorders, motion sickness, adjunctive therapy in anaphylactic reactions, prevention of reactions to blood or plasma, pediatric sedation, parkinsonism, cough due to colds or allergies, acute dystonias, oral anesthesia, insomnia	Topical preparations may cause hypersensitivity reactions; high incidence of drowsiness initially, which decreases with use; monitor blood pressure carefully with parenteral use; very low incidence of GI disturbances; found in several over-the-counter sleeping preparations
Diphenylpyraline (Hispril)	Timed-release capsules—5 mg	Adults—5 mg twice a day Children (over 6 yr)—5 mg daily	Allergic disorders	Do not use in children under 6
Doxylamine (Unisom)	Tablets—25 mg	Adults—25 mg at bedtime	Insomnia	Drowsiness is very common; used as an over-the-counter sleep aid
Meclizine (Antivert, Bonine, Dizmiss, Motion Cure, Wehvert)	Tablets—12.5 mg, 25 mg Chewable tablets—25 mg Chewable capsules—25 mg	Motion Sickness—25 mg to 50 mg 1 hour prior to travel; repeat every 24 hours Vertigo—25 mg to 100 mg daily in divided doses as needed	Motion sickness, vertigo due to vestibular disease	Do not use in pregnancy or young children; commonly causes dry mouth and drowsiness; weak anticholinergic action; tablets are oral or chewable
Methdilazine (Tacaryl)	Chewable tablets—4 mg Tablets—8 mg Syrup—4 mg/5 ml	Adults—8 mg 2 to 4 times/day Children (over 3 yr)—4 mg 2 to 4 times/day	Pruritus, urticaria	Tablets may be chewed (4 mg) or swallowed whole (8 mg); structurally a phenothiazine (see Chap. 22 for possible adverse reactions); drowsiness common

Table 14-1. Antihistamines (continued)

Drug	Preparations	Usual Dosage Range	Major Uses	Remarks
Phenindamine (Nolahist)	Tablets—25 mg	Adults—25 mg every 4 hours to 6 hours Children—(6 yr–12 yr)—12.5 mg every 4 hours to 6 hours	Allergic reactions	Do not exceed 150 mg/24 hr for adults or 75 mg/24 hr for children
Promethazine (Phenergan and various other manufacturers)	Tablets—12.5 mg, 25 mg, 50 mg Syrup—6.25 mg/5 ml, 25 mg/5 ml Suppositories—12.5 mg, 25 mg, and 50 mg Injection—25 mg/ml, 50 mg/ml	Oral: Adults—12.5 mg to 50 mg every 4 hr to 6 hr as necessary Children—6.25 mg to 12.5 mg 3 times/day as needed Rectal: 12.5 mg to 25 mg every 4 hr to 6 hr as necessary Parenteral (usually IM): 12.5 mg to 25 mg individualized to condition (children—0.6–1.2 mg/kg) When used IV—maximum concentration is 25 mg/ml/min	Allergic disorders and reactions to blood and plasma, motion sickness, nausea and vomiting due to anesthesia, drugs or surgery, preoperative and obstetrical sedation, adjunct to analgesics in postoperative or chronic pain, sedation and light sleep, cough	Phenothiazine derivative (see Chap. 22); potent antihistamine and sedative; prolonged effects; avoid intra-arterial injection because severe arteriospasm can result; irritating to tissues if given SC; Reduce dose of analgesics and other sedative–hypnotics if used in combination with promethazine; injection is incompatible with alkaline drugs; good antiemetic, but may mask vomiting caused by other drugs; protect injectable form from light and do not use if cloudy or darkened; available with expectorant either plain or with codeine and/or decongestants
Pyrilamine (Nytol, Sominex, and various other manufacturers)	Tablets—25 mg Capsules—25 mg, 50 mg	Adults—25 mg to 50 mg 3 to 4 times/day Children—12.5 mg to 25 mg 4 times/day	Allergic disorders, cough, insomnia	Not recommended in children under 6; found in several over-the-counter sleep formulations, although degree of drowsiness is slight
Tripelennamine (Pyribenzamine, PBZ)	Tablets—25 mg, 50 mg Long-acting tablets—100 mg Elixir—37.5 mg/5 ml	Adults—25 mg to 50 mg every 4 hours to 6 hours (maximum 600 mg/day) or 100 mg 2 to 3 times/day Children—5 mg/kg/day in 4 to 6 doses (maximum 300 mg/day)	Allergic disorders and reactions to blood or plasma, adjunctive therapy in anaphylactic therapy, pruritus and other topical skin disorders, mucous membrane analgesia and anesthesia in the mouth, cough	Do not use 100-mg sustained-acting form in children; used as mouthwash for herpetic gingivostomatitis in children; caution in elderly, as dizziness, sedation, and hypotension are more likely to occur; possesses some antitussive, antiemetic, and local anesthetic activity
Triprolidine (Actidil)	Tablets—2.5 mg Syrup—1.25 mg/5 ml	Adults—2.5 mg 3 to 4 times/day Children (6 yr–12 yr)—½ adult dose Children (2 yr–6 yr)—0.6 mg to 0.9 mg 3 to 4 times/day Children (under 2 yr)—0.3 mg 3 to 4 times/day	Allergic disorders, prevention of reactions to blood and plasma transfusions	Low degree of drowsiness and most other side-effects; rapid onset of action; may cause paradoxical excitation and irritability; combined with pseudoephedrine as Actifed; this combination is also available with codeine and guaifenesin as Actifed-C; children under 6 should be given syrup only

Common Side-Effects

Sedation, dizziness, epigastric distress, dryness of mouth, thickened bronchial secretions

Significant Adverse Reactions

(Frequency and severity vary among different preparations)

Cardiovascular—hypotension, palpitations, tachycardia, arrhythmias

GI—anorexia, nausea, vomiting, diarrhea or constipation

CNS—confusion, restlessness, impaired coordination, blurred vision, vertigo, tinnitus, heaviness and weakness of the hands, nervousness, tremors, paresthesias, irritability, excitation, insomnia, hysteria

Hematologic—hemolytic anemia, thrombocytopenia, leukopenia, pancytopenia, agranulocytosis

Urinary—urinary frequency or retention, dysuria

Respiratory—wheezing, chest tightness, nasal congestion

Hypersensitivity—urticaria, drug rash, photosensitivity, anaphylactic shock

Other—headache, diplopia, sweating, pallor, stinging or burning at site of injection

With overdosage—fever, ataxia, hallucinations, convulsions, coma, cardiovascular and respiratory collapse (children are especially susceptible)

Contraindications

Asthma, narrow-angle glaucoma, peptic ulcer, prostatic hypertrophy, GI or bladder obstruction, premature or nursing infants, elderly or debilitated patients, pregnant or nursing women, patients on MAO inhibitor therapy; in addition, phenothiazine antihistamines (methdilazine, promethazine, trimeprazine) are contraindicated in comatose patients, states of CNS depression due to drug overdosage, jaundice, bone marrow depression, and acutely ill or dehydrated children.

Interactions

1 Sedative effects may be enhanced by concurrent use of other CNS depressants (*e.g.,* alcohol, barbiturates, narcotics, antianxiety drugs).

2 Atropine-like side-effects (*e.g.,* dryness of mouth, blurred vision, urinary retention, constipation) are potentiated by other anticholinergics, tricyclic antidepressants, and MAO inhibitors.

3 Effects of epinephrine can be increased by several antihistamines (*e.g.,* diphenhydramine, chlorpheniramine).

▶ NURSING ALERTS

▷ 1 Warn users of the danger of engaging in activities requiring mental alertness (*e.g.,* driving, operating machinery) while taking antihistamines.

▷ 2 Use with caution in presence of convulsive disorders, hyperthyroidism, cardiovascular or renal disease, hypertension, urinary retention, diabetes, acute or chronic respiratory impairment (especially in children).

▷ 3 Caution patients about the additive effects of antihistamines and other CNS depressants (*e.g.,* alcohols, sedatives, hypnotics).

▷ 4 Be aware that in children, antihistamines may produce paradoxical excitation or reduce mental alertness. Overdosage in children may result in hallucinations, convulsions, and possibly death.

▷ 5 Do not use antihistamines in lower respiratory tract diseases (*e.g.,* asthma) because their drying effects may cause thickening of secretions and impair expectoration.

▷ 6 Although there is still insufficient information to definitely implicate all antihistamines in cases of fetal damage, avoid their use in pregnancy if at all possible, especially the anti-motion sickness drugs (*e.g.,* cyclizine, meclizine).

▷ 7 Recognize that topical application of antihistamine-containing preparations can produce serious hypersensitivity reactions. Discontinue use at earliest signs of dermatologic toxicity.

▷ 8 Be aware that antihistamines are much more prone to produce dizziness, sedation, confusion, and hypotension in the elderly or debilitated.

▷ 9 When using drug parenterally, administer IM rather than SC because many solutions are irritating. Realize that hypersensitivity reactions are more likely to occur with parenteral rather than with oral administration.

▶ NURSING CONSIDERATIONS

▷ 1 Although antihistamines are found in many cough preparations, recognize that they have a drying effect on mucosal surfaces and may cause thickening of bronchial secretions, making expectoration more difficult.

▷ 2 Advise user that drowsiness will usually lessen or disappear with continued usage of the drug. Provide necessary assistance in walking and other activities while drowsiness is present.

▷ 3 Discontinue use before skin testing for allergies because drug may mask positive results.

▷ 4 Advise patients with severe allergies to carry identification as to type of allergy, medication being used, and name of physician.

▷ 5 Administer drugs with meals or milk to decrease GI irritation when necessary.

▷ 6 Suggest that individuals on long-term therapy have periodic blood counts.

▷ 7 When drug is used for motion sickness, give first dose of drug at least 30 minutes prior to travel and several times a day during travel if necessary, preferably before meals.

▷ 8 Do not apply topical preparations to broken, exposed, or weeping skin area.

▷ 9 Tell patient to report any side-effects, since many can be eliminated by simply reducing the dose or changing to a different antihistamine.

▷ 10 Closely observe patient during parenteral use. Inform him that a stinging sensation may occur briefly. Discontinue use if any other untoward reactions develop.

B H₂ Receptor Antagonists

As previously noted, the designation *antihistamine* is generally used synonymously with H₁ receptor antagonists. A second series of compounds have been developed which act as competitive antagonists of histamine specifically at those receptor sites designated as H₂ receptors. These H₂ reactive sites mediate the gastric acid secretory effects and the cardiac stimulatory action of histamine. Because H₂ antagonists can effectively and almost completely block the secretion of gastric hydrochloric acid in response to most stimuli, it appears that histamine plays a major role in acid secretion from gastric mucosal parietal calls. Clinical studies show substantial reductions in gastric secretory volume, total acidity, and pepsin activity following administration of an H₂ blocker. Therefore, these substances have an important role in the therapeutic management of peptic ulcers and various gastric hypersecretory states.

▶ cimetidine
Tagamet

Mechanism
Selective antagonism of the actions of histamine at H₂ receptor sites in the gastric mucosa; reduces daytime and nocturnal basal gastric acid secretion 90% to 100%, as well as acid secretion stimulated by food, caffeine, pentagastrin, and insulin; increases gastric pH to 5 or greater for 3 hours to 4 hours; decreases total pepsin output.

Uses
1 Treatment of gastric and duodenal ulcers
2 Reduction of acid levels in acute or recurrent gastric hypersecretory conditions (*e.g.,* stress ulcers in hospitalized patients)
3 Prevention of recurrence of ulcers in high risk patients
4 Treatment of pathologic hypersecretory conditions (*e.g.,* Zollinger–Ellison syndrome, systemic mastocytosis, multiple endocrine adenomas)

Dosage
Oral
Duodenal Ulcer—Initially 300 mg 4 times/day for 4 weeks to 8 weeks; reduce to 200 mg to 300 mg 1 to 4 times/day or preferably 400 mg at bedtime for maintenance therapy as necessary to prevent recurrence
Hypersecretory conditions—300 mg 4 to 6 times/day to a maximum of 2400 mg/day

Parenteral
IM injection—300 mg every 6 hours
IV injection—300 mg diluted to 20 ml in saline and injected over 1 minute to 2 minutes every 6 hours
IV infusion—300 mg in 100 ml 5% Dextrose infused over 15 minutes to 20 minutes every 6 hours (maximum 2400 mg/day)

Fate
Rapidly absorbed orally and parenterally; peak serum levels in 45 minutes to 90 minutes; half-life about 2 hours; effects last at least 4 hours to 6 hours; excreted through the kidney largely as unchanged drug and sulfoxide metabolite

Common Side-Effects
Mild diarrhea; transient pain at IM injection site

Significant Adverse Reactions
Dizziness, muscle pain, rash, confusion, gynecomastia, alopecia, increased plasma creatinine and serum transaminase, galactorrhea, impotence, decreased sperm count, bradycardia, arrhythmias with IV administration; rarely, blood dyscrasias

Interactions
1 Cimetidine may potentiate the effects of oral anticoagulants.
2 Antacids may impair absorption of cimetidine if administered simultaneously.
3 Cimetidine may increase the half-life of benzodiazepine drugs (such as chlordiazepoxide and diazepam), theophylline, salicylates, phenytoin, propranolol, caffeine, and other drugs metabolized in the liver by reducing their rate of metabolism.

▶ NURSING ALERT
▷ 1 Use cautiously in pregnant or nursing women, in the elderly and children, and in patients with endocrine abnormalities or impaired renal function.

▶ NURSING CONSIDERATIONS
▷ 1 Give antacids during therapy to provide additional relief of pain, but allow at least 1 hour between cimetidine and antacid administration.
▷ 2 Note that injectable form is stable at room temperature for 48 hours, but that the drug is incompatible with aminophylline and barbiturates in IV solution.
▷ 3 In patients with renal failure, reduce dose to 300 mg every 12 hours.
▷ 4 Be aware that while cimetidine is very effective in healing duodenal ulcers, relapse following discontinuation of therapy is common.

▶ ranitidine
Zantac

Ranitidine is a long acting H₂ antagonist used for treatment of duodenal and gastric ulcers. Unlike cimetidine, its oral absorption is not impaired by antacids, it possesses no antiandrogenic activity, there is no observable potentiation of warfarin-type anticoagulants, and drug-metabolizing activity of liver enzymes is not impaired.

Mechanism
Competitive inhibition of the action of histamine at H₂ receptor sites, including those on the gastric parietal cells; reduces daytime and nocturnal gastric acid secretion; does

not affect pepsin secretion or fasting or postprandial gastrin serum levels; reduces hepatic blood flow slightly

Uses
1 Short-term treatment of active gastric or duodenal ulcers
2 Treatment of pathologic hypersecretory conditions (*e.g.,* Zollinger–Ellison syndrome, systemic mastocytosis)

Dosage
150 mg twice a day; up to 6 g/day have been used in severe pathologic hypersecretory states.

Fate
Peak serum levels occur in 2 hours to 3 hours following oral administration; effects persist 8 hours to 12 hours; absorption is *not* impaired by food or antacids; largely excreted in the urine, approximately one half as unchanged drug

Common Side-Effects
Headache

Significant Adverse Reactions
Dizziness, constipation, nausea, abdominal pain, rash, malaise, and increased serum transaminases

▶ NURSING ALERT
▷ 1 Use with caution in pregnant or nursing women, in young children, and in patients with impaired renal or hepatic function.

▶ NURSING CONSIDERATIONS
▷ 1 Note that ranitidine may be given without regard to meals and may be prescribed with antacids.
▷ 2 Be aware that false-positive tests for urine protein may occur with Multistix during therapy with ranitidine.

II Antiserotonin Agents

Many antihistamine drugs exert varying degrees of serotonin-blocking activity, although in most cases this activity is too weak to be clinically significant. A few drugs, however, have been shown to exert considerable serotonin antagonism, and they are employed in various disease states in which overactivity of serotonin may be the primary etiologic factor. It is important to recognize, however, that drugs classified as antiserotonin agents possess many other pharmacologic actions as well (*e.g.,* antihistamine, anticholinergic, local anesthetic, oxytocic, vasoconstrictor), and that their clinical effects cannot always be ascribed solely to their serotonin-blocking action. Antiserotonin drugs are primarily used for symptomatic management of allergic conditions, for prophylaxis of migraine and other vascular headaches, and to reduce diarrhea and abdominal cramping in the treatment of the carcinoid syndrome.

▶ cyproheptadine
Periactin

Mechanism
Competitive antagonism of serotonin, histamine, and possibly acetylcholine at postsynaptic receptor sites; structural analog of the phenothiazines; exhibits mild CNS depressant activity and may stimulate the appetite, possibly by an action on the hypothalamus

Uses
1 Relief of various allergic disorders, especially rhinitis, allergic conjunctivitis, and allergic skin manifestations (*e.g.,* cold urticaria, pruritus, angioedema)
2 Prevention or reduction of allergic reactions to blood and plasma
3 Adjunctive therapy for anaphylactic reactions
4 Relief of pruritus resulting from drug or serum reactions, physical allergies, or insect bites
5 Prophylaxis of migraine
6 Stimulate appetite (investigational)
7 Treatment of carcinoid syndrome

Dosage
Adults: 4 mg 3 to 4 times/day (usual range is 12 mg–16 mg/day; maximum dose 32 mg/day)
Children: (2 yr–6 yr) 2 mg 2 to 3 times/day (maximum 12 mg/day); (7 yr–14 yr) 4 mg 2 to 3 times/day (maximum 16 mg/day)

Fate
Absorption is adequate; onset of action is within 60 minutes; duration 4 hours to 6 hours

Common Side-Effects
Sedation; dryness of mouth, nose, and throat; dizziness; gastric distress; and thickening of bronchial secretions

Significant Adverse Reactions
Urinary difficulty, skin rash, excitation, impaired coordination, tremor, irritability, confusion, ataxia (CNS effects occur especially in children), hypotension, and tachycardia

Contraindications
Urinary retention, bladder obstruction, lower respiratory disease, narrow-angle glaucoma, peptic ulcer, prostatic hypertrophy, elderly or debilitated patients, newborn or premature infants, nursing mothers, and combination with MAO inhibitors

Interactions
1 MAO inhibitors or anticholinergics may intensify many of the side-effects

▶ NURSING ALERTS
▷ 1 Caution patient to avoid activities requiring alertness and coordination in the early stages of therapy, because drowsiness is common, but usually disappears in several days.

▷ 2 Warn users that the drug has additive CNS depressant effects with other depressants (*e.g.,* alcohols, narcotics, barbiturates).

▷ 3 Use with caution in patients with bronchial asthma, glaucoma, hypertension, hyperthyroidism, and cardiovascular disease.

▷ 4 Give to pregnant women only when apparent benefit clearly outweighs potential risks (*i.e.,* fetal damage).

▶ **NURSING CONSIDERATIONS**

▷ 1 Be aware that use in children may result in an excitatory state (*e.g.,* agitation, confusion, possibly hallucinations), and watch for early signs of stimulation.

▷ 2 Individualize dosage carefully based on patient's needs and responses. Use liquid form in small children because dosage adjustment is easier.

▷ 3 Watch for signs of dizziness, and hypotension especially in elderly individuals.

▶ **ergotamine**

Ergomar, Ergostat, Gynergen, Medihaler–Ergotamine, Wigrettes

Ergotamine is an ergot alkaloid considered to be a *specific* drug for relief of pain associated with vascular headaches. Other ergot alkaloids include ergonovine (Chap. 39), bromocriptine (Chap. 26), methysergide (see below), and LSD (Chap. 81).

Because prolonged use of ergotamine is not recommended, and migraine is usually a chronically recurring condition, it is important to attempt to identify the underlying psychological and physical abnormalities that contribute to the etiology of a migraine attack. Drug therapy, *per se,* is rarely curative and often dangerous, due to a wide range of drug-induced adverse reactions. Other measures such as relaxation and avoidance of stressful situations may be more acceptable and equally effective in reducing the incidence and severity of migraine and other vascular headaches.

Mechanism

Direct spasmogenic effect on smooth muscle of cerebral arteries; constricts the vessels and therefore decreases the pressure on sensory nerve endings resulting from the increased pulsations of the dilated arteries; also exhibits an alpha-adrenergic blocking and a serotonin-blocking action; not a true analgesic and only specific for the pain of vascular headaches; large doses have an oxytocic effect on the myometrium.

Uses

1 Relief of pain associated with vascular headaches, such as migraine and histamine cephalgia (most effective if given early in an attack)

Dosage

Oral, sublingual—2 mg to 6 mg per attack (maximum 10 mg weekly)

Inhalation—1 inhalation (0.36 mg) 5 minutes apart until pain is relieved (maximum 6 inhalations/day)

Fate

Incompletely and erratically absorbed from GI tract; sublingual absorption is more predictable; prolonged duration of action, up to 24 hours; metabolized in the liver and excreted in the bile

Common Side-Effects

Numbness or tingling in extremities, muscle weakness, GI discomfort (oral use), and diarrhea.

Significant Adverse Reactions

Hypertension, bradycardia, angina-like pain, intermittent claudication, depression. Prolonged use of high doses can lead to ergotism, with vomiting, convulsions, weak pulse, confusion, cold and cyanotic skin, or gangrene.

Contraindications

Occlusive or vasospastic peripheral vascular disease, hepatic or renal disease, hypertension, severe pruritus, sepsis, infectious states and malnutrition, pregnancy, and young children

Interactions

1 Vasoconstriction may be increased by other vasoconstrictors (*e.g.,* vasopressor amines, beta-blockers).

▶ **NURSING ALERTS**

▷ 1 Avoid prolonged use of the drug or administration of very high doses, because circulatory impairment can occur. Vasoconstriction can be overcome by a vasodilator such as nitroprusside (Nipride).

▷ 2 Counsel patients to watch for onset of early signs of drug-induced vascular insufficiency, such as numbness, coldness, and weakness in extremities, or tingling sensation. Stopping the drug for 2 to 3 days usually overcomes circulatory problems.

▷ 3 Instruct patients that drug is more effective if taken early in an attack. Alert patient to early symptoms of vascular headaches (visual impairment, paresthesias, possible nausea), and advise that the initial dose be taken right away.

▷ 4 Use with caution in elderly patients and in nursing mothers.

▶ **NURSING CONSIDERATIONS**

▷ 1 Suggest that sublingual tablets be used early in an attack because onset of action is more rapid than with oral or parenteral administration.

▷ 2 Caution patients not to increase dosage beyond recommended limit, because adverse reactions are much more common at high dose levels.

▷ 3 Suggest that individual lie down in a dark, quiet room following drug administration, if possible, because relief of pain is often expedited under such conditions.

▷ 4 Assist patient to identify, where possible, underlying

emotional or physical stresses that may precipitate headaches. Advise practicing relaxation techniques, avoiding stressful situations whenever possible, and obtaining adequate rest.
▷ 5 Note that diagnosis of a vascular origin for severe headaches can be confirmed by relief of pain following IM injection of 1 ml (0.5 mg) ergotamine.
▷ 6 Be aware that ergotamine is available in combination with caffeine (*e.g.,* Cafergot), another cerebral vasoconstrictor, and pentobarbital (Cafergot PB), a sedative. These combinations may be more effective than ergotamine alone in some patients, but also increase the incidence of side-effects.

▶ dihydroergotamine
D.H.E. 45

An ergot alkaloid possessing pharmacologic and toxicologic properties similar to those of ergotamine, with a weaker vasoconstrictive and oxytocic action and a slightly lower incidence of nausea and vomiting; given IM in a dose of 1 mg (1 ml), repeated at 1-hour intervals to a total dose of 3 mg, or IV for a more rapid onset in a dose of 1 mg, to be repeated once. Effects occur within 15 minutes to 30 minutes following IM injection, and persist for up to 4 hours.

▶ methysergide
Sansert

Mechanism
Potent blockade of serotonin receptor sites, and weak vasoconstrictor and oxytocic actions; mechanism of action in preventing migraine attacks has not been definitely established; may prolong serotonin-induced constriction of cerebral arteries, thereby reducing pulsations

Uses
1 Prevention or reduction in frequency of vascular (migraine-type) headaches, especially if frequency exceeds one per week or if severity is intense

Dosage
(Not for use in children)
Adult dose: 4 mg to 8 mg daily in divided doses (if no response in 3 weeks, effects are unlikely to develop)
Discontinue drug for 3-week to 4-week intervals every 6 months in patients on long-term therapy.

Fate
Well absorbed orally; onset of optimal effect is 1 to 2 days; metabolic fate not clearly established

Common Side-Effects
GI distress, abdominal pain, drowsiness, lightheadedness, flushing, muscle and joint pains

Significant Adverse Reactions

Fibrotic complications—retroperitoneal fibrosis (associated with fatigue, weight loss, fever, backache, urinary obstruction, lower limb vascular insufficiency), pleural fibrosis (dyspnea, chest tightness, pleural effusion), and cardiac fibrosis (thickening of aortic root, aortic and mitral valves)

Cardiovascular—chest or abdominal pain, numbness in extremities, paresthesias, peripheral edema, postural hypotension, tachycardia, thrombophlebitis, claudication
GI—nausea, vomiting, constipation, increased gastric acid
CNS—insomnia, euphoria, feelings of dissociation, hallucinations, nightmares (may be related to vascular headache and not the drug)
Dermatologic/hematologic—nonspecific rash, telangiectasia, alopecia, neutropenia, eosinophilia
Other—weight gain, weakness, scotomas

Contraindications
Peripheral vascular disease, phlebitis, arteriosclerosis, hypertension, coronary artery disease, pulmonary disease, impaired liver or renal function, collagen diseases, valvular heart disorders, pregnancy, debilitated states, and serious infections

Interactions
1 May decrease the effectiveness of narcotic analgesics
2 Antimigraine effects may be antagonized by cerebral vasodilators (*e.g.,* nylidrin, papaverine)

▶ NURSING ALERTS
▷ 1 Recognize that this is a very dangerous drug, and that fibrotic complications (formation of scar tissue) can occur in any patient on long-term therapy. Use the drug only in very severe or frequent vascular headaches and under strict and intense medical supervision.
▷ 2 Insist that users report the first sign of coldness or numbness in extremities; leg cramps; edema; girdle, flank, or chest pain; dysuria; or other early signs of developing toxicity.
▷ 3 Carefully monitor cardiac status, renal function, blood picture, and pulmonary function during therapy since adverse effects are usually reversible if drug is discontinued early enough.
▷ 4 Do *not* use methysergide for management of acute migraine attacks; it is only a prophylactic agent.
▷ 5 Allow a drug-free interval of 3 weeks to 4 weeks at least every 6 months.
▷ 6 Withdraw drug *gradually* over a 2 week to 3 week period because abrupt discontinuation may cause headache rebound.

▶ NURSING CONSIDERATIONS

▷ 1 Administer drug with meals to reduce GI distress.

▷ 2 Advise patients how to check for edema, and to maintain a low salt intake and adjust caloric intake if weight gain or edema is noticed.

▷ 3 Instruct user to rise slowly from supine position, as orthostatic hypotension can cause dizziness or fainting. Suggest patient lie down with legs elevated if faintness occurs.

▷ 4 Stress the importance of adjunctive measures (*e.g.,* relaxation, proper exercise, sleep, avoidance of stressful situations) in dealing with migraine-type headaches.

▶ trimeprazine
Temaril

Mechanism

Antagonism of the receptor actions of histamine and serotonin; structurally related to the phenothiazines (see Chap. 22); exerts some anticholinergic activity

Uses

1 Relief of pruritus in urticaria and other dermatologic disorders

2 Preoperative sedation in children (investigational)

Dosage

Adults: 2.5 mg 4 times/day or 5 mg every 12 hours

Children: (Over 3 yr) 2.5 mg 3 times/day as needed (½ yr to 3 yr) 1.25 mg 3 times/day)

Fate

Onset of action in 1 hour to 2 hours; sustained-release forms persist for 8 hours to 12 hours; excreted in the urine as metabolites and intact drug

Common Side-Effects

Drowsiness, dryness of the mouth, blurred vision, GI distress, and weakness

Significant Adverse Reactions

Allergic skin reactions, extrapyramidal reactions, orthostatic hypotension, tachycardia, urinary difficulty, blurred vision, respiratory difficulties; see phenothiazines (Chap. 22)

Contraindications

Excess CNS depression, bone marrow depression, newborn or premature infants, pregnancy, acutely ill or dehydrated children

Interactions

1 Anticholinergic effects are intensified by MAO inhibitors, tricyclic antidepressants, thiazide, diuretics.

2 Phenothiazine-related adverse effects may be intensified by reserpine, nylidrin, oral contraceptives, progesterone.

3 Drug may potentiate depressant and analgesic effects of narcotics, barbiturates, alcohol, etc.

▶ NURSING ALERTS

▷ 1 Caution patients to avoid hazardous activities because drug produces marked drowsiness, especially during first few days.

▷ 2 Warn users that depressive effects of other drugs can be potentiated by trimeprazine.

▷ 3 Be alert for possibility of phenothiazine-related toxic effects (see Chap. 22) because drug is a structural analog of the phenothiazines.

▷ 4 Do not use in children with acute illnesses (flu, measles, chicken pox), because danger of adverse effects (especially dystonias) is increased.

▷ 5 Use cautiously in the presence of asthma, narrow-angle glaucoma, cardiovascular disease, liver impairment, ulcers, prostatic hypertrophy, bladder obstruction, and in elderly patients and young children.

▶ NURSING CONSIDERATIONS

▷ 1 Do not use more than the prescribed dose in children because adverse reactions can easily occur.

▷ 2 Be aware that use in elderly patients may produce hypertension, syncope, confusion, and excess sedation.

▷ 3 Use lowest effective dose, because many side-effects appear to be dose-related. Avoid long-acting capsules in children under 6 years of age.

Summary. Antihistamine–Antiserotonin Drugs

Drug	Preparations	Usual Dosage Range
H₁ Receptor Antagonists		
See Table 14-1		
H₂ Receptor Antagonists		
Cimetidine (Tagamet)	Tablets—200 mg, 300 mg, 400 mg	Oral—300 mg 4 to 6 times/day (maximum 2400 mg/day)
	Liquid—300 mg/5 ml	Maintenance—200 mg to 300 mg 1 to 4 times/day or 400 mg at bedtime
	Injection—300 mg/2 ml	

(continued)

Summary. Antihistamine–Antiserotonin Drugs *(continued)*

Drug	Preparations	Usual Dosage Range
		IV injection—300 mg diluted to 20 ml with saline and injected every 6 hr
		IV infusion—300 mg in 100 ml 5% Dextrose every 6 hr (infused over 15 min to 20 min)
Ranitidine (Zantac)	Tablets—150 mg	Adults—150 mg twice a day
Antiserotonin Agents		
Cyproheptadine (Periactin)	Tablets—4 mg Syrup—2 mg/5 ml	Adults—4 mg 3–4 times/day (usual range 12–16 mg/day; maximum 32 mg/day)
		Children—(2 yr–6 yr) 2 mg 2 to 3 times/day; maximum 12 mg/day (7 yr–14 yr) 4 mg 2 to 3 times/day; maximum 16 mg/day
Ergotamine (Ergomar, Ergostat, Gynergen, Medihaler–Ergotamine, Wigrettes)	Tablets—1 mg Sublingual tablets—2 mg Aerosol—9 mg/ml (0.36 mg/dose)	Oral, sublingual—2 mg to 6 mg per attack (maximum 10 mg/week)
		Inhalation—1 inhalation (0.36 mg) 5 minutes apart until pain is relieved (maximum 6 inhalations/day)
Dihydroergotamine (D.H.E. 45)	Injection—1 mg/ml	IM—1 mg at 1-hour intervals to a total of 3 mg
		IV—1 mg; repeat if needed (maximum 2 mg)
Methysergide (Sansert)	Tablets—2 mg	Adults only—4 mg to 8 mg/day (if no effects in 3 weeks, discontinue drug)
		Allow 3 weeks to 4 weeks drug-free interval every 6 months.
Trimeprazine (Temaril)	Tablets—2.5 mg Sustained-release capsules—5 mg Syrup—2.5 mg/5 ml	Adults—2.5 mg 4 times/day or 5 mg every 12 hours
		Children—(over 3 yr) 2.5 mg 3 times/day; (½ yr to 3 yr) 1.25 mg 3 times/day

Skeletal muscle activity can be affected by a diverse group of pharmacologic agents capable of acting either at the neuromuscular junction or at various levels within the spinal cord and brain stem. Those agents that interfere with transmission of cholinergic impulses at the neuromuscular junction generally produce *paralysis* of the skeletal muscles involved. Those drugs that act either directly on the contractile mechanism of the skeletal musculature or on transmission within spinal cord motor reflex pathways primarily elicit varying degrees of skeletal muscle *relaxation.* The agents in the former group are employed principally as adjuncts to general anesthetics and in minor surgical procedures or shock therapy, whereas the agents in the latter group are used to afford a degree of relief from muscle spasms and hyperreflexia resulting from conditions such as inflammation, anxiety, stress, and neurologic disorders.

Based on their site of action, skeletal muscle relaxants may be classified in the following manner:

I. Peripherally acting muscle relaxants
   A. Neuromuscular blocking agents
       1. Antidepolarizing blockers (*e.g.,* tubocurarine, atracurium, gallamine)
       2. Depolarizing blockers (*e.g.,* succinylcholine)
   B. Direct myotropic acting agents
     (*e.g.,* dantrolene)
II. Centrally acting muscle relaxants
    (*e.g.,* carisoprodol, methocarbamol)

Skeletal Muscle Relaxants

15

I Peripherally Acting Muscle Relaxants

A Neuromuscular Blocking Agents

Drugs in this category interfere with the transmission of cholinergic impulses between somatic motor neurons and skeletal muscle fibers—that is, at the neuromuscular junction. Two mechanisms may be involved in the inhibition of transmission at this junction, both involving the postsynaptic receptor site. One group of drugs, typified by d-tubocurarine, functions as *antidepolarizing* agents, competitively antagonizing the action of acetylcholine at the receptor site and preventing depolarization of the postsynaptic membrane. The second group of drugs, exemplified by succinylcholine, acts as *depolarizing* agents, producing an initial activation (depolarization) of the receptor followed by a persistent occupation that markedly delays repolarization, thus blocking further receptor stimulation. These mechanisms are essentially similar to those displayed by the various ganglionic blocking agents, where both antidepolarizing (*e.g.,* trimethaphan) and depolarizing (*e.g.,* nicotine) blocking actions are evident as well.

Neuromuscular blocking agents are essentially anticholinergic agents; however, their specificity for the neuromuscular junction is realized only at normal therapeutic doses. If present in excessive amounts, their cholinergic antagonism may extend to other sites as well, namely autonomic ganglia and postganglionic parasympathetic (atropine-sensitive) endings. This overlapping of effects is responsible for certain untoward reactions exhibited by these drugs at high dose levels (*e.g.,* cardioacceleration, arrhythmias, hypotension). On the other hand, these drugs do not effectively penetrate the blood–brain barrier at therapeutic concentrations, so their CNS effects are minimal. Finally, these agents release histamine from intracellular stores, and the increased levels of circulating histamine may cause varying degrees of bronchospasm, salivary and mucosal secretions, hypotension, and other unwanted effects.

The skeletal muscles are not all equally susceptible to the paralytic effects of neuromuscular blocking agents. The smaller muscles of the eye and eyelids, along with the muscles involved in talking and swallowing, are the first to be affected, followed by progressive weakening of the muscles of the neck and extremities. Fortunately, the muscles of respiration (intercostals, diaphragm) are the most resistant. However, differences in sensitivity among many of the muscles are very slight, and the margin between the effective dose and potentially toxic dose of most neuromuscular blocking drugs is quite small. Therefore, these drugs should only be used by individuals trained and experienced in their use.

Because there is a very small margin between the dose eliciting clinically useful skeletal muscle relaxation and the dose producing muscle paralysis, a slight overdose can result in serious impairment of respiration and marked hypotension. Overdosage with neuromuscular blocking agents is therefore treated by artificial respiration with oxygen and use of vasopressors (*e.g.,* levarterenol). Cholinesterase inhibitors (*e.g.,* edrophonium) can also be employed in cases of poisoning with *anti*depolarizing blockers (tubocurarine, gallamine, metocurine, pancuronium) to overcome the competitive blockade, but the inhibitors are contraindicated in cases of overdosage with depolarizing blockers (*e.g.,* succinylcholine) because they would further stimulate the cholinergic receptors, and thus may intensify the muscle paralysis.

1 Antidepolarizing Blockers

Drugs belonging to the group classified as antidepolarizing blocking agents are also known as nondepolarizing, stabilizing, or curariform drugs. This latter designation derives from the fact that the first antidepolarizing muscle relaxant was the alkaloid d-tubocurarine, the active principle of a group of South American arrow poisons collectively called curare. Several synthetic products have since been developed that all possess, like d-tubocurarine, two quaternary nitrogen molecules approximately 14 Angstrom units apart. These quaternary nitrogen compounds function as reversible competitive antagonists of ACh at the postsynaptic, neuromuscular cholinergic (NII) receptor sites. Skeletal muscle contraction in response to somatic nerve stimulation is therefore blocked, and a temporary state of muscle paralysis develops.

▶ atracurium
(Tracrium)

Mechanism
Blocks cholinergic neurotransmission at the neuromuscular junction by competitively binding to cholinergic receptor sites on the motor end plate; less likely to release histamine than metocurine or d-tubocurarine, and hypotensive effect is less marked

Uses
1 Relaxation of skeletal muscles during surgery, as an adjunct to general anesthesia
2 Facilitation of endotracheal intubation or mechanical ventilation

Dosage
Initially, 0.4 mg/kg to 0.5 mg/kg as an IV bolus injection; maintenance doses during prolonged surgical procedures are 0.08 mg/kg to 0.10 mg/kg given every 20 minutes to 45 minutes

Fate
Maximum neuromuscular blockade occurs within 2 minutes to 5 minutes of IV injection; recovery begins within 20 minutes to 30 minutes and is nearly complete within 1 hour after injection. Time of onset decreases and duration of effect increases with increasing doses; repeated doses have no cumulative effect on the duration of neuromuscular blockade if recommended dosage intervals are followed; rapidly inactivated in the plasma, with an elimination half-life of about 20 minutes; half-life is *not* altered by impaired renal function

Common Side-Effects
(Especially at high doses) Flushing, mild hypotension

Significant Adverse Reactions
(Mostly due to histamine release at high doses) Erythema, itching, urticaria, wheezing, hypotension, tachycardia. Rarely, apnea and cyanosis

Interactions
1 The muscle relaxing action of atracurium can be enhanced by halothane, enflurane, isoflurane, aminoglycosides, polymyxins, lithium, magnesium salts, quinidine, procainamide
2 The muscle relaxing effects of atracurium may be antagonized by cholinergic drugs, cholinesterase inhibitors, and potassium
3 Concurrent administration of succinylcholine with atracurium may accelerate the onset and increase the depth of neuromuscular blockade

▶ NURSING ALERTS
▷ 1 Recognize that atracurium should be used only by personnel skilled in respiratory management. Equipment for endotracheal intubation and respiratory assistance must be readily available.
▷ 2 Administer only with an adequate analgesia, because drug has no effect on consciousness or pain threshold.

▷ 3 Use with caution in patients with conditions in which histamine release may prove hazardous (*e.g.,* bronchial asthma, cardiovascular disease, systemic allergies), in patients with electrolyte disturbances or bradycardia, and in pregnant or nursing women.

▷ 4 Do not administer drug IM, because severe tissue irritation can result.

▶ **NURSING CONSIDERATIONS**

▷ 1 Reduce initial dose by one third if atracurium is first administered under isoflurane or enflurane anesthesia.

▷ 2 Do not give before unconsciousness has been attained.

▷ 3 Note that dosage adjustments are *not* required for children (over 2 years of age); however, more frequent maintenance doses may be required.

▷ 4 Do not mix injection solution with alkaline solutions (*e.g.,* barbiturates) in the same syringe or administer simultaneously during IV infusion through the same needle, because atracurium may be inactivated.

▶ **gallamine**

Flaxedil

Mechanism

Competitive antagonism of ACh at the neuromuscular junction; less potent than d-tubocurarine but has no significant effect on the bronchioles, autonomic ganglia, GI tract, or blood pressure, and does not release histamine

Uses

1 Production of skeletal muscle relaxation as an adjunct to general anesthesia

2 Facilitate management of patients undergoing mechanical ventilation

3 Reduce intensity of muscle contractions during electro- or chemoshock therapy

Dosage

1 mg/kg IV to a maximum of 100 mg; may be reinjected after 30 minutes to 40 minutes at a dose of 0.5 mg/kg to 1 mg/kg depending on patient status

Fate

Onset of action is immediate; maximal effect in 2 minutes to 3 minutes; duration is 20 minutes; drug may accumulate in the body; excreted largely unchanged in urine

Common Side-Effects

Tachycardia, dizziness

Significant Adverse Reactions

(Usually an extension of its pharmacologic action) Profound muscle weakness, respiratory depression, apnea, and hypersensitivity reactions

Contraindications

Myasthenia gravis, shock, impaired renal function, cardiac disease, hypertension, hyperthyroidism, sensitivity to iodides (drug is the triethiodide salt), infants under 11 pounds (5 kg)

Interactions

1 Muscle relaxant effects may be potentiated by inhalation anesthetics, aminoglycoside antibiotics, amphotericin, clindamycin, lincomycin, lithium, potassium-depleting diuretics, antiarrhythmics (quinidine, procainamide, propranolol), phenothiazines, diazepam, calcium and magnesium salts, trimethaphan

2 Effects may be antagonized by cholinergic drugs, anticholinesterases, and potassium

3 Tachycardia may be enhanced by anticholinergic agents (*e.g.,* atropine, phenothiazines, antihistamines, tricyclic antidepressants)

▶ **NURSING ALERTS**

▷ 1 Do not use unless experienced in the proper administration of the drug. Have facilities on hand for intubation, artificial respiration, and oxygen as well as proper antidotes (cholinesterase inhibitors, antihistamines, atropine).

▷ 2 Use very cautiously in the presence of impaired pulmonary, renal, or hepatic function; collagen diseases; history of allergies; and in elderly, debilitated, or pregnant patients.

▷ 3 Perform renal function tests and electrolyte determinations before use because effects may be increased in the presence of hypokalemia, hypermagnesia, or decreased renal clearance capacity.

▷ 4 Monitor vital signs continually until recovery from drug effects is complete. Be aware of possibility of residual muscle weakness caused by accumulation of drug in some individuals.

▷ 5 As with all antidepolarizing blockers, treat overdosage with edrophonium or neostigmine (see Chap. 9), fluid replacement and vasopressors if needed, and respiratory assistance.

▶ **NURSING CONSIDERATIONS**

▷ 1 Inform patient if awake that tachycardia may occur immediately following administration but will decline gradually.

▷ 2 If succinylcholine was used prior to a curariform drug, allow time for effects of succinylcholine to dissipate before giving second drug.

▶ **metocurine**

Metubine

Mechanism

Competitive antagonism of ACh at N-II receptor sites on skeletal muscles; between 2 and 3 times more potent than d-tubocurarine; releases histamine upon IV injection less frequently than d-tubocurarine and produces minimal ganglionic blockage

Uses

1 Adjunct to general anesthesia to produce adequate skeletal muscle relaxation

2 Assist patients undergoing mechanical respiration

3 Reduce intensity of muscle contractions during chemo- and electroshock

Dosage

Size of initial dose dependent on general anesthetic used; usual range 1.5 mg to 7 mg by IV injection over 30 seconds to 60 seconds; repeat at 0.5 mg to 1 mg every 60 minutes

Electroshock: 2 mg to 3 mg IV injected slowly

Fate

Onset within 3 minutes; duration of effect 30 minutes to 90 minutes (average 60 minutes); half-life is 3 hours to 4 hours; excreted rapidly by the kidney, approximately 50% unchanged

Common Side-Effects

Dizziness

Significant Adverse Reactions

Bronchospasm, hypotension, profound muscle weakness, respiratory depression, apnea, circulatory depression, hypersensitivity reactions, and increased secretions

Contraindications

Patients in whom histamine release proves a definite hazard (*e.g.,* asthmatic patients, allergic individuals), myasthenia gravis, and sensitivity to iodides

Interactions

See Gallamine. In addition:

1 Precipitate may form whenever drug is combined with thiopental or methohexital because drug is unstable in alkaline solutions

▶ NURSING ALERTS

See Gallamine. In addition:

▷ 1 Have vasopressors and fluid replacement on hand to combat hypotension should it occur.

▶ NURSING CONSIDERATIONS

See Gallamine. In addition:

▷ 1 Recognize that drug can interfere with the physical signs of anesthesia.

▶ pancuronium

Pavulon

Mechanism

Competitive antagonism of ACh at the neuromuscular junction; approximately 5 times as potent as d-tubocurarine; little ganglionic blockade or histamine release; high doses produce tachycardia and mild hypertension

Uses

1 Adjunct to anesthetics during surgery
2 Assist patients receiving mechanical ventilation

Dosage

Initially 0.04 mg/kg to 0.1 mg/kg IV; increments of 0.01 mg/kg given as needed; chilren's dose same as adults, other than neonates, who should receive a test dose of 0.02 mg/kg to measure sensitivity

Fate

Onset about 1 minute; maximal effects in 5 minutes that persist approximately 60 minutes; excreted largely unchanged by the kidneys

Common Side-Effects

Tachycardia, muscle weakness, and salivation

Significant Adverse Reactions

Profound muscle weakness, apnea, acne-like skin rash, and hypertension

Contraindications

Myasthenia gravis, bromide hypersensitivity, severe coronary artery disease, and other conditions in which tachycardia is undesirable

Interactions

See Gallamine. In addition:

1 Use with cardiac glycosides may result in additive cardiotoxic effects

▶ NURSING ALERTS

See Gallamine. In addition:

▷ 1 Use cautiously in children under 10 years. Use a test dose of 0.02 mg/kg initially in the pediatric age group.

▶ NURSING CONSIDERATIONS

See Gallamine. In addition:

▷ 1 Use an anticholinergic to reduce incidence and extent of salivation during anesthesia.

▷ 2 Drug may be used in operative obstetrics, but be aware that reversal of drug's effects may be delayed in patients receiving magnesium sulfate for convulsions, because magnesium enhances neuromuscular blockade.

▶ tubocurarine

Tubocurarine

Mechanism

Antagonism of cholinergic transmission at N-II receptor sites on skeletal muscle, blocking nerve impulse activation of muscle fibers; possesses ganglionic blocking and histamine-releasing effects

Uses

1 Adjunct to general anesthetics to provide adequate muscle relaxation
2 Reduce intensity of muscle contractions during shock therapy
3 Facilitate management of patients undergoing mechanical ventilation
4 Diagnosis of myasthenia gravis (when results of other tests are inconclusive)

Dosage

Anesthesia: 40 to 60 units (6 mg–9 mg) IV at time of incision; supplements of 20 to 30 units (3 mg–4.5 mg) as needed

Shock therapy: 0.5 units/lb of body weight by slow IV injection prior to shock

Diagnosis of myasthenia: $\frac{1}{15}$ to $\frac{1}{5}$ of average adult electroshock dose IV

Fate

Immediate onset of action; duration of paralysis 30 minutes to 90 minutes; has a cumulative effect in the body; half-life is 1 hour to 3 hours; moderately (40%) bound to plasma proteins; irregular and unpredictable absorption when given IM; excreted largely through the kidney, approximately half in unchanged form

Common Side-Effects

Dizziness, muscle weakness

Significant Adverse Reactions

Bronchospasm, hypotension, profound muscle weakness, respiratory and circulatory depression, hypersensitivity reactions, and malignant hyperthermia

Contraindications

Myasthenia gravis, persons in whom release of histamine is a hazard, hyperthermia, and electrolyte imbalance or acidosis

Interactions

See Gallamine. In addition:

1 Combination with diazepam may cause malignant hyperthermia

▶ NURSING ALERTS

See Gallamine. In addition:

▷ 1 Give injection in a syringe separate from that used for thiopental or methohexital because precipitate will form if drugs are mixed in same syringe.

▷ 2 Regulate dosage carefully, to minimize possibility of untoward reactions due to overdose.

▶ NURSING CONSIDERATIONS

See Gallamine. In addition:

▷ 1 Monitor fluid intake and output to determine renal status because renal dysfunction may greatly prolong and intensify drug effects.

▷ 2 Critically observe patient during diagnostic test for myasthenia (positive response is a clinically apparent increase in muscle weakness), because very small doses can produce an exaggerated response. Have antidotal measures on hand.

▷ 3 Do not administer IM because unpredictable absorption occurs.

▶ vecuronium

Norcuron

Vecuronium is a new antidepolarizing skeletal muscle relaxant producing a rapid onset (2 min to 3 min) and exhibiting an intermediate duration of action (25 min to 40 min). It does not appear to produce significant changes in cardiovascular function at recommended doses, and there-fore may be used in surgical procedures for cardiovascular diseases. Adverse reactions are usually minimal. Vecuronium is administered IV, 0.08 mg/kg to 0.1 mg/kg as an initial bolus injection, followed by 0.01 mg/kg to 0.015 mg/kg at 20 minute to 40 minute intervals.

2 Depolarizing Blockers

The action of the depolarizing neuromuscular blocking agents is a biphasic one—an initial depolarization of the muscle end plate, which produces an immediate but short-lived activation (depolarization) of the muscle fibers followed by a persistent occupation of the receptor site; this prevents repolarization and essentially desensitizes the receptor site to ACh. This "second phase" block persists for 10 minutes to 30 minutes depending upon the drug and dose used. During this time, the muscle remains paralyzed to motor nerve stimulation. The major difference between these drugs and the antidepolarizing blockers discussed previously is that due to the initial depolarization phase, transient muscle contractions (fasciculations) occur immediately following administration of the depolarizing drug. Contractions are followed rapidly by a flaccid paralysis similar to that observed with the antidepolarizing agents. There is also some evidence that the neuromuscular blockade following a depolarizing drug may persist beyond the actual presence of the drug at the receptor; this suggests the possibility of desensitization of the receptor caused by conformational changes of the reactive area.

▶ succinylcholine

Anectine, Quelicin, Sucostrin, Sux-Cert

Mechanism

Depolarizing neuromuscular blockade, producing initial muscle contraction (fasciculations), followed quickly by flaccid paralysis; rapidly hydrolyzed by plasma cholinesterase enzyme, limiting duration of action of a single dose to a maximum of 10 minutes

Uses

1 Skeletal muscle relaxation as an adjunct to general anesthesia

2 Reduce the intensity of muscle contractions during shock therapy

3 Facilitate intubation procedures

4 Assist mechanical respiration

Dosage

Adults: 20 mg to 80 mg IV injection (test dose of 10 mg may be given initially to determine patient sensitivity)

IV infusion: (for prolonged procedures) 2.5 mg/min of a 0.1% or 0.2% solution

IM: 2.5 mg/kg to a maximum of 150 mg

Children: 1 mg/kg to 2 mg/kg IV injection

Fate

Onset following IV use within 1 minute; maximum effects last 2 minutes to 4 minutes, and return to normal within 8 minutes to 10 minutes; quickly hydrolyzed by plasma cholinesterases; onset with IM injection 2 minutes to 3 minutes; duration 10 minutes to 20 minutes; excreted through kidneys, both as metabolites and small amounts of unchanged drug

Common Side-Effects
Muscle twitching, bradycardia

Significant Adverse Reactions
Muscle weakness, bronchospasm, apnea, hypotension, arrhythmias, increased salivation, postoperative muscle pain, hyperthermia, rash, increased intraocular pressure, myoglobinemia, enlarged salivary glands, and GI atony

Contraindications
History of malignant hyperthermia, severe respiratory depression, acute narrow-angle glaucoma, penetrating eye injury, and genetically determined deficiency of plasma pseudocholinesterase

Interactions
1   Effects may be prolonged and intensified by drugs that interfere with the action of the cholinesterase enzyme, *e.g.,* cholinesterase inhibitors (see Chap. 9), cyclophosphamide, thiotepa, MAO inhibitors, procaine, and antimalarial drugs
2   Muscle relaxant effects may be enhanced by aminoglycoside antibiotics, amphotericin, beta-blockers, clindamycin, lidocaine, lincomycin, lithium, magnesium salts, oxytocin, quinidine, potassium-depleting diuretics, procainamide, procaine, and trimethaphan
3   Cardiac arrhythmias may develop in the presence of digitalis glycosides
4   Diazepam can reduce the duration of action of succinylcholine

▶ NURSING ALERTS
▷ 1   Be aware that overdosage can cause complete respiratory paralysis for which oxygen with artificial respiration is the only effective antidote. Do *not* use cholinesterase inhibitors in overdosage, because increased muscle paralysis can occur.
▷ 2   Note that the actions of the drug can be intensified by dehydration, hypothermia, renal disease, carcinomas, and electrolyte imbalances (especially potassium, calcium, and magnesium).
▷ 3   Use cautiously in the presence of respiratory depression, impaired renal function, severe burns, fractures, muscle spasms, and in elderly, debilitated, or recently digitalized patients.
▷ 4   Monitor vital signs during and immediately following administration. Keep airway clear of secretions. Be alert for postprocedural muscle weakness, and assist patient as necessary.
▷ 5   Use only freshly prepared solutions; succinylcholine is rapidly hydrolyzed in solution and quickly loses potency.
▷ 6   Use cautiously in the presence of cardiovascular, hepatic, pulmonary, renal, or metabolic diseases, glaucoma, insecticide poisoning, anemia, malnutrition.
▷ 7   Be aware that transient apnea can occur at onset of

maximal effect. If spontaneous respiration does not return within a few minutes, initiate controlled respiration with oxygen.
▷ 8   Do not use together with an antidepolarizing blocker, because prolonged effects can occur.
▷ 9   Do not mix succinylcholine with solutions of barbiturates or other alkaline drugs because incompatibility will result.

▶ NURSING CONSIDERATIONS
▷ 1   Observe for development of tachyphylaxis (loss of drug response) with repeated use.
▷ 2   Inform patient that muscle pain and stiffness may be present for some time following recovery, due to the initial stimulatory response.
▷ 3   Make sure proper facilities are available for treating respiratory distress. Drug should be given only by those trained in its proper usage.
▷ 4   To avoid patient distress, administer only after unconsciousness has been attained with anesthetic.
▷ 5   Monitor body temperature during administration because drug may precipitate malignant hyperthermia, especially in presence of general anesthetics.
▷ 6   Consider measuring plasma cholinesterase levels prior to administration because low levels may potentiate and prolong effects of succinylcholine.
▷ 7   Note that drug is initially metabolized to succinylmonocholine, a weaker-acting blocker. Because this compound is slowly hydrolyzed, it can accumulate following prolonged or high doses and produce prolonged paralysis.
▷ 8   When drug is given IM, inject deep into muscle, preferably the deltoid. A small test dose can be given initially to determine sensitivity to drug.
▷ 9   To enhance and prolong neuromuscular blockade and prevent muscle fasciculations, administer hexafluorenium (see below) prior to succinylcholine.

---

3   Plasma Cholinesterase Inhibitor

▶ hexafluorenium
Mylaxen

Mechanism
Reversible inhibition of plasma cholinesterases; does not affect intracellular cholinesterase as do other cholinesterase inhibitors; exclusively used with succinylcholine to delay enzymatic hydrolysis

Uses
1   Prolong succinylcholine-induced muscle relaxation, and reduce initial muscle fasciculations

Dosage
0.4 mg/kg IV 3 minutes before a dose of succinylcholine (0.2 mg/kg)

In long surgical procedures, may repeat at doses of 0.1 mg/kg to 0.2 mg/kg at necessary intervals, *e.g.,* 60 minutes to 90 minutes

Fate

Onset of action is rapid (2 min–3 min); duration is approximately 30 minutes and is unaffected by general anesthetic

Common Side-Effects

Salivation, slight bradycardia

Significant Adverse Reactions

(Characteristic of cholinesterase inhibitors) Bronchospasm, hypotension, arrhythmias, hyperthermia, increased intraocular pressure, respiratory depression, apnea, and prolonged and profound muscle paralysis

Contraindications

Bromide hypersensitivity

Interactions

1 Effects of other muscle relaxants can be enhanced if hexafluorenium–succinylcholine combination is used

▶ NURSING ALERTS

▷ 1 Do not administer if facilities for artificial respiration, intubation, and oxygen are not immediately available.

▷ 2 Because drug can potentiate succinylcholine, use with caution in all instances in which succinylcholine is hazardous.

▶ NURSING CONSIDERATIONS

▷ 1 Determine plasma cholinesterase prior to administration, and avoid using the drug if titers of cholinesterase are low or pattern is atypical.

▷ 2 Do not exceed 36 mg of hexafluorenium for an initial dose, even if patient's weight is greater than 90 kg (200 lb).

B Direct Myotropic Acting Blocking Agent

A different type of peripherally acting skeletal muscle relaxant is typified by the drug dantrolene; unlike the classical neuromuscular blocking agents, dantrolene does not interfere with transmission of impulses between somatic motor nerves and skeletal muscle. Its action appears to be the consequence of a direct effect on the skeletal muscle fibers to interfere with their contractile mechanisms. Specifically, the drug retards the release of a contraction-activating substance, probably calcium, from its binding sites in the sarcoplasmic reticulum. Dantrolene is available in oral form for treatment of muscle spasticity resulting from chronic neurologic disorders such as cerebral palsy, multiple sclerosis, or stroke, and as an IV injection for the emergency management of malignant hyperthermia such as that resulting from general anesthesia.

▶ dantrolene

Dantrium

Mechanism

Direct relaxation of skeletal muscle fibers, due to interference with the release of calcium ions from the sarcoplasmic reticulum; impairs catabolism within muscle cells by blocking increases in myoplasmic calcium, and therefore prevents the abnormal rise in body temperature; may possess some central nervous system action as well, resulting in drowsiness, dizziness, and weakness

Uses

1 Relief of muscle spasticity associated with chronic neurologic disorders, *e.g.,* cerebral palsy, stroke, spinal cord injury, or multiple sclerosis (most effective where spasticity is painful and limits muscle performance)

2 Emergency treatment of malignant hyperthermia (IV injection)

3 Preoperative prophylaxis of malignant hyperthermia in high-risk patients (orally)

Dosage

Muscle spasticity

Adults: Initially 25 mg orally once daily; increase gradually in 25-mg increments to a maximum of 100 mg 2 to 4 times/day; maintain each dose for 4 to 7 days before increasing

Children: Initially 0.5 mg/kg orally twice a day; increase by 0.5 mg/kg increments to a maximum of 3 mg/kg 2 to 4 times/day

Malignant hyperthermia

Treatment: initially, 1 mg/kg IV; if abnormalities persist or reappear, repeat up to a cumulative dose of 10 mg/kg; usual required dose is 2 mg/kg to 5 mg/kg

Prophylaxis: 4 mg/kg to 8 mg/kg/day orally in 3 to 4 divided doses for 1 to 2 days prior to surgery (last dose given 3 hr to 4 hr before start of surgery)

Fate

Oral absorption is slow and incomplete but consistent; significantly bound to plasma proteins; optimal effects may take several days to become manifest; half-life is 8 hours to 9 hours with oral administration and 5 hours following IV injection; metabolized primarily in the liver, and both metabolites and unaltered drug are excreted in the urine

Common Side-Effects (Oral Use Only)

Drowsiness, dizziness, weakness, malaise, fatigue, and diarrhea

Significant Adverse Reactions (Oral Use Only)

GI—constipation, bleeding, cramping, anorexia, difficulty in swallowing, gastric irritation, severe diarrhea

CNS—headache, lightheadedness, insomnia, visual and speech disturbances, taste alterations, seizures, depression, confusion, nervousness

Cardiovascular—tachycardia, phlebitis, erratic blood pressure

Urinary—urinary frequency, crystalluria, incontinence, nocturia, urinary retention, impotence

Dermatologic—abnormal hair growth, rash, pruritus, urticaria, eczema-like reaction, photosensitization

Other—hepatitis, backache, myalgia, tearing, chills, fever, respiratory distress

Contraindications

Hepatic disease, children under 5, conditions in which spasticity is necessary to sustain upright position or balance

Interactions

1 Estrogens may increase the danger of hepatotoxicity
2 CNS depression may be potentiated by other tranquilizing agents
3 Warfarin and clofibrate reduce the protein binding of dantrolene and may potentiate its effects

▶ NURSING ALERTS

▷ 1 Recognize that the drug has a potential for serious hepatotoxicity, especially with long-term therapy (over 60 days). Use only in conjunction with appropriate and frequent monitoring of hepatic function (e.g., SGOT, SGPT, alkaline phosphatase, total bilirubin).

▷ 2 Urge patients to be alert for appearance of skin rash, itching, black or bloody stools, and yellowish skin discoloration, and report these developments immediately.

▷ 3 Discontinue drug if no observable benefit occurs within 45 days, because the danger of liver damage increases with prolonged use.

▷ 4 Use with caution in the presence of impaired pulmonary function, cardiac impairment caused by myocardial disease, hepatic dysfunction, and in pregnant or lactating women.

▷ 5 Caution patient that drowsiness is likely to occur in early stages of therapy, and to avoid hazardous situations (e.g., driving or operating machinery).

▶ NURSING CONSIDERATIONS

▷ 1 If improvement is subtle, it may be confirmed by withdrawing drug for 2 days to 4 days. Watch for signs of exacerbation of spasticity, an indication that the drug is providing some clinical benefit.

▷ 2 Use the lowest effective dose in all cases, and closely observe the patient for any signs of developing toxicity.

▷ 3 Assist patient in developing a total therapeutic regimen, including an exercise program, and use of proper braces if needed. Provide support and encouragement, inform user that beneficial effects may be delayed 1 week to 2 weeks, but conversely, that side-effects will gradually lessen with time.

▷ 4 Advise patients to avoid prolonged exposure to sunlight, because photosensitivity reactions can occur.

II Centrally Acting Muscle Relaxants

Baclofen	Cyclobenzaprine
Carisoprodol	Metaxalone
Chlorphenesin	Methocarbamol
Chlorzoxazone	Orphenadrine

The aim of the centrally acting skeletal muscle relaxants is to produce decreased muscle tone and involuntary movement without loss of voluntary motor function or consciousness. Many CNS depressants (e.g., alcohol, barbiturates) elicit varying degrees of muscle relaxation but are of little use clinically because they also produce marked sedation and other undesirable effects. Attempts to dissociate this CNS depressant action from the muscle-relaxing effect by synthesis of various centrally acting muscle relaxants has met with very limited success, and all currently useful central muscle relaxants evoke a degree of sedation that makes long-term use of these drugs undesirable.

Agents in this class have been termed *interneuronal* or *polysynaptic* blocking drugs, such designations offering an explanation of their mechanism of action. These compounds act at various levels within the CNS (i.e., brain stem or spinal cord interneurons) to depress synaptic transmission in motor reflex pathways. They appear to exert a weak synaptic blocking action between neurons of these motor circuits, the degree of impairment being proportional to the number of synapses involved in the pathway. Their principal advantage over neuromuscular blockers is their oral efficacy; the major disadvantage, of course, is the sedation and sensorimotor impairment that accompanies their use.

With the exception of baclofen and diazepam (see Chap. 23), the drugs comprising the centrally acting muscle relaxants are remarkably similar in their pharmacology and toxicology. No one agent possesses a significant therapeutic advantage over any other agent, and for the most part, choice of a drug is a personal preference.

Because these drugs share many common properties, they will be discussed as a group. Individual drugs are then described in Table 15-1.

Mechanism

Interference with transmission of impulses in polysynaptic motor reflex pathways at the level of the spinal cord, brain stem, and probably basal ganglia; no effect on contractile mechanism of muscle fibers or on the motor end plate of skeletal muscles; CNS depressant action probably contributes as well to the muscle-relaxant effect; baclofen and diazepam also appear to facilitate the action of GABA, an inhibitory neurotransmitter, in the brain stem and at the level of spinal cord interneurons

Uses

1 Relief of pain and discomfort of muscle spasms associated with acute musculoskeletal disorders, e.g., inflammatory states, peripheral injury (sprains, strains), connective tissue disorders
2 Alleviation of spasticity resulting from multiple sclerosis, spinal cord disease, and other neurologic conditions (baclofen and diazepam only)

Dosage

See Table 15-1.

Fate

Well absorbed orally; maximum effects usually occur in 1 hour to 4 hours, and persist for several hours; most of

Table 15-1. Centrally Acting Skeletal Muscle Relaxants

Drug	Preparations	Usual Dosage Range	Remarks
Baclofen (Lioresal)	Tablets—10 mg, 20 mg	5 mg 3 times/day; increase by 5 mg every 3 days to optimal effect (maximum 80 mg/day)	Primarily used for relief of spasticity due to multiple sclerosis or spinal cord diseases; sedation is usually transient; absorption is variable and reduced at higher doses; may increase urinary frequency; do not use in patients with stroke, or rheumatic disorders, in children under 12, pregnant women, nursing mothers; cautious use in epileptics, and in presence of renal impairment; reduce dose slowly to avoid possibility of hallucinations on abrupt withdrawal; may alter laboratory tests for SGOT, alkaline phosphatase, and blood sugar
Carisoprodol (Rela, Soma, Soprodol)	Tablets—350 mg	350 mg 4 times/day	Also available in combination with aspirin as Soma Compound; contraindicated in acute intermittent porphyria, children under 12, and meprobamate sensitivity; allergic reactions can develop to early doses (rash, erythema, pruritus, eosinophilia); stop drug and treat symptomatically; carefully monitor urine output and avoid overhydration; use cautiously in addiction-prone individuals
Chlorphenesin (Maolate)	Tablets—400 mg	Initially 800 mg 3 times/day; may reduce to 400 mg 3 to 4 times/day if effective	Do not use in pregnancy, children, liver disease, or for periods exceeding 8 weeks; discontinue at first sign of allergic reaction; paradoxical excitation may occur but is usually controlled by dosage reduction
Chlorzoxazone (Paraflex)	Tablets—250 mg	Adults—250 mg to 500 mg 3 to 4 times/day; reduce gradually as improvement is noted. Children—125 mg to 500 mg 3 to 4 times/day; may be crushed and mixed with food or other vehicle	Also available with acetaminophen as Parafon Forte and others; use cautiously in pregnancy, history of drug allergy, hepatic dysfunction; may discolor urine, but is *not* nephrotoxic; give with meals to minimize GI irritation
Cyclobenzaprine (Flexeril)	Tablets—10 mg	10 mg 3 times/day to a maximum of 60 mg/day (not in children under 15)	Do not use for longer than 2 weeks to 3 weeks; *not* effective in spasticity due to cerebral or spinal cord disease or cerebral palsy; contraindicated in hyperthyroidism, arrhythmias, congestive heart failure, acute recovery phase of myocardial infarction, or with MAO inhibitors; similar to tricyclic antidepressants in action (see Chap. 24), and may have similar central effects; high incidence of drowsiness, dry mouth, and dizziness; possesses anticholinergic activity, responsible for atropine-like side effects and interactions (see Chap. 10); caution in glaucoma and urinary retention
Metaxalone (Skelaxin)	Tablets—400 mg	800 mg 3 to 4 times/day (not in children under 12)	Contraindicated in anemia, renal or hepatic impairment, nursing mothers; liver function studies should be done regularly; cautious use in epilepsy, pregnancy, allergic states; GI upset is common as is headache, nervousness and irritability; may interfere with Benedict's and cephalin flocculation tests

(continued)

Table 15-1. Centrally Acting Skeletal Muscle Relaxants (continued)

Drug	Preparations	Usual Dosage Range	Remarks
Methocarbamol (Delaxin, Marbaxin-750, Metho-500, Robaxin)	Tablets—500 mg, 750 mg Injection—100 mg/ml	Oral: Adults—1.5 gm 4 times/day initially; reduce to 750 mg to 1000 mg 4 times a day Children—60 to 75 mg/kg/day IM: 0.5 gm to 1 gm every 8 hours IV: 300 mg/min to a total daily dose of 1 gm to 3 gm for maximum 3 days IV infusion: 1 gm (10 ml) diluted to 250 ml saline or 5% dextrose given by IV drip Tetanus—1 gm to 3 gm directly into IV tubing every 6 hours (Children 15 mg/kg every 6 hours)	IV use may control neuromuscular manifestations of tetanus; substitute oral administration as soon as possible; avoid extravasation, because irritation and thrombophlebitis can result; do *not* give SC; contraindicated in renal dysfunction (vehicle may cause acidosis and urea retention), children under 12, epilepsy (especially IV); keep patient recumbent during and at least 15 minutes after IV usage, to minimize orthostatic hypotension and other side-effects; may interfere with laboratory tests for 5-HIAA and VMA; too-rapid IV injection may cause CNS side-effects (*e.g.*, dizziness, vertigo, syncope, headache, blurred vision) as well as bradycardia, hypotension, flushing, and anaphylactic reaction; cautious use in myasthenia gravis; check IV infusion for proper flow to minimize danger of thrombophlebitis and sloughing; may darken urine; also available with aspirin as Robaxisal
Orphenadrine Citrate (Banflex, Flexon, Flexoject, K-Flex, Marflex, Myolin, Norflex, O'Flex, X-Otag)	Tablets—100 mg Sustained-release tablets—100 mg Injection—30 mg/ml	Oral: 100 mg twice a day IV, IM: 60 mg every 12 hours	Available with aspirin and caffeine as Norgesic; strong anticholinergic with high incidence of atropine-like side effects (see Chap. 10); contraindicated in glaucoma, myasthenia, duodenal obstruction, ulcers, prostatic hypertrophy, bladder obstruction, pregnancy, children; periodic monitoring of blood, urine, and liver function recommended with prolonged use; caution in urinary retention, tachycardia, coronary insufficiency, arrhythmias; also available as the HCl salt (Disipal) for control of parkinsonism (see Chap. 26)

these drugs are metabolized by the liver and are excreted in the urine

Common Side-Effects

Drowsiness, fatigue, dizziness, lightheadedness, dry mouth, and GI upset; in addition, other anticholinergic side-effects (*e.g.*, blurred vision, urinary hesitancy) are common with cyclobenzaprine and orphenadrine.

Significant Adverse Reactions

(Not all effects noted with all drugs)

GI—anorexia, nausea, diarrhea, hiccups, bleeding, abdominal pain

CNS—ataxia, headache, blurred vision, insomnia, confusion, irritability, paresthesias

Cardiovascular—tachycardia, hypotension, flushing, petechiae, thrombophlebitis, chest pain, palpitations, syncope

Urinary—urinary retention, dysuria, enuresis

Hematologic—leukopenia, pancytopenia, thrombocytopenia, agranulocytosis, hemolytic anemia

Hypersensitivity—rash, erythema, pruritus, fever, asthma-like reaction, dermatoses, angioedema, anaphylactic reactions

Hepatic—abnormal liver function tests, jaundice

Respiratory—nasal congestion, dyspnea

Other—dysarthria, dyspepsia, tremors, euphoria, metallic taste, pain or sloughing at site of injection, increased intraocular tension, conjunctivitis, tinnitus, slurred speech

Contraindications

See Table 15-1.

Interactions

1 CNS depressive effects of centrally acting muscle relaxants and other CNS depressants (*e.g.*, alcohol, barbiturates, narcotics, antianxiety agents) are additive

2 MAO inhibitors may increase the toxicity of cyclobenzaprine

3 Atropine-like side-effects can be intensified by use of anticholinergic drugs with cyclobenzaprine and orphenadrine

4 Cyclobenzaprine may interfere with the antihypertensive action of guanethidine and similarly acting compounds

▶ **NURSING ALERTS**

(For additional information, see Table 15-1.)

▷ 1 Caution patients against engaging in any hazardous activity while taking these drugs because drowsiness is common and often marked.

▷ 2 Advise patient to avoid concomitant use of other CNS depressants while taking one of these drugs.

▷ 3 Use drugs cautiously in presence of hepatic or renal dysfunction, respiratory depression, and in young children, pregnant or lactating women, and the elderly or debilitated.

▷ 4 Inform user to immediately report signs of developing hepatotoxicity (*e.g.,* abdominal pain, high fever, nausea, diarrhea) or blood dyscrasias (*e.g.,* fever, sore throat, malaise, mucosal ulceraton, petechiae).

▶ **NURSING CONSIDERATIONS**

(For additional information, see Table 15-1.)

▷ 1 Advise patients to take last dose at bedtime, because drowsiness may aid sleep.

▷ 2 Be aware that due to CNS effects of the compounds, prolonged use may lead to dependence. Abrupt termination of the drug in these patients may evoke withdrawal symptoms (cramping, nausea, chills, weakness).

▷ 3 Note that potency of the drugs is enhanced when given IV or IM. Reduce dosage according to instructions.

Summary. Skeletal Muscle Relaxants

Drug	Preparations	Usual Dosage Range
Peripheral Neuromuscular Blockers		
1. Antidepolarizing Agents		
Atracurium (Tracrium)	Injection—10 mg/ml	Initially—0.4 mg/kg to 0.5 mg/kg IV bolus injection; maintenance dose is 0.08 mg/kg to 0.10 mg/kg at 15 minute to 30 minute intervals as needed
Gallamine (Flaxedil)	Injection—20 mg/ml	1 mg/kg IV (maximum 100 mg); repeat as needed (0.5 mg/kg–1 mg/kg) every 30 minutes to 40 minutes
Metocurine (Metubine)	Injection—2 mg/ml	1.5 mg to 7 mg IV over 30 seconds to 60 seconds depending on anesthetic used; repeat as needed (0.5 mg–1 mg) every 60 minutes
Pancuronium (Pavulon)	Injection—1 mg/ml, 2 mg/ml	Initially—0.04 to 0.1 mg/kg IV; may supplement with 0.01 mg/kg as needed (children other than neonates: same as adults)
Tubocurarine (Tubocurarine)	Injection—3 mg/ml	Anesthesia adjunct—40 to 60 units (6 mg–9 mg) IV initially, followed by supplements of 20 units to 30 units (3 mg to 4.5 mg) as needed
		Electroshock—0.5 unit/lb body weight IV over 60 seconds to 90 seconds prior to shock.
		Diagnosis of myasthenia—$\frac{1}{15}$ to $\frac{1}{5}$ of adult electroshock dose, IV
Vecuronium (Norcuron)	Powder for injection— 10 mg/5 ml vial	Initially—0.08 mg/kg to 0.1 mg/kg as an IV bolus; then 0.01 mg/kg to 0.015 mg/kg at 20 minute to 40 minute intervals
2. Depolarizing Agents		
Succinylcholine (Anectine, Quelicin, Sucostrin, Sux-Cert)	Injection—20 mg/ml, 50 mg/ml, 100 mg/ml Powder—500 mg/unit, 1000 mg/unit	Adults—20 mg to 80 mg IV injection individualized to patient IV infusion—2.5 mg/min of a 0.1% to 0.2% solution IM—2.5 mg/kg to a maximum of 150 mg Children—1 to 2 mg/kg IV injection
3. Cholinesterase Inhibitor		
Hexafluorenium (Mylaxen)	Injection—20 mg/ml	IV—0.4 mg/kg 3 minutes prior to 0.2 mg/kg succinylcholine; repeat at doses of 0.1 mg/kg to 0.2 mg/kg as needed in prolonged surgical procedures, at intervals of 60 minutes to 90 minutes

(continued)

Summary. Skeletal Muscle Relaxants *(continued)*

Drug	Preparations	Usual Dosage Range
Direct Myotropic Acting Blocker		
Dantrolene (Dantrium)	Capsules—25 mg, 50 mg, 100 mg Powder for injection—20 mg/vial	Muscle Spasticity: Adults—Initially 25 mg orally daily; increase to a maximum of 100 mg 2 to 4 times/day in 25-mg increments every 4 to 7 days Children—Initially 1 mg/kg daily; increase by 0.5 mg/kg increments to a maximum of 3 mg/kg 2 to 4 times/day Hyperthermia: Treatment: Initially, 1 mg/kg IV; may repeat up to a cumulative dose of 10 mg/kg Prophylaxis: 4 mg/kg/day to 8 mg/kg/day orally in 3 to 4 divided doses for 1 to 2 days prior to surgery (last dose 3 hr–4 hr before start of surgery)

Centrally Acting Muscle Relaxants

See Table 15-1

Local anesthetic agents have the ability to reversibly block conduction of impulses along all sensory, motor, and autonomic nerve fibers. Loss of sensation may be accompanied by other physiologic changes as well, such as muscle relaxation (motor nerve paralysis) and hypotension (sympathetic nerve blockade). When these agents are administered in the region of mixed nerve fibers, differential effects with respect to onset and recovery are observed, depending on the size and state of myelination of the nerve fibers. In general, small, nonmyelinated C fibers (*e.g.,* dorsal root and sympathetic postganglionic) mediating pain and vasoconstrictor impulses are affected first by local anesthetics, followed by the small, myelinated A-delta fibers mediating pain and temperature. Larger fibers carrying sensory impulses (*e.g.,* A-alpha, A-beta) are blocked next, and finally motor nerves (*e.g.,* A-gamma) are anesthetized, resulting in decreased skeletal muscle tone. Recovery proceeds in the opposite direction—motor function is restored before sensory function.

Although the predominant effects of local anesthetics are confined to the circumscribed area adjacent to the injection or application site, systemic absorption does occur to varying degrees, and may produce undesirable reactions. Large doses or inadvertent *intravascular* injection of local anesthetics may result in cardiovascular effects, such as hypotension or cardiac depression, or central nervous system effects, such as stimulation and convulsions followed by depression. Systemic absorption of local anesthetics can be minimized by addition of a local vasoconstrictor (*e.g.,* 1:200,000 epinephrine) to the injection solution; this constricts the vessels in the immediate area and prevents spread of the administrered anesthetic. Vasoconstrictors also prolong the duration of action of local anesthetics, reduce the amount of drug needed, and may help slow local hemorrhaging if surgery is performed.

A local anesthetic must be able to penetrate the nerve membrane to exert its effects, and therefore must be in the un-ionized state. Because most drugs are injected in the form of water-soluble, cationic salts, they must be converted to the free base (nonionic, lipid-soluble form) before they can reach their sites of action within the nerve fiber. This is facilitated by the *p*H of the extracellular fluid spaces. Evidence now indicates that once the drug is at the site of action, the *active* form of the drug may be the original cationic state, and thus the molecule must revert to this form once again to exert a local anesthetic action. Local anesthetics stabilize the nerve membrane potential by decreasing its permeability to sodium. This action may be accomplished by competing with calcium ions bound to phospholipids for a site in the nerve membrane that controls the passage of sodium across the membrane and into the cell. The drugs thus block the initial event in the generation of an action potential, namely depolarization.

Classification of local anesthetics can be based either on chemical structure or principal clinical usage. Structurally, most local anesthetic drugs belong to one of three categories:

1 Esters of benzoic or aminobenzoic acid (*e.g.,* procaine, tetracaine)
2 Amides (*e.g.,* lidocaine, bupivacaine)
3 Ethers (*e.g.,* pramoxine, dimethisoquin)

Local anesthetics have several clinical applications, both topically and parenterally, and thus can also be classified as follows:

1 *Surface anesthetics* (skin, mucous membrane, eye, ear—*e.g.,* benzocaine, butacaine, cocaine)
2 *Infiltration anesthetics* (local intradermal or subcutaneous injection—*.e.g.,* procaine, lidocaine)
3 *Spinal anesthetics* (subarachnoid injection—*e.g.,* tetracaine, dibucaine)
4 *Epidural anesthetics* (injection into area surrounding the dura mater of spinal cord—*e.g.,* lidocaine, mepivacaine)

The general pharmacology and clinical implications of local anesthetics are discussed as a group. Specific characteristics of individual drugs are then detailed in Table 16-1 along with prescribing information and available preparations.

Local Anesthetics

Benoxinate	Dyclonine
Benzocaine	Etidocaine
Bupivacaine	Hexylcaine
Butamben	Lidocaine
Chloroprocaine	Mepivacaine
Cocaine	Pramoxine
Cyclomethycaine	Prilocaine
Dibucaine	Procaine
Dimethisoquin	Proparacaine
Diperodon	Tetracaine

Mechanism
Stabilization of neurons by blocking passage of sodium ions across the membrane; prevent initial depolarization and generation of nerve action potential; compete with calcium for a site on the nerve membrane controlling the passage of sodium, thus blocking propagation of the nerve impulse

Uses
(See Table 16-1 for indications for individual drugs)
1 Relief of pain, soreness, irritation, and itching associated with various skin and mucous membrane disorders, *e.g.,* minor burns, rashes, wounds, allergic conditions, fungus infections, skin ulcers, hemorrhoids, fissures
2 Production of corneal and conjunctival anesthesia to facilitate ophthalmic procedures, such as tonometry, gonioscopy, removal of foreign bodies, and minor ocular surgery
3 Production of infiltration, nerve block, spinal, epidural, or caudal anesthesia in surgery, obstetrics, or dental work
4 Management of cardiac arrhythmias (see Chap. 30)

Dosage
See Table 16-1.

Fate
(See Table 16-1 for specific information)
Absorption is largely dependent on site of administration, dose, degree of vasoconstriction, and blood flow to the area. Onset of action is usually rapid; duration is variable and following injection may range from 1 hour (procaine) to 4 to 6 hours (bupivacaine). Some agents are rapidly hydrolyzed by plasma cholinesterases (*e.g.,* procaine) or liver enzymes (*e.g.,* lidocaine), while others are more resistant to inactivation. Excreted primarily in the urine mainly as metabolites, but some unchanged drug as well.

Common Side-Effects
Topical—sensitization reactions, stinging or burning in the eyes
Injection—(rare at low doses) slight hypotension, anxiety

Significant Adverse Reactions
(Vary from drug to drug)
Topical—hyperallergenic corneal reaction, keratitis, corneal opacities, allergic contact dermatitis with fissuring of fingertips, urticaria, cutaneous lesions, edema, anaphylactic reactions, urethritis with swelling, irritation, sloughing, and necrosis
Injection—(mainly due to systemic absorption) CNS stimulation (dizziness, blurred vision, confusion, irritability, tinnitus, convulsions, tremors) followed by CNS depression (drowsiness, unconsciousness, respiratory arrest), difficulty in speaking, hearing, swallowing, or breathing, muscle twitching, hypotension, myocardial depression, bradycardia, cardiac arrest
Epidural or caudal injection may provoke spinal block, urinary retention, incontinence, loss of sexual function, paresthesias, headache, or backache.
Spinal anesthesia may cause hypotension, severe headache or backache, respiratory depression, or nerve root damage.

Contraindications
Topical—history of allergic reactions
Injection—history of hyersensitivity, severe infection, and heart block
In addition, prilocaine is contraindicated in methemoglobinemia (see also Table 16-1).

Interactions
1 Certain anesthetic drugs (*e.g.,* lidocaine) may enhance muscle-relaxing effects of neuromuscular blocking agents.
2 Additive cardiac depressant effects may occur when some local anesthetics and other cardiac depressant drugs (*e.g.,* quinidine, propranolol, phenytoin) are given together.
3 Solutions of local anesthetics containing a vasoconstrictor can produce blood pressure alterations in combination with MAO inhibitors, tricyclic antidepressants, phenothiazines, and pressor agents.
4 Vasoconstrictors in local anesthetic solutions may precipitate arrhythmias in combination with halothane and related general anesthetics.

Table 16-1. Local Anesthetics

Drug	Preparations	Usual Dosage Range	Remarks
Benoxinate (Dorsacaine)	Drops—0.4%	Tonometry and removal of sutures and foreign bodies—1 to 2 drops before operation Ophthalmic anesthesia—2 drops 90 seconds apart for 3 instillations	Short acting anesthetic, with possible bacteriostatic action; does not affect pupil size or accommodation, and produces minimal toxicity; low incidence of stinging and burning
Benoxinate and Fluorescein (Fluress)	Drops—0.4% benoxinate and 0.25% sodium fluorescein	Tonometry and removal of sutures and foreign bodies—1 to 2 drops before operation Ophthalmic anesthesia—2 drops 90 seconds apart for 3 instillations	Combination of a short-acting anesthetic and a disclosing agent to highlight abraded, ulcerated or otherwise damaged areas; does not affect pupil size or accommodation and has a low incidence of burning and stinging
Benzocaine (Various manufacturers)	Ointment—1%, 2%, 5%, 20% Cream—1%, 5% Lotion—0.5% Aerosol—2%, 3%, 4.5%, 9.4%, 10%, 13.6%, 20% Liquid—2%, 6.37%, 20% Gel—20%	Apply to area several times a day as required Suppositories and rectal ointment given morning and night, and after each bowel movement Gel used as a lubricant on catheters, specula, and so forth Liquid, gel, or spray for oral mucous membrane anesthesia in dentistry	Slowly absorbed from mucous membranes and exerts a fairly prolonged action; component of many combination products (*e.g.*, oral, anorectal, otic, topical); produces hypersensitivity reactions in some individuals; stop drug at first sign of allergic response; avoid contact with eyes; may be used for temporary relief of toothache and other dental procedures; employed to lubricate catheters, endoscopic tubes, sigmoidoscopes, proctoscopes, and vaginal specula
Bupivacaine (Marcaine, Sensorcaine)	Injection—0.25%, 0.5%, 0.75% alone or with 1:200,000 epinephrine	Infiltration—0.25% Epidural/caudal—0.25% to 0.75% Peripheral nerve block—0.25% to 0.5% Sympathetic block—0.25%; maximum single dose is 200 mg (250 mg with epinephrine)	Onset slower than lidocaine, but more prolonged duration; widely used for nerve block, epidural or caudal for long surgical or obstetrical procedures, and relief of pain during labor; do not use 0.75% concentration for obstetrical epidural anesthesia, because cardiac arrest can occur; maximum dose 400 mg (with epinephrine) in 24 hours; Do not use for spinal block
Butamben (Butesin)	Ointment—1%	Apply 2 to 3 times/day as needed	Used primarily in minor burns and skin irritations
Chloroprocaine (Nesacaine)	Injection—1%, 2%, 3%	Infiltration/nerve block—1% to 2% Caudal/epidural—2% to 3%	Do not use solution with preservatives for caudal or epidural block; more rapid acting and less toxic than procaine; IV use may produce thrombophlebitis
Cocaine (Various manufacturers)	Bulk powder added to solution Soluble tablets—135 mg	Surface anesthesia—1% to 2% Nose/throat—5% to 10%	Class II controlled substance (see Appendix); central stimulant that may cause profound psychological dependence when taken internally; produces vasoconstriction when applied to mucous membrane; not used by injection or in the eyes; onset of action is rapid when applied locally, and duration is about 1 hour to 2 hours; abused either by snuffing powder or injecting substance mixed with other opiates
Cyclomethycaine (Surfacaine)	Ointment—1% Cream—0.5% Jelly—0.75% Suppositories—10 mg	Apply locally 2 to 3 times/day Jelly used to lubricate tubes, cystoscopes, bronchoscopes Suppository—1 twice a day	Used in rectal, vaginal, and urethral examinations and various intubation procedures; less effective on mucous membranes of the mouth, nose, eye, and bronchi than most other agents
Dibucaine (Nupercainal)	Ointment—1% Cream—0.5% Suppositories—2.5 mg Injection—1:200, 1:1500, and 2.5 mg/ml with 5% Dextrose	Apply locally 2 to 3 times/day Suppository—1 to 2/day Injection (spinal anesthesia): 1:200—mixed with spinal fluid; 1:1500—injected without removal of spinal fluid; 2.5 mg/ml (heavy)—for low spinal anesthesia	Approximately 8 to 10 times more potent than procaine and cocaine; onset about 15 minutes, and duration 3 hours to 4 hours; toxic drug when used parenterally, and caution must be exercised; not for SC injection because sloughing and necrosis can occur
Dimethisoquin (Quotane)	Ointment—0.5%	Apply locally as needed	Rapid onset and fairly prolonged duration (2 hr–4 hr); used mainly for burns, itching, irritation, and pain of various dermatoses

(continued)

Table 16-1. Local Anesthetics (continued)

Drug	Preparations	Usual Dosage Range	Remarks
Diperodon (Diothane, Proctodon)	Ointment—1% Suppositories—1%	Apply locally as needed Suppository—1 to 2/day	Potent, prolonged acting agent; suppository contains vitamins A and D in a water-miscible base; topical product is irritating and can cause allergic reactions
Dyclonine (Dyclone)	Solution—0.5%, 1%	Apply topically to skin or mucous membranes	Used prior to endoscopic procedures to block the gag reflex and to relieve pain of oral or anogenital lesions; onset in about 10 minutes; duration approximately 60 minutes; may be used in patients hypersensitive to other local anesthetics
Etidocaine (Duranest)	Injection—1% alone or 1%, 1.5% with 1:200,000 epinephrine	Infiltration—1.0% Nerve block—1% Caudal—1% Central neural block—1.0% to 1.5%	Onset of action 3 minutes to 5 minutes; duration may last 8 hours to 10 hours (caution in ambulatory patients); induces profound motor blockade when given peridurally
Hexylcaine (Cyclaine)	Solution—5%	Apply topically as required	Indicated for topical anesthesia of intact mucous membranes of the respiratory, upper GI, or urinary tract; too toxic for injection
Lidocaine (Xylocaine and various other manufacturers)	Ointment—2.5%, 5% Cream—3% Jelly—2% Solution—2%, 4% Spray—2.5%, 10% Injection—0.5%, 1%, 1.5%, 2%, 4% alone Injection—0.5%, 1%, 1.5%, 2% with epinephrine Injection—1.5% with 7.5% dextrose Injection—5% with 7.5% glucose	Apply topically as needed Solution for pain and inflammation of mouth, throat, pharynx, and urethra, as needed Injection: Infiltration—0.5% to 1% Nerve block: Dental—2% Intercostal—1% Brachial—1.5% Paracervical—1% Epidural: Thoracic—1% Lumbar—1% to 2% Caudal: Obstetric—1% Surgical—1.5% Spinal: 5% with glucose Saddle block: 1.5% with dextrose	More potent than procaine; immediate onset of action, lasting 1 hour to 2 hours; widely used as antiarrhythmic agent (see Chap. 30); IV injection is usually 50 mg to 100 mg at a rate of 25 mg/min to 50 mg/min; maximum 200 mg to 300 mg in 1-hour period; infusion rate normally 20 mcg/kg/min to 50 mcg/kg/min; do *not* use solution with epinephrine for arrhythmias, or solutions with preservatives for spinal or epidural; oral solutions can block swallowing reflex—caution in pediatric and geriatric patients especially; can enhance muscle-relaxing action of neuromuscular blocking agents; contraindicated in persons with blood dyscrasias
Mepivacaine (Carbocaine, Isocaine)	Injection—1%, 1.5%, 2%, 3% Injection—2% with 1:20,000 levonordefrin	Nerve block—1% to 2% Paracervical block—1% Caudal/epidural—1% to 2% Infiltration—1% Analgesia—1% to 2% Dental block—2% to 3%	Twice as potent as procaine, approximately equal in onset, but more prolonged duration than either procaine or lidocaine; possesses some vasoconstrictive action and thus does not usually require a vasoconstrictor; injection containing levonordefrin is used for dental procedures only; not used topically; less drowsiness and depression than observed with lidocaine; caution in renal disease
Pramoxine (Tronothane)	Cream—1% Jelly—1% Rectal suppositories—1% Aerosol foam—1%	Apply topically or rectally 2 to 3 times/day as needed	Not used by injection, or applied to the eye or nasal mucosa; component of many anorectal preparations (*e.g.,* ointments, foams, suppositories); used mainly to relieve pain and itching, and to facilitate endotracheal, intragastric, and rectal intubation procedures
Prilocaine (Citanest)	Injection—1%, 2%, 3%, 4% Injection—4% plain and with 1:200,000 epinephrine	Infiltration—1% to 2% Peripheral nerve block—1% to 3% Epidural—1% to 3% Caudal: Obstetrics—1% Surgery—2% to 3% Dental procedures—4%	Similar to lidocaine in its actions, but slower onset and longer duration; may induce drowsiness and sleepiness; associated with some cases of methemoglobinemia and not widely used for this reason; no more than 600 mg should be administered as a single injection as a precaution against methemoglobinemia

(continued)

Table 16-1. Local Anesthetics *(continued)*

Drug	Preparations	Usual Dosage Range	Remarks
Procaine (Anduracaine, Anuject, Durathesia, Novocain)	Injection—1%, 2%, 10% (plain) Injection—2% with epinephrine Rectal Injection—1.25% with isobutyl p-aminobenzoate (4%) and 1.5% with butyl aminobenzoate (6%)	Infiltration—0.25% to 0.5% Nerve block—0.5% to 2% Spinal—10% Rectal anesthesia—1.25% to 1.5%	Not employed topically; rapidly eliminated, short-acting (30 min–60 min), no central stimulation, and relatively nontoxic, although fairly high incidence of allergic reactions; metabolic product may interfere with actions of sulfonamides, and other local anesthetics should be used in presence of sulfonamide antibiotics. The amide of procaine is an effective antiarrhythmic agent (see Chap. 30).
Proparacaine (Ak-taine, Alcaine, Ophthaine, Ophthetic)	Ophthalmic drops—0.5%	Cataract surgery—1 drop every 5 minutes to 10 minutes Removal of sutures—1 to 2 drops 2 minutes to 3 minutes prior to surgery Foreign bodies—1 to 2 drops prior to extraction Tonometry—1 to 2 drops before measurement	Used in the eye exclusively; produces minimal irritation; may produce allergic contact dermatitis with drying and fissuring of the fingertips
Tetracaine (Anacel, Pontocaine, Zem-Tetra)	Cream—1% Ointment—0.5% Oral solution—2% Ophthalmic ointment—0.5% Ophthalmic solution—0.5% Injection—1% Injection—0.2%, 0.3% with 6% dextrose Powder—20 mg in Niphanoid (snow-like crystals) ampules	Apply locally (0.5% to 2%) as needed for pain, burning, itching Cataract surgery—1 drop (0.5%) every 5 minutes to 10 minutes Suture removal—1 to 2 drops (0.5%) 2 minutes to 3 minutes prior to procedure Foreign bodies—1 to 2 drops prior to operating Tonometry—1 to 2 drops before measurement Ophthalmic inflammation—Apply ointment 2 to 3 times/day Spinal anesthesia—0.2% to 1% Caudal anesthesia—0.2% to 0.3% with dextrose Nasal or pharyngeal anesthesia—2% solution	More potent (8–10 times) and longer acting than procaine, but more toxic as well; onset of action is slow with a duration between 2 hours to 3 hours; employed in rather low concentrations for surface anesthesia of eye, nose, and throat, as well as spinal and caudal anesthesia; produces *prolonged* spinal anesthesia for operations requiring 2 hours to 3 hours; doses exceeding 15 mg are rarely required; do not re-use left over autoclaved ampules because crystals may form.

5 Procaine, chloroprocaine, tetracaine, and piperocaine may retard action of sulfonamide antibiotics.

▶ **NURSING ALERTS**

▷ *Topical*

▷ 1 When there is a possibility of systemic involvement (*e.g.,* large doses, elderly or debilitated patients, debrided or traumatized areas), have resuscitative equipment and antidotal medications on hand (*e.g.,* respirators, vasopressors, IV fluids).

▷ 2 Be alert for early signs of allergic reactions and discontinue drug immediately. Begin appropriate symptomatic therapy.

▷ 3 Instruct patient receiving anesthetic eye drops to avoid touching the eye area until effects have dissipated. Cover eye with a patch, since blink reflex is temporarily absent.

▷ 4 Use cautiously in pregnancy and in patients with known allergies, cardiac diseases, or hyperthyroidism.

Note that prolonged ocular use may produce visual loss and possibly delay local wound healing.

▷ 5 Warn user that if drug is applied to oral mucosa, swallowing may be impeded. Do not administer food or liquids for at least 1 hour following drug.

▷ *Injection*

▷ 1 Have facilities and drugs for respiratory and cardiovascular assistance on hand at all times.

▷ 2 Do not use solutions with preservatives for spinal or epidural injection.

▷ 3 Use lowest dose resulting in effective anesthesia, to minimize danger of systemic effects. Reduce dosage in children, elderly, debilitated, or acutely ill patients.

▷ 4 Give injection slowly to decrease dangers in case of allergic or other systemic reactions. Aspirate syringe first to prevent intravascular injection.

▷ 5 Use caution in giving solutions with vasoconstrictors to patients with peripheral vascular diseases or hypertension.

▷ 6 Administer epidural injections cautiously in patients with neurologic diseases, spinal deformities, septicemia, hypertension, and in the very young.

▷ 7 Fetal bradycardia and acidosis can occur with paracervical block. Monitor fetal heart rate closely and do not exceed recommended dose.

▶ **NURSING CONSIDERATIONS**

▷ *Topical*

▷ 1 Do not touch eyelids with dropper tip, and do not rub eyes during period of anesthesia.

▷ 2 Discontinue drug if sensitivity reactions or irritation develops.

▷ 3 Inform patient that use of anesthetic ear drops can mask symptoms of middle ear infection.

▷ 4 Avoid contact of topical local anesthetics with the eyes (unless ophthalmic solution is used), and do not inhale mist from aerosal spray preparations.

▷ 5 Caution patients against prolonged use of any local anesthetic preparation. Advise them to seek proper treatment for the *cause* of the condition requiring the local anesthetic.

▷ *Injection*

▷ 1 Do not inject local anesthetic into areas of infection because effectiveness is greatly diminished, systemic toxicity may be enhanced, and drug (*e.g.,* procaine) may interfere with action of sulfonamide antibiotics.

▷ 2 Place patient receiving spinal anesthesia in proper position to avoid diffusion of drug toward respiratory muscles.

▷ 3 Be aware that repeated injections of certain slowly metabolized drugs may cause accumulation and prolonged adverse effects.

▷ 4 Counsel patients receiving spinal or epidural anesthesia that sensation in lower areas of the body may not return for an hour or two. Be prepared to assist movement as needed.

▷ 5 Do *not* autoclave solutions of local anesthetics containing epinephrine.

▷ 6 Discard unused portions of solutions not containing preservatives.

Drugs classified as general anesthetics are agents that, in sufficient amounts, are capable of producing analgesia, decreased muscle reflex activity, and ultimately loss of consciousness. General anesthetics have varying degrees of potency, and there exist distinct advantages as well as disadvantages among the many drugs used to induce anesthesia. Consequently, no one drug represents an "ideal" general anesthetic in terms of potency, stability, safety, and efficacy. Rather, several drugs are often used in combination to provide smooth induction, sufficient depth and duration of anesthesia, adequate muscle relaxation, and minimal hazards to the vital systems.

Several interesting theories have been proposed to explain the mechanism of action of the general anesthetics, but no single theory appears adequate to describe the effects observed with all of these agents. Parallels have been observed between the action of general anesthetics and their lipid solubility, their ability to inhibit glucose metabolism in the brain by blocking utilization of high energy compounds such as ATP, and their capacity to combine with cellular water, thereby interfering with cellular function and nerve transmission. It is likely that general anesthetics in some way alter the structure or functioning of nerve cell components, thereby reducing neuronal excitability and increasing the firing threshold.

The primary site of action of these compounds is the reticular formation in the brain stem, which is the first area of the CNS to be affected by the general anesthetics. By reducing the number of impulses that arise from this area of the brain stem to the cerebral cortex, these drugs progressively decrease sensory awareness, and when a sufficient concentration of anesthetic is present, consciousness is lost. Cells of the dorsal horn of the spinal cord are also quite sensitive to general anesthetics, resulting in an interruption of incoming sensory (*e.g.,* pain) impulses.

As anesthesia deepens, various *stages* (I–IV) follow in which certain characteristic signs may be noted; they give an indication of the degree of depression being produced by the anesthetic agent. Surgical procedures are usually performed in stage III, which is further subdivided in four *planes*. Table 17-1 presents a review of the most important pharmacologic effects elicited by a general anesthetic as the patient passes through the various stages of anesthesia. The appearance and duration of the effects noted in each stage vary widely, and depend on the choice of anesthetic, speed of induction, and technique of the anesthesiologist. For example, the early stages are often not seen with the use of an ultrashort-acting barbiturate such as thiopental, because the transition from consciousness to a stage of surgical anesthesia is quite rapid.

Production of safe and efficient general anesthesia depends in part on proper preparation of the patient. In addition to the anesthetic drug itself, several other drugs are used routinely before, during and after surgical procedures.

General Anesthetics 17

A *Preanesthetic Medication*

The purposes of preanesthetic medication and examples of drugs used are the following:

Table 17-1. Stages and Characteristics of Anesthesia

Stage/Plane	Respiration	Cardiovascular	Muscle Tone	Reflexes	Other
Stage I	Regular	Normal	Normal	Normal	Analgesia, euphoria, amnesia
Stage II	Rapid Irregular	↑Heart rate ↑Blood pressure	Tense Struggling	Swallowing Retching Gagging Vomiting	Mydriasis, roving eyeballs, loss of consciousness, decreased eyelid reflex
Stage III					
Plane 1	Regular	Heart rate and blood pressure normal	Smaller muscles relaxed	Lid and pharyngeal (gag) reflex absent	Increased tear secretion, miosis, some eye movement, increased respiration and blood pressure with incision
Plane 2	Regular but shallower	Normal	Large muscles relaxed	Corneal and laryngeal reflex absent	Eyes stilled, miosis, decreased tear secretion, no response to incision
Plane 3	Shallow and mainly abdominal	Blood pressure falls slightly; some tachycardia	Complete relaxation	Pupillary (light) and cough reflex disappear	Mydriasis, decreased tear secretion
Plane 4	Abdominal and very shallow	Hypotension and some tachycardia	Complete relaxation	No reflexes	Mydriasis, no lacrimation
Stage IV	Respiratory paralysis	Marked hypotension and failing circulation	Complete relaxation	No reflexes	Extreme mydriasis, medullary paralysis, and eventual death

1 Relief of anxiety (sedatives)
2 Reduction in salivary and mucous secretions (anticholinergics)
3 Inhibition of undesirable side-effects (*e.g.*, bradycardia and muscle spasms) occurring reflexly due to the anesthetic agent (anticholinergics, peripherally acting skeletal muscle relaxants)

The use of narcotics for preoperative sedation and analgesia is subject to some controversy, inasmuch as they may depress respiration and cough, prolong the anesthetic state, and induce postoperative nausea and vomiting. Their use is largely a matter of physician preference.

B   Adjunctive Anesthetic Medication

Drugs given during the surgical procedure depend upon the type and length of procedure and the patient's status. Neuromuscular blocking agents (*e.g.*, succinylcholine) are commonly administered during the operation while the patient is still at a relatively light level of anesthesia. These agents provide an additional degree of skeletal muscle relaxation and therefore allow a lower dose of general anesthetic to be used, reducing the incidence of untoward reactions. Since they are all relatively short-acting drugs, good control of skeletal muscle activity can be maintained by an experienced anesthetist. For a more complete description of the peripherally acting skeletal muscle relaxants, see Chapter 15.

C   Postoperative Medication

Principal indications for use of drugs postoperatively are the following:
1 Nausea and vomiting (phenothiazines)
2 Abdominal distention and urinary retention (cholinergics)
3 Pain (analgesics)

The clinically useful general anesthetics may be classified in the following manner:
I. Inhalation Anesthetics
   A. Gases
   (*e.g.*, nitrous oxide, cyclopropane)
   B. Volatile Liquids
   (*e.g.*, halothane, methoxyflurane, isoflurane)
II. Intravenous Anesthetics
   A. Ultrashort-Acting Barbiturates
   (*e.g.*, thiopental, methohexital)
   B. Hypnotics
   (*e.g.*, etomidate)
   C. Dissociative Agents
   (*e.g.*, Ketamine, Innovar—may also be given IM)

Although the clinical pharmacology of each general anesthetic drug is reviewed briefly here, anyone handling these drugs on a routine basis should become thoroughly familiar with the advantages and disadvantages of each preparation and the procedures for its proper administration (*i.e.*, open-drop, semi-closed, or complete rebreathing methods) by consulting specific literature sources pertaining to each agent. The following monographs attempt to provide the essential information on the more widely used drugs; however, it should not be viewed as a complete description of the pharmacologic properties and clinical implications of the compounds.

I Inhalation Anesthetics

The inhalation anesthetics include gases and volatile liquids. Both types enter the circulation rapidly upon inhalation and are transported through the blood stream to the CNS. Eventually, most are again returned to the lungs and excreted (exhaled) essentially unchanged. Halothane and methoxyflurane, however, are metabolized to a significant extent in the liver. A potential danger with most of the potent, fat-soluble inhalational anesthetics is malignant hyperthermia, an acute condition characterized by a sudden, marked elevation in body temperature that is often fatal unless treated immediately and vigorously. This condition is also caused by many neuromuscular blocking agents, especially when used concurrently with inhalation anesthetics. When these drugs are used together, the patient must be carefully monitored. Treatment consists of injections of dantrolene (see Chap. 15) or possibly one of the calcium-channel blockers (see Chap. 32).

A Gases

Three gases are currently available for use as general anesthetics, and of these, only nitrous oxide is used extensively. In fact, it is one of the most widely used of all general anesthetics, most often as part of a total anesthetic regimen that also includes sedatives, other anesthetics, narcotics, barbiturates, and muscle relaxants; such a regimen is termed *balanced anesthesia*. This type of drug combination usually produces rapid induction with minimal adverse effects, and it allows a significant reduction in the amount of each drug required.

▶ cyclopropane

Uses
1 Anesthesia, especially in patients with cardiovascular complications, reduced arterial oxygen tension, or impending shock
2 Obstetrical analgesia

Dosage
(Administered in a *closed* system with oxygen)
Induction: 50%
Maintenance: 10% to 20%
For analgesia: 1% to 2% continuous inhalation

Fate
Rapid induction (1 min–2 min); rapid emergence (5 min–10 min) following termination of inhalation; largely eliminated through the lungs; good margin of safety, with low incidence of hypotension

Common Side-Effects
Postoperative nausea, vomiting, and headaches; bradycardia

Significant Adverse Reactions
Respiratory depression, cardiac arrhythmias (in presence of catecholamines), laryngospasm, bronchospasm, malignant hyperthermia

Contraindications
Simultaneous use of adrenergic agents, asthmatic conditions, use of electrocautery equipment during administration (agent is flammable)

Interactions
1 Cardiac arrhythmias may occur in combination with catecholamine-like agents, due to sensitization of the myocardium by the anesthetic.
2 Cyclopropane is explosive in the presence of oxygen.
3 Aminoglycoside antibiotics (*e.g.*, gentamycin, kanamycin, amikacin) may produce apnea if given with cyclopropane.

▶ NURSING ALERTS
▷ 1 Use adequate precautions (*e.g.*, antistatic equipment) to prevent explosion when drug is present.
▷ 2 Be alert for signs of arrhythmias, and have proper materials and equipment on hand to quickly treat arrhythmias if they occur.
▷ 3 Do *not* use any sympathomimetic drug during cyclopropane anesthesia because danger of arrhythmia is increased.

▶ NURSING CONSIDERATIONS
▷ 1 Emergence excitement is common. Consider giving small dose of narcotic before discontinuing anesthetic to reduce excitatory behavior.
▷ 2 Be aware that hypotension can occur following prolonged use of cyclopropane. Monitor blood pressure and heart rate frequently, and have proper drugs on hand to treat hypotension.
▷ 3 Position patient properly to reduce danger of aspiration of vomitus.

▶ ethylene

Infrequently used today, except possibly for obstetrical analgesia in a few cases; possesses a wide safety margin, low toxicity, poor muscle relaxing ability, and rapid induction and recovery. It is similar in many other respects to nitrous oxide. However, unlike nitrous oxide, ethylene is highly explosive and has a very unpleasant odor. Its use should be discouraged with the availability of more potent and safer agents.

▶ **nitrous oxide**
N_2O

Uses
1 Induction (basal) anesthesia
2 Component of *balanced anesthesia* (see introduction)
3 Obstetrical or dental analgesia

Dosage
(Always used in an oxygen mixture)
Induction anesthesia: 70% to 80% N_2O
Maintenance anesthesia: 70% N_2O
Analgesia: 20% to 30% N_2O

Fate
Rapid onset and short duration of action; excreted primarily by the lungs

Significant Adverse Reactions
(Primarily caused by lack of oxygen resulting from improper administration technique; see Nursing Alerts) Confusion, cyanosis, convulsions; bone marrow depression can also occur with prolonged use; malignant hyperthermia is possible

▶ **NURSING ALERTS**
▷ 1 Do not administer undiluted (without oxygen) for more than a few breaths. Hypoxia will result if concentrations of N_2O greater than 80% are employed for any length of time.
▷ 2 Use cautiously in patients with pneumothorax because pulmonary pressure may be elevated with N_2O.

▶ **NURSING CONSIDERATIONS**
▷ 1 Recognize that N_2O is a rather weak anesthetic and muscle relaxant. Use supplemental drugs (muscle relaxants, barbiturates, other general anesthetics) when N_2O is employed in anesthesia.
▷ 2 Inform patient that dizziness, confusion, vivid dreams, and hallucinations may occur with use of N_2O but will disappear upon termination of the drug.
▷ 3 Caution patient receiving N_2O to use care in driving or operating other machinery until effects of the drug have completely disappeared.

B   Volatile Liquids

The volatile liquid anesthetics are administered by inhalation of the vapors given off by the liquid along with adequate amounts of oxygen. The depth of anesthesia can be fairly well controlled by varying the concentration, because these agents are generally short acting. Recovery begins as soon as the drug is removed because most drugs are excreted largely through the lungs. These agents must be used cautiously in patients with pulmonary diseases, because excretion may be impaired and accumulation toxicity can result.

▶ **enflurane**
Ethrane

Anesthesia resembles that produced by halothane, but muscle relaxation is more pronounced and hepatotoxicity and nephrotoxicity have not been reported. Heart rate remains constant and cardiac rhythm is stable; hypotension occurs at deeper levels of anesthesia; releases fluoride ion, and thus may damage kidneys in large amounts; probably superior to halothane for abdominal procedures

Uses
1 Induction and maintenance general anesthesia, usually in combination with minimal amounts of skeletal muscle relaxants
2 Provide analgesia for vaginal delivery or supplement other anesthetics for cesarean section (high levels may relax uterus)

Dosage
Induction: 2.0% to 4.5% for 7 minutes to 10 minutes
Maintenance: 0.5% to 3.0%

Fate
Rapid onset of action and recovery; excreted largely (85%–90%) through the lungs, the remainder metabolized by the liver and excreted in the kidney

Common Side-Effects
Slight hypotension

Significant Adverse Reactions
Decreased myocardial contractility, CNS stimulation with prolonged use, renal damage, and malignant hyperthermia

Interactions
1 Arrhythmias may be produced in combination with sympathomimetic agents (enflurane sensitizes the myocardium).
2 Antidepolarizing neuromuscular blocking agents can be potentiated by enflurane.

▶ **NURSING ALERT**
▷ 1 Use very cautiously in patients with cardiac or renal disease.

▶ **NURSING CONSIDERATIONS**
▷ 1 Muscle relaxation is generally sufficient for most operations. If additional relaxation is desired, use minimal doses of neuromuscular blocking agents.
▷ 2 Do not use sympathomimetic agents during enflurane administration because arrhythmias can result.

▶ ether

Diethyl Ether

The first clinically useful volatile liquid anesthetic, it has a good safety margin and is an excellent muscle relaxant. It is not used very often today because of its slow, unpleasant induction, excessive secretory action, high incidence of postoperative nausea and vomiting, and danger of flammability. It is primarily of historical interest today.

Uses

1 Maintenance anesthesia, usually in prolonged procedures (rarely used)

Dosage

Induction: 5% to 7%
Maintenance: 3% to 5%

Fate

Slow, rather unpleasant induction, marked by excessive salivary and bronchial secretions; prolonged recovery; over 90% excreted unchanged by the lungs

Common Side-Effects

Mucuous membrane irritation and hypersecretion, increased microvascular bleeding, and postoperative nausea and vomiting

Significant Adverse Reactions

Decreased urinary output, hypotension, postoperative abdominal distention and paralytic ileus, and aspiration of mucosal secretions

Contraindications

Renal disease, acidosis, and electrocautery procedures

Interactions

1 Muscle-relaxant effect of ether may be enhanced by aminoglycoside antibiotics
2 Adrenergic blocking agents may significantly decrease blood pressure or cardiac output during ether anesthesia

▶ NURSING ALERTS

▷ 1 Use additional muscle relaxants very cautiously with ether to avoid excessive paralysis because the drug has good muscle relaxant actions of its own.

▶ NURSING CONSIDERATIONS

▷ 1 Always pretreat patients with anticholinergic agents prior to ether anesthesia to reduce the volume of secretions produced by the anesthetic.
▷ 2 During recovery, nausea and vomiting are common. Turn patient's head toward one side to avoid aspiration of the vomitus.
▷ 3 As with any general anesthetic, remember that the sense of hearing is one of the *earliest* to return during recovery. Avoid remarks that may be upsetting to the patient during this time, even though he may still be unconscious.
▷ 4 Use only unopened, sealed containers of ether for anesthesia.

▶ halothane

Fluothane

One of the best and most widely used inhalation anesthetics; it is four times as potent as ether, with rapid induction and recovery, little irritation, and low incidence of nausea and vomiting. It is a weak muscle relaxant and is generally administered with a neuromuscular blocking agent. Halothane has been associated with liver dysfunction (hepatitis, jaundice), especially in persons with prior hepatic disease or previous exposure to halothane.

Uses

1 Induction and maintenance anesthesia

Dosage

(Usually with oxygen or oxygen–nitrous oxide mixture)
Induction: 1% to 4%
Maintenance: 0.5% to 1.5%

Fate

Quickly absorbed; largely excreted by the lungs, but up to 20% may be converted to metabolites and excreted in the urine

Common Side-Effects

Hypotension, rapid and shallow respiration

Significant Adverse Reactions

Arrhythmias (in presence of sympathomimetic agents), vomiting, hypoxia, respiratory difficulty, postoperative shivering, bradycardia, liver damage, increased intracranial pressure, and malignant hyperthermia

Contraindications

Obstetrical anesthesia (drug is a potent uterine relaxant), severe hepatic or biliary disease

Interactions

1 Halothane may potentiate the effects of antidepolarizing muscle relaxants (*e.g.,* curare, gallamine) and ganglionic blocking agents.
2 Arrhythmias may be produced by the combination of halothane and catecholamines.

▶ NURSING ALERTS

▷ 1 Do not use a second time in individuals who show evidence of liver damage (fever, anorexia, nausea, vomiting) following halothane. Incidence of serious hepatic damage increases with progressive use. Although not absolutely contraindicated, administration of halothane in patients with pre-existing liver disease should be undertaken cautiously.

▷ 2 Use cautiously in patients with severe cardiac disease, and during pregnancy.

▶ **NURSING CONSIDERATIONS**
▷ 1 Be aware that the uterine-relaxant effect of halothane may not respond to ergot drugs or oxytocin.
▷ 2 Have on hand atropine to treat bradycardia, and vasopressors (*e.g.,* ephedrine, phenylephrine) to treat marked hypotension resulting from halothane.
▷ 3 Keep patient warm postoperatively, to minimize shivering.

▶ **isoflurane**
Forane

A volatile liquid anesthetic structurally similar to enflurane, isoflurane has a rapid onset and quick recovery. It does not sensitize the heart to catecholamines, and produces good muscle relaxation. CNS excitation is minimal, but respiratory depression may be significant, and blood pressure progressively decreases with depth of anesthesia.

Uses
1 Induction and maintenance of general anesthesia

Dosage
Induction: 1.5% to 3% for 5 minutes to 10 minutes
Maintenance: 1.0% to 2.5% with nitrous oxide

Fate
Induction and recovery are rapid; less than 1% of the total dose absorbed systemically is metabolized; primarily excreted through the lungs

Common Side-Effects
Mild hypotension

Significant Adverse Reactions
Respiratory depression, tachycardia, malignant hyperthermia

Interactions
1 The muscle relaxant effect of isoflurane can be increased by concomitant use of other skeletal muscle relaxants.
2 Increased respiratory depression can occur in combination with barbiturates, narcotics, and other respiratory depressants.

▶ **NURSING ALERTS**
▷ 1 Monitor respiration closely, because drug is a potent respiratory depressant. Have respiratory assistance immediately available.

▶ **NURSING CONSIDERATIONS**
▷ 1 Use only small doses of neuromuscular blocking agents to provide additional muscle relaxation, because isoflurane has considerable muscle relaxing action itself.

▷ 2 Have vasopressors available to treat hypotension should it develop.

▶ **methoxyflurane**
Penthrane

A very potent inhalation anesthetic, with slow onset and recovery, it produces fair muscle relaxation and significant analgesia at light levels of anesthesia; produces low incidence of arrhythmias, but elicits profound circulatory depression at higher concentrations. The drug is associated with liver and especially kidney damage.

Uses
1 Surgical anesthesia of less than 4-hour duration (usually with nitrous oxide and oxygen)
2 Production of analgesia in obstetrics and minor surgical procedures

Dosage
Analgesia: 0.3% to 0.8% (may be used with hand-held inhalers, *e.g.,* Analgizer, Cyprane)
Anesthesia:
Induction—up to 2% for 2 minutes to 5 minutes
Maintenance—0.1% to 2.0% with at least 50% nitrous oxide
(Use lowest effective concentration at all times)

Fate
Slow onset often associated with excitement; prolonged emergence if not discontinued 30 minutes to 40 minutes before end of surgery due to high lipid solubility; up to 70% of the drug is metabolized in the liver; remainder is excreted through lungs and kidneys

Common Side-Effects
Mild hypotension, nausea

Significant Adverse Reactions
Renal dysfunction, hepatic dysfunction (jaundice, necrosis), respiratory depression, prolonged postoperative sedation, delirium, malignant hyperthermia, and cardiac arrest (rare)

Contraindications
Renal disease, vascular surgery near the renal vessels, patients receiving the drug within the previous month, cirrhosis, viral hepatitis, and patients showing jaundice or unexplained fever with other inhalation anesthetics

Interactions
1 Use of methoxyflurane with certain nephrotoxic antibiotics (*e.g.,* tetracycline, aminoglycosides, amphotericin) may result in fatal renal toxicity.
2 Muscle-relaxing action of antidepolarizing neuromuscular blocking agents may be augmented by methoxyflurane. Reduce dose of each accordingly.

NURSING ALERTS

▷ 1 Nephrotoxicity with methoxyflurane is dose related, probably due to liberation of the fluoride ion as a metabolic product. Always use lowest effective dose to minimize danger of renal damage.

▷ 2 Carefully monitor urinary output and other laboratory signs of possible renal dysfunction (*e.g.,* creatinine, electrolytes).

▷ 3 Do not attempt to produce adequate muscle relaxation with methoxyflurane alone because overdose can result. Always use additional skeletal muscle relaxants (*e.g.,* succinylcholine).

▷ 4 Use cautiously if at all in pregnancy, diabetes, hepatic impairment, and for surgical procedures lasting beyond 4 hours.

▷ 5 Use catecholamines or related drugs carefully because arrhythmias can develop in the presence of methoxyflurane.

NURSING CONSIDERATIONS

▷ 1 When giving barbiturates or narcotics as adjunctive medication, use conservative doses to avoid additive respiratory depression.

▷ 2 For rapid induction, preferably use another anesthetic such as N_2O or thiopental rather than giving large doses of methoxyflurane for prolonged periods.

▷ 3 Reduce usual dose of muscle relaxant by half when given in combination with methoxyflurane.

II Intravenous Anesthetics

The general anesthetics administered IV include three *ultrashort-acting* barbiturates that are used mainly for induction of anesthesia, but may also be employed as the sole anesthetic agent in short surgical procedures associated with minimal pain, and for supplementing other anesthetic agents during longer procedures.

They are rapidly taken up by the brain following IV injection and are almost as rapidly redistributed to other parts of the body. Therefore, within 5 minutes after injection, the brain level of the barbiturate has declined to about one half of its peak attained shortly (30 sec–45 sec) after injection, and only about one tenth of the initial concentration remains in the brain at 30 minutes following injection because the drug has been redistributed to other fatty stores in the body. Emergence occurs during this period of declining brain levels, even though the rate of metabolism and excretion of the drug from the body is quite constant and rather slow (10%–15%/hr).

A rapid-acting nonbarbiturate hypnotic, etomidate, is also available for IV use as an induction anesthetic and for supplementing other anesthetics, such as nitrous oxide. It is reviewed below.

Two other drugs that can be administered either IV or IM are categorized as *dissociative* anesthetics because they induce a neuroleptic-like effect that is characterized by analgesia, quietude, and detachment from the environment *without* loss of consciousness. These two drugs, ketamine

and Innovar, differ slightly in some of their pharmacologic properties, and are discussed separately below.

A Ultrashort-Acting Barbiturates

The barbiturates employed in general anesthesia are those having an extremely rapid onset and relatively short duration (15 min–30 min) of action. The response of the CNS to these drugs is essentially the same as that following an inhalation anesthetic—in succeeding order, loss of consciousness, diminished reflexes, loss of motor tone, and ultimately failure of the vital medullary centers. Recovery proceeds in the reverse direction.

The major advantages of the IV barbiturates compared to many inhalation anesthetics are the rapidity and smoothness of onset, absence of salivation, greater patient acceptance (no occlusive face mask), short duration (allowing better control), speedy recovery, nonflammability, lower degree of irritation, and little danger of arrhythmias.

Disadvantages of the IV anesthetics include higher incidences of respiratory and circulatory depression, laryngospasm, bronchospasm, and if leakage occurs, the danger of tissue necrosis. Prolonged or repeated administration may result in cumulative toxicity, because the drugs are removed slowly from the body.

▶ methohexital
Brevital

Uses
1 Induction anesthesia
2 Short surgical procedures with minimal painful stimuli
3 Supplementation of other anesthetics
4 Induction of a hypnotic state

Dosage
Induction: 5 ml to 12 ml of a 1% solution at a rate of 1 ml/5 sec
Maintenance: 2 ml to 4 ml of a 1% solution every 4 minutes to 7 minutes (continuous drop—0.2% at a rate of 1 drop/sec)

Fate
Very rapid onset (30 sec) and extremely short duration (5 min–8 min); quickly redistributed in the body and slowly excreted through the kidneys; accumulation in fatty tissues is significant

Common Side-Effects
Respiratory depression, mild hypotension, and hiccups

Significant Adverse Reactions
Headache, vomiting, salivation, delerium upon emergence, pain at injection site, muscle twitching, shivering, laryngospasm, apnea, bronchospasm, thrombophlebitis, allergic reactions (pruritus, urticaria, rhinitis, dyspnea), abdominal pain, peripheral vascular collapse, circulatory or myocardial depression, and arrhythmias

Contraindications
Latent or manifest porphyria, absence of suitable veins for IV administration

Interactions
1 CNS depressant effects may be additive to those of other depressants, including alcohol, sedatives, and narcotics.
2 Orthostatic hypotension may be elicited by combined use with bumetanide, furosemide, or ethacrynic acid.

▶ NURSING ALERTS
▷ 1 Repeated or continuous injection may cause accumulation and lead to prolonged sedation and severe cardiovascular and respiratory depression. Always have appropriate resuscitative measures (*e.g.,* endotracheal tube, suction, oxygen) available.
▷ 2 Use cautiously in pregnant or debilitated patients, in *status asthmaticus,* and in impaired circulatory, respiratory, renal, hepatic, or endocrine function.
▷ 3 Do not use lactated Ringer's solution for dilution. Solutions are incompatible.

▶ NURSING CONSIDERATIONS
▷ 1 Use only clear, colorless dilutions.
▷ 2 Be alert for signs of excess pain or swelling at injection site, indication of extravasation, and danger of tissue necrosis. Procaine (1%) can be injected locally to alleviate pain.
▷ 3 Stock solutions must be diluted before injection. Follow diluting instructions carefully; do not use diluents containing bacteriostatic agents. Sterile Water for Injection is the preferred diluent.
▷ 4 Note that solutions in Sterile Water are stable for up to 6 weeks at room temperature, but solutions in saline or dextrose are stable only for 24 hours.
▷ 5 Closely monitor patient postoperatively because drug may have extended action due to slow metabolism.

▶ thiamylal
Surital

Uses
See Methohexital.

Dosage
Induction: 3 ml to 6 ml of a 2.5% solution at a rate of 1 ml/5 sec
Maintenance: 2.5% solution by intermittent IV injection as needed; alternately, continuous drip (0.3% solution) sufficient to maintain desired depth

Fate
Very rapid onset and short duration (10 min–30 min)

Common Side-Effects
Respiratory depression, hypotension

Significant Adverse Reactions
See Methohexital.

Contraindications
See Methohexital.

Interactions
See Methohexital.

▶ NURSING ALERTS
See Methohexital. In addition:
▷ 1 Do not mix solutions of atropine, d-tubocurarine, or succinylcholine with thiamylal solution prior to injection. Give separately.
▷ 2 Do not heat solutions for sterilization.

▶ NURSING CONSIDERATIONS
See Methohexital. In addition:
▷ 1 Do not reconstitute thiamylal with Ringer's Solution or solutions containing bacteriostatic or buffer agents because precipitate can occur.
▷ 2 When preparing dilute solutions for IV drip, use 5% Dextrose or saline rather than sterile water to avoid extreme hypotonicity and danger of hemolysis.
▷ 3 Use solutions stored in a refrigerator within 6 days, and those at room temperature within 24 hours.

▶ thiopental
Pentothal

Uses
See Methohexital. In addition:
1 Control of convulsive states during and following general or local anesthesia or other causes
2 Aid to narcoanalysis and narcosynthesis in psychiatric disorders

Dosage
(Must be individualized according to age, sex, and body weight)
Injection (doses represent average range)
Anesthesia:
Induction—2 ml to 3 ml of a 2.5% solution at 20-second and 40-second intervals; maintenance—1 ml to 2 ml as needed (continuous IV drip—0.2% to 0.4%)
Convulsive States: 3 ml to 5 ml of a 2.5% solution
Psychiatric Disorders: 4 ml/min of a 2.5% solution until drowsy but still coherent (IV drip—0.2% at a rate not to exceed 50 ml/min)
("Test" dose of 1 ml to 3 ml of a 2.5% solution is often given to determine sensitivity prior to giving larger dose.)
Rectal
1 g/75 lb; (30 mg/kg); total dosage should not exceed 1.5 g for children or 4 g for adults over 200 lb

Fate
Rapid onset (30 sec) of hypnosis with IV injection, and rapid recovery; readily absorbed rectally when administered as a suspension, with onset of action about 10 minutes; rapidly redistributed into fatty tissue and slowly metabolized by the liver

Common Side-Effects
Respiratory depression, sneezing, and coughing

Significant Adverse Reactions
See methohexital; in addition, necrosis and sloughing of tissues on extravasation, arteriospasm upon inadvertent intra-arterial injection, skeletal muscle hyperactivity; rectal administration can result in irritation, diarrhea, cramping and bleeding.

Contraindications
Latent or manifest porphyria, status asthmaticus, absence of suitable veins, severe cardiovascular disease, hypotension, shock, Addison's disease, hepatic or renal dysfunction, myxedema, increased blood urea, severe anemia, increased intracranial pressure, asthma, and myasthenia gravis. Rectal solution should not be used in the presence of inflammatory, ulcerative, bleeding, or neoplastic lesions of the lower bowel or in patients undergoing rectal surgery.

Interactions
See Methohexital.

▶ NURSING ALERTS
▷ 1 Have appropriate resuscitative equipment and respiratory aids on hand in case of extreme respiratory depression.
▷ 2 Observe vital signs continually during administration, and, if possible, give small test dose initially to determine sensitivity.
▷ 3 If shivering or facial twitching occurs, warm patient with blankets, maintain room temperature near 26°C, and administer chlorpromazine or methylphenidate if needed.
▷ 4 Should extravasation occur, inject 1% procaine and apply heat to area to reduce pain and minimize irritation.
▷ 5 Because thiopental solution contains no bacteriostatic agent, use aseptic technique in preparing and handling solution to prevent contamination. Do *not* sterilize by heating.

▶ NURSING CONSIDERATIONS
▷ 1 Prepare solutions promptly using sterile water, saline, or 5% Dextrose. Do not use sterile water for solutions less than 2% due to danger of hemolysis. Discard unused portions within 24 hours.
▷ 2 Do not mix solutions of acidic (low) *p*H with thiopental solution, because likelihood of precipitation is increased.

B Nonbarbiturate Hypnotic

▶ etomidate
Amidate

Etomidate is a rapid acting hypnotic that is primarily used IV for induction of general anesthesia. The drug has minimal

effects on heart rate, cardiac output, or peripheral circulation but produces frequent myoclonic muscle movements and transient venous pain upon injection.

Uses
1 Induction of general anesthesia
2 Supplemental anesthesia during short operative procedures

Dosage
Induction: 0.2 mg/kg to 0.6 mg/kg IV over 30 seconds to 60 seconds
Maintenance: 0.1 mg/kg to 0.3 mg/kg as needed in combination with nitrous oxide and oxygen

Fate
Onset is usually within 1 minute, and effects persist for 3 minutes to 5 minutes; rapidly metabolized in the liver and primarily excreted by the kidney; highly lipid soluble and widely distributed in the body

Common Side-Effects
Transient venous pain, myoclonic skeletal muscle movements, tonic muscle activity, eye movements

Significant Adverse Reactions
Hypotension, tachycardia, arrhythmias, hyperventilation, transient apnea, laryngospasm, and hiccough

Interactions
1 An additive CNS depressant effect can occur in combination with narcotics, sedatives, and other depressants.

▶ NURSING ALERTS
▷ 1 Be alert for development of myoclonic (and occasionally tonic) skeletal muscle activity following injection.
▷ 2 Note that drug is not recommended for use in children under 10. Cautious use is indicated in pregnant or nursing mothers, and in the presence of respiratory disease.

▶ NURSING CONSIDERATIONS
▷ 1 Advise patient that pain at the injection site may occur but is usually transient.
▷ 2 Be aware that etomidate is compatible with most commonly used preanesthetic medications.

C Dissociative Agents

Two drugs, ketamine and Innovar, can be used in certain situations in which an anesthetic-like state is desired, but unconsciousness might prove disadvantageous. These agents are employed alone for certain indications or combined with other anesthetics or analgesics. They differ sufficiently in their actions and pharmacologic properties; thus, they will be discussed separately.

▶ ketamine

Ketaject, Ketalar

A rapid-acting anesthetic producing a state of *dissociation,* characterized by profound analgesia, normal skeletal muscle tone and laryngeal reflexes, and variable cardiovascular and respiratory stimulation. The patient is awake but does not respond to pain nor remember the experience. Ketamine's actions are presumed to result from an interruption of *association* pathways in the brain prior to an effect on specific *sensory* pathways. Blood pressure is usually elevated within a few minutes after injection but returns to normal within 15 minutes. Ketamine possesses a rather wide margin of safety and is compatible with commonly used general and local anesthetics. Emergence from ketamine anesthesia is prolonged (several hours), and in 10% to 15% of patients is marked by psychological manifestations ranging from pleasant (dream-like states, vivid imagery) to quite disagreeable (nightmare-like effects, hallucinations). These may be accompanied by confusion, excitement, and irrational behavior.

Uses

1 Diagnostic and short surgical procedures not requiring skeletal muscle relaxation, *e.g.,* treatment of burns
2 Induction of anesthesia before administration of other general anesthetics
3 Supplementation of low-potency agents such as nitrous oxide

Dosage

Induction: 1 mg/kg to 4.5 mg/kg IV injection over 60 seconds, or 6.5 mg/kg to 13 mg/kg IM. Alternately, 1 mg/kg to 2 mg/kg by slow IV injection (0.5 mg/kg/min) in combination with diazepam (2 mg–5 mg IV over 60 sec) in a separate syringe
Maintenance: increments of one half to full-induction doses repeated as needed, titrated to patient's needs

Fate

Onset of surgical anesthesia is 30 seconds with IV injection and 3 minutes to 4 minutes for IM; duration lasts 5 minutes to 10 minutes IV and 15 minutes to 25 minutes IM. Recovery time is dose-dependent; metabolites are excreted primarily in the urine.

Common Side-Effects

Elevated blood pressure, tachycardia, and respiratory stimulation

Significant Adverse Reactions

Pain at injection site, laryngospasm, rash, diplopia, nystagmus, intensified muscle tone (tonic or clonic convulsions); large doses may produce respiratory depression, hypotension, or arrhythmias. Upon recovery, CNS effects such as hallucinations, vivid dreams; or nightmares, confusion, and irrational behavior can occur. See Nursing Alerts.

Contraindications

Individuals for whom an elevation in blood pressure may prove dangerous

Interactions

1 Barbiturates or narcotics may prolong ketamine recovery time.
2 Severe hypertension and tachycardia can occur in the presence of thyroid drugs.

▶ NURSING ALERTS

▷ 1 During the recovery period, minimize verbal, visual, and tactile stimulation to reduce the danger of irrational behavior and other disturbing psychological manifestations. A rapid-acting barbiturate can be given to control severe emergence reactions.

▷ 2 Continually monitor blood pressure and respiration during ketamine use. Be prepared to provide assistance with mechanical ventilation if respiratory depression occurs.

▷ 3 Do *not* use without additional muscle relaxants in surgical or diagnostic procedures involving the pharynx, larynx, or bronchial tree.

▷ 4 Use with caution in the alcoholic, in patients with hypertension and elevated cerebrospinal fluid pressure, and in pregnant women.

▷ 5 Administer drug slowly IV (over 1 min) to avoid excessive respiratory depression and hypertension. Do not inject 100 mg/ml concentration IV without dilution in sterile water, saline, or dextrose.

▶ NURSING CONSIDERATIONS

▷ 1 Note that disturbing emergence reactions are less likely to occur in very young (under 15) and elderly (over 65) patients, and when the drug is used IM rather than IV.

▷ 2 Do not mix ketamine with barbiturates in the same syringe, because chemical incompatibility will result.

▷ 3 Be aware that tonic–clonic movements may occur during ketamine anesthesia. These do *not* signify a light plane of anesthesia and do *not* indicate a need for additional drug.

▷ 4 Use atropine, scopolamine, or other antisecretory drugs prior to administration of ketamine.

▷ 5 Read product literature for specific recommendations for application of ketamine. These recommendations are quite numerous and encompass many different types of procedures.

▶ Innovar

A combination of a narcotic analgesic (fentanyl) and a neuroleptic or major tranquilizer (droperidol), producing an effect termed *neuroleptanalgesia,* characterized by general quiescence, reduced motor activity, and profound analgesia; complete loss of consciousness usually does not occur with Innovar alone. It produces mild to moderate hypotension and bradycardia, respiratory depression, and muscle rigidity.

Uses

1 Production of tranquilization and analgesia for diagnostic and minor surgical procedures
2 Induction of anesthesia or anesthetic premedication
3 Adjunct for the maintenance of general and regional anesthesia

Dosage

(1 ml contains 0.05 mg fentanyl and 2.5 mg droperidol)

Premedication: 0.5 ml to 2.0 ml IM 45 minutes to 60 minutes prior to surgery (Children—0.25 ml/20 lbs IM)

Induction: 1 ml/20 lb to 25 lb by slow IV injection (3 min–5 min), or 10 ml/250 ml 5% Dextrose by IV drip. (Children—0.5 ml/20 lb IM)

Diagnostic: 0.5 ml to 2.0 ml IM 45 minutes to 60 minutes before procedure; increments of 0.5 ml to 1.0 ml IV may be used for prolonged procedures as needed. Dosage must be individualized and adjusted according to need. Vital signs must be monitored during administration.

Fate

The drug combination exhibits a fairly slow onset and prolonged duration, although each component has different characteristics. Fentanyl possesses an onset of 5 minutes to 10 minutes and a duration of 30 minutes to 60 minutes. Droperidol has a slower onset (30 min) and prolonged action (up to 6 hr).

Common Side-Effects

Respiratory depression, muscle rigidity, hypotension, and postoperative drowsiness

Significant Adverse Reactions

Extrapyramidal symptoms (see Chap. 22), dizziness, laryngospasm, bronchospasm, shivering, tachycardia, vomiting, delirium, and hallucinations

Contraindications

Presence of MAO inhibitors, children under 2 and parkinsonism

Interactions

1 CNS depressants (*e.g.,* barbiturates, narcotics, alcohol) may have additive CNS effects with Innovar.

▶ NURSING ALERTS

▷ 1 Because one component of the drug is a narcotic capable of causing severe respiratory depression, have appropriate resuscitative equipment and narcotic antagonists (Naloxone) on hand.
▷ 2 Reduce the initial dose in elderly, debilitated, and other poor-risk patients.
▷ 3 Use cautiously in patients with arrhythmias, chronic obstructive pulmonary disease, and liver or kidney dysfunction.
▷ 4 Give IV injection *slowly* to minimize the occurrence of muscle rigidity. If it should occur, use respiratory assistance and a neuromuscular blocking drug.

▶ NURSING CONSIDERATIONS

▷ 1 Recognize that fluids and pressor agents may be needed to manage hypotension, and have these agents available.
▷ 2 Note that when Innovar is used for procedures such as bronchoscopy, appropriate topical anesthesia is still needed.

Summary. General Anesthetics

Drug	Preparations	Usual Dosage Range
Inhalation Gases		
Cyclopropane	Orange cylinders	Induction—50%
		Maintenance—10% to 20%
		Analgesia—1% to 2%
Ethylene	Red cylinders	Anesthesia—80%
Nitrous oxide	Blue cylinders	Induction—70% to 80%
		Maintenance—70%
		Analgesia—20% to 30%
Volatile Liquids		
Enflurane (Ethrane)	125-ml, 250-ml bottles	Induction—3.5% to 4.5%
		Maintenance—1.5% to 3.0%
Ether	Containers of various sizes	Induction—5% to 7%
		Maintenance—3% to 5%
Halothane (Fluothane)	125-ml, 250-ml containers	Induction—1% to 4%
		Maintenance—0.5% to 2%
Isoflurane (Forane)	100-ml, 125-ml, 250-ml bottles	Induction—1.5% to 3% for 5 minutes to 10 minutes
		Maintenance—1.0% to 2.5% with nitrous oxide

(continued)

Summary. General Anesthetics *(continued)*

Drug	Preparations	Usual Dosage Range
Methoxyflurane (Penthrane)	15-ml, 125-ml bottles	Induction—3% Maintenance—0.2% to 0.4% Analgesia—0.3% to 0.8%

Intravenous

Ultrashort-Acting Barbiturates

Drug	Preparations	Usual Dosage Range
Methohexital (Brevital)	Powder for injection— 500 mg, 2.5 g, 5 g in ampules or vials	Induction—5 ml to 12 ml of a 1% solution at 1 ml/5 sec Maintenance—2 ml to 4 ml of a 1% solution every 4 minutes to 7 minutes (IV drip—0.2% at a rate of 1 drop/sec)
Thiamylal (Surital)	Powder for injection—1- g, 5-g, 10-g vials	Induction—1 ml/5 sec of a 2.5% solution Maintenance—2.5% solution as needed (IV drip—0.3% solution)
Thiopental (Pentothal)	Injection—250-mg, 400- mg, 500-mg syringes 500-mg, 1-g vials 1-g, 2.5-g, 5-g kits (2.5%) 2.5-g, 5-g kits (2.0%) Rectal suspension: 400 mg/g, in 2.0-g syringe with applicator	*Anesthesia* Induction—2 ml to 3 ml of 2.5% solution at 20-second to 40-second intervals Maintenance—1 ml to 2 ml 2.5% solution as needed (IV drip 0.2%–0.4%) *Convulsions*—3 ml to 5 ml of 2.5% solution *Psychiatry*—4 ml/min of 2.5% solution (IV drip—0.2% at a rate of 50 ml/min) *Rectal*—1 g/50 lb to 75 lb to a maximum of 1.5 g for children and 4 g for adults.

Nonbarbiturate Hypnotic

Drug	Preparations	Usual Dosage Range
Etomidate (Amidate)	Injection—2 mg/ml	0.2 mg/kg–0.6 mg/kg IV over 30 seconds to 60 seconds

Dissociative Agents

Drug	Preparations	Usual Dosage Range
Ketamine (Ketaject, Ketalar)	Injection—10 mg/ml, 50 mg/ml, 100 mg/ml	Induction—1 mg/kg to 4.5 mg/kg IV over 60 seconds or 6.5 mg/kg to 13 mg/kg IM Maintenance—half full induction dose repeated as needed
Innovar	Injection—2-ml, 5-ml ampules (0.05 mg fentanyl and 2.5 mg droperidol per ml)	Premedication—0.5 ml to 2.0 ml IM 45 minutes to 60 minutes prior to surgery (Children—0.25 ml/20 lb IM) Induction—1 ml/20 lb to 25 lb by slow IV injection (IV drip—10 ml/250 ml 5% dextrose) Diagnosis—0.5 ml to 2.0 ml IM 45 minutes to 60 minutes before procedure Increments of 0.5 ml to 1.0 ml IV as required

The narcotic analgesics encompass a group of both naturally occurring and synthetic agents capable of relieving severe pain in the conscious state. Because the prototype of these drugs is morphine, which is obtained from the seeds of the opium poppy, these compounds are often termed *opiates*. The naturally occurring alkaloids of opium (morphine, codeine) are themselves commonly used, or they may be modified chemically to form semisynthetic derivatives that are significantly more potent in some cases than the two natural alkaloids. In addition, a group of purely synthetic opiate compounds have been prepared that produce many pharmacologic effects similar to those of morphine but differ slightly in some of their actions.

Most opiates possess only an agonistic action at the narcotic receptor sites; however, a few drugs exhibit not only a receptor activating action but a partial antagonistic action at certain narcotic receptors as well. These latter compounds are termed narcotic agonist–antagonist analgesics, and are claimed to have a lower abuse potential and less respiratory depression in large doses than the pure opiate agonists. (See Classification of Narcotic Analgesics, below.) When administered in equivalent analgesic amounts, principal differences among the narcotic agents are seen in onset and duration of action. Table 18-1 lists the approximate oral and parenteral dosage equivalents of the important narcotic analgesics. It is important to recognize that addiction liability, a major problem inherent in the repeated use of narcotics, closely parallels potency, and habituation is an almost inescapable consequence of prolonged use of the potent opiates. The topic of drug addiction is discussed more fully in Chapter 81.

The sites and mechanisms of narcotic-induced analgesia are multiple and complex. These drugs are known to modify cholinergic, adrenergic, and serotonergic mechanisms; however, the importance of these effects to the analgesic activity of the compounds is still unclear, because no single neurotransmitter can account for the varied effects of the opiates.

Narcotic analgesics have the ability to modify both the actual sensation of pain through an effect on pain pathways in the spinal cord and brain, as well as the perception of the noxious sensation by the patient through an effect on higher cortical areas. Thus, the transmission of the painful stimuli from the site of origin to the sensory cortex is reduced, while at the same time the painful sensation is perceived as being less intense or bothersome. The resultant tranquility and release from tension often lead to a state of euphoria and an exaggerated sense of well-being, and it is this euphoric state that is frequently responsible for the desire to repeat the drug, ultimately leading to habituation in many chronic users.

The opiate drugs exert their effects by combining with specific narcotic receptor sites in the CNS. Sites of high receptor concentration include the dorsal horn of the spinal cord and several subcortical brain areas, such as the periaqueductal gray, hypothalamus, thalamus, locus coeruleus, and raphe. At least three different types of opiate receptors (mu, kappa, sigma) have been characterized, and they are differentiated primarily by the responses which each receptor

Narcotic Analgesics and Antagonists

18

Table 18-1. Comparable Potencies of Opiates

Drug	Equivalent Dosage Ranges (SC, IM)	(Oral)
Morphine	10 mg	60 mg
Fentanyl	0.1 mg–0.2 mg	
Hydromorphone	1 mg–2 mg	8 mg
Oxymorphone	1 mg–1.5 mg	6 mg
Levorphanol	2 mg–3 mg	4 mg
Butorphanol*	2 mg–4 mg	
Methadone	7 mg–10 mg	20 mg
Nalbuphine*	10 mg	
Oxycodone	15 mg	30 mg
Pentazocine*	30 mg–60 mg	150 mg
Alphaprodine	45 mg	
Meperidine	75 mg–100 mg	300 mg
Codeine	120 mg	200 mg

* Narcotic agonist–antagonist

mediates. Table 18-2 lists the various narcotic receptors and the pharmacologic effects associated with each receptor type.

The narcotic agonists bind to the different receptors with varying affinities, although their principal effects are exerted at the mu receptors. The narcotic agonists–antagonists likewise have a differential effect at the various receptor sites. They appear to be partial antagonists at the mu sites, but are more active agonists at the kappa sites than are the pure narcotic agonists. This may help explain their lower abuse potential.

A major development in the opiate field has been the isolation of endogenous morphine-like compounds (endorphins and enkephalins) from various subcortical brain areas. The principal endorphin is beta-endorphin, a polypeptide found in largest amounts in the pituitary. It is one of the most potent endogenous opiate-like substances known. The major enkephalins are methionine–enkephalin and leucine–enkephalin, pentapeptides that differ only in the terminal amino acid. These compounds are structural subunits of beta-endorphin (i.e., their structure is contained within the larger beta-endorphin molecule), but they are probably not derived by fragmentation of beta-endorphin

Table 18-2. Opiate Receptors

Receptor	Pharmacologic Effects
mu (μ)	Supraspinal analgesia Euphoria Respiratory depression Addiction
kappa (κ)	Spinal analgesia Sedation Miosis
sigma (σ)	Dysphoria Hallucinations Respiratory/vasomotor stimulation

but rather synthesized in another manner. The enkephalins are particularly abundant in the brainstem, spinal cord and basal ganglia, where they are believed to act by modifying impulse transmission in pain pathways by combining with opiate receptor sites in a manner similar to the narcotic drugs. They may be released in response to various stimuli and also by the presence of a narcotic analgesic. Although both the endorphins and enkephalins can mimic the action of narcotic drugs in various pharmacologic test systems, they are of little clinical value inasmuch as they are not absorbed orally and are rapidly degraded by metabolizing enzymes in the brain, blood, and other tissues. Their precise function in central adaptation to pain and stress as well as their role in the analgesic and addictive properties of the narcotic drugs remain to be established definitively. The development of synthetic analogs of these endogenous substances that would retain their analgesic action while conferring oral effectiveness and resistance to rapid inactivation would be a major development in the area of pain management.

The pharmacologic effects of therapeutic doses of the narcotic analgesics extend to many different systems of the body. The more important actions of the opiates are outlined in Table 18-3. However, not all of these effects are exhibited to the same degree by all of the narcotic agents. Moreover, most of the actions are dose dependent, and therefore are more marked at high dose levels.

Table 18-3. Pharmacologic Effects of Narcotic Analgesics

CNS

Analgesia
Sedation
Euphoria
Emesis (antiemetic at very high doses)
Depressed cough reflex
Respiratory depression (depression of medullary respiratory center)

Cardiovascular

Orthostatic hypotension (depression of medullary vasomotor center; peripheral vascular dilation)

GI Tract

Decreased peristalsis and stomach motility
Delayed gastric emptying time
Constipation

Smooth Muscle

Increased tone of most nonvascular smooth muscle (e.g., GI, urinary, biliary)

Urinary System

Urinary tract spasm
Contraction of urinary sphincter
Release of antidiuretic hormone

Eye

Miosis

The principal acute toxic effect of morphine and related narcotic agonists is respiratory depression, characterized by slow, shallow, irregular respiration and cyanosis. Other important adverse effects include hypotension, decreased urinary output, and hypothermia. Treatment includes artificial respiration and use of a narcotic antagonist. Use of narcotic agonists–antagonists results in some sedation at normal doses. Higher doses may elicit sweating, nausea and dizziness, but the extent of respiratory depression is less at elevated doses than with comparable doses of pure narcotic agonists.

Chronic use of opiate drugs invariably results in development of tolerance, habituation, and eventually physical dependence. Useful diagnostic signs of dependence are miosis, constipation, superficial infections, itching and, of course, needle marks, scars, and abscesses in the abuser. Further attention is directed to the problem of narcotic abuse in Chapter 81.

Classification of Narcotic Analgesics

Narcotic analgesics may be classified into one of two broad categories, the narcotic agonists and the narcotic agonists–antagonists. The former group comprises those clinically useful opiates that possess only an agonistic action at narcotic receptor sites, whereas the latter group is composed of those compounds that have both an agonistic and a partial antagonistic action at certain receptors, as outlined above. Within each of these broad categories of opiate drugs, a subclassification exists that is based on chemical structure of the individual drugs. Even within each subclass, different potencies and toxicities are noted among the representative drugs. For example, while morphine and codeine belong to the same chemical grouping (*i.e.,* phenanthrenes), the former is quite potent and highly addicting, while the latter is much less potent and habituating.

The various classes of narcotic analgesics are listed below:
I. Narcotic agonist analgesics
   A. Phenanthrenes
      1. Naturally occurring opium alkloids (morphine, codeine)
      2. Semisynthetic derivatives of morphine (hydromorphone, oxymorphone)
      3. Semisynthetic derivatives of codeine (oxycodone)
   B. Methadones (methadone, propoxyphene)
   C. Morphinans (levorphanol)
   D. Phenylpiperidines (alphaprodine, fentanyl, meperidine)
II. Narcotic agonist–antagonist analgesics
   A. Phenanthrenes (nalbuphine)
   B. Morphinans (butorphanol)
   C. Benzomorphans (pentazocine)

Most of the narcotic drugs exhibit qualitatively the same actions and adverse effects; they differ primarily in potency, onset, and duration of action. The pharmacology of the opiate drugs, therefore, is discussed as a group, with the exception of the narcotic antagonists. Specific information relating to each narcotic agonist is provided in Table 18-3. The two narcotic antagonists are reviewed together at the conclusion of the chapter.

Narcotic Analgesics

Alphaprodine	Methadone
Butorphanol	Morphine
Codeine	Nalbuphine
Fentanyl	Opium
Hydrocodone	Oxycodone
Hydromorphone	Oxymorphone
Levorphanol	Pentazocine
Meperidine	Propoxyphene

Mechanism
Complex and incompletely understood; elevate the pain threshold, alter the perception of pain, reduce the anxious or fearful reaction to the presence of pain, and induce sedation or hypnosis. Effects are probably due to several mechanisms, including direct activation of opiate receptor sites in the spinal cord, brain stem, and subcortical brain areas, and perhaps increased release of endogenous opiates. Activate descending spinal cord pathways, thus interfering with incoming sensory pain pathways at various levels; may reduce calcium influx into neuronal cells, impairing release of norepinephrine, dopamine, serotonin, and possibly substance P; decrease sensitivity of medullary respiratory center to carbon dioxide, resulting in dose-dependent respiratory depression; depress responsiveness of alpha-adrenergic receptors, leading to visceral pooling of blood and orthostatic hypotension; reduce GI peristalsis by direct relaxant effect on intestinal smooth muscle; increase tone of urinary bladder sphincter; stimulate chemoreceptor trigger zone in brain stem, causing nausea and vomiting

Uses
1 Relief of moderate to severe pain (*e.g.,* myocardial infarction, carcinomas, burns, fractures, postsurgical trauma)
2 Preoperative medication to reduce anxiety and to enhance effects of general anesthetics
3 Relief of persistent cough (especially codeine)
4 Relief of severe diarrhea and cramping
5 Relief of dyspnea associated with pulmonary edema or left ventricular failure
6 Detoxification treatment of narcotic addiction (*methadone only*)
7 Obstetrical analgesia

Dosage
See Table 18-4.

(*Text continues on p. 154.*)

Table 18-4. Narcotic Analgesics

Drug	Preparations	Usual Dosage Range	Remarks
Phenanthrenes			
Morphine (Morphine Sulfate, RMS, Roxanol)	Tablets—10 mg, 15 mg, 30 mg Injection—2 mg/ml, 4 mg/ml, 8 mg/ml, 10 mg/ml, 15 mg/ml Oral solution—10 mg/5 ml, 20 mg/5 ml Concentrated oral solution—20 mg/ml Suppositories—5 mg, 10 mg, 20 mg	Oral—10 mg to 30 mg every 4 hours SC, IM— (Adults) 5 mg to 20 mg every 4 hours (Children) 0.1 to 0.2 mg/kg IV—4 mg/5 ml to 10 mg/5 ml injected over 4-minute to 5-minute period	Principal opium alkaloid, and standard to which other opiates are compared; most effective parenterally because GI availability is limited; commonly produces drowsiness and relief from anxiety; large doses induce deep sleep and profound respiratory depression; concentrated oral solution (Roxanol) is used in cancer patients and others with severe chronic pain. (Schedule II)
Codeine (Codeine Phosphate, Codeine Sulfate)	Hypodermic tablets—15 mg, 30 mg, 60 mg Tablets—15 mg, 30 mg, 60 mg Injection—30 mg/ml, 60 mg/ml	Analgesia Adults—15 mg to 60 mg 4 times/day, orally, SC, IM, or IV Children—3 mg/kg daily in 6 divided doses, orally, SC, or IM Antitussive Adults—10 mg to 20 mg every 4 hours to 6 hours to a maximum of 120 mg/24 hours Children—(6 yr–12 yr) 5 mg to 10 mg every 4 hours to 6 hours (maximum 60 mg/day) (2 yr–6 yr) 2.5 mg to 5 mg every 4 hours to 6 hours (maximum 30 mg/day)	Less potent and less abuse potential than morphine; widely used in cough medications; suppresses cough by direct depressant effect on medullary cough center; as an analgesic, most frequently used in combination with aspirin, acetaminophen or other analgesics; high doses (e.g., 60 mg) may cause restlessness and excitement; rapid onset of action following oral administration (10 min–15 min) and effects persist for up to 6 hours; used in combination with centrally acting muscle relaxants for pain of muscle spasm and rigidity (Schedule II)
Hydromorphone (Dilaudid)	Tablets—1 mg, 2 mg, 3 mg, 4 mg Injection—1 mg/ml, 2 mg/ml, 4 mg/ml 10 mg/ml Suppositories—3 mg	SC, IM—2 mg to 4 mg every 4 hours to 6 hours, up to 10 mg Oral—2 mg every 4 hours to 6 hours Rectal—1 suppository every 6 hours to 8 hours	Very potent (8×–10× morphine) analgesic, producing less sedation, vomiting, and nausea than morphine; elicits marked respiratory depression; therefore, use smallest dose possible; 10 mg/ml injection (Dilaudid-HP) used in severe, chronic pain. Suppositories give prolonged effect; high abuse potential and popular "street drug" due to extreme potency and lack of hypnotic effect (Schedule II)
Oxycodone (Oxycodone)	Tablets—5 mg Oral solution—5 mg/5 ml	5 mg to 10 mg every 6 hours	Moderately potent, orally effective narcotic, commonly used in fixed combinations with aspirin (Percodan, Codoxy) or acetaminophen (Percocet)
Oxymorphone (Numorphan)	Injection—1 mg/ml, 1.5 mg/ml Suppositories—5 mg	SC, IM—1 mg to 1.5 mg every 4 hours to 6 hours IV—0.5 mg as needed Rectal—5 mg every 4 hours to 6 hours Analgesia during labor—0.5 mg to 1 mg IM every 4 hours to 6 hours	Rapid acting (5 min–10 min), potent (5×–10× morphine) analgesic. High incidence of nausea, vomiting, and euphoria; little constipation or antitussive action; Not recommended in children under 12; cautious use in pregnancy (other than during labor) (Schedule II)
Opium (Paregoric, Pantopon)	Injection (Pantopon) 20-mg opium alkaloids hydrochlorides/ml = 15 mg morphine Tincture 10% opium in 19% alcohol	Injection IM, SC—5 mg to 20 mg every 4 hours to 5 hours *Tincture* 0.6 ml (6 mg morphine) every 4 hours	Activity primarily due to morphine content; use has been largely replaced by morphine or other narcotics, except for paregoric, which is widely used for cramps, diarrhea, and teething pain in infants (topical application);

Table 18-4. Narcotic Analgesics (continued)

Drug	Preparations	Usual Dosage Range	Remarks
	Camphorated Tincture (Paregoric) 2 mg morphine equivalent/5 ml	*Camphorated tincture* Adults—5 ml to 10 ml (2 mg to 4 mg morphine) 2 to 4 times/ day Children—0.25 to 0.5 ml/kg	discontinue drug once diarrhea has been controlled, to prevent excessive dosage; do not confuse paregoric (camphorated opium tincture containing 2 mg morphine/5 ml) with opium tincture itself (50 mg morphine/5 ml); absorption of drug from GI tract is improved if diluted in a little water; injection and tincture as Schedule II and camphorated tincture is Schedule III
Nalbuphine (Nubain)	Injection—10 mg/ml	SC, IM, IV—10 mg/70 kg individual; repeat every 3 hours to 6 hours as necessary; maximum 160 mg/day	Chemically related to oxycodone and naloxone, and possesses both agonist and weak antagonistic properties; analgesia equivalent to morphine on a mg basis with somewhat lower abuse potential; may precipitate withdrawal symptoms in patients on chronic narcotic therapy; use one-fourth normal dose initially in these patients; high incidence of sedation; does not increase systemic vascular resistance like other narcotic agonist–antagonists; duration of analgesia ranges from 3 hours to 6 hours; do not use in pregnant women or children under 18 years of age.
Methadones			
Methadone (Dolophine)	Injection—10 mg/ml Tablets—5 mg, 10 mg Oral solution—1 mg/ml, 2 mg/ml Dispersible tablets—40 mg (for detoxification only)	Analgesia IM, SC, orally—2.5 mg to 10 mg every 3 hours to 4 hours (children 0.7 mg/kg/ day) Narcotic detoxification (highly individualized depending on severity of withdrawal symptoms) 15 mg to 20 mg orally (up to 40 mg) to suppress symptoms; treatment not to exceed 21 days during which time the dose is gradually reduced Maintenance Therapy 20 mg to 120 mg daily, individualized to control abstinence symptoms but not produce sedation or respiratory depression	May be used to relieve severe pain, preferably IM; long-acting and less sedating than morphine; one-half as potent orally as parenterally; exerts a similar degree of respiratory depression and addiction liability as morphine; not recommended for obstetrics or as an analgesic in young children; principal use is detoxification and maintenance of narcotic addiction in approved programs; administered orally on a daily basis; abstinence syndrome is qualitatively similar to morphine, but onset is slower, course is more prolonged, and symptoms are less severe; with prolonged oral use, most side-effects disappear, but constipation and sweating often persist; euphoria is much less prominent with methadone, and addict may eventually overcome compulsive need for the narcotic "high"; should be used in combination with other psychiatric and social counseling, See Chapter 81. (Schedule II)
Propoxyphene (Darvon, Dolene, Pargesic 65, Profene 65, SK-65)	Capsules—32 mg, 65 mg Tablets—100 mg Suspension—10 mg/ml	Adults—65 mg to 100 mg every 4 hours *Note:* 65 mg of the HCl salt is equivalent to 100 mg of the napsylate salt.	Very *weak* analgesic, structurally related to methadone; little antitussive activity; has many of the side-effects of narcotics and can produce habituation and

(continued)

Table 18-4. Narcotic Analgesics (continued)

Drug	Preparations	Usual Dosage Range	Remarks
			physical dependence to approximately the same degree as codeine; restlessness, tremor, and mild euphoria commonly occur; usually administered in fixed combination with aspirin and caffeine (e.g., Bexophene, Darvon Compound, SK-65 Compound), acetaminophen (e.g., Darvocet), or aspirin (e.g., Darvon w/ASA); will potentiate CNS depressant effects of alcohol and tranquilizers; symptoms of overdosage resemble those of narcotics, with the addition of convulsions; treatment consists of respiratory assistance, narcotic antagonists, anticonvulsants, and circulatory support (fluids, vasopressors); use with caution, and avoid prolonged or excessive dosage; maximum recommended doses are 390 mg/day of the HCl salt and 600 mg/day of the napsylate salt (Schedule IV)
Morphinans			
Levorphanol (Levo-Dromoran)	Injection—2 mg/ml Tablets—2 mg	2 mg to 3 mg orally or SC every 4 hours to 6 hours	Very potent analgesic (4×–5× morphine); almost as effective orally as parenterally; used preoperatively to potentiate and prolong general anesthesia, and to shorten recovery time; also is a useful supplement to nitrous oxide–oxygen anesthesia; low incidence of nausea, vomiting, and constipation, but strong sedative and respiratory depressant; slow onset of peak effect (60 min–90 min) but prolonged duration (6 hr–8 hr); reduce dose in pediatric and geriatric population and in poor-risk patients (Schedule II)
Butorphanol (Stadol)	Injection—1 mg/ml, 2 mg/ml	IM—2 mg every 3 hours to 4 hours (maximum 4 mg/dose) IV—1 mg every 3 hours to 4 hours	Potent analgesic (4×–7× that of morphine on a weight basis); respiratory depression with 2-mg dose is equivalent to that observed with 10 mg of morphine, but does not increase appreciably at 4 mg; possesses weak narcotic antagonistic activity; thus, do not use in patients dependent on narcotics because withdrawal symptoms can occur; most frequent side-effect is sedation; peak analgesia occurs in 1 hour with IM use and persists for 3 hours to 4 hours; not recommended in children under 18
Phenylpiperidines			
Meperidine (Demerol, Pethadol)	Injection—25 mg/ml, 50 mg/ml, 75 mg/ml, 100 mg/ml Tablets—50 mg, 100 mg	Analgesia IM, SC, Orally—50 mg to 150 mg every 3 hours to 4 hours	Moderately potent analgesic (1/10 morphine) with weak antitussive activity; much less spasmogenic and constipating than most other

Table 18-4. Narcotic Analgesics (continued)

Drug	Preparations	Usual Dosage Range	Remarks
	Elixir—50 mg/5 ml	Children—1 mg/kg to 2 mg/kg IM, SC, or orally every 3 hours to 4 hours Preoperative Medication Adults—50 mg to 100 mg IM or SC 30 minutes to 90 minutes before anesthesia Children—1 mg/kg to 2 mg/kg IM or SC Obstetrical Analgesia 50 mg to 100 mg IM or SC; repeat at 1-hour to 3-hour intervals	narcotics; more rapid onset and shorter duration of action (2 hr–4 hr) compared to morphine; significantly less effective orally than parenterally; frequent dizziness and occasional tremors, uncoordinated muscle movements, and other signs of CNS excitation can occur; used for moderate or severe pain, often associated with diagnostic procedures, minor surgical procedures or obstetrics; also for preanesthetic medication and by slow IV infusion (1 mg/ml) for support of anesthesia; elixir should be diluted with water to minimize local anesthesia of mucous membranes; solutions of meperidine and barbiturates are incompatible (Schedule II)
Fentanyl (Sublimaze)	Injection—0.05 mg/ml	Preoperative 0.05 mg to 0.1 mg IM General Anesthesia Induction—0.05 mg to 0.1 mg IV (repeat at 2-min–3-min intervals) Maintenance—0.025 mg to 0.05 mg IV or IM as needed *Adjunct to General Anesthesia* 0.002 mg/kg to 0.05 mg/kg as needed Postoperative 0.05 mg to 0.1 mg IM every 1 hour to 2 hours for pain, tachypnea, and delirium Children (2 yr–12 yr)—0.02 mg to 0.03 mg/20 lb to 25 lb	Very potent (100× morphine) analgesic that is used for short durations (*e.g.*, preoperative, during surgery or postoperative), to relieve pain and anxiety and as an anesthetic agent with oxygen in selected high-risk patients (*e.g.*, open-heart surgery, complicated neurologic procedures); rapid onset (10 min–15 min IM) and short duration (1 hr–2 hr); respiratory depression often outlasts analgesia; have antidotal measures (*e.g.*, oxygen, endotracheal tube, narcotic antagonist, muscle relaxant) on hand; rapid IV administration may cause muscle spasm or rigidity; also available in combination with the neuroleptic droperidol as Innovar, which is used to produce analgesia and tranquilization (neuroleptanalgesia) for short surgical and diagnostic procedures (see Chapter 17); combination may result in restlessness, hallucinations, extrapyramidal symptoms, and postoperative drowsiness. Vital signs should be monitored continuously during use. (Schedule II)
Alphaprodine (Nisentyl)	Injection—40 mg/ml, 60 mg/ml	Analgesia 0.4 mg/kg to 0.6 mg/kg IV or 0.4 mg/kg to 1.2 mg/kg SC Obstetrics 40 mg to 60 mg SC after cervical dilation has begun; repeat every 2 hours as needed Minor surgery 40 mg SC or 20 mg IV Preoperatively 20 mg to 40 mg SC or 10 mg to 20 mg IV	Rapid acting narcotic with a short duration; primarily used for minor surgery of brief duration, urologic procedures, obstetrics, and pediatric dental procedures; excessive doses can result in convulsions. Onset of action SC is within 10 minutes and effects last for 1 hour to 2 hours; IV injection produces analgesia within 1 minute to 2 minutes, which persists for 30 minutes to 90 minutes; when administered for pediatric dental procedures,

(continued)

Table 18-4. Narcotic Analgesics (continued)

Drug	Preparations	Usual Dosage Range	Remarks
		Pediatric dentistry 0.3 mg/kg to 0.6 mg/kg submucosally	effects should be reversed with naloxone following completion of the procedure; use in children for other than dental procedures is not recommended.
Benzomorphan			
Pentazocine (Talwin)	Tablets—50 mg Injection—30 mg/ml	Oral 50 mg every 3 hours to 4 hours (maximum dose 600 mg/day) IM, SC, IV 30 mg every 3 hours to 4 hours (maximum dose 360 mg/day) Obstetrics 30 mg IM or 20 mg IV every 2 hours to 3 hours	One third as potent as morphine parenterally; possesses some narcotic antagonist activity as well; therefore, can antagonize the effects of other opiates and may elicit withdrawal symptoms in patients who have been taking other narcotics regularly; onset is 15 minutes to 30 minutes after IM, SC, or oral use and 2 minutes to 3 minutes IV; duration from 2 hours to 3 hours parenterally and up to 5 hours with oral use. Has sedative activity and widely used preoperatively and in obstetrics as well as for moderate and severe pain; addiction liability about equal to codeine; tablets are marketed as Talwin-Nx and contain 0.5 mg of naloxone, a potent narcotic antagonist; although inactive orally, naloxone has profound antagonistic actions against narcotics when injected, and its inclusion in the tablet is intended to curb a form of pentazocine abuse in which the tablets are dissolved and injected; can induce tachycardia, hypertension, confusion, hallucinations, bizarre thought processes, and other CNS effects in large doses. Abrupt discontinuation of drug may result in muscle cramping, chills, restlessness, anxiety, and other symptoms of narcotic withdrawal. Do not mix with soluble barbiturates because a precipitate will form. Rotate injection sites if used chronically to minimize sclerosis of skin and subcutaneous tissues. Severe respiratory depression is treated with naloxone and other supportive measures. (Schedule IV)

Fate

GI absorption with orally effective derivatives is usually complete but variable in rate. Many drugs undergo significant first-pass hepatic metabolism after absorption. Onset of action following oral administration is approximately 30 minutes, and from 5 minutes to 30 minutes when used IM or SC. Peak effect occurs in 30 minutes to 90 minutes and is maintained for up to 6 hours (average 3 hr–5 hr). IV administration produces rapid onset and more pronounced peak effects but shorter duration of action. Widely distributed in the body; metabolized largely in the liver and up to 90% excreted in the urine within 24 hours in a conjugated form. Small amounts are recovered in the feces, derived almost entirely from the bile.

Common Side-Effects

Dizziness, lightheadedness, sedation, nausea, sweating, and flushing

Significant Adverse Reactions

CNS—euphoria or dysphoria, headache, agitation, tremor, disorientation, delirium, uncoordinated movements, and transient hallucinations

Cardiovascular—bradycardia, palpitations, hypotension, syncope, and phlebitis (IV injection only)

GI—dry mouth, anorexia, constipation, vomiting, biliary tract spasm

Respiratory—respiratory depression (observed in fetus and newborn as well)

Genitourinary—urinary hesitancy or retention, dysuria, antidiuretic effect, loss of potency or libido

Hypersensitivity—urticaria, pruritus, sneezing, edema, hemorrhagic urticaria, wheal and flare at IV injection site

Other—pain at injection site, local tissue irritation, porphyria

Acute overdose—extreme miosis, hypothermia, oliguria, bradycardia, hypotension, deep sleep, marked respiratory depression, pulmonary edema, coma, cardiac arrest

Contraindications

Convulsive states, severe respiratory depression, acute asthma, undiagnosed acute abdominal conditions, severe ulcerative colitis, and hepatic cirrhosis

Interactions

1 CNS depressant effects of narcotics may be potentiated or prolonged by concurrent use of other CNS depressants (*e.g.*, barbiturates, alcohol, anesthetics,, phenothiazines, sedatives, tricyclic antidepressants).

2 Muscle relaxation and respiratory depression may be intensified by concurrent use of narcotics and neuromuscular blocking agents (*e.g.*, succinylcholine).

3 Symptoms of acute narcotic overdose, possibly causing death, may occur with use of *meperidine* within 14 days of a MAO inhibitor.

4 Withdrawal symptoms may occur in patients addicted to narcotics if the narcotic agonist–antagonists *nalbuphine, pentazocine* or *butorphanol* are added, because they may antagonize the effects of the pure agonists.

5 *Meperidine* has anticholinergic effects that may be additive with those of other drugs (*e.g.*, atropine-like agents, tricyclic antidepressants, quinidine).

▶ NURSING ALERTS

▷ 1 Be aware that narcotic drugs may produce drug dependence upon repeated administration. Always give smallest effective dose over the shortest period of time that will adequately provide the patient with the necessary relief of pain.

▷ 2 Recognize that maximal analgesic effect is attained if drug is given *prior to* development of intense pain.

▷ 3 Use narcotics with extreme caution in patients with head injuries or elevated intracranial pressure, chronic obstructive pulmonary disease, prostatic hypertrophy. Addison's disease, hypothyroidism, acute alcoholism,

delirium tremens, cardiovascular disease (especially supraventricular tachycardia), diabetic acidosis, severe obesity, hepatic or renal failure, and in elderly, debilitated, pregnant, or lactating patients.

▷ 4 When used IV, give a dilute solution by *slow* injection because with rapid injection toxic effects can occur quickly and be severe (*e.g.*, respiratory depression, hypotension, circulatory collapse, cardiac arrest). Always have a narcotic antagonist and measures for respiratory assistance on hand.

▷ 5 Observe patients for early signs of toxicity (respiratory rate below 12/min, miosis, deep sleep). Stop drug, advise physician, and prepare to administer a narcotic antagonist.

▷ 6 Caution patient that drug may impair mental or physical abilities, making tasks involving use of machinery (*e.g.*, driving) hazardous.

▷ 7 Advise patient that orthostatic hypotension can occur. Urge gradual rising to a sitting and standing position to minimize dizziness.

▷ 8 Carefully monitor intake/output ratio and bowel function since drugs can cause urinary retention and fecal impaction. Encourage frequent voiding and check for abdominal or bladder distention.

▷ 9 In the drug-dependent individual, realize that administration of an antagonist will likely produce severe acute withdrawal symptoms. Have supportive measures (*e.g.*, oxygen, IV fluids, vasopressors) on hand, and use smallest dose of antagonist possible.

▷ 10 Use with caution in obstetrics because drugs easily cross the placental barrier and can produce respiratory depression in the fetus and neonate.

▶ NURSING CONSIDERATIONS

▷ 1 Use good judgment in evaluating a patient's need for a narcotic analgesic. Administer a nonaddictive analgesic drug when possible and provide reassurance and supportive care to patients in pain; if a narcotic is needed, note onset and duration of response, and record frequency of administration.

▷ 2 Observe patients carefully for developing dependence (*e.g.*, more frequent requests for medication, feigning pain to obtain drug), and advise physician.

▷ 3 Encourage deep breathing, frequent position changes, and purposeful coughing to prevent atelectasis and other respiratory difficulties in postoperative patients receiving narcotics. Drugs will depress cough and sigh reflexes.

▷ 4 When using IM or SC, aspirate syringe before injection to avoid direct IV injection because toxic effects can be markedly increased.

▷ 5 Advise patient that ambulation is likely to increase incidence of dizziness, transient hypotension, nausea, and vomiting. Assist early ambulation.

▷ 6 Reassure patient that symptoms such as flushing, sweating, itching, feelings of warmth, visual and auditory distortions, and dysphoria are not uncommon, and that they will disappear shortly and are not a cause for anxiety. Keep patient quiet and reduce sensory stimulation as much as possible.

▷ 7 Observe patient (especially postsurgical) for signs that pain is present, for which an analgesic may be needed (*e.g.,* elevated respiratory rate and pulse, grimacing, restlessness).

▷ 8 Keep proper records of all narcotic drugs used, and do not dispense without proper authorization. Learn regulations governing handling and dispensing of all classes of narcotics as listed in Table 18-3 (see Appendix).

Narcotic Antagonists

Drugs capable of reversing many of the effects of the narcotic analgesics, particularly the respiratory depressant effects, are termed *narcotic antagonists.* Of the two currently available drugs in this category, levallorphan is classified as a mixed agonist–antagonist, and naloxone as a *pure* antagonist. When used alone, levallorphan exhibits effects similar to the opiates themselves (*e.g.,* analgesia, sedation, respiratory depression, bradycardia) due to its narcotic-like (agonistic) activity. However, levallorphan is of little clinical value as an analgesic because its use is associated with many unpleasant symptoms, ranging from restlessness and anxiety to dysphoria, delirium, hallucinations, and psychotic reactions. In comparison to morphine and other narcotics, levallorphan possesses stronger receptor attraction but weaker activity at the receptor site. Therefore, in the presence of severe narcotic overdose, levallorphan is capable of *displacing* molecules of the narcotic drug from the receptor site, and lessening the effects of the narcotic poisoning.

The other drug used as a narcotic antagonist, naloxone, exhibits *no* intrinsic activity of its own at narcotic receptor sites, so it is referred to as a *pure* antagonist. For this reason, it is usually considered the drug of choice in most cases of narcotic overdosage.

Narcotic antagonists are specific for poisoning with opiate drugs, and will not reverse the respiratory depression induced by other types of CNS depressants (*e.g.,* barbiturates, anesthetics). The narcotic antagonists are relatively short-acting drugs (*i.e.,* 15 min–30 min) and must be administered at frequent intervals in the severely intoxicated patient. Because levallorphan is a partial agonist, its use is restricted to cases of *severe* opiate-induced respiratory depression, because if it is administered in cases of mild opiate overdose, or in respiratory depression induced by other classes of CNS depressant drugs, levallorphan may further depress respiration due to its agonistic action. This problem, of course, is not associated with naloxone.

▶ levallorphan

Lorfan

Mechanism

Reversible, competitive antagonism of narcotics at the opiate receptor; displaces narcotic from receptor site because of higher affinity; may exert a morphine-like (agonistic) ac-

tion in the absence of severe narcotic overdose and can worsen mild respiratory depression

Uses

1 Treatment of *severe* narcotic-induced respiratory depression, both in adults and neonates secondary to narcotic use in the mother

Dosage

Adults: 1 mg IV, followed at 10-minute to 15-minute intervals by additional doses of 0.5 mg IV (maximum dose—3 mg)

Neonates: 0.05 mg to 0.1 mg IM, SC, or preferably into the umbilical vein immediately after delivery.

Fate

Rapid acting (1 minute–2 minutes); effects persist for 2 hours to 5 hours; easily crosses blood–brain barrier and placental barrier

Common Side-Effects

Miosis, drowsiness, dizziness, sweating, GI upset, heaviness in the limbs, mild respiratory depression

Significant Adverse Reactions

(Usually occur with high doses) Bizarre dreams, visual hallucinations, disorientation, dysphoria; respiratory depression may be enhanced; in neonates, irritability and excessive crying.

Contraindications

Mild respiratory depression, either narcotic-induced or due to other types of drug overdose (*e.g.,* barbiturates, anesthetics, hypnotics), narcotic addiction

Interactions

1 Respiratory depression may be increased if drug is given in presence of other narcotic or CNS depressants. (*e.g.,* barbiturates, anesthetics).

2 Severe withdrawal symptoms can occur in the presence of other narcotics that have been used on a regular basis.

▶ NURSING ALERTS

▷ 1 Do not administer in the presence of respiratory depression due to other than a narcotic drug because the depression can be worsened.

▷ 2 Do not use unless respiratory depression is severe. Mild respiratory depression can be increased by levallorphan.

▷ 3 In cases of severe narcotic overdose, use artificial respiration, oxygen, and other necessary supportive measures with the narcotic antagonist.

▶ NURSING CONSIDERATIONS

▷ 1 Monitor vital signs during use. Observe patient closely for recurrence of respiratory depression following termination of antagonist's action. Duration of narcotic action often outlasts that of the antagonist.

▷ 2 Be alert to appearance of early withdrawal symptoms (*e.g.,* restlessness, sweating, mydriasis, lacrimation) after administration of antagonist. Advise physician and be prepared to begin supportive treatment (*e.g.,* respiratory assistance, vasopressors).

▶ naloxone
Narcan

Mechanism
Competitive antagonism of narcotic drugs at opiate receptor sites; prevents or reverses respiratory depression, sedation, hypotension, and analgesia seen with opiates; can also reverse the dysphoric effects of agonist–antagonist narcotic drugs, such as pentazocine; when administered in the absence of narcotics, produces no analgesia, respiratory depression, miosis, or other effects noted with narcotic drugs; no tolerance or dependence has been reported

Uses
1 Treatment of respiratory depression and other untoward effects induced by narcotic agonists and narcotic agonists–antagonists
2 Diagnosis of suspected narcotic overdosage

Dosage
Narcotic overdosage (known or suspected)
Adults: 0.4 mg to 2.0 mg IV, IM, or SC; may be repeated IV at 2-minute to 3-minute intervals for 2 to 3 doses, then at 1-hour to 2-hour intervals as needed
Children and Neonates: 0.01 mg/kg IV, IM, or SC initially; may repeat with 0.1 mg/kg if needed
Postoperative narcotic depression: 0.1 mg to 0.2 mg IV at 2-minute to 3-minute intervals until desired degree of reversal is attained

Fate
Onset of action 2 minutes to 5 minutes; duration of action is variable depending on dose and route of administration, but effects generally last from 1 hour to 4 hour; metabolized in the liver and excreted as conjugated products in the urine

Significant Adverse Reactions
(Occur with excessive dose or too rapid reversal of narcotic depression) Nausea, vomiting, hypertension, tachycardia, hyperventilation, and tremors

Contraindications
Respiratory depression due to nonnarcotic drugs

▶ NURSING ALERTS
▷ 1 Note that large doses of naloxone may reverse the analgesic effects of narcotics as well as the respiratory depression. Dose should be titrated according to patient response. If clinical signs of pain (*e.g.,* sweating, tachycardia, grimacing, vomiting) are noted, the antagonist should be stopped.

▷ 2 Ensure that other supportive measures (*e.g.,* respiratory assistance, vasopressors) are available when drug is used.
▷ 3 Use cautiously in patients with cardiac instability, during pregnancy, and in known or suspected narcotic addicts.
▷ 4 Administer diagnostic test for narcotic addiction only in presence of a physician, and inform patients of risks involved and possible untoward reactions.
▷ 5 Recognize that severity of withdrawal symptoms will depend on the amount and type of narcotic used by the addict. They are particularly severe in methadone addicts. Conversely, habituation to extremely large doses of meperidine (1.6 g or more per day) is necessary to result in withdrawal symptoms when a narcotic antagonist is administered.

▶ NURSING CONSIDERATIONS
▷ 1 For initial reversal of respiratory depression, inject drug IV at 2-minute to 3-minute intervals until the desired degree of reversal is attained (*i.e.,* adequate ventilation and alertness without significant pain or discomfort).
▷ 2 Due to prolonged action of some narcotics, repeat injections of naloxone IM at 1-hour to 2-hour intervals as needed to maintain antagonistic effects.
▷ 3 Be aware that failure to obtain significant improvement in patients condition after 3 doses of naloxone suggests that depressants effects may be partly or wholly due to drugs other than narcotics (*e.g.* barbiturates).

Summary. Narcotic Antagonists

Drug	Preparations	Usual Dosage Range
Levallorphan (Lorfan)	Injection—1 mg/ml	Adults—1 mg IV; repeat in 10 minutes to 15 minutes with 0.5 mg to a maximum of 3 mg
		Neonates—0.05 mg to 0.1 mg into umbilical vein after delivery
Naloxone (Narcan)	Injection—0.02 mg/ml, 0.4 mg/ml, 1.0 mg/ml	Narcotic overdosage (known or suspected)
		Adults—0.4 mg–2.0 mg IV, IM, or SC; repeat IV at 2-minute to 3-minute intervals for 2 to 3 doses
		Children and neonates—0.01 mg/kg IV, IM, or SC
		Postoperative narcotic depression
		0.1 mg to 0.2 mg IV at 2-minute to 3-minute intervals until desired degree of reversal is attained

Non-Narcotic Analgesic and Anti-Inflammatory Drugs

19

A large group of drugs possess analgesic and/or antiinflammatory actions but are devoid of many of the undesirable effects (*e.g.,* respiratory depression, habituation) of the narcotic agents and are called *non-narcotic* analgesics. These compounds have a variety of uses, principally relief of mild to moderate pain, reduction of elevated body temperatures (antipyresis), reduction in the symptoms of inflammation, and prevention or relief of the manifestations of gout. In addition, certain of these agents (*e.g.,* salicylic acid, methyl salicylate) are employed topically as keratolytics, counterirritants, and astringents.

Aspirin (acetylsalicyclic acid) is the most widely used, easily obtained, and least expensive of the non-narcotic analgesics. Due to its easy availability, however, aspirin is responsible for more instances of untoward reactions than is generally recognized. In fact, aspirin is the leading cause of drug poisoning in young children, and only barbiturates, alcohol, and carbon monoxide are responsible for more accidental fatalities among the general population. Other non-narcotic analgesics (*e.g.,* acetaminophen) may offer some advantages over aspirin (*e.g.,* decreased GI irritation, reduced effect on blood coagulation) and are frequently used in its place, especially in small children and in aspirin-intolerant persons. However, no single agent represents the "ideal" analgesic, and each drug possesses certain distinct disadvantages for different drug-taking populations.

The large number of chemically diverse agents possessing analgesic and anti-inflammatory action makes classification of these drugs quite arbitrary. This chapter considers these compounds in the following order:

  I. Salicylates
     (*e.g.,* aspirin, choline salicylate)
 II. Para-aminophenol derivative
     (*e.g.,* acetaminophen)
III. Pyrazolones
     (*e.g.,* phenylbutazone, oxyphenbutazone)
 IV. Nonsteroidal anti-inflammatory agents
     (*e.g.,* ibuprofen, naproxen, tolmetin)
  V. Gold compounds
     (*e.g.,* aurothioglucose)
 VI. Penicillamine
VII. Anti-gout drugs
     (*e.g.,* colchicine, probenecid, allopurinol)
VIII. Miscellaneous
     (*e.g.,* ethoheptazine)

I Salicylates

Aspirin	Salicylamide
Choline salicylate	Salicyclic acid
Diflunisal	Salsalate
Magnesium salicylate	Sodium salicylate
Methyl salicylate	Sodium thiosalicylate

Drugs in this category are derivatives of salicylic acid and possess analgesic, antipyretic, and anti-inflammatory actions. In addition, some of these drugs are capable of inhibiting platelet aggregation, and in large doses can decrease prothrombin production and can impair renal tubular reabsorption of uric acid.

Aspirin is the most commonly used of the salicylates and therefore is discussed in detail. Other related drugs are then reviewed in Table 19-1.

▶ aspirin
Acetylsalicylic Acid, ASA

Mechanism

1 Analgesia—blocks prostaglandin synthesis, thus decreasing sensitivity of peripheral pain receptors to mechanical or chemical activation; may enhance reabsorption of fluid from swollen, inflamed tissues and interfere with transmission of pain impulses at subcortical brain centers (*e.g.,* thalamus)

2 Antipyresis—reduces outflow of vasoconstrictor impulses from hypothalamus, thus promoting vasodilation, sweating, and heat loss; decreases release of prostaglandin E in response to endogenous pyrogens

3 Anti-inflammatory—decreases capillary permeability and leakage of fluid into surrounding tissues; interferes with release of tissue-destructive lysosomal enzymes; inhibits synthesis of prostaglandin E, an endogenous substance thought to mediate the inflammatory reaction by causing swelling and sensitizing peripheral pain receptors.

4 Decreased platelet aggregation—blocks formation of platelet thromboxane A_2, a prostaglandin derivative that facilitates platelet aggregation and causes vasoconstriction. Platelet aggregation appears to be inhibited by aspirin but not to a significant extent by other salicylates; this difference may be due to the acetyl group in the aspirin molecule. This effect is irreversible and persists for the life of the platelet. Low doses of aspirin are apparently more effective in reducing platelet aggregation than are higher doses. This is probably due to a more selective inhibitory action on the formation of platelet thromboxane A_2 than on the formation of vessel wall prostacyclin (a prostaglandin vasodilator and inhibitor of platelet aggregation). The *precise dose* of aspirin that is most effective in blocking platelet aggregation remains to be definitively established, however. The effects on platelet aggregation suggest a potential clinical value for these compounds in protecting against certain thrombotic events thought to be associated with cerebrovascular and ischemic heart diseases.

5 Other actions include inhibition of prothrombin formation (high doses only), decreased excretion of uric acid (small doses), increased excretion of uric acid (high doses), hyperglycemia, and decreased glucose tolerance.

Uses

1 Relief of mild to moderate pain, especially that associated with inflammatory states (*e.g.,* myalgia, neuralgia, cephalgia)

2 Reduction of elevated body temperature

3 Symptomatic treatment of various inflammatory conditions (*e.g.,* rheumatoid and osteoarthritis, bursitis, rheumatic fever); large doses (3 g–7 g/day) are usually necessary

4 Prophylaxis of thromboembolic complications (*e.g.,* venous emboli, cerebral ischemia) associated with cardiovascular disorders and reduction in the risk of recurrent transient ischemic attacks (*no* benefit in treating completed strokes)

Dosage
Adults:
Pain, fever—325 mg to 650 mg (5 gr–10 gr) every 4 hours
Inflammation—2.6 g to 7.8 g/day
Prophylaxis of ischemic attacks—40 mg/day to 80 mg/day
Children:
65 mg/kg/day in divided doses for pain or fever and 90 mg/kg/day to 130 mg/kg/day for inflammation

Fate
Absorbed essentially intact from stomach and upper intestine; rapidly hydrolyzed to salicylic acid, which is excreted either free or as conjugates in the urine; rate of excretion is inversely related to blood level, larger doses being eliminated more slowly than small doses; salicylic acid is highly (70%–90%) protein bound; alkalinization of the urine increases the rate of excretion of salicylates by favoring ionization in the renal tubules, which decreases reabsorption.

Common Side-Effects
Gastric distress, heartburn, and occasional nausea

Significant Adverse Reactions

Warning: Use of salicylates, especially aspirin, in children with influenzae or chickenpox has been associated with occasional development of Reye's syndrome, an acute, life-threatening condition, marked by initial severe vomiting and lethargy and progressing to delirium, coma, and death. Mortality rate is 20% to 30% and permanent brain damage frequently occurs in survivors. Although a *definite* causal relationship to salicylates has not been confirmed, aspirin and other salicylates should not be given to children with influenzae or chickenpox.

(Generally dose related—more common at high doses or with prolonged use). Salicylism (headache, nausea, tinnitus, dizziness, confusion, sweating, palpitations, hyperventilation, diarrhea, impaired hearing or vision); idiosyncratic hypersensitivity reactions (bronchoconstriction, urticaria, edema, asthma-like attacks, shock); renal or hepatic impairment; GI bleeding or ulceration; anemia; anorexia; and elevations in serum amylase, SGOT, SGPT, and CO_2 levels

Severe intoxication may lead to CNS stimulation (delirium, hallucinations), respiratory alkalosis followed by aci-

(*Text continues on p. 162.*)

Table 19-1. Salicylates

Drug	Preparations	Usual Dosage Range	Remarks
Aspirin (various manufacturers)	Tablets—65 mg, 81 mg, 325 mg, 487 mg, 650 mg Gum tablets—210 mg Enteric-coated tablets—325 mg, 650 mg, 975 mg Timed-release tablets (Measurin, Zorprin)—650 mg, 800 mg Capsules—325 mg Suppositories—65 mg, 130 mg, 195 mg, 300 mg, 325 mg, 600 mg, 650 mg, 1200 mg	See general discussion of aspirin	See general discussion of aspirin
Choline salicylate (Arthropan)	Liquid—870 mg/5 ml (870 mg equivalent to 650 mg aspirin)	1 teaspoonful (870 mg) every 3 hours to 4 hours to a maximum of 6 times/day For rheumatoid arthritis—1 tsp to 2 tsp up to 4 times/day	Liquid preparation giving more rapid absorption and less gastric irritation than aspirin; useful in patients with difficulty in swallowing tablets or capsules, in patients who experience gastric distress with regular aspirin, and in patients who should avoid sodium-containing salicylates; taste may be objectionable; drug can be mixed with fruit juice or other vehicle if desired; do not give with antacids.
Diflunisal (Dolobid)	Tablets—250 mg, 500 mg	Pain—1 g initially, followed by 500 mg every 8 hours to 12 hours Osteoarthritis—500 mg to 1000 mg daily in 2 divided doses (maximum 1500 mg/day)	A salicylic acid derivative *not* metabolized to salicylic acid; used for mild to moderate pain and osteoarthritis; long-acting (used twice a day) analgesia comparable in potency to aspirin or acetaminophen at a dose of 500 mg and equivalent to acetaminophen + codeine at a dose of 1000 mg; nonhabituating; platelet inhibitory effect is transient and reversible; anti-inflammatory efficacy equal to 2 g to 3 g/day of aspirin, with less GI distress in some patients; do not use in children under 12; use cautiously in patients with impaired cardiac function or hypertension, as fluid retention can occur; do not take aspirin, acetaminophen, or nonsteroidal anti-inflammatory drugs with diflunisal
Magnesium Salicylate (Durasal, Doans Pills, Efficin, Magan, Mobidin, MSG-600)	Tablets—325 mg, 480 mg, 500 mg, 545 mg, 600 mg	500 mg to 600 mg 3 to 4 times/day; increase to 3.6 to 4.8 g/day at 3-hour to 6-hour intervals as needed; up to 9.6 g/day have been used in rheumatic fever	Not recommended for children under 12; a sodium-free salicylate having a somewhat lower incidence of GI upset than regular aspirin; contraindicated in chronic renal insufficiency
Methyl salicylate (Oil of Wintergreen)	10% to 50% in ointment and liniments	Applied topically as a counter-irritant to relieve pain associated with muscular and rheumatic conditions	Significant absorption can occur through the skin and may produce untoward effects; very toxic if orally ingested, especially by children; liquids containing more than 5% methyl salicylate must be in child-resistant containers; use cautiously on irritated skin.

Table 19-1. Salicylates (continued)

Drug	Preparations	Usual Dosage Range	Remarks
Salicylamide (Uromide)	Tablets—325 mg, 650 mg, 667 mg	Adults—325 mg to 650 mg 3 to 4 times/day Children—65 mg/kg/day in 6 divided doses	An amide of salicylic acid that is less effective than aspirin, but also slightly less toxic; shorter-acting than other salicylates, because it is largely metabolized before entering systemic circulation; may be useful in aspirin-allergic individuals; drowsiness and dizziness can occur; no significant anti-inflammatory action
Salicylic Acid (Calicylic, Compound W, Hydrisalic, Keralyt, Mediplast, Off-Ezy, Salacid, Salonil, Wart-off)	Cream—10%, 25% Ointment—25%, 40%, 60% Gel—6%, 17% Soap—3.5% Liquid—17% Plaster—40%	Apply to affected area, usually at night, and wash off in the morning	Primarily used topically as a keratolytic agent for conditions such as psoriasis, acne, fungal infections, or any other condition requiring removal of excessive dead skin; skin should be hydrated at least 5 minutes prior to use with wet packs or soaks; may cause irritation and burning of skin; systemic absorption can occur to a significant extent; also may be applied as an ether–alcohol (Off-Ezy) or colloidian (Wart-Off) solution for removal of corns, warts, and calluses; use cautiously in children under 12; avoid contact with eyes or mucous membranes.
Salsalate (Disalcid, Mono-Gesic)	Tablets—325 mg, 500 mg, 750 mg Capsules—500 mg	325 mg to 1000 mg 2 to 3 times/day	Primarily for relief of signs and symptoms of rheumatoid arthritis and other rheumatic conditions; does not inhibit platelet aggregation; hydrolyzed to 2 molecules of salicylic acid; drug is insoluble in gastric juice and not absorbed until it reaches small intestine; low incidence of GI upset; not for use in children under 12; avoid other salicylates during salsalate therapy.
Sodium Salicylate (Uracel)	Tablets—325 mg, 650 mg Enteric-coated tablets—325 mg, 650 mg Injection—1 g, 1.5 g/10 ml	325 mg to 650 mg every 4 hours to 6 hours as needed	Less effective than an equal dose of aspirin; irritating to GI mucosa because free salicylic acid is liberated; use cautiously in renal dysfunction or in individuals on a low-sodium diet; sodium bicarbonate given concurrently may reduce gastric irritation, but increases rate of excretion as well; when giving injection, avoid extravasation, because drug will cause sloughing and necrosis of tissues.
Sodium thiosalicylate (Arthrolate, Asproject, Jecto-Sal, Nalate, Rexolate, Thiocyl, Thiodyne, Thiosal, Thiosul, TH-Sal, Tusal)	Injection—50 mg/ml	Analgesia—50 mg to 100 mg daily Arthritis—100 mg daily Rheumatic fever—100 mg to 150 mg every 4 hours to 6 hours for 3 days, then 100 mg twice/day Acute gout—100 mg every 3 hours to 4 hours for 2 days, then 100 mg/day	Readily absorbed following IM administration; primarily used in inflammatory conditions and acute stages of rheumatic fever

dosis, acid–base disturbances, petechial hemorrhaging, hyperthermia, hypokalemia, oliguria, convulsions, respiratory failure, and coma.

Contraindications

History of severe GI disorders (ulcer, hemorrhage, gastritis), severe anemia, deficiency of vitamin K, and hemophilia

Interactions

1 Effects of aspirin may be enhanced or prolonged by drugs that acidify the urine (*e.g.,* ammonium chloride, ascorbic acid) and may be decreased by urinary alkalinizers (*e.g.,* absorbable antacids, sodium bicarbonate).
2 By competing for protein binding sites, *large* doses of aspirin may enhance the actions of oral anticoagulants, heparin, oral antidiabetics, phenytoin, indomethacin, methotrexate, sulfonamide antibiotics, and penicillins.
3 Aspirin in small doses can inhibit the uricosuric effects of probenecid and sulfinpyrazone.
4 Furosemide may decrease aspirin excretion, resulting in toxicity at lower doses.
5 The incidence of GI bleeding with aspirin can be increased by alcohol, corticosteroids, indomethacin and pyrazolones (*e.g.,* phenylbutazone).

▶ NURSING ALERTS

▷ 1 Use aspirin cautiously in patients on anticoagulant therapy. A decrease in the anticoagulant dose may be required. Observe patients carefully for appearance of mucous membrane bleeding, bruising and petechiae, signs of increased anticoagulant effects. Periodic prothrombin and hemoglobin tests are indicated.

▷ 2 Be alert to the possibility of development of hypersensitivity reactions. Use with extreme caution in patients with asthma, nasal polyps, or a history of allergic reactions. Have epinephrine, antihistamines, and other supportive measures (*e.g.,* oxygen, respiratory aids) on hand.

▷ 3 When high doses of aspirin are used, counsel patients to be alert for early signs of overdose (*i.e.,* tinnitus, dizziness, impaired vision or hearing), and inform physician of their occurrence.

▷ 4 Warn patient that continual self-medication with aspirin for fever or pain may obscure more serious underlying conditions. Advise against prolonged use of aspirin unless directed by a physician.

▷ 5 Be aware of measures which should be used in cases of aspirin intoxication, *i.e.,* prompt emesis or gastric lavage, use of fluids and electrolytes, oxygen with artificial respiration, and dialysis in cases of *severe* intoxication.

▷ 6 Note that children with fever and dehydration may be especially prone to develop toxic effects with even small doses of aspirin. Administer carefully to such children, do not give for prolonged period of time, and keep drug out of reach of all children at all times. See Warning under Significant Adverse Reactions.

▶ NURSING CONSIDERATIONS

▷ 1 Recognize that commercially buffered aspirin is probably no less irritating to the gastric mucosa than taking plain aspirin with food, milk, or a full glass of water.

▷ 2 Note that although effervescent aspirin preparations (*e.g.,* Alka Seltzer) may be more rapidly absorbed and less irritating to the GI tract, they can alkalinize the urine, and their high sodium content may be hazardous in cardiac patients if used repeatedly.

▷ 3 Advise patients taking large doses of aspirin for its anti-inflammatory effects to maintain a constant dosage schedule to minimize fluctuations in plasma levels.

▷ 4 Recognize that combinations of aspirin, phenacetin, and caffeine (APC) are probably no more effective than aspirin alone, and have been associated with a higher incidence of renal damage. Such combinations should be avoided.

▷ 5 Caution individuals with aspirin hypersensitivity to read labels of over-the-counter medications (*e.g.,* cold preparations) carefully, because many contain aspirin or other salicylates.

▷ 6 Inform patients who experience GI upset with aspirin, even when taken with food or milk, that enteric-coated tablets are available (*e.g.,* Easpirin, Ecotrin), that resist breakdown in the stomach and therefore may eliminate much gastric distress.

▷ 7 Keep aspirin tablets in a cool dry place. Exposure to moisture or excessive heat will hasten hydrolysis and cause loss of potency. Do not use tablets if a vinegar-like odor is detectable.

▷ 8 Consider use of suppositories if the patient is vomiting or is otherwise incapable of taking the drug orally. Keep in mind that absorption from suppository is more variable than with the oral route.

II Para-Aminophenol Derivatives

There are two important compounds in this category, phenacetin and N-acetyl-p-aminophenol (acetaminophen). Previously, phenacetin was employed in many analgesic drug combinations, principally with aspirin and caffeine as APC. The advantage of the combination, that is, APC over aspirin alone as a pain reliever, is subject to question. Moreover, phenacetin use has been associated with anemia, acidosis, methemoglobinemia, and kidney damage. However, because phenacetin is almost always used in combination with other drugs, it is difficult to implicate it as the sole toxic ingredient. Nevertheless, the use of phenacetin combinations should be strongly discouraged because other equally effective and less toxic analgesics and antipyretics exist. Phenacetin now has been removed from virtually all commercially available preparations, and those few remaining must now carry a warning against the dangers of kidney damage with chronic use of the drug.

In the body, phenacetin is converted largely to acetaminophen, which is a very popular analgesic agent itself, widely used as an aspirin substitute and much less toxic

than the related phenacetin. In comparison to aspirin, acetaminophen has the following advantages:
1 Lower incidence of GI upset and bleeding
2 Lower incidence of hypersensitivity reactions
3 No significant interaction with oral anticoagulants or uricosuric drugs
4 Availability in a palatable liquid form for pediatric use
The principal disadvantage of acetaminophen relative to aspirin is that acetaminophen possesses no significant anti-inflammatory action, presumably due to its lack of inhibitory effect on prostaglandin synthesis in the periphery. Excessive doses of acetaminophen can cause hepatotoxicity, and liver damage may occur with normal doses in chronic alcoholics and patients with impaired hepatic function (see Significant Adverse Reactions).

▶ acetaminophen

Datril, Tempra, Tylenol, and various other manufacturers

Mechanism
Elevates the pain threshold and reduces sympathetic outflow from hypothalamic temperature-regulating center; may also inhibit action of an endogenous pyrogen on the heat-regulating center in the CNS; weak antidiuretic action; exerts *no* significant anti-inflammatory or uricosuric effect, and does not produce gastric erosion, inhibition of platelet aggregation, or prothrombin depression at therapeutic dose levels; Analgesic and antipyretic potency approximately equivalent to aspirin

Uses
1 Relief of mild to moderate pain of various origins, *e.g.,* musculoskeletal, headache, toothache, teething, dysmenorrhea, "flu," tonsillectomy, and so forth
2 Reduction of elevated temperatures associated with colds and other bacterial and viral infections

Dosage
Adults: 325 mg to 650 mg 3 to 4 times/day (maximum 4.0 g/day for short-term therapy)
Children: 7 yr to 12 yr—162.5 mg to 325 mg 3 to 4 times/day (maximum 1.3 g/day)
3 yr to 6 yr—120 mg to 240 mg 3 to 4 times/day (maximum 480 mg/day)

Fate
Well absorbed from the GI tract; onset 15 minutes to 30 minutes; duration 3 hours to 5 hours; metabolized in the liver and approximately 80% excreted in the urine as conjugated acetaminophen; bound to variable degrees (20%–50%) to plasma proteins, especially in cases of acute intoxication

Common Side-Effects
None with occasional usage

Significant Adverse Reactions
(Usually with chronic use of high doses) Urticaria, hypoglycemia, CNS stimulation, cyanosis, methemoglobinemia, hemolytic anemia, leukopenia, kidney damage, and psychological changes; *acute* poisoning characterized by chills, diarrhea, emesis, fever, skin eruptions, palpitations, weakness, sweating, and CNS stimulation (excitement, delirium, toxic psychosis) followed by CNS depression, vascular collapse, convulsions, and coma

Hepatoxicity can occur with overdosage or chronic high dosage, especially in adults. Initial signs are nausea, vomiting, malaise, sweating, diarrhea, and abdominal pain. Plasma acetaminophen levels can be used to predict the degree of hepatic damage in overdosage (see Nursing Alerts).

Contraindications
Glucose-6-phosphate dehydrogenase deficiency

Interactions
1 May *slightly* increase the effects of oral anticoagulants, necessitating a minimal dosage adjustment
2 Oral absorption may be reduced by anticholinergics, antacids, and narcotics.

▶ NURSING ALERTS
▷ 1 Caution against indiscriminate, excessive, or prolonged use of the drug. Keep away from children because many liquid preparations are pleasantly flavored, and may be consumed in large amounts.
▷ 2 If ingestion of a toxic dose is suspected, person should be hospitalized and observed carefully for signs of hepatic damage (nausea, vomiting, abdominal pain, diarrhea). Note that hepatic damage may not be evident for several days.
▷ 3 Determine serum half-life of acetaminophen to assess degree of liver damage. If greater than 4 hours, hepatic necrosis is probable; if greater than 12 hours, hepatic coma is likely. Hepatic damage can be prevented by oral methionine (2.5 g every 4 hr) or acetylcysteine (70 mg/kg–140 mg/kg every 4 hr) if given within 10 hours to 12 hours of ingestion.

▶ NURSING CONSIDERATIONS
▷ 1 Do not use in very small children or for periods greater than 10 days unless directed by a physician.
▷ 2 Use cautiously in arthritis or rheumatic conditions because drug lacks anti-inflammatory action. If pain persists for more than 10 days or if redness is present, consult physician, because additional medication is indicated.
▷ 3 Observe prolonged users of the drug for possible signs of methemoglobinemia (cyanosis, dyspnea, vertigo, weakness, anginal-like pain); hemolytic anemia (pallor, palpitations); and kidney damage (albuminuria, hematuria).

III Pyrazolones

The pyrazolones are currently represented by three drugs (phenylbutazone, oxyphenbutazone, and sulfinpyrazone) that have pharmacologic effects similar to those of the salicylates, but are more potent anti-inflammatory agents. Sulfinpyrazone, however, is a much more effective uricosuric drug than it is an anti-inflammatory agent and is employed in the maintenance therapy of gout.

Phenylbutazone and oxyphenbutazone are very effective anti-inflammatory agents, but they are highly toxic compounds. Therefore, their use should be restricted to short-term therapy of severe acute inflammatory conditions not benefited by other less toxic agents such as the salicylates. Although they possess analgesic and antipyretic actions as well, the pyrazolones should never be used in place of aspirin or acetaminophen as a general-purpose pain reliever or fever reducer.

Phenylbutazone and its metabolite oxyphenbutazone are quite similar in their actions and are reviewed together. Sulfinpyrazone, on the other hand, is primarily indicated for the chronic treatment of gout and is discussed with other anti-gout drugs at the end of this chapter.

▶ phenylbutazone

Azolid, Butazolidin

▶ oxyphenbutazone

Oxalid, Tandearil

Mechanism

Not completely established; interferes with the synthesis of prostaglandins and mucopolysaccharides in cartilage; inhibits leucocyte migration and activity of lysosomal enzymes; exerts a weak blocking effect on uric acid reabsorption by renal tubular cells; produces significant retention of sodium and water; inhibits enzymes of the Krebs' cycle

Uses

1 Relief of acute symptoms of active rheumatoid arthritis, ankylosing spondylitis, osteoarthritis, psoriatic arthritis, and painful shoulder conditions (*e.g.,* peritendinitis, bursitis, capsulitis)
2 Symptomatic treatment of acute superficial thrombophlebitis
3 Short-term treatment of acute attacks of degenerative joint disease of the hips and knees
4 Treatment of acute gout (short-term use only; not for maintenance therapy)

Dosage (for both drugs)

Arthritis, spondylitis, painful shoulder: Initially—300 mg to 600 mg in divided doses (maximum 600 mg/day)
Maintenance dose—100 mg to 400 mg/day
Acute gout: 400 mg initially, then 100 mg every 4 hours for up to 4 days

Fate

Rapidly and completely absorbed from GI tract; onset of action in 30 minutes; highly bound (90%–98%) to plasma proteins with a half-life of 75 hours to 85 hours; therefore prolonged duration (3 days–5 days); slowly metabolized in the liver and excreted in the urine

Common Side-Effects

Nausea, vomiting, gastric discomfort, skin rash, diarrhea, vertigo, insomnia, nervousness, blurred vision, water and electrolyte retention

Significant Adverse Reactions

GI—ulceration of the esophagus, stomach, small intestine, and bowel; occult GI bleeding, gastritis; abdominal distention; hematemesis
Hematologic—blood dyscrasias, bone marrow depression
Allergic/dermatologic—(requires prompt withdrawal of drug) petechiae, toxic pruritus, erythema nodosum, erythema multiforme, exfoliative dermatitis, Stevens–Johnson syndrome (see Chap. 6), serum sickness, polyarteritis, urticaria, arthralgia, fever, anaphylactic shock
Renal/metabolic—proteinuria, hematuria, oliguria, anuria, glomerulonephritis, renal stones, tubular necrosis, ureteral obstruction, sodium and chloride retention, edema, metabolic acidosis, hyperglycemia, thyroid hyperplasia, toxic goiter
Cardiovascular—hypertension, pericarditis, myocarditis with muscle necrosis, cardiac decompensation
Ocular/otic—diplopia, optic neuritis, retinal hemorrhage, retinal detachment, hearing loss
CNS (seen primarily with overdose)—agitation, confusion, lethargy, depression, hallucinations, convulsions, psychosis, hyperventilation

Contraindications

GI inflammation; ulceration or persistent dyspepsia; blood dycrasias; hypertension; thyroid disease; renal, hepatic, or cardiac dysfunction; temporal arteritis; polymyalgia rheumatica; patients receiving anticoagulants or potent chemotherapeutic agents; children under 14 years; senile patients

Interactions

1 Pyrazolones may potentiate the effects of other protein-bound drugs (oral anticoagulants, sulfonamides, phenytoin, oral hypoglycemics, other anti-inflammatory drugs such as salicylates and indomethacin).
2 Pyrazolones may decrease the effects of digitoxin.
3 Effects of pyrazolones may be decreased by tricyclic antidepressants and by cholestyramine, which inhibits pyrazolone absorption.
4 The effects of insulin can be enhanced by pyrazolones.

▶ NURSING ALERTS

▷ 1 Do *not* begin therapy before a detailed history and complete physical and laboratory examinations have been performed. Repeat laboratory examinations at regular, frequent intervals during therapy.
▷ 2 Caution patients not to exceed recommended dosage, because incidence of adverse effects increases *sharply* at high dose levels. If no therapeutic effect is observed within 1 week, discontinue drug. If improvement is noted, attempt to decrease dosage to lowest effective level as quickly as possible.

▷ 3 Advise patients to report the appearance of early signs of blood dyscrasias (fever, sore throat, mouth ulceration), as well as epigastric pain, unusual bruising or bleeding, black or tarry stools, skin rash, blurred vision, pruritus, and significant edema or weight gain. Discontinue the drug immediately.

▷ 4 Monitor blood picture frequently during prolonged therapy, especially in patients over 40. Discontinue drug if any marked change in white cell count occurs. Observe blood picture for several weeks following discontinuation of therapy because blood dyscrasias may appear for some time after termination of the drug.

▷ 5 Use with extreme caution during pregnancy or lactation, in patients over 40 years, and in individuals with glaucoma.

▶ **NURSING CONSIDERATIONS**

▷ 1 Advise user to take drug with meals or milk to minimize gastric irritation.

▷ 2 Because drugs induce sodium retention, restrict salt intake to avoid edema, especially in hypertensive individuals.

▷ 3 Teach patient to check for signs of edema and to examine stools for presence of blood. Report any changes immediately.

▷ 4 Attempt to reduce dosage to lowest effective level once a significant response has been observed. Caution patient to follow dosage schedule closely.

▷ 5 Do not use these drugs as *first choice* in inflammatory states. They are indicated only when other less toxic agents are ineffective or poorly tolerated.

▷ 6 In individuals with suspected GI ulceration, use oxyphenbutazone, because it has less ulcerogenic activity than phenylbutazone.

▷ 7 In severe inflammatory conditions, consider use of adjunctive measures with these drugs, such as anticoagulants (reduce dose of each drug proportionately), pressure bandages, limb elevation, and bed rest.

IV Nonsteroidal Anti-Inflammatory Agents

In a search for effective anti-inflammatory drugs that might prove less toxic than many of the older, established agents, several organic acids were shown to have a somewhat lower incidence of side-effects (*e.g.,* tinnitus, GI distress) than comparably effective doses of the salicylates or pyrazolones. These compounds have been termed the *nonsteroidal* anti-inflammatory agents, and they are approximately equal to aspirin in relieving most types of inflammation. Of these substances, indomethacin is the most toxic and is discussed separately. The remaining drugs may be slightly better tolerated by some people than are repeated high doses of aspirin, but the drugs are essentially equivalent in most other respects. They are therefore discussed as a group.

These compounds possess analgesic and antipyretic activity but should *not* be used for the relief of minor headache pain or reduction of elevated body temperature in place of more commonly prescribed drugs (aspirin, acetaminophen). However, with the exception of indomethacin and meclofenamate, they may be employed for relieving other types of mild to moderate pain such as dysmenorrhea, postextraction dental pain, postsurgical episiotomy, and soft-tissue athletic injuries, in addition to their use as anti-inflammatory drugs. Their action in inflammatory states is to reduce joint swelling, pain, and stiffness, and to increase the functional capacity of the joint; however, they do *not* alter the progressive course of the underlying disease state.

While the nonsteroidal anti-inflammatory drugs may be somewhat more effective than aspirin in treating ankylosing spondylitis, acute gouty arthritis and psoriatic arthropathy, their effectiveness in managing the common forms of rheumatoid and osteoarthritis is comparable to that of aspirin.

These compounds are expensive, so there is little justification for their use in treating inflammatory states in compliant persons who can tolerate the large daily doses of salicylates needed to control inflammation. Rather, the compounds are logical alternatives to the salicylates in patients unable to take large doses of aspirin-like drugs on a continual basis, and certainly should be employed as aspirin substitutes instead of the more toxic pyrazolones and corticosteroids. The fact that several of the nonsteroidal anti-inflammatory drugs have a long duration of action permits single- or twice-daily dosing, another advantage over the multiple daily doses of aspirin.

These drugs (other than indomethacin and meclofenamate) exhibit a somewhat lower incidence of the *milder* forms of GI distress that commonly occur with high-dose salicylate use. It must be noted, however, that most of the other untoward reactions and drug interactions associated with large doses of aspirin and related compounds are also evident to a similar degree with the nonsteroidal, anti-inflammatory agents. In addition, aspirin itself should not be given with these nonsteroidal drugs because it can decrease the blood level and activity of the nonaspirin drugs. Likewise, combinations of the nonsteroidal drugs with low doses of corticosteroids are probably not significantly more effective than either drug alone, in most patients.

▶ **indomethacin**

Indocin

An effective anti-inflammatory agent (potency somewhat greater than high doses of aspirin) with a high incidence of adverse reactions, indomethacin is indicated only where other less toxic agents are unsuitable or have become ineffective. It produces relief of symptoms of acute gouty arthritis, but should only be used for a maximum of 5 days.

Mechanism

Not definitively established; probably acts in part by inhibiting prostaglandin synthesis; decreases capillary permeability and migration of polymorphonuclear leukocytes; no effect on the pituitary–adrenal system

Uses

1 Treatment of moderate to severe rheumatoid arthritis, ankylosing (rheumatoid) spondylitis, and osteoarthritis of large joints (*e.g.,* hip, shoulder)
2 Symptomatic relief of acute gouty arthritis (short-term use *only*)
3 Assist closure of persistent patent ductus arteriosus in premature infants (investigational use only)

Dosage

Chronic: 25 mg 2 to 3 times/day; increase by 25 mg to 50 mg weekly to a maximum of 200 mg/day; for maintenance therapy, 75-mg sustained-release capsule can be used once or twice a day depending on dosage requirements.

Acute gout: 50 mg 3 times/day until pain is tolerable; decrease dose rapidly over next 3 to 5 days until cessation of therapy; do *not* use 75-mg sustained-release dosage form.

Patent ductus arteriosus: 0.3 mg/kg as a single dose *via* retention enema or orogastric tube.

Fate

Readily absorbed and widely distributed in the body, onset of action is 1 hour to 2 hours; half-life about 4½ hours; highly protein-bound (90%) in the plasma; metabolized in the liver and kidney, and excreted in the urine (60%) as conjugates and unchanged drug; remainder is eliminated through bile in the feces

Common Side-Effects

Headache, dizziness, nausea, dyspepsia, epigastric pain, heartburn, and diarrhea

Significant Adverse Reactions

GI—anorexia; bloating; ulceration; perforation and hemorrhage of the esophagus, stomach and small intestine; gastroenteritis; proctitis; rectal bleeding

CNS—fatigue, depression, anxiety, confusion, muscle weakness, syncope, involuntary movements, psychic disturbances, convulsions, peripheral neuropathy, depersonalization

Hematologic—leukopenia, bone marrow depression, anemia secondary to bleeding, aplastic anemia, agranulocytosis, thrombocytopenic purpura

Cardiovascular—hypertension, tachycardia, chest pain, palpitations

Eye/ear—retinal changes including macula, corneal deposits, blurred vision, hearing disturbances, tinnitus

Dermatologic—pruritus, rash, urticaria, petechiae, alopecia, exfoliative dermatitis

Allergic—hypotension, angioedema, respiratory distress, asthmalike attack

Other—epistaxis, vaginal bleeding, hematuria, and increased BUN, SGOT, SGPT, alkaline phosphatase and serum amylase

Contraindications

Aspirin allergy, nasal polyps associated with angioedema, GI lesions, pregnancy, nursing mothers, children under 14

Interactions

1 GI bleeding due to indomethacin can be intensified by use of corticosteroids, salicylates, and pyrazolones.
2 Indomethacin may interfere with the action of furosemide (Lasix) and thiazide diuretics, and decrease the antihypertensive effect of beta-adrenergic blockers.
3 Large doses of aspirin may decrease indomethacin blood levels.
4 Probenecid may increase plasma levels of indomethacin.
5 Indomethacin may alter oral anticoagulant requirements, either by decreasing plasma protein binding, therefore elevating anticoagulant blood levels, or by causing excessive bleeding due to GI ulceration.
6 Lithium excretion may be impaired by indomethacin, possibly leading to lithium toxicity.
7 Indomethacin and triamterene together can result in acute reversible renal faliure.

▶ **NURSING ALERTS**

▷ 1 Because the drug is potentially quite toxic, instruct patient to observe carefully for any untoward reaction and report immediately. Use lowest effective dose at all times and discontinue drug as soon as possible.
▷ 2 Perform periodic blood counts, renal and hepatic function tests, ophthalmoscopic examinations, and hearing tests on patients using the drug for prolonged periods of time.
▷ 3 Use with caution in patients with psychotic disturbances, epilepsy, parkinsonism, severe infections, renal or hepatic dysfunction, and coagulation defects, and in elderly persons.
▷ 4 Observe user carefully for indications of improvement. If no significant changes occur within 2 weeks to 3 weeks, discontinue drug.
▷ 5 Advise patient to use caution in activities requiring alertness or motor coordination because drug may cause drowsiness or dizziness.
▷ 6 In treatment of acute gouty arthritis, do not use drug more than 5 days. Relief of pain and tenderness usually occurs in 24 hours to 36 hours and swelling disappears in 3 days to 5 days.

▶ **NURSING CONSIDERATIONS**

▷ 1 Always administer drug with food, milk, or antacids to minimize GI distress.
▷ 2 In patients with persistent night pain or morning stiffness, give largest portion of the dose (maximum 100 mg) at bedtime.
▷ 3 Do not give aspirin with indomethacin because reduced therapeutic effect can occur, and incidence of GI complications is increased.
▷ 4 Determine if patient has an aspirin allergy prior to administration of indomethacin. Do not give to aspirin-intolerant patients.

▶ **fenoprofen**

Nalfon

▶ **ibuprofen**
Motrin

▶ **meclofenamate**
Meclomen

▶ **mefenamic acid**
Ponstel

▶ **naproxen**
Anaprox, Naprosyn

▶ **piroxicam**
Feldene

▶ **sulindac**
Clinoril

▶ **tolmetin**
Tolectin

▶ **zomepirac**
Zomax

Nonsteroidal, anti-inflammatory drugs having a pharmacologic spectrum of action similar to aspirin, with a slightly lower incidence of milder GI side-effects (except meclofenamate), and less of an inhibitory action on platelet aggregation. They are used principally for symptomatic management of rheumatoid and osteoarthritis, except mefenamic acid and zomepirac, which are employed primarily as analgesics.

Mechanism
Not completely established; block synthesis and possibly release of prostaglandins; lower sensitivity of temperature-regulating center in the hypothalamus; decrease contractions of the myometrium due to prostaglandin inhibition in the uterus

Uses
1 Relief of symptoms of rheumatoid arthritis and osteoarthritis (not recommended in class IV disease, where patient is incapacitated, largely bedridden, and capable of little or no self-care)
2 Relief of mild to moderate pain associated with dysmenorrhea, dental extractions, episiotomy, and athletic injuries such as strains and sprains (except meclofenamate)

Dosage
See Table 19-2.

Fate
Rapidly and almost completely absorbed; food generally delays absorption; however, except for zomepirac, does not affect total amount absorbed. Peak serum levels are usually attained within 2 hours to 3 hours, except piroxicam (3 hr–5 hr) and tolmetin (0.5 hr–1 hr). Half-lives vary widely (see

Table 19-2), with piroxicam having longest duration of action (24 hr), followed by naproxen and sulindac (8 hr–12 hr). All drugs are highly bound to plasma proteins and are excreted largely as metabolites through the kidney. Some biliary excretion also occurs.

Common Side-Effects
GI upset, dizziness, headache, tinnitus, and constipation

Significant Adverse Reactions
(Incidence and severity vary among different drugs; see Table 19-2.)
GI—nausea, vomiting, cramping, diarrhea, bloating, epigastric pain, peptic ulceration, ulcerative stomatitis, bleeding, proctitis
Allergic—pruritus, skin rash, urticaria, erythema multiforme (rare), purpura (rare)
CNS—drowsiness, nervousness, insomnia, confusion, depression, tremor, muscle weakness
Eye/ear—blurred vision, diplopia, decreased hearing
Cardiovascular—palpitation, tachycardia, edema, prolonged bleeding time, arrhythmias, chest pain
Hepatic—cholestatic hepatitis, jaundice

Contraindications
Aspirin sensitivity, active peptic ulcer; in addition, mefenamic acid is contraindicated in patients with ulceration or chronic inflammation of the GI tract and in those with significantly impaired renal function.

Interactions
1 Effects of other protein-bound drugs (*e.g.,* hydantoins, sulfonamides, oral hypoglycemics, oral anticoagulants, pyrazolones) may be increased by nonsteroidal anti-inflammatory drugs.
2 GI adverse reactions may be intensified by concurrent administration of indomethacin, pyrazolones, salicylates, and corticosteroids.
3 Aspirin and other salicylates may decrease the blood level of nonsteroidal drugs.
4 Barbiturates may decrease the effects of fenoprofen by promoting its metabolism by the liver.
5 Plasma levels of nonsteroidal anti-inflammatory drugs can be increased by probenecid.

▶ **NURSING ALERTS**
▷ 1 Use very cautiously in patients with impaired renal function; monitor creatinine clearance closely in these individuals.
▷ 2 Observe patients with a history of GI problems for signs of gastric intolerance to these drugs (*e.g.,* dyspepsia, epigastric pain, nausea, cramping). Stop drug if symptoms persist.
▷ 3 Advise patient to report signs of GI bleeding, blurred vision, skin rash, and edema immediately. Drug regimen should be reviewed and adjusted as necessary.
▷ 4 Caution patient that drowsiness, dizziness, or light-headedness can occur and may impair ability to perform mechanical tasks.

Table 19-2. Nonsteroidal Anti-inflammatory Agents

Drug	Preparations	Usual Dosage Range	Remarks
Fenoprofen (Nalfon)	Capsules—200 mg, 300 mg Tablets—600 mg	Arthritis—300 mg to 600 mg 4 times/day (maximum 3200 mg/day) Mild to moderate pain—200 mg every 4 hours to 6 hours	Administer 30 minutes before or 2 hours after meals unless GI distress occurs, then give with milk; perform periodic auditory function tests during chronic therapy; *not* recommended for children under 14; periodic liver function tests are advised, as drug can elevate serum transaminase, LDH, and alkaline phosphatase; drowsiness and headache are common.
Ibuprofen (Advil, Motrin, Nuprin)	Tablets—200 mg, 300 mg, 400 mg, 600 mg	Arthritis—initially, 600 mg 3 to 4 times/day (maximum 2400 mg/day) Maintenance—600 mg twice a day Mild to moderate pain—400 mg every 4 hours to 6 hours	If blurred or diminished vision occurs, discontinue drug; perform periodic ophthalmologic examination; at a dose of 600 mg, slightly more effective than aspirin as an anti-inflammatory drug and for relief of dysmenorrhea; minimal interaction with oral anticoagulants; 200-mg tablets are available over-the-counter for relief of minor pain (*e.g.*, headache, backache, and menstrual cramps) and for reduction of fever; not recommended in children under 12
Meclofenamate (Meclomen)	Capsules—50 mg, 100 mg	200 mg to 400 mg/day in 3 to 4 divided doses	Not recommended for children under 14; should not be used as initial therapy for rheumatoid arthritis or osteoarthritis, due to high incidence of diarrhea (10%–30%), vomiting (10%–12%), and other GI disorders (10%); take with meals, milk, or antacids; periodic hemoglobin/hematocrit determinations are recommended during extended therapy.
Mefenamic acid (Ponstel)	Capsules—250 mg	Initially, 500 mg; then 250 mg every 6 hours	Short-acting drug used to relieve moderate pain of brief duration and to treat symptoms of primary dysmenorrhea; diarrhea occurs frequently, and necessitates discontinuation of therapy; administer with food and do not exceed 1 week of treatment; maximum duration for dysmenorrhea is 3 to 4 days; do not use in patients with a history of renal impairment or chronic inflammation or ulceration of the GI tract; discontinue drug if skin rash, petechiae, dark stools or hematemesis are noted; contraindicated in children under 14
Naproxen (Naprosyn) Naproxen sodium (Anaprox)	Tablets—250 mg, 275 mg, 375 mg, 500 mg (275-mg tablet is the sodium salt, equivalent to 250-mg naproxen base)	Arthritis—250 mg to 375 mg twice a day (maximum 1000 mg/day) Mild to moderate pain—550 mg (sodium salt) initially, then 275 mg every 6 hours to 8 hours Acute gout—750 mg followed by 250 mg every 8 hours until attack has subsided	Prolonged half-life (13 hr) in the body allows only twice-a-day administration, which may aid patient compliance; sodium salt is more quickly absorbed giving a faster onset of action; duration of action is equal to base, however; drug may have to be used for up to one month to obtain a significant clinical response; readily crosses placental barrier and is excreted in significant concentrations in breast milk
Piroxicam (Feldene)	Capsules—10 mg, 20 mg	Initially, 20 mg once daily; maintenance dosage is 10 mg to 20 mg once daily	Long-acting drug used in rheumatoid and osteoarthritis; steady state plasma levels are generally attained within 1 week to 2 weeks; antacids do not affect plasma levels, but aspirin can reduce blood levels of piroxicam to 80% of normal; GI side-effects are experienced by 20% of patients; not recommended for use in children

Table 19-2. Nonsteroidal Anti-inflammatory Agents *(continued)*

Drug	Preparations	Usual Dosage Range	Remarks
Sulindac (Clinoril)	Tablets—150 mg, 200 mg	150 mg to 200 mg twice a day (maximum 400 mg/day)	Long-acting drug used twice a day; useful in rheumatoid arthritis, osteoarthritis and gouty arthritis, spondylitis, and acute painful shoulder; may allow a gradual reduction in corticosteroid dosage if used concurrently; liver function test abnormalities can occur; not indicated for use in children; high incidence (10%) of GI pain and other GI symptoms; administer with food
Tolmetin (Tolectin)	Tablets—200 mg Capsules—400 mg	Adults—Initially, 400 mg 3 times/day (maximum 2000 mg/day); maintenance doses are 600 mg to 1800 mg/day in 3 or 4 divided doses. Children (over 2 yr)—20 mg/ kg/day in 3 to 4 divided doses (maximum 30 mg/kg/ day)	May be used in juvenile rheumatoid arthritis in children over 2; minimal interaction with oral anticoagulants; if GI intolerance occurs, give with food, milk or antacids other than sodium bicarbonate; sodium and water retention can occur; caution in cardiac patients; headache is observed in 10% of patients
Zomepirac (Zomax)	Tablets—100 mg	50 mg to 100 mg every 4 hours to 6 hours depending on severity of pain	Indicated for relief of mild to moderately severe pain; analgesic efficacy of 100-mg tablet is comparable to two tablets of either aspirin or acetaminophen with 30 mg of codeine; not recommended for inflammatory conditions as the sole therapeutic agent; do not administer to aspirin-hypersensitive patient; fatal anaphylactic reactions have occurred; drug was temporarily withdrawn from the market, but is being remarketed with stringent prescribing guidelines; GI symptoms are the most common adverse reactions, with nausea, diarrhea, and abdominal pain occurring most frequently; prolongs bleeding time but does *not* alter warfarin protein binding; not recommended in children or pregnant or nursing mothers due to rat tumorigenicity findings

▶ **NURSING CONSIDERATIONS**

▷ 1 Observe for improvement in patient's condition, which should be evident within 2 weeks. Review dosage at that time and decrease gradually to lowest effective level.

▷ 2 Caution user against self-medication with aspirin or other salicylates, because they may reduce the non-steroidal drug's effectiveness. However, acetaminophen can be used without significant problems in this regard.

▷ 3 In patients with compromised cardiac function or hypertension, observe carefully for signs of developing edema and fluid retention.

▷ 4 Note that additional therapeutic benefit can be obtained with these drugs in combination with gold salts, but usually not with salicylates or corticosteroids.

▷ 5 Recognize that some patients may respond only to one of the several available nonsteroidal agents. Try different derivatives at 2 week to 3 week intervals before concluding that this type of drug is ineffective.

V Gold Compounds

Injectable preparations containing approximately 50% elemental gold have been used for many years as part of the regimen for treating severe rheumatoid arthritis. Aurothioglucose and gold sodium thiomalate are two preparations used primarily in active arthritis that progresses despite adequate rest, physical therapy, and other drug treatment. These drugs can temporarily arrest the progression of the disease in involved joints if therapy is initiated early enough. Gold compounds are highly toxic substances, so persons receiving them must be carefully and continually observed for adverse reactions.

Injections are normally given at weekly or longer intervals for prolonged periods of time, occasionally with rest periods if remission has occurred. Because of the long course of therapy, repeated injections, and the necessity of periodic laboratory tests to detect toxicity, patient compliance with this form of therapy is often poor.

Auranofin is an orally effective gold compound that is presently experimental, although marketing is expected in the near future. It appears to retain the clinical efficacy of injectable gold preparations with a reduced incidence of untoward reactions and improved patient acceptance.

Due to a similar pharmacologic profile, the two injectable gold preparations are discussed together.

▶ **aurothioglucose**

Solganal

▶ **gold sodium thiomalate**

Myochrysine

Mechanism

Largely speculative; in animals, gold reduces macrophage phagocytosis, increases collagen cross-linkages, inhibits lysosomal enzymes, decreases formation of glucosamine-6-phosphate in connective tissue, prevents prostaglandin synthesis, interferes with tryptophan binding to plasma proteins, and suppresses the anaphylactic release of histamine.

Uses

1 Adjunctive treatment of active adult and juvenile rheumatoid arthritis (greatest benefit in the early, active stages)
2 Symptomatic treatment of nondisseminated lupus erythematosus and pemphigus (investigational)

Dosage

Aurothioglucose

Adults: Weekly IM injections; first week, 10 mg; second and third week, 25 mg; thereafter 50 mg. If improvement is noted, continue with 50-mg injections at 2-week to 4-week intervals as necessary. Cessation of treatment depends on individual response.

Children (6 yr–12 yr): Proportional to adult dose on a weight basis; maximum 25 mg/week to children under 12

Gold sodium thiomalate

Adults: weekly injections; first week, 10 mg; second week, 25 mg; third and subsequent weeks, 25 to 50 mg until major clinical improvement or toxicity occurs. Injections of 25 mg to 50 mg may be given every third or fourth week indefinitely if clinical improvement remains stable.

Children: 1 mg/kg, not to exceed 50 mg on a single injection; schedule is same as for adults.

Fate

Fairly slow absorption from IM sites; peak gold plasma levels occur in 4 hours to 6 hours; well distributed throughout the body; highly bound (95%) to plasma proteins; plasma half-life is between 3 days and 7 days with a 50-mg dose; excreted in the urine (60%–90%) and feces (10%–40%) slowly over prolonged periods, so danger of accumulation in tissues exists, resulting in cumulation toxicity.

Common Side-Effects

(25%–50% incidence) Erythema, dermatitis, pruritus, stomatitis, metallic taste, flushing, dizziness, sweating, and proteinuria

Significant Adverse Reactions

Dermatologic—papular, vesicular, or exfoliative dermatitis; alopecia, chrysiasis

Mucous membrane—gingivitis, pharyngitis, gastritis, colitis, upper respiratory tract inflammation, vaginitis

Hematologic—blood dyscrasias (rare)

Renal—glomerulitis, hematuria, nephritis

Allergic—syncope, bradycardia, angioedema, difficulty in swallowing or breathing, anaphylactic shock

Other—GI distress (nausea, cramping, vomiting, colic), iritis, corneal ulcers (rare), hepatitis, acute yellow atrophy, peripheral neuritis, synovial destruction, EEG abnormalities, pulmonary fibrosis

Contraindications

Uncontrolled diabetes, renal disease, hepatic dysfunction, severe hypertension, cardiac failure, systemic lupus, history of blood dyscrasias, eczema, colitis, severely debilitated states, recent radiation therapy, elderly patients, and pregnancy

Interactions

1 Incidence of blood dyscrasias or hematologic toxicity may be increased by concurrent use of pyrazolones, antimalarial drugs (*e.g.,* hydroxychloroquine), immunosuppressants (*e.g.,* azathioprine), or cytotoxic drugs.
2 Corticosteroids can reduce the effectiveness and increase the toxicity of gold salts.

▶ **NURSING ALERTS**

▷ 1 Carefully explain to patients the kind of toxicity that might develop, and advise them to report promptly any signs of developing toxic reactions.

▷ 2 Use with caution in individuals with a history of allergies, compromised cerebral or coronary circulation, or moderate hypertension.

▷ 3 Perform differential, white blood cell, erythrocyte, and platelet counts, hemoglobin determination, and urinalysis before initiating therapy and after every second injection. Discontinue drug if proteinuria or hematuria is present, if hemoglobin is markedly reduced, if leukopenia occurs or if platelet count decreases below 100,000/cu ml.

▷ 4 Counsel patient to be aware of early signs of developing gold toxicity (mouth sores, pruritus, GI upset, dermatitis, rash, bleeding gums, petechiae, fever, chills, weakness, sore throat, dysphagia), and report to physician immediately.

▷ 5 Have dimercaprol (BAL) available as a specific antidote to gold overdosage.

▶ **NURSING CONSIDERATIONS**

▷ 1 Shake vial well and do not use if color is darker than pale yellow. Inject deep into gluteal muscle with patient lying down, and instruct patient to remain lying for 20 minutes after injection to eliminate possible dizziness.

▷ 2 Advise patient that beneficial effects may take several months to become evident but will be of prolonged duration once they occur.

▷ 3 Urge oral hygiene to reduce risk of stomatitis and other mouth disorders.

▷ 4 Be aware that toxic effects can occur for months after cessation of drug therapy. Advise continual close observation for possible adverse effects.

▷ 5 Avoid exposure to sunlight as much as possible during therapy because dermatologic toxicity may be increased.

VI Penicillamine (Cuprimine, Depen)

Penicillamine is a chelating agent that has been successfully used to remove excess copper in patients with Wilson's disease, and to increase cystine excretion in cystinuria. It is also approved for the treatment of severe forms of rheumatoid arthritis. Because of its potential to elicit *serious* adverse effects, however, its use should be restricted to those patients with progressive rheumatoid disease that is unresponsive to other less toxic anti-inflammatory agents.

Mechanism
Largely unknown; may inhibit lysosomal enzyme release in connective tissue; suppresses T-cell activity *in vitro,* and lowers IgM rheumatoid factor titer. Other actions ascribed to penicillamine are degradation of collagen, inhibition of lymphocyte transformation, and reduction of circulating immune complexes.

Uses
1 Treatment of severe, active rheumatoid arthritis resistant to other conventional forms of therapy, including rest, exercise, salicylates, nonsteroidal anti-inflammatory drugs, and corticosteroids
2 Promotion of copper excretion in patients with Wilson's disease (hepatolenticular degeneration)
3 Promotion of cystine excretion in patients with cystinuria
4 Investigational uses include treatment of primary biliary cirrhosis and scleroderma

Dosage
Rheumatoid arthritis: initially, 125 mg to 250 mg/day for 4 weeks; increase at 4-week to 12-week intervals by 125 mg to 250 mg/day depending on response and tolerance; maximum 1000 mg to 1500 mg/day for 3 months to 4 months; if no response at this level, discontinue drug; usual maintenance range is 500 mg to 750 mg/day
Wilson's disease: Initially, 250 mg 4 times/day, increased to 500 mg 4 times/day as needed

Cystinuria: Adults: 250 mg to 500 mg 4 times/day
Children: 30 mg/kg/day

Fate
Well absorbed orally if given on an empty stomach; peak plasma level in 1 hour to 2 hours; excreted in the urine, almost completely within 24 hours.

Common Side-Effects
Loss of sense-of-taste, indigestion, rash, pruritus, and proteinuria

Significant Adverse Reactions
GI—epigastric pain, vomiting, diarrhea, oral ulceration, activation of peptic ulcer
Hematologic—leukopenia, thrombocytopenia, bone marrow depression, agranulocytosis, aplastic anemia
Allergic—arthralgia, lymphadenopathy, pemphigoid reaction, urticaria, exfoliative dermatitis, colitis, synovitis, thyroiditis
Renal/hepatic—hematuria, hepatic dysfunction, cholestatic jaundice, pancreatitis, glomerulonephritis (Goodpasture's syndrome)
CNS—tinnitus, optic neuritis
Other—thrombophlebitis, myasthenia-like reaction, hyperpyrexia, polymyositis, systemic lupus-like syndrome, mammary hyperplasia, epidermal necrolysis, alveolitis, obliterative bronchiolitis

Contraindications
Renal insufficiency; pregnancy; young children; history of penicillin sensitivity or blood dyscrasias; concurrent use with other anti-inflammatory drugs (pyrazolones, gold compounds), anti-malarials, or cytotoxic agents

Interactions
1 Penicillamine may potentiate the neurotoxicity of isoniazid.
2 Effects of penicillamine can be decreased by the presence of iron, antacids, or food that can decrease absorption.
3 Risk of blood dyscrasias and renal toxicity may be increased by concomitant use of antimalarial drugs, antineoplastics, gold compounds, or pyrazolones.

▶ **NURSING ALERTS**
▷ 1 Perform urinalysis, differential blood cell counts, hemoglobin determinations, and direct platelet counts every 2 weeks for the first 6 months of therapy, and monthly thereafter. WBC counts below 3500 or platelet counts below 100,000 indicate that therapy should be discontinued.
▷ 2 Observe carefully for proteinuria and hematuria, possible early signs of developing glomerulonephritis. Discontinue drug if proteinuria exceeds 2 g/24 hours, or if gross or persistent microscopic hematuria develops.
▷ 3 Advise patients to promptly report possible early signs of developing blood dyscrasias (*e.g.,* fever, sore throat,

chills, bruising, abnormal bleeding, malaise), and perform blood studies immediately. Drug-induced fever is an indication for discontinuing the drug.

▷ 4 Be alert for appearance of allergic manifestations (*e.g.,* fever, arthralgia, lymphadenopathy, rash, intense pruritus), and advise physician immediately. Decrease in dosage and use of antihistamines can usually eliminate early rash and pruritus.

▷ 5 Note that onset of therapeutic response is delayed up to 3 months. Avoid frequent dosage increments (see dosage), to allow sufficient time for clinical effects to become apparent and to avoid excessive untoward reactions.

▶ **NURSING CONSIDERATIONS**

▷ 1 Watch for signs of increasing muscle weakness because drug can cause a myasthenia-like syndrome. Symptoms will usually disappear following drug withdrawal.

▷ 2 Administer drug on an empty stomach, at least 1 hour apart from any other drug, food, antacid, or milk.

▷ 3 Consider a gradual dosage reduction (125 mg–250 mg/day at 3-month intervals) if patient has been in remission for at least 6 months.

▷ 4 Be aware that because the drug increases soluble collagen, there may be increased skin friability, especially at pressure points (*e.g.,* elbows, knees, buttocks). External bleeding or vesicles containing blood may appear, and skin wrinkling can occur. These effects are not progressive and do not require discontinuance of the drug; they may disappear with dosage reduction.

VII Anti-Gout Drugs

Gout is a metabolic disorder of purine metabolism characterized by an excess of uric acid in the blood (hyperuricemia) that results from either overproduction or a defect in elimination. When uric acid begins to precipitate out of the blood and is deposited in joints, skin, kidney, and other tissues, the symptoms of acute gout appear—pain, swelling, tenderness, and other signs of inflammation. The pharmacotherapy of gout, therefore, involves controlling the serum levels of uric acid to prevent attacks, and providing relief of the symptoms of an acute attack of gouty arthritis. Drugs used as anti-gout agents may be classified as one of the following:

1 *Anti-inflammatory agents*—relieve the pain and inflammation associated with an acute attack of gout

2 *Hypouricemic (uricosuric) agents*—reduce the blood levels of uric acid on a chronic basis

The drugs that may be used to relieve the symptoms of an acute attack are indomethacin, phenylbutazone, oxyphenbutazone, naproxen, sulindac, and colchicine. The first five have been discussed previously in this chapter, because they are also used to control symptoms of rheumatoid arthritis and osteroarthritis. Colchicine is reviewed in detail in this section.

Hypouricemic agents are drugs that either interfere with the synthesis of uric acid (*e.g.,* allopurinol) or promote the urinary excretion of uric acid by blocking its renal tubular reabsorption (*e.g.,* probenecid, sulfinpyrazone). These drugs are also discussed in this section.

▶ **colchicine**

An alkaloid capable of dramatically relieving pain and inflammation associated with acute attacks of gouty arthritis within 12 hours to 24 hours, colchicine is also useful but somewhat less effective in the treatment of chondrocalcinosis (pseudogout). It is nonanalgesic and nonuricosuric, and is specific for the symptoms of gout, being effective in up to 90% of patients if given at the first sign of an attack. Although once it was exclusively the drug of choice, colchicine has now been largely replaced by indomethacin, sulindac, or phenylbutazone because of its extremely high incidence of GI side-effects.

Mechanism
Reduces lactic acid production by leukocytes, thereby decreasing acid deposition, and impairs phagocytic breakdown of white blood cell membrane and release of tissue damaging enzymes; also binds to microtubular cellular proteins, thereby arresting mitosis at metaphase and interfering with movement of mobile cells (*e.g.,* leukocytes)

Uses
1 Relief of pain and inflammation of acute gout and pseudogout
2 Limit the destruction of joint cartilage and reduce the incidence of acute attacks (not an approved indication)
3 Other experimental uses include symptomatic treatment of leukemia, adenocarcinoma, sarcoid arthritis, mycosis fungoides, acute calcium-dependent tendinitis, and familial Mediterranean fever.

Dosage
Oral: 1 mg to 1.2 mg initially, followed by 0.5 mg to 0.6 mg every hour until pain is relieved or diarrhea occurs. (4 mg–8 mg total dose usually required for acute attack; prophylaxis—0.5 mg to 0.6 mg orally 3 to 4 times/ week (severe cases—0.5 mg–1.8 mg daily)
IV: 1 mg to 2 mg initially, followed by 0.5 mg every 6 hr (maximum 4 mg/24 hr)

Fate
Rapidly absorbed orally; relatively short-acting (half-life 20 min); partially metabolized in the liver; both metabolites and unchanged drug are recycled into the GI tract through the bile and intestinal secretions; mainly eliminated in the feces, with 10% to 20% excreted in the urine; drug may persist for up to 9 days in leukocytes after single IV dose.

Common Side Effects
Nausea, vomiting, abdominal pain, and diarrhea

Significant Adverse Reactions

(Usually observed at high doses or with hepatic dysfunction) Severe diarrhea, muscle weakness, dermatitis, hematuria, oliguria, generalized vascular damage, alopecia; prolonged use may lead to agranulocytosis, aplastic anemia, and peripheral neuritis. Overdose may be characterized by vomiting, diarrhea, (profuse and bloody), burning in the throat, stomach or skin, hematuria, shock due to extensive vascular damage, marked muscle weakness, delirium, and convulsions.

Contraindications

Severe renal, GI, cardiac, or hepatic disease; IV use contraindicated with vascular damage.

Interactions

1 Effects of colchicine are enhanced by alkalinizing agents (*e.g.,* sodium bicarbonate) and inhibited by acidifying agents (*e.g.,* ascorbic acid).
2 Colchicine may increased the response to CNS depressants and sympathomimetics.
3 Prolonged use of colchicine may reduce GI absorption of vitamin B_{12}.

▶ NURSING ALERTS

▷ 1 Instruct patients to note signs of early toxicity (nausea, vomiting, diarrhea, abdominal discomfort, weakness). Drug should be discontinued until symptoms subside, then carefully resumed.
▷ 2 Allow 3 days between courses of therapy for acute attacks to prevent cumulative toxicity.
▷ 3 Use with caution in elderly or debilitated patients, especially in the presence of renal, hepatic, GI, or heart disease.
▷ 4 Administer IV only, not SC or IM. Observe for signs of localized irritation (pain, swelling, erythema) at site of injection. Be aware of danger of thrombophlebitis.
▷ 5 Note early signs of bone marrow depression (sore throat, bleeding gums, fever, weakness) and discontinue drug.

▶ NURSING CONSIDERATIONS

▷ 1 Initiate therapy with colchicine at earliest sign of acute attack because drug is most effective if begun early.
▷ 2 Take drug with meals or milk to reduce GI irritation.
▷ 3 During acute attack, instruct patient to immobilize affected joints and avoid use of heat or pressure to area involved.
▷ 4 Consider using IV route if oral administration is associated with excessive GI toxicity. Note, however, that overdose occurs more commonly with IV use, and that extravasation can cause pain and necrosis of tissues.
▷ 5 Monitor intake and output, and maintain a high urine output (at least 2000 ml/day) to promote urate excretion and reduce danger of uric acid deposition in kidneys and ureters.
▷ 6 Counsel patients on proper adjunctive measures (*e.g.,* diet control, weight reduction, increased fluid intake,

avoidance of alcoholic beverages in large amounts) that may help reduce the incidence and severity of attacks.
▷ 7 Note that colchicine may be needed in the *initial stages* of therapy with uricosuric agents because these drugs can mobilize large quantities of uric acid and thus increase the incidence of acute attacks during the early phase of therapy.
▷ 8 Administer 0.5 mg to 0.6 mg 3 times a day for 3 days before and after any surgical procedure (including dental), because an acute attack of gout may be precipitated by the surgery.
▷ 9 Note that colchicine is available in fixed combination with probenecid (Col-Benemid, Proben-C) for treating chronic gouty arthritis complicated by frequent, recurrent acute attacks.

▶ probenecid

Benemid, Probalan, SK-Probenecid

A uricosuric agent that enhances the excretion of uric acid through the kidneys, probenecid has no analgesic or anti-inflammatory action, and thus is of no value in treating acute attacks. The drug also inhibits renal tubular *secretion* of penicillins and cephalosporins, and is often used to increase the plasma level of penicillins by two to four times, thus enhancing their effects.

Mechanism

Inhibits the renal tubular reabsorption of urates, increasing excretion of uric acid and reducing plasma uric acid levels; decreased serum urate concentration retards further urate deposition and increases resorption of urate deposits in tissues; competitively inhibits tubular secretion (*i.e.,* plasma to renal tubule) of many weak organic acids, especially penicillins

Uses

1 Treatment of hyperuricemia associated with gout and gouty arthritis
2 Adjuvant to therapy with penicillins and cephalosporins to elevate and prolong antibiotic plasma levels

Dosage

Gout: 0.25 g twice a day for 1 week, then 0.5 g twice a day thereafter; may increase if necessary by 0.5 g/day every 4 weeks to a maximum of 2 g/day
Penicillin therapy:
Adult—2 g daily in divided doses
Children—40 mg/kg/day in divided doses; (over 50 kg—adult dosage may be given)
Gonorrhea: 1 g probenecid given together with 4.8 million units of penicillin G or 3.5 g ampicillin

Fate

Completely absorbed orally; peak effects in 2 hours to 4 hours; half-life is 8 hours to 10 hours; highly bound to plasma protein (85%–95%); metabolized in the liver; slowly excreted in urine primarily as metabolites and some unchanged drug; excretion increased by alkalinization of the urine

Common Side-Effects

GI irritation, nausea, skin rash, headache, and worsening of symptoms of acute gout for first few days

Significant Adverse Reactions

Abdominal discomfort, diarrhea, sore gums, urinary frequency, flushing, dizziness, hypersensitivity reactions (dermatitis, fever, pruritus, anaphylaxis), anemia, hepatic necrosis, nephrotic syndrome, and aplastic anemia are rare

Contraindications

Children under 2 years, blood dyscrasias, uric acid kidney stones, an acute gouty arthritis attack, severe renal impairment

Interactions

1 Probenecid prolongs the action of penicillins and cephalosporins, and may enhance the action of methotrexate, clofibrate, oral anticoagulants, oral hypoglycemics, naproxen, indomethacin, sulfinpyrazone, sulfonamides, and thiazide diuretics.
2 Salicylates can antagonize the uricosuric effect of probenecid, especially in small analgesic doses.
3 Xanthines (*e.g.,* caffeine, theophylline) and pyrazinamide may antagonize the uricosuric effect of probenecid.

▶ NURSING ALERTS

▷ 1 Caution patient to follow prescribed dosage regimen carefully. Reduction in dose level may result in sharp elevation of serum uric acid levels and precipitation of acute attacks.
▷ 2 Be aware that frequency of acute attacks may increase during first few months of therapy with probenecid. Prophylactic doses of colchicine or indomethacin may be indicated during initial stages of probenecid therapy (colchicine and probenecid are available together as Col-Benemid or Proben-C).
▷ 3 Use cautiously in patients with intermittent porphyria, history of peptic ulcers, or glucose-6-phosphatase deficiency.

▶ NURSING CONSIDERATIONS

▷ 1 Do not initiate therapy with probenecid during an acute attack because symptoms may be worsened. If an attack occurs while the patient is taking the drug, however, do not discontinue but add colchicine or indomethacin as necessary.
▷ 2 Take drug with milk or meals to minimize GI upset.
▷ 3 Maintain high fluid intake (3 liters/day) and alkalinize the urine (*e.g.,* sodium bicarbonate, potassium citrate) to help retard formation of uric acid kidney stones.
▷ 4 Warn patients of the dangers of taking aspirin or related drugs while on probenecid therapy because clinical effects of the uricosuric drug may be greatly reduced.

▷ *Dietary precautions*
▷ 1 Although there is no firm evidence that excessive dietary intake of purines is a primary cause of gout, high-purine foods such as liver, meat extracts, peas, meat soups, broth, and alcohol should be prudently restricted during early stages of therapy, at least until uric acid levels have stabilized.

▶ sulfinpyrazone
Anturane

A pyrazolone derivative with relatively weak anti-inflammatory action, indicated primarily for the maintenance therapy of hyperuricemia, the drug also inhibits platelet aggregation, and some studies suggest that it is effective in reducing the incidence of cardiac death in patients with recent myocardial infarction. This effect may result from an inhibition of platelet thromboxane A_2 synthesis, protection of the vascular endothelium from injury, and diminished release of ADP and possibly serotonin.

Mechanism

Inhibits the active renal tubular reabsorption of uric acid, thereby increasing its urinary excretion and reducing serum urate levels; decreases platelet aggregation, although the mechanism is not completely established (see above); very small doses may interfere with active tubular *secretion* of uric acid (transport from blood to renal tubule) thereby causing retention of serum urates.

Uses

1 Maintenance therapy in hyperuricemia to reduce the incidence and severity of acute attacks of gouty arthritis
2 Prevention of cerebrovascular and ischemic heart disease, and transient ischemic attacks, and reduction in fatalities following myocardial infarction (experimental use only)

Dosage

Initially 200 mg to 400 mg daily in divided doses; increase gradually to an optimal dose (maximum 800 mg/day); continue without interruption, even during an acute attack, which can be treated with colchicine, phenylbutazone, or indomethacin.

To decrease platelet aggregation, a dose of 200 mg 4 times/day is recommended.

Fate

Well absorbed orally; onset in 30 minutes to 60 minutes; duration 4 hours to 6 hours, perhaps up to 10 hours; highly bound to plasma proteins (98%–99%); excreted primarily unchanged (90%) in the urine.

Common Side-Effects

Nausea, epigastric pain, burning, and dyspepsia

Significant Adverse Reactions

Activation of peptic ulcer, dizziness, tinnitus, skin rash, fever, blood dyscrasias, jaundice, precipitation of acute gout (early stages of therapy), urolithiasis, and renal colic

Contraindications

Active peptic ulcer or GI inflammation

Interactions

1 Sulfinpyrazone may potentiate the effects of antico-agulants, sulfonylurea hypoglycemic agents, sulfon-amides, penicillins, insulin, allopurinol, indomethacin, and nitrofurantoin.
2 The uricosuric effects of sulfinpyrazone may be re-duced by salicylates (low doses) and xanthines (*e.g.,* caffeine, theophylline).
3 Serum urate levels may be elevated by diuretics, al-cohol, diazoxide, and mecamylamine, necessitating higher sulfinpyrazone dosage.
4 Incidence of blood dyscrasias may be increased with combined use of sulfinpyrazone and colchicine, other pyrazolones, or indomethacin.

▶ NURSING ALERTS

▷ 1 Be alert for appearance of fever, sore throat, mucosal lesions, malaise, joint pains, sudden bleeding, or skin rash. These are often early signs of blood dyscrasias, and drug should be discontinued.
▷ 2 Consider use of prophylactic doses of colchicine dur-ing early stages of sulfinpyrazone therapy, because incidence of acute attacks is often temporarily in-creased due to mobilization of large amounts of uric acid.
▷ 3 Perform periodic blood counts and renal function tests in patients on long-term therapy to prevent blood dys-crasias and renal colic.
▷ 4 Use with caution in impaired renal function, unex-plained GI pain, and pregnancy.

▶ NURSING CONSIDERATIONS

▷ 1 Caution patients to avoid aspirin-containing medica-tions because effects of sulfinpyrazone may be reduced.
▷ 2 Administer drug with food or milk to reduce GI ir-ritation.
▷ 3 Advise maintaining a fluid intake of at least 2000 ml/day to reduce danger of urate deposition and alkalinize the urine (*e.g.,* sodium bicarbonate, potassium citrate) to increase uric acid solubility.
▷ 4 Inform patient that rigid adherence to dosage schedule is important, because *minor* fluctuations in serum lev-els can result in untoward reactions.
▷ 5 Instruct patient not to alter sulfinpyrazone dosage schedule during an acute attack. Colchicine or other anti-inflammatory drugs should be *added to* the reg-imen.
▷ 6 Monitor prothrombin times carefully in patients taking sulfinpyrazone and oral anticoagulants. Adjustment in dosage may be needed.

▶ allopurinol

Lopurin, Zyloprim

The drug of choice for controlling hyperuricemia resulting from *overproduction* of uric acid, it is especially effective in preventing development of uric acid stones. By reducing the serum urate level, reabsorption of deposits of urate crys-tals from tissues is enhanced. Use of allopurinol must be undertaken cautiously because the incidence of untoward reactions, some rather severe, is fairly high.

Mechanism

Competitively inhibits the action of xanthine oxidase, the enzyme responsible for converting the natural purine hy-poxanthine to xanthine, and xanthine to uric acid; substan-tially reduces both serum and urinary levels of uric acid even in the presence of renal damage; has no analgesic, anti-inflammatory, or uricosuric activity

Uses

1 Treatment of gout, either primary or secondary to the hyperuricemia associated with blood dyscrasias and their treatment
2 Treatment of primary or secondary uric acid nephrop-athy
3 Treatment of recurrent uric acid stone formation
4 Prevention of urate deposition and uric acid nephrop-athy in patients receiving cancer chemotherapy (see Nursing Alerts) or radiation for leukemia and other malignancies

Dosage

200 mg to 600 mg/day in divided doses depending on severity of condition; prevention of uric acid nephrop-athy during cancer chemotherapy—600 mg to 800 mg/day for 2 to 3 days with high fluid intake; reduce slowly to minimum effective maintenance levels.
Children (hyperuricemia secondary to malignancy only): 6 years to 10 years—300 mg/day; under 6 years–150 mg/day

Fate

Fairly rapidly absorbed; peak plasma levels in 2 hours to 6 hours; short half-life (2 hr–3 hr) of the parent compound in plasma; widely distributed in body, except for the brain; largely converted to oxypurinol (also a xanthine oxidase inhibitor) that is slowly excreted in the urine (half-life of 18 hr–30 hr); small amounts excreted unchanged in urine (10%–30%) and feces (10%–20%)

Common Side-Effects

Skin rash, pruritus

Significant Adverse Reactions

Hypersensitivity reactions (fever, chills, malaise, nausea, muscle pain, eosinophilia, leukopenia, reversible acute in-terstitial nephritis)
Dermatologic—exfoliative, urticarial, or purpuric skin le-sions; erythema multiforme; alopecia; dermatitis
Hematologic—blood dyscrasias, bone marrow depres-sion, vasculitis, necrotizing angiitis
GI—vomiting, diarrhea, abdominal pain
Other—peripheral neuritis, cataract formation, acute gouty attacks (early in therapy), hepatotoxicity, drowsiness, vertigo

Contraindications

Children other than those with hyperuricemia secondary to malignancy, and nursing mothers

Interactions

1 Allopurinol may potentiate the action of oral anticoagulants, oral antidiabetics, azathioprine, and 6-mercaptopurine. The drug is a *nonspecific* enzyme inhibitor, and therefore can potentially alter the metabolism of a wide range of drugs dependent on hepatic metabolism for clearance.

2 The effects of allopurinol may be reduced by thiazide and loop diuretics, salicylates, sulfinpyrazone, probenecid, and xanthines.

3 Allopurinol may increase iron absorption and hepatic iron stores. Do not administer oral iron to patients taking allopurinol or use the two drugs together.

4 Increased incidence of skin rash may occur with combinations of ampicillin (and possibly other penicillins) and allopurinol.

5 Allopurinol may increase serum levels of theophylline.

▶ **NURSING ALERTS**

▷ 1 Warn patients to *continually* observe for signs of skin rash, often an early sign of hypersensitivity. Rash can be followed by severe hypertension or more serious dermatologic disorders (*e.g.,* exfoliative dermatitis, Stevens–Johnson syndrome, toxic epidermal necrolysis). Therefore, upon development of a rash, discontinue drug and advise physician.

▷ 2 Perform blood counts and liver and kidney function tests before initiating therapy and periodically during therapy, particularly in patients with preexisting liver disease.

▷ 3 Caution users against engaging in activities requiring alertness, because drug may cause drowsiness and vertigo during early stages of therapy.

▷ 4 Use cautiously in individuals with liver disease, impaired renal function, and during pregnancy.

▷ 5 Although allopurinol is employed during cancer chemotherapy to prevent hyperuricemia and uric acid nephropathy resulting from certain antineoplastic drugs, note that when it is used with purine analogs (*e.g.,* 6-mercaptopurine), allopurinol will retard inactivation of these particular antineoplastic drugs and thus increase their toxicity.

▶ **NURSING CONSIDERATIONS**

▷ 1 Use colchicine during early stages of allopurinol therapy to minimize occurrence of acute gouty attacks due to urate mobilization.

▷ 2 Maintain a fluid intake volume of at least 2000 ml/day, and keep the urine alkaline to prevent urate deposition and possible kidney damage. Be alert for reduced urinary output and advise physician.

▷ 3 Inform patients that effects may take several weeks to develop, and caution against changing dosage levels unless instructed.

▷ 4 When transferring from a uricosuric agent to allopurinol, do so *gradually* by reducing the dosage of the uricosuric slowly and simultaneously increasing the dose of allopurinol over several weeks.

▷ *Dietary precautions*

▷ 1 Suggest that patient restrict certain high-purine foods (*e.g.,* kidney, liver, dried beans, meat extracts) and reduce weight as adjunctive measures to control hyperuricemia. Recognize, however, that dietary intake of purines has *not* been firmly linked to the etiology of gout.

Summary. Non-Narcotic Analgesics

Drug	Preparations	Usual Dosage Range
Salicylates	See Table 19-1	
Para-aminophenols		
Acetaminophen (various manufacturers)	Tablets—300 mg, 325 mg, 500 mg, 650 mg	Adults—325 mg to 650 mg 3 to 4 times/day
	Capsules—325 mg, 500 mg	Children:
	Chewable tablets—80 mg	7 years to 12 years—162.5 mg to 325 mg 3 to 4 times/day (maximum 1.3 g/day)
	Wafers—120 mg	3 years to 6 years—120 mg 3 to 4 times/day (maximum 480 mg/day)
	Suppositories—120 mg, 125 mg, 130 mg, 300 mg, 325 mg, 600 mg, 650 mg	
	Elixir—120 mg, 130 mg, 160 mg, 325 mg/5 ml	
	Syrup—120 mg/5 ml	
	Drops—60 mg/0.6 ml, 100 mg/ml, 120 mg/2.5 ml	
Pyrazolones		
Oxyphenbutazone (Oxalid, Tandearil)	Tablets—100 mg	Initially—300 mg to 600 mg daily in divided doses
		Maintenance—100 mg to 400 mg daily
Phenylbutazone (Azolid, Butazolidin)	Tablets—100 mg	Initially—300 mg to 600 mg daily in divided doses (maximum 600 mg/day)
	Capsules—100 mg	Maintenance—100 mg to 400 mg daily

Summary. Non-Narcotic Analgesics (*continued*)

Drug	Preparations	Usual Dosage Range
Nonsteroidal Anti-inflammatory Agents		
Indomethacin (Indocin)	Capsules—25 mg, 50 mg Sustained-release capsules—75 mg	Arthritis, spondylitis—25 mg 2 to 3 times/day; increase by 25 mg to 50 mg weekly (maximum 200 mg/day) Acute gout—50 mg 3 times/day; decrease rapidly over 3 to 5 days until cessation
Fenoprofen (Nalfon) Ibuprofen (Motrin) Meclofenamate (Meclomen) Mefenamic acid (Ponstel) Naproxen (Anaprox, Naprosyn) Piroxicam (Feldene) Sulindac (Clinoril) Tolmetin (Tolectin) Zomepirac (Zomax)	See Table 19-2	
Gold Compounds		
Aurothioglucose (Solganal)	Injection—50 mg/ml	IM—10 mg first week; 25 mg second and third week; 50 mg on subsequent weeks until benefit is observed; continue with 25 mg to 50 mg every 2 weeks to 4 weeks as patient's condition warrants
Gold sodium thiomalate (myochrysine)	Injection—10 mg/ml, 25 mg/ml, and 50 mg/ml	Adults—10 mg IM first week, 25 mg second week, then 25 mg to 50 mg thereafter at weekly intervals until significant clinical improvement or toxicity Children—1 mg/kg/week, not to exceed 50 mg on a single injection
Penicillamine		
Penicillamine (Cuprimine, Depen)	Capsules—125 mg, 250 mg Tablets—250 mg	Rheumatoid arthritis—initially 125 mg to 250 mg/day for 4 weeks; increase by 125 mg to 250 mg/day at 4-week to 12-week intervals to maximally tolerated dose; do not exceed 1000 mg to 1500 mg/day for longer than 4 months; usual maintenance dose 500 mg to 750 mg/day Wilson's disease: Adults—250 mg 4 times/day Children—250 mg/day Cystinuria: Adults—250 mg to 500 mg 4 times/day Children—30 mg/kg/day
Anti-gout Drugs		
Colchicine	Tablets—0.5 mg to 0.6 mg Enteric-coated tablets—0.432 mg Granules—0.5 mg Injection—1 mg/2 ml	Acute Attack: Oral—1 mg to 1.2 mg initially; repeat with 0.5 mg to 0.6 mg every hour until pain is relieved or diarrhea occurs (control usually accomplished with 4 mg–8 mg total dose). IV—1 mg to 2 mg initially, followed by 0.5 mg every 6 hours (total dose 4 mg/24 hr) (maintenance 1 mg–2 mg daily for several days) Prophylaxis: Oral—0.5 mg to 0.6 mg 3 to 4 times/week (severe cases 0.6 mg–1.8 mg daily)

(continued)

Summary. Non-Narcotic Analgesics *(continued)*

Drug	Preparations	Usual Dosage Range
Probenecid (Benemid, Probalan, SK-Probenecid)	Tablets—0.5 g	Gout—0.25 g twice a day for 1 week, then 0.5 g twice a day; increase to a maximum of 2 g/day Penicillin therapy—2 g daily in divided doses (Children under 50 kg—40 mg/kg/day in divided doses) Gonorrhea—1 g given with 4.8 million units penicillin G or 3.5 g ampicillin
Sulfinpyrazone (Anturane)	Tablets—100 mg Capsules—200 mg	Initially 200 mg to 400 mg/day in divided doses Maintenance—200 mg to 800 mg/day adjusted to patients needs (do not interrupt during acute attacks)
Allopurinol (Lopurin, Zyloprim)	Tablets—100 mg, 300 mg	Control of Gout—200 mg to 600 mg/day in divided doses Prevention of Uric Acid Nephropathy: Adults—600 mg to 800 mg/day for 2 to 3 days; reduce to effective maintenance levels based on serum urate levels Children (6 yr–10 yr)—300 mg/day Children (under 6)—150 mg/day

Many drugs are capable of eliciting varying degrees of CNS depression, and one such group of agents are commonly referred to as sedative–hypnotics. With increasing doses, these drugs produce a range of central effects from mild sedation through hypnosis (induction of sleep) to complete loss of consciousness or anesthesia. Drugs possessing these actions are generally classified into two broad categories: (1) barbiturates—derivatives of barbituric acid, and (2) non-barbiturates—a group of drugs structurally unrelated to barbituric acid but possessing many of the pharmacologic actions of barbiturates. The next two chapters address the barbiturate and nonbarbiturate sedative–hypnotics, respectively.

Barbiturates were one of the first effective hypnotics to be introduced into medicine around the turn of the 20th century. They elicit a general CNS depression, the magnitude of which is largely dependent on the dose. Although occasionally employed in small doses for daytime sedation in anxiety states, barbiturates are principally used at full therapeutic dose for the induction of sleep. Certain individual barbiturates are also indicated as antiepileptics (see Chap. 25), general anesthetics (see Chap. 17), and in certain types of psychoanalysis.

The major pharmacologic action of these drugs is a reduction in overall CNS alertness. They appear to act at several levels of CNS, and with increasing dosage can depress many centrally mediated functions, including motor activity and respiration. All are effective anticonvulsants in large doses, and the longer acting derivatives are employed as specific antiepileptic drugs as well (see Chap. 25). Barbiturates are not effective analgesics in subanesthetic doses and generally do not produce significant hypnosis in severely painful conditions. Conversely, when combined with an analgesic, they are capable of markedly potentiating its ability to relieve pain.

The most important adverse reactions occur with either overdose or prolonged use of the drugs. *Overdose* is characterized by marked respiratory depression, lowered body temperature, circulatory collapse, and eventually coma, and is an acute medical emergency. Conversely the principal danger associated with *prolonged* use of the barbiturates is habituation and addiction. Withdrawal from barbiturates should be accomplished gradually because sudden withdrawal can result in severe anxiety, tremors, marked excitement, convulsions, and delirium. Repeated use of barbiturates also decreases the time spent in the REM (rapid eye movement) phase of sleep, the phase associated with dreaming. Personality changes have been noted in persons deprived of REM sleep for long periods of time, and signs of irritability, confusion, aggressiveness, and decreased attention may be observed with prolonged use of barbiturates.

The clinically useful barbiturates have been categorized into one of four groups based upon their duration of action. These groups are

1 *Long-Acting* (6 hr–8 hr)—mephobarbital, metharbital, phenobarbital
2 *Intermediate-Acting* (4 hr–6 hr)—amobarbital, aprobarbital, butabarbital, talbutal
3 *Short-Acting* (2 hr–4 hr)—pentobarbital, secobarbital
4 *Ultrashort-Acting* (10 min–30 min)—methohexital, thiamylal, thiopental

Barbiturate

Sedative–

Hypnotics

20

While this represents a convenient means of classification, it must be noted that differences in duration of action among the first three categories depend on several factors other than the drug itself, such as dosage form, route of administration, presence of disease states (*e.g.,* liver or kidney dysfunction), and length of treatment.

The ultrashort-acting barbiturates are indicated primarily as induction anesthetics and have been discussed in Chapter 17. The remaining barbiturates are reviewed as a group, and specific information relating to each drug will then be given in Table 20-1.

Barbiturates

Amobarbital	Metharbital
Aprobarbital	Pentobarbital
Butabarbital	Phenobarbital
Hexobarbital	Secobarbital
Mephobarbital	Talbutal

Mechanism

Act at several sites in the CNS; interfere with the transmission of impulses at synapses in the reticular formation of the brain stem and thalamus, thereby decreasing overall impulse transmission to the cortex; increase the threshold for electrical excitation of the motor cortex; produce no analgesia alone, and may intensify reaction to painful stimuli in small doses; reduce analgesic requirements by approximately 50% when combination of barbiturate and analgesic are used together; minimal effects on autonomic or cardiovascular system in normal therapeutic doses; depress the respiratory center in a dose-dependent fashion

Uses

1 Daytime sedative for the relief of anxiety, tension, and nervousness (infrequent use)
2 Short-term treatment of insomnia
3 Control of acute convulsive states (IV, IM)
4 Treatment of various forms of epilepsy
5 Pre- and postoperative sedation
6 Induction anesthesia and brief, minor surgical procedures (ultrashort- and short-acting drugs)
7 Aid in psychoanalysis (narcoanalysis and narcotherapy)
8 Management of catatonic and manic reactions (IV, IM)

Dosage

See Table 20-1.

Fate

Well absorbed from GI tract and IM injection sites; soluble sodium salts are absorbed more rapidly than free bases, especially on an empty stomach; widely distributed in the body and bound to plasma proteins to varying degrees; lipid solubility is a major determinant of distribution; highly lipid-soluble drugs more readily penetrate body tissues; thus, drugs with low lipid solubility (*e.g.,* phenobarbital) have a slow onset and long duration and *vice versa.* However, lipid-soluble drugs are quickly redistributed from active CNS sites to fatty tissue stores, from where the drug may be slowly released. Because the pharmacologic effects often disappear before the drug is totally eliminated from the body, too-frequent dosing can result in cumulation toxicity. Most drugs are metabolized in the liver and excreted in the urine, principally as metabolites, except for aprobarbital and phenobarbital, which are excreted in part unchanged.

Common Side-Effects

Drowsiness, hangover, and ataxia

Significant Adverse Reactions

Oral—skin rash, vertigo, lethargy, nausea, diarrhea, jaundice (rare), hypersensitivity reactions (fever, urticaria, hives, serum sickness), muscle and joint pain. Paradoxical excitation occasionally seen, especially in children and older people. Prolonged use may lead to tolerance, habituation and addiction.

IV—see Oral; in addition, respiratory depression, coughing, hiccoughing, laryngospasm, bronchospasm, hypotension, pain at injection site, thrombophlebitis, and blood dyscrasias (rare)

Overdose—respiratory depression, hypothermia, depressed reflexes, anuria, rapid pulse, pulmonary edema, anoxia, cyanotic skin, stupor, and coma

Contraindications

Latent or manifest porphyria, marked liver impairment, severe respiratory disease or obstruction, uncontrolled pain, impaired renal function, and early pregnancy

Interactions

1 Barbiturates may potentiate the CNS and respiratory-depressant effects of alcohol, narcotic analgesics, other sedative–hypnotics, phenothiazine and other antipsychotic drugs, antihistamines, anesthetics, antidepressants, antianxiety agents, centrally acting muscle relaxants, and reserpine.
2 Barbiturates increase the activity of liver metabolic enzymes and therefore may decrease the effects of drugs metabolized by those enzymes, such as oral anticoagulants, corticosteroids, diphenhydramine, digitalis glycosides, methyldopa, lidocaine, griseofulvin, estrogens, progestogens, androgens, pyrazolones, tricyclic antidepressants, and tetracyclines.
3 The effects of barbiturates may be increased by MAO inhibitors, chloramphenicol, valproic acid, sulfonamides, acidifying agents, anticholinesterase drugs, and disulfiram.
4 Barbiturates may inhibit GI absorption of griseofulvin.
5 Concurrent administration of barbiturates and furosemide can produce or aggravate orthostatic hypotension.
6 Chloramphenicol may impair the metabolism of phenobarbital.

▶ **NURSING ALERTS**

▷ 1 Be aware that use for prolonged periods of time, even at therapeutic levels, is associated with a high inci-

Table 20-1. Barbiturates

Drug	Preparations	Usual Dosage Range	Remarks
Short-Acting			
Pentobarbital (Nembutal)	Capsules—30 mg, 50 mg, 100 mg Elixir—20 mg/5 ml Suppositories—30 mg, 60 mg, 120 mg, 200 mg Injection—50 mg/ml	Oral: Sedation— (Adults) 30 mg 3 to 4 times/day (Child) 2 mg/kg to 6 mg/kg/day in divided doses Hypnosis— (Adults) 100 mg Rectal: Adults—120 mg to 200 mg Child—30 mg to 120 mg based on age and weight IM: Adults—150 mg to 200 mg Child—25 mg to 80 mg IV: Adults—100 mg initially; repeat at 50-mg to 100-mg increments to a maximum of 500 mg	Used for preoperative sedation, for minor diagnostic or surgical procedures, and for emergency control of convulsions; hypnotic effects show rapid tolerance; parenteral solution is highly alkaline; avoid extravasation as necrosis can occur; do not give more than 5 ml at one IM site; administer slowly IV, and wait at least 1 minute before giving subsequent injections; potent respiratory depressant; can produce bronchospasm, hypotension, and apnea if injection is too rapid; IM injections should be made deep into large muscle mass (*e.g.,* gluteus) (Schedule II)
Secobarbital (Seconal)	Capsules—50 mg, 100 mg Tablets—100 mg Elixir—22 mg/5 ml Suppositories—30 mg, 60 mg, 120 mg, 200 mg Injection—50 mg/ml	Oral: Sedation— (Adults) 30 mg to 50 mg 3 times/day (Child) 6 mg/kg/day Preoperative— (Adults) 200 mg to 300 mg (Child) 50 mg to 100 mg Hypnosis— Adult 100 mg Rectal: Adults—120 mg to 200 mg Child—15 mg to 120 mg based on age and weight IM: Hypnosis— (Adults) 100 mg to 200 mg (Child) 3 mg/kg to 5 mg/kg IV Convulsions—5.5 mg/kg at a rate of 50 mg/15 sec; repeat every 3 hours to 4 hours as needed IV Anesthesia—50 mg/15 sec slow IV injection until effect is attained (maximum 250 mg)	Used for insomnia, to provide basal hypnosis for anesthesia, in the emergency control of convulsions, and for dental and minor surgical procedures; tolerance develops quickly (within 2 wk) to the hypnotic effect; aqueous solutions for injection must be freshly prepared with Sterile Water for Injection; make sure drug dissolves completely, and use solution within 30 minutes because it is very unstable; injectable form is also available in a more stable aqueous-polyethylene glycol vehicle that should be refrigerated; use of this latter vehicle is contraindicated in patients with renal dysfunction or insufficiency because it is very irritating to the kidneys; give *slowly* IV and monitor patient continually (Schedule II)
Intermediate-Acting			
Amobarbital (Amytal)	Tablets—15 mg, 30 mg, 50 mg, 100 mg Capsules—65 mg, 200 mg (sodium salt) Elixir—44 mg/5 ml Powder for injection—250 mg, 500 mg powder with diluent	Oral: Sedation—30 mg to 50 mg 2 to 3 times/day Hypnosis—100 mg to 200 mg Preoperative—200 mg 1 hour to 2 hours before surgery Convulsive disorders—65 mg 2 to 4 times/day Labor—200 mg to 400 mg initially; repeat at 1-hour to	Used as sedative, hypnotic, preanesthetic medication, anticonvulsant, and for the management of catatonic or manic reactions; prepare solutions with sterile water, and use within 30 minutes after opening vial; do not use if solution is not clear; inject deeply IM or slow IV (1 ml/min maximum IV rate) (Schedule II)

(continued)

Table 20-1. Barbiturates *(continued)*

Drug	Preparations	Usual Dosage Range	Remarks
		3-hour intervals to a maximum of 1 g. IM and IV: Individualized based on condition, age, weight; usual adult range is 65 mg to 500 mg by deep IM injection or slow IV injection	
Aprobarbital (Alurate)	Elixir—40 mg/5 ml	Sedation—40 mg 3 times/day Hypnosis—40 mg to 160 mg depending on severity	Only used orally for daytime sedation or relief of insomnia (Schedule II)
Butabarbital (Butalan, Butatran, Buticaps, Butisol, Sarisol)	Tablets—15 mg, 30 mg, 50 mg, 100 mg Capsules—15 mg, 30 mg Elixir—30 mg, 33.3 mg/5 ml	Sedation: Adults—15 mg to 30 mg 3 to 4 times/day Child—7.5 mg to 30 mg/day Hypnosis: Adults—50 mg to 100 mg Child—based on age and weight	Used as mild sedative, for insomnia, and preoperatively; similar to phenobarbital in most respects (Schedule III)
Talbutal (Lotusate)	Tablets—120 mg	120 mg 15 minutes to 30 minutes before bedtime	Used for relief of insomnia (Schedule III)

Long-Acting

Drug	Preparations	Usual Dosage Range	Remarks
Mephobarbital (Mebaral, Mephohab)	Tablets—32 mg, 50 mg, 100 mg, 200 mg	Sedation: Adults—32 mg to 100 mg 3 to 4 times/day Child—16 mg to 32 mg 3 to 4 times/day Epilepsy: Adults—400 mg to 600 mg/day Child—16 mg to 64 mg 3 to 4 times/day depending on age	Used for daytime sedation in various anxiety states, and primarily as adjunctive treatment of grand mal and petit mal epilepsy (see Chap. 25); similar to phenobarbital in most respects but very weak hypnotic, and produces minimal drowsiness; dosage alterations should be made gradually in epileptic states, to avoid precipitation of convulsions (Schedule IV)
Metharbital (Gemonil)	Tablets—100 mg	Epilepsy: Adults—initially 100 mg 1 to 3 times/day; increase to optimal level Child—5 mg to 15 mg/kg/day based on age and weight	Used in various forms of epilepsy (grand and petit mal, myclonic, and mixed seizures), either alone or more frequently combined with other drugs; not as effective as phenobarbital and produces more sedation (See Chap. 25) (Schedule III)
Phenobarbital (various manufacturers)	Tablets—8 mg, 15 mg, 16 mg, 30 mg, 32 mg, 65 mg, 100 mg Capsules—16 mg Timed-release capsules—65 mg Elixir—20 mg/5 ml Liquid—15 mg/5 ml Drops—16 mg/ml Injection—30 mg, 60 mg, 65 mg, 130 mg/ml Powder for injection—120 mg/vial	Oral: Sedation— (Adults) 16 mg to 32 mg 2 to 4 times/day (Child) 1 mg to 3 mg/kg/day Hypnosis— (Adults) 100 mg to 320 mg Epilepsy— (Adults) 100 mg to 300 mg/day (Child) 4 mg to 6 mg/kg/day IV: 30 mg to 60 mg/minute until an optimal effect is obtained (maximum dose 600 mg) IM: 100 mg to 320 mg/day (maximum 600 mg/day)	Widely used for sedation and in grand mal and focal seizures, either alone or combined with other antiepileptic drugs; used IV in acute convulsive states (see Chap. 25); solutions should be freshly prepared with Sterile Water for Injection, and used within 30 minutes after preparation; do not use if solution is not clear after 5 minutes of mixing; some injectable forms contain alcohol and propylene glycol, and are more stable than aqueous solutions; drug has a long half-life (2 days–5 days), and too frequent dosing can cause accumulation toxicity (Schedule IV)

dence of habituation and addiction. Discourage use of any barbiturate for chronic daytime sedation.

▷ 2 Recognize that barbiturates generally lose effectiveness as hypnotics within 2 weeks of continued usage, and dosage should *not* be increased in an attempt to regain effectiveness.

▷ 3 Warn patient against abruptly discontinuing therapy following chronic use of a barbiturate. Withdrawal symptoms may occur and can be quite serious (*e.g.,* tremors, convulsions, delirium).

▷ 4 Caution patients against engaging in any hazardous occupation during barbiturate therapy because drowsiness and impaired motor coordination often are present.

▷ 5 Counsel chronic users to note and report the appearance of sore throat, fever, superficial bleeding, bruising, rash and jaundice symptoms, signs of possible hematologic toxicity.

▷ 6 Use very cautiously in pediatric, elderly, debilitated, or nursing patients or in the presence of fever, hyperthyroidism, diabetes, hepatic, renal, or cardiac impairment, as well as severe anemia and alcoholism.

▷ 7 When giving IV, administer *slowly* to prevent respiratory depression, laryngospasm, and hypotension, and monitor vital signs continually. Have resuscitative equipment and other supportive measures (*e.g.,* IV fluids, vasopressors) on hand in case respiratory or circulatory depression occurs. Observe site of injection for evidence of extravasation (swelling, pain).

▷ 8 Caution patients using barbiturates at home *not* to keep more than one night's supply by the bed at night. Drowsiness may cause the patient to forget he took a dose of the drug, and mistaken repeated dosage may result in accidental overdose if large quantities of medication are readily available at the bedside.

▷ 9 Recognize that barbiturates given to patients in severe pain may produce anxiety and restlessness and may intensify the person's reaction to the painful stimuli. Always give in combination with an analgesic in the presence of pain.

▶ NURSING CONSIDERATIONS

▷ 1 Advise patients of the dangers of additive CNS depressant effects if barbiturates are combined with alcohol, antihistamines, tranquilizers, and other central depressants.

▷ 2 Be alert for signs of excessive dosage (*e.g.,* mental clouding, impaired coordination), and reduce dosage accordingly.

▷ 3 Use adjunctive measures where possible (*e.g.,* warm bath, back rub, quiet atmosphere, mild analgesic, avoidance of coffee at night) to aid in sleep induction.

▷ 4 Observe patients for signs of developing tolerance and habituation (*e.g.,* more frequent usage, use of larger doses, decreased drug effects). Advise physician and consider *gradual* drug withdrawal.

▷ 5 Advise patients using oral contraceptives that their efficacy may be reduced by prolonged use of barbiturates. Counsel patients on other possible methods of contraception.

▷ 6 Be prepared to deal with an initial period of excitement or confusion in some patients given barbiturates, especially the very young and elderly. Attempt to calm the patient and prevent injury.

▷ 7 Inform patients that "hangover" effects are common with barbiturates. Suggest rising slowly from bed and walking cautiously until equilibrium is established.

▷ 8 Because barbiturates are all controlled substances, learn regulations for handling and dispensing each agent (see Appendix).

Nonbarbiturate Sedative– Hypnotics

21

In addition to the barbiturates, a variety of other drugs are used for many of the same indications, such as daytime sedation and relief of insomnia. Much confusion exists, however, about the terminology used to describe these other sedative–hypnotic drugs. For the purposes of our discussion, drugs reviewed in this chapter will be termed *nonbarbiturate sedative–hypnotics* because they are occasionally employed to provide temporary relief from preoperative anxiety, but are primarily used for short-term treatment of insomnia. A distinction can be made between most of these nonbarbiturate sedative–hypnotics and the minor tranquilizers or antianxiety agents, to be discussed in Chapter 23, primarily on the basis of clinical indications and certain pharmacologic properties. Table 21-1 presents a general comparison of these two groups of drugs. It is important to recognize, however, that the differences cited may not be as clearly defined for individual drugs in the two groups, especially with the three benzodiazepine hypnotics (see discussion of these drugs below).

In general, the nonbarbiturate sedative–hypnotics induce sleep in therapeutic doses and produce significant drowsiness and motor retardation in small doses. The difference between the calming or sedative dose and the hypnotic or sleep-inducing dose is often minimal, and likewise the difference between the therapeutic (hypnotic) dose and the toxic dose is quite small. Therefore, most of these drugs, again with the exception of the benzodiazepine hypnotics, offer no advantage over the barbiturates in terms of either efficacy or safety. Habituation and addiction are as much a problem with continued use of these drugs as with the barbiturates, with only occasional exceptions that are noted below.

Classification of nonbarbiturate sedative–hypnotics is difficult, owing to the variety of chemical structures possessed by these agents. However, they all share a common action— that is, the ability to depress the CNS in a dose-related fashion. The mechanism of this action, however, is not completely understood in all cases. Several older drugs, once frequently used, have been rendered essentially obsolete by development of more effective agents, and these older drugs are addressed only briefly in this chapter. A detailed account, however, is given of those drugs currently used on a more frequent basis.

In addition to the nonbarbiturate sedative–hypnotics to be reviewed in this chapter, several antihistamines are found in various over-the-counter sleep aids, where they provide a small degree of drowsiness to assist the user in falling asleep. The recommended doses are 25 mg to 50 mg pyrilamine maleate (*e.g.,* Sominex, Somnicaps), 50 mg diphenhydramine (*e.g.,* Compoz, Nytol, Sleep-Eze, Sominex Formula 2, Twilite), and 25 mg doxylamine (*e.g.,* Unisom). Maximum recommended dosages are 100 mg/24 hours. Use of antihistamine-containing sleep aids is recommended for short periods of time only (7 days–10 days). These preparations should not be given to children, pregnant women, or patients with asthma, prostate enlargement, or glaucoma.

▶ **acetylcarbromal**
Paxarel

Table 21-1. Comparison Between Nonbarbiturate Sedative–Hypnotics and Antianxiety Drugs

	Nonbarbiturates	Antianxiety Agents
Major Indications	Insomnia	Stress, tension, and other psychoneuroses
Sedative/hypnotic ratio	Low	High
Drowsiness, psychomotor impairment, and confusion	Moderate to severe	Mild
Dependence liability	High	Moderate to high
Central skeletal muscle-relaxing effect	No	Yes

A derivative of urea with short-acting sedative–hypnotic properties, acetylcarbromal acts by releasing free bromide ion and therefore can give rise to bromide intoxication (see discussion of bromides later in the chapter). Acetylcarbromal is largely an obsolete drug that provides no advantage over most other sedative–hypnotics. Large doses may cause excessive drowsiness, narcosis, and respiratory depression. Prolonged use may result in decreased reflexes, stupor, skin rash, joint pain, and psychotic behavior. Toxicity is best treated by intake of large amounts of sodium chloride and water to promote bromide excretion. The drug is habit forming and should not be used chronically.

Benzodiazepine Hypnotics

▶ flurazepam
Dalmane

▶ temazepam
Restoril

▶ triazolam
Halcion

Most benzodiazepine drugs are used for the relief of simple anxiety (see Chap. 23). The above three benzodiazepines, however, are primarily intended for the short-term management of insomnia and should not be given during the day to control anxiety states. Because their pharmacology is similar, they are discussed as a group, and are then listed individually in Table 21-2.

Mechanism
Exact site and mechanism unknown; drugs are benzodiazepine derivatives, similar in structure and most pharmacologic properties to related agents such as diazepam (Valium) (see Chap. 23); produce good hypnosis, skeletal muscle relaxation (probably centrally mediated), and an-

Table 21-2. Benzodiazepine Hypnotics

Drug	Preparations	Usual Dosage Range	Remarks
Flurazepam (Dalmane)	Capsules—15 mg, 30 mg	15 mg to 30 mg at bedtime (15 mg in elderly or debilitated patients)	Longest acting benzodiazepine hypnotic; major metabolite is N-desalkyl-flurazepam, which is an active hypnotic with prolonged half-life (50 hours–100 hours); daytime carry-over effects can include decreased alertness, impaired coordination, confusion and subtle personality changes; maximum hypnotic effectiveness may not be achieved for several nights; residual effects can persist for days following discontinuation of therapy; not recommended in children under 15; do not discontinue drug abruptly after prolonged usage
Temazepam (Restoril)	Capsules—15 mg, 30 mg	15 mg to 30 mg at bedtime (15 mg in elderly or debilitated patients)	Intermediate acting benzodiazepine (plasma half-life of 9 hours–12 hours); no accumulation of metabolites; hangover effects are minimal and early morning wakening is reduced; use in children under 18 is not recommended; transient sleep disturbances can occur for several nights following discontinuation of therapy
Triazolam (Halcion)	Tablets—0.25 mg, 0.5 mg	0.25 to 0.5 mg at bedtime (0.125 mg–0.25 mg in elderly or debilitated patients)	Short-acting hypnotic; plasma half-life is 1.5 hours to 3 hours; metabolites are inactive; elicits few daytime hangover effects, but may lead to increased wakefulness during the last third of the night; not recommended for children under 18

ticonvulsive action; exert little suppression of REM sleep, and display a good safety margin and fairly low abuse potential; minimal hangover effects reported with shorter acting drugs; drugs do not appear to induce hepatic microsomal enzymes.

Uses
1 Short-term relief of insomnia

Dosage
See Table 21-2.

Fate
Oral absorption is good; sleep usually occurs within 15 minutes to 45 minutes with all drugs; peak plasma levels are attained at 30 minutes to 60 minutes with flurazepam, 2 hours to 3 hours with temazepam, and 1 hour to 1.5 hours with triazolam. Flurazepam is converted to an active metabolite with a half-life of 50 hours to 100 hours; thus, it has the longest duration of action and can elicit a prolonged "hangover" effect. Temazepam exhibits a plasma half-life of 9 hours to 12 hours and is metabolized to inactive compounds in the liver. Triazolam is also converted to inactive metabolites, and has a plasma half-life of only 1.5 hours to 3 hours; therefore, it is very short acting and early morning awakening has occurred. All three drugs are excreted largely in the urine.

Common Side-Effects
Occasional drowsiness, dizziness, headache (especially triazolam), ataxia, and lightheadedness (more common in elderly)

Significant Adverse Reactions
(Rare at normal dose levels) Lethargy, disorientation, slurred speech, faintness, confusion, anorexia, nervousness, apprehension, weakness, irritability, palpitation, joint pain, nausea, vomiting, diarrhea, heartburn, abdominal and urinary discomfort, memory impairment, and depression

Contraindications
Pregnancy

Interactions
1 Possible additive effect with other CNS depressants, especially with the longer acting derivatives

▶ NURSING ALERTS
▷ 1 Use cautiously in patients with hepatic or renal diseases, depression, a history of drug habituation, and in elderly, debilitated, pregnant, or nursing patients.
▷ 2 Caution patients to use care in driving or performing hazardous tasks until effects of the drug have been determined.

▶ NURSING CONSIDERATIONS
▷ 1 Recognize that sedative effects of long-acting drugs may persist for several days after use of the drug is terminated. Daytime carry-over effects are enhanced by alcohol, antianxiety drugs, and other CNS depressants.

▷ 2 Reduce initial dose in the elderly to minimize sedation and dizziness.
▷ 3 Perform periodic blood counts and liver and kidney function tests in patients on chronic therapy.
▷ 4 Although addiction potential is lower than with most similar drugs, be aware that tolerance and habituation may occur with repeated use, especially of larger doses. Drugs are classified in schedule IV (see Appendix).

Bromides

Inorganic bromide salts were one of the earliest known sedative–hypnotic agents and were once widely used for their sedative, hypnotic, and anticonvulsant effects. Today, they are only infrequently employed, largely due to the availability of other more effective and less toxic agents. Both sodium and potassium bromide powders are still available and are occasionally prescribed for the treatment of generalized seizures where other anticonvulsants are inappropriate or ineffective. Because the bromide ion is excreted slowly through the kidneys, it should never be used in patients with renal dysfunction because accumulation toxicity easily can occur, possibly leading to severe psychotic reactions. The most frequent untoward effects are generalized skin rash, drowsiness, and GI disturbances. Normal adult dosage is 1 g to 2 g 3 times a day. Chloride intake should be kept low during bromide therapy because high plasma chloride levels will accelerate bromide excretion.

▶ chloral hydrate
Aquachloral Supprettes, Noctec, Oradrate

Mechanism
Depressant effect on cerebral cortex, with minimal involvement of lower brain centers regulating respiration and blood pressure; metabolized quickly to trichloroethanol, considered to be the active metabolite; little "hangover" or depressant after-effects, and good safety margin; no suppression of REM sleep

Uses
1 Temporary relief of insomnia
2 Pre- and postoperative sedation
3 Aid to obtaining sleep EEG recordings
4 Daytime sedation

Dosage
Adults:
Hypnosis—500 mg to 1000 mg at bedtime
Sedation—250 mg 3 times/day
Children:
Hypnosis—50 mg/kg (maximum 1000 mg)
Sedation—25 mg/kg/day in divided doses

Fate
Quickly absorbed orally or rectally, and converted to trichloroethanol; onset of effect in 30 minutes to 60 minutes;

duration is 4 hours to 8 hours; metabolite is conjugated in the liver and excreted chiefly in the urine, and in lesser amounts in the bile.

Common Side-Effects

Unpleasant taste, gastric distress, and lightheadedness

Significant Adverse Reactions

Drowsiness, vertigo, motor incoordination, allergic reactions (erythema, urticaria, dermatitis), nightmares, paradoxical excitement and delirium, reduction in white cell count; chronic use—gastritis, skin eruptions, renal damage, habituation, and addiction

Contraindications

Hepatic or renal impairment, gastritis, severe cardiac disease, history of allergic reactions, and nursing mothers

Interactions

1 Effects of other CNS depressants may be potentiated by chloral hydrate.
2 May potentiate the action of acidic, protein-bound drugs (*e.g.,* anticoagulants, salicylates, oral hypoglycemics) by displacing them from protein-binding sites.
3 Chloral hydrate may interfere with the action of steroids.
4 Effects of chloral hydrate can be potentiated by MAO inhibitors and phenothiazines.
5 Use of IV furosemide with chloral hydrate may result in sweating, tachycardia, and hypertension, due to displacement of thyroid hormone from its bound state.

▶ NURSING ALERTS

▷ 1 Caution patient to avoid alcohol while taking drug, because combination can produce flushing, tachycardia, hypotension, headache, and loss of consciousness.
▷ 2 Be aware that patients using the drug chronically may suddenly exhibit "intolerance," resulting in hypotension, respiratory depression, and possibly death. Advise against prolonged use.
▷ 3 Use cautiously in patients with cardiac arrhythmias, asthma, history of drug dependence, and during pregnancy.
▷ 4 Do not use alone in patients with severe pain; may cause delirium and excitement.
▷ 5 Advise patients to avoid hazardous activities while taking the drug because it may cause excessive drowsiness.

▶ NURSING CONSIDERATIONS

▷ 1 Administer drug in capsules or well-diluted liquid form with meals, to minimize GI irritation.
▷ 2 Observe for signs of chronic intoxication (*e.g.,* gastritis, skin eruptions), and begin supervised *gradual* withdrawal. Have supportive treatment available if needed (*e.g.,* respiratory aids, pressor agents).
▷ 3 Note drug is classified as schedule IV controlled substance (see Appendix).

▶ ethchlorvynol

Placidyl

Mechanism

Not established; short-acting hypnotic, with anticonvulsant and muscle-relaxing effects

Uses

1 Short-term treatment of insomnia (most effective in patients having difficulty falling asleep rather than having frequent awakenings)

Dosage

500 mg to 1000 mg at bedtime; a single 100-mg to 200-mg supplement may be given if awakening occurs (not recommended for children)

Fate

Rapidly absorbed orally; onset in 15 minutes to 30 minutes; duration usually 4 hours to 5 hours; widely distributed and localized in body lipids; less than 0.1% of the dose excreted in the urine within the first 24 hours; extensively metabolized by the liver, and slowly excreted

Common Side-Effects

Dizziness, blurred vision, unpleasant aftertaste, and mild hangover

Significant Adverse Reactions

Nausea, facial numbness, hypotension, skin rash, urticaria, jaundice (rare), ataxia, and giddiness if absorption is rapid, idiosyncratic reactions (excitement, hysteria, prolonged hypnosis, muscle weakness, syncope); chronic use—tremors, incoordination, confusion, slurred speech, hyperreflexia, diplopia, and muscle weakness

Contraindications

Porphyria, early pregnancy (first 6 months), and children

Interactions

1 Additive depressant effects may occur if used with other CNS depressants or MAO inhibitors.
2 Drug may reduce the effects of oral anticoagulants.
3 Delirium can occur if used in combination with tricyclic antidepressants.

▶ NURSING ALERTS

▷ 1 Advise patients to avoid activities requiring alertness while taking the drug and to avoid concomitant use of alcohol, because excessive drowsiness can occur.
▷ 2 Use cautiously in depressed patients and those with a history of or potential for drug abuse.
▷ 3 Do not give alone to patients with pain; control pain with analgesics first.
▷ 4 Administer carefully to patients with renal or hepatic disease, to elderly or debilitated patients, during the third trimester of pregnancy, and to nursing mothers.
▷ 5 Observe for signs of dependence, and discontinue drug *slowly* in patients on prolonged therapy. Abrupt

withdrawal may precipitate barbiturate-like withdrawal symptoms.

▶ **NURSING CONSIDERATIONS**
▷ 1 Avoid use of the drug as a daytime sedative because its duration of action is short.
▷ 2 Administer with food or milk to slow absorption, and to prevent giddiness and ataxia resulting from rapid absorption.
▷ 3 Follow proper handling procedures because drug is a class IV substance (see Appendix).

▶ **ethinamate**
Valmid

Mechanism
Nonspecific central depressive action of unknown mechanism; exhibits anticonvulsant activity as well; little or no hangover

Uses
1 Short-term treatment of insomnia (especially where difficulty is in falling asleep rather than remaining asleep)

Dosage
500 mg to 1000 mg at bedtime (not recommended for children)

Fate
Quickly absorbed; onset in 20 minutes to 30 minutes; duration is 3 hours to 5 hours; partly metabolized by the liver, conjugated and excreted by the kidney

Common Side-Effects
Drowsiness, nausea

Significant Adverse Reactions
Skin rash, GI distress, excitement, and thrombocytopenic purpura

Interactions
1 May enhance the sedative effects of other CNS depressants

▶ **NURSING ALERTS**
See Ethchlorvynol.

▶ **NURSING CONSIDERATIONS**
▷ 1 Inform patient to report development of fever because it may be a sign of developing toxicity.
▷ 2 Note that drug is a class IV substance (see Appendix).

▶ **glutethimide**
Doriden

Mechanism
Depressive effects are similar to those of the barbiturates, including decreased REM sleep; has no analgesic or anticonvulsant actions; possesses significant anticholinergic activity, most pronounced in the iris (mydriasis), but also affecting the GI tract (decreased motility) and salivary glands (reduced secretions); little respiratory depression in normal doses

Uses
1 Insomnia (all types)
2 Sedation during early stages of labor or preoperatively

Dosage
Insomnia: 250 mg to 500 mg at bedtime; may repeat once if necessary; maximum dose is 1000 mg/night
Preoperative: 500 mg to 1000 mg
Early labor: 500 mg at onset; may repeat once

Fate
Erratically absorbed orally because of poor water solubility; onset usually within 30 minutes; duration is 4 hours to 8 hours; about 50% is bound to plasma proteins; distributed to most body tissues; less than 2% excreted unchanged; most is metabolized by the liver, where it is conjugated and then slowly excreted in the urine; plasma half-life is about 10 hours

Common Side-Effects
(Generally infrequent) Skin rash, hangover, dizziness, ataxia, blurred vision, and osteomalacia with long term use

Significant Adverse Reactions
Anorexia, nausea, vomiting, urticaria, exfoliative dermatitis, hypotension, hypersensitivity reactions, blood dyscrasias, peripheral neuropathy, and porphyria.
Acute overdose—CNS depression (possibly coma), shock, hypothermia (may be followed by fever), depressed reflexes, bladder atony, cyanosis, tachycardia, and sudden apnea; requires immediate treatment (see Nursing Alerts)
Chronic overdose—ataxia, tremors, irritability, slurred speech, hyporeflexia, memory impairment, confusion, delirium; withdraw drug *gradually*

Contraindications
Intermittent porphyria, pregnancy, and children under 12

Interactions
1 Effects of other CNS depressants (*e.g.,* alcohol, barbiturates) may be enhanced.
2 Drug induces liver microsomal enzyme activity, so that effects of anticoagulants, antihistamines, corticosteroids, griseofulvin, meprobamate, phenytoin, and other drugs metabolized by these enzymes may be reduced.
3 May exert an additive anticholinergic effect with tricyclic antidepressants, and other anticholinergic drugs.

▶ **NURSING ALERTS**

See Ethchlorvynol. In addition:

▷ 1 Be prepared to perform gastric lavage (1:1 mixture of castor oil and water) immediately in cases of overdose. Forced diuresis and urinary alkalinization are not recommended. Have adjunctive measures at hand, including vasopressors and mechanical respiratory aids. Do not use analeptic drugs to treat overdose.

▷ 2 Recognize that a lethal dose in some individuals is as low as 5 g; drug is highly lipid soluble, and can persist in the body for long periods of time; as drug is removed from the bloodstream (*e.g.,* dialysis), more drug is gradually released from fat storage back into the bloodstream, and can prolong the symptoms of overdosage or cause them to recur after dialysis is terminated.

▷ 3 Use cautiously in patients with glaucoma, prostatic hypertrophy, stenosing peptic ulcer, bladder obstruction, and arrhythmias.

▶ **NURSING CONSIDERATIONS**

▷ 1 Observe for appearance of skin rash, and discontinue drug.

▷ 2 Ensure that regular bowel and urinary function is present, because drug may reduce intestinal motility and cause urinary retention. Provide fluids and roughage as needed.

▷ 3 Do not administer less than 4 hours before expected arising, because residual effects may persist during the day.

▷ 4 Caution patients against prolonged or excessive usage because danger of psychological and physical dependence is high (schedule III drug—see Appendix).

▶ **methyprylon**

Noludar

Mechanism

Largely speculative; may increase brain stem firing threshold; similar to glutethimide in most aspects; suppresses REM sleep and induces hepatic microsomal enzymes

Uses

1 Insomnia of all types

Dosage

Adults: 200 mg to 400 mg at bedtime
Children (over 12 years): 50 mg to 200 mg at bedtime

Fate

Onset of action is 30 minutes to 45 minutes, and duration lasts 5 hours to 8 hours; almost completely metabolized in the liver and 60% excreted in the urine, mostly as conjugated metabolites

Common Side-Effects

(Usually infrequent) Hangover, GI upset, and dizziness

Significant Adverse Reactions

(Usually rare) Vomiting, diarrhea, skin rash, paradoxical excitation, esophagitis, neutropenia, and thrombocytopenia
Overdose—Confusion, somnolence, hypotension, pulmonary edema, respiratory depression, miosis, elevated body temperature, shock, and coma

Contraindications

Porphyria, children under 3 months

Interactions

See Glutethimide.

▶ **NURSING ALERTS**

See Ethchlorvynol. In addition:

▷ 1 Do not exceed 400 mg daily because there are no additional hypnotic benefits, but danger of toxicity is increased.

▷ 2 Treat overdose with gastric lavage, assisted respiration, IV fluids, and pressor agents. If excitement is present, a rapid-acting barbiturate can be given. Closely monitor vital signs and urinary output. Hemodialysis may be performed if necessary.

▶ **NURSING CONSIDERATIONS**

▷ 1 Advise periodic blood counts for individuals on prolonged use.

▷ 2 Warn of rebound REM (nightmares, insomnia, hallucinations) when prolonged use of drug is discontinued.

▷ 3 Observe for early signs of fever, rash, sore throat, petechiae (early signs of possible blood dyscrasia), and discontinue drug gradually.

▷ 4 Be aware that drug is classified as Schedule III. Observe appropriate handling procedures (see Appendix).

▶ **paraldehyde**

Paral

Mechanism

Nonspecific CNS depression, with minimal effects on respiration and blood pressure

Uses

1 General sedative and hypnotic
2 Emergency treatment of tetanus, eclampsia, status epilepticus, and poisoning with convulsive drugs
3 Basal anesthesia, especially in children (rectally)

Dosage

1 ml liquid or injection equals 1 g paraldehyde
Adults:
Sedative—2 ml to 5 ml IM or 5 ml IV diluted with 100 ml sodium chloride at a rate of 1 ml/minute
Hypnotic—4 ml to 8 ml orally or rectally, 10 ml IM (5 ml per injection site) or 10 ml/200 ml sodium chloride IV at a rate of 1 ml/minute

Anticonvulsant—5 ml IM or 3 ml to 5 ml/100 ml sodium chloride IV at a rate of 1 ml/minute
Children:
Sedative—0.15 ml/kg IM
Hypnotic—0.3 ml/kg IM

Fate
Well absorbed by all routes; onset of sleep is within 10 minutes to 15 minutes; duration is 6 hours to 10 hours; largely metabolized by the liver (70%–80%) or exhaled unchanged through the lungs (11%–28%)

Common Side-Effects
Mucosal irritation, unpleasant taste and odor on breath, and pain at IM injection site

Significant Adverse Reactions
Metabolic acidosis, GI irritation, skin rash, necrosis or sterile abscess at injection site; IV use may cause severe coughing.
Overdose—Respiratory difficulty, pulmonary edema, marked hypotension, gastritis, renal and hepatic damage (albuminuria, oliguria, nephrosis, azotemia, toxic hepatitis, fatty liver), right-side heart dilatation, and cardiovascular collapse

Contraindications
Bronchopulmonary disease, GI ulceration, and hepatic insufficiency

Interactions
1 Effects of other CNS depressants may be potentiated by paraldehyde.
2 Paraldehyde may antagonize the antibacterial activity of sulfonamides by increasing their rate of metabolism, which may result in crystalluria.
3 Tolbutamide (Orinase) may potentiate the hypnotic action of paraldehyde.
4 Disulfiram (Antabuse) used with paraldehyde may result in a toxic reaction due to excessive blood levels of acetaldehyde.

▶ NURSING ALERTS
▷ 1 Administer IV only in emergencies, and then inject diluted solution very slowly. Discontinue at onset of coughing, which is an early indication of pulmonary toxicity.
▷ 2 Avoid the vicinity of nerve trunks when injecting IM, because drug may cause nerve injury and paralysis. Use upper outer quadrant of buttocks, and inject *deeply*. IM injections are usually painful.
▷ 3 Do not withdraw drug rapidly after prolonged use, because delirium, hallucinations, and tremors can occur.
▷ 4 Do not use in presence of pain; drug may produce delirium or excitement.
▷ 5 Never administer solution if it has a brownish color or an odor of acetic acid, indications of decomposition. Fatal poisoning or extreme tissue damage can result.

Discard unused portion of open container within 24 hours.

▶ NURSING CONSIDERATIONS
▷ 1 When injecting drug, use a *glass* syringe because paraldehyde is incompatible with most plastics.
▷ 2 Give oral drug well chilled in fruit juice or milk, to mask objectionable odor and taste and to reduce GI irritation.
▷ 3 Dilute drug to be administered rectally in 2 volumes of olive or cottonseed oil (retention enema) or in normal saline to reduce mucosal irritation.
▷ 4 Keep room well ventilated to minimize odor. Inform patient that his breath will have the characteristic odor for several hours after administration.
▷ 5 Note that the drug may produce false positive plasma and urinary ketone levels, and can interfere with urinary steroid measurements.
▷ 6 Follow proper handling procedures as drug is a Schedule IV agent (see Appendix).

▶ propiomazine
Largon

Mechanism
Not established; derivative of phenothiazines with sedative, antiemetic, and antihistamine effects

Uses
1 Sedative for relief of apprehension and restlessness preoperatively or during surgery
2 Adjunct to analgesics for relief of apprehension during labor

Dosage
(IM or IV only)
Preoperatively: 20 mg to 40 mg, usually with 50 mg meperidine
During local or spinal anesthesia: 10 mg to 20 mg
Obstetrics: 20 mg to 40 mg with 50 mg meperidine; may repeat at 3-hour to 4-hour intervals
Children, preoperatively: 0.25 mg to 0.5 mg/lb

Fate
Absorbed quickly IM; peak effect in 15 minutes to 30 minutes IV and 30 minutes to 60 minutes IM; duration lasts 4 hours to 6 hours

Common Side-Effects
(Usually rare) Dry mouth, tachycardia, and GI distress

Significant Adverse Reactions
(High doses) Respiratory depression, hypotension, restlessness, dizziness, and confusion; IV injection may cause thrombophlebitis

Interactions
1 May intensify the effects of other CNS depressants and narcotic analgesics

2 May reduce or reverse the pressor response to epinephrine

▶ **NURSING ALERTS**

▷ 1 Administer cautiously to ambulatory patients, and advise against operating hazardous machinery shortly after receiving the drug.

▷ 2 Do not administer subcutaneously because tissue irritation is likely. Intra-arterial injection can cause vascular spasm.

▶ **NURSING CONSIDERATIONS**

▷ 1 Do not use if the solution is cloudy or contains a precipitate.

▷ 2 Note that elderly patients may experience dizziness and confusion. Observe them carefully following administration, and assist ambulation as required.

▷ 3 Use norepinephrine if a pressor agent is required because of excessive hypotension. Epinephrine should not be used, because increased hypotension (epinephrine reversal) can occur.

▷ 4 Use cautiously during pregnancy, especially in the first trimester.

▶ **triclofos**
Triclos

Rapidly hydrolyzed in the body to trichloroethanol, the active metabolite of chloral hydrate. Therefore, the pharmacology and toxicology of triclofos are similar to chloral hydrate; however, it is claimed to produce less gastric irritation, and does not have the disagreeable taste of chloral hydrate. The adult hypnotic dose is 1500 mg taken 15 minutes to 30 minutes before bedtime, and the drug is effective in all forms of insomnia. It is not recommended in children under 12.

Summary. Nonbarbiturate Sedative-Hypnotics

Drug	Preparations	Usual Dosage Range
Acetylcarbromal (Paxarel)	Tablets—250 mg	250 mg to 500 mg up to 4 times/day
Benzodiazepine hypnotics	See Table 21-2	
Chloral Hydrate (Aquachloral Supprettes, Noctec, Oradrate)	Capsules—250 mg, 500 mg Syrup—250, 500 mg/5 ml Elixir—500 mg/5 ml Suppositories—325 mg, 500 mg, 650 mg	Adults: Hypnosis—500 mg to 1000 mg hs Sedation—250 mg 3 times/day Children: Hypnosis—50 mg/kg hs Sedation—25 mg/kg/day
Ethchlorvynol (Placidyl)	Capsules—100 mg, 200 mg, 500 mg, 750 mg	Hypnosis—500 mg to 1000 mg hs as required; supplement of 100 mg to 200 mg may be given once nightly upon awakening
Ethinamate (Valmid)	Capsules—500 mg	Hypnosis—500 mg to 1000 mg hs
Glutethimide (Doriden)	Tablets—250 mg, 500 mg Capsules—500 mg	Hypnosis—250 mg to 500 mg hs (may repeat if needed) Preoperative—500 mg to 1000 mg 1 hour before surgery Labor (first stage)—500 mg at onset of labor
Methyprylon (Noludar)	Tablets—50 mg, 200 mg Capsules—300 mg	Hypnosis: Adult—200 mg to 400 mg hs Child—50 mg to 200 mg hs
Paraldehyde (Paral)	Oral or rectal liquid—30 ml Injection—1 g/ml	Hypnosis: Adult—4 ml to 8 ml orally or rectally; 10 ml IM; 10 ml/200 ml sodium chloride IV at a rate of 1 ml/min Child—0.3 ml/kg IM Sedation: Adult—2 ml to 5 ml IM or 5 ml IV Child—0.15 ml/kg IM Anticonvulsant: 5 ml IM; 3 ml to 5 ml/100 ml sodium chloride IV

(continued)

Summary. Nonbarbiturate Sedative-Hypnotics *(continued)*

Drug	Preparations	Usual Dosage Range
Propiomazine (Largon)	Injection—20 mg/ml	Preoperatively—20 mg to 40 mg IM or IV
		During regional anesthesia—10 mg to 20 mg IM or IV
		Obstetrics—20 mg to 40 mg IM or IV with 50 mg meperidine; repeat at 3-hour to 4-hour intervals
Triclofos (Triclos)	Tablets—750 mg Liquid—1.5 g/15 ml	Hypnosis—1500 mg hs (Children under 12—0.1 ml/lb)

The antipsychotic drugs, represented by several chemically distinct groups of compounds, are capable of improving the mood and calming the disturbed behavior of psychotic patients without causing marked sedation or habituation. Although the term *tranquilizer* is often used to describe these drugs, it is a misnomer because these agents fundamentally are *not* CNS depressants. Rather, they appear to act principally at lower brain centers to improve the disturbed thought processes of the psychotic individual and therefore create a more favorable mental state for other forms of psychotherapy. In fact, the development of effective antipsychotic drugs revolutionized the institutional practice of psychiatry and saved countless thousands of patients from lives of confinement in locked psychiatric wards.

Distinction must be made between antipsychotic drugs, used to treat acute and chronic psychoses, and antianxiety drugs or minor tranquilizers (see Chap. 23) indicated primarily for the relief of anxiety and tension associated with psychoneurotic or psychosomatic disorders. Antipsychotic drugs are significantly more potent than antianxiety agents in their actions on the CNS and are considerably more toxic as well. Yet, despite the greater potency and toxicity of these drugs, prolonged use of antipsychotic drugs is not associated with development of habituation or addiction—a major problem with chronic use of the antianxiety agents.

Chemically, the antipsychotic drugs may be divided into five groups (Table 22-1). In addition, lithium is often categorized along with these other drugs, inasmuch as it is used to control the manic phase of manic–depressive psychoses. Lithium is also reviewed in this chapter.

A comparison of the potencies and incidence of common side-effects among the various classes of antipsychotic drugs is presented in Table 22-1. Although distinct *quantitative* differences in milligram potency and toxicologic properties are evident among the different groups, no significant *qualitative* differences exist regarding the effectiveness of each drug; that is, when the drugs are used in therapeutically equivalent doses, their clinical efficacy is essentially equal. Choice of an antipsychotic drug, therefore, is based largely upon the desire to minimize particular types of side-effects in different psychotic populations (*e.g.,* reduced sedative effects in persons operating machinery, or reduced hypotensive effects in older patients).

The pharmacologic actions of the antipsychotic agents are quite complex. In addition to their behavior-modifying effects, the agents have a range of other central and peripheral effects, the extent of which differs among the various chemical groups. An outline of the principal pharmacologic actions of the antipsychotic drugs is presented in Table 22-2.

The *phenothiazines* constitute the largest and most widely used group of antipsychotic drugs. Based on their structural configuration, they are divided into three groups: (1) aliphatics, (2) piperazines, and (3) piperidines. These groups differ in certain respects, outlined in Table 22-1. The piperazines are the most potent derivatives and have the highest incidence of extrapyramidal side-effects, whereas the aliphatics and piperidines possess the greatest sedative and hypotensive action. Antiemetic potency generally parallels antipsychotic potency, the only major exception being thioridazine, which is a potent antipsychotic essentially devoid

Antipsychotic Drugs

22

Table 22-1. Antipsychotic Drugs—Comparison of Effects

	Approximate Potency Relative to Chlorpromazine	Relative Incidence of Side Effects			
		Extrapyramidal Symptoms	Sedation	Hypotension	Anticholinergic
Phenothiazines					
Aliphatic					
Chlorpromazine	1	++	+++	++	+++
Promazine	0.5	++	++	++	+++
Triflupromazine	4	++	+++	++	+++
Piperazine					
Acetophenazine	5	+++	++	+	+
Fluphenazine	50	+++	+	+	+
Perphenazine	12	+++	+	+	+
Prochlorperazine	10	+++	++	+	+
Trifluoperazine	25	+++	+	+	+
Piperidine					
Mesoridazine	2	+	+++	++	++
Piperacetazine	10	+	++	+	++
Thioridazine	1	+	+++	++	+++
Thioxanthenes					
Chlorprothixene	1	++	+++	+++	++
Thiothixene	25	+++	+	++	+
Butyrophenone					
Haloperidol	50	+++	+	+	+
Indolone					
Molindone	5	++	++	++	++
Dibenzoxazepine					
Loxapine	5	+++	++	+	+

+++—frequent
++—occasional
+—infrequent

of antiemetic activity. The aliphatics exhibit the greatest anticholinergic activity of the phenothiazines, whereas the piperazines are only weak anticholinergics. Anticholinergic activity results in a wide range of side-effects (xerostomia, blurred vision, urinary hesitancy), but also may reduce the incidence of extrapyramidal reactions.

Thioxanthene derivatives are chemically and pharmacologically similar to the phenothiazines, so the two classes can be used interchangeably. Clinical evidence of an antidepressant action for the thioxanthenes suggests that these agents might be more beneficial than phenothiazines in certain types of withdrawn, retarded, or apathetic psychotic states.

Haloperidol, a butyrophenone derivative, is a potent antipsychotic agent providing an alternative to the phenothiazines in psychotic states characterized by agitation, aggressiveness, or hostility. Its toxicity is quite high, comparable to that of the piperazine group of phenothiazines, but it is only a weak anticholinergic.

Newer drugs used to control psychotic symptoms are chemically unrelated to other antipsychotic drugs, but are pharmacologically and toxicologically similar. *Molindone*

and *Loxapine* may provide alternatives to the other antipsychotics in unresponsive or intolerant patients but have no distinct advantages over any of the older compounds, except in a somewhat lower incidence of certain side-effects.

Because many similarities are evident among the antipsychotic drugs, they are reviewed as a group. Specific information pertaining to individual drugs is then given in Table 22-3. Finally, a few antipsychotic-related drugs (*e.g.,* droperidol, methotrimeprazine) with different indications are considered at the end of the chapter.

Antipsychotic Drugs

Acetophenazine	Perphenazine
Carphenazine	Piperacetazine
Chlorpromazine	Prochlorperazine
Chlorprothixene	Promazine
Fluphenazine	Thioridazine
Haloperidol	Thiothixene
Loxapine	Trifluoperazine
Mesoridazine	Triflupromazine
Molindone	

Table 22-2. Antipsychotic Drugs—Pharmacologic Effects

I. Central Nervous System

1. Antipsychotic effect—reduced agitation, emotional quieting, decreased paranoid ideation, and lessening of hallucinations and disturbed thought processes.
2. Antiemetic effect—decreased sensitivity of chemoreceptor trigger zone (CTZ) in medulla to activation by drugs or toxins and direct depression of brain stem vomiting center in large doses
3. Impaired temperature regulation—hypothermia caused by increased heat loss and decreased compensatory heat production
4. Endocrine effects—inhibition of FSH and LH release, and increased release of LTH (prolactin), resulting in abnormal lactation. Hormonal effects are due to the blocking action of antipsychotic drugs on dopamine receptors either in the hypothalamic–pituitary pathway or on anterior pituitary cells themselves.
5. Motor effects—increased involuntary muscle activity (*e.g.,* tremors, dyskinesias, akathisias) caused by dopamine blockade in motor-integrating areas of the CNS

II. Peripheral Nervous System

1. Antiadrenergic effects—blockade of alpha receptors, and inhibition of catecholamine uptake by nerve endings, leading to orthostatic hypotension and reflex tachycardia
2. Anticholinergic/antihistamine effects—blockade of cholinergic (largely muscarinic) and histaminergic activity

III. Other

1. Antiarrhythmic effects—quinidine-like depressant action on the myocardium, and local anesthetic action
2. Diuretic effect—depression of ADH release, and inhibition of water and electrolyte reabsorption (weak effect)

Mechanism

Complex and not completely understood; act primarily at several subcortical brain sites, including the limbic system, hypothalamus, and brain stem; among the known effects of the drugs are reduction of intraneuronal levels of cyclic AMP in brain regions associated with emotion and behavior, and decreased cortical sensory input from ascending spinal tracts by way of collateral nerves to the reticular formation. Biochemical mechanisms of action may include dopamine receptor blockade, increased dopamine turnover, inhibition of neuronal uptake of norepinephrine and serotonin, and suppression of acetylcholine release. No appreciable direct cortical depression is evident. They produce varying degrees of sedation, antiemesis, hypothermia, and altered pituitary hormone release in addition to an antipsychotic action. Other peripheral actions that are responsible for many of the observed side-effects include antiadrenergic (alpha-blocking effect) and anticholinergic activity, as well as some degree of antiserotonergic, local anesthetic, and a quinidine-like cardiac depressant effect.

Uses

(See Table 22-3 for specific indications of each drug)
1 Management of acute and chronic psychoses, either organic or drug-induced
2 Control of the manic phase of manic–depressive psychoses (lithium)
3 Relief of severe nausea and vomiting
4 Control of intractable hiccoughs
5 Relief of anxiety, apprehension, and agitation associated with a variety of somatic disorders, or prior to surgery
6 Facilitation of alcohol withdrawal
7 Adjunctive treatment of tetanus and acute intermittent porphyria
8 Control of aggressiveness in disturbed children
9 Control of tics and vocal utterances of Gilles de la Tourette's disease (haloperidol)

Dosage

See Table 22-3.

Fate

Adequately absorbed orally, and well absorbed parenterally; widely distributed to most body tissues, and found in high concentrations in the brain; onset and duration of action largely dependent on dosage form and route of administration; clinical effects may not be attained for several weeks after intiation of therapy; most drugs are significantly protein-bound, and metabolism and excretion are generally slow; metabolized by the liver and excreted in both the urine and feces; many metabolites are biologically active and contribute to the prolonged effects of some drugs. Enzyme inducers (*e.g.,* barbiturates, meprobamate) can accelerate phenothiazine metabolism. Excretion is by way of the kidney and the enterohepatic circulation.

Common Side-Effects

(Most common in early stages of therapy) Drowsiness, orthostatic hypotension (dizziness, weakness), dry mouth, blurred vision, constipation, nasal stuffiness, and palpitations

Significant Adverse Reactions

(Incidence varies among different drugs)
CNS—hyperpyrexia, lowering of convulsive threshold, hyperactivity, confusion, bizarre dreams, insomnia, depression, cerebral edema
Neuromuscular—extrapyramidal reactions, akathisia (motor restlessness), dystonias (muscle spasms of the face or throat, difficulty in speech or swallowing, extensor rigidity of the back muscles, upward rotation of the eyeballs), pseudoparkinsonism, tardive dyskinesia (involuntary orofacial movements such as chewing, protrusion of the tongue, puffing of the cheeks and puckering of the mouth), hyperreflexia
Cardiovascular—tachycardia, fainting, ECG changes, cardiac arrest (rare)
Hematologic—blood dyscrasias (agranulocytosis, leukopenia, leukocytosis, anemias, thrombocytopenic purpura, pancytopenia)
Hypersensitivity—urticaria, itching, eczema, photosensitivity, contact dermatitis, angioneurotic edema, anaphylactic reaction, exfoliative dermatitis, cholestatic jaundice
Endocrine—abnormal lactation, breast engorgement, gynecomastia, changes in libido, amenorrhea, glycosuria and hyperglycemia, increased appetite

(*Text continues on p. 200.*)

Table 22-3. Antipsychotic Drugs

Drug	Preparations	Usual Dosage Range	Remarks
Phenothiazines			
Aliphatic			
Chlorpromazine (Thorazine and various other manufacturers)	Tablets—10 mg, 25 mg, 50 mg, 100 mg, 200 mg Sustained-release capsules—30 mg, 75 mg, 150 mg, 200 mg, 300 mg Syrup—10 mg/5 ml Concentrate—30 mg/ml, 100 mg/ml Suppositories—25 mg, 100 mg Injection—25 mg/ml	Adults: Psychoses Oral—30 mg to 200 mg/day IM—25 mg to 50 mg 3 times/day (Severe psychoses—500 mg to 1000 mg/day) Nausea/vomiting Oral—10 mg to 25 mg every 4 hours to 6 hours IM—25 mg to 50 mg every 3 hours to 4 hours Rectal—50 mg to 100 mg every 6 hours to 8 hours Preoperative sedation Oral—25 mg to 50 mg IM—12.5 mg to 25 mg Porphyria Oral—25 mg to 50 mg 3 to 4 times/day IM—25 mg 3 to 4 times/day Tetanus IM, IV—25 mg to 50 mg 3 to 4 times/day Hiccoughs Oral—25 mg to 50 mg 3 to 4 times/day IM—25 mg to 50 mg IV—25 mg to 50 mg diluted in 500 to 1000 ml saline by infusion Children: Oral—0.25 mg/lb 2 to 4 times/day Rectal—0.5 mg/lb every 6 hours to 8 hours IM—0.125 mg to 0.25 mg/lb every 6 hours to 8 hours IV—0.25 mg/lb	Used in acute and chronic psychoses, manic phase of manic–depressive psychoses, for pre- and postoperative sedation, intractable hiccoughs, acute intermittent porphyria, tetanus and control of severe nausea and vomiting resulting from drugs, surgery, or toxins; plasma levels following IM injection are several times higher than following oral administration; duration of action ranges from 3 hours to 6 hours; high incidence of drowsiness, dizziness, and hypotension, especially during first few weeks of therapy and in older patients; IV solution should be diluted to 1 mg/ml in saline and administered at a rate of 1 mg/min; doses in excess of 1000 mg/day for prolonged periods are not recommended
Promazine (Sparine)	Tablets—10 mg, 25 mg, 50 mg, 100 mg, 200 mg Syrup—10 mg/5 ml Concentrate—30 mg/ml Injection—25 mg/ml, 50 mg/ml	Adults: Initially—50 mg to 150 mg IM Maintenance—10 mg to 200 mg every 4 hours to 6 hours orally or IM as required Children (over 12): 10 mg to 25 mg every 4 hours to 6 hours	Used primarily for management of psychotic disorders; the preferred parenteral route is IM; IV administration is recommended only in hospitalized patients; when used IV, injections should be given slowly in diluted solutions (25 mg/ml or less); concentrate for oral use should be diluted in fruit juice or other flavored vehicle (2 tsp of diluent for every 25 mg of drug); less potent and equally toxic compared to chlorpromazine.
Triflupromazine (Vesprin)	Tablets—10 mg, 25 mg, 50 mg Suspension—50 mg/5 ml Injection—10 mg/ml, 20 mg/ml	Adults: Psychoses Oral—100 mg to 150 mg/day IM—60 mg to 150 mg/day Nausea/vomiting Oral—20 mg to 30 mg/day IM—5 mg to 15 mg every 4 hours	Effective in psychotic disorders (other than psychotic depression) and for control of nausea and vomiting; sedation and extrapyramidal reactions are common, especially with parenteral use and in the elderly and debilitated; has been used as an adjunct for pre- and postoperative management

Table 22-3. Antipsychotic Drugs *(continued)*

Drug	Preparations	Usual Dosage Range	Remarks
		IV—1 mg to 3 mg	
		Children (over 2 yr):	
		Psychoses Oral—2 mg/kg (maximum 150 mg/day)	
		IM—0.2 to 0.25 mg/kg (maximum 10 mg)	
		Nausea/vomiting 0.2 to 0.25 mg/kg orally or IM (maximum 10 mg)	
Piperazines			
Acetophenazine (Tindal)	Tablets—20 mg	Adults: 20 mg 3 times/day (80 mg to 120 mg/day in hospitalized patients) Children 0.8 to 1.6 mg/kg/day	Used for management of psychotic disorders. In patients with insomnia, last tablet should be taken 1 hour before bedtime Higher degree of sedation but fewer extrapyramidal reactions than other similar derivatives
Fluphenazine (Permitil, Prolixin)	Tablets—0.25 mg, 1 mg, 2.5 mg, 5 mg, 10 mg Elixir—2.5 mg/5 ml Concentrate—5 mg/ml Injection HCL—2.5 mg/ml Enanthate—25 mg/ml Decanoate—25 mg/ml	Oral: Initially—2.5 mg to 10 mg/day; (maximum 20 mg) Maintenance—1 mg to 5 mg/day IM: HCl—1.25 mg 2 to 4 times/day (range 2.5 mg to 10 mg/day in divided doses) Enanthate/Decanoate (esters in a sesame oil vehicle)—12.5 mg to 25 mg every 2 weeks to 3 weeks (may also be given SC); range—12.5 mg to 100 mg at 1-week to 3-week intervals	Used for control of psychotic manifestations; oral dosage forms and HCl injection are rapid acting and can be used initially to stabilize patient; enanthate and decanoate salts are released slowly from tissue sites and thus have a prolonged effect (1 wk–4 wk); indicated for maintenance therapy in patients who cannot be relied upon to follow a regular oral dosage schedule; if given cautiously in low doses, may be useful in patients who are hypersensitive to other phenothiazines; very potent drug with high incidence of extrapyramidal reactions and mental depression; decanoate may have a lower incidence of extrapyramidal side-effects than other dosage forms; monitor renal function and blood picture periodically in patients on long-term therapy; protect solutions from light, and use dry syringe and needle for injection because moisture may cloud the solution; avoid use of antacids with oral dosage forms, because GI absorption is impaired; due to prolonged effects of enanthate and decanoate salts, advise patients to report appearance of side-effects *immediately;* not indicated in children
Perphenazine (Trilafon)	Tablets—2 mg, 4 mg, 8 mg, 16 mg Repeat-action tablets—8 mg Concentrate—16 mg/5 ml Injection—5 mg/ml	Oral: Psychoses—8 mg to 16 mg 2 to 4 times a day (maximum 64 mg/day) initially; reduce to 4 mg to 8 mg 3 times a day for maintenance Anxiety and tension states—2 mg to 4 mg 3 times/day Nausea and vomiting—8 mg to 16 mg/day in divided doses IM—Initially 5 mg to 10 mg; repeat every 6-hours (maximum 30 mg/day); switch to oral therapy as soon as possible	Effective in psychoses and in the control of severe nausea and vomiting due to surgery or other acute situations; may also be effective in the management of anxiety and tension due to severe neuroses; do not use in children under 12; high incidence of extrapyramidal reactions; transient hypotension can occur, especially IV; keep patient recumbent, and monitor pulse and pressure; oral concentrate should be diluted (2 oz diluent/5 ml concentrate) with fruit juice, milk, carbonated beverage, or other liquid (tea is not recommended)

(continued)

Table 22-3. Antipsychotic Drugs *(continued)*

Drug	Preparations	Usual Dosage Range	Remarks
		IV (severe vomiting only)—1 mg/minute infusion of an 0.5 mg/ml dilution (maximum 5 mg)	
Prochlorperazine (Compazine)	Tablets—5 mg, 10 mg, 25 mg Capsules—(sustained-release) 10 mg, 15 mg, 30 mg Concentrate—10 mg/ml Syrup—5 mg/5 ml Suppositories—2.5 mg, 5 mg, 25 mg Injection—5 mg/ml	Adults: Psychoses Oral—10 mg 3 to 4 times/day, increased gradually until maximum effect (usually 100 mg to 150 mg/day) IM—10 mg to 20 mg initially; repeat in 2 hours to 4 hours Switch to oral form as soon as possible Nausea/vomiting Oral—5 mg to 10 mg 3 to 4 times/day Rectal—25 mg 2 times/day IM—5 mg to 10 mg; repeat every 3 hours to 4 hours to a maximum of 40 mg/day IV (severe vomiting)—5 mg to 10 mg IV injection or 20 mg added to 1 liter of IV infusion 15 minutes to 30 minutes before induction of anesthesia Children: (over 2 yr and 20 lb): Psychoses Oral/rectal—2.5 mg 2 to 3 times/day IM—0.06 mg/lb Nausea/vomiting Oral/rectal—2.5 mg to 5 mg 1 to 2 times a day based on weight IM—0.06 mg/lb	Used for control of psychotic manifestations in adults and children over 2 years and for relief of nausea and vomiting; widely used pre- and postoperatively; do not use in short-term vomiting in children or for vomiting of unknown cause; do not give oral concentrate to children, as they are more prone to develop extrapyramidal reactions at high doses; discontinue if signs of restlessness or excitement occur; inject deeply IM (avoid SC use), and do not mix solution with other agents in same syringe; do not confuse *2.5-mg* child suppository with *25-mg* adult suppository; dilute oral concentrate dose in 60 ml of vehicle immediately before administration (liquid or semisolid food may be used); use cautiously in the elderly or debilitated and in children who are dehydrated or who have an acute illness because extrapyramidal reactions are common; monitor blood pressure during IV use, because hypotension is likely to occur; supervise ambulation following parenteral use
Trifluoperazine (Stelazine, Triazine)	Tablets—1 mg, 2 mg, 5 mg, 10 mg Concentrate—10 mg/ml Injection—2 mg/ml	Adults: Oral—Initially 2 mg to 5 mg twice a day (maximum 40 mg/day); maintenance—1 mg to 2 mg twice a day IM—1 mg to 2 mg every 4 hours to 6 hours (maximum 10 mg/day) Children: (over 6 yr): Oral—1 mg 1 to 2 times/day (maximum 15 mg/day in older children) IM—1 mg 1 to 2 times/day	Indicated for treatment of psychotic disorders and for controlling manifestations of severe psychoneuroses; very potent agent with high incidence of extrapyramidal reactions; maximum response may be delayed 2 weeks to 3 weeks; increase dosage very slowly in elderly or debilitated patients; prolonged action of the drug allows once-a-day dosage in many less severe cases; dilute concentrate in 60 ml of appropriate vehicle (liquid or semisolid) to aid palatability; do not give IM injections more frequently than every 4 hours because of danger of cumulation
Piperidines Mesoridazine (Serentil)	Tablets—10 mg, 25 mg, 50 mg, 100 mg Concentrate—25 mg/ml Injection—25 mg/ml	Psychoses Oral—Initially 25 mg to 50 mg 3 times/day (range 100 mg to 400 mg/day) IM—25 mg; repeat in 30 minutes to 60 minutes if necessary (range 25 mg to 200 mg/day)	Used for treatment of schizophrenia, chronic brain syndrome, and psychoneuroses, and as adjunctive therapy in acute and chronic alcoholism; weak antiemetic; low incidence of extrapyramidal reactions but very sedating; may reduce hyperactive behavior associated with

Table 22-3. Antipsychotic Drugs (continued)

Drug	Preparations	Usual Dosage Range	Remarks
		Neuroses Oral—10 mg 3 times/day (range 30 mg to 150 mg/day) Alcoholism 25 mg twice a day (range 50 mg to 200 mg/day)	mental deficient states; Not recommended in children under 12; concentrate should be diluted prior to use
Piperacetazine (Quide)	Tablets—10 mg, 25 mg	Initially 10 mg 2 to 4 times/day; increase gradually to an optimal dose (maximum 160 mg/day)	Used for management of chronic psychoses; do not use in children under 12; marked drowsiness can occur, especially early in therapy; avoid hazardous tasks during this time
Thioridazine (Mellaril)	Tablets—10 mg, 15 mg, 25 mg, 50 mg, 100 mg, 150 mg, 200 mg Concentrate—30 mg/ml, 100 mg/ml Suspension—25 mg/5 ml, 100 mg/5 ml	Adults: Psychoses Initially—50 mg to 100 mg 3 times/day; maintenance 200 mg to 800 mg/day in 2 to 4 divided doses Depressive neuroses Initially—25 mg 3 times/day Maintenance—20 mg to 200 mg/day in 3 to 4 divided doses Children (over 2 yr): 0.5 to 3.0 mg/kg/day depending on severity of condition	Indicated for psychotic disorders and short-term treatment of depressive neuroses; possibly useful in hyperactive or aggressive children, alcohol withdrawal, intractable pain, and senility; low incidence of extrapyramidal reactions and no antiemetic action, but strong anticholinergic effect and highly sedating; frequently produces dryness of the mouth, constipation, urinary retention, and impotence in early stages of therapy; discontinue drug or reduce dosage if visual changes (reduced or brownish vision, impaired night vision) occur; periodic blood and liver function tests should be performed during prolonged therapy; dilute oral concentrate immediately prior to use with fruit juice or water
Thioxanthenes			
Chlorprothixene (Taractan)	Tablets—10 mg, 25 mg, 50 mg, 100 mg Concentrate—20 mg/ml Injection—12.5 mg/ml	Adults: Oral—Initially 25 mg to 50 mg 3 to 4 times/day; increase to optimal level (maximum 600 mg/day) IM—25 mg to 50 mg 3 to 4 times/day; substitute oral therapy as soon as possible Children: Oral—10 mg to 25 mg 3 to 4 times/day IM—over 12 years, same as adult dose	Effective in acute and chronic schizophrenia; produces significant sedation and orthostatic hypotension; when used IM, keep patient recumbent during administration; do not give IM in children under 12, or orally in children under 6; anticholinergic side-effects are prominent; no advantage over chlorpromazine
Thiothixene (Navane)	Capsules—1 mg, 2 mg, 5 mg, 10 mg, 20 mg Concentrate—5 mg/ml Injection—2.5 mg/ml	Oral—Initially 2 mg to 5 mg 2 to 3 times/day; maintenance 20 mg to 60 mg/day in divided doses IM—4 mg 2 to 4 times/day (usual range 16 mg to 20 mg/day)	Used for management of acute and chronic schizophrenia; not for use in children under 12; high incidence of extrapyramidal reactions and drowsiness in early stages of therapy; therapeutic effects may take several weeks to develop with oral administration; do not withdraw drug abruptly because delirium can occur; dosage may need to be adjusted when switching from IM to oral administration
Butyrophenone			
Haloperidol (Haldol)	Tablets—0.5 mg, 1 mg, 2 mg, 5 mg, 10 mg, 20 mg Concentrate—2 mg/ml Injection—5 mg/ml	Oral—0.5 mg to 5 mg 2 to 3 times/day depending on symptoms (maximum 100 mg/day)	Indicated in psychotic disorders, manic phase of manic–depressive psychoses, and for management of tics and vocal utterances of Gilles de la Tourette'

(continued)

Table 22-3. Antipsychotic Drugs (continued)

Drug	Preparations	Usual Dosage Range	Remarks
		IM—2 mg to 5 mg; repeat at 4-hour to 8-hour intervals as needed	disease; very potent antipsychotic with high incidence of extrapyramidal reactions; strong antiemetic; less sedation and hypotension than many other similar drugs; do not use in children under 12 or in parkinsonian patients (drug is a potent dopamine-blocking agent); use cautiously in epileptic individuals because drug may lower convulsive threshold; when used for manic episodes, be alert for reversal to severe depression which may invite suicidal attempts; concomitant use with lithium may elicit dyskinesias, parkinsonian-like symptoms, or dementia; observe patients closely, and provide emotional support as necessary; perform periodic liver function and blood studies
Indolone			
Molindone (Moban)	Tablets—5 mg, 10 mg, 25 mg, 50 mg, 100 mg Concentrate—20 mg/ml	Initially—50 mg to 75 mg/day Maintenance—5 mg to 25 mg 3 to 4 times a day depending on symptoms (maximum 225 mg/day)	Used for control of schizophrenia; not recommended in children under 12; provides an alternative drug to the phenothiazines and thioxanthenes in unresponsive patients, although actions are essentially identical to other classes of antipsychotics; high degree of initial drowsiness; resumption of menses in previously amenorrheal women has been reported; no ophthalmologic complications have occurred; tablet contains calcium, which may interfere with GI absorption of phenytoin and tetracyclines
Dibenzoxazepine			
Loxapine (Loxitane)	Capsules—5 mg, 10 mg, 25 mg, 50 mg Concentrate—25 mg/ml Injection—50 mg/ml	Initially 10 mg orally twice a day; increase to optimal levels (usually 60 mg to 100 mg/day) (maximum 250 mg/day) IM—12.5 mg to 50 mg every 4 hours to 6 hours to control acutely agitated patients	Indicated for manifestations of schizophrenia; elicits strong sedation in early therapy, lowers convulsive threshold, produces hypotension, and is an anticholinergic of moderate potency; has antiemetic activity and may produce ocular toxicity; not recommended in children under 16; produces frequent extrapyramidal reactions, usually parkinsonian-like in nature; no endocrine abnormalities have been reported; concentrate should be mixed with orange or grapefruit juice before administration

Autonomic—fecal impaction, adynamic ileus, urinary retention, enuresis, incontinence, impotence

Ocular—ptosis, photophobia, pigmentary retinopathy, lens opacities

Respiratory—laryngospasm, bronchospasm, dyspnea

Other—skin pigmentation, polydipsia, aggravation of peptic ulcers, fever, systemic lupus-like reaction, psychotic flare-up

Contraindications

Bone marrow depression, blood dyscrasias, parkinsonism, jaundice, liver damage, renal insufficiency, cerebral arteriosclerosis, coronary disease, circulatory collapse, mitral insufficiency, severe hypotension, chronic alcoholism, comatose states, and subcortical brain damage

Interactions

1 Antipsychotic drugs may potentiate the effects of other CNS depressants (e.g., alcohol, barbiturates, general anesthetics, antianxiety agents, narcotic analgesics).

2 Additive anticholinergic effects may be observed with concomitant use of antipsychotic drugs and other agents having anticholinergic activity (e.g., antihistamines, tricyclic antidepressants, antiparkinsonian drugs).

3 Effects of antipsychotics may be enhanced by estrogens, progestins, anticholinesterases, furazolidone, and MAO inhibitors.

4 Hypotensive action of antipsychotic drugs can be increased by antihypertensives, epinephrine, thiazide diuretics, and tricyclic antidepressants.

5 Antipsychotic drugs may decrease the effectiveness of amphetamines, oral anticoagulants, heparin, anticonvulsants (lowering of seizure threshold), oral hypoglycemics, levodopa, and other antiparkinsonian drugs.

6 The hypoglycemic effect of insulin may be potentiated by antipsychotics.

7 Absorption of antipsychotic agents can be impaired by antacids and antidiarrheal preparations.

8 Lithium and other antipsychotic drugs may exert additive hyperglycemic effects.

9 The combination of antipsychotic drugs and griseofulvin may precipitate acute porphyria.

10 Narcotic analgesics may increase the respiratory-depressant action of the antipsychotics.

11 Antipsychotics can reduce the effectiveness of guanethidine by interfering with its neuronal uptake.

12 Antipsychotic drugs can potentiate muscle relaxants, possibly resulting in prolonged apnea.

13 Additive cardiac depressant effects may occur with quinidine and antipsychotic drugs.

14 Antipsychotic-induced extrapyramidal effects can be intensified by anticholinergic antiparkinsonian drugs and piperazine, and can be reduced by diphenhydramine.

▶ **NURSING ALERTS**

▷ 1 Use these drugs very cautiously in patients with glaucoma, prostatic hypertrophy, epilepsy, diabetes, severe hypertension, ulcers, cardiovascular disease, chronic respiratory disorders, liver impairment, in pregnant or lactating women, in children under 6 months of age, and in persons exposed to extreme heat, phosphorus insecticides, or pesticides.

▷ 2 Caution against operating dangerous machinery during initial stages of therapy because drowsiness is common.

▷ 3 Observe carefully for early signs of blood dyscrasias (fever, sore throat, mucosal ulceration, fatigue, upper respiratory infection), and advise physician.

▷ 4 Note signs of developing jaundice (fever, abdominal pain, rash, itching, diarrhea, yellowing of skin), and consult physician.

▷ 5 Caution against *abrupt* stoppage of therapy, particularly with high doses, because gastritis, vomiting, dizziness, tremors, insomnia, and psychotic behavior may occur. Withdraw drug gradually over several weeks (*e.g.,* 10% to 25% reduction in dosage every 2 weeks).

▷ 6 Be alert for complaints of decreased visual acuity, photophobia, and brownish discoloration of visual objects. Advise immediate ophthalmologic examination.

▷ 7 Critically observe for appearance of fine, worm-like movements of the tongue, an early sign of tardive

dyskinesia, which usually develops after long-term (6 mo–24 mo) treatment. Because the symptoms (see Significant Adverse Reactions) are difficult to treat, prompt cessation of therapy at the initial sign of the developing syndrome can prevent worsening of symptoms. Be aware that antiparkinsonian drugs do *not* alleviate these symptoms and may, in fact, worsen them.

▷ 8 Monitor renal function of patients on long-term therapy. If serum creatinine is elevated, discontinue the drug.

▷ 9 Advise periodic breast examination in patients on chronic therapy, especially those with previous breast cancer or a family history of breast cancer.

▷ 10 Observe for signs of dizziness and weakness, indications of orthostatic hypotension. Monitor blood pressure before each dose during the initial treatment period. Advise patient to change position gradually, sit up slowly, and lie down immediately if dizziness occurs. Caution against prolonged standing and lengthy hot showers or baths because hypotension is likely to develop.

▷ 11 Keep patient recumbent for at least 1 hour after parenteral administration, and monitor blood pressure closely. Marked hypotension can be treated by placing patient in head-low position and if necessary, by using volume expanders and pressor agents such as levarterenol or dopamine. Do *not* use epinephrine because reversal of effects can occur, leading to worsened hypotension.

▶ **NURSING CONSIDERATIONS**

▷ 1 Periodically evaluate patients on long-term therapy, and make dosage adjustments as necessary. Doses should be kept as low as possible, and drug-free periods should be employed where possible to minimize incidence of untoward reactions, particularly dyskinesias and other involuntary movement episodes.

▷ 2 Reassure patients that many side-effects (drowsiness, dry mouth, decreased salivation) are common early in therapy and usually disappear. Others such as orthostatic hypotension, extrapyramidal reactions, and sedation may be minimized by selection of proper agent.

▷ 3 Be alert for the onset of acute dystonic reactions. These reactions are very frightening to many patients. Remain with the patient to provide reassurance, and notify the physician promptly.

▷ 4 Do not use antiparkinsonian medication to *prevent* extrapyramidal reactions. If symptoms appear during antipsychotic therapy, attempt to eliminate by dosage reduction first. If unsuccessful, titrate dose of antiparkinsonian drug carefully so that the smallest dose to relieve the extrapyramidal symptoms is employed (see Chap. 26).

▷ 5 Caution patients to avoid direct sunlight while taking these drugs, because photosensitivity reactions can occur. Use of sunscreen lotions is recommended.

▷ 6 Note that children with acute illnesses (*e.g.,* mumps,

measles, severe infections) or who are dehydrated are more susceptible than adults to development of dystonias (*i.e.,* neck spasms, eye rolling, dysphagia, convulsions). Be prepared to discontinue drug and consult physician.

▷ 7 Monitor fluid intake and output and bowel function during prolonged therapy, and observe for abdominal distention. Urinary retention and constipation can occur. Increase fluid intake and roughage in the diet. Consider reduced dosage or change in drug if above conditions persist. Avoid use of proprietary laxatives unless prescribed because many contain anticholinergics and may interact with phenothiazines.

▷ 8 Observe diabetic patients for signs of altered carbohydrate metabolism such as glycosuria, weight loss, and polyphagia. Dosage alterations or dietary changes may be warranted.

▷ 9 Alert patients to the possible occurrence of endocrine changes caused by the antipsychotic drug. Menstrual irregularities, gynecomastia, breast engorgement, impotence, and altered libido are possible. Provide reassurance to the patient, and attempt to minimize changes by dosage adjustment or use of an alternate drug.

▷ 10 Encourage frequent rinsing of the mouth, adequate fluid intake, and use of gum or hard candy to alleviate mouth dryness. Stress meticulous oral hygiene to prevent development of oral candidiasis, especially with use of the oral concentrate.

▷ 11 Warn patients that drug may discolor the urine (pink to red brown). This is not serious and does not necessitate interruption of therapy.

▷ 12 Emphasize the need to maintain a regular dosage schedule, especially during initial stages, because beneficial effects sometimes require several weeks to become manifest. Periodically reevaluate the patient's status, and stress the need for regular follow-up care.

▷ 13 Avoid drug contact with skin or mucous membranes, because contact dermatitis can occur.

▷ 14 Dispense oral liquid preparations in dark bottles, because solutions are light sensitive.

▷ 15 Do not use discolored injectable solutions or mix other solutions in same syringe. Inject deeply IM. Avoid SC injections because tissue irritation is common.

▷ 16 Note that phenothiazines may interfere with laboratory tests for pregnancy, I^{131} uptake, urinary catecholamines, urine ketones, bilirubin, and steroids.

▶ droperidol

Inapsine

A butyrophenone producing tranquilization, sedation, and mild peripheral vascular dilation, droperidol has a strong antiemetic effect and can potentiate the action of other CNS depressants. It is principally used in combination with a narcotic analgesic (fentanyl) as Innovar (see Chap. 17) for the production of neuroleptanalgesia, which is a state of quietude, reduced motor activity, and indifference to pain. Alone, droperidol is given to provide tranquilization and reduce nausea and vomiting during surgical and diagnostic procedures.

Mechanism
Not completely established; has alpha-adrenergic and dopaminergic-blocking activity

Uses
1 Reduces the incidence of nausea and vomiting associated with minor surgical and diagnostic procedures
2 Adjunct in the maintenance of general and regional anesthesia and for preanesthetic medication to provide a state of tranquilization
3 Neuroleptanalgesia, in combination with fentanyl, a narcotic analgesic

Dosage
Adults:
Premedication—2.5 mg to 10 mg IM 30 minutes to 60 minutes preoperatively
Adjunct to general anesthesia—2.5 mg/20 lb to 25 lb IV during induction
Maintenance—1.25 mg to 2.5 mg IV
Diagnostic procedures—2.5 mg to 10 mg IM 30 minutes to 60 minutes before procedure, then 1.25 mg to 2.5 mg IV as needed
Children (2 yr–12 yr):
1 mg to 1.5 mg/20 lb to 25 lb for premedication or induction of anesthesia

Fate
Onset of action with IM or IV use is 3 minutes to 10 minutes; duration lasts 2 hours to 4 hours; altered consciousness may persist up to 12 hours; metabolized in the liver and excreted largely in the urine, mostly as metabolites, but some unchanged drug

Common Side-Effects
Hypotension, tachycardia, and drowsiness

Significant Adverse Reactions
Dizziness, anxiety, restlessness, extrapyramidal reactions, chills, shivering, laryngo- and bronchospasm; rarely, hallucinations and mental depression; when used with fentanyl, respiratory depression, muscular rigidity and apnea can occur.

Contraindications
Parkinsonism, marked hypotension

Interactions
1 May enhance or prolong the depressant effects (including respiratory depression) of other CNS depressant drugs, *e.g.,* barbiturates, narcotics, alcohol, general anesthetics.
2 Effects may be increased by MAO inhibitors.
3 Hypotension resulting from spinal or epidural anes-

thetics may be intensified by pretreatment or concurrent treatment with droperidol.

▶ NURSING ALERTS
▷ 1 Monitor vital signs closely during use. Have fluids, vasopressors, and other necessary measures on hand to manage hypotension should it occur. Do *not* use epinephrine because reversal of pressor effect can occur, worsening the hypotension.
▷ 2 Use cautiously in elderly, debilitated, and other poor-risk patients; during pregnancy; in children under 2 years; and in the presence of liver, kidney, or cardiac dysfunction.
▷ 3 Use narcotics or other CNS depressants in reduced doses in the presence of droperidol, because additive depressant effects can occur.
▷ 4 When drug is used with fentanyl (as Innovar), be alert for early signs of respiratory depression (dyspnea, restlessness, rigidity), especially if rapid IV injection is given. Be prepared to provide respiratory assistance, and have necessary resuscitative equipment available (*e.g.,* endotracheal tube, oxygen, suction apparatus).

▶ NURSING CONSIDERATIONS
▷ 1 Exercise care in moving and positioning the patient following a dose of droperidol because orthostatic hypotension may develop.
▷ 2 Reduce initial dose in elderly or debilitated patients. Observe reaction to initial small dose carefully, and give incremental doses depending on response.
▷ 3 Watch for development of extrapyramidal side-effects, which may occur up to 1 to 2 days after administration. They can usually be controlled with an antiparkinsonian agent.
▷ 4 Postoperative drowsiness is common. Assist ambulation and other activities until drowsiness disappears.

▶ lithium
Cibalith-S, Eskalith, Lithane, Lithobid, Lithonate, Lithotabs

An alkali metal ion effective in the control of the manic phase of manic–depressive psychoses, lithium is capable of calming the agitated patient and "smoothing out" the wide swings in mood between mania and depression. Its toxicity is very closely related to its serum levels, and the effective therapeutic dose in many instances is near the toxic level. Therefore, repeated and accurate serum lithium levels should be determined in all patients taking the drug (see Dosage).

Mechanism
Specific mechanism for control of mania is unknown. The drug can alter sodium transport at the nerve ending, thereby changing the electrophysiologic characteristics of nerve cells. It promotes neuronal uptake of norepinephrine and serotonin, thereby causing their more rapid inactivation, and may also reduce norepinephrine release and inhibit catecholamine-activated cyclic AMP formation.

Uses
1 Controls acute mania symptoms, *i.e.,* motor hyperactivity, talkativeness, restlessness, poor judgment, gradiose ideation, aggressiveness, and possibly hostility
2 Prophylaxis of recurrent manic–depressive episodes
3 Improves neutrophil count in patients with neutropenia due to cancer chemotherapy (investigational use)

Dosage
Acute mania: 600 mg 3 times/day (desired serum level is 1 mEq/liter–1.5 mEq/liter); adjust oral dosage to optimal clinical response as well as desired serum level; clinical effects begin to appear within 4 days to 7 days
Prophylaxis: 300 mg 3 to 4 times/day (serum levels 0.6 mEq/liter–1.4 mEq/liter)

Fate
Rapidly absorbed orally; peak serum levels in 1 hour to 2 hours, although optimal clinical response may take a week or more to develop; widely distributed in the body; very little is protein-bound; crosses blood–brain barrier; excreted through the kidneys (half-life about 24 hr), the rate being directly proportional to its plasma concentration; excretion is diminished by low sodium levels, for example, those resulting from diminished salt intake or concomitant diuretic therapy.

Common Side-Effects
Fine hand tremors, nausea, thirst, polyuria, fatigue, and mild muscle weakness

Significant Adverse Reactions
(Usually observed at serum levels above 1.5 mEq/liter)
Neuromuscular—lack of coordination, ataxia, muscle hyperirritability and twitching, choreiform movements, extrapyramidal-like symptoms
CNS—drowsiness, dizziness, restlessness, confusion, slurred speech, tinnitus, incontinence, psychomotor retardation, epileptic-like seizures, stupor, coma
Autonomic—dry mouth, blurred vision
Cardiovascular—hypotension, arrhythmias, circulatory collapse
GI—anorexia, vomiting, diarrhea, abdominal pain
Urinary—albuminuria, glycosuria, oliguria
Dermatologic—rash, pruritus, thinning of hair, folliculitis, topical anesthesia, acneiform eruptions, cutaneous ulceration
Other—hypothyroidism, transient hyperglycemia, excessive weight gain, leucocytosis, scotomas, flattening and inversion of the T-wave, worsening of psoriasis

Contraindications
Severe renal or cardiovascular disease, organic brain syndrome, sodium depletion (low-salt diet, diuretic therapy, dehydration), early pregnancy, and children under 12

Interactions

1 Effects of lithium may be decreased by acetazolamide, alkalinizing agents (*e.g.,* sodium bicarbonate, antacids), aminophylline, caffeine, excess sodium chloride, and urea, all substances that increase its excretion.
2 Toxic effects of lithium may be intensified by use of diuretics (sodium loss), methyldopa, and antipsychotic drugs, phenytoin, carbamazepine, mazindol and indomethacin.
3 Combinations of lithium and haloperidol may produce severe encephalopathic symptoms such as parkinsonism, dyskinesias, and dementia.
4 Profound hypothermia may occur with simultaneous use of benzodiazepines (*e.g.,* Valium, Librium) and lithium.
5 Lithium may reduce the effects of amphetamine-like drugs.
6 Lithium may prolong the effects of neuromuscular blocking agents.

▶ **NURSING ALERTS**

▷ 1 Recognize that toxic effects frequently develop when the serum levels rise above 1.5 mEq/liter. Perform periodic blood tests (at least monthly in stabilized outpatients, but as frequently as every other day during the initial dosing phase) to determine precise serum levels.
▷ 2 Warn patients to consult physician immediately should signs of toxicity appear, such as diarrhea, vomiting, drowsiness, muscle weakness, ataxia, or tremor.
▷ 3 Stress the importance of adequate salt and fluid intake during lithium therapy (2500 ml–3000 ml/day). Reduced fluid intake can slow lithium excretion, resulting in increased toxicity.
▷ 4 Caution person about engaging in activities requiring alertness until reaction to lithium has been established. The drug may cause significant drowsiness and impaired coordination.
▷ 5 Dosage needs are much greater during acute phase of treatment. Reduce dosage proportionately as therapeutic effects become evident, to minimize toxicity.
▷ 6 Use cautiously in elderly, debilitated, or dehydrated patients, and in the presence of thyroid disease and epilepsy.

▶ **NURSING CONSIDERATIONS**

▷ 1 Draw blood samples 8 hours to 12 hours after the previous dose of lithium. Patient evaluation should consist of both laboratory and clinical observations.
▷ 2 Be aware that optimum therapeutic effects usually occur 7 to 14 days after initiation of treatment. Do not prolong therapy past 4 weeks if no response is evident.
▷ 3 Test urine periodically for specific gravity, and note signs of polydipsia and polyuria. These are common in the elderly and do not seem to be dose related; if severe, therapy may need to be discontinued.
▷ 4 Provide supplemental fluid and salt in cases of prolonged sweating or diarrhea.

▷ 5 Note symptoms of developing hypothyroidism (*e.g.,* fatigue, weight gain, cold intolerance, puffy face). Symptoms are reversible upon cessation of therapy but may be controlled by supplemental thyroxine without discontinuation of lithium therapy.
▷ 6 Check patient regularly for signs of edema (*e.g.,* puffy ankles), and report any sudden weight gain.
▷ 7 Give drug with meals or use sustained-release forms or smaller, more frequent divided doses to minimize GI irritation. Ensure that consistent serum levels are being maintained, however.

▶ **methotrimeprazine**
Levoprome

A phenothiazine derivative having a profound CNS-depressant effect, methotrimeprazine is characterized by sedation, reduced motor activity, increased pain threshold, and amnesia. Analgesia is comparable to that elicited by morphine but is *not* accompanied by signs of dependence or addiction, even with prolonged use. It rarely produces respiratory depression and does not alter the cough reflex; high incidence of orthostatic hypotension and sedation, but most other phenothiazine-related side-effects (*e.g.,* extrapyramidal symptoms, anticholinergic effects) occur less frequently than with other antipsychotic drugs.

Mechanism
Elevates the sensory pain threshold by an undetermined action on possibly several subcortical areas (limbic system, reticular formation, thalamus); has anticholinergic, antihistaminic, and antiadrenergic effects.

Uses

1 Relief of moderate to marked pain in nonambulatory patients
2 Pre- and postoperative sedation and analgesia
3 Obstetrical analgesia, where respiratory depression should be avoided

Dosage
Analgesia: 10 mg to 20 mg IM every 4 hours to 6 hours (5 mg–10 mg in elderly patients)
Obstetrical analgesia: 15 mg to 20 mg IM; repeat as needed
Preanesthetic sedation: 10 mg to 20 mg IM 1 hour to 3 hours before surgery
Postoperative: 2.5 mg to 7.5 mg IM

Fate
Maximum analgesia occurs within 20 minutes to 40 minutes following IM injection; duration is 4 hours to 5 hours; metabolized and conjugated in the liver, and excreted largely in the urine with small amounts in the feces

Common Side-Effects
Orthostatic hypotension (dizziness, faintness, weakness), sedation, and pain at injection site

Significant Adverse Reactions

Abdominal discomfort, nausea and vomiting, disorientation, urinary hesitancy, chills, local inflammation and swelling at injection site, agranulocytosis (rare), and jaundice (rare)

Because the drug is a phenothiazine derivative, the potential for producing any adverse effect associated with phenothiazines is present. See the general discussion on antipsychotic drugs earlier in this chapter.

Contraindications

Severe myocardial, renal, or hepatic disease; with antihypertensive agents or in the presence of significant hypotension; comatose states; and children under 12 years

Interactions

1 An additive depressive effect may occur with other CNS depressants (*e.g.,* narcotics, barbiturates, meprobamate, anesthetics, alcohol).
2 Exaggerated hypotensive effects may occur in combination with antihypertensive drugs and MAO inhibitors.
3 Methotrimeprazine may increase the action and toxicity of anticholinergics, skeletal muscle relaxants, antipsychotic drugs, and analgesics.
4 A reversal of the vasopressor action of epinephrine may occur with methotrimeprazine, leading to profound hypotension.

▶ NURSING ALERTS

▷ 1 Administer by deep IM injection only. Avoid SC use because severe tissue irritation can occur.
▷ 2 Keep patient recumbent for at least 6 hours following administration to avoid orthostatic hypotension. Supervise ambulation and provide assistance when needed.
▷ 3 Monitor blood pressure and pulse frequently until response stabilizes. If vasopressors are needed to combat hypotension, use methoxamine or phenylephrine. Do not give epinephrine, because reversal can occur.
▷ 4 Use cautiously in elderly or debilitated patients with heart disease, during early pregnancy, and in patients with a history of convulsive disorders.

▶ NURSING CONSIDERATIONS

▷ 1 Do not use longer than 30 days, except where narcotics are contraindicated or in terminal illnesses. When used for prolonged periods, regular liver function tests and blood studies should be performed.
▷ 2 With repeated use, rotate injection sites to minimize pain and inflammation.
▷ 3 Advise patients receiving the drug for prolonged periods that tolerance will develop to the hypotensive and sedative effects of the drug.
▷ 4 Do not mix in the same syringe with other drugs (except atropine or scopolamine) as incompatibility can result.

Summary. Antipsychotic Drugs

Drug	Preparations	Usual Dosage Range
Antipsychotic Agents		
See Table 22-3		
Droperidol (Inapsine)	Injection—2.5 mg/ml	Adults: Preanesthetic medication—2.5 mg to 10 mg IM Adjunct to general anesthesia—1.25 mg to 2.5 mg/20 lb to 25 lb IV Diagnostic procedures—2.5 mg to 10 mg IM initially; repeat with 1.25-mg to 2.5-mg increments Children (2 yr–12 yr): 1 mg to 1.5 mg/20 lb to 25 lb
Lithium (Cibalith-S, Eskalith, Lithane, Lithobid, Lithonate, Lithotabs)	Tablets—300 mg Slow-release tablets—300 mg, 450 mg Capsules—300 mg Syrup—300 mg/5 ml	Acute mania: 600 mg 3 times/day; adjust to optimal response Prophylaxis: 300 mg 3 to 4 times/day, or 300-mg slow-release tablets twice a day
Methotrimeprazine (Levoprome)	Injection—20 mg/ml	Analgesia: 10 mg to 20 mg IM every 4 hours to 6 hours (5 mg–10 mg in elderly) Preanesthetic medication: 10 mg to 20 mg IM 1 hour to 3 hours before surgery Postoperative analgesia: 2.5 mg to 7.5 mg IM

Antianxiety Drugs

23

Several groups of drugs have the ability to induce mild sedation and therefore reduce anxiety and tension in doses that do not markedly impair mental alertness or psychomotor performance. Such drugs have been designated as antianxiety agents, and have become a widely used and often abused class of drugs.

Pharmacologically, these compounds are difficult to distinguish from the barbiturates; however, their principal advantage relative to the barbiturates is their significantly higher sedative/hypnotic ratio. In other words, the margin between the calming, tension-relieving dose and the hypnotic, sleep-inducing dose is much greater with the antianxiety agents than with the barbiturates. Likewise, their safety margin— therapeutic/toxic dose levels— is wider than that observed with barbiturates. Their primary use, therefore, is to provide a degree of relief from emotional symptoms (such as agitation, anxiety, muscle tension, and motor hyperactivity) associated with psychoneurotic and psychosomatic disorders. They are rarely satisfactory alone for controlling severely disturbed psychotic patients, but have been employed in conjunction with antipsychotic drugs in treating acute psychotic episodes.

In contrast to the antipsychotic drugs, antianxiety agents have a rather low incidence of adverse reactions when administered in normal therapeutic doses. Moreover, their central skeletal muscle relaxant action may contribute to their effectiveness in treating emotional disorders compounded by excessive muscular tension or spasm. However, their prolonged use is associated with development of tolerance, and a significant potential for habituation and abuse exists with these compounds, whereas it is highly unlikely with the more potent antipsychotic drugs.

Most antianxiety agents also have clinically significant anticonvulsant activity when administered IV, and can effectively control acute convulsive states such as status epilepticus or those associated with acute alcohol withdrawal. Moreover, their use is not accompanied by extrapyramidal or autonomic side-effects.

The currently available antianxiety agents can be conveniently classified into one of three groups:

1 *Benzodiazepines*—alprazolam, chlordiazepoxide, clorazepate, diazepam, halazepam, lorazepam, oxazepam, prazepam
2 *Carbamates*—meprobamate
3 *Miscellaneous*—chlormezanone, hydroxyzine

I Benzodiazepines

Alprazolam	Halazepam
Chlordiazepoxide	Lorazepam
Clorazepate	Oxazepam
Diazepam	Prazepam

The benzodiazepines are the most widely used antianxiety agents; in fact, diazepam, the most popular of the benzodiazepines, is one of the most prescribed drugs in this country. Much of their popularity is due to their demonstrated effectiveness at dose levels that are not associated with the high risk of untoward reactions or with development of physical dependence that is characteristic of chronic barbiturate consumption. The drugs in this group that are discussed in this chapter are indicated primarily for the relief of situational anxiety. Other benzodiazepines have somewhat different indications and are found elsewhere in the book. Flurazepam (Dalmane), triazolam (Halcion), and temazepam (Restoril) are effective nonbarbiturate hypnotics used to relieve insomnia and are reviewed in Chapter 21. Clonazepam (Clonopin) is used in certain forms of epilepsy and is discussed in Chapter 25.

The effectiveness of benzodiazepines in relieving symptoms of anxiety over prolonged periods has not been conclusively established; these drugs should not be used for longer than 3 months to 4 months unless careful patient reassessment establishes a definite need for continued treatment.

Although all of the clinically useful benzodiazepines share many common pharmacologic properties (mild sedation, skeletal-muscle relaxation, anticonvulsant action) and vary little in their clinical efficacy, they differ significantly in their duration of action, depending upon whether they are converted to an active metabolite or an inactive conjugate. Table 23-1 lists the usual doses, metabolic activity, and elimination half-lives of the benzodiazepine drugs. The benzodiazepines are first discussed as a group; characteristics of each individual agent are outlined in Table 23-2.

Mechanism

Not completely understood; appear to alter neurotransmission in subcortical brain areas, especially the limbic system, possibly by augmenting the activity of GABA, an inhibitory neurotransmitter; may also have a direct GABA-like action at receptor sites; exert a centrally mediated skeletal muscle-relaxing action, and increase the seizure threshold, again presumably by a GABA-like action; little effect on respiration or circulation in normal therapeutic doses

Uses

1 Symptomatic relief of anxiety, tension, and irritability associated with neuroses, psychoneuroses, and psychosomatic disorders (short-term use only)
2 Symptomatic relief of the symptoms of acute alcohol withdrawal (chlordiazepoxide, clorazepate, diazepam, oxazepam)
3 Preoperative sedation
4 Relief of muscle hypertonicity associated with anxiety or tension states
5 Control of acute (*e.g.,* status epilepticus) or severe, recurrent convulsive seizure states (diazepam IV)
6 Adjunctive treatment prior to cardioversion or endoscopic procedures to lessen anxiety and reduce recall (diazepam IV, IM)
7 Control of nocturnal enuresis and "night terrors" (experimental use only)

Dosage
See Table 23-2.

Fate
Generally well absorbed orally although rates differ widely; IM absorption of lorazepam is rapid and complete, but that of chlordiazepoxide and diazepam is erratic; onset of action ranges from 30 minutes to 60 minutes orally (diazepam has quickest onset of action) and 15 minutes to 30 minutes IM. Most drugs have long half-lives, and metabolites may be clinically active as well (see Table 23-1); excreted as both unchanged drug and metabolites, largely through the kidney; elimination may occur in two stages; a rapid (within several hours) phase followed by a slower (within days) phase. Danger of accumulation exists with chronic use.

Common Side-Effects
Drowsiness, fatigue, lethargy, and ataxia (most common during early stages of therapy)

(*Text continues on p. 210.*)

Table 23-1. Benzodiazepine Metabolism

Drug	Usual Daily Dosage Range	Activity of Metabolites	Elimination Half-Life
Alprazolam (Xanax)	0.75 mg to 1.5 mg	Inactive	10 hours to 15 hours
Chlordiazepoxide (Librium)	15 mg to 100 mg	Active	5 hours to 30 hours
Clorazepate (Tranxene)	15 mg to 60 mg	Active	30 hours to 90 hours
Diazepam (Valium)	4 mg to 40 mg	Active	20 hours to 50 hours
Halazepam (Paxipam)	80 mg to 160 mg	Active	12 hours to 15 hours
Lorazepam (Ativan)	2 mg to 8 mg	Inactive	10 hours to 15 hours
Oxazepam (Serax)	30 mg to 120 mg	Inactive	5 hours to 15 hours
Prazepam (Centrax)	20 mg to 60 mg	Active	60 hours to 120 hours

Table 23-2. Benzodiazepines

Drug	Preparations	Usual Dosage Range	Remarks
Alprazolam (Xanax)	Tablets—0.25 mg, 0.5 mg, 1.0 mg	Initially, 0.25 mg to 0.5 mg 3 times/day; maximum total dose is 4 mg/day Elderly—0.25 mg 2 to 3 times/day	Metabolized to an inactive compound, thus has a short half-life (12 hr–15 hr) and relatively brief duration of action; possesses some antidepressant activity, particularly at higher doses; drowsiness and lightheadedness are common during early stages of therapy (Schedule IV)
Chlordiazepoxide (A-poxide, Libritabs, Librium, Murcil, Reposans-10, Sereen, SK-Lygen, Tenax)	Capsules—5 mg, 10 mg, 25 mg Tablets—5 mg, 10 mg, 25 mg Powder for Injection—100 mg/5 ml	**Oral** Adults: Anxiety—5 mg to 10 mg 3 to 4 times/day up to 25 mg 4 times/day Alcohol withdrawal—50 mg to 100 mg up to 300 mg/day Children (over 6 yr)—5 mg to 10 mg 2 to 4 times/day as needed **Parenteral** Adults—50 mg to 100 mg IM or IV Children (over 12 yr)—25 mg to 50 mg IM or IV	Less potent than diazepam and has less anticonvulsive activity; excreted slowly by the kidneys, so danger of accumulation exists; prepare IM solution immediately before administration and discard unused portion; do not use IM diluent if hazy or opalescent; IM solution should *not* be given IV because of air bubbles that form in solution; inject slowly and deeply IM; IV solution can be prepared with Sterile Water or saline; give IV injection slowly over 1 minute; do *not* inject IV solution IM because pain is common; do not add to IV infusion, because solution is unstable and quickly deteriorates; sterilization by heating should not be attempted; available in combination with amitriptyline as Limbitrol for treatment of anxious depressions (Schedule IV)
Clorazepate (Tranxene)	Capsules—3.75 mg, 7.5 mg, 15 mg Tablets—3.75 mg, 7.5 mg, 15 mg Long-acting tablets—11.25 mg, 22.5 mg	Anxiety—15 mg to 60 mg daily in divided doses or 11.25 mg to 22.5 mg once a day Elderly—7.5 mg to 15 mg/day Adjunct to anticonvulsants— Adults: 7.5 mg 3 times/day initially; increase gradually Children: 7.5 mg twice a day; increase gradually. Alcohol withdrawal— Day 1: 30 mg initially, then 30 mg to 60 mg in divided doses Day 2: 45 mg to 90 mg in divided doses Day 3: 22.5 mg to 45 mg in divided doses Day 4: 15 mg to 30 mg in divided doses	Slower onset (about 60 min) and longer duration (up to 24 hr) than diazepam; active metabolite is desmethyldiazepam; single daily dose is usually given at bedtime; recommended in children only as adjunct to other anticonvulsant drugs; Effects parallel those of diazepam (Schedule IV)
Diazepam (Valium, Valrelease)	Tablets—2 mg, 5 mg, 10 mg Capsules (sustained release)—15 mg Injection—5 mg/ml	**Oral** Adults: Anxiety—2 mg to 10 mg 2 to 4 times/day or 15 mg to 30 mg/day sustained-release capsules Alcohol withdrawal—10 mg 3 to 4 times/day initially, followed by 5 mg 3 to 4 times/day	Effects occur within 20 minutes to 30 minutes with oral administration, 15 minutes to 30 minutes IM, and immediately IV; when using IV, inject slowly (5 mg/min) and avoid small veins to reduce danger of thrombophlebitis and local swelling and irritation; do not mix or dilute with other solutions or add to IV fluids; IM

Table 23-2. Benzodiazepines *(continued)*

Drug	Preparations	Usual Dosage Range	Remarks
		Adjunct in muscle spasm and convulsive states—2 mg to 10 mg 2 to 4 times/day or 15 mg to 30 mg once daily Children (over 6 months): 1 mg to 2.5 mg 3 to 4 times/ day; may increase gradually as required Parenteral Adults: Psychoneuroses—2 mg to 10 mg IM or IV every 3 hours to 4 hours as necessary depending on severity of symptoms Alcohol withdrawal—5 mg to 10 mg IM or IV; repeat every 3 hours to 4 hours Preoperative and minor surgical procedures (*e.g.,* endoscopy)—5 mg to 10 mg IM or 10 mg IV prior to procedure Convulsive states—5 mg to 10 mg IV; repeat at 10-minute to 15-minute intervals to a maximum of 30 mg Cardioversion—5 mg to 15 mg IV 5 minutes to 10 minutes before procedure Children: Tetanus—2 mg to 10 mg IM or slow IV every 3 hours to 4 hours Status epilepticus—Under 5 years: 0.2 mg to 0.5 mg by slow IV every 2 minutes to 5 minutes Over 5 years: 1 mg every 2 minutes to 5 minutes	injection should be made deeply and slowly into a large muscle, such as the gluteus; when used to control convulsions, be prepared to readminister drug if seizures recur, as duration of action with IV use is rather short; use cautiously in patients with chronic lung disease or unstable cardiovascular status; facilities for respiratory assistance should be present when drug is given parenterally; use of diazepam for endoscopic procedures has been associated with coughing, dyspnea, hyperventilation, laryngospasm, and pain in the throat and chest; use a topical anesthetic, and have counter-measures available (*e.g.,* respiratory assistance); reduce dose of narcotic analgesic by one third when used with diazepam (Schedule IV)
Halazepam (Paxipam)	Tablets—20 mg, 40 mg	20 mg to 40 mg 3 or 4 times/ day Elderly—20 mg 1 to 2 times/ day	Long-acting benzodiazepine; maximum plasma levels are attained in 1 hr to 3 hr; Highly protein-bound; Do not use in children under 18 (Schedule IV)
Lorazepam (Ativan)	Tablets—0.5 mg, 1 mg, 2 mg Injection—2 mg/ml, 4 mg/ml	Oral Anxiety—1 mg to 2 mg 2 to 3 times/day Insomnia—2 mg to 4 mg at bedtime IM Preoperative medication—0.05 mg/kg 2 hours before procedure (maximum 4 mg) IV Acute anxiety—2 mg to 4 mg	Short-acting drug used for anxiety, preanesthetic medication and temporary relief of insomnia; not recommended in children less than 12 years; dosage must be individually titrated; increase dose gradually to minimize adverse effects; elderly or debilitated persons should receive an initial dose of 1 mg to 2 mg/day; less danger of accumulation than with other derivatives because no active metabolites are formed; inject IM deep into muscle mass; dilute in appropriate diluent for IV administration; do not use if discolored (Schedule IV)

(continued)

Table 23-2. Benzodiazepines *(continued)*

Drug	Preparations	Usual Dosage Range	Remarks
Oxazepam (Serax)	Capsules—10 mg, 15 mg, 30 mg Tablets—15 mg	Adults—10 mg to 30 mg 3 to 4 times/day Elderly or debilitated—10 mg 3 to 4 times/day	Shorter duration of action than diazepam, and produces a lower incidence of side-effects; not recommended in children under 6 years of age; paradoxical excitation may occur in first 2 weeks of therapy; reduce dose until symptoms subside (Schedule IV)
Prazepam (Centrax)	Tablets—10 mg Capsules—5 mg, 10 mg	Adults—20 mg to 60 mg/day in divided doses Elderly—10 mg to 15 mg/day	Not indicated in patients under 18 years of age; can be used as a single daily dose (20 mg–40 mg) at bedtime; similar to diazepam in actions and toxicity (Schedule IV)

Significant Adverse Reactions
(Not all reactions observed with every drug)

CNS—confusion, disorientation, agitation, slurred speech, headache, syncope, vertigo, depression, hyporeactivity, stupor, tremor; paradoxical excitement (hostility, rage, muscle spasticity, irritability, vivid dreams, euphoria, insomnia, hallucinations) can occur, especially in psychotic patients

Autonomic—dry mouth, constipation, urinary retention, blurred vision, diplopia

Cardiovascular/hematologic—bradycardia, hypotension, edema and weight gain, cardiovascular collapse, agranulocytosis, neutropenia

Hypersensitivity—skin rash, urticaria, fever, angioneurotic edema, bronchial spasm

Other—changes in libido, menstrual irregularities, salivation, hiccoughs, difficulty swallowing, hepatic dysfunction (jaundice), pain or thrombophlebitis on IV injection

Contraindications
Severe psychoses, narrow-angle glaucoma, shock, children under 6 years (except diazepam—children under 6 months)

Interactions
1 May enhance the CNS-depressant effects of alcohol, barbiturates, antihistamines, phenothiazines, opiates, and other CNS-depressant drugs.
2 The effects of phenytoin may be potentiated by benzodiazepines.
3 An increased muscle relaxant effect can occur with combinations of benzodiazepines and other centrally and peripherally acting muscle relaxants.
4 The effects of levodopa may be antagonized by benzodiazepines.
5 The effects of benzodiazepines may be lessened in individuals who smoke.
6 Antacids or food may slow oral absorption of some benzodiazepines.
7 The half-life of some benzodiazepines, but not lorazepam or oxazepam, can be prolonged by cimetidine.

▶ NURSING ALERTS
▷ 1 Caution patients about engaging in potentially hazardous activities during early stages of therapy, because drowsiness and ataxia can occur.
▷ 2 Warn patients to avoid excessive use of other CNS depressants (*e.g.,* alcohol, antihistamines, hypnotics) because increased sedation can occur.
▷ 3 Observe carefully for signs of excessive drug usage (*e.g.,* ataxia, dizziness, slurred speech), and note frequency of requests for medication. Habituation can occur quite easily with prolonged or excessive drug consumption.
▷ 4 Do not use alone in primary depressions or psychotic disorders.
▷ 5 Warn women of childbearing potential of the possibility of congenital malformations if the drugs are ingested during early pregnancy. Discourage their use during this period.
▷ 6 Use cautiously in addiction-prone patients, during lactation, and in the presence of liver or kidney disease.
▷ 7 Administer the injectable dosage forms very carefully in elderly, seriously ill, or debilitated patients or in those with limited pulmonary reserve. Do not use injectable dosage forms in patients in shock, coma, or acute alcohol intoxication with depression of vital signs.
▷ 8 When given parenterally, drugs may produce marked muscle weakness, respiratory depression, and hypotension, especially in the presence of narcotics. Observe the patient carefully, monitor vital signs, and have resuscitative equipment available.
▷ 9 Be alert for possible development of paradoxical excitatory effects. Discontinue drug if they occur, and provide appropriate supportive care.
▷ 10 Caution patient against abrupt cessation of therapy after long-term treatment because withdrawal symp-

toms (*e.g.,* vomiting, cramping, sweating, tremor, convulsions) can occur and persist for several days. Treat symptomatically as needed.

▷ 11 Watch for early signs of developing jaundice (nausea, diarrhea, abdominal pain, rash) or blood dyscrasias (sore throat, fever, weakness, mucosal ulceration), and discontinue drug.

▶ NURSING CONSIDERATIONS

▷ 1 Carefully regulate dosage in elderly or debilitated patients, because they generally require smaller, less frequent doses.

▷ 2 Consider use of a short-acting derivative (*e.g.,* lorazepam, oxazepam) when therapy must be continued for extended periods of time to lessen the danger of accumulation toxicity.

▷ 3 Periodically reassess the patient's status and drug responsiveness. Long-term therapy with these drugs (greater than 4 mo–5mo) is undesirable in most cases.

▷ 4 Perform periodic blood cell counts and liver function tests during prolonged therapy.

▷ 5 If possible, closely supervise the pattern of drug-taking behavior, especially in persons with a history of drug abuse.

▷ 6 Attempt to show understanding and concern for the anxious, agitated, or fearful patient. Provide emotional support, and encourage relaxation and avoidance of stressful situations where possible.

▷ 7 Following IV administration, monitor blood pressure, keep patient supine for several hours, elevate slowly, and provide assistance in ambulation.

▷ 8 Be aware that benzodiazepines are Schedule IV drugs. Proper handling and dispensing procedures must be followed.

II Carbamates

Only one carbamate antianxiety drug remains in clinical practice, namely meprobamate. Its CNS-depressant actions are similar to those of the barbiturates but are generally shorter in duration. Other effects produced by meprobamate include skeletal muscle relaxation and, in large doses, an anticonvulsant action. It also reduces REM sleep time. Prolonged use can result in habituation and dependence, and meprobamate is more dangerous in this regard than the benzodiazepines.

▶ meprobamate
Equanil, Miltown, and various other manufacturers

Mechanism
Not well established; appears to act at several subcortical loci, including the limbic system and thalamus; no specific depressant effects on the reticular activating system or the autonomic nervous system; suppresses REM sleep and exerts a skeletal muscle relaxing effect, probably resulting in part from its sedative action

Uses
1 Short-term relief of anxiety and tension associated with various disease states
2 Promote sleep in anxious or agitated patients (short-term basis only)

Dosage
Adults—1200 mg to 1600 mg/day in divided doses
Children (6 yr–12 yr)—100 mg to 200 mg 2 to 3 times/day

Fate
Well absorbed orally; onset of effect within 1 hour orally and 15 minutes IM. Plasma half-life is 10 hours; uniformly distributed in the body; metabolized in the liver and largely excreted in the urine mainly as inactive metabolites; meprobamate induces liver microsomal enzymes; readily crosses placental barrier

Common Side-Effects
Drowsiness, ataxia, and rash

Significant Adverse Reactions
CNS—dizziness, vertigo, slurred speech, weakness, paresthesias, headache, depression, confusion, paradoxical excitation, euphoria, hyperactivity
Hypersensitivity—pruritus, urticaria, fever, edema, petechiae, ecchymoses, adenopathy, bronchospasm, anaphylaxis, exfoliative dermatitis
Hematologic—leukopenia, agranulocytosis, thrombocytopenic purpura, aplastic anemia, pancytopenia
Cardiovascular—hypotension, flushing, syncope, palpitations, tachycardia, arrhythmias
GI—nausea, vomiting, diarrhea, dry mouth, glossitis
Other—exacerbation of porphyria, increased incidence of grand mal attacks, pain at IM injection site

Contraindications
Acute intermittent porphyria, renal insufficiency (IM use), and children under 6

Interactions
1 Additive depressant effects can occur between meprobamate and other CNS depressants (*e.g.,* alcohol, barbiturates, phenothiazines).
2 Meprobamate may augment the metabolism of oral anticoagulants and steroid hormones, thereby reducing their pharmacologic effects.

▶ NURSING ALERTS
See Benzodiazepines. In addition:

▷ 1 Note development of sore throat, rash, or fever, and discontinue drug. These are possible early indications of blood dyscrasias.

▶ **NURSING CONSIDERATIONS**

See Benzodiazepines. In addition:

▷ 1 Withdraw drug *gradually* over 1 week to 2 weeks following prolonged therapy. Sudden withdrawal may precipitate symptoms such as vomiting, tremors, muscle twitching, hyperactivity, confusion, and possibly convulsions.

▷ 2 Use cautiously in epileptics because seizures may be exacerbated.

III   Miscellaneous Antianxiety Agents

Two additional drugs showing an antianxiety action are largely unrelated to the benzodiazepines and carbamates. These compounds, hydroxyzine and chlormezanone, are reviewed briefly below.

▶ **chlormezanone**

Trancopal

An infrequently used antianxiety drug for the treatment of mild anxiety and tension states, chlormezanone's usual dosage range is 100 mg to 200 mg, 3 to 4 times/day for adults, and 50 mg to 100 mg 3 to 4 times/day in children 5 years to 12 years of age. Its onset of action is 15 minutes to 30 minutes, and effects persist for up to 6 hours. Adverse reactions can include dizziness, rash, drowsiness, dryness of the mouth, muscle weakness, edema, and depression.

The warnings, precautions, and nursing considerations discussed previously in connection with the benzodiazepines generally pertain to the use of chlormezanone as well. The drug has no particular advantage over the other antianxiety agents and is simply an alternative drug.

▶ **hydroxyzine**

Atarax, Vistaril, and various other manufacturers

Hydroxyzine is a diphenylmethane derivative having a mild CNS-depressant action, together with anticholinergic, antihistaminic, local anesthetic, antiemetic, antispasmodic, antisecretory, and skeletal muscle relaxant effects. It has a wide safety margin, and exerts a rapid-acting calming effect.

Mechanism

Not completely established; may suppress activity in subcortical brain areas but appears to have little effect on the cortex; blocks action of histamine and exerts both a direct and an indirect (through its sedative action) skeletal muscle relaxant effect.

Uses

1 Symptomatic treatment of psychoneurotic states characterized by anxiety, tension, hostility, and motor hyperactivity

2 Adjunctive preoperative and prepartum therapy to help reduce anxiety and lessen narcotic analgesic requirements

3 Relieve symptoms of anxiety associated with organic disturbances such as digestive disorders, allergic conditions (*e.g.,* urticaria, dermatoses, asthma), senility, menopause, alcoholism, and behavioral problems, especially in children

4 Adjunctive treatment of alcohol withdrawal or delirium tremens (IM)

Dosage
Oral:
Adults: 25 mg to 100 mg 3 to 4 times/day
Children (over 6): 50 mg to 100 mg/day in divided doses
Children (under 6): 50 mg/day in divided doses
IM: Psychiatric emergencies; acute alcoholism: 50 mg to 100 mg at once; repeat every 4 hours to 6 hours as needed
Preoperative medication: Adults: 50 mg to 100 mg; Children: 0.6 mg/kg

Fate
Rapidly absorbed orally and parenterally; onset of action within 15 minutes to 30 minutes; effects last for up to 6 hours

Common Side-Effects
Transitory drowsiness, dry mouth

Significant Adverse Reactions
Involuntary motor activity, dizziness, rare hypersensitivity reactions (urticaria, skin eruptions, erythema multiforme)

Contraindications
Early pregnancy

Interactions
1 May exert additive effects with other CNS depressants (*e.g.,* alcohol, hypnotics, narcotics)

▶ **NURSING ALERTS**

▷ 1 Caution patients against driving or operating machinery during early stages of therapy because drowsiness can occur.

▷ 2 Avoid drug during pregnancy, especially the first trimester, because fetal abnormalities have been observed in experimental animals.

▷ 3 When administering preoperatively in combination with barbiturates or narcotics, reduce dose of each drug appropriately, as additive effects are likely to occur.

▷ 4 Do not administer IM solution SC or IV.

▶ NURSING CONSIDERATIONS

▷ 1 Suggest frequent rinsing of the mouth or use of hard candies to relieve dryness.

▷ 2 Note that hydroxyzine is often a preferred antianxiety drug in cardiac patients because it allays anxiety and does not interfere with the effects of digitalis glycosides.

▷ 3 Inject IM deeply into a large muscle mass (*e.g.,* gluteus in adults and midlateral thigh in children). Rotate injection sites.

Summary. Antianxiety Drugs

Drug	Preparations	Usual Dosage Range
Benzodiazepines		
See Table 23-2		
Carbamates		
Meprobamate (Equanil, Miltown, and various other manufacturers)	Tablets—200 mg, 400 mg, 600 mg Capsules—400 mg Sustained-release capsules—200 mg, 400 mg	Oral Adults—1200 mg to 1600 mg/day in divided doses (maximum 2400 mg/day) Child (6 yr–12 yr)—100 mg to 200 mg 2 to 3 times/day
Miscellaneous		
Chlormezanone (Trancopal)	Tablets—100 mg, 200 mg	Adults—100 mg to 200 mg 3 to 4 times/day Child (5 yr–12 yr)—50 mg to 100 mg 3 to 4 times/day
Hydroxyzine (Atarax, Vistaril, and various other manufacturers)	Tablets—10 mg, 25 mg, 50 mg, 100 mg Capsules—25 mg, 50 mg, 100 mg Syrup—10 mg/5 ml, 25 mg/5 ml Injection—25 mg/ml, 50 mg/ml Injection—75 mg/dose, 100 mg/dose	Oral Adults—25 mg to 100 mg 3 to 4 times/day Child (over 6 yr)—50 mg to 100 mg daily in divided doses Child (under 6 yr)—50 mg daily IM Adults—25 mg to 100 mg as required Child—0.6 mg/kg

Antidepressants 24

Drug treatment of depression is a confusing and somewhat controversial area of pharmacotherapy. The rather high "placebo" response rate in certain types of depressions—the apparent clinical benefit without active drug—suggests that great reliance should not be placed solely on drug therapy to the exclusion of other forms of treatment, including psychotherapy, environmental changes, and electroconvulsive therapy.

Nevertheless, in some types of depressions, significant therapeutic benefit has been obtained with many antidepressant drugs. Optimal clinical responses depend mainly upon an accurate diagnosis of the depressive state, and it is here that much controversy still exists. One useful, though not universally accepted, classification of depressions, based primarily upon their etiology, categorizes them as follows:

1 Endogenous, psychotic depressions
2 Anxious, neurotic depressions
3 Situational, reactive depressions
4 Manic–depressive disorders

Endogenous, psychotic depressions are characterized by absence of pleasure, emotional withdrawal, motor retardation, and sleep disturbances, among other signs, and do not seem to have an external precipitating factor. Central neurohormonal imbalances are likely present in these types of depressions, and they can usually be treated with antidepressant drugs.

Anxious, neurotic depressions are marked by anxiety, tension, "overreactiveness" to disappointment or losses, and signs of irritability, anger, hostility, and even helplessness. Classic antidepressant drugs are usually not very effective in these depressive states, yet they often respond to antianxiety or antipsychotic agents.

The situational, reactive types of depression are generally precipitated by stressful or grief-producing external factors, such as death of a loved one, serious illness, or loss of employment. Because the cause *is* external, the depressive reaction is frequently self-limiting, and remission is often seen in a matter of weeks. Drug therapy is usually not indicated unless the disorder becomes severe or chronic and interferes with normal functioning.

Manic–depressive disorders are characterized by excessive and sometimes violent mood swings that tend to recur regularly. Treatment generally is effected with lithium (see Chap. 22) and possibly an antidepressant, for example, maprotiline.

Severe depressions, in which agitation is a predominant feature or in which risk of suicide is high, are often best treated initially with electroconvulsive therapy (ECT). Rapid and dramatic improvement is frequently noted in severely depressed persons following ECT, making these patients more amenable to subsequent drug therapy. Concurrent use of antidepressants during ECT may increase the hazards, and such therapy should be avoided. Patients receiving tricyclic antidepressants who are to undergo ECT should have the drugs discontinued for 24 hours to 48 hours prior to the ECT.

Successful outpatient treatment of depression requires accurate diagnosis, critical dosage adjustment, and careful observation of the patient for untoward reactions, and is a difficult task at best. The available antidepressant drugs are both effective and potentially hazardous substances; they must be prescribed and monitored with care and attention. Moreover, depressed patients need emotional support perhaps as much as they need the proper drugs, and lack of support can negate the beneficial effects of any antidepressant drug.

The two principal theories of depression, the catecholamine and serotonin hypotheses, ascribe most depressive symptoms to a central biochemical deficit of functional norepinephrine and serotonin, respectively. Although the theories are probably oversimplistic, there is evidence to suggest that a reduced functioning of these central monoamine neurohormones does occur in many forms of depression; therefore, potentiation of their action in the CNS is associated with significant improvement in many depressed persons. All currently useful antidepressants act to enhance the activity of one or more central neurotransmitters.

Drugs capable of relieving the symptoms of depressive disorders include several tricyclic antidepressants, a tetracyclic derivative, a chemically unrelated antidepressant (trazodone), monoamineoxidase (MAO) inhibitors, and psychomotor stimulants such as amphetamine and methylphenidate. The latter category of drugs are of benefit only in *mild* depression and are infrequently used because of their potential for abuse and their limited therapeutic effectiveness. Their other clinical indications are reviewed in Chapter 27. The remaining drugs (tricyclics, tetracyclics, trazodone, and the MAO inhibitors) are potent and effective antidepressants and are discussed in detail below.

I Tricyclic Antidepressants

Amitriptyline	Maprotiline (tetracyclic
Amoxapine	derivative)
Desipramine	Nortriptyline
Doxepin	Protriptyline
Imipramine	Trimipramine

Tricyclic antidepressants are so named because of their characteristic three-ring nuclear structure. Some newer compounds (*e.g.,* maprotiline) possess a four-ring nuclear structure, and while similar in most respects to the tricyclic drugs, may have a lower incidence than the tricyclics of some undesirable side-effects. The discussion that follows uses the term *tricyclic* as a matter of convention; however, the information refers to the tetracyclic compounds as well. Differences among the various drugs are noted throughout the discussion where appropriate.

The tricyclic antidepressant agents are the most widely used drugs for the treatment of depression. In comparison to MAO inhibitors, they are consistently more effective and potentially less toxic. Either advantage alone warrants preference for them. The currently available tricyclic antidepressants are structurally analagous to the phenothiazine antipsychotic agents, and there are many similarities in the pharmacologic and toxicologic spectrum of action of these

two classes of drugs (*e.g.,* sedation, anticholinergic action, orthostatic hypotension). The tricyclics are characterized by their *specific* blocking action on the uptake of biogenic amines at the nerve ending, which accounts for at least a part of the drugs' antidepressant action. Selective differences exist among the different tricyclic drugs, however, in their relative potency in blocking norepinephrine *versus* serotonin uptake. These differences, outlined below, may account for the varying degrees of effectiveness among tricyclics observed in different depressed populations.

Most tricyclic compounds have a sedative action in addition to their antidepressant effect, and all derivatives exert a central and peripheral anticholinergic action and can induce orthostatic hypotension, especially in the elderly. Differences in amine-uptake blocking action among the tricyclic compounds are reflected not only in variations in their clinical effectiveness but also in the type and intensity of the various side-effects (*e.g.,* sedation, hypotension) that may occur with each drug. The relationship of amine-uptake blocking activity to the occurrence of the major side-effects encountered with each tricyclic drug is outlined in Table 24-1. Those drugs having a marked sedative action (*e.g.,* amitriptyline) appear to effectively block serotonin uptake to a greater extent than norepinephrine uptake; they may be more effective in agitated, anxious, or hostile depressions rather than in retarded depressions.

As noted earlier, endogenous depressions are often characterized by either a predominant norepinephrine or serotonin deficiency. Patients with a norepinephrine deficiency, as determined by low urinary levels of 3-methoxy-4-hydroxy phenyl glycol (MHPG), the major norepinephrine metabolite, may respond well to tricyclics that block norepinephrine uptake to a significant extent (*i.e.,* desipramine, nortriptyline, imipramine). Conversely, low urinary levels of 5-hydroxyindoleacetic acid (5-HIAA), the serotonin metabolite, suggest a relative serotonergic deficiency, and tricyclics with strong serotonin-uptake blocking activity (*i.e.,* amitriptyline) appear to be the logical drugs of choice in this situation.

It is important to realize that blockade of biogenic amine uptake into nerve endings is not the sole mechanism of the antidepressant action of the tricyclics. In fact, clinical observations suggest it may not even be the *principal* mechanism of action. It is well known that the therapeutic benefit—the relief of depressive symptoms—of the tricyclics is evident only after several weeks of continual therapy with most of the drugs, whereas the blocking effect of these drugs on amine uptake occurs almost immediately. Therefore, it is difficult to explain the latency of clinical action in view of the immediacy of the biochemical action. Tricyclics also have been shown to exert a blocking action at presynaptic alpha-adrenergic receptors (alpha-2 sites) regulating norepinephrine release. Presynaptic alpha-blockade results in increased norepinephrine release, because normal activation of these receptors is responsible for inhibiting release of norepinephrine through a negative feedback effect. Increased presynaptic neurohormone release leads to a persistent occupation of postsynaptic receptor sites, which then become fewer in number and *hypo*sensitive. Loss of receptor sensitivity, termed *down regulation,* is slow in developing

Table 24-1. Tricyclic Antidepressants—Pharmacologic Characteristics

	Blockade of Amine Pump		Sedation	Anticholinergic Action
	Norepinephrine	*Serotonin*		
Amitriptyline	+	+++	+++	+++
Amoxapine	++	++	++	++
Desipramine	+++	+	+	+
Doxepin	(−)	(−)	+++	+++
Imipramine	++	++	++	++
Maprotiline*	++	0	++	+
Nortriptyline	++	+	++	++
Protriptyline	(−)	(−)	0	++
Trimipramine	(−)	(−)	+++	++

* *tetracyclic derivative*
+++—strong effect
++—moderate effect
+—weak effect
0—no significant effect
(−)—variable, inconsistent effect (studies are inconclusive)

when a patient is started on a tricyclic antidepressant, and the time course of the receptors' down regulation closely corresponds to the onset of antidepressant activity. Therefore, it may play a major role in the therapeutic efficacy of the tricyclic antidepressants.

Differences in amine-uptake blockade notwithstanding, the overall pharmacologic profile of all tricyclic antidepressants is similar, and these drugs are reviewed as a group. Selective differences among the drugs are then presented in Table 24-2.

Mechanism

Inhibit neuronal uptake of biogenic amines (norepinephrine, serotonin) into presynaptic endings, blocking a major mechanism for their inactivation, and thereby potentiating their effects. Exert a blocking effect at presynaptic alpha-adrenergic receptor sites to increase release of neurotransmitters, especially norepinephrine and serotonin. The increased receptor activation that results at postsynaptic adrenergic and serotonergic receptor sites gradually decreases their number and sensitivity. The clinical efficacy of these agents is thought to be the result of this *down regulation* of adrenergic and serotonergic receptors. Drugs possess anticholinergic, antihistaminic, and quinidine-like action, and produce peripheral vasodilation and mild hypotension.

Uses

1   Relief of the symptoms of depression, especially of the endogenous types
2   Control of anxiety associated with depressive states (especially doxepin)
3   Treatment of depression in patients with manic–depressive disorders (especially maprotiline)
4   Treatment of childhood enuresis (especially imipramine)
5   Investigational uses include enhanced control of pain (in combination with narcotic analgesics) and prevention of migraine attacks

Dosage

See Table 24-2.

Fate

Well absorbed from the GI tract; peak plasma concentrations attained within 3 hours to 4 hours; widely distributed in the body, and highly bound to plasma proteins (90%–95%); long plasma half-life (several days), and wide individual variation in plasma levels caused by variability in liver metabolic activity; metabolized in the liver, often to therapeutically active compounds (*e.g.,* imipramine to desipramine); hydroxylated metabolites excreted in the urine, along with small amounts of unchanged drug

Common Side-Effects

Sedation; anticholinergic effects (dryness of the mouth, blurred vision, tachycardia, constipation, urinary hesitancy); headache; muscle twitching; and weight gain

In children—nervousness, insomnia, lethargy, and GI disturbances

Significant Adverse Reactions

CNS—anxiety, restlessness, agitation, irritability, fever, insomnia, nightmares, disorientation, confusion, delusions, hypomania, hallucinations, dizziness, tinnitus, numbness and tingling in extremities, ataxia, tremors, extrapyramidal symptoms, paresthesias, seizures

Cardiovascular—orthostatic hypotension, arrhythmias, palpitations, congestive heart failure, infarction, heart block, stroke; EEG changes include prolongation of the P–R and Q–T intervals, reduction of the T-wave and formation of a prominent U-wave.

Allergic—skin rash, pruritus, urticaria, petechiae, photosensitization, edema, fever

GI—nausea, anorexia, vomiting, diarrhea, cramping, epigastric distress, stomatitis

Endocrine—galactorrhea, gynecomastia, testicular and breast swelling, altered libido, delayed ejaculation or impotence, altered blood sugar levels

Table 24-2. Tricyclic–Tetracyclic Antidepressants

Drug	Preparations	Usual Dosage Range	Remarks
Amitriptyline (Amitril, Elavil, Endep, SK-Amitriptyline)	Tablets—10 mg, 25 mg, 50 mg, 75 mg, 100 mg, 150 mg Injection—10 mg/ml	Oral Initially 75 mg to 150 mg/day Maintenance—50 mg to 100 mg/day in divided doses or at bedtime IM 20 mg to 30 mg 4 times/day initially; replace with oral form as soon as possible	Most effective in endogenous depressions, especially those accompanied by anxiety, or in patients over 50 years of age; investigational uses include prevention of migraine headaches and control of chronic pain, especially in combination with potent narcotics; sedative effect is prominent, especially early in therapy; give drug at bedtime to minimize daytime drowsiness; plasma half-life is 20 hours to 40 hours
Amoxapine (Asendin)	Tablets—25 mg, 50 mg, 100 mg, 150 mg	Initially 50 mg 3 times/day; increase to 100 mg 3 times/day on the third day Once effective dose is established, may be given in a single bedtime dose	Used in a wide range of depressions; exhibits a moderate sedative action; clinical effects are usually observed within 7 days; may be used on a once-daily basis at bedtime; highly bound (90%) to plasma proteins, so interactions with other protein-bound drugs can occur; serum half-life is 8 hours, but converted to an active metabolite with a half-life of 30 hours; do not use in children under 16 years of age; most frequent adverse reactions (10%–15%) are sedation, dry mouth, and constipation
Desipramine (Norpramin, Pertofrane)	Tablets—25 mg, 50 mg, 75 mg, 100 mg, 150 mg Capsules—25 mg, 50 mg	25 mg to 50 mg 3 to 4 times/day (maximum 200 mg/day) 25 mg to 100 mg/day in geriatric patients	Active metabolite of imipramine, with essentially the same uses and adverse effect; not recommended in children; slightly lower incidence of sedation and anticholinergic action than imipramine; increased psychomotor activity may occur in first few weeks of therapy; orthostatic hypotension is common early in treatment; caution against rapid position changes; improvement is usually apparent within 1 week to 2 weeks
Doxepin (Adapin, Sinequan)	Capsules—10 mg, 25 mg, 50 mg, 75 mg, 100 mg, 150 mg Oral concentrate—10 mg/ml	10 mg to 50 mg 3 times/day (maximum 300 mg/day) Do not use in children under 12 years	Indicated for relief of depression and anxiety associated with psychotic or psychoneurotic disorders; antianxiety effects occur within several days, but antidepressant action requires several weeks; sedation is marked during initial stage of treatment; effects of alcohol may be enhanced; dilute oral concentrate with 4 oz of water, juice, or milk prior to administration
Imipramine (Janimine, SK-Pramine, Tofranil)	Tablets—10 mg, 25 mg, 50 mg Long-acting capsules (Tofranil-PM)—75 mg, 100 mg, 125 mg, 150 mg Injection—25 mg/2 ml	Depression Oral Initially—100 mg to 200 mg/day Maintenance—50 mg to 150 mg/day IM 100 mg/day in divided doses Enuresis Initially—25 mg to 50 mg/night, orally Alternately 25 mg in midafternoon and 25 mg at bedtime	Used for relief of symptoms of endogenous depressions and for reducing enuresis in children 6 years of age and older; decreases time spent in deep phases of sleep associated with bedwetting; may be administered in a single nightly dose (Tofranil-PM) for depression; do *not* use the PM (pamoate salt) dosage form in enuresis; plasma half-life is 10 hours to 25 hours.

(continued)

Table 24-2. Tricyclic–Tetracyclic Antidepressants (continued)

Drug	Preparations	Usual Dosage Range	Remarks
Maprotiline (Ludiomil)	Tablets—25 mg, 50 mg, 75 mg	Initially—75 mg/day in single or divided doses; adjust to desired maintenance range, usually 75 mg to 225 mg/day (maximum 300 mg/day)	A *tetracyclic* antidepressant with a slightly lower incidence of cardiovascular reactions and fewer anticholinergic side-effects than most tricyclic compounds; may have a rapid response (within 1 wk) in some patients; used in manic–depressive disorders; most common side-effects are dry mouth and drowsiness; not indicated in children under 18 years; reduce dosage in elderly patients, and during prolonged maintenance therapy
Nortriptyline (Aventyl, Pamelor)	Capsules—10 mg, 25 mg, 75 mg Liquid—10 mg/5 ml	25 mg 3 to 4 times a day (maximum 100 mg/day) 30 mg to 50 mg/day in geriatric patients	Primarily effective in endogenous depressions; not recommended in children under 12 years; drug is a metabolite of amitriptyline and is similar to imipramine in most of its pharmacologic effects
Protriptyline (Vivactil)	Tablets—5 mg, 10 mg	5 mg to 10 mg 3 to 4 times/day (maximum 60 mg/day) 5 mg 3 times/day in geriatric patients	Most effective in endogenous depressions in withdrawn and anergic patients; use is associated with less sedation, but drug has more CNS-stimulatory, cardiovascular, and anticholinergic action than other tricyclics; caution in cardiac patients or in those with insominia; not recommended in children under 12 years; last dose should be taken not later than midafternoon, to avoid excessive stimulation at bedtime
Trimipramine (Surmontil)	Capsules—25 mg, 50 mg, 100 mg	Initially—75 mg to 150 mg/day in divided doses. Maintenance—50 mg to 150 mg/day at bedtime 50 mg to 150 mg/day in geriatric patients.	Possesses significant sedative action; similar to amitriptyline in most respects; not recommended in children

Hematologic—blood dyscrasias (agranulocytosis, eosinophilia, leukopenia, thrombocytopenia), bone marrow depression

Other—altered liver function (including jaundice), alopecia, parotid gland enlargement, flushing, sweating, chills, nocturia

Contraindications

Acute recovery phase of myocardial infarction, severe renal or hepatic impairment, concomitant use of MAO inhibitors, narrow-angle glaucoma

Interactions

1 Tricyclics may enhance the effects of other CNS depressants (*e.g.,* alcohol, barbiturates, benzodiazepines, hypnotics, phenothiazines); catecholamines; other adrenergic drugs (*e.g.,* ephedrine, amphetamine); anticholinergics; narcotic analgesics; thyroid drugs; disulfiram; anticoagulants; vasodilators; and centrally acting muscle relaxants.

2 Tricyclics may antagonize the action of antihypertensives (*e.g.,* guanethidine, clonidine); beta-blockers; anticonvulsants (increase incidence of seizures); phenylbutazone; and cholinergic drugs.

3 Effects of tricyclics may be potentiated by phenothiazines, methylphenidate, amphetamines, furazolidone, acetazolamide, MAO inhibitors, and urinary alkalinizers (*e.g.,* sodium bicarbonate).

4 Tricyclics should not be administered within 14 days of MAO inhibitors because hypertension, hyperpyresis, and convulsions can occur.

5 Reserpine and tricyclic antidepressants can result in a "stimulating effect," possibly leading to mania.

6 Therapeutic effects of tricyclics may be reduced by barbiturates (enzyme induction) and urinary acidifiers such as ammonium chloride and ascorbic acid (decreased renal tubular reabsorption), and oral contraceptives.

7 Increased cardiovascular toxic effects may be seen with thyroid drugs, quinidine, or procainamide in combination with tricyclic antidepressants.

▶ **NURSING ALERTS**

▷ 1   Carefully observe severely depressed patient during initial improvement phase. Suicide tendency may be increased as depression and psychomotor retardation are lessened.

▷ 2 Perform baseline blood and liver function studies and an ECG prior to beginning treatment, and monitor vital functions frequently during early phase of therapy, especially in patient receiving high doses.

▷ 3 Note appearance of early signs of cholestatic jaundice (fever, rash, nausea, abdominal pain); if they exist withhold drug, and advise physician.

▷ 4 Be alert for signs of developing blood dyscrasias (fever, sore throat, mucosal ulceration, weakness) and should they appear, discontinue drug upon physician's advice.

▷ 5 Use cautiously in patients with a history of seizure disorders, cardiovascular disease, urinary dysfunction, or narrow-angle glaucoma. Also give cautiously in the presence of pregnancy, lactation, hepatic or renal impairment, prostatic hypertrophy, hyperthryoidism, schizophrenia, or other psychoses.

▷ 6 Warn patients of the dangers of excessive sedation during the early stages of treatment. Caution against driving or operating other machinery.

▷ 7 Instruct patients to change positions gradually because orthostatic hypotension can produce dizziness and syncope. Assist ambulation if necessary.

▷ 8 Withdraw drugs gradually. Abrupt discontinuance can result in nausea, muscle aching, insomnia, and irritability.

▷ 9 Note that concurrent tricyclic therapy with ECT may increase the hazards involved. Use combination only when deemed essential.

▷ 10 Do not administer tricyclic in conjunction with or within 2 weeks of MAO inhibitor therapy unless patient is hospitalized and proper antidotal measures are on hand. Severe adverse reactions, including hypertensive crises, can result.

▶ NURSING CONSIDERATIONS

▷ 1 Advise patient that effects may take several weeks to become manifest, although some newer drugs (*e.g.,* maprotiline) claim a quicker onset of action (5 days–7 days). Stress adherence to the prescribed regimen, and urge avoidance of all other nonprescribed drugs (including over-the-counter medications) while taking tricyclics.

▷ 2 Provide necessary emotional supportive care during drug therapy. Encourage patient to participate in physical and mental activities on a regular basis. Observe carefully for development of side-effects, and should they appear advise physician; dosage adjustment may be necessary.

▷ 3 Tailor dose to patient's needs, if possible. For example, consider single daily bedtime dose of a highly sedating derivative, or morning dosage of a stimulating derivative in an insomniac patient. Reduce dose in elderly and adolescent patients.

▷ 4 Monitor fluid intake and output, and watch for signs of urinary retention or constipation. Dosage adjustment or adjunctive therapy may be necessary (*e.g.,* laxatives, increased fluids).

▷ 5 Advise patient that effects of alcohol and other depressants are augmented by tricyclics, and that loss of motor coordination can occur.

▷ 6 Suggest frequent mouth rinsing or use of gum or candy to alleviate dryness, which is common in early therapy.

▷ 7 Avoid excessive exposure to sunlight with tricyclic drugs because photosensitivity may occur.

▷ 8 Discontinue drugs several days prior to elective surgery, to reduce operative risks (*e.g.,* excessive hypotension or respiratory depression).

▷ 9 Do not use in children under 12 years of age except for treatment of enuresis in children 6 years to 12 years; see Table 24-2.

▷ 10 If no improvement is observed within 8 weeks, discontinue drug and seek alternate therapy.

▷ 11 Monitor blood sugar of diabetics closely during therapy, because both hypo- and hyperglycemia have been reported.

▷ 12 Use lowest effective dose for maintenance therapy, and observe patient carefully for continued clinical progress. Gradually taper dosage after symptoms have been controlled for some time (at least 3 months), but be alert for possible relapse.

▶ trazodone
Desyrel

Trazodone is an effective antidepressant chemically unrelated to tricyclics, tetracyclics, or MAO inhibitors. Its use is associated with minimal anticholinergic and cardiac conductive effects. However, arrhythmogenic incidences have occurred with trazodone, particularly at high doses. Symptomatic improvement is often noted within 1 week.

Mechanism
Selectively inhibits serotonin uptake in the brain; does not elicit CNS stimulation

Uses
1 Treatment of depression, with or without accompanying anxiety

Dosage
Initially, 150 mg/day in divided doses; increase by 50 mg/day increments every 3 to 4 days until optimal effect is attained

Maximum dose is 400 mg/day in outpatients and 600 mg/day in inpatients.

Fate
Well absorbed orally; peak plasma levels occur in 1 hour if taken on an empty stomach and within 2 hours if taken with food. Clinically significant therapeutic response is seen within 2 weeks in 75% of responders.

Common Side-Effects
Drowsiness, dizziness, lightheadedness, fatigue, and dry mouth

Significant Adverse Reactions

(See also general discussion of tricyclic antidepressants)

Cardiovascular—hypotension, syncope, tachycardia

CNS—confusion, headache, insomnia, nervousness, disorientation, reduced concentration, malaise

Autonomic—blurred vision, constipation

GI—nausea, vomiting

Neurologic—incoordination, paresthesias, tremors

Other—allergic skin conditions; myalgia; sinus congestion; tinnitus; weight gain; tired, itching eyes; sweating; bradycardia; dyspnea; decreased libido

Interactions

See general discussion of tricyclic antidepressants. In addition:

1 Increased serum levels of digoxin and phenytoin have been reported with trazodone therapy.

▶ **NURSING ALERTS**

See general discussion of tricyclic antidepressants. In addition:

▷ 1 Recognize that although the drug is claimed to produce few clinically significant ECG changes, such changes have been observed in some patients; thus, as with all antidepressants, use trazodone cautiously in patients with cardiovascular disease.

▷ 2 Perform regular white blood cell and differential counts during therapy. Discontinue drug if WBC or absolute neutrophil counts fall below normal.

▷ 3 Do not administer drug concurrently with ECT or during initial recovery phase following myocardial infarction.

▶ **NURSING CONSIDERATIONS**

See general discussion of tricyclic antidepressants. In addition:

▷ 1 Administer drug during or shortly following a meal or snack, because total drug absorption is greater in the presence of food in the stomach.

▷ 2 Note that trazodone is not recommended in children under 18.

II Monoamineoxidase (MAO)

Inhibitors

Isocarboxazid	Tranylcypromine
Phenelzine	

Drugs that can form stable complexes with and therefore inhibit the action of the enzyme monoamineoxidase (MAO) have been employed for many years as antidepressants. MAO is an enzyme system that catalyzes the deamination, or inactivation, of several naturally occurring biogenic amines, most notably norepinephrine, epinephrine, and serotonin, in numerous body tissues, especially the liver, kidney, intestines, and nerve endings. It is found within the mitochondria of cells comprising these tissues, and its principal role in neuronal transmission is the regulation of *intra*cellular neurotransmitter levels. Inhibition of MAO in adrenergic nerve endings increases the amounts of free norepinephrine available for release after the arrival of a nerve impulse. By blocking a major means for intraneuronal catecholamine (and serotonin) breakdown, MAO inhibitors can increase the synaptic actions of these amine neurohormones, thereby alleviating the biochemical deficit thought to be present in depression.

Although MAO inhibitors were the first clinically effective antidepressants to be introduced, their relatively low therapeutic effectiveness coupled with their high toxicity have severely restricted their usefulness in favor of the more effective and less toxic tricyclic antidepressants. Today, MAO inhibitors are employed principally in a hospital setting in patients refractory to or intolerant of the tricyclics. Their use in outpatients must be carefully and continually monitored, and necessary precautions must be taken to avoid precipitation of serious adverse reactions and drug interactions.

These agents require several weeks for optimal antidepressant action to develop. Likewise, their effects persist for up to 2 weeks following termination of therapy, because they irreversibly inhibit MAO, requiring the synthesis of new enzyme for the restoration of function. This prolonged duration of action makes it difficult to maintain a stable level of symptomatic improvement without the danger of serious toxicity. Moreover, when severe untoward reactions do occur, they may persist for a disturbingly long period of time. It is imperative, then, that both clinicians and patients be fully aware of the potential hazards associated with MAO inhibitor therapy.

There are four currently available MAO inhibitors, of which three are indicated as alternate drugs for the treatment of severe depression resistant to tricyclic therapy. The fourth MAO inhibitor, pargyline, is not indicated for depression, but is occasionally used as an antihypertensive agent and is considered in Chapter 31.

Mechanism

Inhibit the monoamineoxidase enzyme system by forming an irreversible (stable) complex with the enzyme; consequently, intraneuronal breakdown of catecholamines and serotonin is inhibited, and their concentration rises in various body tissues, including the CNS, heart, blood, and intestine. The increased availability of these neurohormones (especially norepinephrine) in certain brain areas is believed to be responsible for relieving symptoms of depression. Likewise, increased neurohormone availability in other body tissues is thought to underlie many of the toxic reactions elicited by these agents. These drugs also inhibit hepatic microsomal drug-metabolizing enzymes, thereby prolonging the action of many other drugs.

Uses

1 Management of severe endogenous, exogenous (atypical), or reactive depressions resistant to treatment with tricyclic antidepressants, ECT, or other adjunctive psychotherapy

2 Control of the depressive phase of manic–depressive psychoses

Dosage
See Table 24-3.

Fate
Readily absorbed orally; enzyme inhibition occurs rapidly, but clinical effects take several weeks to develop, except with tranylcypromine (10 days–14 days); termination of drug effect following administration of irreversible inhibitors (isocarboxazid, phenelzine) depends largely on regeneration of MAO enzyme, a process taking several weeks; tranylcypromine effects decline within 3 days to 5 days following discontinuation of therapy; drugs are metabolized in the liver and excreted in the urine as metabolites and some unchanged drug.

Common Side-Effects
Orthostatic hypotension, dizziness, weakness, fatigue, jitteriness, hyperactivity, insomnia, GI disturbances, headache, disturbances in cardiac rate and rhythm, dry mouth, blurred vision, and hyperhidrosis

Significant Adverse Reactions
CNS—vertigo, tremors, hypomania, euphoria, confusion, memory impairment, drowsiness, ataxia, excessive sweating, delirium, hallucinations, convulsions

Autonomic/Cardiovascular—dysuria, incontinence, impotence, palpitations, edema, and weight gain

Hematologic/Dermatologic—leukopenia, hypochromic anemia, skin rash, hepatocellular jaundice

Other—anorexia, peripheral neuritis, photosensitivity reactions, nystagmus, sodium retention, hypoglycemia, galactorrhea, glaucoma, optic damage

Overdose—restlessness, tachycardia, hypotension, respiratory depression, confusion, incoherence, convulsions, shock

Contraindications
Children under 16 years of age, congestive heart failure, liver disease, pheochromocytoma, hyperthyroidism, hypertension, cardiovascular or cerebrovascular disease, and elderly or debilitated patients

Interactions
1 Effects of sympathomimetic drugs (*e.g.,* amphetamines, catecholamines, l-dopa, ephedrine, phenylephrine, methylphenidate) may be potentiated, resulting in severe hypertension, headache, and possibly cerebrovascular hemorrhage.
2 Hypertensive reactions can occur in patients taking MAO inhibitors who ingest foods containing tyramine, a pressor substance (*e.g.,* cheeses, sour cream, beer, red wines, yeasts, yogurt, pickled herring, chicken livers, aged meats, fermented sausages, tenderizers, licorice), as well as caffeine and chocolate.
3 Concurrent use of MAO inhibitors and tricyclic antidepressants (or within 10 days of each other) can result in marked hypertension, convulsions, fever, sweating, delirium, tremor, circulatory collapse, and coma, although some tricyclic antidepressants have been employed safely in conjunction with MAO inhibitors.
4 MAO inhibitors may increase the toxic effects of barbiturates and phenothiazines by decreasing their metabolism by the liver.
5 Effects of antihypertensive drugs may be potentiated by MAO inhibitors (increased orthostatic hypotension). However, severe *hypertension* can occur with parenteral use of reserpine or guanethidine, due to release of large amounts of catecholamines.
6 Hypotension, respiratory arrest, shock, and coma can occur if MAO inhibitors are used in combination with CNS depressants such as alcohol, anesthetics, narcotics (especially meperidine), and sedative–hypnotics.
7 Increased hypoglycemic effects have occurred with combined use of MAO inhibitors and either insulin or oral hypoglycemics.

Table 24-3. Monoamineoxidase Inhibitors

Drug	Preparations	Usual Dosage Range	Remarks
Isocarboxazid (Marplan)	Tablets—10 mg	Initially—30 mg/day; reduce to maintenance levels (usually 10 mg to 20 mg/day) as soon as possible	Administer with meals to reduce gastric upset; adjust dosage critically, based upon careful patient observation; note that although therapeutic effects may take several weeks to develop, toxic interactions can occur within hours; may be administered either as a single dose or in divided doses
Phenelzine (Nardil)	Tablets—15 mg	Initially—15 mg 3 times/day; reduce slowly to maintenance levels, usually 15 mg every 1 to 2 days	Effective in moderate to severe depressive states, especially accompanied by anxiety and agitation; do not exceed 75 mg a day
Tranylcypromine (Parnate)	Tablets—10 mg	Initially—20 mg to 30 mg/day; reduce to 10 mg to 20 mg/day as needed With concurrent electroconvulsive therapy, 10 mg 1 to 2 times/day	Incidence of hypertensive reactions is higher than with other MAO-inhibitors; latency of therapeutic effect is generally shorter (3–5 days) than with other similar drugs; it is a structural analog of amphetamine and probably exerts a direct receptor activation, as well as MAO inhibition

8 Muscle-relaxing action of succinylcholine may be increased because MAO inhibitors interfere with plasma pseudocholinesterase, the enzyme that inactivates succinylcholine.

9 MAO inhibitors reduce convulsive seizure threshold and may reduce the efficacy of antiepileptic drugs.

10 Effects of anticholinergic, antihistamine, and antiparkinsonian drugs may be potentiated by MAO inhibitors, which decrease their rate of metabolism.

▶ NURSING ALERTS

▷ 1 Carefully explain to patient the dangers associated with use of MAO inhibitors, especially the possibility of hypertensive crisis. Advise patient to note and report early signs of an impending hypertensive reaction (headache, palpitations, neck stiffness, sweating, nausea, photophobia).

▷ 2 Advise patients to rise from a supine position gradually, because orthostatic hypotension is common and may result in dizziness and fainting. Avoid prolonged standing in one position, hot showers or baths, or anything that may cause a fall in blood pressure.

▷ 3 Use cautiously in patients with epilepsy, diabetes, depression accompanying drug or alcohol addiction, chronic brain syndromes, history of anginal attacks, impaired renal function, and during pregnancy and lactation.

▷ 4 Be alert for development of hypomania, especially in patients whose hyperkinetic symptoms have been masked by the concurrent depression. Relief of depression by MAO inhibitors can precipitate agitation, delusion, and exaggeration of feelings. Use of sedatives is indicated.

▷ 5 Note development of hepatic complications, marked by jaundice-like reactions (*e.g.,* rash, abdominal pain, pruritus, yellowing of skin). Discontinuation of the drug is advisable. Periodic liver function tests should be performed in all patients on MAO inhibitor drugs.

▷ 6 Instruct patients to report immediately any visual disturbances, especially changes in red–green color vision, because these are often the initial signs of drug-induced ocular damage.

▷ 7 Caution patients, especially those with a history of heart disease, to avoid exertion. MAO inhibitors suppress anginal pain and may therefore mask the warning signs of an ischemic attack.

▷ 8 Remember that toxic effects and drug interactions with MAO inhibitors may occur up to several weeks after termination of therapy. Advise patient to avoid all foods and drugs that may be hazardous for at least several weeks after the last dose of MAO inhibitor has been taken.

▷ 9 Avoid rapid withdrawal of the drug, especially after prolonged or high dosage, because excitability, hallucinations, and possibly severe depression can occur.

▶ NURSING CONSIDERATIONS

▷ 1 Determine pretreatment blood pressure level, and monitor the patient's pressure repeatedly during therapy.

▷ 2 Perform baseline liver function studies and blood cell counts prior to initiation of therapy and at regular intervals thereafter.

▷ 3 Monitor intake–output ratio, and note signs of edema and weight gain. Advise physician of any changes because renal impairment may result in greatly increased toxicity.

▷ 4 Observe diabetic patients carefully for signs of hypoglycemia, and adjust dosage of insulin or oral antidiabetics as necessary.

▷ 5 Consider discontinuing MAO inhibitors at least 1 week before elective surgery to reduce the danger of interaction with anesthetic agents.

▷ 6 Suggest use of candy or gum and frequent mouth rinsing to relieve dryness.

▷ 7 If no significant clinical response has occurred within 4 weeks, re-evaluate patient and consider alternate forms of treatment.

▷ 8 Impress upon patient the necessity of *closely* following the prescribed drug regimen and diet to minimize the danger of untoward reactions.

▷ *Dietary precaution*

▷ 1 The following foods should be avoided by patients taking MAO inhibitors, due to the danger of hypertensive reactions resulting from the tyramine content of the food: aged cheeses, sour cream, imported beers and ales, red wines (especially chianti), yogurt, yeasts, pickled herring, aged meats and tenderizers, and chicken livers. Chocolate and caffeine have also been implicated in blood pressure elevations with MAO inhibitors.

Summary. Antidepressants

Drug	Preparations	Usual Dosage Range
Tricyclic–tetracyclic derivatives	See Table 24-2	
Trazodone (Desyrel)	Tablets—50 mg, 100 mg	Initially, 150 mg/day in divided doses; increase by 50 mg/day every 3 days to 4 days until optimal effect is achieved; maximum dose is 400 mg/day
Monoamine oxidase inhibitors	See Table 24-3	

Epilepsy is a chronic CNS disorder estimated to afflict between 0.5% and 1.5% of the population. Although attempts have been made to classify the epilepsies according to the type of seizure manifestation, complete agreement is lacking. Certain characteristics, however, such as EEG alterations and localized or generalized muscular hyperactivity can aid in distinguishing among the major types of epilepsies and can assist the physician in making the proper diagnosis and prescribing appropriate drug therapy.

Several agents (including barbiturates and diazepam) that are employed in the emergency control of acute convulsive states resulting from trauma, hyperthermia of infection, or drug overdosage have already been reviewed. The drugs to be considered here are used primarily to treat the various forms of epilepsy and therefore may be regarded, in most cases, as specific antiepileptic agents.

Most forms of epilepsy are idiopathic (without demonstrable cause). Manifestations may include generalized tonic–clonic seizures (grand mal); cessation of activity or absence seizures (petit mal); or partial seizures having a local origin and accompanied by bizarre actions and impairment of consciousness (psychomotor seizures). Less frequently, focal partial seizures involving motor disturbances (Jacksonian seizures) and generalized atonic, akinetic, or myclonic seizures are observed. Although many theories have attempted to explain the etiology of the various seizure patterns, the exact cause of most epileptic attacks remains unknown. A general review of common seizure types and their appropriate management are illustrated in Table 25-1.

Anticonvulsant drugs are effective in controlling the various manifestations of the epilepsies, but critical dosage regulation is of paramount importance for optimal seizure control. Drugs and doses must be individualized according to a particular patient's needs. Some antiepileptic drugs are not only ineffective in certain types of seizure disorders, they may actually worsen certain aspects of these conditions. Successful therapy, therefore, depends upon accurate diagnosis, careful selection of drugs, and critical adjustment of dosage.

Therapy usually is initiated with a single agent, but complete control of most seizure types generally requires addition of a second and often a third drug. Frequent dosage alterations or too-rapid shifting among anticonvulsant drugs should be avoided. The essential requirement of any antiepileptic drug is that it control the seizures without causing undue sedation and with minimal adverse drug effects. While many agents possess significant anticonvulsant activity at doses associated with disabling side-effects, the clinically useful antiepileptic drugs provide adequate control of most seizure types without subjecting the patient to frequent and debilitating adverse reactions. Although the drugs do not *cure* the affliction, they do allow the epileptic patient to function in a productive manner.

Stabilization of epileptic patients is a difficult task in most cases, and once attained, patients should be advised of the dangers inherent in altering the prescribed drug regimen or in subjecting themselves to physical and emotional stresses that might compromise their stable conditions. Patients should be taught to observe their conditions and to report any unusual symptoms that occur during therapy,

Table 25-1. Review of Seizure Classification and Management

Seizure Type	Usual Age at Onset	EEG Pattern	Effective Drugs
Tonic–clonic (Grand Mal)	Any age (generally before 20)	Multifocal spikes (storm pattern)	Phenytoin Primidone Carbamazepine Phenobarbital
Simple absence (Petit Mal)	3 years to 10 years	3/sec, spike–wave	Ethosuximide Trimethadione Valproic acid Clonazepam
Complex partial motor seizures (Psychomotor)	Young adults	Temporal lobe discharges	Carbamazepine Primidone Phenacemide Phenytoin
Focal motor or sensory seizures	Any age	Unilateral spike and/or wave	Carbamazepine Phenytoin
Generalized myclonic jerks	5 years to 20 years	Mixed spike and slow wave	Phenobarbital Clonazepam
Atonic/akinetic seizures	1 year to 5 years	Slow spike–wave (petit mal variant)	Diazepam Clonazepam
Status epilepticus	Any age	Diffuse, continuous spiking	Diazepam Phenobarbital Phenytoin

because these may indicate early manifestations of serious toxicity. Drugs should be discontinued *gradually* whenever necessary, and changes in medication should be accomplished slowly over several weeks. Abrupt discontinuance or alteration in drug therapy can precipitate *status epilepticus,* a series of rapid, repetitive seizures that may be fatal unless terminated quickly.

I Anticonvulsant Barbiturates

Mephobarbital　　　　　Phenobarbital
Metharbital

Although all barbiturates can abolish seizure activity at doses sufficient to produce anesthesia, only three barbiturates, phenobarbital, metharbital and mephobarbital, appear to be particularly suited for chronic treatment of epilepsy. They are effective at nonsedating doses, exert a prolonged action, and tend to be well tolerated during extended drug therapy.

Mechanism
Reduce excitability of nerve cells by increasing their firing threshold; block the active transport of ions across the nerve cell membrane

Uses
1　Infantile spasms
2　Generalized tonic–clonic seizures (grand mal); used alone in infants and young children, and most often in combination with phenytoin in adults
3　Generalized myclonic jerks

4　Complex absences with autonomic manifestations
5　Status epilepticus (IV)

Dosage
See Table 25-2.

Fate
Well absorbed orally; onset following oral administration ranges from 30 minutes (phenobarbital) to 2 hours (metharbital); effects are evident in 10 minutes to 15 minutes with IV injection; duration lasts from 6 hours to 10 hours; partly metabolized in the liver, and excreted both as metabolites and unchanged drug in the urine

Common Side-Effects
Lethargy, dizziness, and irritability

Significant Adverse Reactions
Nausea, vomiting diarrhea, skin rash (2% of patients), muscle and joint pain, respiratory depression, paradoxical excitation (especially in children and elderly), and megaloblastic anemia

Contraindications
Latent or manifest porphyria, respiratory obstruction

Interactions
See Chapter 20.

▶ **NURSING ALERTS**
(See also Chap. 20)
▷ 1　Note that drugs may impair mental and physical abilities required for performance of many tasks (*e.g.,* driving).

Table 25-2. Anticonvulsant Barbiturates

Drug	Preparations	Usual Dosage Range	Remarks
Mephobarbital (Mebaral)	Tablets—32 mg, 50 mg, 100 mg, 200 mg	Adults—400 mg to 600 mg/day Children (over 5 yr)—32 mg to 64 mg 3 to 4 times/day; (under 5 yr) 16 mg to 32 mg 3 to 4 times day	Similar to phenobarbital in most respects, producing somewhat less sedation; largely converted to phenobarbital within 24 hours; used as a single daily dose at bedtime for nocturnal seizures; withdraw slowly when necessary, and reduce dose of other antiepileptics when added to the regimen (Schedule IV)
Metharbital (Gemonil)	Tablets—100 mg	Adults—Initially 100 mg 1 to 3 times/day; adjust to optimal level Children—5 to 15 mg/kg/day	Less effective than phenobarbital, and possesses somewhat greater sedative action; usually used in combination with other antiepileptic drugs for grand mal, petit mal, myclonic or mixed seizures (Schedule III)
Phenobarbital (various manufacturers)	Tablets—8 mg, 15 mg, 16 mg, 30 mg, 32 mg, 65 mg, 100 mg Capsules—16 mg, 65 mg Elixir—20 mg/5 ml Drops—16 mg/ml Injection—30 mg/ml, 60 mg/ml, 65 mg/ml, 130 mg/ml	Oral Adults—50 mg to 100 mg 2 to 3 times/day Children—Initially, 4 mg/kg to 6 mg/kg/day for 7 to 10 days; adjust to blood level of 10 mcg/ml to 15 mcg/ml IV Initially, 30 mg to 130 mg at rate of 30 mg to 60 mg/min (maximum dose 600 mg) IM Adults—200 mg to 300 mg; repeat in 6 hours Children—3 mg/kg to 5 mg/kg/dose	Very effective alone for treatment of grand mal (especially in children) and as part of the drug regimen in most other forms of epilepsy; also used IV or IM for status epilepticus and other acute convulsive states; following IV injection, 15 minutes or more may be required to attain peak CNS concentration. Thus, give drug *intermittently,* even though convulsions persist. Continuous injection can result in excessive CNS levels of drug after convulsions have ceased, possibly leading to respiratory depression. Solutions should be prepared in Sterile Water for Injection and should not be used if not completely clear after 5 minutes of mixing. Inject drug within 30 minutes after preparation of solution. Drowsiness is common in early stages of therapy but diminishes with continued use. Frequency of IV administration is determined by patient's response. Discontinue drug as soon as desired response is obtained (Schedule IV)

▷ 2 Use cautiously in patients with pulmonary, hepatic, or renal disease, status asthmaticus, hyperthyroidism, diabetes, and in elderly or debilitated patients.

▷ 3 Be aware that drugs may reduce the levels of vitamin K-dependent clotting factors produced in the liver, resulting in neonatal hemorrhage. Vitamin K can be given prophylactically at birth.

▷ 4 Do not administer IV in acute convulsive states without adequate resuscitative measures immediately at hand. Give slowly and monitor vital signs closely.

▶ **NURSING CONSIDERATIONS**
(See also Chap. 20)

▷ 1 Recognize that drugs may increase vitamin D requirements by stepping up its metabolism, occasionally leading to rickets or osteomalacia with prolonged use.

▷ 2 Be aware that prolonged use, even in rather low doses, can lead to tolerance and habituation. Watch for signs of tolerance and if necessary, withdraw drug *slowly* to avoid possibility of delirium, tremors, and convulsions.

▷ 3 Carefully weigh benefit *versus* risk in pregnant women. Although a small incidence of fetal damage has been reported with these drugs, discontinuing them may result in increased seizure activity and fetal anoxia.

▷ 4 Be alert for occurrence of paradoxical excitatory reactions, especially in the elderly and young children.

▷ 5 Note that metharbital is a Schedule III drug and that phenobarbital and mephobarbital are Schedule IV drugs (see Appendix).

II Primidone (Mysoline)

Although not a true barbiturate, primidone is structurally related to phenobarbital and has a similar profile of action.

It is metabolized to phenobarbital and phenylethylmalon-amide, both active anticonvulsants.

Mechanism

Not established, but probably similar to phenobarbital

Uses

(May be given alone or with other anticonvulsants)
1 Grand mal seizures
2 Psychomotor seizures
3 Complex partial motor seizures (Jacksonian)
4 Benign familial (essential) tremor (investigational use)

Dosage

Adults: Initially 250 mg/day; increase by 250-mg increments to optimal level (usually 250 mg 3 to 4 times/day); maximum 2 g/day

Children (under 8 yr): 500 mg to 750 mg/day in divided doses

Fate

Well absorbed orally; peak serum levels attained in 3 hours to 4 hours; prolonged action caused by conversion to active metabolites; excreted through kidney, approximately one fourth as unchanged drug

Common Side-Effects

Lethargy, ataxia, vertigo, and irritability

Significant Adverse Reactions

Nausea, anorexia, vomiting, fatigue, allergic reactions, severe skin rash (macropapular and morbilliform), lymph gland enlargement, megaloblastic anemia (rare), visual disturbances, impotence, personality disorders, drowsiness, blood dyscrasias (leukopenia, thrombocytopenia), and systemic lupus-like reaction

Contraindications

Latent or manifest porphyria

Interactions

See Anticonvulsant Barbiturates

▶ NURSING ALERTS

(See also Anticonvulsant Barbiturates)

▷ 1 Observe for early signs of lymph gland enlargement or appearance of fever, sore throat, bruising, and weakness—possible indications of blood dyscrasias.

▷ 2 Caution patient to avoid hazardous activities during early stages of therapy because incidence of drowsiness is quite high.

▷ 3 Watch for symptoms of folic acid deficiency (drug may impair folate absorption) such as anemia, mental dysfunction, neuropathy, and psychiatric disturbances. Use of folic acid (15 mg/day) or vitamin B_6 may be necessary to prevent megaloblastic anemia.

▷ 4 Consider administration of prophylactic vitamin K one month prior to and during delivery to prevent neonatal hemorrhage because drug may reduce production of vitamin K-dependent clotting factors in neonatal liver.

▶ NURSING CONSIDERATIONS

▷ 1 Watch for development of hyperexcitability, especially in children and elderly patients.

▷ 2 Note signs of early overdosage (e.g., incoordination, slurred speech, blurring of vision) and gradually decrease dose.

▷ 3 Make dosage adjustments gradually and readjust dosage of other antiepileptics if primidone is added to the regimen.

▷ 4 Recognize that patients allergic to barbiturates will probably be allergic to primidone.

▷ 5 During prolonged therapy, perform a complete blood count at 6-month intervals.

III Hydantoins

Ethotoin   Phenytoin
Mephenytoin

The hydantoin group of antiepileptic agents generally are the most effective drugs for the treatment of grand mal seizures, and can be used in the control of psychomotor epilepsy as well. These drugs, unlike barbiturates, are not CNS depressants and do not interfere with normal sensory function. There are three currently marketed hydantoins, of which phenytoin is the most frequently prescribed.

Mechanism

Inhibit spread of seizure activity to neurons surrounding seizure focus in the motor cortex by raising the threshold of excitability of these neurons; promote sodium efflux from neuronal cells, thereby blocking development of post-tetanic potentiation, which prevents focal seizure activity from spreading to adjacent cortical areas; may shorten duration of afterdischarges and increase release of GABA, an inhibitory neurotransmitter in the central nervous system.

Uses

1 Grand mal seizures (may be combined with primidone or carbamazepine)
2 Focal, Jacksonian, or psychomotor seizures, either alone or in combination with primidone
3 Alcohol withdrawal syndrome
4 Trigeminal neuralgia
5 Cardiac arrhythmias (especially ventricular arrhythmias due to digitalis intoxication—see Chap. 30)
6 Status epilepticus and seizures during neurosurgery (IV) or IM).

Dosage

See Table 25-3.

Fate

(Discussion applies to phenytoin, the only hydantoin whose pharmacokinetics has been extensively studied)

Generally slowly absorbed orally; rate and extent of phenytoin absorption varies widely among the different available

Table 25-3. Hydantoins

Drug	Preparations	Usual Dosage Range	Remarks
Ethotoin (Peganone)	Tablets—250 mg, 500 mg	Adults—250 mg 4 times/day initially; increase to optimal levels (usually 2 g–3 g/day) Children—750 mg/day initially; Maintenance 500 mg to 1000 mg/day based on age and weight	Administer with food, and begin therapy at small dose levels; compatible with most other anticonvulsants (dosage must be adjusted) except phenacemide (danger of paranoid reactions); less effective than phenytoin, but somewhat less toxic as well; not used as an antiarrhythmic
Mephenytoin (Mesantoin)	Tablets—100 mg	Adults—Initial dose 50 mg to 100 mg/day; increase gradually to optimal levels (usual range 200 mg–600 mg/day) Children—100 mg to 400 mg/day based on age, weight, and severity of seizures	Most toxic of the hydantoins; reserved for patients refractory to less toxic anticonvulsants; may be useful in Jacksonian seizures; possesses a strong sedative action; blood counts should be performed every 2 weeks to 4 weeks; more rapidly absorbed than other hydantoins with an onset of action in 30 minutes
Phenytoin (Dilantin Infatab, Dilantin-30 Pediatric, Dilantin-125) Phenytoin Sodium, Extended (Dilantin Kapseals) Phenytoin Sodium, Prompt (Diphenylan, Ditan) Phenytoin Sodium, Parenteral (Dilantin)	Chewable tablets—50 mg Suspension—30 mg, 125 mg/5 ml Capsules—30 mg, 100 mg Capsules—30 mg, 100 mg Injection—50 mg/ml	Oral Adults—Initially, 100 mg 3 times/day; usual range is 300 mg to 400 mg/day Children—Initially 5 mg/kg/day in 2 or 3 divided doses Usual maintenance range is 4 to 8 mg/kg/day in children under 6 Parenteral IV Status Epilepticus 150 mg to 250 mg; repeat in 30 minutes with 100 mg to 150 mg if necessary (Children—250 mg/m² body surface area) Arrhythmias 100 mg every 5 minutes until arrhythmia is abolished (maximum 1000 mg) IM Neurosurgery 100 mg to 200 mg every 4 hours during surgery and postoperative period (maximum 1000 mg/day)	*Extended* phenytoin sodium capsules (Dilantin) can be used on a more convenient once daily basis when seizure control has been established with divided doses initially due to their slower dissolution rate; do not administer IM in status epilepticus, because sufficient plasma levels cannot be attained due to erratic absorption; an IM dose 50% greater than the oral dose is necessary to maintain stable plasma levels; margin between the effective and toxic IV dose is very small; administer slowly, and carefully monitor vital signs; effective against digitalis-induced arrhythmias (see Chap. 30); phenytoin is also available in combination with phenobarbital (Dilantin-Pb capsules)

preparations, the sodium salt being the best absorbed; bioavailability also differs markedly (20%–90%) among products of different manufacturers; oral phenytoin sodium *extended* (Dilantin) attains peak plasma levels in 5 hours to 6 hours; phenytoin sodium *prompt* (other clinically available preparations) achieves peak serum levels in 2 hours to 3 hours; erratically absorbed following IM injection; peak blood levels occur at varying times up to 24 hours and are significantly lower than blood levels obtained with oral or IV administration; highly bound (85%–95%) to plasma proteins; metabolized in the liver and excreted largely as conjugated metabolites in the urine; elimination half-life ranges from 8 hours to 60 hours

Common Side-Effects

Sluggishness, ataxia, nystagmus, confusion, slurred speech; less commonly—dizziness, insomnia, nervousness, fatigue, and irritability

Significant Adverse Reactions

GI—nausea, vomiting, diarrhea, abdominal pain, dysphagia

CNS—headache, depression, tremors, behavioral disturbances

Dermatologic—skin rashes (morbilliform, maculopapular, scarlatiniform), urticaria, keratosis, hirsutism, lupus erythematosus, exfoliative dermatitis (rare)

Hematopoietic—blood dyscrasias, anemias, lymphadenopathy, bone marrow depression

Other—gingival hyperplasia (20%–30% incidence, especially children), periodontal infection, polyarthropathy, hepatitis, liver damage, alopecia, hyperglycemia, edema, chest pain, numbness, photophobia, pulmonary fibrosis, osteomalacia

Contraindications

Hematologic disorders, hepatic dysfunction, incomplete heart block; IV phenytoin is contraindicated in sinus bradycardia, sinoatrial block, second and third degree A–V block, and Adams–Stokes syndrome

Interactions

1 Phenytoin may increase the effects of oral anticoagulants, antihypertensives, thyroid hormones, sedatives and hypnotics, propranolol, and methotrexate.
2 Phenytoin may diminish the effects of corticosteroids, oral contraceptives, disopyramide, quinidine, digitalis glycosides, and tetracyclines (by increasing their liver metabolism).
3 Phenytoin effects may be increased by coumarin anticoagulants, cimetidine, chloramphenicol, disulfiram, isoniazid, salicylates, pyrazolones, minor tranquilizers, phenothiazines, methylphenidate, estrogens, and sulfonamides. These drugs can slow phenytoin metabolism.
4 Phenytoin effects may be diminished by alcohol, antacids, barbiturates (clinically significant interactions unlikely between antiepileptic barbiturates and phenytoin), antihistamines, calcium, carbamazepine, oxacillin, and folic acid.
5 Tricyclic antidepressants may precipitate seizures, so phenytoin dosage should be adjusted accordingly. Valproic acid and phenytoin may result in breakthrough seizures.
6 Phenytoin can impair the absorption of furosemide.
7 Concomitant administration of phenytoin and dopamine may lead to hypotension and bradycardia.

▶ NURSING ALERTS

▷ 1 Perform periodic blood counts and urinalyses during hydantoin therapy, and be alert for early symptoms of developing blood dyscrasias (*e.g.,* fever, sore throat, mucosal ulceration, malaise) or hepatic dysfunction (dark urine, abdominal cramps, jaundice).
▷ 2 Discontinue drugs if a skin rash appears. If rash is marked by scaling or desquamation, do not re-institute therapy with these drugs. Otherwise, drugs may be resumed when symptoms disappear.
▷ 3 Observe for lymph node enlargement and if present, consider placing the patient on alternate antiepileptic medication.
▷ 4 Be alert for nystagmus, confusion, ataxia, dysarthria, and unresponsive pupils—signs of overdosage. Readjust dosage carefully.
▷ 5 Consider benefit *versus* risk ratio in pregnant women. Although fetal damage has been reported (cleft palate), discontinuance of therapy may precipitate status epilepticus with resulting hypoxia to the fetus. Carefully weigh all factors when using these drugs during pregnancy.
▷ 6 Do not alter dosage or discontinue medication abruptly, as convulsions may occur. Do not use hydantoins in seizures due to hypoglycemia.
▷ 7 Do not interchange brands of phenytoin unless serum concentrations are carefully monitored, because bioavailability among different preparations varies markedly (see *Fate*). Note that *only Dilantin* products are

approved for once daily use due to prolonged absorption. All other phenytoin products are classified as *prompt* acting and are used 2 to 4 times a day.
▷ 8 Use carefully in elderly or debilitated patients and in the presence of impaired hepatic or renal function, hypotension, myocardial insufficiency, or impending heart failure.
▷ 9 Recognize that hydantoins may interfere with folic acid availability. Observe for signs of folic acid deficiency (anemia, neuropathy, psychiatric disorders, mental dysfunction), and consider supplemental folic acid as needed. Note, however, that additional folic acid can increase phenytoin metabolism and may increase seizure frequency. Adjust dose accordingly.
▷ 10 When administering IV, give *slowly* to avoid bradycardia and hypotension, and monitor blood pressure, ECG, and respiration. Have appropriate antidotal measures on hand (*e.g.,* vasopressors, oxygen, respiratory aids).
▷ 11 Stress oral hygiene, regular gum massage, and frequent brushing to minimize the severity of gingival hyperplasia, especially in children where the incidence is much higher than in adults.

▶ NURSING CONSIDERATIONS

▷ 1 Consider use of vitamin K prophylactically during latter stages of pregnancy because drugs can reduce levels of vitamin K-dependent clotting factors produced by the liver.
▷ 2 Monitor the patient's blood sugar levels because drugs may inhibit insulin release, leading to hyperglycemia. Carefully adjust hydantoin dosage in the diabetic.
▷ 3 Note that hydantoins are ineffective in petit mal seizures and may worsen the symptoms. Combined drug therapy is indicated when mixed seizure types are present.
▷ 4 Advise patient that excessive use of alcohol or other CNS depressants may reduce the efficacy of hydantoins.
▷ 5 Counsel patient on the importance of proper diet, avoidance of fatigue, stress, or illness, and maintenance of prescribed dosage regimen for good seizure control.
▷ 6 Individualize dosage schedule in each patient to minimize toxicity. In some patients, peak blood levels after full dosage may be associated with transient signs of CNS toxicity (*e.g.,* ataxia, nystagmus, confusion), and these adverse effects may be reduced by multiple smaller doses.
▷ 7 Use parenteral solutions immediately after mixing, and do not add to any IV infusion because solubility may be altered by *p*H differences. Shake suspension thoroughly to obtain correct dosage. Avoid continuous infusion of hydantoin solutions.
▷ 8 Administer slowly IV (50 mg/min into running IV). Do not give IM in status epilepticus because sufficient plasma levels cannot be attained in most cases.
▷ 9 Follow each IV injection by an injection of sterile saline through the same needle or catheter to avoid local venous irritation caused by alkalinity of the drug solution.

▷ 10 Inform patient that hydantoins may harmlessly color urine pink to reddish-brown.
▷ 11 Give oral drugs with meals if possible to minimize gastric irritation because drug is strongly alkaline.
▷ 12 Provide emotional support to the patient. Instruct family members and close associates in the proper methods for dealing with a seizure episode. Urge patient to carry an identification card with pertinent medical information.

▷ *Dietary precaution*
▷ 1 Ensure adequate intake of vitamin D-containing foods to prevent hypocalcemia, because hydantoins can accelerate metabolism of this vitamin.

IV Oxazolidinediones

Paramethadione   Trimethadione

The oxazolidinediones are effective drugs for the control of petit mal seizures, but elicit a rather high incidence of untoward reactions. They are largely reserved for patients intolerant of or unresponsive to other less toxic agents. The two currently available drugs, trimethadione and paramethadione, differ only slightly in their pharmacologic properties; thus, they are reviewed together, and are then listed separately in Table 25-4.

Mechanism
Complex and incompletely understood; prolong the recovery period of postsynaptic neurons in those CNS systems (primarily thalamocortical) where repetitive discharges produce absence attacks through a negative feedback mechanism; other central effects include elevating the threshold for seizure discharge in the thalamus and interference with the propagation of seizure activity from a cortical focus to the thalamus; possess little sedative or hypnotic action, but may exert an analgesic effect

Uses
1 Petit mal (simple absence) seizures refractory to other drugs

Dosage
See Table 25-4.

Fate
Readily absorbed from GI tract; peak plasma concentrations in 30 minutes to 60 minutes; uniformly distributed and not bound to plasma proteins; metabolized in liver to an active metabolite with an extended half-life; slowly excreted in the urine

Common Side-Effects
Drowsiness, GI distress, hiccoughs, and photophobia

Significant Adverse Reactions

Warning: Fetal malformations and serious side-effects have occurred during therapy with oxazolidinediones. Use only where other less toxic drugs are ineffective.

GI—nausea, vomiting, abdominal pain, anorexia
CNS—vertigo, irritability, personality changes, headache, paresthesias, precipitation of grand mal seizures
Ocular—diplopia, scotomata, hemeralopia (day blindness), retinal hemorrhage
Hematologic—epistaxis, mucosal bleeding (*e.g.,* gums, vagina), blood dyscrasias (especially neutropenia), changes in blood pressure
Dermatologic—skin rash (acneiform, morbilliform), exfoliative dermatitis, erythema multiforme
Other—albuminuria, alopecia, lymphadenopathy, systemic lupus-like reaction, myasthenia gravis-like reaction, nephrosis, hepatitis

Table 25-4. Oxazolidinediones

Drug	Preparations	Usual Dosage Range	Remarks
Paramethadione (Paradione)	Capsules—150 mg, 300 mg Solution—300 mg/ml	Adults—300 mg to 600 mg 3 to 4 times/day (initial dose 900 mg/day; increase by 300 mg/wk to above range) Children—300 mg to 900 mg/day in 3 to 4 divided doses	Less effective but slightly less toxic than trimethadione; no myasthenic-like reactions have occurred, but sedation is common; oral solution contains 65% alcohol and should be diluted with water before administration to children
Trimethadione (Tridione)	Chewable tablets—150 mg Capsules—300 mg Solution—40 mg/ml	Adults—Initially 300 mg 3 times/day; usual maintenance dose 900 mg to 2400 mg/day in divided doses Children—300 mg to 900 mg/day in 3 to 4 divided doses	Plasma level of dimethadione, the active metabolite of trimethadione may be used as a dosage guide; this level should be maintained about 700 mcg/ml for optimal control of petit mal attacks in patients receiving trimethadione; alkalinization of the urine will increase excretion of this metabolite.

Contraindications

Hepatic and renal disease, blood dyscrasias

Interactions

1 CNS depression induced by oxazolidinediones may be augmented by other depressants, oral anticoagulants, and p-aminosalicylic acid.

▶ **NURSING ALERTS**

▷ 1 Observe closely for early signs of hematologic toxicity (*e.g.,* sore throat, mucosal ulceration, fever, malaise, petechiae), and discontinue drug.

▷ 2 Withdraw drug upon the occurrence of skin rash, neutrophil depression (see below), jaundice, albuminuria, scotomas, lymph node enlargement, or myasthenia symptoms because severe toxicity can ensue.

▷ 3 Perform complete blood counts, liver function tests, and urinalysis prior to and at regular intervals during therapy. Discontinue therapy if neutrophil count drops below 2500/mm^3.

▷ 4 Advise patient to report immediately any development of ocular side-effects (*e.g.,* glaring, dark spots, blurring), and reduce dose. Retinal damage may occur if dose is too high.

▷ 5 Use cautiously in patients with diseases of the retina or optic nerve and during pregnancy and lactation.

▷ 6 Withdraw gradually to prevent development of simple absence attacks, which have occurred upon abrupt discontinuation.

▶ **NURSING CONSIDERATIONS**

▷ 1 Inform patient that incidence of petit mal attacks may *increase* during first few days of therapy. Provide reassurance that clinical benefit will occur within several days.

▷ 2 Stress the importance of rigid adherence to prescribed regimen, to minimize untoward reactions.

▷ 3 Advise patient that drowsiness will diminish with continued use. A mild stimulant (*e.g.,* caffeine) may be employed in the early stages of therapy to reduce excessive drowsiness.

▷ 4 Do not use alone in mixed seizure forms because oxazolidinediones can worsen grand mal symptoms. Combination therapy is indicated where more than one seizure pattern is evident.

V Succinimides

Ethosuximide	Phensuximide
Methsuximide	

Although slightly less effective than the oxazolidinediones in the treatment of simple absence seizures including petit mal, the succinimides remain the drugs of choice for these conditions primarily because of their low toxicity. Because they may increase the frequency of grand mal attacks, however, their use in mixed seizure patterns must be accompanied by other antiepileptics capable of controlling tonic–clonic seizures. Three succinimides are currently available, offering little in the way of significant differences among them. They are discussed as a group, then listed individually in Table 25-5.

Mechanism

Remains to be definitively established; in laboratory tests, their effects generally resemble those of the oxazolidinediones, and they are known to suppress the three-per-second spike–wave EEG pattern characteristic of absence seizures; evidence suggests a depressant effect on the motor cortex and possible elevation of the firing threshold of cortical neurons.

Uses

1 Petit mal (simple absence)
2 Psychomotor and other minor motor seizures (methsuximide *only*)

Table 25-5. Succinimides

Drug	Preparations	Usual Dosage Range	Remarks
Ethosuximide (Zarontin)	Capsules—250 mg Syrup—250 mg/5 ml	Adults—Initially 500 mg/day; increase by 250 mg every 4 to 7 days until control is achieved (maximum 1500 mg/day) Children—250 mg/day increased slowly to optimal level	Inform patient that drug may color urine pink to reddish-brown; appearance of frequent GI distress, dizziness, ataxia, or other neurologic disorders signifies need for dosage adjustment; administer with meals to reduce GI upset; long half-life; therefore, do not exceed recommended dosage as danger of accumulation exists
Methsuximide (Celontin)	Capsules—150 mg, 300 mg	Initially 300 mg/day for 1 week; may increase by 300 mg weekly to a maximum of 1200 mg	Equally effective in petit mal as ethosuximide but somewhat more toxic, especially to the CNS (*e.g.,* severe depression, confusion); may be useful in certain cases of psychomotor epilepsy
Phensuximide (Milontin)	Capsules—500 mg	Adults—500 mg to 1000 mg 2 to 3 times/day (range 1 g to 3 g/day) Children—600 mg to 1200 mg 2 to 3 times/day	Slightly less effective and less toxic than other succinimides; may color urine reddish-brown

Dosage

See Table 25-5.

Fate

Well absorbed orally; peak serum levels in 1 hour to 3 hours; not bound to plasma proteins; short half-life (2 hr–4 hr) except ethosuximide (30 hr–60 hr); metabolized by the liver and excreted primarily in the urine as both active and inactive metabolites

Common Side-Effects

GI distress (nausea, upset, cramping, pain, diarrhea), drowsiness, ataxia, dizziness

Significant Adverse Reactions

CNS—irritability, nervousness, euphoria, aggressiveness, hyperactivity, confusion, lethargy, fatigue, depression, sleep disturbances, night terrors, inability to concentrate, hiccoughs, insomnia

Ocular—blurred vision, myopia, photophobia, periorbital edema

Hematologic—blood dyscrasias

Dermatologic—urticaria, erythematous rashes, erythema multiforme, systemic lupus erythematosus, Stevens–Johnson syndrome (see Chap. 6)

Genitourinary—urinary frequency, hematuria, albuminuria, renal damage (rare)

Other—alopecia, vaginal bleeding, hyperemia, swelling of the tongue, muscular weakness, hirsutism

Contraindications

Severe liver or renal damage

Interactions

1 Absorption of ethosuximide may be reduced by amphetamine.

2 Increased libido may result if ethosuximide is combined with other anticonvulsants.

▶ **NURSING ALERTS**

▷ 1 Caution against engaging in any hazardous activity during initial stages of therapy, because drowsiness is common.

▷ 2 Administer cautiously to patients with liver disorders, and perform periodic liver function tests and urinalysis.

▷ 3 Note that in the presence of mixed seizure patterns, succinimide drugs may increase the frequency of grand mal seizures. Always employ combination drug therapy in such instances.

▷ 4 Be alert for development of behavior changes (*e.g.*, depression, aggressiveness), and withdraw drug slowly.

▷ 5 Inform physician if skin rash, dizziness, fever, blurred vision, joint pain, bruising, or bleeding occur, because these symptoms may indicate developing toxicity.

▷ 6 Perform periodic blood counts, because various blood dyscrasias have been reported with use of succinimides.

▶ **NURSING CONSIDERATIONS**

▷ 1 Stress the importance of carefully noting the development of untoward reactions while taking these drugs. Most adverse effects can be minimized or eliminated by a dosage adjustment if detected early.

▷ 2 Always make dosage adjustments gradually, because abrupt changes may precipitate increased seizure activity.

VI Carbamazepine (Tegretol)

Carbamazepine is structurally related to the tricyclic antidepressants, and has a spectrum of action similar to phenytoin. It has been employed to successfully treat the pain of trigeminal neuralgia (tic douloureux). The drug is a highly toxic agent usually restricted to the treatment of grand mal and psychomotor seizures in patients not responding satisfactorily to other less toxic drugs.

Mechanism

Increases latency, decreases responsivity, and suppresses afterdischarges in polysynaptic pathways associated with cortical and limbic function; may reduce post-tetanic potentiation; has anticholinergic, antidepressant, and muscle-relaxing action (interferes with neuromuscular transmission)

Uses

1 Psychomotor seizures (alone or with primidone or phenytoin)

2 Grand mal (with phenytoin)

3 Mixed seizures

4 Relief of pain associated with trigeminal neuralgia

5 Termination of intractable hiccoughs (experimental use)

Dosage

Epilepsy

Adults and children over 12: Initially 200 mg twice a day; increase by 200 mg/day in divided doses until optimal response is achieved; maximum 1200 mg/day; usual maintenance range is 800 mg to 1200 mg/day

Children 6 to 12: Initially, 100 mg twice a day; increase by 100 mg/day until optimal response is achieved; usual maintenance level is 400 mg to 800 mg daily

Trigeminal Neuralgia

Initially 100 mg twice a day; increase by 100 mg/12 hours; usual maintenance range is 400 mg to 800 mg/day

Fate

Oral absorption is slow but complete; peak plasma levels in 4 hours to 6 hours; widely distributed and highly protein-bound; serum half-life 15 hours to 30 hours; metabolized in the liver (epoxide metabolite has anticonvulsant activity), and excreted as several metabolites and some unchanged drug through the kidney

Common Side-Effects

Drowsiness, dizziness, ataxia, nausea, blurred vision, and diplopia

Significant Adverse Reactions

Warning: Serious and sometime fatal blood dyscrasias have occurred with carbamazepine. Early detection is vital, because in some patients aplastic anemia is irreversible. See Nursing Alerts.

CNS—confusion, incoordination, speech disturbances, involuntary movements, dysphasia, visual hallucinations, tinnitus, depression, peripheral neuritis, paresthesias, nystagmus

Dermatologic—rash, sweating, urticaria, photosensitivity reactions, alopecia, exfoliative dermatitis, erythema multiforme, abnormal pigmentation

Hematologic—blood dyscrasias, (aplastic anemia, leukopenia, agranulocytosis, eosinophilia, leukocytosis, thrombocytopenia)

Genitourinary—urinary frequency, albuminuria, glycosuria, urinary retention, oliguria, impotence

GI—diarrhea, vomiting, abdominal pain, anorexia, xerostomia, glossitis

Cardiovascular—hypotension, syncope, arrhythmias, aggravation of coronary artery disease and hypertension, thrombophlebitis, A–V block, congestive heart failure

Other—abnormal liver function, jaundice, muscle aching, fever, chills, lenticular opacities, adenopathy

Contraindications

History of bone marrow depression, severe hypertension, and concomitant use of MAO inhibitors

Interactions

1 Carbamazepine may accelerate the metabolism and therefore decrease the effects of other anticonvulsants (phenobarbital, phenytoin, primidone), oral anticoagulants, and tetracyclines.

2 Concurrent use of carbamazepine with MAO inhibitors or tricyclic antidepressants is not recommended because toxicity may be increased.

3 Carbamazepine is highly protein-bound and therefore may potentiate other protein-bound drugs (*e.g.,* salicylates, oral hypoglycemics, anticoagulants, anti-inflammatory agents) by displacing them from protein-binding sites.

4 Cimetidine, isoniazid, erythromycin, and propoxyphene can elevate serum levels of carbamazepine, leading to increased toxicity.

5 Carbamazepine can result in breakthrough bleeding in women taking oral contraceptives.

▶ **NURSING ALERTS**

▷ 1 Perform complete blood counts, liver function tests, urinalysis, and BUN determination prior to initiating therapy. Repeat at regular intervals during therapy,

and discontinue drug if findings are abnormal or if any evidence of bone marrow depression develops.

▷ 2 Counsel patient to observe for early signs of hematologic toxicity (sore throat, mucosal ulceration, petechiae, bruising, malaise), and advise physician immediately.

▷ 3 Use cautiously in patients with renal, hepatic, or cardiac disease, hypertension, glaucoma, and in elderly, pregnant, or nursing patients.

▷ 4 Withdraw drug or make dosage adjustments slowly. Abrupt changes may provoke seizures or status epilepticus.

▷ 5 Advise patient to avoid hazardous tasks until reaction to the drug has been determined. Drowsiness and dizziness are common in initial stages of therapy.

▶ **NURSING CONSIDERATIONS**

▷ 1 Note that confusion, agitation, and behavioral disturbances occur more commonly in the elderly. Supervised ambulation may be necessary.

▷ 2 Advise periodic ophthalmologic examinations because drug can produce ocular damage.

VII Phenacemide (Phenurone)

A structural analog of the hydantoins, phenacemide is useful in severe epileptic states, especially mixed forms of psychomotor seizures refractory to other medications. It is generally employed as a last resort, however, because of its extreme toxicity.

Mechanism

Essentially unknown; elevates threshold for experimental electroshock seizures in animals

Uses

1 *Severe* epileptic states, especially mixed forms of psychomotor seizures refractory to other drugs.

Dosage

Adults: 250 mg to 500 mg 3 times/day (usual maintenance range 2 g–3 g/day); maximum 5 g/day

Children (5 yr–10 yr): One half adult dose

Fate

Well absorbed from the GI tract; onset in 30 minutes to 60 minutes; duration 4 hours to 6 hours; metabolized by the liver and excreted in the urine as inactive metabolites

Common Side-Effects

Anorexia, nausea, ataxia, drowsiness, dizziness, weakness, and headache

Significant Adverse Reactions

Paresthesias, skin rash, bone marrow depression (possible *fatal* aplastic anemia or agranulocytosis), CNS disturbances (marked personality changes, paranoid psychotic states, melancholia with suicidal tendencies), hepatitis, and nephritis

Contraindications
Pregnancy, severe personality disorders

Interactions
1 Concomitant use of other anticonvulsants (especially ethotoin) may increase incidence of untoward reactions.

▶ NURSING ALERTS
▷ 1 Use with extreme caution in patients with personality disorders, and carefully observe for behavioral changes (*e.g.,* depression, apathy, aggressiveness, paranoia). Withdraw drug under medical supervision if these changes are noted.
▷ 2 Perform complete blood counts and liver function tests before and at regular intervals during drug therapy. Discontinue drug if symptoms of jaundice or hepatitis appear or if blood picture is abnormal.
▷ 3 Advise patient to report early evidence of hematologic toxicity (*e.g.,* sore throat, fever, malaise, mucosal ulceration) or liver damage (*e.g.,* pruritus, yellow skin, frothy amber urine, petechiae). Withdraw drug slowly as indicated.
▷ 4 Do not use in women of childbearing age, during lactation, or in patients with a history of allergy. Discontinue at first sign of skin rash or other allergic manifestation.

▶ NURSING CONSIDERATIONS
▷ 1 Impress upon patient the potential toxicity of the drug and the importance of immediate reporting of *any* untoward reaction.
▷ 2 Suggest taking the drug with food or milk to minimize GI irritation.

VIII Clonazepam (Klonopin)

Clonazepam is a benzodiazepine derivative having a wide application in various seizure manifestations. Its use is associated with a significant degree of CNS depression and can result in psychological dependence. As many as 50% of users develop tolerance within 12 months, necessitating a dosage adjustment.

Mechanism
Not well established; may potentiate inhibitory mechanisms in subcortical brain structures; has been shown to suppress the spike–wave discharge characteristic of absence seizures, and to decrease the frequency, duration, amplitude, and spread of minor motor seizure discharges

Uses
1 Petit mal variant (Lennox–Gastaut syndrome)
2 Myclonic and akinetic seizures
3 Simple absence seizures refractory to succinimides (may be used alone or as an adjunct; some evidence of benefit in psychomotor and focal seizures in combination with other drugs)
4 Status epilepticus (IV)

Dosage
Adults: Initially 0.5 mg 3 times/day; increase by 0.5 mg to 1.0 mg every 3 days until optimal effect is achieved (maximum 20 mg/day)
Children: Initially 0.01 mg/kg to 0.03 mg/kg/day; increase by 0.25 mg to 0.5 mg every 3 days (usual range 0.1 mg/kg–0.2 mg/kg/day)

Fate
Onset following oral administration in 30 minutes to 60 minutes; maximum plasma levels occur in 1 hour to 2 hours; duration 6 hours to 12 hours; half-life varies from 20 hours to 40 hours; metabolized in the liver and primarily excreted in the urine

Common Side-Effects
Drowsiness, ataxia, and disturbed or abnormal behavior

Significant Adverse Reactions
CNS—confusion, insomnia, depression, hysteria, headache, hypotonia, involuntary movements, slurred speech, tremor, vertigo, nystagmus, hallucinations, psychosis
GI—anorexia, constipation, dry mouth, gastritis, nausea, sore gums, hepatomegaly, coated tongue
Respiratory—rhinorrhea, shortness of breath, hypersecretion
Dermatologic—rash, ankle edema, hirsutism
Urinary—dysuria, enuresis, nocturia
Other—palpitations, muscle weakness, fever, lymphadenopathy, dehydration, blood dyscrasias (rare), diplopia, abnormal eye movements, increased salivation

Contraindications
Liver disease, narrow-angle glaucoma

Interactions
1 CNS depressive effects may be enhanced by other drugs having a depressant action, *e.g.,* alcohol, narcotics, sedatives, phenothiazines, barbiturates, and so forth.
2 Phenytoin and phenobarbital can reduce serum clonazepam levels.
3 Combined use of clonazepam and valproic acid may elicit absence seizures.

▶ NURSING ALERTS
▷ 1 Caution patients against performing hazardous tasks during clonazepam therapy because incidence of drowsiness is quite high.

▷ 2 Use cautiously in patients with renal dysfunction, respiratory disease (drug increases secretions), behavioral disturbances, in children and addiction-prone patients, and during pregnancy and lactation.

▷ 3 Do not use alone in presence of mixed seizures. Drug may worsen tonic–clonic seizures or precipitate grand mal seizures. Appropriate anticonvulsants should be combined with clonazepam.

▷ 4 Be aware that paradoxical increases in seizure activity can occur with this drug. Do not discontinue abruptly because marked exacerbation of seizures or status epilepticus can result.

▶ NURSING CONSIDERATIONS

▷ 1 Perform periodic blood counts and liver function tests during prolonged therapy.

▷ 2 Because tolerance is common, periodically review dosage and make adjustments as necessary. Be alert, however, for signs of dependence, and discontinue drug slowly if necessary to avoid withdrawal symptoms.

IX Diazepam (Valium)

Diazepam is a benzodiazepine widely used for control of simple anxiety states. It may be useful orally as an adjunct in the management of convulsive disorders, but it rarely is effective alone. Its principal indication is parenterally (IV) for the treatment of status epilepticus and other severe recurrent convulsive seizures. Diazepam may also be used for convulsions accompanying acute alcohol withdrawal. The drug is discussed fully in Chapter 23; thus, only those aspects relating to its use as an antiepileptic will be reviewed here.

Mechanism

Not established; suppresses polysynaptic neuronal activity in the spinal cord and mesencephalic reticular formation; may function like an inhibitory neurotransmitter by activating GABA-like receptor sites (see valproic acid)

Uses

1 Adjunctive treatment of convulsive disorders, especially minor motor seizures
2 Control of status epilepticus and other acute convulsive seizures (IV)
3 Treatment of convulsions associated with acute alcohol withdrawal (IV)

Dosage

Oral

Adults: 2 mg to 10 mg 2 to 4 times/day (reduce dose in geriatric or debilitated patients)

Children (over 6 mo): 1 mg to 2.5 mg 3 to 4 times/day

IV

Adults: 5 mg to 10 mg initially; repeat if necessary at 10-minute to 15-minute intervals to a maximum of 30 mg

Children (up to 5 yr): 0.2 mg to 0.5 mg every 2 minutes to 5 minutes to a maximum of 5 mg

Children (over 5 yr): 1 mg every 2 minutes to 5 minutes to a maximum of 10 mg

▶ NURSING ALERTS

(See also Chap. 23)

▷ 1 Be prepared to re-administer diazepam IV as necessary to control acute seizure episodes because effects of drug are short-lived, and many patients experience recurrent seizure episodes.

▷ 2 Do not administer IV to patients with petit mal or petit mal variants, because status epilepticus can be *precipitated* in these patients.

▷ 3 IV diazepam may cause venous thrombosis, swelling, or phlebitis. To prevent this, inject very slowly (5 mg/min) and do not use small veins (*e.g.,* dorsum of the hand or wrist).

▷ 4 Use IV route if at all possible. If severe convulsions prevent this, drug may be given IM deeply into a large muscle mass.

X Valproic Acid Derivatives

▶ **valproic acid**
   Depakene

▶ **sodium valproate**
   Depakene

▶ **divalproex sodium**
   Depakote

Although chemically unrelated to other anticonvulsants, valproic acid, its sodium salt, and a stable compound composed of equal parts valproic acid and sodium valproate (*i.e.,* divalproex sodium) generally provide improved seizure control when added to the drug regimen of refractory patients with multiple seizure types. They are most effective against simple and complex absence seizures. Divalproex is an enteric-coated dosage form and has a slightly lower incidence of GI side-effects.

Mechanism

Elicit a consistent elevation in the functional levels of GABA (an inhibitory neurotransmitter) in the CNS; the contribution of this effect to the antiepileptic efficacy of the drug remains to be established.

Uses

1 Simple and complex absence seizures, including petit mal (alone or in combination with other anticonvulsants)
2 Adjunct in the treatment of multiple seizure types

3 Investigational uses include grand mal seizures, myclonic seizures, infantile spasms, and prevention of recurrent febrile seizures.

Dosage
(Dosage is expressed in valproic acid equivalents) Initially, 15 mg/kg/day; increase by 5 mg/kg to 10 mg/kg weekly until seizures are controlled (maximum 60 mg/kg/day)

Fate
Valproic acid and sodium valproate are rapidly absorbed orally; divalproex is enteric coated and absorption is delayed 1 hour, but is uniform and consistent; peak serum levels occur within 15 minutes to 30 minutes with sodium valproate and within 1 hour to 4 hours with the other dosage forms; widely distributed and highly (90%) protein-bound; drug is primarily metabolized in the liver and is excreted in the urine, almost entirely as conjugated metabolites.

Common Side-Effects
Nausea, vomiting, indigestion, sedation, and elevated serum transaminase

Significant Adverse Reactions

Warning: Fatal hepatic failure has occurred in patients receiving valproic acid, usually during the first 6 months of treatment. Frequent liver function tests are required, especially during the initial months of therapy.

Diarrhea, abdominal cramps, lenticular opacities, nystagmus, visual disturbances, diplopia, dizziness, incoordination, tremor, dysarthria, skin rash, petechiae, alopecia, depression, aggression, hyperactivity, behavioral disturbances, altered bleeding time (drug inhibits platelet aggregation), muscle weakness, blood dyscrasias (rare), hepatotoxicity

Note: Because the drug has been used mostly in combination with other antiepileptic medication, it is difficult to ascribe the above adverse effects solely to valproic acid.

Contraindications
Hepatic disease or dysfunction

Interactions
1 Valproic acid may potentiate the depressant effects of other CNS depressant drugs, *e.g.,* barbiturates, narcotics, alcohol.
2 Serum phenobarbital levels may be elevated by valproic acid.
3 Simultaneous use of valproic acid and clonazepam may *induce* absence seizures, and combinations of valproic acid and phenytoin may result in breakthrough seizures.
4 Valproic acid interferes with platelet aggregation and

therefore may enhance the action of anticoagulants, dipyridamole, and salicylates.

▶ NURSING ALERTS
▷ 1 Perform liver function tests prior to and at frequent intervals during therapy, because hepatic failure has occurred with use of valproic acid. Discontinue drug at first sign of hepatic dysfunction, as indicated by either serum biochemistry or clinical evaluation.
▷ 2 Caution patient against the use of alcohol or other depressants with valproic acid, and advise against engaging in hazardous activities because drowsiness and dizziness can occur.
▷ 3 Instruct patient to report any visual disturbances immediately, because ocular toxicity has been noted.
▷ 4 Use cautiously in pregnant or nursing women, or in the presence of renal disease.

▶ NURSING CONSIDERATIONS
▷ 1 Advise periodic blood counts during drug therapy because reports of platelet dysfunction and blood dyscrasias have appeared.
▷ 2 Instruct patient to swallow capsule whole to avoid local mouth and throat irritation. Administer with food to minimize GI irritation.
▷ 3 Note that drug is excreted in part as a ketone-containing metabolite, which can interfere with urine tests for ketone bodies.

XI Acetazolamide (Ak-Zol, Diamox)

Acetazolamide is a carbonic anhydrase inhibitor used as an *adjunct* in the control of petit mal and other absence or nonlocalized seizures, but seldom alone. The drug has also been employed as a mild diuretic, for relief of migraine headaches, and chronic open-angle glaucoma (reduces formation of aqueous humor).

Mechanism
Inhibits the enzyme carbonic anhydrase, reducing formation of H^+ and HCO_3^- ions; appears to retard excessive or abnormal discharges from central neurons, although the mechanism of this effect is not well understood; beneficial effects may be largely a consequence of the slight acidosis produced by the drug

Uses
1 Adjunctive treatment of petit mal or other absence seizures; may be helpful in grand mal, myclonic, or mixed seizures as well

Dosage
8 mg/kg to 30 mg/kg/day in divided doses; usual range is 400 mg to 1000 mg/day, in combination with other anticonvulsants

Fate

Rapidly absorbed orally; onset in 20 minutes to 30 minutes; duration 6 hours to 12 hours; primarily excreted unchanged through the kidneys (80% within 24 hr)

Common Side-Effects

Paresthesias of face and extremities

Significant Adverse Reactions

Polyuria, hematuria, glycosuria, acidosis, drowsiness, confusion, myopia, urticaria, rash, hepatic dysfunction, and flaccid paralysis

Drug is a sulfonamide derivative; see Chapter 59 for adverse effects caused by sulfonamides; these effects can also occur with acetazolamide.

Contraindications

Renal or hepatic dysfunction, adrenal insufficiency, acidosis, narrow-angle glaucoma, severe pulmonary obstruction, sulfa allergy, and early pregnancy

Interactions

See Carbonic Anhydrase Inhibitors (Chap. 37)

▶ **NURSING ALERT**

▷ 1 Caution patient to report signs of hypokalemia (muscle weakness, cramping, cardiac irregularities) and metabolic acidosis (nausea, weakness, malaise, vomiting, abdominal pain, dehydration), and adjust dosage as needed.

▶ **NURSING CONSIDERATIONS**

▷ 1 Use parenteral solution within 24 hours after reconstitution, because it contains no preservative.

▷ 2 Observe diabetic patients closely because acetazolamide may alter antidiabetic drug requirements by increasing blood glucose levels.

XII   Magnesium Sulfate

Magnesium, in the form of magnesium sulfate, is an effective anticonvulsant in seizures associated with the toxemia of pregnancy and other clinical situations characterized by abnormally low levels of plasma magnesium. The drug may be used IV or IM, depending on the speed of action desired although IV use is significantly more hazardous. Other clinical applications for magnesium sulfate are its use orally as a cathartic, topically as an antipruritic, and parenterally to control uterine tetany, paroxysmal atrial tachycardia, hypertension, and cerebral edema. It has also been employed as an adjunct in hyperalimentation and for replacement therapy in acute magnesium deficiency.

Mechanism

Not completely understood; has CNS depressant action and may decrease release of acetylcholine from motor nerve terminals, thereby reducing neuromuscular transmission

Uses

1 Control convulsions associated with epilepsy, toxemia of pregnancy, hypothyroidism, and other clinical situations characterized by reduced magnesium levels

Dosage

IM: 1 g to 2 g of a 25% to 50% solution
IV: 1.5 ml of a 10% solution per minute until desired effect is attained

Fate

Immediate onset with IV; effects persist about 30 minutes; following IM administration, onset in about 1 hour and duration 3 hours to 4 hours; eliminated almost entirely by the kidney

Common Side-Effects

Flushing

Significant Adverse Reactions

(Dependent on plasma magnesium levels) Hypotension, cardiac depression, sedation, confusion, hypothermia, respiratory depression, and circulatory collapse

Contraindications

Heart block, myocardial insufficiency, and severe renal disease

Interactions

1 Additive CNS effects may occur with other CNS depressants.
2 Drug may potentiate neuromuscular blocking agents.

▶ **NURSING ALERTS**

▷ 1 Have IV calcium on hand as an antidote, along with appropriate respiratory assistance when using magnesium parenterally.

▷ 2 Note appearance of early signs of magnesium toxicity (thirst, feeling of warmth, confusion, depressed tendon reflexes, muscle weakness), and discontinue drug.

▶ **NURSING CONSIDERATIONS**

▷ 1 Monitor blood pressure and pulse repeatedly during IV therapy, as well as intake and output ratio during extended use. Discontinue if output falls below 100 ml/4 hours preceding each dose.

▷ 2 Determine plasma magnesium levels during parenteral treatment. Plasma levels above 4 mEq/liter are usually associated with untoward reactions.

Summary. Anticonvulsants

Drug	Preparations	Usual Dosage Range
Barbiturates		
See Table 25-2		
Primidone (Mysoline)	Tablets—50 mg, 250 mg Suspension—250 mg/5 ml	Adults—Initially 250 mg/day; increase by 250 mg increments to an optimal level (maximum 2 g/day) Children (under 8 yr)—500 mg to 750 mg/day in divided doses
Hydantoins		
See Table 25-3		
Oxazolidinediones		
See Table 25-4		
Succinimides		
See Table 25-5		
Carbamazepine (Tegretol)	Tablets—200 mg Chewable tablets—100 mg	Epilepsy Adults—200 mg twice a day, increased by 200 mg/day to optimal response (maximum 1200 mg/day) Children 6 yr–12 yr—100 mg twice a day; increase by 100 mg/day until desired response is achieved; maximum 1000 mg/day Trigeminal Neuralgia 100 mg twice a day, increased by 100 mg/12 hours; usual range 400 mg to 800 mg/day
Phenacemide (Phenurone)	Tablets—500 mg	Adults—250 mg to 500 mg 3 times/day (usual range is 2 g to 3 g/day) Children (5 yr–10 yr)—one half adult dose
Clonazepam (Klonopin)	Tablets—0.5 mg, 1 mg, 2 mg	Adults—0.5 mg 3 times/day increased by 0.5 mg to 1 mg every 3 days (maximum 20 mg/day) Children—0.01 mg/kg to 0.03 mg/kg/day; increase to a maintenance range of 0.1 mg/kg to 0.2 mg/kg/day
Diazepam (Valium, Val-Release)	Tablets—2 mg, 5 mg, 10 mg Sustained-release capsules—15 mg Injection—5 mg/ml	Oral Adults—2 mg to 10 mg 2 to 4 times/day Children—1 mg to 2.5 mg 3 to 4 times/day IV Adults—5 mg to 10 mg initially; repeat at 10-minute to 15-minute intervals to a maximum of 30 mg Children—0.2 mg to 1 mg every 2 minutes to 5 minutes based on age and weight

(continued)

Summary. Anticonvulsants *(continued)*

Drug	Preparations	Usual Dosage Range

Valproic acid derivatives
Valproic acid
  (Depakene)
Sodium valproate
  (Depakene)
Divalproex sodium
  (Depakote)
	Capsules—250 mg
	Syrup—250 mg/5 ml
	Enteric-coated tablets—250
	  mg, 500 mg
		Initially 15 mg/kg/day; increase
		  by 15 mg/kg weekly until
		  optimal effect is noted
		  (maximum 60 mg/kg/day).

Acetazolamide
  (Ak-Zol, Diamox)
	Tablets—125 mg, 250 mg
	Injection—500 mg/vial
		8 to 30 mg/kg/day in divided
		  doses (usual range 400 mg to
		  1000 mg/day)

Magnesium sulfate
  (various manufacturers)
	Injection—10%, 12.5%, 50%	1 g to 2 g IM or IV; IV rate not
		  to exceed 1.5 ml of 10%
		  solution/min

Parkinson's disease, or *paralysis agitans,* is a chronic progressive disorder of the CNS, the etiology of which is largely unknown. *Parkinsonism* is a term used to describe the symptom complex that may result from either the normal course of the disease itself or from administration of certain groups of drugs (*e.g.,* phenothiazines) that produce similar symptoms. However, the terms are usually used interchangeably. Although the symptoms vary depending on the stage of the disease—which becomes progressively more disabling—the three cardinal manifestations of Parkinson's disease are the following:

1 *Akinesia*—a lack of or difficulty in initiating voluntary muscle movement; advanced disease states are characterized by "frozen" muscles, resulting in mask-like facial expression, impairment of postural reflexes, and inability to adequately care for oneself

2 *Rigidity*—usually of the "plastic" type; the affected area usually can be moved without great difficulty but often remains fixed once again in its new position

3 *Tremor*—coarse (3 cycles/sec–7 cycles/sec), repetitive muscle activity, usually worse when the person is at rest; commonly manifested as a "pill-rolling" motion of the hands and a bobbing of the head

Besides the principal symptoms of the disease, afflicted patients may show disturbances in gait or posture, impaired speech, muscular weakness, and autonomic hyperactivity such as salivation and seborrhea. Advanced stages, however, are frequently characterized by autonomic *insufficiency,* resulting in severe orthostatic hypotension, which may be exacerbated by the anticholinergic drugs used in treatment.

Onset usually occurs in middle age, and during the early stages symptoms frequently are much worse on one side of the body. Diagnosis is largely symptomatic, although definite biochemical changes are present in the CNS. The most characteristic pathologic feature of parkinsonism is a degeneration of dopaminergic neurons having their cell bodies in the substantia nigra. Because motor regulatory areas such as the corpus striatum receive their dopamine supply from the substantia nigra, degeneration of these nigral–striatal neurons decreases the functional amount of dopamine available to the nuclei of the corpus striatum (*i.e.,* caudate nucleus, putamen). This upsets the normal balance between the inhibitory transmitter dopamine and the excitatory transmitter acetylcholine in these brain regions, and therefore allows an excitatory predominance on lower motor centers by the intact cholinergic pathways.

Although striatal dopamine deficiency provides a common basis for the various manifestations of parkinsonism, the only *true* symptom resulting from low striatal dopamine is akinesia. As such, akinesia is the abnormality most benefitted by dopamine-replacement therapy. The other symptoms probably reflect the effects of the abnormal neurotransmitter ratio *triggered* by the dopamine deficit, and involve alterations in more complex pathways among central motor regulatory structures. Therefore, tremor and rigidity may be more effectively controlled by both dopamine replacement *and* cholinergic antagonism.

Because parkinsonism largely results from a functional lack of dopamine in the CNS, symptoms resembling the disease also can occur as a consequence of therapy with

Antiparkinsonian Drugs 26

dopamine-blocking drugs such as phenothiazines and other antipsychotic agents. These adverse effects have been reviewed in Chapter 22, and are treated by many of the same drugs used for the control of Parkinson's disease.

Drug therapy of parkinsonism is directed either toward augmentation of central dopaminergic function or reduction of central cholinergic activity. Drugs effective in the control of Parkinson's disease may be grouped as follows:

I. *Dopaminergic agents*
1. Dopamine precursor (*e.g.*, levodopa)
2. Dopamine releasing agent (*e.g.*, amantadine)
3. Dopamine receptor agonist (*e.g.*, bromocriptine)

II. *Anticholinergic/antihistaminergic agents* (*e.g.*, benztropine, ethopropazine)

In addition to proper drug treatment, which of course is not curative but simply palliative, adjunctive therapy for parkinsonism should include physical therapy to delay disability and emotional support to help lessen feelings of helplessness and inadequacy as the disease inexorably progresses and limits the patient's activities.

I Dopaminergic Agents

Three types of drugs are available that can enhance dopaminergic functioning in the motor regulatory centers of the CNS. *Levodopa* (l-DOPA) is the metabolic precursor of dopamine, and its use results in increased concentrations of dopamine in the corpus striatum. It is used rather than dopamine itself because l-DOPA readily passes the blood–brain barrier, whereas dopamine does not and therefore does not reach sufficient levels in the CNS following systemic administration. l-DOPA is used either alone or in a fixed-ratio combination with carbidopa, the latter being an inhibitor of peripheral dopa decarboxylase, the enzyme responsible for converting dopa to dopamine. Peripheral inhibition of this enzyme allows a greater fraction of intact l-DOPA to penetrate the CNS, thereby increasing the amount of dopamine formed in central motor areas. Thus, much smaller doses of l-DOPA may be employed, thereby reducing the incidence of side-effects.

In addition to being available in two fixed dosage ratios with l-DOPA (1:4, 1:10), carbidopa is also marketed alone in 25-mg tablets (Lodosyn) that allow the clinician to more carefully titrate the dosage ratio to obtain better symptom control. Carbidopa is only indicated for use with l-DOPA because carbidopa has no therapeutic effect of its own in parkinsonism.

Another drug employed to potentiate the effects of dopamine in the CNS is *amantadine*. Originally developed as an antiviral agent against the Asian (A) influenza strain, amantadine was demonstrated to have a beneficial action in certain parkinsonian patients to whom it was administered. It apparently increases the release of dopamine from presynaptic nerve endings. Therefore, its effectiveness is limited to those patients having functional stores of dopamine present in striatal brain areas.

The third type of dopaminergic drug is *bromocriptine*,

a dopamine receptor agonist. It finds its principal clinical application in cases of parkinsonism refractory to conventional therapy as an adjunct to levodopa/carbidopa treatment. Bromocriptine can provide additional therapeutic benefit in those patients whose condition has begun to deteriorate and may allow a reduction in levodopa dosage, thus reducing the incidence of side-effects associated with prolonged levodopa therapy. However, patients unresponsive to levodopa are not likely to benefit from bromocriptine.

▶ levodopa

Dopar, Larodopa

Mechanism

Crosses blood–brain barrier intact, then is decarboxylated to dopamine, thereby evaluating functional levels of dopamine in motor regulatory areas depleted of the neurohormone; most effective in relieving akinesia

Uses

1 Treatment of parkinsonism, whether idiopathic, postencephalitic, or secondary to injury or cerebral arteriosclerosis

Dosage

Highly individualized; initially 0.5 g to 1 g/day in 2 or more divided doses; increase gradually in increments of 0.75 g every 3 to 7 days; maximum dose is 8 g/day

Fate

Well absorbed from GI tract; peak plasma levels occur in 1 hour to 2 hours; significant amounts are metabolized to dopamine in the stomach, intestines, and liver; relatively small fraction of administered dose reaches CNS unchanged (1%–2%); dopamine metabolites are rapidly and almost completely excreted in the urine.

Common Side-Effects

Nausea, vomiting, anorexia, orthostatic hypotension, salivation, dry mouth, dysphagia, ataxia, headache, confusion, dizziness, weakness, fatigue, hand tremor, insomnia, anxiety, euphoria, choreiform and other involuntary movements, nightmares, and agitation

Significant Adverse Reactions

GI—diarrhea, GI bleeding, ulceration
Cardiovascular—palpitations, tachycardia, arrhythmias, phlebitis, hemolytic anemia
Neurologic/psychiatric—bradykinetic episodes ("on-off" phenomena—see Nursing Alerts); muscle twitching; grinding of the teeth; convulsions; paranoid ideation; psychotic reactions; depression; dementia
Ocular—spasmodic winking (blepharospasm), diplopia, blurred vision
Other—urinary retention, bitter taste, skin rash, sweating, hot flashes, edema, alopecia, leukopenia
Drug may elevate BUN, SGOT, SGPT, LDH, bilirubin, alkaline phosphatase, and PBI; may also reduce WBC, hemoglobin, and hematocrit.

Contraindications

Narrow-angle glaucoma, undiagnosed skin lesions or history of melanoma, acute psychoses, and patients on MAO inhibitor therapy

Interactions

1 Effects of levodopa may be *decreased* by antipsychotics, phenytoin, papaverine, pyridoxine, reserpine, phenylbutazone, benzodiazepines (*e.g.,* diazepam).
2 Levodopa may enhance the hypotensive effect of methyldopa, guanethidine, diuretics, and possibly other antihypertensive drugs.
3 Therapeutic effects of l-DOPA may be potentiated by propranolol, methyldopa, and anticholinergics.
4 Cardiovascular effects of sympathomimetic drugs such as amphetamines, ephedrine, and epinephrine can be increased by levodopa.
5 Diabetic control with oral hypoglycemic drugs may be adversely affected by l-DOPA.

▶ NURSING ALERTS

▷ 1 Use cautiously in patients with severe cardiovascular, pulmonary, renal, hepatic, or endocrine disease; peptic ulcer; chronic wide-angle glaucoma; diabetes; psychiatric disturbances (including depression); a history of myocardial infarction with residual arrhythmias; and in pregnant or lactating women.
▷ 2 Inform patients that orthostatic hypotension is common during early months of therapy, and is often asymptomatic. Advise caution in hazardous occupations because of the possibility of dizziness or ataxia, and urge gradual position changes.
▷ 3 Observe for appearance of muscle twitching and blepharospasm (intermittent winking), early signs of overdosage.
▷ 4 Be alert for *sudden* worsening of symptoms (*e.g.,* extreme weakness, bradykinesia) during prolonged high-dosage therapy, the so-called "on-off" phenomenon. Condition usually lasts for several hours, and is apparently due to temporarily excessive l-DOPA levels, perhaps resulting from altered metabolism.
▷ 5 Note that prolonged use often leads to development of abnormal involuntary movements, especially of the face, mouth, tongue, and head. Attempt to reduce dose to lowest effective level to minimize these effects.

▶ NURSING CONSIDERATIONS

▷ 1 Advise patients to avoid multiple vitamin preparations containing vitamin B_6 (pyridoxine) because this will reduce the effects of l-DOPA by increasing its *peripheral* conversion to dopamine.
▷ 2 Carefully observe patient's response to and tolerance of l-DOPA. Dosage adjustments should be made slowly to minimize adverse effects; vital signs need to be monitored during the period of early dosage regulation.
▷ 3 Perform periodic tests on hepatic, renal, and cardiovascular function during prolonged drug therapy.
▷ 4 Observe diabetic patients for loss of control following levodopa administration. Check blood sugar frequently during therapy. Note that levodopa may cause false negative with Clinistix and false positive with Clinitest.
▷ 5 Inform patient that urine and sweat may be darkened by levodopa.
▷ 6 Administer drug with food to lessen GI irritation.
▷ 7 Advise patients that some improvement generally occurs within 2 weeks to 3 weeks, but may take several months in some cases.

▶ carbidopa/levodopa
Sinemet

A fixed ratio (1:4, 1:10) combination of carbidopa and l-DOPA; carbidopa competes for the enzyme dopa decarboxylase, thereby retarding the *peripheral* breakdown of l-DOPA. This allows a greater fraction of the administered l-DOPA dose to pass the blood–brain barrier, resulting in higher dopamine levels in central motor regulatory centers. Carbidopa itself does not cross the blood–brain barrier and therefore does not interfere with conversion of l-DOPA to dopamine in the CNS. Levodopa dosage requirements are reduced approximately 75% by combination with carbidopa, because plasma levels and plasma half-life are increased. Consequently, much less dopamine is formed peripherally than with the use of l-DOPA alone, resulting in a lower incidence of many systemic side-effects, especially nausea, vomiting, and cardiovascular disturbances. However, adverse *CNS* effects (*e.g.,* dyskinesias) may occur sooner and at lower doses of l-DOPA when combined with carbidopa than when given alone, because more levodopa is reaching the brain to be converted there to dopamine. Carbidopa also prevents the antagonism of l-DOPA by vitamin B_6 (pyridoxine).

The pharmacologic and toxicologic properties of carbidopa/levodopa are similar to those of levodopa in most respects. However, the fixed ratio combinations allow use of lower doses of l-DOPA, provide a smoother response, and permit more rapid dosage adjustments than can be obtained with l-DOPA alone. Untoward reactions, contraindications, and drug interactions observed with carbidopa/levodopa are essentially the same as those noted with levodopa itself, although blood levels of urea nitrogen, uric acid, and creatinine are lower during carbidopa/levodopa administration than during treatment with levodopa alone.

Levodopa must be discontinued at least 8 hours prior to initiating therapy with carbidopa/levodopa, which should be substituted at a dosage level that will provide approximately 25% of the previous levodopa dose. The combination is not recommended in children under 18.

The dosage of carbidopa/levodopa, like that of levodopa itself, is highly individualized. Tablets are available in a fixed ratio of either 10 mg carbidopa/100 mg levodopa, 25 mg carbidopa/100 mg levodopa, or 25 mg carbidopa/250 mg levodopa. Dosage schedules are as follows:

A. *Patients not receiving levodopa*—Initially, 1 tablet (10/100 or 25/100) 3 times/day; increase by 1 tablet daily until 6 tablets/day. If more l-DOPA is necessary, substitute 1 tablet (25/250) 3 to 4 times/day; increase by ½ to 1 tablet/day to a maximum of 8 tablets (25/250) per day.

B. *Patients receiving levodopa*—(Discontinue l-DOPA for at least 8 hr) Initially, 1 tablet (25/250) 3 to 4 times/day in patient previously requiring 1500 mg or more of levodopa alone per day. Otherwise, 1 tablet (10/100) 3 to 4 times/day. Adjust by ½ to 1 tablet a day until control is obtained.

Patients should be closely observed for development of involuntary movements or blepharospasm, which are often early indications that the dosage may be excessive. For other clinical alerts and considerations, see Levodopa. In addition, carbidopa (Lodosyn) is available alone as 25-mg tablets to be used *only* with l-DOPA. Individual dosing of the two drugs allows separate titration of each agent, and may result in better control of the symptoms and a lower incidence of side-effects than with use of the fixed-dosage combinations. Although most parkinsonian patients can be managed adequately with the carbidopa/levodopa combination (Sinemet), certain patients may require individual titration of each drug, especially when nausea and vomiting are prominent.

▶ amantadine
Symmetrel

A synthetic antiviral agent originally used for prophylaxis against the Asian (A) strain of influenza, Amantadine can also effectively relieve symptoms of parkinsonism (especially akinesia and rigidity) in many patients. It is less effective than l-DOPA but elicits fewer adverse effects, and often produces a more rapid clinical improvement. Amantadine is somewhat more effective than anticholinergics, but its efficacy tends to diminish with time. Improvement may persist from several months to several years. The drug is usually given in combination with l-DOPA, resulting in an additive effect.

Mechanism
Not completely understood; may enhance release of dopamine from presynaptic nerve endings; effectiveness is greatly reduced in the absence of functional dopamine stores in the corpus striatum; no anticholinergic activity

Antiviral action has been attributed to prevention of the release of viral nucleic acid into host cells; does not interfere with the influenza A viral vaccine (see Chap. 73)

Uses
1 Symptomatic treatment of parkinsonism and drug-induced extrapyramidal reactions
2 Prophylaxis against Asian (A) influenza virus strains, especially in high-risk patients (see Chap. 73)
3 Symptomatic management of respiratory disease caused by Asian (A) influenza virus (see Chap. 73)

Dosage
Parkinsonism—100 mg 1 to 2 times/day (maximum 400 mg/day)
Drug-Induced Extrapyramidal Reactions—100 mg twice a day (maximum 300 mg/day)

Influenza
Adults: 100 mg twice a day
Children (1 yr–9 yr): 2 mg to 4 mg/lb/day (maximum 150 mg/day)

Fate
Well absorbed orally; peak plasma levels in 2 hours to 4 hours; long duration of action (half-life 18 hr–24 hr); not metabolized to any extent and excreted almost entirely intact through the kidneys; excretion is enhanced in an acid urine.

Common Side-Effects
Irritability, anxiety, nausea, dizziness, ataxia, confusion, mild depression, constipation, urinary retention, peripheral edema, and livedo reticularis (skin mottling)

Significant Adverse Reactions
Orthostatic hypotension, vomiting, headache, weakness, fatigue, insomnia, dyspnea, tremors, visual disturbances, skin rash, dermatitis, congestive heart failure, psychotic reactions, leukopenia, and neutropenia

Contraindications
Nursing mothers

Interactions
1 Amantadine may worsen the side-effects of anticholinergics (*e.g.*, hallucinations, confusion).
2 Excessive CNS stimulation may occur with other stimulants.

▶ NURSING ALERTS
▷ 1 Use cautiously in patients with a history or evidence of epilepsy, congestive heart failure, or peripheral edema. Also in patients with dermatitis, hypotension, psychotic disturbances, liver or kidney disease, and in elderly patients.
▷ 2 Caution patient that dizziness, drowsiness, and blurred vision resulting from drug use may impair ability to drive or operate machinery.
▷ 3 Do not discontinue drug *abruptly* because marked worsening of symptoms can occur. Taper dosage gradually.

▶ NURSING CONSIDERATIONS
▷ 1 Avoid administering last dose close to bedtime because insomnia can result.
▷ 2 Inform patient that livedo reticularis (skin mottling, usually of lower extremities) may occur, particularly if patient is exposed to cold. Effect generally appears early in therapy and will subside once drug is discontinued or possibly when dose is reduced.
▷ 3 Note that if the drug becomes ineffective, beneficial effects may be regained by increasing the dose or discontinuing the drug briefly, then resuming.
▷ 4 Advise patients to make position changes slowly, especially arising from bed, because orthostatic hypotension may occur.
▷ 5 Observe patient closely during therapy because therapeutic effectiveness of the drug is unpredictable and

may decrease abruptly. Advise physician of any change in patient's status.

▶ bromocriptine
Parlodel

Bromocriptine is primarily used orally as adjunctive therapy to provide additional therapeutic benefits in patients, currently maintained on l-DOPA, who are beginning to show signs of deterioration in their condition. Due to the progressive degenerative nature of parkinsonism, even persons receiving maximum doses of l-DOPA, in combination with carbidopa, are eventually susceptible to breakthrough effects. These are sometimes referred to as "late l-DOPA failures." Examples of such conditions are return of tremor or rigidity, "end-of-dose" failure (appearance of akinesia between dosing), and "on-off" phenomena (abrupt loss of mobility). Bromocriptine may delay the onset of late l-DOPA failure and may also ameliorate the symptoms (e.g., dyskinesias) that result from excessive l-DOPA levels by allowing a dosage reduction.

Bromocriptine functions as a dopamine receptor agonist and is employed in several other ways in addition to its adjunctive use in parkinsonism. Among the other indications for bromocriptine, discussed in Chapter 80, are treatment of amenorrhea–galactorrhea and control of postpartum lactation. Only those aspects of its usage that pertain to its applicability to parkinsonism are considered here.

Initial dosage is one half of a 2.5-mg tablet twice daily, in conjunction with carbidopa/levodopa at their previously employed doses, unless increased side-effects necessitate a dosage reduction. Bromocriptine dosage may be increased by 2.5-mg increments every 2 weeks to 4 weeks until satisfactory control has been attained.

Adverse reactions to bromocriptine are similar to those of l-DOPA, but the incidence of nausea, confusion, hypotension, and dizziness appears to be somewhat higher with bromocriptine than with l-DOPA. Bromocriptine is contraindicated in nursing mothers, because it prevents lactation, and its safety has not been determined in children under 15.

II Anticholinergic/Antihistaminergic Agents

Benztropine	Ethopropazine
Biperiden	Orphenadrine
Cycrimine	Procyclidine
Diphenhydramine	Trihexyphenidyl

The first drugs used for the treatment of Parkinson's disease were the belladonna alkaloids, atropine and scopolamine, and for many years these were the only effective drugs available for this disease. These agents, although still occasionally employed, have been supplanted by a group of synthetic drugs having central anticholinergic (and in some instances antihistaminergic) activity.

These agents are useful on their own in patients with mild symptoms, and the agents appear to be most effective in relieving rigidity and occasional tremor. They are commonly prescribed in combination with levodopa, to obtain more efficient control of the condition than either drug alone is capable of providing. The usefulness of these compounds is mainly limited by their side-effects, which, although not usually serious, are frequent and annoying (e.g., blurred vision, dizziness, dysuria). Moreover, large doses are associated with development of CNS toxicity resembling atropine intoxication, characterized by confusion, ataxia, delirium, and hallucinations.

In addition to their use in parkinsonism, these drugs are also widely employed to control the extrapyramidal manifestations (akinesia, dystonias, akathisia, tremor) characteristic of treatment with the antipsychotic agents.

The anticholinergic/antihistaminergic drugs used in Parkinson's disease are pharmacologically and toxicologically similar, and are reviewed as a group. Most of the individual drugs have been mentioned previously, either in Chapter 10 (anticholinergics) or Chapter 14 (antihistamines). They are listed again here in Table 26-1, where specific information is provided relating to their use in parkinsonism and extrapyramidal disorders.

Mechanism
Exhibit a blocking effect on central cholinergic excitatory pathways that normally exert increasing effect as dopaminergic inhibition is reduced due to lack of functional dopamine; also retard re-uptake of dopamine into presynaptic nerve endings, thereby blocking its inactivation; some agents may have a direct relaxing effect on smooth muscle.

Uses
1 Sole or adjunctive treatment of parkinsonian symptoms, especially rigidity
2 Prevention and relief of extrapyramidal reactions resulting from antipsychotic drug therapy

Dosage
See Table 26-1.

Fate
Generally well absorbed orally; onset usually in 30 minutes to 60 minutes; duration of action is variable (average 4 hr–6 hr), except for sustained-release preparations (8 hr–12 hr); excreted primarily by the kidney, both as metabolites and intact drug

Common Side-Effects
Dryness of mouth, blurred vision, dizziness, nausea, nervousness, drowsiness, and urinary hesitancy

Significant Adverse Reactions
(Usually due to excessive dosage) Confusion, agitation, delirium, hallucinations, depression, memory loss, vomiting, constipation, paralytic ileus, dilatation of the colon, skin rash, flushing, decreased sweating, tachycardia, palpitation,

Table 26-1. Anticholinergic/Antihistaminergic Drugs Used For Parkinsonism

Drug	Preparations	Usual Dosage Range	Remarks
Benztropine (Cogentin)	Tablets—0.5 mg, 1 mg, 2 mg Injection—1 mg/ml	Parkinsonism 1 mg to 2 mg/day (range 0.5 mg–6 mg) Extrapyramidal rections 1 mg to 4 mg 1 to 2 times/day	IM injection used for rapid response in acute dystonic reactions (onset 15 min); do not use in children under 3; effects are cumulative and may take several days to develop; usually not effective against tremors
Biperiden (Akineton)	Tablets—2 mg Injection—5 mg/ml	Parkinsonism 2 mg 3 to 4 times/day Extrapyramidal reactions Oral—2 mg 1 to 3 times/day IM, IV—2 mg; may repeat every 30 minutes to a total of 4 doses	Most effective against akinesia and rigidity; effectively reduces salivation and seborrhea; may produce mood elevation or temporary euphoria, especially parenterally; IV injection can cause hypotension and incoordination
Diphenhydramine (Benadryl and others; see Chap. 14)	Capsules—25 mg, 50 mg Tablets—25 mg, 50 mg Elixir—12.5 mg/5 ml Syrup—12.5, 13.3 mg/5 ml Injection—10, 50 mg/ml	Oral—50 mg 3 to 4 times/day IV, IM—10 mg to 50 mg (maximum 400/day)	Effective in mild parkinsonism and extrapyramidal reactions (especially dystonias); often combined with other anticholinergics or l-DOPA; see Chapter 14 for adverse effects, contraindications, and interactions
Ethopropazine (Parsidol)	Tablets—10 mg, 50 mg	Initially 50 mg 1 to 2 times/day Increase gradually to a maximum of 600 mg/day in severe cases	A phenothiazine derivative with significant anticholinergic activity; effectively controls most symptoms, including tremor; does *not* potentiate other CNS depressants; high incidence of side-effects and poorly tolerated by many older patients; used for treatment of extrapyramidal reactions, even though it is a phenothiazine itself
Orphenadrine HCl (Disipal)	Tablets—50 mg	Parkinsonism 50 mg 3 times/day (maximum 250 mg/day)	Antihistamine that is also a centrally acting muscle relaxant; relieves rigidity and controls autonomic manifestations as well; minimal drowsiness, but high incidence of other atropine-like side-effects; use with chlorpromazine has resulted in hypoglycemic coma; may decrease the effects of barbiturates, phenylbutazone, and griseofulvin; also available as the citrate for relief of musculoskeletal disorders (see chap. 15)
Procyclidine (Kemadrin)	Tablets—2 mg, 5 mg	Parkinsonism 2 mg to 2.5 mg 3 times/day; increase gradually to a maximum of 20 mg/day Extrapyramidal reactions 2 mg to 2.5 mg 3 times/day (usual range 10 mg–20 mg/day)	Anticholinergic and smooth muscle antispasmodic; most effective against rigidity; controls excessive salivation as well; may temporarily worsen tremor as rigidity is relieved; be alert for confusion, agitation, and behavioral changes, which are common in the elderly with hypotension; Similar to trihexyphenidyl
Trihexyphenidyl (Artane, Tremin, Trihexane, Trihexidyl, Trihexy)	Tablets—2 mg, 5 mg Capsules—5 mg (sustained-release) Elixir—2 mg/5 ml	Parkinsonism Iniitally 1 mg; increase by 2-mg increments every 3 to 5 days to a maximum of 15 mg/day Usual range 6 mg to 10 mg/day, in 3 to 4 divided doses or 5 mg sustained-release once or twice a day Extrapyramidal Reactions Initially 1 mg; increase by 1 mg every few hours until control is obtained Usual range 5 mg to 15 mg/day in divided doses	Anticholinergic and smooth muscle relaxant; do *not* use sustained-release capsules for initial therapy because they do not allow enough flexibility in dosage regulation; major effect is on rigidity, although most symptoms improve to some extent; effects may be potentiated by MAO inhibitors

weakness, mild orthostatic hypotension, parasthesia, numbness in extremities, muscle cramping, elevated temperature, mydriasis, diplopia, headache, and increased intraocular pressure

Contraindications
Acute narrow-angle glaucoma

Interactions
1 Combined use with other drugs having an anticholinergic action (*e.g.,* phenothiazines, tricyclic antidepressants) may result in increased toxicity.
2 May potentiate the sedative action of other CNS depressants (*e.g.,* alcohol, barbiturates, narcotics).
3 Psychotic episodes may be precipitated by use of centrally acting anticholinergics with antipsychotic drugs.

▶ NURSING ALERTS
▷ 1 Use with extreme caution in patients with glaucoma; pyloric, duodenal, or bladder neck obstruction; prostatic hypertrophy; myasthenia gravis; peptic ulcer; cardiac, liver, or kidney disorders; and in small children, elderly or debilitated patients; alcoholics, and pregnant or nursing women.
▷ 2 Caution patients that drugs may impair physical and mental abilities, especially during early therapy. Advise care in driving and operating machinery.
▷ 3 Be alert for impaired sweating ability, especially during hot weather, which may interfere with maintenance of heat equilibrium. Consider dosage reduction if problem is present, and counsel patient to avoid exertion as much as possible.
▷ 4 Be alert for development of abdominal pain, distention, and constipation, which are possible signs of developing paralytic ileus. Advise physician.

▶ NURSING CONSIDERATIONS
▷ 1 Stress need for periodic ophthalmic examinations for patients on prolonged therapy.
▷ 2 Note that dosage requirements are quite variable and may change as condition deteriorates. Observe patient's response closely, and make dosage adjustments as situation warrants to minimize side-effects.
▷ 3 Monitor urinary output and bowel function during prolonged therapy, and advise physician of any changes.
▷ 4 Advise patients that clinical improvement may take several days or even weeks to occur. Stress the importance of rigid adherence to prescribed dosage levels.
▷ 5 Suggest use of hard candy, gum, or frequent sips of water to alleviate dryness of the mouth.
▷ 6 When adding drugs to an established antiparkinsonian regimen, do so gradually and taper the dose of other drugs slowly.
▷ 7 Give drugs with or following meals to minimize gastric irritation.

Summary. Antiparkinsonian Drugs

Drug	Preparations	Usual Dosage Range
Dopaminergic Agents		
Levodopa (Dopar, Larodopa)	Tablets—100 mg, 250 mg, 500 mg Capsules—100 mg, 125 mg, 250 mg, 500 mg	Initially 0.5 g to 1 g/day; increase by 0.75 g/3 to 7 days to a maximum of 8 g/day
Carbidopa/Levodopa (Sinemet)	Tablets—10 mg carbidopa and 100 mg levodopa, 25 mg carbidopa and 100 mg levodopa, or 25 mg carbidopa and 250 mg levodopa	Initially 1 tablet (10:100 or 25:100) 3 times/day; increase by 1 tablet daily to 6 tablets/day; alternately 1 tablet (25:250) 3 to 4 times/day; increase by ½ to 1 tablet to 8 tablets/day depending on response
Carbidopa (Lodosyn)	Tablets—25 mg	12.5 mg to 25 mg as needed with carbidopa/levodopa combination to provide improved symptom control or to reduce side-effects
Amantadine (Symmetrel)	Capsules—100 mg Syrup—50 mg/5 ml	Parkinsonism—100 mg 1 to 2 times/day (maximum 400 mg/day) Extrapyramidal Reactions—100 mg twice a day (maximum 300 mg/day)

(continued)

Summary. Antiparkinsonian Drugs *(continued)*

Drug	Preparations	Usual Dosage Range
		Influenza: Adults—100 mg twice a day
		Children (1 yr–9 yr)—2 mg to 4 mg/lb/day (maximum 150 mg/day)
Bromocriptine (Parlodel)	Tablets—2.5 mg Capsules—5 mg	Initially, 1.25 mg twice a day; increase by 2.5 mg/day every 2 weeks to 4 weeks until optimal response is achieved

Anticholinergic/Antihistaminergic Agents

See Table 26-1

Although a large number of pharmacologic agents have a stimulating effect on the central nervous system (CNS), the number of drugs actually employed clinically for this purpose is quite small. A useful classification of the therapeutically effective CNS stimulants is as follows:

I. Respiratory stimulants (analeptics)
   (*e.g.,* doxapram)
II. Caffeine
III. Amphetamines
   (*e.g.,* dextroamphetamine, methamphetamine)
IV. Anorexiants
   (*e.g.,* phentermine, diethylpropion)
V. Methylphenidate
VI. Pemoline

The analeptics are used primarily as physiologic antagonists of respiratory depression due to overdosage with CNS depressants. Analeptics are considered in detail in Chapter 57.

Caffeine is the most widely used CNS stimulant, largely because it is consumed in coffee, tea, soda, and many over-the-counter drug combinations. In small amounts, it is a relatively weak stimulant that aids in maintaining mental alertness. It can also be employed parenterally as a respiratory stimulant, and may relieve the pain of vascular headaches by virtue of its constricting action on cerebral blood vessels.

The amphetamines are potent CNS stimulants with a high potential for abuse. They have been used to treat obesity, although their usefulness is restricted to a short-term basis (several weeks). A group of amphetamine-related drugs, termed anorexiants, are used in the therapy of obesity, with most of the same restrictions and limitations as amphetamine itself. Other approved indications for the amphetamines are the treatment of narcolepsy and minimal brain dysfunction (MBD).

The remaining drugs listed above are primarily indicated as alternatives to amphetamine for the treatment of the minimal brain dysfunction syndrome in children.

Central Nervous System Stimulants

27

I Analeptics

Analeptic drugs are termed medullary stimulants because their effects are primarily exerted on the respiratory and vasomotor centers in the medulla. Their major action is reversal of the respiratory depression induced by large doses of CNS depressant drugs. Because these agents primarily affect respiratory function, they are discussed with other drugs acting on the respiratory system in Section VII of this book.

II Caffeine (Caffedrine, Kirkaffeine, NōDōz, Quick Pep, Tirend, Vivarin)

Caffeine is a xanthine derivative possessing relatively weak CNS-stimulant, smooth-muscle relaxant, vasodilatory, diuretic, and myocardial stimulant actions. However, it constricts cerebral arteries and enhances the contraction of skeletal muscles. CNS stimulant effects are exerted mainly on the cortex in small doses, relieving fatigue and improving sensory awareness. Larger doses can further excite lower brain centers (*e.g.*, vasomotor, respiratory, vagal).

Mechanism

Increases the concentration of cyclic AMP in tissues by inhibiting the phosphodiesterase enzyme that inactivates cyclic AMP; may also increase release of calcium from the sarcoplasmic reticulum, increasing skeletal muscle tone; stimulates all levels of the CNS, produces cardiac stimulation, augments gastric acid secretion, and constricts cerebral blood vessels

Uses

1　Allays fatigue and increases sensory awareness (orally)
2　Treatment of mild to moderate respiratory depression caused by overdosage with CNS depressants such as morphine or alcohol (parenterally)
3　Relieves pain associated with vascular headaches or spinal puncture (orally or parenterally, often with ergotamine)

Dosage

Oral: 100 mg to 250 mg every 3 hours to 4 hours
IM: (caffeine and sodium benzoate)—500 mg; repeat as necessary (maximum single dose—1000 mg)
IV: 500 mg in respiratory failure

Fate

Readily absorbed following injection; well absorbed orally; readily crosses the blood–brain barrier; half-life is 3 hours to 6 hours; minimally protein-bound; partially demethylated and oxidized in the liver; excreted largely through the kidney, 10% as unchanged drug

Common Side-Effects

Nervousness, insomnia, and gastric irritation

Significant Adverse Reactions

(Usually with large doses) Nausea, vomiting, hematemesis, restlessness, irritability, excitement, tinnitus, scotomas, tremors, flushing, palpitation, tachycardia, extrasystoles, diuresis, hypotension, delirium, and respiratory distress

Interactions

1　Caffeine may cause hypertensive reactions in combination with MAO inhibitors.
2　Caffeine can increase CNS stimulation due to propoxyphene overdosage, resulting in convulsions.

▶ NURSING ALERTS

▷　1　Administer caffeine and sodium benzoate slowly. Do not exceed 1000 mg per dose, because increased respiratory depression may result.
▷　2　Use carefully in patients with gastric ulcers, myocardial infarction, respiratory depression, and diabetes.

▶ NURSING CONSIDERATIONS

▷　1　Advise heavy caffeine users that headache, dizziness, palpitations, and nervousness can occur either during use or upon abrupt withdrawal.
▷　2　Have a short-acting barbiturate on hand when giving IM or IV, to counteract excessive CNS stimulation.

III　Amphetamines

Amphetamine	Dextroamphetamine
Amphetamine complex	Methamphetamine

The amphetamines are synthetic sympathomimetic amines with marked CNS-stimulatory action. They increase alertness and concentration, temporarily elevate mood, and stimulate motor activity. Amphetamines can induce varying degrees of euphoria depending on the dose as well as the personality of the user. Major peripheral effects of the components include elevation of blood pressure, relaxation of bronchiolar smooth muscle, contraction of the urinary sphincter, and mydriasis.

Prolonged oral use of amphetamines often leads to irritability, insomnia, and dizziness. The stimulation resulting from amphetamine usage is invariably followed by an equally intense depression, usually accompanied by fatigue and listlessness. The desire to overcome this poststimulatory depression often leads to repetitive amphetamine dosing, and in the emotionally unstable person, this can evolve into a vicious circle culminating in habituation and addiction. Large, repeated doses of amphetamines have brought about a behavioral state that is difficult to distinguish clinically from paranoid schizophrenia. Obviously, the danger is greatly increased when these agents are abused parenterally (IV) as "spree drugs." The acute behavioral changes that ensue with IV injection include extreme disorientation, hallucinations, and paranoid ideation; users are given to violent outbursts that can endanger themselves and others (see Chap. 81 for a discussion of amphetamine abuse).

Approved clinical indications for amphetamines are few; use of these drugs must be undertaken cautiously, and patients closely observed. The amphetamines are discussed as a group, then are listed individually in Table 27-1.

Mechanism

Promote release of catecholamines from presynaptic nerve terminals, and prevent their re-uptake into these nerve endings; net effect is potentiation of endogenous catecholamine activity; may exert a direct-activating effect on adrenergic receptor sites and interfere with the functioning of monoamine oxidase (MAO), an enzyme responsible for intracellular breakdown of monoamines such as norepinephrine, dopamine, and serotonin; stimulant effect thought to be caused by an action on the cortex and possibly reticular formation; anorexiant action may be caused by an inhibitory effect on hypothalamic feeding centers as well as elevation of mood. Usefulness in minimal brain dysfunction has been related to potentiation of dopamine action in the CNS.

Table 27-1. Amphetamines

Drug	Preparations	Usual Dosage Range	Remarks
Amphetamine sulfate	Tablets—5 mg, 10 mg Sustained-release capsules—15 mg	**Narcolepsy** 5 mg to 60 mg/day in divided doses **Minimal brain dysfunction** 3 years to 5 years—2.5 mg/day; increase by 2.5 mg/week over 6 years—5 mg 1 to 2 times/day; increase by 5 mg/week **Obesity** 5 mg to 30 mg/day in divided doses	Note development of insomnia or anorexia, and reduce dose; give first dose on awakening and last dose 4 hours to 6 hours before bedtime if possible; attempt to provide "drug-free" periods in children with minimal brain dysfunction, especially during periods of reduced stress (*e.g.,* summer vacations, holidays); be aware that response is more variable in children than in adults, and observe more closely (Schedule II)
Amphetamine complex (Biphetamine)	Capsules—12½ mg, 20 mg (contain 6.25 mg and 10 mg each of dextroamphetamine and amphetamine, respectively)	**Obesity** 1 capsule daily in the morning	Indicated only for *short-term* adjunctive treatment of exogenous obesity; high potential for abuse; should be prescribed cautiously and patient's consumption monitored carefully (Schedule II)
Dextroamphetamine sulfate (Dexampex, Dexedrine, Ferndex, Oxydess II, Spancap No. 1)	Tablets—5 mg, 10 mg Capsules—15 mg Capsules—(sustained-release) 5 mg, 10 mg, 15 mg Elixir—5 mg/5 ml	**Narcolepsy** 5 mg to 60 mg/day in divided doses **Obesity** 2.5 mg to 10 mg 1 to 3 times/day **Minimal brain dysfunction** (over 3 yr)—2.5 mg to 5 mg/day; increase gradually to optimal effect (maximum 40 mg/day)	More potent CNS stimulant than amphetamine, but less of an effect on the cardiovascular and peripheral nervous systems; give last dose at least 6 hours before bedtime; tolerance usually develops within several weeks; possesses the same pharmacologic properties and hazards as amphetamine, and should be used sparingly and cautiously (Schedule II)
Methamphetamine (Desoxyn, Methampex)	Tablets—5 mg, 10 mg Long-acting tablets—5 mg, 10 mg, 15 mg	**Obesity** 5 mg 3 times/day (long-acting—1 tablet daily) **Minimal brain dysfunction** (over 6 yr)—Initially, 5 mg 1 to 2 times/day; increase by 5 mg/week to optimal level (usual range 20 mg to 25 mg/day)	CNS effects slightly greater than amphetamine; do not use long-acting tablets to initiate dosage; give 30 minutes before meals and last dose at least 6 hours before bedtime; large doses may result in cardiac stimulation; tolerance develops quickly, so drug has high abuse potential; commonly called *speed* among abusers; has caused severe psychotic reactions following repeated injections of dissolved tablets (Schedule II)

Uses

1 *Short*-term adjunct in the treatment of obesity, as an aid to a total weight control program (potential benefit does *not* outweigh inherent risks—see below)
2 Treatment of narcolepsy
3 Treatment of minimal brain dysfunction syndrome in children

Dosage

See Table 27-1.

Fate

Rapidly absorbed from GI tract and widely distributed in the body; high concentrations are found in the brain and cerebrospinal fluid; onset of action is usually in 30 minutes to 60 minutes; plasma half-life is approximately 4 hours to 6 hours but effects may persist for up to 24 hours; partially metabolized in the liver, and excreted in the urine as both metabolites and unchanged drug

Common Side-Effects

Nervousness, palpitations, insomnia, dryness of the mouth, and unpleasant taste

Significant Adverse Reactions

CNS—dizziness, euphoria or dysphoria, headache, chills, tremor; large doses may cause confusion, hallucinations, panic, aggressiveness, and psychotic episodes
Cardiovascular—tachycardia, hypertension, arrhythmias
GI—nausea, vomiting, diarrhea, anorexia and weight loss, cramping
Other—impotence, urticaria, delayed or difficult urination; large doses can cause dyspnea, anginal pain, syncope, convulsions, and coma

Contraindications

Cardiovascular disease, hypertension, hyperthyroidism, arteriosclerosis, glaucoma, agitated states, severe endogenous depression, history of drug abuse, children under 3, and pregnancy

Interactions

1 Amphetamines may reduce the antihypertensive effects of guanethidine, methyldopa, hydralazine, and possibly other antihypertensive drugs.
2 Effects of amphetamines can be potentiated by acetazolamide, cocaine, furazolidone, propoxyphene, tricyclic antidepressants, MAO inhibitors, and by sodium bicarbonate and other substances that alkalinize the urine.
3 Amphetamines may be antagonized by acidifying agents (ascorbic acid, methenamine, reserpine, glutamic acid, fruit juices), lithium, haloperidol, and phenothiazines.
4 Amphetamines may delay the effects of phenytoin, ethosuximide, and related anticonvulsants by impairing their GI absorption.

▶ NURSING ALERTS

Note: The risk of dependence with amphetamines is considerable; thus, it is probably *not* appropriate to prescribe them for weight reduction.

▷ 1 Use amphetamines for weight control only after other weight reduction programs have failed. Do not give for more than a few weeks, and observe patients closely for signs of tolerance. Discontinue the drug rather than increase the dose.
▷ 2 Caution the patient that ability to drive or operate machinery may be impaired by the drug.
▷ 3 Warn users that there may be a poststimulatory depression reaction, and stress the need for proper rest and avoidance of hazardous activities during this period as well.
▷ 4 Carefully screen potential users for a history of drug abuse or altered behavior patterns. Prescribe cautiously in such persons and closely monitor drug-taking practices.
▷ 5 Do not give concurrently or within 14 days of treatment with MAO inhibitors, because hypertensive crisis can occur.
▷ 6 Do not discontinue drug abruptly following prolonged therapy because extreme fatigue or depression can occur, as well as psychotic behavior.

▶ NURSING CONSIDERATIONS

▷ 1 Administer last dose at least 6 hours before bedtime, if possible, to minimize insomnia.
▷ 2 Inform diabetic patients that insulin or dietary requirements may be altered by amphetamines. Urge patients to report any symptomatic changes.
▷ 3 Note that amphetamines are class II substances. Learn regulations governing their handling (see Appendix).

▷ 4 When used for minimal brain dysfunction in children, provide appropriate educational, psychological, and social intervention along with drug therapy.
▷ 5 Attempt to determine *lowest* effective dose for each patient to minimize danger of adverse effects and habituation.

▷ *Dietary precautions*
▷ 1 When used for weight reduction, stress the importance of rigid adherence to dietary program, to obtain maximal benefit.
▷ 2 Avoid excessive use of foods high in tyramine (*e.g.,* cheese, beer, chianti wine, liver, salted fish, broad beans, avocados) because an excessive rise in blood pressure can occur with amphetamines.

IV   Anorexiants

Benzphetamine	Phendimetrazine
Diethylpropion	Phenmetrazine
Fenfluramine	Phentermine
Mazindol	Phenylpropanolamine

A group of drugs related structurally to amphetamine have been used in the treatment of exogenous obesity. These agents, termed *anorexiants, anorectics,* or *anorexigenics,* possess essentially the same spectrum of pharmacologic and toxicologic actions as amphetamine. With the exception of fenfluramine, which produces CNS depression, all these drugs evoke varying degrees of stimulation that appear to be a major component of their anorectic action. They are primarily indicated for the temporary, adjunctive management of obesity in conjunction with a carefully supervised program of caloric restriction and proper exercise. Although none of these agents is superior to amphetamine in effectiveness, some do have less potential for habituation than the amphetamines and may be preferable for short-term therapy. It is important to recognize, however, that *all* of these drugs can become habituating with continued use. Since their therapeutic benefit is restricted to a few weeks at best, because of developing tolerance, there is significant danger in their prolonged consumption.

In addition to the prescription-only anorexigenic drugs discussed below, the decongestant *phenylpropanolamine* is available over-the-counter as a diet aid, either alone or in combination with caffeine. A weak CNS stimulant, phenylpropanolamine is recommended for the short-term management of obesity, although its efficacy is subject to considerable doubt. Moreover, because it stimulates alpha-adrenergic receptors and releases norepinephrine, it can significantly elevate blood pressure, and should not be taken by anyone with even mild hypertension. Severe hypertensive episodes have occurred during concomitant administration of phenylpropanolamine and propranolol or indomethacin. Contraindications to phenylpropanolamine include hypertension, diabetes, kidney disease, arteriosclerosis, symptomatic cardiovascular disease, and hyperthyroidism. Recommended doses of phenylpropanolamine are 25 mg 3 times/day or 75 mg (sustained-release) once daily. Strict supervision is necessary whenever these nonprescription diet aids are used.

The anorexigenic drugs are discussed as a group, followed by a tabular listing of the agents indicating significant differences in their actions. As with amphetamines, the potential benefit to be derived from these agents does not justify the risks associated with their use.

Mechanism

Probably similar to amphetamine; exert a CNS-stimulant effect on the cortex, and may activate hypothalamic satiety center regulating food intake to decrease appetite

Uses

1 Short-term (8 wk–12 wk) adjunctive management of exogenous obesity in conjunction with caloric restriction

Dosage

See Table 27-2.

Fate

Most are quickly and completely absorbed orally; onset of action occurs within 1 hour, and effects generally persist 4 hours to 6 hours; sustained-release formulations may have prolonged action (12 hr–18 hr). Tolerance develops within several weeks; metabolized by the liver and excreted both as unchanged drug and metabolites by the kidney.

Common Side-Effects

Nervousness, irritability, insomnia, dryness of the mouth, and palpitations

Significant Adverse Reactions

Cardiovascular—tachycardia, hypertension, precordial pain, arrhythmias, syncope

CNS—anxiety, dizziness, headache, euphoria, tremors, confusion, incoordination; occasionally depression, dysphoria, dysarthria

GI—nausea, vomiting, unpleasant taste, cramping, constipation, glossitis, stomatitis

Genitourinary—dysuria, polyuria, diuresis, cystitis, impotence, menstrual irregularities, changes in libido, gynecomastia

Other—rash, urticaria, erythema, mydriasis, blurred vision, muscle pain, chills, flushing, fever, sweating, alopecia, blood dyscrasias (rare)

Contraindications

See Amphetamines.

Interactions

See Amphetamines. In addition:

1 Fenfluramine may augment the effects of other CNS depressants (*e.g.,* alcohol, narcotics, barbiturates) and may potentiate the action of antihypertensive drugs.

2 Anorexiants may reduce diabetic drug requirements, by increasing glucose uptake by skeletal muscle cells, necessitating dosage adjustment.

▶ NURSING ALERTS

▷ 1 Do not exceed recommended dose in an attempt to increase anorectic effect. Discontinue therapy after several weeks to avoid development of tolerance and possible habituation.

▷ 2 Caution patients to avoid activities requiring mental alertness and coordination because dizziness and confusion can occur with these drugs.

▷ 3 Do not discontinue drug abruptly if used for prolonged periods of time because extreme fatigue and depression may ensue.

▷ 4 Use cautiously in pregnant or lactating women, and in patients with glaucoma, diabetes, anxiety neuroses, and epilepsy.

▶ NURSING CONSIDERATIONS

▷ 1 Take last dose of medication at least 6 hours before bedtime, if possible, to minimize insomnia. Recognize, however, that much overeating occurs at night; therefore, consider the benefits and disadvantages of giving a dose in the evening.

▷ 2 Emphasize the importance of careful adherence to the *total* treatment regimen (*i.e.,* drugs, diet, exercise) if weight control is to be successful. Stress the danger of overreliance on the drug as the answer to the obesity problem.

▷ 3 Advise the patient to swallow whole the delayed or sustained-action dosage forms. Chewing or crushing the tablets may release large quantities of medication too quickly.

▷ 4 Be aware that drugs are classified in either Schedule II, III, or IV. Note individual classification, and follow proper handling and dispensing procedures for each drug (see Appendix).

▷ 5 Watch for signs of excessive stimulation (tachycardia, dizziness, restlessness, hypertension), and notify physician immediately.

▷ *Dietary precautions*

▷ 1 Outline the proper dietary restrictions that must accompany drug therapy to obtain maximal benefit.

▷ 2 Caution against excessive use of foods high in tyramine (*e.g.,* meat or yeast extracts, cheeses, beef or chicken liver, dried fish, broad beans, beer, vermouth, chianti wine) because increases in blood pressure can occur.

V Methylphenidate (Ritalin)

A CNS stimulant with a pharmacologic profile of action similar to that of amphetamine, but having a more marked effect on mental rather than physical or motor activities at normal doses, methylphenidate shares the same potential for habituation and psychological addiction as the amphetamines,

Table 27-2. Anorexiant Drugs

Drug	Preparations	Usual Dosage Range	Remarks
Benzphetamine (Didrex)	Tablets—25 mg, 50 mg	Initially 25 mg to 50 mg/day; increase as necessary (usual range 50 mg to 150 mg/day)	Usually given as single daily dose, mid-morning or mid-afternoon (Class III)
Diethylpropion (Depletite, Tenuate, Tepanil)	Tablets—25 mg Tablets (sustained-release)— 75 mg	25 mg 3 times/day 1 hour before meals and in mid-evening if needed, *or* 75 mg daily in the morning	Less effective but somewhat less hazardous than amphetamines; caution in epileptics because drug has been shown to increase convulsions; may alter ECG (T-wave changes) (Class IV)
Fenfluramine (Pondimin)	Tablets—20 mg	Initially 20 mg 3 times/day before meals; increase by 20 mg/week to a maximum of 120 mg/day	Differs from other anorexiants because it often produces CNS *depression*; may enhance glucose uptake by skeletal muscles; use cautiously in depression and diabetes; diarrhea is often noted early in therapy; reduce dose or discontinue if severe; do not discontinue abruptly because severe depression can ensue; avoid use in alcoholics, because psychiatric symptoms can develop; may potentiate effects of both CNS stimulants and CNS depressants (Class IV)
Mazindol (Sanorex)	Tablets—1 mg, 2 mg	1 mg 3 times/day before meals, or 2 mg daily before lunch	Take with food if necessary, to reduce GI discomfort; may alter diabetic drug requirements by lowering blood glucose levels; elicits CNS and cardiovascular stimulation, and appears to alter mood by an action on the limbic system (Class III)
Phendimetrazine (Various manufacturers)	Tablets—35 mg Capsules—35 mg Sustained-release capsules— 105 mg	35 mg 2 to 3 times/day 1 hour before meals, or 105 mg once a day	Similar to amphetamine in action but somewhat less potent (Class III)
Phenmetrazine (Preludin)	Tablets—25 mg Tablets (sustained-release)— 50 mg, 75 mg	25 mg 2 to 3 times/day 1 hour before meals, or 50 mg to 75 mg daily in the morning	Blood pressure may be elevated by drug; monitor pressure periodically; congenital malformations have occurred but a causal relationship has not been proven; sustained-release forms are no more effective than regular tablets and may be more hazardous if taken in excess; more intense CNS stimulation than most other anorexiants, and greater incidence of abuse
Phentermine (Ionamin and various other manufacturers)	Tablets—8 mg Tablets (long-acting)— 37.5 mg Capsules—15 mg, 30 mg Capsules (long-acting)— 15 mg, 30 mg	8 mg 3 times/day before meals or 15 mg to 37.5 mg daily in the morning	Less potent stimulant of CNS and cardiovascular activity than amphetamine; available as a resin-complex capsule (15 mg, 30 mg) providing prolonged action (10 hr–15 hr); do not use resin complex if patient has diarrhea because effectiveness is lost (Class IV)

although its central excitatory effects are weaker. In usual therapeutic dosage, it does not elevate the blood pressure, heart rate, or respiratory rate; however, in large doses, signs of generalized CNS excitation can occur (*e.g.,* tremors, tachycardia, hyperpyrexia, confusion). It is most widely used as an adjunct in the therapy of minimal brain dysfunction in children, where its effectiveness equals that of the amphetamines.

Mechanism

Not definitively established but probably similar to amphetamine; major action appears to be on the cerebral cortex;

increases release of catecholamines from presynaptic nerve endings

Uses
1 Adjunctive therapy of minimal brain dysfunction syndrome (attention deficit disorder) in children
2 Treatment of narcolepsy
3 Relief of mild depression and apathetic or withdrawn senile behavior

Dosage
Adults: Initially 10 mg 2 to 3 times/day (usual range—20 mg–40 mg/day)

Children (over 6 yr): Initially 5 mg 2 times/day; increase by 5 mg to 10 mg/week to optimal dose (maximum 60 mg/day)

Fate
Absorbed well from GI tract; distributed throughout the body, including CNS; onset of action occurs in 30 minutes to 60 minutes and peak blood levels are achieved in 1 hour to 3 hours; effects persist up to 6 hours with oral administration; excreted through the kidneys, largely as metabolites

Common Side-Effects
Nervousness, insomnia; in children, anorexia, mild weight loss, and tachycardia are also frequent.

Significant Adverse Reactions
CNS—nausea, dizziness, drowsiness, headache, dyskinesia, agitation, toxic psychoses

Cardiovascular—palpitations, blood pressure changes, tachycardia, anginal attacks, arrhythmias

Allergic—skin rash, fever, urticaria, arthralgia, erythema multiforme, necrotizing vasculitis, exfoliative dermatitis

Other—visual disturbances, alopecia, abdominal pain, anemia

Contraindications
Marked tension, anxiety or agitated states, glaucoma, seizure disorders, and *severe* depression

Interactions
1 Methylphenidate may increase the effects of oral anticoagulants, anticonvulsants, tricyclic antidepressants, and phenylbutazone by inhibiting their metabolism.
2 Hypertensive reactions may occur with vasopressors, MAO inhibitors, and furazolidone.
3 Methylphenidate decreases the antihypertensive action of guanethidine.
4 Effects of methylphenidate can be antagonized by phenothiazines and propoxyphene.

▶ NURSING ALERTS
▷ 1 Use cautiously in patients with hypertension, in patients with a history of drug dependence or alcoholism, and during pregnancy.

▷ 2 Carefully supervise drug-taking patterns, especially in emotionally unstable persons, because chronic abuse can occur.

▷ 3 Withdraw drug gradually, to avoid precipitation of severe depressive episodes or psychotic behavior. Do not use in severely depressed patients.

▶ NURSING CONSIDERATIONS
▷ 1 Monitor blood pressure and weight regularly during therapy, and perform periodic blood counts during extended periods of treatment.

▷ 2 Advise patients that nervousness and insomnia may occur early in therapy but generally lessen with time; however, dosage reduction may be required.

▷ 3 Do not administer last dose later than 4 hours to 5 hours prior to bedtime to minimize insomnia.

▷ 4 In treating minimal brain dysfunction, temporarily discontinue drug periodically to assess the patient's condition. If improvement is not noted within approximately 1 month, terminate drug.

▷ 5 Recognize that drug therapy is not indicated in all children with minimal brain dysfunction, and that greatest benefit is usually obtained with appropriate educational and psychological counseling in addition to proper drug treatment.

▷ 6 Be aware that the drug is a class II substance, and handle accordingly (see Appendix).

▷ *Dietary precautions*
See Amphetamine.

VI Pemoline (Cylert)

A chemically unique CNS stimulant having minimal sympathomimetic effects, pemoline is otherwise pharmacologically comparable to amphetamine and methylphenidate. It appears to have a lower abuse potential than most other CNS stimulants.

Mechanism
Not established; increases alertness and motor activity and induces a mild euphoria, probably by an action on the cortex; may increase dopaminergic transmission in CNS structures

Uses
1 Adjunctive therapy of minimal brain dysfunction (attention deficit disorder) in children
2 Treatment of narcolepsy and excessive sleepiness

Dosage
Children (over 6 yr): Initially 37.5 mg/day as single morning dose; increase by 18.75 mg/week until optimal effects are noted; maximum dose—112.5 mg/day

Fate

Absorbed from GI tract, with peak blood levels in 2 hours to 4 hours; effects last 8 hours to 10 hours; plasma half-life approximately 12 hours; metabolized by the liver, and excreted in the urine both as unchanged drug (45%) and various conjugated metabolites

Common Side-Effects

Insomnia, anorexia

Significant Adverse Reactions

Nausea, diarrhea, dizziness, headache, drowsiness, irritability, nystagmus, dyskinesias, abdominal pain, skin rash, jaundice, convulsive movements, and hallucinations

Contraindications

Children under 6

Interactions

1 May enhance the effects of other CNS stimulants (*e.g.,* caffeine, amphetamines)

▶ **NURSING ALERTS**

▷ 1 Use cautiously in patients with impaired renal or hepatic function, in those with a history of drug abuse, and in pregnant or lactating women.

▷ 2 Perform periodic liver function tests during prolonged therapy and discontinue drug if SGOT, SGPT, or serum LDH levels are significantly elevated.

▶ **NURSING CONSIDERATIONS**

▷ 1 Administer drug once a day in the morning to minimize insomnia.

▷ 2 Monitor weight of children on prolonged therapy because growth suppression and weight loss can occur.

▷ 3 Periodically interrupt therapy to assess effectiveness of drug treatment.

▷ 4 Provide appropriate emotional and educational assistance in addition to drug therapy in minimal brain dysfunction children.

▷ 5 Note drug is a class IV controlled substance (see Appendix).

Summary. CNS Stimulants

Drug	Preparations	Usual Dosage Range
Analeptics		
See Chapter 57		
Caffeine (Caffedrine, Kirkaffeine, Nō Dōz, Quick-Pep, Tirend, Vivarin)	Tablets—100 mg, 150 mg, 200 mg, 250 mg	Oral—100 mg to 250 mg every 3 hours to 4 hours
	Timed-release capsules—200 mg, 250 mg	IM—500 mg; repeat as necessary (maximum single dose is 1000 mg)
	Injection—250 mg/ml (caffeine and sodium benzoate)	IV—500 mg in emergency respiratory failure
Amphetamines		
See Table 27-1		
Anorexiants		
See Table 27-2		
Methylphenidate (Ritalin)	Tablets—5 mg, 10 mg, 20 mg	Adults—10 mg to 40 mg/day in divided doses
	Sustained-release tablets—20 mg	Children (over 6)—Initially 5 mg 2 times/day; increase by 5 mg to 10 mg/week (maximum 60 mg/day)
Pemoline (Cylert)	Tablets—18.75 mg, 37.5 mg, 75 mg	Initially 37.5 mg/day in the morning; increase by 18.75 mg/week (maximum 112.5 mg/day)
	Chewable tablets—37.5 mg	

Drugs Acting on the Cardiovascular System

The cardiovascular system functions as a highly integrated unit to establish and maintain, within a wide range of conditions, the hemodynamic state necessary to meet the moment-to-moment needs of each body tissue.

The rhythmic pumping action of the heart establishes blood flow at an adequate level of pressure. The elastic recoil of the aorta and large arteries transforms the intermittent output of the heart into a relatively steady peripheral flow of blood. Unidirectional flow of blood is maintained by suitable pressure gradients and is aided by strategically placed valves. Blood pressure is maintained by delicate reflex mechanisms, and blood flow to individual body tissues is controlled by local metabolic needs as well as central integrating mechanisms.

Cardiovascular Physiology— A Review

28

The Heart

The human heart is a four-chambered, highly muscular organ lying within the mediastinum enclosed by a double-layered pericardium (Fig. 28-1). The heart wall is composed of three layers: an outer thin transparent *epicardium* (visceral pericardium); a thick middle muscular *myocardium;* and an inner serous lining, or *endocardium.* In addition to lining the chambers of the heart, the endocardium covers the valves of the heart and is continuous with the endothelium of the blood vessels.

The thin-walled superior chambers, or *atria,* function primarily as reservoirs for blood returning to the heart. The right atrium receives systemic venous blood from the superior and inferior venae cavae and coronary venous blood chiefly through the coronary sinus. The left atrium receives oxygenated blood from the lungs by way of four pulmonary veins. Because no true valves separate the great veins near the heart from the atrial chambers, elevations in right atrial pressure are reflected backward into the systemic venous circulation, while elevations in left atrial pressure lead to pulmonary congestion.

The inferior chambers or *ventricles* are thick walled, being formed by three indistinct layers of muscle arranged in a complex spiral fashion. During contraction, the myocardium of each ventricle generates a force sufficient to overcome the existing pressure in the receiving artery. The right ventricle ejects its contents into the pulmonary artery, while the left ventricle pumps oxygenated blood into the aorta. Because the pulmonary circulation is maintained at a considerably lower pressure than the systemic circulation, the thickness of the right ventricular wall is approximately one third that of the left, reflecting the lighter work load of the right ventricle.

Unidirectional blood flow through the heart is maintained by two types of valves: the *atrioventricular* (AV) valves and the *semilunar* valves. The AV valves separate the atria from the ventricles. Each valve is composed of leaflets or cusps that attach to the papillary muscles of the ventricles by way of chordae tendinae. A *tricuspid* valve separates the right atrium from the right ventricle, while a *bicuspid* or mitral valve is found between the left atrium and left ventricle.

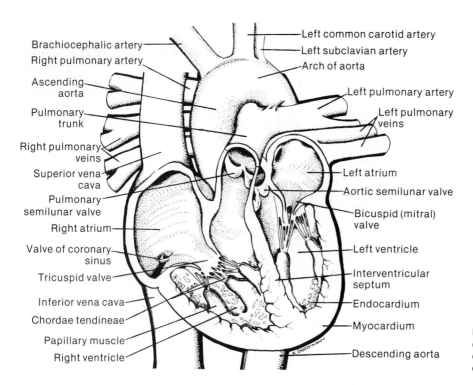

Figure 28–1 The human heart contains four chambers and is enclosed by a double-layered pericardium.

The semilunar valves consist of three symmetrical cup-like cusps secured onto a fibrous ring. The *pulmonic* valve is situated between the right ventricle and the pulmonary artery, while the *aortic* valve is located between the left ventricle and the aorta. Immediately above the free margins of the aortic valve are the sinuses of Valsalva and the openings of the coronary arteries.

Coronary Circulation

The myocardium is richly vascularized, its blood supply coming by way of the coronary circulation. The coronary vessels course around the heart in two external anatomical grooves: the atrioventricular groove and the interventricular groove.

The coronary arteries arise from the ascending aorta immediately above the free margins of the aortic semilunar valve. They form a crown around the heart and provide branches to supply the atrial and ventricular myocardium.

The right coronary artery, with its marginal and posterior interventricular branches, supplies the right atrium, right ventricle, and a portion of the left ventricle. The left coronary artery and its major branches, the circumflex and anterior interventricular, supply the left atrium, left ventricle, and part of the right ventricle. Anastomoses between arterial branches exist and serve as potential routes for collateral circulation if gradual occlusion of a vessel occurs. Coronary veins accompany the coronary arteries. The most significant myocardial venous return occurs by way of the coronary sinus, which opens into the right atrium near the orifice of the inferior vena cava.

Blood flow through the coronary arteries occurs primarily during ventricular relaxation (*diastole*) because ventricular contraction (*systole*) compresses the arteries and impedes arterial flow. The reduced time in diastole that occurs at rapid heart rates can markedly decrease coronary arterial perfusion, a potentially critical situation in coronary patients.

Coronary perfusion is primarily controlled by local metabolites and is minimally affected by autonomic nervous system activity. Coronary vessels dilate in response to increased acidity (reduced *p*H), increased carbon dioxide, and diminished oxygen availability in the blood.

If a coronary artery is partially occluded by a plaque or embolus, the vasodilation that automatically occurs distal to the block may provide sufficient blood flow to meet the needs of a resting heart. However, during exercise or emotional stress, such vasodilation may not be sufficient to meet the increased demand on the heart, and ischemia may result. The characteristic substernal thoracic pain, which occasionally radiates along the medial aspect of the left arm, and results from moderate inadequacy of coronary perfusion, is termed *angina pectoris*. Angina pectoris is usually relieved by rest and vasodilators such as nitroglycerin. Severe and prolonged ischemia of the myocardium results in irreversible damage to the heart. This state, termed *myocardial infarction*, is characterized by severe substernal oppression, and may result in shock, arrhythmias, cardiac dysfunction, or sudden death.

The Conduction System

The myocardium exhibits the physiologic properties of excitability, conductivity, contractility, and autorhythmicity. The heart spontaneously and rhythmically generates impulses

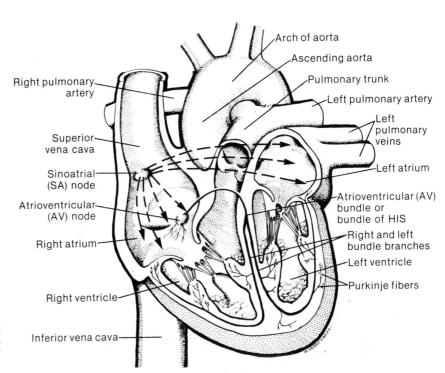

Figure 28-2 A highly specialized conduction system maintains the rhythmic synchronized activity of the heart.

Labels on figure: Arch of aorta; Ascending aorta; Pulmonary trunk; Left pulmonary artery; Left pulmonary veins; Left atrium; Atrioventricular (AV) bundle or bundle of HIS; Right and left bundle branches; Left ventricle; Purkinje fibers; Right pulmonary artery; Superior vena cava; Sinoatrial (SA) node; Atrioventricular (AV) node; Right atrium; Right ventricle; Inferior vena cava

that are distributed along specialized conduction pathways to all parts of the myocardium, permitting synchronous contraction of the ventricular myocardium. Like all excitable tissues, the myocardium exhibits refractory periods. During such times of decreased reactivity, the myocardium is unresponsive to a second stimulus.

The rhythmic synchronized activity of the heart is maintained by a spontaneously active, highly specialized conduction system illustrated in Figure 28-2.

The cardiac impulse normally originates in the *sino-atrial (SA) node,* a small mass of modified myocardial tissue located in the posterior wall of the right atrium, below the opening of the superior vena cava.

A second specialized mass of conduction tissue, the *atrioventricular (AV) node,* lies in the posterior right side of the interatrial septum near the opening of the coronary sinus. The AV node is continuous with a tract of conducting tissue termed the *atrioventricular (AV) bundle* or the *bundle of His.* Descending along the interventricular septum, the AV bundle divides into right and left bundle branches that descend along opposite sides of the interventricular septum and ultimately terminate in an extensive network of fine branches known as *Purkinje fibers.*

The spread of the cardiac impulse over the Purkinje fibers is extremely rapid, thereby ensuring virtually simultaneous excitation of the entire ventricular myocardium. Adjacent myocardial cells approximate at specialized junctions of low resistance, called *intercalated discs.* These intercalated discs facilitate the rapid spread of excitation from cell to cell, thereby allowing the heart to function as a *syncytium.*

The SA node initiates a wave of depolarization that spreads rapidly throughout the atria. Upon reaching the AV node, the impulse is delayed briefly (0.08 sec–0.12 sec) to allow completion of atrial contraction. Excessive delay or failure of impulse conduction at the AV node results in heart block.

Following the normally brief delay at the AV node, the cardiac impulse then proceeds along the bundle of His and its right and left bundle branches to the rapidly depolarizing fibers of the Purkinje network. The impulse sweeps through the ventricular myocardium from the endocardial (inner) to the epicardial (outer) surface.

While all parts of the conduction system can rhythmically discharge cardiac action potentials, the cells of the SA node intrinsically depolarize at the highest frequency (60–100 times per min), thereby setting the pace or rhythm of the heart. Hence the SA node is commonly termed the cardiac *pacemaker.* The discharge rate of the SA node may be affected extrinsically by the autonomic nervous system, as well as by certain hormones, drugs, and even temperature changes. If the SA node fails to generate rhythmic cardiac impulses, other sites, such as the AV node or AV bundle, may assume a pacemaker role.

Disturbances of normal cardiac rhythm, or arrhythmias, result from altered myocardial electrophysiology. Cardiac arrhythmias may result from abnormal sites of impulse formation (ectopic foci), abnormal rates of impulse formation, or abnormal rates or routes of impulse conduction (see Chap. 30). A shortened myocardial refractory period may also contribute to the development of cardiac arrhythmias. Other predisposing factors include cardiac ischemia, electrolyte imbalance, excessive autonomic stimulation, and drug toxicity.

The Electrocardiogram

The electrocardiogram (ECG or EKG) is a graphic record of the electrical activity of the heart. A typical ECG (lead II tracing) is shown in Figure 28-3. The *P wave* depicts atrial depolarization, the *QRS* complex depicts ventricular depolarization, and the *T wave* depicts ventricular repolarization.

The P–R interval (normally 0.12 sec–0.20 sec) indicates conduction time through the atria and includes the delay at the AV node. Abnormal prolongation of the P–R interval indicates first-degree heart block.

The Q–T interval encompasses both ventricular depolarization and repolarization. The Q–T interval may be prolonged by some antiarrhythmic drugs such as quinidine.

The T wave may be flattened or inverted by digitalis overdosage. Hyperkalemia causes peaking and elevation of the T wave. To a skilled reader, the ECG offers valuable information about cardiac rhythm (atrial and ventricular rates), conduction rate, chamber hypertrophy, presence of infarction, ionic imbalance, and drug effects.

Cardiac Cycle

The cardiac cycle consists of an orderly sequence of interdependent electrical and mechanical events associated with one complete cycle of contraction (systole) and relaxation (diastole) of the heart. Electrical excitation of the heart precedes contraction.

During diastole, the atrial and ventricular chambers are relaxed and the semilunar valves are closed. Blood that has entered the atria through the great veins flows passively from the atria to the ventricles through the open atrioventricular (AV) valves. The period of slow ventricular filling is termed *diastasis,* and it occurs in mid-diastole. During late diastole, a wave of depolarization (P wave) sweeps through the atria, leading to contraction of the atrial musculature. Atrial contraction (atrial systole) contributes approximately 30% to the ventricular blood volume.

Ventricular contraction follows the wave of depolarization through the ventricular conduction system and myocardium (QRS complex). When the ventricular pressures exceed the atrial pressures, the atrioventricular (AV) valves close, generating the first heart sound. During this phase of ventricular systole, the arterial pressures within the aorta and pulmonary artery exceed the ventricular pressures, thereby keeping the semilunar valves closed and maintaining the ventricular volumes constant (period of isovolumetric contraction). Eventually the sustained ventricular contraction generates sufficient ventricular pressure to exceed the arterial pressure. At this point the semilunar valves open, and the ventricles eject the blood into the pulmonary artery and aorta.

A wave of repolarization (T wave) sweeps through the ventricles, causing the ventricular myocardium to relax. As the ventricles relax, the ventricular pressures drop below the arterial pressures of the pulmonary artery and aorta, causing the semilunar valves to close and generating the second heart sound.

With continued ventricular relaxation, the ventricular pressures fall below the atrial pressures, causing the atrioventricular (AV) valves to open. The venous blood that has

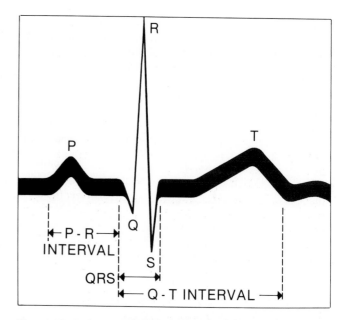

Figure 28-3 A typical electrocardiogram includes the following features: the P wave (depicting atrial depolarization), the QRS complex (depicting ventricular depolarization), and the T wave (depicting ventricular repolarization).

been accumulating in the atria during ventricular systole now rapidly flows through the open atrioventricular valves into the ventricles. At rest, approximately 70% of ventricular filling takes place during this period of early diastole.

Cardiac Output

The work of the heart may be expressed in terms of *cardiac output,* that is, the volume of blood ejected from each ventricle in 1 minute. Cardiac output is the product of stroke volume and heart rate. The cardiac output of a resting adult falls in the range of 4.5 liters to 5 liters per minute; however, during exercise an average adult may achieve a cardiac output of 15 liters to 20 liters per minute.

Multiple factors contribute to the control of cardiac output. The *stroke volume* (the volume of blood ejected from a ventricle during a single contraction) is equal to the difference between the end-diastolic and end-systolic volumes. The end-diastolic volume represents the degree of ventricular filling, and it is determined by factors such as ventricular filling time, atrial contraction, myocardial distensibility, and the effective filling pressure. Normally, the bulk of ventricular filling occurs during early diastole, so that ventricular filling time is inversely related to the heart rate. At very rapid heart rates, the ventricular filling time is substantially reduced. In this case, atrial contraction may contribute significantly to the ventricular volume.

The effective filling pressure is directly related to the venous return, which is determined largely by the circulating blood volume and venous tone. Venous return to the heart is enhanced by the thoracico-abdominal pump and by skeletal muscle contraction. The pressure within the thorax is negative with respect to atmospheric pressure, whereas the pressure within the abdominal cavity is slightly positive. This pressure gradient, which becomes even greater during inspiration, favors the return of blood from the abdomen to the thorax. According to Starling's Law of the Heart, there is, within physiologic limits, a direct relationship between myocardial fiber length and the force of ventricular contraction. The degree of stretch of myocardial fibers before contraction is termed *preload,* and it is determined largely by the end-diastolic ventricular volume.

Increased preload will, within physiologic limits, increase the force of ventricular contraction and thereby increase the stroke volume. *Excessive* stretching of myocardial fibers will, however, ultimately lead to cardiac failure.

The end-systolic volume is primarily determined by the afterload and the contractility of the myocardium. The term *afterload* refers to the amount of tension that a ventricle must develop during systole in order to open the semilunar valve and to eject blood into the receiving artery. Afterload is a function of arterial pressure and ventricular size. As the size of a ventricle increases, the ventricle must develop a greater tension in order to generate a given pressure. Therefore, a dilated ventricle would have to develop a greater tension than a normal ventricle to generate the same systolic pressure.

Elevations in arterial pressure will also increase resistance to the outflow of blood from a ventricle, thereby necessitating an increase in ventricular tension. Chronic or excessive increases in afterload will adversely affect the cardiac output by elevating end-systolic volume, thereby reducing stroke volume.

The contractility of the myocardium is affected by a multitude of factors, including the metabolic state of the myocardium, physical and mechanical factors (Starling's Law of the Heart), nervous activity, hormones, and pharmacologic agents.

Factors that enhance the contractility of the myocardium are said to have a positive inotropic effect on the heart. Sympathetic stimulation, epinephrine, and isoproterenol, for example, enhance the contractile force of the myocardium and thereby increase the stroke volume and cardiac output. Cardiac output may also be altered by changes in heart rate.

Heart rate is responsive to extrinsic control by the autonomic nervous system. The sino-atrial (SA) and atrioventricular (AV) nodes are richly innervated by sympathetic and parasympathetic nerve fibers. The atria receive some innervation from each division of the autonomic nervous system, while the ventricles are innervated principally by sympathetic fibers. Sympathetic stimulation, through the release of norepinephrine from adrenergic nerve terminals, accelerates the heart rate and speed of cardiac impulse conduction. Sympathetic activation also can markedly enhance the force of myocardial contractility.

Parasympathetic nerves to the heart are anatomically vagal and functionally cardio-inhibitory. Vagal stimulation, through mediation of the neurotransmitter acetylcholine, produces a notable decrease in heart rate and speed of impulse conduction, and a slight reduction of cardiac contractility.

Blood Flow—Hemodynamics

The cardiovascular system forms a continuous closed circuit for the distribution of blood to all body tissues. With each contraction, the left ventricle ejects the blood with a force sufficient to propel it through the entire systemic circuit. The elasticity of the aorta and large arteries transforms the intermittent output of the heart into a relatively steady peripheral blood flow. Blood flows through the arteries, arterioles, capillaries, venules, and veins according to existing pressure gradients, the progressive drop in pressure across the systemic circuit promoting undirectional forward flow.

According to Poiseuille's law, blood flow is directly proportional to the driving pressure and inversely proportional to the resistance. Resistance to blood flow is directly related to the viscosity of blood, and is inversely related to the vascular radius. The viscosity of blood depends upon the hematocrit, the rate of flow, and the diameter of the vessel. With a constant hematocrit, the viscosity changes over normal ranges of flow are insignificant. The variable resistance to blood flow is determined largely by the radius of the blood vessels, notably the small muscular arteries and arterioles (resistance vessels). Because the vascular resistance to flow varies inversely as the fourth power of the vascular radius, even a small change in the caliber of a blood vessel can produce a pronounced change in blood flow.

Blood flow varies widely among the various organs and tissues of the body. The brain and kidneys, which represent only a small fraction of the total body mass, receive a generous blood supply; skeletal muscle, despite its large mass, receives only a small percentage of the cardiac output at rest.

Distribution of the cardiac output among the various organs and tissues is determined by individual metabolic requirements of the tissue as well as by neural and humoral factors. Due to the ever-changing needs of individual body tissues, blood flow must continually be adjusted. Blood flow to a given organ may be enhanced by increasing the cardiac output or by shunting blood from other body tissues. Distribution of the cardiac output is controlled by intrinsic as well as extrinsic mechanisms, which will now be examined in greater detail.

Intrinsic Control of Blood Flow

Local metabolic conditions and individual tissue requirements play an important role in the regulation of regional blood flow. Factors involved in the intrinsic control of blood flow include tissue oxygen requirements and availability, rate of tissue metabolism, and presence of certain tissue metabolites. The vascular smooth muscle of the microcirculation (arterioles, precapillaries, and precapillary sphincters) is highly sensitive to lack of oxygen. The vascular response to tissue ischemia is vasodilation. Local increases in carbon dioxide and hydrogen ions also produce vasodilation and increased blood flow independently of nervous reflexes. Local control of perfusion is particularly evident in the heart and brain.

In addition to changes in pH and gas tension, endogenous vasodilators such as bradykinin, histamine, adenosine, and potassium ions may act locally to increase blood flow, possibly during times of tissue injury or inflammation. The precise role and importance of these vasodilators and of other vasoactive substances such as prostaglandins, angiotensin, serotonin, and acetylcholine in the regulation of regional blood flow probably vary from tissue to tissue, and remain to be clarified.

Autoregulation of blood flow assumes the inherent ability of a vascular bed to maintain a constant flow rate despite fluctuations in arterial pressure. Central to the mechanism of autoregulation is the ability of vascular smooth muscle to respond to distention caused by increased intraluminal pressure with appropriately graded contraction. Chemical influences have also been implicated in the mechanism of autoregulation.

Extrinsic Control of Blood Flow

The walls of small arteries and arterioles are abundantly innervated by autonomic vasomotor fibers, the majority of which are sympathetic. Sympathetic vasoconstrictor nerves play an important role in the regulation of peripheral resistance. Arteriolar vasomotor tone changes in accordance with the level of sympathetic activity. Increased sympathetic discharge of vasoconstrictor fibers produces a reduction in vascular caliber and therefore an increase in peripheral resistance to blood flow. All vasoconstrictor fibers are adrenergic.

Vasodilator nerves are of minor functional significance in most vascular beds, with the exception of skeletal muscle. In addition to possessing sympathetic adrenergic vasoconstrictor fibers, the vasculature of skeletal muscle is uniquely equipped with sympathetic cholinergic vasodilator nerves that produce vasodilation in response to stress or exercise. Parasympathetic vasodilator nerves (also cholinergic) innervate only certain organs such as the salivary glands, bladder, and external genitalia. These vasodilator fibers do not significantly influence peripheral vascular resistance. Rather, their specific and limited distribution suggests a more specialized physiologic role.

In addition to neural regulation, humoral agents such as epinephrine and angiotensin extrinsically influence peripheral vascular resistance and blood flow.

Arterial Blood Pressure

The arterial blood pressure serves as the driving force for blood flow through the vascular system. The magnitude of

arterial blood pressure changes throughout the cardiac cycle. The maximum pressure (*systolic pressure*) occurs at the peak of ventricular contraction or systole. The magnitude of systolic pressure may be altered by changes in cardiac output or arterial distensibility. An increase in stroke volume, and hence cardiac output, will elevate systolic pressure, as will a reduction in arterial distensibility such as that occurring in arteriosclerosis.

The lowest pressure (*diastolic pressure*) occurs during diastole, just before ventricular contraction. Changes in peripheral resistance alter the level of diastolic pressure.

The difference between the systolic and diastolic pressures is termed *pulse pressure*. Pulse pressure is directly related to the stroke volume, and is inversely related to the heart rate and peripheral resistance.

The mean arterial pressure is generally assumed to equal the diastolic pressure plus one third of the pulse pressure. At rapid heart rates, the times spent in systole and diastole are more nearly equal, and mean arterial pressure equals approximately one half of the sum of systolic and diastolic pressures.

The mean arterial pressure equals the product of cardiac output and peripheral resistance. Any factor or condition that alters either or both of these variables will therefore affect the blood pressure.

The arterial blood pressure must be constantly and carefully regulated to provide a driving force sufficient to distribute blood to all body tissues without imposing an excessive load upon the heart and blood vessels. Several control mechanisms exist for the continuous and precise regulation and integration of cardiovascular functions.

Within the medulla of the brain stem are cardiovascular (cardiac and vasomotor) control centers that receive and integrate input from various sensory receptors. Homeostatically, the most important of these are the pressure-sensitive baroreceptors located in the carotid sinus and aortic arch. Associated with the baroreceptors are branches of the glossopharyngeal (IX) and vagus (X) nerves, which serve as "buffer" nerves for the physiologic regulation and maintenance of systemic arterial pressure.

In response to blood pressure changes detected by the baroreceptors, afferent (sensory) impulses travel along the glossopharyngeal (sinus) and vagus (aortic) nerves to the cardiovascular integrating centers of the medulla. Activation of autonomic sympathetic and parasympathetic efferent nerves to the heart and blood vessels produces appropriate changes in cardiac output and peripheral resistance for the homeostatic restoration of blood pressure.

Efferent responses to an elevated blood pressure include the following: (1) a slowing of the heart (bradycardia) resulting from increased parasympathetic and decreased sympathetic activity, (2) reduced myocardial contractility caused by decreased sympathetic discharge, and (3) vasodilation resulting from decreased sympathetic tone. The reduction in cardiac output (resulting from a decreased heart rate and stroke volume) and the decreased peripheral vascular resistance restore the blood pressure toward normal.

The activity of the medullary cardiovascular integrating centers may also be influenced by afferent impulses from

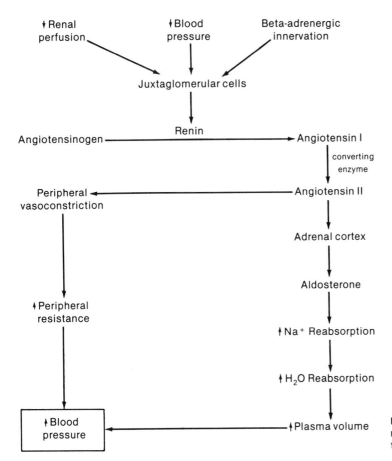

Figure 28-4 Renin–angiotensin–aldosterone mechanism for blood pressure regulation. See text for explanation.

higher brain centers such as the hypothalamus and cerebral cortex. It is through such afferent input that emotional responses, for example, fear or rage, alter blood pressure.

A peripheral mechanism operative in the control of blood pressure is the renin–angiotensin–aldosterone system, which is outlined in Figure 28-4. Renin is released from renal juxtaglomerular cells (see Fig. 36-3) in response to a number of stimuli, including hypotension, reduced renal perfusion pressure, and beta-adrenergic stimulation. Renin acts upon the plasma protein angiotensinogen to form the decapeptide angiotensin I, which is then converted by endothelial cell and plasma enzymes into the physiologically active angiotensin II. Angiotensin II is a potent vasopressor that acts through several mechanisms, but primarily by direct stimulation of vascular smooth muscle, to produce intense vasoconstriction and increased peripheral resistance. Angiotensin II also stimulates release of aldosterone from the

adrenal cortex. Aldosterone stimulates renal tubular reabsorption of sodium, thereby promoting water reabsorption and increasing blood volume. The increased blood volume and the increased peripheral resistance both contribute to the elevation of blood pressure.

The contribution of the renin–angiotensin–aldosterone system to hypertension, other than those cases resulting from renal dysfunction or renovascular stenosis, has yet to be definitively established. Although it does not appear that abnormalities of this system are a *consistent* factor in the development of most forms of hypertension, a number of different compounds that reduce the formation of angiotensin II have shown promise as antihypertensive drugs under a wide variety of circumstances. In addition, several currently used antihypertensives reduce the release of renin, presumably because of a beta-blocking action, and this action may contribute to their efficacy in reducing blood pressure.

29 Cardioactive Glycosides

The cardioactive glycosides encompass a group of both naturally occurring and semisynthetic steroidal compounds having qualitatively similar effects on cardiac function. Most of the commonly used drugs are derived from the leaves of either *Digitalis purpurea* or *Digitalis lanata,* both species of the foxglove plant. Because digitalis is the name of the principal botanical source of these agents, they are frequently referred to collectively as the digitalis glycosides.

While all the cardiac glycosides have similar pharmacologic effects on the heart, they differ with respect to onset and duration of action (due to differences in absorption, biotransformation, and extent of protein binding) as well as mode of administration. The drugs can be divided arbitrarily into three groups according to their routes of administration: oral only, parenteral only, and both oral and parenteral. The major characteristics of the currently available cardioactive glycosides, grouped according to their methods of administration, are listed in Table 29-1.

The digitalis glycosides increase myocardial contractility in both normal and failing hearts. Consequently, there is significant improvement in cardiovascular performance and an associated decrease in the size of the ventricles. Although there is some increase in oxygen demand because of increased contractility, this is more than compensated for by the reduced oxygen demand that occurs as ventricular size is reduced. Therefore, in the failing heart, there is an overall increase in efficiency (work performed/energy required).

The overall cardiodynamic effects of the digitalis agents are quite complex, being a combination of direct actions on the myocardium as well as indirect actions that alter the normal electrophysiologic properties of the heart (automaticity, conductivity, refractoriness). Moreover, the benefits of the digitalis drugs, as we have seen, are significantly greater in the failing heart than in the normal heart; this is a further indication that the drugs are acting to correct the hemodynamic imbalances associated with heart failure.

The direct action of the cardiac glycosides on the myocardium is largely responsible for the increased force of contraction (positive inotropic effect) noted with these drugs. On the other hand, their effects on the heart's electrical properties play an essential role in their ability to alter the rate and rhythm of the heartbeat. This latter action is responsible for both the therapeutic effect of the drugs in managing certain supraventricular arrhythmias, and their toxic effects on the heart, namely the development of many other types of arrhythmias. A review of the major cardiovascular actions of the digitalis glycosides is found in Table 29-2.

The progressive AV block seen with increasing dosage can lead to a major manifestation of digitalis toxicity—disturbances in cardiac rhythm. The arrhythmias that develop following toxic doses of these drugs also are attributable to a shortened AV refractory period, suppression of normal pacemaker activity, and increased ventricular automaticity. Many factors can predispose the heart to digitalis toxicity, the most important being hypokalemia (reduced serum potassium levels), hypercalcemia (elevated serum calcium levels), catecholamine depletion, concurrent use of quinidine, systemic alkalosis, and renal or hepatic impairment.

Following administration, digitalis glycosides are dis-

Table 29-1. Characteristics of Digitalis Glycosides

	Onset		Maximum Effect		Plasma Half-life	Extent of GI Absorption	Protein Binding
	IV	*PO*	*IV*	*PO*			
Parenteral							
Deslanoside	10 minutes to 30 minutes		60 minutes to 90 minutes		30 hours to 36 hours		20% to 30%
Oral/Parenteral							
Digitoxin	30 minutes to 90 minutes	2 hours to 3 hours	6 hours to 8 hours	6 hours to 12 hours	5 to 7 days	90% to 100%	95% to 97%
Digoxin	10 minutes to 30 minutes	1 hour to 2 hours	2 hours to 4 hours	4 hours to 8 hours	32 hours to 40 hours	60% to 90%	20% to 30%
Oral							
Digitalis leaf		3 hours to 4 hours		12 hours to 24 hours	5 to 7 days	40%	Significant
Digitalis glycosides mixture		1 hour to 2 hours		8 hours to 12 hours	5 to 7 days	Variable	Significant
Gitalin		2 hours to 4 hours		8 hours to 10 hours	3 to 6 days	Variable	

tributed widely in the body, into both inactive reservoir (binding) sites and active receptor sites in the myocardium. Therefore, it is necessary to administer sufficient drug to saturate the reservoir of nonspecific binding sites in order to achieve the desired effect at the active myocardial receptor sites. In *acute* congestive failure, large loading doses of drug may be administered rapidly to achieve the desired effect quickly. This process is termed *digitalization,* and carries the risk of serious toxicity if the loading dose is excessive. Therefore, in less acute conditions, the patient should be loaded (digitalized) more slowly to reduce the risk of potential toxicity. Such slow loading can often be effectively accomplished by simply administering the small recommended maintenance doses from the beginning of therapy.

The *maintenance* dose is the amount of drug sufficient to replace the amount of drug eliminated between dosing, and therefore maintain a steady-state plasma level of the drug. Maintenance doses, therefore, are smaller than rapid loading doses and must be individualized based on the patient's condition and the type of digitalis preparation used (long- or short-acting). Periodic clinical assessment is necessary to ensure that the optimal maintenance dose of the cardiac glycoside is being used, and that adverse reactions are kept at a minimum. Because there is often a substantial difference between the digitalizing and maintenance doses of some agents, both dosage ranges will be given for each drug throughout the chapter.

The digitalis glycosides will be reviewed as a group because they have similar pharmacologic properties; characteristics of individual drugs are then given in Table 29-3.

Table 29-2. Cardiovascular Actions— Digitalis Glycosides

A. Excitability of myocardium
   Small doses—0 (↑)
   Large doses—↓
B. Conduction velocity
   AV conduction system—↓ (dose-dependent)
   Cardiac muscle—0 (↑)
C. Refractory period
   AV conduction system—↑ (dose-dependent)
   Cardiac muscle—↓
D. Heart rate—↓
E. Force of contraction—↑
F. Cardiac output—↑
G. Blood pressure
   Venous—↓
   Systolic—slight ↑
   Diastolic—slight ↓
H. ECG
   P–R interval—↑
   Q–T interval—↓
   S–T segment—↓
   T wave—↓
I. Diuretic action
   Renal blood flow and glomerular filtration—↑
   Aldosterone release (deactivation of renin–angiotensin mechanism)—↓
   Sodium reabsorption in renal tubules—↓

0—no effect
↑—increased or prolonged
↓—decreased or shortened

Digitalis Glycosides

Deslanoside	Digitoxin
Digitalis Glycosides Mixtures	Digoxin
Digitalis Leaf	Gitalin

Table 29-3. Cardioactive Glycosides

Drug	Preparations	Usual Dosage Range Digitalizing	Maintenance	Remarks
Deslanoside (Cedilanid-D)	Injection—0.2 mg/ml	IV—1.6 mg as 1 injection or in 0.8-mg portions IM—0.8 mg at each of two sites		Rapid-acting glycoside used for emergency treatment of acute pulmonary edema and supraventricular arrhythmias; maintenance therapy with an oral glycoside may be instituted within 12 hours after deslanoside
Digitalis *glycosides mixture* (Digiglusin)	Tablet—1 unit	Normal—2 units twice a day for 4 days Rapid—6 units initially, 4 units 4 hours to 6 hours later, then 2 units every 4 hours to 6 hours until full effect is noted	0.5 to 3 units/day	Infrequently used preparation
Digitalis leaf (Digifortis)	Tablets—100 mg Capsules—100 mg	1.2 g total dose in several equal parts administered every 6 hours	100 mg to 200 mg/day (range 30 mg–400 mg daily)	Extract of leaves of *Digitalis purpurea,* consisting mainly of gitalin, gitoxin, and digitoxin, the latter component primarily responsible for the therapeutic action of the mixture
Digitoxin (Crystodigin, Purodigin)	Tablets—0.05 mg, 0.1 mg, 0.15 mg, 0.2 mg Injection—0.2 mg/ml	Oral: Rapid—0.6 mg initially, followed by 0.4 mg, then 0.2 mg at intervals of 4 hours to 6 hours Slow—0.2 mg twice a day for 4 days IV Adults—Total dose 1.2 mg to 1.6 mg; initially 0.6 mg, followed by 0.4 mg in 4 hours to 6 hours, then 0.2 mg every 4 hours to 6 hours until digitalized Children— Premature/newborn—0.022 mg/kg Under 1 year—0.045 mg/kg 1 year to 2 years—0.04 mg/kg Over 2 years—0.03 mg/kg divided into 3 or 4 portions given every 4 hours to 6 hours	Oral: 0.05 mg to 0.3 mg/day (usual—0.1 mg/day) Children—one-tenth digitalizing dose	Long-acting, potent glycoside mainly employed for maintenance rather than digitalizing therapy; slow onset and extremely long half-life makes digitalization difficult; danger of accumulation toxicity is high with this drug; do *not* give full digitalizing doses to patients receiving other digitalis glycosides within the preceding 3 weeks; rarely used IM because injections are often very painful; if employed, inject deep into gluteal muscle
Digoxin (Lanoxin, Lanoxicaps)	Tablets—0.125 mg, 0.25 mg, 0.5 mg Capsules—0.05 mg, 0.1 mg, 0.2 mg Elixir (pediatric)—0.05 mg/ml Injection—0.1, 0.25 mg/ml	Oral Adults Rapid—0.5 mg to 0.75 mg initially, followed by 0.25 mg to 0.5 mg every 6 hours to 8 hours to a total of 1 mg to 1.5 mg	Oral/IV: Adults—0.125 mg to 0.5 mg/day (average 0.25 mg/day) Children—20% to 30% of the total digitalizing dose daily	Widely used for both rapid digitalization and maintenance therapy; little danger of accumulation because drug is rapidly excreted; capsules have greater bioavailability than tablets; therefore, 0.2-mg

Table 29-3. Cardioactive Glycosides (continued)

Drug	Preparations	Usual Dosage Range		Remarks
		Digitalizing	Maintenance	
		Slow—0.125 mg to 0.25 mg daily for 7 days Children Newborn—40 mcg/kg to 60 mcg/kg 1 month to 2 years—60 mcg/kg to 80 mcg/kg 2 years to 10 years—40 mcg/kg to 60 mcg/kg IV Adults—0.25 mg to 0.5 mg initially, then 0.25 mg every 4 hours to 6 hours to a total of 1 mg Children—25 mcg/kg to 50 mcg/kg in divided doses		capsule is equivalent to 0.25-mg tablet and 0.1-mg capsule is equivalent to 0.125-mg tablet; drug can be given IM but absorption is erratic; do not give full digitalizing dose if patient has received a more slowly excreted cardiac glycoside within the last 2 weeks; administration with food slows rate of absorption but does not affect the total amount absorbed; closely monitor patients with renal insufficiency because drug is primarily excreted unchanged through the kidney; dosage may need to be decreased in patients receiving quinidine (see interactions)
Gitalin (Gitaligin)	Tablets—0.5 mg	Rapid: Initially 2.5 mg, followed by 0.75 mg every 6 hours until digitalized Slow: 1.5 mg/day for 4 to 6 days	0.5 mg/day (range 0.25 mg–1.25 mg daily)	Mixture of glycosides from *Digitalis purpurea*; maintenance dose is given in the morning

Mechanism

Inhibit $Na^+ - K^+$ membrane ATPase, the enzyme responsible for breakdown of ATP to supply energy for the $Na^+ - K^+$ pump; therefore, electrical properties of the myocardium are altered, and intracellular sodium and extracellular potassium concentrations are elevated. Increased intracellular levels of free calcium occur, perhaps due to transmembrane exchange with sodium or liberation of calcium ions from binding sites on the sarcoplasmic reticulum. Therefore, cardiac contraction is enhanced and cardiac output is increased. Heart rate is slowed by both vagal and extravagal mechanisms. Vagally, the drugs stimulate medullary vagal nuclei and increase sensitivity of pacemaker cells to the action of acetylcholine; extravagally, the drugs decrease AV conduction and increase the AV refractory period. Diuretic effect is primarily caused by increased renal blood flow and glomerular filtration rate secondary to increased cardiac output, but may also involve decreased aldosterone release, and possibly direct interference with sodium reabsorption in renal tubules.

Uses

1 Treatment of congestive heart failure, especially low-output failure associated with depressed left ventricular function
2 Treatment of certain cardiac arrhythmias, including atrial fibrillation, atrial flutter, and paroxysmal atrial tachycardia
3 Treatment of cardiogenic shock accompanied by pulmonary edema

Dosage

See Table 29-3.

Fate

Variable rates of absorption, onset of action, and duration of effect are observed among the different digitalis glycosides (see Table 29-1). Digitoxin is highly lipid soluble and extensively absorbed orally. Digoxin is somewhat less well absorbed. The digitalis glycosides are widely distributed in peripheral tissues. Most oral preparations are bound to varying degrees by plasma proteins and are excreted through the kidneys, either as unchanged drug (*e.g.,* digoxin, deslanoside) or as hepatic metabolites (*e.g.,* digitoxin).

Common Side-Effects

Anorexia, nausea, slow or irregular pulse, and altered color perception (yellow or green vision)

Significant Adverse Reactions

(Generally result from overdosage)
GI—vomiting, diarrhea, abdominal pain
CNS—weakness, lethargy, disorientation, headache, confusion, depression, paresthesias, amblyopia, diplopia, visual disturbances (*e.g.,* flashes, halos, white dots), neuralgia-like pain, delirium

Cardiac—arrhythmias (all types are possible); most common are ventricular premature beats and paroxysmal atrial tachycardia

Other—thromboembolism, pruritus, urticaria, fever, facial edema, joint pain, gynecomastia

Contraindications

Ventricular tachycardia or fibrillation, severe myocarditis

Interactions

1 Absorption of digitalis drugs may be reduced by antacids, anticholinergics, cholestyramine resin, laxatives, metoclopramide, neomycin and possibly other aminoglycosides.

2 Effects of digitalis drugs can be reduced by agents that increase their metabolism, such as anticonvulsants, antihistamines, barbiturates, oral hypoglycemics, and pyrazolones.

3 Toxic effects of cardiac glycosides (especially arrhythmias) may be *increased* by adrenergics, amphotericin, calcium salts, corticosteroids, diuretics (except potassium-sparing drugs), glucose, insulin, magnesium, pancuronium, reserpine, succinylcholine, and thyroid preparations.

4 Marked bradycardia may develop if digitalis drugs are given in combination with carbamazepine, guanethidine, phenytoin, propranolol, and reserpine.

5 Digitalis drugs may decrease the effects of oral anticoagulants and heparin.

6 Quinidine can increase serum levels of digoxin, possibly by displacement from tissue binding sites or reduced renal clearance.

7 Increased plasma levels of digitalis drugs can result from combined use with potassium-sparing diuretics or propantheline.

8 Calcium channel blocking drugs can increase the serum levels of digoxin, possibly by decreasing its renal clearance.

▶ **NURSING ALERTS**

▷ 1 Recognize that the margin between the therapeutic dose and the toxic dose of cardiac glycosides is extremely narrow. Closely observe patient for early signs of impending toxicity (weakness, nausea, vomiting, diarrhea, blurred vision, diplopia, halos, dizziness, precordial pain, palpitations, anxiety, and facial pain) and advise physician immediately.

▷ 2 Be aware that ventricular arrhythmias may occur in the absence of other signs of digitalis toxicity, especially in patients with advanced heart failure, severe pulmonary disease, rheumatic carditis, or Wolff–Parkinson–White syndrome.

▷ 3 Note that in children, nausea, vomiting, and neurological and visual disturbances are rare, and that atrial arrhythmias are often the most reliable indication of developing toxicity.

▷ 4 Watch for any changes in pulse rate (*e.g.,* sudden increase above 120 when pulse has been slowing) or rhythm or a fall in ventricular rate below 60/minute, which are signs of possible overdose, and advise physician.

▷ 5 Use cautiously in patients with Adams–Stokes syndrome, acute myocardial infarction, severe pulmonary disease, advanced heart failure, myxedema, incomplete AV block, chronic constrictive pericarditis, or hypertrophic subaortic stenosis. Also in the presence of hypoxia, hypomagnesemia, hypokalemia, hypercalcemia, renal or hepatic insufficiency, and in elderly, debilitated, pregnant, or nursing patients.

▷ 6 Note that premature, immature, and newborn infants are particularly sensitive to digitalis drugs. Digitalize very cautiously. Watch for disturbances of rhythm in children with rheumatic carditis because arrhythmias occur very frequently.

▷ 7 Because hypokalemia greatly increases the incidence of digitalis toxicity, be alert for early signs of potassium deficiency (*e.g.,* drowsiness, paresthesias, muscle weakness, anorexia, depressed reflexes, orthostatic hypotension, polyuria), especially in patients on potassium-wasting diuretics such as thiazides and loop diuretics. Consider potassium supplementation (KCl liquid, orange juice, bananas).

▷ 8 Never use digitalis preparations for adjunctive treatment of obesity; they are ineffective and potentially hazardous.

▷ 9 Recognize that many symptoms associated with conditions for which digitalis is used (*e.g.,* nausea and vomiting due to heart failure, arrhythmias) also indicate digitalis intoxication. A careful determination of the cause (*i.e.,* disease *versus* digitalis overdose) is essential to proper management.

▷ 10 Caution patients against taking an "extra" dose of medication to compensate for a missed dose. The possibility of toxicity is increased if doses are taken too close together, due to danger of accumulation.

▶ **NURSING CONSIDERATIONS**

▷ 1 Determine patient's baseline data (*i.e.,* clinical symptoms, serum electrolytes, vital signs) before initiating therapy, and take apical and radial pulse for 1 minute immediately before giving drug. In patients with atrial fibrillation, also determine pulse deficit (apical minus radial pulse).

▷ 2 Check with physician as to what pulse rates (both high and low) should be used as indicators for withholding therapy.

▷ 3 Monitor intake–output ratio regularly, and note weight changes and signs of edema. Dosage adjustments may be necessary to improve renal function.

▷ 4 Perform renal and liver function tests periodically, as well as ECG and serum electrolyte determinations.

▷ 5 If nausea and vomiting are present, give drug after meals; if symptoms do not subside, it may indicate digitalis toxicity through central emetic action. Advise physician immediately.

▷ 6 Provide patients with a checklist of body functions

they can monitor themselves (*e.g.,* pulse rate, urinary output, weight fluctuations) to determine if therapy is appropriate. Instruct patients how to take these readings. Counsel them to report untoward reactions immediately because toxicity can develop rapidly.

▷ 7 Advise patients that protracted diarrhea or vomiting can alter electrolyte balance and possibly lead to digitalis toxicity. Physician should be notified at once.

▷ 8 Impress upon the individual the importance of strict observance of the prescribed dosage regimen, avoidance of extra doses to make up for missed ones, and close adherence to the recommended diet, in order to obtain maximal benefit and minimal toxicity.

▷ 9 Give drugs parenterally only when oral administration is not feasible (*e.g.,* need for *rapid* digitalization, severe vomiting, unconsciousness).

▷ 10 Recommend cautious use of over-the-counter drugs high in sodium (*e.g.,* Alka Seltzer, Bromo Seltzer, Bisodol).

▷ *Dietary precautions*

▷ 1 Advise a reduction in overall salt intake. High-salt foods (*e.g.,* lunch meats, smoked meats and fish, chinese foods, processed cheese, salted snacks) should be avoided as well as any extra table salt.

▷ 2 Caution patients against consuming large quantities of licorice, as it contains glycyrrhizic acid, which is capable of causing salt and water retention, hypokalemia, and other symptoms of congestive heart failure.

▷ 3 Encourage an overall reduction in caloric intake to produce a weight reduction, to lessen the demands upon the cardiovascular system.

30 Antiarrhythmic Drugs

Cardiac arrhythmias can be regarded as any deviation from the normal rate and rhythm of contractions of the heart. Excessive slowing of the heart rate—*bradyarrhythmias*—usually result from a depressed rate of depolarization in normal pacemaker cells of the SA node, and generally respond to therapy with anticholinergic or adrenergic drugs such as atropine or isoproterenol. Most antiarrhythmic agents are used in the treatment of the various *tachyarrhythmias,* in which there is an abnormally rapid rate of atrial or ventricular contraction.

Cardiac arrhythmias arise from electrophysiologic disturbances of cardiac function. The two principal alterations are the following:

1 *Disorders of impulse formation*—impulses arise in areas of the heart other than the normal SA pacemaker; often termed *ectopic beats.*

2 *Disorders of impulse conduction*—impulses spread throughout the heart by abnormal pathways, *i.e.,* other than by the AV conduction system. Common examples are the "circus movement" of an impulse around an area of damaged myocardium, and "re-entry excitation," a complex phenomenon in which impulses re-enter an area of the myocardium from a direction opposite to normal flow, re-activating the fibers.

While certainly serious, *atrial arrhythmias* are usually not life-threatening if normal ventricular function is maintained. Conversely, disturbances in *ventricular* rhythm of even a few minutes' duration can be fatal, and therefore require immediate and vigorous therapy. The purposes of antiarrhythmic drug treatment, therefore, are twofold: (1) to restore normal cardiac rhythm, and (2) to prevent recurrence or extension of an existing arrhythmia.

Antiarrhythmic drugs have traditionally been grouped into categories according to their electrophysiologic actions on the heart. However, some newer antiarrhythmic drugs do not fit well into any one of these groups because of their diverse pharmacologic actions. Another useful means of classifying these drugs, into which most available drugs can be compartmented, is as follows:

I. *Membrane stabilizers*—(slow ventricular conduction and prolong refractory period of myocardium) *e.g.,* quinidine, procainamide, disopyramide

II. *Sodium channel blockers*—(enhance conduction, decrease refractory period duration) *e.g.,* lidocaine

III. *Sympathomimetic blockers*—(slow AV conduction, decrease SA nodal rate, and reduce adrenergic activity) *e.g.,* propranolol, bretylium

IV. Calcium channel blockers—(slow AV conduction, decrease SA nodal rate) *e.g.,* verapamil

Selection of an appropriate antiarrhythmic agent depends on the type of arrhythmia present as well as the characteristics of the drugs themselves—their onset, duration, type, and incidence of side-effects, in addition to other factors.

The major pharmacokinetic properties as well as the electrophysiologic effects of the principal antiarrhythmic drugs are listed in Table 30-1.

Drugs used in treating arrhythmias alter the heart's basic electrical properties, including excitability, conduction velocity, refractory period, and automaticity. These, then, are

Table 30-1. Pharmacokinetic and Electrophysiologic Properties of Antiarrhythmic Drugs

	Pharmacokinetics				Electrophysiology			
	Onset (min)	Duration (hr)	Plasma Half-Life (hr)	Protein Binding	AV Conduction Velocity	Effective Refractory Period	SA Nodal Rate	Ectopic Pacemakers
Quinidine	30	6–12	6	60%–80%	↓	↑	0 (↓)	↓
Procainamide	30	3–4	2–4	10%–20%	↓	↑	0 (↓)	↓
Disopyramide	30	5–6	4–8	30%–60%	0 (↓)	↑	0 (↓)	↓
Lidocaine (IV)	1–2	0.2–0.4	1–2	40%–80%	0 (↑)	0 (↓)	0	↓
Phenytoin	30–60	24	24–36	85%–95%	0 (↑)	0 (↓)	0	↓
Propranolol	30	3–6	4–6	90%–95%	↓	↑	↓	↓
Bretylium (IV)	1–2	6–8	6–12		0	↑	↕	↕
Verapamil (IV)	2–5	1–2	3–6	90%	↓	↑	↓	↓

0 = no effect; ↑ = increase; ↓ = decrease; 0 (↑), 0 (↓) = slight change; ↕ = variable effect

potentially dangerous drugs. Because not all arrhythmias require drug therapy, careful diagnosis of the type of disordered rhythm present is essential for effective and safe management of these conditions. Since the overall pharmacology and toxicology of the different drugs vary to a significant degree, they will be discussed individually in this chapter.

▶ **bretylium**

Bretylol

Mechanism

Complex and incompletely understood; prolongs the effective refractory period of Purkinje fibers and ventricular muscle fibers; increases ventricular fibrillation threshold, action potential duration, and spontaneous firing rate of pacemaker tissue; initially releases norepinephrine from adrenergic nerve endings, then blocks release in response to nerve stimulation; may also interfere with uptake of neurohormones into adrenergic nerve endings

Uses

1 Treatment of life-threatening ventricular arrhythmias that have not responded to lidocaine or procainamide (use is restricted to intensive or coronary-care units with appropriate facilities for continuous monitoring of cardiac function)

Dosage

Acute

Ventricular fibrillation:

IV—5 mg/kg (undiluted) by rapid injection; may repeat at 10 mg/kg every 15 minutes to 30 minutes to a total dose of 30 mg/kg

Ventricular arrhythmias:

IV—5 mg/kg to 10 mg/kg of a diluted solution by IV infusion over a period of at least 8 minutes to 10 minutes.

Dilution—10 ml (500 mg) diluted to a minimum of 50 ml with dextrose or sodium chloride injection.

IM—(do not dilute) 5 mg/kg to 10 mg/kg; may repeat in 1 hour to 2 hours, then every 6 hours to 8 hours thereafter (maximum injection volume is 5 ml)

Maintenance

5 mg/kg to 10 mg/kg of diluted solution infused over 8 minutes to 10 minutes every 6 hours, or 1 mg/kg to 2 mg/kg of diluted solution by constant infusion

Fate

Adequately absorbed IM; peak plasma concentrations in 60 minutes to 90 minutes; however, maximum antiarrhythmic effects are not seen for 6 hours to 9 hours; effects of a single dose persist for 6 hours to 8 hours; onset following IV injection within minutes; excreted largely unchanged by the kidney, approximately 70% to 80% of a dose within 24 hours

Common Side-Effects

Hypotension, nausea and vomiting (especially with rapid IV injection), and lightheadedness

Significant Adverse Reactions

Vertigo, syncope, bradycardia, transitory hypertension, increased arrhythmias (initially), anginal attacks, substernal pressure and pain

Other (cause–effect relationship has not been definitively established): diarrhea, flushing, hyperthermia, dyspnea, anxiety, abdominal pain, erythematous rash, diaphoresis, confusion, nasal congestion, renal dysfunction

Contraindications

There are no absolute contraindications to use in treating life-threatening ventricular arrhythmias; use in less serious arrhythmias is contraindicated in severe pulmonary hypertension or in aortic stenosis and in patients with fixed cardiac output.

Interactions

1 May increase digitalis toxicity by releasing norepinephrine

2 Peripheral vasodilation occurring in patients already receiving procainamide or quinidine may be increased by bretylium.

▶ **Nursing Alerts**

▷ 1 Keep patient supine until tolerance to the hypotensive action of the drug has developed, which often does not occur for several days. Assist ambulation as needed.

▷ 2 Reduce dosage in patients with impaired renal function to prevent accumulation toxicity because drug is excreted primarily through the kidney.

▷ 3 Do not use in atrial arrhythmias or in asymptomatic ventricular ectopic beats because effectiveness has not been demonstrated.

▷ 4 Do not initiate therapy concurrently with digitalis because increased incidence of arrhythmias can occur.

▷ 5 Use cautiously during pregnancy and in children.

▷ 6 Monitor cardiac function closely during therapy, and have appropriate equipment and drugs (*e.g.,* dopamine) on hand to treat adverse effects such as hypotension

▶ NURSING CONSIDERATIONS

▷ 1 Note that transient hypertension and arrhythmias may develop during *early* stages of therapy because of initial release of catecholamines. Monitor closely and advise physician if effects are severe or prolonged.

▷ 2 Rotate IM injection sites, and limit volume of injection at any one site to 5 ml.

▷ 3 Discontinue drug (under electrocardiographic monitoring) and substitute alternate antiarrhythmic as needed within 3 to 5 days.

▶ disopyramide

Norpace, Norpace CR

Mechanism

Decreases the rate of diastolic depolarization (phase 4) in myocardial cells, and decreases up-stroke velocity of the action potential (phase 0); increases action potential duration and effective refractory period of the atria and ventricles, thereby decreasing automaticity and conduction velocity; minimal effect on AV conduction or AV nodal refractory period; possesses significant anticholinergic activity, which may contribute to its antiarrhythmic activity.

Uses

1. Suppression and prevention of recurrence of the following arrhythmias:
   a. Unifocal premature (ectopic) ventricular contractions
   b. Premature (ectopic) ventricular contractions of multifocal origin
   c. Paired premature ventricular contractions
   d. Episodes of ventricular tachycardia

Dosage

Initially, 300 mg loading dose, followed by 150 mg every 6 hours; controlled-release capsules (Norpace CR) may be given every 8 hours; usual dose is 400 mg to 800 mg/day

In patients weighing less than 50 kg, or in those with hepatic or mild renal insufficiency—200 mg loading dose followed by 100 mg every 6 hours

In patients with cardiomyopathy or cardiac decompensation—100 mg every 6 hours with *no* loading dose

Pediatric dosage (divided doses every 6 hr):

1 yr to 4 yr—10 mg/kg to 20 mg/kg/day

4 yr to 12 yr—10 mg/kg to 15 mg/kg/day
12 yr to 18 yr—6 mg/kg to 15 mg/kg/day

Fate

Rapidly and almost completely absorbed; onset within 30 minutes; peak serum levels occur within 2 hours to 3 hours; duration approximately 6 hours; plasma half-life 4 hours to 8 hours; approximately 50% protein-bound; excreted mainly in the urine, one half as unchanged drug; remainder is excreted as metabolites, either through the kidney or in the feces; renal excretion is independent of urinary *p*H

Common Side-Effects

Dry mouth, urinary hesitancy, nausea, bloating, GI pain, constipation, blurred vision, fatigue, headache, and malaise

Significant Adverse Reactions

Urinary retention, dizziness, muscle weakness, anorexia, diarrhea, vomiting, rash, dermatoses, dyspnea, chest pain, hypotension, syncope, edema, arrhythmias, depressed myocardial contractility and cardiac output, precipitation or aggravation of congestive heart failure, impotence, hypoglycemia; rarely, insomnia, psychotic episodes, depression, dysuria, numbness, AV block, elevated BUN and creatinine, cholestatic jaundice, respiratory difficulty, agranulocytosis, and anaphylactic reaction

Contraindications

Cardiogenic shock, second- or third-degree AV block, uncompensated congestive heart failure or hypotension, and nursing mothers

Interactions

1 Effects of disopyramide may be enhanced by concurrent use of other antiarrhythmic drugs, beta-adrenergic blockers and calcium channel blockers

2 Plasma levels can be increased by the presence of other protein-bound drugs (*e.g.,* sulfonamides, anti-inflammatory agents, oral anticoagulants, oral hypoglycemics).

3 Therapeutic effects may be reduced by the presence of hypokalemia (*e.g.,* diuretic therapy).

4 Effects of cholinesterase inhibitors in relieving myasthenia gravis may be impaired by disopyramide.

5 Plasma levels of disopyramide may be lowered by the presence of enzyme inducers, such as phenytoin, barbiturates, and glutethimide.

▶ NURSING ALERTS

▷ 1 Monitor blood pressure and cardiac functioning closely. Be alert for development of excessive widening of QRS complex, hypotension, conduction disturbances, bradycardia and worsening of congestive heart failure—these are all signs of developing toxicity.

▷ 2 If first-degree heart block occurs, reduce dosage. If block persists, weigh benefits of continuing therapy against risk of causing higher degrees of heart block.

▷ 3 Watch for signs of cardiac decompensation, especially in patients with marginally compensated heart failure. Treat progressive congestive failure with cardiac glycosides and diuretics.

▷ 4 Use cautiously in patients with glaucoma, urinary retention, prostatic hypertrophy, sick sinus syndrome, Wolff–Parkinson–White syndrome, bundle branch block, renal impairment, hepatic dysfunction, and in children and pregnant women.

▷ 5 In patients with atrial flutter or fibrillation, digitalize prior to administering disopyramide to ensure that the drug-induced increase in AV conduction does not result in unacceptably rapid ventricular rates.

▶ **NURSING CONSIDERATIONS**

▷ 1 Individualize dosage in each patient based upon clinical response and tolerance.

▷ 2 If no response occurs within 48 hours after initiation of therapy, either discontinue drug or hospitalize patient for careful observation while higher-than-recommended doses (250 mg–300 mg every 6 hr) are tried. Do not administer these doses to outpatients without a previous hospital trial.

▷ 3 Caution patient against driving until effects of the drug are known because lightheadness and dizziness can occur.

▷ 4 Suggest use of candy, gum, or frequent rinsings to relieve mouth dryness that often accompanies disopyramide use.

▷ 5 Monitor intake and output because urinary retention can occur; advise physician if output decreases.

▷ 6 Review patient's medication profile, including over-the-counter drugs, and advise caution in the use of drugs having sympathomimetic effects (*e.g.,* cough or cold preparations, nasal decongestants) because they may alter cardiac stability.

▶ **lidocaine**

Lidopen, Xylocaine

Mechanism

Increases the electrical stimulation threshold of the ventricle during diastole; suppresses automaticity of ectopic pacemaker, shortens the refractory period, and decreases the duration of the action potential in Purkinje fibers, thereby slowing spontaneously firing ectopic ventricular rhythms; little effect on atrial muscle, AV conduction, systolic arterial pressure, myocardial contractility, and cardiac output; has a local anesthetic action (see Chap. 16)

Uses

1 Management of acute ventricular arrhythmias such as those resulting from myocardial infarction, cardiac surgery or catheterization, and digitalis intoxication

Dosage

(Loading dose is given initially, followed by a maintenance infusion to maintain a therapeutic plasma level of 2 mcg/ml–5 mcg/ml)

IV injection: 1 mg/kg at a rate of 25 mg to 50 mg/minute; may repeat at one third to one half initial dose in 5 minutes; maximum is 300 mg/hour

IV infusion: 20 mcg/kg to 50 mcg/kg/minute (1 mg–4 mg/min) of a 0.1% solution (1 g lidocaine in 1 liter 5% Dextrose in Water)

IM: 300 mg in an average 70-kg individual (approximately 4.3 mg/kg); may repeat in 60 minutes to 90 minutes; use only 10% solution, or LidoPen Auto-Injector (300 mg/3 ml)

Fate

Onset with IV injection is immediate and duration is 10 minutes to 20 minutes; following IM injection, onset is 5 minutes to 15 minutes and duration is approximately 60 minutes to 90 minutes. Plasma half-life is 1 hour to 2 hours; although the initial distribution half-life from the plasma is 5 to 10 minutes; widely distributed in the body and significantly bound to plasma proteins (40%–80%); largely (90%) metabolized in the liver and excreted in the urine

Common Side-Effects

Drowsiness; lightheadedness; sensations of heat, cold, or numbness; and paresthesias

Significant Adverse Reactions

CNS—dizziness, impaired hearing or vision, slurred speech, anxiety, apprehension, euphoria, vomiting, muscle twitching, tremors, convulsions, respiratory depression

Cardiovascular—hypotension, bradycardia, cardiovascular collapse, cardiac arrest (overdosage)

Dermatologic—urticaria, peripheral edema, cutaneous lesions

Other—pain at IM injection site, excessive perspiration, local thrombophlebitis (IV infusion)

Contraindications

Adams–Stokes syndrome; Wolff–Parkinson–White syndrome; severe SA, AV, or intraventricular block; hypersensitivity to local anesthetics

Interactions

1 Cardiac depression may increase if lidocaine is used along with other antiarrhythmic drugs, especially phenytoin or propranolol.

2 Concurrent administration of procainamide may result in additive neurologic effects.

3 Muscle relaxant effects of neuromuscular blocking agents (*e.g.,* succinylcholine, aminoglycosides) may be increased by lidocaine.

4 Lidocaine inhibits the antibacterial action of sulfonamides.

5 Barbiturates may decrease the action of lidocaine through enzyme induction.

▶ **NURSING ALERTS**

▷ 1 Observe patients carefully for symptoms of CNS toxicity (*e.g.,* confusion, paresthesias, excitement, tremors), particularly during IV infusion. CNS effects are especially a problem in patients with congestive heart failure. Advise physician and be prepared to administer diazepam or a rapid-acting barbiturate to control convulsions.

▷ 2 Have resuscitative equipment (*e.g.,* respiratory aids) and drugs (*e.g.,* IV fluids, vasopressors, muscle relaxants) on hand to treat adverse reactions involving the CNS, cardiovascular, or respiratory systems.

▷ 3 Monitor cardiac function and blood pressure closely, and discontinue infusion if signs of cardiac depression (*e.g.,* prolonged P–R interval, widened QRS complex) or increased arrhythmias develop.

▷ 4 In patients with sinus bradycardia or incomplete heart block, acceleration of the heart beat with isoproterenol or electric pacing should be accomplished prior to administering lidocaine to avoid precipitation of more frequent or serious ventricular arrhythmias or complete heart block.

▷ 5 Do not use lidocaine solutions containing either preservatives or epinephrine for treating arrhythmias.

▷ 6 Lidocaine has short duration of action, so IV flow rate must be closely monitored to ensure maintenance of adequate plasma levels.

▷ 7 Do *not* add lidocaine to transfusion assemblies.

▷ 8 Use cautiously in the presence of liver or kidney disease, congestive heart failure, severe respiratory depression, hypovolemia, shock, or myasthenia gravis.

▶ **NURSING CONSIDERATIONS**

▷ 1 Terminate IV infusion as soon as cardiac rhythm is stable (or signs of toxicity develop). Patients should be changed to oral antiarrhythmic as soon as possible for maintenance, usually within 24 hours.

▷ 2 Give IM injections into deltoid muscle, because therapeutic blood levels occur sooner, and peak blood level is higher than with other IM injection sites.

▷ 3 Note that IM use may result in increased creatine phosphokinase (CPK) levels, which can interfere with enzyme diagnostic test for myocardial infarction.

▶ **phenytoin**

Dilantin, Diphenylan, Ditan

(Although not an approved indication, phenytoin has been employed in treating certain arrhythmias, particularly those resulting from digitalis toxicity.)

Mechanism

Depresses ectopic pacemaker activity and shortens action potential duration in isolated Purkinje tissue; improves AV and intraventricular conduction in the digitalis-depressed heart; increases membrane responsiveness in Purkinje fibers; slightly impairs force of contraction and has little effect on arterial pressure; exerts an anticonvulsant activity (see Chap. 25), and is widely used in grand mal seizures.

Uses

1 Treatment of paroxysmal atrial tachycardia, particularly if associated with digitalis intoxication
2 Treatment of ventricular ectopic rhythms, especially those resulting from digitalis overdosage

Dosage

IV injection: 100 mg every 5 minutes to 10 minutes until arrhythmia is abolished or toxicity appears (maximum dose is 1000 mg/24 hr)
Oral: Initially 1000 mg first day in divided doses, then 500 mg to 600 mg on second and third days; maintenance is 100 mg 2 to 4 times/day; usual serum level is 10 mcg/ml to 20 mcg/ml

Fate

(See also Chap. 25)
Onset of action orally is 30 minutes to 60 minutes; plasma half-life is 24 hours to 36 hours; highly protein-bound (85%–95%); metabolized by the liver and excreted largely by the kidney as conjugated metabolites

Common Side-Effects

Nystagmus, diplopia, nausea, and GI upset (see also Chap. 25)

Significant Adverse Reactions

(See also Chap. 25)
Cardiovascular—bradycardia, hypotension, cardiac arrest
CNS—confusion, nervousness, ataxia, drowsiness, tremors, visual disturbances

Contraindications

Severe bradycardia, second-degree or complete heart block

Interactions

See Chapter 25.

▶ **NURSING ALERTS**

(See also Chap. 25)

▷ 1 Closely monitor cardiac function during IV administration. Have atropine available to reverse bradycardia or heart block.

▷ 2 Observe patient for development of hypotension, and be prepared to administer IV fluids and vasopressors as needed.

▷ 3 Do not administer drug IM (erratic absorption). IV infusion may be accomplished with a dilute solution (1 g/liter of Dextrose in Water) given over 2 hours to 4 hours; however, IV infusion carries a danger of phlebitis and is very painful.

▶ **NURSING CONSIDERATIONS**

(See also Chap. 25)

▷ 1 Note that achievement of steady-state plasma levels requires 6 to 12 days of oral drug therapy (because of prolonged half-life). This time can be shortened by administering larger loading doses initially.

▷ 2 Advise taking drug with food or milk to reduce GI irritation.

▷ 3 Recognize that most arrhythmias that respond to phenytoin do so at plasma concentrations below the toxic levels. Cautious therapy will eliminate most adverse effects.

▷ 4 Refer to Chapter 25 for discussion of adverse effects that can be expected when drug is given orally for prolonged periods. Limit therapy to the shortest period of time that is feasible.

▶ procainamide
Procan SR, Promine, Pronestyl, Pronestyl-SR, Sub-Quin

Mechanism
Essentially identical to quinidine in pharmacologic actions; decreases cardiac excitability (screening out weaker ectopic impulses), slows conduction in the atria, ventricles, and bundle of His, and prolongs the refractory period of the atria; little effect on contractility or cardiac output; may elicit tachycardia because of its anticholinergic (*i.e.,* vagal blocking) action; produces peripheral vasodilation (especially IV) and hypotension; large doses can result in progressive AV block and ventricular extrasystoles.

Uses
1 Treatment of premature ventricular contractions (PVCs), ventricular tachycardia, paroxysmal atrial tachycardia, and atrial fibrillation
2 Treatment of arrhythmias associated with surgery or general anesthesia

Dosage
Oral

Ventricular tachycardia—initially, 1-g loading dose, then 50 mg/kg/day in divided doses every 3 hours (every 6 hr with sustained-release tablets)

Atrial fibrillation and paroxysmal atrial tachycardia—initially, 1.25 g, followed in 1 hour by 0.75 g; then, 0.5 g to 1 g every 2 hours until arrhythmia is interrupted; maintenance dose 0.5 g to 1 g.

IM: 0.5 g to 1 g every 4 hours to 8 hours; switch to oral therapy as soon as possible (for arrhythmias during anesthesia or surgery, 0.1 g–0.5 g IM)

IV injection: 100 mg every 5 minutes by slow IV injection (25–50 mg/min) to a maximum of 1 g; usual serum level 4 mcg/ml to 8 mcg/ml

IV infusion: (extreme emergencies only) 20 mg to 25 mg/minute of a diluted solution over 30 minutes to a maximum of 600 mg with continual ECG monitoring; if necessary, change to a second infusion (2–6 mg/min) for maintenance

Fate
Well absorbed orally, except in patients with severely compromised cardiovascular function; onset is 30 minutes and duration is 3 hours to 4 hours; peak plasma levels occur in 60 minutes; onset following IM or IV administration is immediate; maximum plasma levels in 15 minutes to 30 minutes; half-life is 2 hours to 4 hours; minimal protein binding (10%–20%); slowly hydrolyzed by plasma liver esterases, approximately one fourth converted to n-acetylprocainamide, an active metabolite with a 6-hour half-life; primarily (60%–70%) excreted by the kidneys, at least half as the unchanged drug

Common Side-Effects
Anorexia, nausea (orally); hypotension (IV)

Significant Adverse Reactions
Orally—vomiting, diarrhea, urticaria, angioedema, maculopapular rash, weakness, depression, psychotic behavior, agranulocytosis, systemic lupus-like reaction (fever, rashes, muscle and joint pain, pericarditis, pleural effusion, hepatomegaly, hemolytic anemia, thrombocytopenia)
IV—flushing, ventricular asystole, ventricular fibrillation

Contraindications
Myasthenia gravis, second- or third-degree AV block, and hypersensitivity to local anesthetics (drug is a derivative of procaine)

Interactions
1 Procainamide may potentiate the muscle relaxing action of neuromuscular blocking agents and those antibiotics (especially aminoglycosides) having a skeletal muscle relaxant effect.
2 Additive effects on the heart may occur with combinations of procainamide and other antiarrhythmic or digitalis-like drugs.
3 Procainamide may increase the hypotensive effects of antihypertensives and diuretics.
4 Effects of procainamide can be potentiated by agents that alkalinize the urine and reduce urinary excretion, such as acetazolamide, sodium lactate, and sodium bicarbonate.
5 The action of cholinesterase inhibitors in treating myasthenia gravis can be antagonized by procainamide.

▶ NURSING ALERTS
▷ 1 During IV infusion, keep patient supine, and monitor ECG and blood pressure continually. If blood pressure falls more than 15 mm Hg or if ventricular rate slows significantly without development of regular AV conduction, discontinue infusion. Have pressor agent (*e.g.,* levarterenol or dopamine) available to combat extreme hypotension.
▷ 2 Stop infusion when arrhythmia is terminated, or if excessive widening of QRS complex or prolongation of P–R interval occurs. Arrhythmias are usually abolished within minutes following IV infusion.
▷ 3 In treatment of atrial arrhythmias, be alert for sudden development of ventricular tachycardia when rapid atrial rate is slowed during drug infusion, allowing 1:1 AV conduction. Prior digitalization will reduce this danger.
▷ 4 In patients receiving large oral doses over prolonged periods, observe carefully for signs of possible lupus-like reaction (*e.g.,* fever, arthralgia, skin lesions, pericarditis, chest pain, coughing, pleural effusions), and

periodically measure antinuclear antibody titers. Discontinue drug if clinical signs of lupus appear or if titer rises (quinidine may be substituted), and initiate steroid therapy if symptoms persist or worsen.

▷ 5 Watch for indications of developing agranulocytosis (fever, sore throat, mucosal ulceration, respiratory tract infection), and perform leukocyte count. Discontinue medication if values are abnormal.

▷ 6. Use cautiously in patients with liver or kidney disease because accumulation can occur. Advise patient to report possible signs of renal dysfunction (*e.g.,* dysuria, oliguria)

▶ NURSING CONSIDERATIONS

▷ 1 Perform periodic ECG determinations and blood counts in patients on prolonged therapy.

▷ 2 Administer oral drug with meals or milk to reduce GI upset.

▷ 3 Inform patients that drug may cause lightheadedness and dizziness due to hypotensive effect; advise caution in driving or operating machinery.

▷ 4 Note that drug does not appear to increase effects of oral anticoagulants as does quinidine, and therefore may be used in patients taking oral anticoagulants without necessitating dosage alterations.

▷ 5 Stress caution in the use of other medications that can alter cardiac stability (*e.g.,* sympathomimetics, anticholinergics) during chronic therapy with procainamide.

▷ *Dietary precaution*

▷ 1 Consult physician as to whether intake of caffeine-containing beverages should be curtailed.

▶ propranolol

Inderal

Propranolol is a beta-adrenergic blocking agent used in several disease states, including arrhythmias. The drug is discussed fully in Chapter 12, and mention is made here only of those properties pertaining specifically to its application as an antiarrhythmic agent.

Mechanism

Competitively antagonizes the action of adrenergic agents at beta-receptor sites; specifically, on the heart, it reduces rate, force of contraction, irritability, AV conduction, and automaticity of the SA node and ectopic pacemakers. Large doses exert a direct quinidine-like depressant effect on the myocardium, suppressing overall cardiac functioning.

Uses

1 Treatment of arrhythmias, especially tachyarrhythmias resulting from digitalis intoxication, thyrotoxicosis, or excessive catecholamine action, as during anesthesia or surgery

Dosage

Oral: 10 mg to 30 mg 3 to 4 times/day

IV: 1 mg to 3 mg at a rate of 1 mg/minute; a second dose can be given after 2 minutes.

Fate

(Orally—see Chap. 12.) With IV administration, onset is 1 minute to 2 minutes and duration lasts 3 hours to 6 hours.

▶ NURSING ALERTS

See Chapter 12. In addition:

▷ 1 Be alert for development of a severe bradycardia with IV propranolol administration, especially in patients with digitalis intoxication. Have atropine injection available, and monitor ECG closely.

▷ 2 Recognize that effects of propranolol and digitalis are additive in depressing AV conduction; use of propranolol in digitalis overdosage may further depress myocardial contractility and can lead to cardiac failure. Closely monitor patient on combined therapy, and withdraw propranolol if signs of cardiac failure persist.

▶ quinidine

Cardioquin, Cin-Quin, Duraquin, Quinaglute Dura-Tabs, Quinatime, Quinidex Extentabs, Quinora, Quin-Release

Mechanism

Complexes with lipoproteins in myocardial cell membrane, thereby decreasing sodium influx during depolarization and potassium efflux during repolarization; depresses cardiac excitability (elevates firing threshold to screen out weak ectopic impulses), slows conduction velocity, and reduces myocardial contractility; prolongs effective refractory period of the myocardium; slows phase O (depolarization) and prolongs phase 4 (diastolic depolarization) of the ventricular action potential; exerts anticholinergic (decreases vagal tone and prevents cardiac slowing due to vagal activation) and skeletal muscle relaxant effects, resulting in peripheral vasodilation in high doses

Uses

1. Treatment of the following arrhythmias:
   a. Paroxysmal supraventricular tachycardia
   b. Atrial flutter and fibrillation
   c. Premature atrial and ventricular contractions
   d. Paroxysmal AV junctional rhythm
   e. Paroxysmal ventricular tachycardia not associated with complete heart block.
2. Maintenance therapy after electrical conversion of atrial flutter or fibrillation

Dosage

Oral: usual 10 mg/kg to 20 mg/kg/day in 4 to 6 divided doses (200 mg–300 mg 4 times/day) individualized to patient's response

Paroxysmal supraventricular tachycardia—400 mg to 600 mg every 2 hours to 3 hours until paroxysm is terminated

Premature atrial and ventricular contractions—200 mg to 300 mg 3 to 4 times/day

Atrial fibrillation—200 mg every 2 hours to 3 hours for 5 to 8 doses; increase gradually until sinus rhythm is restored (maximal daily dose is 3 g–4 g)

Maintenance—200 mg to 300 mg 3 to 4 times/day (sustained-release forms—1 to 2 tablets 2 to 3 times/day)

IM: 600 mg gluconate salt initially, then 400 mg every 2 hours as needed

IV: 200 mg to 750 mg gluconate salt or equivalent by slow IV infusion of a dilute (800 mg gluconate/50 ml 5% glucose) solution at a rate of 1 ml (16 mg) per minute.

Fate

Completely absorbed orally; maximum effects occur in 1 hour to 3 hours, and action persists for at least 6 hours to 8 hours (8 hr–12 hr with sustained-release forms); widely distributed in the body and significantly bound (60%–80%) to plasma proteins; metabolized in the liver and excreted through the kidney both as metabolites (80%) and unchanged (20%); elimination half-life is 6 hours.

Common Side-Effects

Nausea, diarrhea, abdominal distress, lightheadedness, tinnitus, headache

Significant Adverse Reactions

GI—vomiting, cramping

CNS—fever, vertigo, impaired hearing, blurred vision, altered color perception, photophobia, diplopia, scotomas, excitement, confusion, delirium, syncope

Cardiovascular—ventricular ectopic beats, cardiac asystole, hypotension, severe bradycardia, atrial or ventricular flutter and fibrillation, arterial embolism

Hematologic/dermatologic—acute hemolytic anemia, thrombocytopenic purpura, leukopenia, agranulocytosis (rare), flushing, urticaria, angioedema, pruritus, sweating

Other—arthralgia, dyspnea, respiratory depression, asthmatic episodes

IV use—sweating, nervousness, vomiting, cramping, urge to urinate or defecate

Contraindications

AV conduction defects or complete AV block, ectopic impulses and rhythms due to escape mechanisms, thrombocytopenic purpura, and acute rheumatic fever

Interactions

1 Quinidine may increase the effects of oral anticoagulants, antihypertensives, neuromuscular blocking agents, anticholinergics, digitalis, and other antiarrhythmics.

2 Blood levels of quinidine can be elevated by substances that alkalinize the urine (*e.g.*, sodium bicarbonate, antacids, carbonic anhydrase inhibitors), thereby retarding quinidine excretion.

3 Effects of cholinergic drugs (*e.g.*, neostigmine, edrophonium) may be antagonized by quinidine.

4 Additive cardiac depressant effects may occur with use of propranolol or phenothiazines with quinidine.

5 Administration of phenytoin, rifampin, or barbiturates may reduce the serum half-life of quinidine because of enzyme induction.

6 Quinidine may elevate blood levels of digoxin by reducing its tissue binding or by retarding its renal clearance.

▶ **NURSING ALERTS**

▷ 1 In patients with atrial flutter or fibrillation, pretreat with digitalis prior to administering quinidine to retard AV conduction and to reduce the danger of ventricular tachycardia resulting from a progressive reduction in the degree of AV block to a 1:1 ratio.

▷ 2 Closely monitor patients receiving quinidine (especially parenterally or in large oral doses), and note evidence of developing cardiotoxicity (widening of QRS complex greater than 25%, ventricular extrasystoles, abolition of P waves). Discontinue drug and advise physician immediately.

▷ 3 Advise patient to be alert for signs of quinidine overdosage, collectively termed *cinchonism*. These signs include tinnitus, impaired vision, dyspnea, palpitations, nausea, headache, and chest tightness. Physician should be informed and dosage reduced.

▷ 4 During parenteral therapy, monitor ECG, pulse rate, rhythm, and blood pressure. Have available sodium lactate, vasopressors, and cardiopulmonary resuscitative equipment.

▷ 5 Use cautiously in the presence of incomplete heart block, digitalis intoxication, congestive heart failure, hypotension, respiratory disorders, potassium imbalance (*e.g.*, diuretic therapy), and impaired renal or hepatic function.

▷ 6 Keep patient supine during IV administration and watch for development of severe hypotension. Perform frequent determinations of serum quinidine levels during IV use, to prevent cardiac toxicity that is often noted at levels greater than 8 mg/liter.

▶ **NURSING CONSIDERATIONS**

▷ 1 Administer drug with food to minimize GI distress.

▷ 2 Advise patient that diarrhea is common early in therapy and should disappear. If diarrhea persists, consult physician, because dosage adjustment may be required.

▷ 3 Perform periodic blood counts, serum electrolyte determinations, and liver and kidney function tests in patients on prolonged therapy.

▷ 4 Use prolonged-acting forms of quinidine (*i.e.*, Quinaglute Dura-Tabs, Quinidex Extentabs) only for maintenance therapy. Make appropriate dosage adjustments when changing preparations (Quinaglute Dura-Tabs are 62% base; Quinidine sulfate is 82% base).

▷ 5 If time permits, administer a preliminary test dose (200 mg PO or IM) to determine if hypersensitivity to quinidine is present, especially in patients receiving the drug for the first time.

▷ 6 Counsel patient to report immediately feelings of dizziness or faintness, which are possible indications of ventricular arrhythmias and depressed cardiac output.

▷ *Dietary precautions*

▷ 1 Advise moderation in the consumption of excessive caffeine or alcohol during quinidine therapy, and caution against heavy smoking, which can alter the irritability of the heart.

▷ 2 Be aware that consumption of large amounts of citrus fruits can alkalinize the urine, resulting in retention of quinidine.

▶ verapamil
Calan, Isoptin

Verapamil is termed a calcium channel blocker or calcium antagonist because it inhibits the movement of calcium ions across the cell membrane through the so-called slow calcium channels. Together with the other calcium channel blockers diltiazem and nifedipine, it is used orally for the treatment of angina (this application is reviewed in Chap. 32). In addition, verapamil is also indicated for the treatment of supraventricular tachyarrhythmias because it has a much greater effect on SA and AV nodal function than do the other calcium blockers. Its use as an antiarrhythmic is discussed below.

Mechanism
Inhibits influx of calcium ions through slow channels into cells of the cardiac conductile system; AV conduction is slowed and the effective refractory period of the AV node is prolonged, thus reducing elevated ventricular rate, interrupting AV nodal impulse re-entry, and restoring normal sinus rhythm in supraventricular tachycardias; decreases myocardial contractility and reduces aortic impedance to left ventricular ejection (*i.e.,* afterload); may transiently lower systemic arterial pressure, and raise left ventricular filling pressure

Uses
1 Treatment of supraventricular tachyarrhythmias, such as paroxysmal atrial tachycardia
2 Control of excessive ventricular rate in patients with atrial flutter or atrial fibrillation

Dosage
(Given by slow IV injection)
Adults: initially, 5 mg to 10 mg over 2 minutes to 3 minutes; repeat with 10 mg 30 minutes after first dose if initial response is inadequate
Children: 0 to 1 yr—0.75 mg to 2 mg over 2 min; 1 yr–15 yr—2 mg to 5 mg over 2 minutes; may repeat initial dose in 30 minutes, if necessary

Fate
Effects are usually noted within 2 minutes to 5 minutes of injection. Duration of action of a single injection is 30 minutes to 45 minutes. Elimination half-life is 3 hours to 8 hours. Verapamil is rapidly metabolized in the liver and metabolites are excreted in the urine (70%) and feces (15%–20%). It is highly protein-bound (90%).

Common Side-Effects
Transient hypotension and dizziness; bradycardia

Significant Adverse Reactions
(Infrequent)
Cardiovascular—tachycardia, marked hypotension, asystole, AV block, congestive heart failure
CNS—headache, depression, vertigo, fatigue, nystagmus
GI—nausea, abdominal discomfort
Other—diaphoresis, muscle weakness

Contraindications
Severe hypotension, cardiogenic shock, second- or third-degree AV block, severe congestive heart failure, sick sinus syndrome, concurrent administration of IV beta-blocker or disopyramide

Interactions
1 Verapamil may be potentiated by other strongly protein-bound drugs, such as oral anticoagulants, antiinflammatory drugs, and sulfonamides.
2 The desired effects of verapamil may be reduced by administration of supplemental calcium.
3 The depressant action of verapamil on the myocardium and AV node can be enhanced by simultaneous use of an IV beta-blocking drug or disopyramide.
4 Excessive bradycardia or AV block can occur if verapamil is given together with a digitalis drug. Chronic verapamil therapy increases serum digoxin levels.
5 Verapamil can enhance the blood pressure lowering action of antihypertensive drugs.

▶ NURSING ALERTS
▷ 1 Ensure that complete monitoring and proper resuscitative equipment is available when verapamil is first administered because some patients have responded with rapid ventricular rate or, conversely, with marked hypotension and extreme bradycardia. Cardioversion, lidocaine, or procainamide are effective in treating rapid ventricular rate; norepinephrine or metaraminol may be used to treat hypotension and isoproterenol or atropine is indicated to reverse bradycardia or AV block.
▷ 2 Closely monitor patients receiving verapamil along with digitalis drugs, beta-blockers, or other antiarrhythmics because adverse effects can be increased.

▶ NURSING CONSIDERATIONS
▷ 1 Administer IV injection over at least 3 minutes in older patients to minimize the possibility of adverse reactions. Keep patient recumbent for 1 hour after injection to minimize hypotension.
▷ 2 Advise patients on prolonged therapy to refrain from

using over-the-counter products containing calcium, because effectiveness of verapamil may be impaired.

▷ 3 Monitor urinary output, because impaired renal function can prolong the duration of action of verapamil.

▷ 4 Be aware that during conversion to normal sinus rhythm, complexes resembling premature ventricular contractions can occur. These events have no clinical significance.

Summary. Antiarrhythmic Agents

Drug	Preparations	Usual Dosage Range
Bretylium (Bretylol)	Injection—50 mg/ml	IV injection—5 mg/kg undiluted solution by rapid IV injection; may repeat at 10 mg/kg to a total dose of 30 mg/kg IV infusion—5 mg/kg to 10 mg/kg of a diluted solution over at least 8 minutes to 10 minutes IM—5 mg/kg to 10 mg/kg undiluted solution; repeat in 1 hour to 2 hours, then every 6 hours to 8 hours thereafter
Disopyramide (Norpace, Norpace CR)	Capsules—100 mg, 150 mg Sustained-release capsules—100 mg, 150 mg	Initially 300 mg, then 150 mg every 6 hours (every 8 hr with sustained-release capsules); usual range is 400 mg to 800 mg/day Pediatric—6 mg/kg–20 mg/kg/day in divided doses every 6 hours depending on age
Lidocaine (LidoPen, Xylocaine)	Injection—10 mg, 20 mg, 40 mg, 100 mg, 200 mg/ml IV infusion—2 mg, 4 mg, 8 mg/ml in 5% Dextrose	IV injection—1 mg/kg at a rate of 25 mg to 50 mg/minute; may repeat in 5 minutes IV infusion—20 mcg/kg to 50 mcg/kg/minute (1 mg–4 mg/min) of a 0.1% solution IM—300 mg in a average-size patient (4.3 mg/kg); may repeat in 60 minutes to 90 minutes
Phenytoin (Dilantin, Diphenylan, Ditan)	Chewable tablets—50 mg Capsules—30 mg, 100 mg, 250 mg Suspension—30 mg, 125 mg/5 ml Injection—50 mg/ml	IV injection—100 mg every 5 minutes to 10 minutes until arrhythmia is abolished or toxicity appears Oral—initially 1000 mg first day, then 500 mg to 600 mg second and third days; maintenance dose 100 mg 2 to 4 times/day
Procainamide (Procan SR, Promine, Pronestyl, Pronestyl-SR, Sub-Quin)	Capsules—250 mg, 375 mg, 500 mg Tablets—250 mg, 375 mg, 500 mg Sustained-release tablets—250 mg, 500 mg, 750 mg Injection—100 mg, 500 mg/ml	Oral—initially 1 g; then 50 mg/kg/day in divided doses every 3 hours IM—0.5 g to 1 g every 6 hours (arrhythmias during surgery or anesthesia—0.1 g to 0.5 g IM) IV infusion—20 mg to 50 mg/min to a maximum of 1 g
Propranolol (Inderal)	Tablets—10 mg, 20 mg, 40 mg, 60 mg, 80 mg, 90 mg Sustained-release capsules—80 mg, 120 mg, 160 mg Injection—1 mg/ml	Oral—10 mg to 30 mg 3 to 4 times/day IV—1 mg to 3 mg at a rate of 1 mg/minute Repeat in 2 minutes if necessary
Quinidine (Cardioquin, Cin-Quin, Duraquin, Quinaglute Dura-Tabs, Quinatime, Quinidex Extentabs, Quinora, Quin-Release)	Tablets—100 mg, 200 mg, 300 mg Sustained-release tablets—300 mg, 324 mg, 330 mg Capsules—200 mg, 300 mg Injection—80 mg, 200 mg/ml	Oral—usually 200 mg to 600 mg 4 times/day individualized to patient's response Maximal daily dose 3 g to 4 g Maintenance—200 mg to 300 mg 3 to 4 times/day or 1 to 2 sustained-acting tablets 2 to 3 times/day

(continued)

Summary. Antiarrhythmic Agents *(continued)*

Drug	Preparations	Usual Dosage Range
		IM—(gluconate) 600 mg initially, then 400 mg every 2 hours as needed
		IV—(gluconate or sulfate) 200 mg to 750 mg by slow IV infusion (800 mg/50 ml 5% glucose at a rate of 1 ml/min or 16 mg/min)
Verapamil (Calan, Isoptin)	Tablets—80 mg, 120 mg Injection—2.5 mg/ml	Adults—5 mg to 10 mg IV over 2 to 3 minutes; repeat with 10 mg 30 minutes after the first dose
		Children—0.75 mg to 5 mg IV over 2 to 3 minutes depending on age; repeat in 30 minutes if necessary

Drug therapy of hypertension is directed towards reducing elevated arterial pressure, which is believed to be the primary cause of vascular degeneration and other complications that impair health and reduce life expectancy. The etiology of most cases of hypertension is unknown, thus treatment is essentially palliative—that is, directed at lowering the elevated systolic and diastolic pressures. The currently available antihypertensive drugs neither prevent nor cure the basic underlying hemodynamic disturbances.

Nevertheless, judicious use of one or more of the available antihypertensive agents can provide excellent control of blood pressure for extended periods of time. The agents can also markedly delay the onset of vascular damage and can significantly prolong the life of the hypertensive patient. Drug therapy, however, is only one aspect of a complete therapeutic regimen that should also include proper rest, exercise, and reduced caloric and salt intake.

The wide range of antihypertensive medications in clinical use today allows the physician to carefully tailor drug therapy to the needs of each hypertensive patient. Milder forms of hypertension frequently can be controlled by diuretic therapy alone, whereas more elevated pressures may require one or more additional antihypertensive agents in the regimen. Combination drug therapy enhances the pharmacologic effects of each drug, allowing use of smaller individual doses, which thereby reduces the incidence and severity of untoward reactions. Control of all degrees of blood pressure can therefore be attained, in most instances, with minimal untoward effects on the patient. Controversy exists about the necessity for drug treatment of mild or labile hypertension (diastolic pressure 90 mm Hg to 100 mm Hg), especially where other risk factors are absent (*e.g.,* if there is lack of tissue or organ damage, no familial history of hypertension, and the patient is not young, male, or black). Elimination of certain contributory factors (*e.g.,* stress, overweight, smoking, dietary salt) is often sufficient to adequately control the arterial pressure in this labile hypertensive population. On the other hand, there is clear indication for the use of antihypertensive medications in patients who exhibit sustained diastolic pressures above 100 mm Hg, or in high-risk patients (*e.g.,* presence of diabetes or hypercholesterolemia, young black males, genetic predisposition toward hypertension) whose diastolic pressures are consistently above 90 mm Hg.

Clinically effective antihypertensive drugs act at many sites in the body and through numerous mechanisms. They have a wide range of potencies, side-effects, and potential interactions. Choice of a suitable antihypertensive drug depends on many factors, such as the degree of hypertension being treated, the presence of other disease states (*e.g.,* reserpine is contraindicated in active hepatic disease), the presence of other drugs (*e.g.,* antidepressants reduce guanethidine's effectiveness), and a patient's acceptance of the mild yet often inescapable side-effects of many agents. Although many antihypertensive drugs have more than one site or mechanism of action, they can be conveniently grouped according to their *principal sites* of action, recognizing, however, that these may not be the only active sites for many of the compounds. Such a grouping is presented in Table 31-1.

Antihypertensive Drugs

31

**Table 31-1. Antihypertensive Drugs—
Principal Sites of Action**

I. CNS
  A. Cortex
    1. Reserpine and rauwolfia derivatives
  B. Cardiovascular centers (hypothalamus, medulla)
    1. Clonidine/Guanabenz
    2. Methyldopa
    3. Beta-adrenergic blockers (*e.g.,* propranolol)
II. Sympathetic Ganglia
  A. Ganglionic blocking agents (*e.g.,* trimethaphan)
III. Adrenergic Nerve Endings
  A. Alpha-adrenergic blockers (*e.g.,* phentolamine, prazosin)
  B. Beta-adrenergic blockers (*e.g.,* propranolol)
  C. Reserpine and rauwolfia derivatives
  D. Guanethidine/guanadrel
  E. Metyrosine
  F. Pargyline
IV. Vascular Smooth Muscle
  A. Hydralazine
  B. Diazoxide
  C. Minoxidil
  D. Nitroprusside
  E. Diuretics
  F. Calcium channel blockers
V. Kidney and Afferent Arteriole
  A. Diuretics
  B. Beta-adrenergic blockers (*e.g.,* propranolol)
VI. Renin–Angiotensin System
  A. Captopril

Another means of classifying the various available antihypertensive drugs is based on a suggested progressive drug regimen that treats all stages of hypertension, from mild to

**Table 31-2. Stepped-Care Approach
to Treating Hypertension**

Step 1 (Mild Hypertension)

Diuretics
  Thiazides/sulfonamides (most frequently used)
  Indapamide
  High-ceiling (loop) drugs
  Potassium-sparing drugs
Beta-blockers

Step 2 (Mild to Moderate Hypertension)

Beta-blockers
Clonidine/guanabenz
Guanadrel
Methyldopa
Prazosin
Reserpine (infrequently used)

Step 3 (Moderate Hypertension)

Captopril
Hydralazine

Step 4 (Severe Hypertension)

Captopril
Guanethidine
Minoxidil

Hypertensive Emergencies

Diazoxide
Nitroprusside
Trimethaphan

severe. This so-called "stepped-care approach" is widely followed, and despite some minor disagreements on the placement of certain drugs, is generally regarded as the preferred approach for managing the hypertensive patient. A typical stepped-care classification is presented in Table 31-2. Mild hypertension is usually treated initially with a diuretic (step 1) although beta-blockers have been recommended as suitable alternatives, especially in younger patients with a high pulse pressure (*i.e.,* systolic minus diastolic) and rapid heart beat, and in patients with arrhythmias, angina, or hyperuricemia. Adrenergic inhibitors are usually added next (step 2), when maximally tolerated doses of diuretics fail to provide sufficient control; however, the diuretic is most often continued in lower doses. However, significant differences in mechanisms and profile of side-effects among the antiadrenergic drugs mandate that careful selection be made among the drugs to optimize the therapeutic benefit. Several different step-2 drugs should be tried before adding a third drug. Vasodilators, such as hydralazine or angiotensin converting enzyme inhibitors, like captopril, may provide adequate control in patients refractory to or intolerant of a combination of step-1 and step-2 drugs. Severe refractive hypertension may require that one of the step-4 drugs be used, although the incidence of untoward reactions with these agents is substantial.

Hypertensive emergencies are best managed by IV sodium nitroprusside or diazoxide, both vascular smooth muscle relaxants, or trimethaphan, a ganglionic blocking agent. Pheochromocytoma, a catecholamine secreting tumor of chromaffin tissue (*e.g.,* adrenal medulla), leads to marked elevations in blood pressure. Metyrosine or possibly phentolamine can be used to reduce the excessively high blood pressure in pheochromocytoma.

Several classes of antihypertensive agents have been discussed in previous chapters (*e.g.,* alpha- and beta-adrenergic blocking agents, ganglionic blocking agents); only those aspects relating to their antihypertensive action will be mentioned here. Likewise, diuretics are reviewed in detail in Chapter 37 and are not considered in this chapter. Calcium channel blockers are potentially useful antihypertensive agents because of their peripheral vasodilating action; these drugs are discussed in Chapter 32.

▶ **atenolol**
  Tenormin

A long-acting beta-adrenergic blocking agent with a relative specificity for beta-1 receptors in the heart, atenolol is indicated for the management of mild to moderate hypertension, either alone or combined with other antihypertensive drugs, particularly diuretics. Its long elimination half-life allows for once daily dosing and its beta-1 selectivity permits its cautious use in patients with bronchospastic disorders (refer to Chap. 12 for a complete discussion of atenolol and the other beta-blockers).

Dosage

Initially, 50 mg as a single daily dose; increase to 100 mg as a single dose if an optimal response is not achieved within 2 weeks. Further dosage increases are unlikely to result in improved clinical effects.

▶ **captopril**

Capoten

Mechanism

Captopril suppresses the functioning of the renin–angiotensin–aldosterone mechanism by inhibiting angiotensin converting enzyme (ACE) in the plasma and vascular endothelium. Thus, conversion of inactive angiotensin I to active angiotensin II is blocked, and formation of aldosterone is impaired; it may also interfere with breakdown of bradykinin, an endogenous peptide that elicits vasodilation. Plasma renin activity increases due to loss of negative feedback, and serum potassium may rise due to absence of aldosterone activity. There is no significant change in cardiac output; renal blood flow is increased. In patients with heart failure, captopril decreases systemic vascular resistance and pulmonary capillary wedge pressure and increases cardiac output.

Uses

1 Management of moderate to severe hypertension, combined with a diuretic, in patients who fail to respond to or cannot tolerate multiple drug regimens (not a first-line antihypertensive drug)
2 Adjunctive therapy of congestive heart failure, in combination with digitalis drugs and diuretics
3 Treatment of mild to moderate hypertension, as a step-2 drug in lowered doses (investigational use)

Dosage

Hypertension

Initially, 25 mg 3 times/day; may increase to 50 mg 3 times/day in 1 week to 2 weeks if satisfactory response is not attained; may increase further in 50-mg increments in combination with a diuretic; usual maintenance range is 25 mg to 150 mg 3 times/day; maximal daily dose is 450 mg

Congestive Heart Failure

Initially, 12.5 mg to 25 mg 3 times/day; increase gradually in 25-mg increments; usual dosage range is 50 mg to 100 mg 3 times/day in conjunction with a diuretic and digitalis; maximum dose is 450 mg/day

Fate

Rapidly absorbed orally (absorption is impaired by food); peak serum levels occur within 1 hour; approximately 25% to 30% bound to plasma proteins; elimination half-life is 2 hours to 3 hours; metabolized and excreted as both unchanged drug (40%–50%) and conjugated metabolites in the urine

Common Side-Effects

Rash (usually maculopapular), pruritus, and altered taste perception

Significant Adverse Reactions

Cardiovascular—tachycardia, chest pain, palpitations, flushing, hypotension, angina, congestive heart failure, myocardial infarction (rare)

GI—nausea, gastric irritation, abdominal pain, diarrhea, peptic ulcer

CNS—dizziness, malaise, insomnia, headache

Hematologic—neutropenia, agranulocytosis, eosinophilia, hemolytic anemia

Dermatologic—photosensitivity, angioedema, paresthesias, flushing, pallor

Renal—proteinuria, oliguria, polyuria, urinary frequency, renal insufficiency

Other—dry mouth, dyspnea, lymphadenopathy, Raynaud's disease, laryngeal edema

Interactions

1 The hypotensive effects of captopril may be increased by diuretics and other antihypertensive drugs and by severe salt restriction.
2 Serum potassium levels can be markedly elevated by the combination of captopril with potassium-sparing diuretics or potassium supplements.
3 Vasodilators (*e.g.,* nitrites) may be potentiated by captopril.

▶ **NURSING ALERTS**

▷ 1 Perform urinary protein estimates prior to therapy and at monthly intervals thereafter. If proteinuria exceeds 1 g/day, drug should be discontinued unless benefits clearly outweigh risks.

▷ 2 Obtain white blood cell and differential counts prior to beginning therapy and at 2-week intervals during early months of treatment. Urge patients to report any signs of infection (fever, sore throat), possible signs of neutropenia, and withdraw drug if white cell count is abnormal.

▷ 3 Use cautiously in patients with renal impairment, systemic lupus or other auto-immune disease; in patients receiving other drugs that may affect the white cell count; in children under 15 years; and in pregnant or nursing mothers.

▷ 4 Notify physician if mouth sores, swelling of hands or feet, irregular heart beat, or chest pains occur.

▶ **NURSING CONSIDERATIONS**

▷ 1 Discontinue other antihypertensive drugs at least 1 week before beginning captopril, if possible.

▷ 2 Recognize that the blood pressure lowering effects of captopril and diuretics appear to be *additive* but that those of captopril and beta-blockers are less than additive.

▷ 3 Note that several weeks of therapy may be required to achieve optimal therapeutic results. Make dosage adjustments gradually during this period.

▷ 4 Caution patients that excessive perspiration and dehydration (*e.g.,* due to diarrhea, vomiting) may lead to excessive reductions in blood pressure during captopril therapy.

▷ 5 Administer drug 1 hour before meals.

▷ *Dietary precaution*
▷ 1 Advise patients to maintain the same salt intake as prior to therapy, because salt restriction can lead to a precipitous drop in pressure with initial doses of captopril.

▶ clonidine
Catapres

▶ guanabenz
Wytensin

Clonidine and guanabenz are similar, orally active antiadrenergic agents that are indicated in the treatment of mild to moderate hypertension. They are centrally acting antihypertensive drugs with a very low incidence of serious toxicity; principal side-effects are drowsiness and dry mouth.

Mechanism
Activation of presynaptic adrenergic alpha-2 receptors in cardiovascular integrating centers in the brain stem, resulting in a decreased outflow of sympathetic vasoconstrictor and cardioaccelerator impulses; moderate reduction in pulse rate and cardiac output; decrease in plasma renin activity; initially, may stimulate peripheral alpha-adrenergic receptors, causing transient vasoconstriction

Uses
1 Treatment of mild to moderate degrees of hypertension, either alone or with a diuretic or another antihypertensive drug
2 Investigational uses for clonidine include prophylaxis of migraine, treatment of episodes of menopausal flushing, symptomatic management of opiate detoxification, and treatment of Gilles de la Tourette's disease.

Dosage
Clonidine
Initially 0.1 mg twice a day; increase by 0.1 mg to 0.2 mg/day to desired response; usual range is 0.2 mg to 0.8 mg/day in divided doses; maximum 2.4 mg/day; may be effective as a single daily dose
  Opiate withdrawal: 10 mcg/kg to 17 mcg/kg/day in divided doses (experimental use only)
  Gilles de la Tourette's disease: 0.05 mg to 0.6 mg/day

Guanabenz
Initially, 4 mg twice a day; increase in increments of 4 mg to 8 mg/day every 1 week to 2 weeks; maximum dose is 32 mg a day in divided doses

Fate
Onset for both drugs in 30 minutes to 60 minutes following oral administration; maximum effect in 2 hours to 4 hours; duration 6 hours to 8 hours; plasma half-life is 12 hours to 16 hours for clonidine and 6 hours to 8 hours for guanabenz; metabolized by the liver and excreted in the urine (60%–70%) and feces (20%) both as metabolites and unchanged drug

Common Side-Effects
Dry mouth, drowsiness, sedation, constipation, dizziness, headache, fatigue

Significant Adverse Reactions
GI—anorexia, nausea, vomiting, parotid pain, liver function test abnormalities
CNS—insomnia, nervousness, anxiety, depression, vivid dreams or nightmares
Dermatologic—rash, angioedema, urticaria, hives, hair loss, pruritus
Cardiovascular—Raynaud's phenomenon (pallor, cyanosis, pain in extremities); palpitation; flushing; congestive heart failure (rare)
Other—weight gain, hyperglycemia, gynecomastia, urinary retention, impotence, itching or burning of eyes, pallor, dryness or nasal mucosa.

Interactions
1 Clonidine and guanabenz may intensify the CNS-depressant effects of alcohol, barbiturates, narcotics, and other depressants.
2 Effects of clonidine and guanabenz may be antagonized by tricyclic antidepressants (except doxepin) and tolazoline.
3 Excessive bradycardia can occur when clonidine or guanabenz is used in combination with digitalis agents, propranolol, or guanethidine.

▶ NURSING ALERTS
▷ 1 Use cautiously in patients with coronary insufficiency, recent myocardial infarction, cerebrovascular disease, chronic renal failure, thromboangiitis obliterans, history of depression, and in pregnant women and young children.
▷ 2 Advise patient to make positional changes slowly and to lie down if faintness occurs because postural hypotension has been reported (although less frequent than with many other antihypertensive drugs).
▷ 3 Caution against engaging in activities that require mental alertness, especially in early stages of therapy, because drowsiness is quite common.
▷ 4 Discontinue drugs slowly over a period of several days. *Abrupt* termination of therapy can produce headache, agitation, and a rapid rise in blood pressure; these can be treated by reinstituting clonidine or use of both an alpha- and beta-adrenergic blockers.

▶ NURSING CONSIDERATIONS
▷ 1 Closely observe patients with a prior history of mental depression because clonidine and guanabenz can evoke depressive episodes.
▷ 2 Advise patients to undergo periodic eye examinations during prolonged therapy because retinal degeneration has been noted in animal studies.
▷ 3 Counsel patients to avoid over-the-counter cough, cold,

or allergy medications containing sympathomimetic agents because blood pressure control can be adversely affected.

▷ 4 Be alert for development of tolerance to effects of clonidine or guanabenz. Re-evaluate therapy, and consider addition of other antihypertensive medications.

▷ 5 Urge patients to report any changes in pattern of urination because drugs can produce urinary hesitancy.

▷ *Dietary precaution*

▷ 1 Inform patients that drugs may increase sensitivity to alcohol.

▶ **diazoxide, parenteral**

Hyperstat IV

Mechanism

Direct relaxation of arteriolar smooth muscle, resulting in vasodilation; reflexly increases heart rate, stroke volume, and cardiac output; renal blood flow is increased; causes sodium and water retention, and inhibits tubular secretion of uric acid; elicits hyperglycemia by inhibiting insulin secretion from the pancreas, and elevates serum free fatty acids

Uses

1 Acute treatment (IV) of hypertensive emergencies
2 Management of hypoglycemia caused by hyperinsulinism (*e.g.,* islet cell carcinoma); available in *oral* form as Proglycem—see Chapter 42

Dosage

1 mg/kg to 3 mg/kg (maximum 150 mg) by IV push within 30 seconds or less; repeat at intervals of 5 minutes to 15 minutes until a satisfactory response is attained, then at 4-hour to 24-hour intervals until a regimen of oral antihypertensive drug becomes effective

Fate

Onset usually within 1 minute to 2 minutes, with maximal blood pressure decrease in 5 minutes; duration is 2 hours to 12 hours; extensively bound to serum proteins (90%); excreted slowly through the kidney

Common Side-Effects

(Usually seen with repeated injections) Sodium and water retention, hyperglycemia

Significant Adverse Reactions

Cardiovascular—hypotension, dizziness, myocardial and cerebral ischemia, palpitations, arrhythmias, sweating, flushing, supraventricular tachycardia

CNS—(secondary to blood flow changes in the brain) confusion, headache, lightheadedness, somnolence, hearing impairment, euphoria, convulsions, paralysis

GI—abdominal pain, nausea, vomiting, anorexia, parotid swelling, salivation, dry mouth, constipation or diarrhea, ileus

Dermatologic/hypersensitivity—rash, fever, leukopenia

Respiratory—cough, dyspnea, choking sensation

Other—pancreatitis, weakness, lacrimation, cellulitis, pain along injected vein, back pain, nocturia, hyperuricemia

Contraindications

Hypersensitivity to thiazide diuretics, coronary artery disease, compensatory hypertension (*e.g.,* aortic coarctation, arteriovenous shunt), and dissecting aortic aneurysm

Interactions

1 Combined use of diuretics with diazoxide may intensify its hyperglycemic, hyperuricemic, and antihypertensive effects.
2 Diazoxide may potentiate the action of other highly protein-bound drugs (*e.g.,* oral anticoagulants, anti-inflammatory agents, sulfonamides, phenytoin, quinidine, propranolol) by displacing them from binding sites.
3 Chlorpromazine and furosemide may potentiate the hyperglycemic effect of diazoxide.
4 An increased hypotensive response can occur when diazoxide is used along with other antihypertensive drugs such as vasodilators (*e.g.,* nitrites, hydralazine), catecholamine-depleting drugs (*e.g.,* reserpine), beta-blockers, or centrally acting agents.

▶ **NURSING ALERTS**

▷ 1 Be alert for development of marked hypotension when drug is administered. Have vasopressors (*e.g.,* metaraminol) on hand to treat extreme blood pressure reductions.

▷ 2 Administer carefully to, and monitor closely, patients with edema, diabetes, impaired cerebral or cardiac circulation, renal dysfunction, or history of gout; use cautiously in pregnant or nursing mothers and children.

▷ 3 With repeated injections, observe patient for signs of developing congestive heart failure (cough, dyspnea, edema, distended neck veins, rales), and renal or bowel dysfunction (urinary hesitancy, decreased urine output, constipation, abdominal distention). Advise physician.

▷ 4 Administer only in a peripheral vein, and avoid extravasation because solution is alkaline and very irritating. Never inject SC.

▶ **NURSING CONSIDERATIONS**

▷ 1 Perform blood glucose and electrolyte determinations at start of therapy, and then frequently during repeated dosing.

▷ 2 Keep patient recumbent during injection and for at least 30 minutes after injection. Monitor blood pressure closely until stabilized, then hourly thereafter during expected duration of effect. Check blood pressure with patient in upright position before ending surveillance.

▷ 3 Be aware that smaller than recommended doses can be given by IV injection with less danger of sharp pressure drop. IV infusion may be effective if patient is receiving other antihypertensive drugs concurrently.

▷ 4 Note that concomitant use of a diuretic will prevent sodium and water retention elicited by diazoxide, and will also increase the antihypertensive effect. When diuretics are used, keep patient supine for 8 hours to 10 hours because of added hypotensive effect.

▷ 5 Consider use of a beta-blocker (*e.g.,* propranolol) if the reflex tachycardia and increased cardiac output become clinically significant.

▷ 6 Be aware that diazoxide-induced hyperglycemia is usually transient, reversible, and clinically insignificant in most nondiabetic patients; however, dosage adjustments of antidiabetic drugs may be necessary in the diabetic patient.

▶ guanadrel
Hylorel

▶ guanethidine
Ismelin

Guanadrel and guanethidine are two antihypertensive drugs that impair sympathetic nerve functioning by inhibiting norepinephrine release from nerve endings. However, in spite of their similar pharmacologic profile, guanadrel is recommended for step-2 therapy, whereas guanethidine is usually reserved for step-4 treatment of severe hypertension.

Mechanism
Accumulate in peripheral adrenergic nerve endings, and interfere with release of norepinephrine from these nerve endings; also deplete intraneuronal stores of norepinephrine, resulting in a prolonged decrease in heart rate and peripheral vascular resistance and decreased venous return; may also reduce plasma renin activity and inhibit cardiovascular reflexes; elicit a high incidence of orthostatic hypotension, and fluid retention frequently occurs

Uses
1 Treatment of moderate to severe hypertension not adequately controlled by other antihypertensive agents (guanethidine)
2 Treatment of mild to moderate hypertension in patients not adequately responding to a diuretic (guanadrel)

Dosage

Guanadrel
Initially 10 mg/day: increase gradually until optimal effect is seen; usual dosage range is 20 mg to 75 mg in twice daily doses

Guanethidine
Ambulatory patients: initially 10 mg/day; increase gradually every 5 to 7 days to achieve optimal response; usual dose is 25 mg to 50 mg/day in a single dose
Hospitalized patients: initially 10 mg to 50 mg, depending on other antihypertensive drugs being used; increase by 10 mg to 25 mg every 2 to 4 days until desired response is obtained

Fate
Guanethidine is poorly but consistently absorbed orally; peak effect occurs within 8 hours of a single dose; half-life is 5 days, so drug accumulates slowly; partially metabolized by the liver, and excreted as active drug and inactive metabolites primarily by the kidney; guanadrel is rapidly absorbed orally and attains peak plasma concentration in 1.5 hours to 2 hours; effects are noted within 2 hours and maximal blood pressure decreases occur within 4 hours to 6 hours; excreted primarily in the urine, approximately 40% as unchanged drug

Common Side-Effects
Fatigue, headache, faintness, drowsiness, nocturia, urinary urgency, increased bowel movements, diarrhea, shortness of breath on exertion, palpitations, bradycardia, fluid retention, and ejaculation disturbances

Significant Adverse Reactions
Nausea, vomiting, paresthesias, incontinence, dermatitis, anorexia, constipation, leg cramps, hair loss, nasal congestion, blurred vision, asthma, chest pains, myalgia, tremor, depression, and cardiac irregularities

Contraindications
Pheochromocytoma, congestive heart failure not caused by hypertension, and concurrent use with MAO inhibitors

Interactions
1 The antihypertensive effects of guanethidine and guanadrel may be antagonized by amphetamines, antidepressants, antihistamines, antipsychotics (*e.g.,* phenothiazines, thioxanthenes, haloperidol), cocaine, diethylpropion, ephedrine, MAO inhibitors, methylphenidate, oral contraceptives, and sympathomimetic agents.
2 Enhanced hypotensive effects may be observed when guanethidine or guanadrel is given in combination with alcohol, diuretics, hydralazine, levodopa, methotrimeprazine, propranolol, quinidine, reserpine, and vasodilator drugs.
3 Excessive bradycardia can occur if guanethidine or guanadrel is used in combination with digitalis drugs.
4 Guanethidine or guanadrel may impair the hyposecretory effect of anticholinergics.
5 Guanethidine or guanadrel may exert an additive hypoglycemic effect with insulin or oral antidiabetic drugs.
6 Increased responses to adrenergic agents (*e.g.,* catecholamines, phenylephrine, metaraminol) may occur with guanethidine or guanadrel.

▶ NURSING ALERTS
▷ 1 Caution patient to sit or lie down immediately upon onset of dizziness or weakness. Orthostatic hypotension is most common upon arising, and is accentuated by alcohol, hot weather, exercise, or prolonged standing. Advise patient to change positions gradually, and inform physician if episodes of faintness persist.

▷ 2 Inform physician of development of persistent diarrhea

or sudden weight gain or edema. Dosage adjustment or additional medication may be required.

▷ 3 Use cautiously in patients with fever, bronchial asthma, renal disease, coronary insufficiency, recent myocardial infarction, cerebral vascular disease, congestive heart failure, colitis, peptic ulcer, and during pregnancy.

▷ 4 Be aware that hypotensive effect is greater in upright *versus* supine position. Monitor pressure both ways during period of dosage adjustment. Caution patients not to arise from bed without assistance during period of dosage titration because dizziness and syncope are common.

▷ 5 Inform patients that use of over-the-counter products (*e.g.,* cough or cold remedies, allergy medications, nasal sprays) containing sympathomimetic ingredients can result in a hypertensive reaction in the presence of guanethidine or guanadrel. Suggest that patient consult physician or pharmacist before taking any additional medication.

▶ **NURSING CONSIDERATIONS**

▷ 1 Caution patient against discontinuing medication unless directed by the physician. Stress the importance of adjunctive measures (*e.g.,* weight control, salt restriction, reduction of stress, limiting of caffeine) to the total therapeutic regimen.

▷ 2 Recognize that these drugs have a prolonged duration of action. Make dosage adjustments carefully and allow sufficient time between dosage changes (*e.g.,* 3–5 days) for effects to become manifest.

▷ 3 Note that a diuretic is often given concurrently to minimize sodium and water retention as well as to enhance the hypotensive response.

▷ 4 Monitor patients on antidiabetic medication carefully, because guanethidine or guanadrel may have additive hypoglycemic effects.

▷ 5 If possible, withdraw drugs 48 hours to 72 hours before use of general anesthetics to reduce the possibility of vascular collapse and cardiac arrest. Have oxygen, vasopressors, volume expanders, and other necessary resuscitative equipment on hand.

▷ 6 Recommend that patients on prolonged therapy have periodic blood counts and liver and kidney function tests, and that they be alert for development of adverse reactions such as edema, urinary hesitancy or retention, weakness, and bradycardia, and that they promptly report these effects.

▷ *Dietary precautions*

▷ 1 Urge moderation in the use of salt-containing foods and in ingestion of caffeine-containing beverages.

▷ 2 Warn patients that alcohol may intensify the hypotensive reaction.

▶ **hydralazine**

Apresoline

Mechanism

Direct relaxation of vascular smooth muscle, primarily arteriolar, leading to decreased peripheral resistance; little

effect on venous capacitance vessels; diastolic pressure is usually lowered more than systolic; no change or possibly an increase in renal and cerebral blood flow; reflex increase in heart rate, stroke volume, and cardiac output

Uses

1 Management of moderate forms of hypertension, sometimes alone but more commonly in combination with other antihypertensive medications

2 Short-term treatment of severe essential hypertension (IV or IM)

Dosage

Oral: initially 10 mg 4 times/day for 2 to 4 days; increase to 25 mg 4 times/day for balance of week; for second and subsequent weeks, increase to 50 mg 4 times/day; adjust to lowest effective levels for maintenance; twice daily dosage may be adequate

IM, IV: 20 mg to 40 mg repeated as necessary

Fate

Well absorbed orally; peak plasma levels in 1 hour to 2 hours; half-life is 2 hours to 6 hours; effects last for at least 6 hours; highly protein bound (85%–90%); onset following IM injection is 10 minutes to 15 minutes and duration lasts 3 hours to 4 hours; IV administration results in immediate onset, with maximal response in 1 hour; metabolized by the liver and rapidly excreted, largely in the feces

Common Side-Effects

Headache, nausea, vomiting, diarrhea, sweating, palpitations, and tachycardia

Significant Adverse Reactions

Paresthesias, numbness and tingling in extremities, anginal pain, tremors, disorientation, anxiety, depression, flushing, lacrimation, conjunctivitis, urticaria, pruritus, fever, chills, nasal congestion, muscle cramping, arthralgia, eosinophilia, constipation, difficulty in micturition, dyspnea, and paralytic ileus

Reduced hemoglobin, leukopenia, agranulocytosis, and purpura

Systemic lupus-like syndrome (high doses) marked by fever, dermatoses, myalgia, arthralgia, anemia, splenomegaly, edema, and lymphadenopathy

Contraindications

Rheumatic heart disease, coronary artery disease, and systemic lupus erythematosus

Interactions

1 Hypotensive action of hydralazine can be antagonized by amphetamines, ephedrine, and other sympathomimetic agents, and the incidence of tachycardia and anginal pain increased.

2 Additive hypotensive effects can occur with combined use of hydralazine and anesthetics, antidepressants, other antihypertensives, diuretics, quinidine, and procainamide

▶ **NURSING ALERTS**

▷ 1 Observe patients receiving large amounts of hydralazine very closely for signs of developing lupus-like reaction (*e.g.,* fever, myalgia, dermatoses, arthralgia, anemia, skin lesions); discontinue drug, and use alternate antihypertensive medication if signs develop. Do not exceed 400 mg/day. Most symptoms regress when drug is withdrawn, but residual effects may persist for years.

▷ 2 During prolonged hydralazine therapy, perform periodic blood counts, LE (*i.e.,* lupus erythematosus) cell preparations, and antinuclear antibody titer determinations.

▷ 3 Advise patients to make positional changes slowly, because orthostatic hypotension can occur, resulting in dizziness and fainting. Urge caution in operating machinery.

▷ 4 Use cautiously in patients with renal impairment, ischemic heart disease, cerebrovascular accidents, and in pregnant women.

▶ **NURSING CONSIDERATIONS**

▷ 1 Observe for changes in patient's mental acuity because this may indicate cerebral ischemia. Notify physician should these occur.

▷ 2 Advise patient that headache and palpitations may occur during early stages of therapy, but generally disappear.

▷ 3 Note that a beta-blocker (*e.g.,* propranolol) is commonly used with hydralazine to prevent reflex tachycardia and increased cardiac output.

▷ 4 Withdraw drug slowly to avoid a possible sudden rise in blood pressure.

▷ 5 If signs of hydralazine-induced peripheral neuritis occur (paresthesias, numbness, tingling), consider use of pyridoxine (vitamin B_6) to alleviate these symptoms.

▷ 6 Suggest that drug be taken with meals because bioavailability has been reported to be *enhanced* by concurrent ingestion of food, which may decrease first-pass hepatic metabolism.

▷ 7 Check for edema, and monitor intake and output, especially when drug is used parenterally and in patients with renal dysfunction. Advise patient to report any changes in urinary pattern or body weight.

▷ 8 During hydralazine therapy, caution patients against use of over-the-counter medications containing sympathomimetic agents without consulting physician.

▷ 9 Note that hydralazine is available in three strengths in fixed combination with hydrochlorothiazide as Apresazide and Hydral.

▶ **mecamylamine**

Inversine

Mecamylamine is an orally effective ganglionic blocking agent very infrequently used to manage moderate to severe hypertension. It is discussed in Chapter 13.

Dosage

Initially 2.5 mg twice a day; increase by 2.5 mg every 2 days until desired response is attained; average dose is 25 mg/day in 2 to 4 divided doses; usually given after meals, with the larger fraction of the dose administered later in the day

▶ **methyldopa**

Aldomet

Mechanism

Inhibits the enzyme aromatic-amino-acid-decarboxylase by competitive antagonism, and is itself converted to alpha-methyl norepinephrine, which functions as an activator of central alpha-2 adrenergic receptors. Stimulation of brain stem alpha receptors results in a decreased outflow of sympathetic vasoconstrictor and cardio-accelerator impulses, thereby producing vasodilation and bradycardia; may reduce plasma renin activity, but does not significantly affect renal blood flow; cardiac output is usually decreased; diurnal blood pressure variations occur rarely; has a sedative action, and promotes sodium and water retention

Uses

1 Treatment of sustained moderate to severe hypertension, either alone or more commonly with other antihypertensive agents

2 Treatment of acute hypertensive crises (methyldop*ate* ester, IV); infrequently used due to slow onset of action

Dosage

Oral

Adults—Initially 250 mg 2 to 3 times/day; adjust dosage by increments at intervals of not less than 2 days until desired response occurs; usual maintenance dosage 500 mg to 2000 mg/day in 2 to 4 divided doses (maximum 3 g/day)

Children—10 mg/kg/day in 2 to 4 divided doses adjusted to desired level; maximum dose 65 mg/kg or 3 g daily.

IV infusion

Adults—250 mg to 500 mg at 6-hour intervals (dose is added to 100 ml 5% Dextrose Injection and infused over 30 min to 60 min); maximum dose 1 g every 6 hours

Children—20 mg to 40 mg/kg in divided doses every 6 hours; maximum dose 3 g/day

Fate

Oral absorption is variable (average 50%); peak effect occurs in 4 hours to 6 hours; duration may persist for 24 hours even though elimination half-life is 2 hours to 3 hours; following IV infusion, maximal effects are seen in 4 hours to 8 hours and last 12 hours to 16 hours; appears rapidly in the urine, predominately in unaltered form

Common Side-Effects

Sedation, headache, weakness, dry mouth, weight gain, and positive direct Coombs' test

Significant Adverse Reactions

Cardiovascular—bradycardia, anginal pain, orthostatic hypotension, edema, myocarditis, paradoxical pressor response with IV use

CNS—dizziness, paresthesias, parkinsonian-like symptoms, choreo-athetoid movements, psychoses, depression, nightmares, memory impairment

GI—nausea, vomiting, constipation, "black" tongue, abdominal distention, pancreatitis, sialadenitis

Hematologic—hemolytic anemia, leukopenia, thrombocytopenia, granulocytopenia

Hepatic—jaundice, liver dysfunction

Other—fever, myalgia, arthralgia, dermatoses, rash, nasal congestion, breast enlargement, gynecomastia, lactation, impotence, decreased libido

Laboratory test variations—abnormal liver function tests; positive tests for antinuclear antibody, LE (*i.e.*, lupus erythematosus) cells, and rheumatoid factor; rise in BUN; falsely high urinary catecholamines

Contraindications

Active hepatic disease, pheochromocytoma, and blood dyscrasias

Interactions

1 Additive hypotensive effects can occur with methyldopa and anesthetics, alcohol, diuretics and other antihypertensive drugs, narcotics, methotrimeprazine, levodopa, quinidine, and vasodilators.
2 Hypotensive action of methyldopa can be antagonized by amphetamines, catecholamines (except levodopa), tricyclic antidepressants, MAO inhibitors, phenothiazines, sympathomimetics, and vasopressors.
3 Methyldopa can potentiate the hypoglycemic action of tolbutamide.
4 Elevated serum lithium levels can occur with methyldopa.
5 Psychiatric disturbances can result from combined use of methyldopa and haloperidol.
6 Phenoxybenzamine and methyldopa together have resulted in reversible urinary incontinence.

▶ NURSING ALERTS

▷ 1 Be aware that a positive Coombs' test, as well as hemolytic anemia and liver disorders, can occur with methyldopa therapy, potentially leading to fatal complications. A positive Coombs' test is observed in approximately 20% of patients on chronic therapy, is dose-dependent, and may persist for 3 months to 18 months after drug is withdrawn. In most cases, it is *not* clinically significant in the absence of other complications (*e.g.*, anemia, hepatitis). A positive Coombs' test may not revert to normal until weeks or months after therapy is stopped.
▷ 2 Perform a complete blood count and direct Coombs' test prior to initiating therapy and periodically during drug treatment. If positive Coombs' test develops, determine whether hemolytic anemia exists. Positive direct Coombs' test is not in itself an indication for stopping therapy; however, if Coombs'-positive hemolytic anemia occurs or if non-dose-dependent drug fever or hepatitis is noted, discontinue drug immediately.
▷ 3 Reversible methyldopa hepatotoxicity can occasionally occur, especially during first few months of therapy.

Be alert for development of fever, chills, headache, pruritus, rash, arthralgia, and enlarged liver; if present, perform liver function tests. If fever, jaundice, or liver function abnormalities appear, discontinue drug.
▷ 4 Warn patients that drowsiness and sedation are common during initial stages of therapy or periods of dosage adjustment. Urge caution in operating machinery or performing other tasks requiring mental alertness.
▷ 5 Use cautiously in patients with impaired liver function, angina, and in pregnant or nursing mothers.
▷ 6 Be alert for development of paradoxical pressor response with IV use of methyldopate ester.
▷ 7 During IV administration, check blood pressure repeatedly until stabilized, and monitor urinary output.

▶ NURSING CONSIDERATIONS

▷ 1 Watch for appearance of involuntary movements and advise physician. If these occur, drug should be discontinued.
▷ 2 Inform patients (particularly the elderly or those with renal dysfunction) that orthostatic hypotension can occur (although less frequently than with most other antihypertensive drugs) and that dizziness and lightheadedness may ensue. Advise slow positional changes and prolonged standing in one position.
▷ 3 During period of dosage adjustments, take blood pressure of patient in upright and supine positions.
▷ 4 Inform patient that methyldopa may darken urine because of a breakdown product. This effect is not harmful.
▷ 5 Consider adding a diuretic to methyldopa (combination available as Aldoril) to reduce sodium and water retention and enhance blood pressure lowering effect.

▶ metoprolol
Lopressor

Metoprolol is a beta-adrenergic blocking agent with a preferential, although not exclusive, effect on beta-1 receptors in cardiac muscle. In equivalent doses, it has much less effect on bronchiolar and vascular beta responses than does propranolol. Its antihypertensive action is not completely established, but probably involves reduced outflow of central sympathetic impulses, suppression of renin activity, and possibly reduced cardiac output. Refer to the discussion on beta-blockers in Chapter 12 for a complete review of metoprolol as well as propranolol, which shares many of the same properties as metoprolol.

Dosage

Initially 100 mg/day in a single dose or 2 divided doses; increase at weekly intervals until optimal blood pressure reduction is attained; usual maintenance range is 100 mg to 450 mg/day; once daily administration may not provide 24-hour control, especially with lower doses; larger or more frequent doses may be necessary

▶ metyrosine
Demser

Mechanism

Inhibits tyrosine hydroxylase, the enzyme that catalyzes the conversion of tyrosine to DOPA, which is the initial reaction in the biosynthesis of the catecholamines dopamine, norepinephrine, and epinephrine. Therefore, catecholamine production is reduced.

Uses

1. Symptomatic treatment of patients with pheochromocytoma (a tumor of the sympathetic nervous system, usually of the adrenal medulla)
   a. Preoperative preparation
   b. Management of patients when surgery is contraindicated
   c. Chronic therapy of malignant pheochromocytoma

Dosage

Initially 250 mg 4 times/day; increase by 250 mg to 500 mg every day as needed to a maximum of 4 g/day in divided doses

Common Side-Effects

Sedation; extrapyramidal symptoms (drooling, fine tremor, speech difficulties); and diarrhea

Significant Adverse Reactions

Anxiety, depression, hallucinations, confusion, headache, nasal congestion, decreased salivation, vomiting, dry mouth, abdominal pain, impotence, galactorrhea, breast swelling, crystalluria, dysuria, hematuria, hypersensitivity reactions (urticaria, rash, pharyngeal edema)

Interactions

1 Extrapyramidal effects may be intensified by concurrent use of phenothiazines or other antipsychotic drugs.
2 Metyrosine may have additive effects with alcohol or other CNS depressants.

▶ NURSING ALERTS

▷ 1 Ensure that adequate intravascular fluid volume is maintained postoperatively in patients receiving metyrosine, to avoid hypotension and reduced perfusion of vital organs.
▷ 2 Continually monitor blood pressure and ECG during surgery because arrhythmias can occur. Be prepared with lidocaine and a beta-adrenergic blocking agent.
▷ 3 Use cautiously in patients with impaired renal or hepatic function, and in pregnant or nursing women.
▷ 4 Advise physician at first sign of drooling, speech difficulty, fine tremors, diarrhea, disorientation, or jaw stiffness.

▶ NURSING CONSIDERATIONS

▷ 1 Urge patients to maintain water intake sufficient to achieve a daily urine volume of 2000 ml or more to minimize the danger of the drug crystallizing in the urine.

▷ 2 Be aware that the drug can interfere with urinary catecholamine measurements.
▷ 3 If patient is not adequately controlled with metyrosine, consider adding an alpha-adrenergic blocking drug to the regimen.

▶ minoxidil

Loniten

Mechanism

Direct relaxation of vascular smooth muscle possibly due to blockade of calcium uptake *via* the cell membrane, thus decreasing peripheral vascular resistance; microcirculatory blood flow is maintained in all systemic vascular beds; does not enter CNS or interfere with vasomotor reflexes; therefore, does not elicit orthostatic hypotension; reflexly increases heart rate and cardiac output, renin secretion, and salt and water retention

Uses

1 Treatment of severe hypertension not manageable by maximum doses of a diuretic plus two other antihypertensive drugs; usually given together with a diuretic or a beta-blocker, or both. Methyldopa and clonidine have also been used concurrently.

Dosage

Adults: initially 5 mg/day as a single dose; increase stepwise to 40 mg/day in divided doses, or until optimal control is attained; usual range is 10 mg to 40 mg/day (maximum is 100 mg/day)
Children (under 12): initially, 0.2 mg/kg/day as a single dose; increase in 50% to 100% increments until optimal control is attained; usual range is 0.25 mg/kg to 1.0 mg/kg/day (maximum is 50 mg/day)

Fate

Well absorbed from the GI tract; maximum plasma levels occur within 60 minutes; half-life is approximately 4 hours; almost completely metabolized in the liver, and excreted principally in the urine; does not bind to plasma proteins

Common Side-Effects

Hypertrichosis (elongation, thickening, and enhanced pigmentation of fine body hair—80% of patients within 3 wk–6 wk), temporary edema, ECG (*i.e.*, T-wave) changes not associated with other symptoms

Significant Adverse Reactions

Warning: Use only in severe hypertension because serious adverse reactions have occurred. Pericardial effusion, occasionally progressing to tamponade, has been reported, and anginal symptoms may be exacerbated.

Nausea; vomiting; fatigue; headache; pericardial effusion; tamponade; reflex tachycardia; breast tenderness; temporary decreases in hemoglobin, hematocrit, and erythrocytes; increases in alkaline phosphatase and serum creatinine; hypersensitivity reactions

Contraindications
Pheochromocytoma

Interactions
1 Minoxidil may markedly worsen the degree of orthostatic hypotension caused by guanethidine.

▶ NURSING ALERTS
▷ 1 Administer only under close supervision to patients with severe hypertension who have not responded to a diuretic plus two other antihypertensive drugs, and closely monitor these patients for development of adverse reactions.
▷ 2 Give concomitantly with a diuretic to reduce salt and fluid retention, and with a beta-blocker to prevent reflux tachycardia.
▷ 3 When drug is used in patients already receiving guanethidine, hospitalize the patient and continually monitor blood pressure following minoxidil administration, to detect a too-large or a too-rapid drop in blood pressure.
▷ 4 Observe patients closely for any suggestion of a pericardial disorder and perform echocardiographic studies if such a disorder is suspected. Pericardial effusion occurs in about 3% of treated patients not on dialysis, especially those with reduced renal function.
▷ 5 Use with caution in patients with any cardiac disease, renal or hepatic insufficiency, and in pregnant or nursing mothers and small children.

▶ NURSING CONSIDERATIONS
▷ 1 Monitor fluid and electrolyte balance, intake–output ratio, and body weight.
▷ 2 Allow at least 3 days between dosage adjustments to permit the full response to a given dose to become manifest.
▷ 3 Stress the importance of taking other antihypertensive medications (*i.e.,* diuretics, beta-blockers) exactly as prescribed along with minoxidil to increase the drug's effectiveness and to reduce untoward reactions. Do not discontinue any other drugs without consulting physician.
▷ 4 Inform patients that increased growth and darkening of fine body hair will probably occur within 3 weeks to 6 weeks (80% incidence with minoxidil). While bothersome, it is not associated with hormonal changes and is probably not dangerous. It is first noticeable in the area of the temple, eyebrows, and sideburns, later extending to the back, arms, and legs. Condition will regress and eventually disappear within 2 months to 6 months after cessation of treatment.
▷ 5 Be alert for increased pulse rates (20 or more beats per minute over normal), rapid weight gain or swelling in the extremities, dyspnea, and dizziness or chest

pain, and inform physician. Dosage adjustment is then indicated.

▶ nadolol
Corgard

Nadolol is a nonselective beta-adrenergic blocking agent resembling propranolol in most respects. It possesses a relatively long half-life (20 hr–24 hr), so it is effective in once daily dosing. Nadolol exhibits little direct myocardial depressant activity, and unlike propranolol, it does not display an anesthetic-like membrane stabilizing action. Consult the discussion on beta-blockers in Chapter 12 for additional information concerning the pharmacology and toxicology of nadolol.

Dosage
Initially, 40 mg once daily; increase gradually in 40-mg to 80-mg increments until optimal effect is noted; usual maintenance range is 80 mg to 320 mg/day in a single dose; also available in fixed combination with bendroflumethiazide (5 mg) as Corzide.

▶ nitroprusside
Nipride, Nitropress

Mechanism
Direct relaxation of arteriolar and venular smooth muscle, resulting in marked reduction of arterial pressure, slight reflex increase in heart rate, and a small decrease in cardiac output; renin activity is markedly increased. In patients with left ventricular failure, there is an increase in cardiac output, a decrease in ventricular filling pressure, a reduction of pulmonary wedge pressure, and no significant effect on heart rate.

Uses
1 Emergency treatment of hypertensive crises
2 Production of controlled hypotension during surgery or anesthesia
3 Investigational uses include adjunctive therapy of severe, refractory congestive heart failure, treatment of lactic acidosis due to reduced peripheral perfusion, and attenuation of the vasoconstrictor effects of norepinephrine and dopamine.

Dosage
Adults and Children: used only by IV infusion; 3 mcg/kg/minute (range 0.5 mcg/kg–10 mcg/kg/min) of a 50 mg in 250 ml to 1000 ml of 5% Dextrose in Water dilution.

Fate
Onset of effect is almost immediate, and duration lasts only as long as infusion is maintained; nitroprusside is rapidly metabolized to cyanmethemoglobin and also to free cyanide ion, which in turn is converted to thiocyanate in the liver. Thiocyanate is readily excreted by patients with normal renal

function. Blood pressure reaches its pretreatment level in 2 minutes to 10 minutes after infusion is terminated.

Common Side-Effects

(Usually result of too-rapid infusion) Nausea, sweating, headache, restlessness, muscle twitching, palpitations, dizziness, substernal discomfort

Significant Adverse Reactions

(Usually due to thiocyanate accumulation, especially in patients with impaired renal function) Blurred vision, hypothyroidism, delirium, and convulsions

Contraindications

Compensatory hypertension (arteriovenous shunt, aortic coarctation), and inadequate cerebral circulation

Interactions

1 Enhanced hypotension can occur if nitroprusside is given to patients receiving other antihypertensive medications, circulatory depressants, and volatile liquid anesthetics.
2 Tolbutamide may decrease the effects of nitroprusside.

▶ NURSING ALERTS

▷ 1 Use *only* by slow IV infusion. Determine blood pressure frequently, and adjust rate of flow to produce desired response. Do not allow systolic pressure to go below 70 mm Hg.

▷ 2 Use cautiously in patients with hepatic insufficiency, renal impairment, hypothyroidism, and in elderly, debilitated, and poor-risk surgical patients.

▷ 3 Note that nitroprusside is metabolized to cyanide, then to thiocyanate. If treatment is continued longer than 2 to 3 days, determine thiocyanate blood levels and discontinue drug if levels exceed 10 mg/100 ml. Have sodium nitrite and sodium thiosulfate injections on hand to treat cyanide intoxication in cases of overdosage. Inject 2.5 ml to 5 ml/minute of 3% sodium nitrite to a total of 15 ml, then give sodium thiosulfate, 12.5 g/50 ml of 5% Dextrose over 10 minutes by IV infusion. Repeat at one half above doses if signs of overdose reappear.

▶ NURSING CONSIDERATIONS

▷ 1 Do not exceed 10 mcg/kg/minute as infusion rate. If pressure is not reduced within 10 minutes at this dose, discontinue drug. Reduce dose in patients already receiving antihypertensive medication.

▷ 2 When using drug for controlled hypotension during surgery, correct any pre-existing anemia or hypovolemia prior to administering nitroprusside.

▷ 3 Note that freshly prepared solutions have a faint brownish tinge. Discard any solution that is strongly colored, and use solutions within 4 hours after preparation. Cover infusion container with opaque material to exclude light, which can increase rate of decomposition to cyanide ion.

▷ 4 Observe infusion site for signs of extravasation (*e.g.,*

swelling, pain) because irritation may occur; readjust infusion as necessary.

▷ 5 Change patient to oral antihypertensive medication as soon as possible. Oral drug may be started while pressure is being brought under control by nitroprusside.

▷ 6 Do not add other drugs or preservatives to infusion solution.

▶ pargyline
Eutonyl

Mechanism

Antihypertensive mechanism is largely unknown; drug is an MAO inhibitor (see Chap. 24), and its hypotensive action is predominantly orthostatic in nature; may form a ''false neurotransmitter'' in adrenergic nerve endings, and may elevate central catecholamine levels, interfering with sympathetic venoconstriction; may also modify ganglionic transmission; often effective at reduced dosage when used with a thiazide diuretic (see Dosage)

Uses

1 Treatment of moderate to severe essential hypertension, usually in combination with other antihypertensive drugs (infrequently used)

Dosage

Initially, 25 mg daily in single dose; increase by 10 mg/week until desired response; Maximum dose 200 mg/day
Added to antihypertensive regimen (e.g., thiazide diuretic)—initially 10 mg to 25 mg/day; usual maintenance range is 50 mg to 75 mg/day

Fate

Onset of action in 3 to 4 days; maximum response occurs within 2 weeks to 3 weeks; effects persist for several weeks after drug is withdrawn; excreted primarily unchanged by the kidney

Common Side-Effects

Dry mouth, insomnia, nervousness, fluid retention and weight gain, orthostatic hypotension (weakness, palpitations, dizziness, syncope), impotence, mild constipation, sweating, headache, muscle twitching, blurred vision, and rash

Significant Adverse Reactions

Extrapyramidal symptoms, nightmares, hypoglycemia, arthralgia, and congestive heart failure; in addition, see Chapter 24

Contraindications

Mild or labile hypertension or that controlled by other antihypertensive drugs, malignant hypertension, children under 12, pheochromocytoma, schizophrenia, hyperthyroidism, renal failure, pregnancy, acute febrile episodes, hyperactive or hyperexcitable patients, parkinsonism

Interactions

See Chapter 24.

▶ **NURSING ALERTS**

See Chapter 24. In addition:

▷ 1 Do not combine pargyline with methyldopa or guanethidine because severe CNS stimulation and hypertension can occur.

▶ **NURSING CONSIDERATIONS**

See Chapter 24. In addition:

▷ 1 Monitor blood pressure of patient in the standing position to determine need for dosage adjustments, because drug exerts a strong orthostatic effect.

▷ 2 Instruct patients to notify physician immediately if faintness, dizziness, palpitation, or weakness occur; dosage adjustment is indicated to alleviate orthostatic hypotension

▷ 3 Recognize that pargyline should only be employed where all other less toxic antihypertensive agents have proven ineffective or intolerable. Closely observe patients on pargyline therapy because risk of severe untoward reactions is considerable.

▶ **phenoxybenzamine**

Dibenzyline

An orally effective, long-acting alpha-adrenergic blocking agent indicated for the control of episodes of hypertension and sweating associated with pheochromocytoma. Phenoxybenzamine produces a "chemical sympathectomy," interrupting impulse transmission through alpha-adrenergic receptor sites, which results in reduced blood pressure and increased blood flow to the skin, mucosa, and abdominal organs. In addition to its use in pheochromocytoma, it is also rated "possibly effective" for symptomatic treatment of vasospastic peripheral vascular disease. Phenoxybenzamine is discussed in detail in Chapter 12.

Dosage

Initially 10 mg/day; increase by 10 mg every 4 days until desired response is achieved; usual dosage range is 20 mg to 60 mg/day.

Note: At last 2 weeks are generally required to attain significant improvement, and possibly several more weeks are required for full benefits.

▶ **pindolol**

Visken

Pindolol is an orally effective, nonselective beta-adrenergic blocker indicated for the management of mild to moderate hypertension. The drug also exhibits a partial agonistic activity at beta receptor sites, and thus possesses intrinsic sympathomimetic activity (ISA) in addition to its beta-blocking activity. ISA is manifested as a smaller reduction in resting heart rate and cardiac output than that observed with the other beta-blockers; however, the clinical significance of this action is probably minimal. Pindolol is reviewed together with the other beta-blockers in Chapter 12.

Dosage

Initially 10 mg twice a day (or 5 mg 3 times/day), alone or in combination with other antihypertensive drugs; adjust dose in increments of 10 mg/day at 2-week to 3-week intervals until optimal response is reached; maximum dose 60 mg/day

▶ **phentolamine**

Regitine

Phentolamine is an alpha-adrenergic blocking agent that can be used orally or parenterally, mainly for the diagnosis and control of symptoms of pheochromocytoma, and to prevent necrosis and sloughing following extravasation of solutions of norepinephrine. It is more rapid acting and shorter acting than phenoxybenzamine, and it exerts a direct relaxing effect on vascular smooth muscle in addition to its alpha-blocking activity. Phentolamine is likewise reviewed in Chapter 12.

Dosage

Oral

Adults—50 mg 4 to 6 times/day
Children—25 mg 4 to 6 times/day

Parenteral:

Hypertension—IV, IM, 5 mg (adults); 1 mg (children)
Necrosis/sloughing—10 mg/liter of IV infusion solution, or 5 mg to 10 mg/10 ml saline injected into area of extravasation

▶ **prazosin**

Minipress

Mechanism

Selectively blocks postsynaptic alpha-1 receptor sites; may also have a direct relaxant effect on vascular smooth muscle; dilates both resistance (*i.e.,* arterioles) and capacitance (*i.e.,* veins) vessels; therefore, little change in cardiac output, heart rate, renal blood flow, or glomerular filtration rate; blood pressure is lowered in both supine and standing positions, and effects are most pronounced on the diastolic pressure; reduces venous return (preload) and aortic impedance to left ventricular ejection (afterload)

Uses

1 Treatment of mild to moderate hypertension, either alone or with a diuretic or other antihypertensive agent
2 Adjunctive treatment of severe, refractive congestive heart failure

Dosage

Initially 1 mg 2 to 3 times/day; increase slowly to optimal response, up to 20 mg/day; usual maintenance range is 6 mg to 15 mg/day in 2 or 3 divided doses

Fate

Rapidly and completely absorbed orally; peak plasma concentrations are attained in 2 hours to 3 hours; extensively bound (95–98%) to plasma proteins; plasma half-life is 2 hours to 3 hours, but effects last considerably longer; metabolized in the liver, and excreted mainly (90%–95%) in the bile and feces

Common Side-Effects

Dizziness, headache, malaise, drowsiness, weakness, palpitations, and nausea

Significant Adverse Reactions

(Causal relationships not established in all cases)

GI—vomiting, constipation, abdominal pain

Cardiovascular—tachycardia, angina, syncope, edema, orthostatic hypotension

CNS—nervousness, paresthesias, vertigo, depression

Other—urinary frequency or incontinence, impotence, rash, pruritus, dyspnea, blurred vision, tinnitus, dry mouth, nasal congestion, epistaxis, diaphoresis, arthralgia, leukopenia, drug-induced lupus-like syndrome (rare)

Interactions

1 Enhanced hypotensive effects can occur in combination with other antihypertensive drugs, especially propranolol.
2 Effects of prazosin may be potentiated by other highly protein-bound drugs.

▶ NURSING ALERTS

▷ 1 Caution patients that fainting caused by excessive orthostatic hypotension can occur shortly after small, initial doses of prazosin. This is termed the *first-dose phenomenon.* Patients should avoid hazardous activities during the early stages of therapy until effects of the drug have been determined.

▷ 2 Advise patients to arise slowly, to avoid sudden postural changes, and to lie down immediately upon feeling faint or weak, in order to minimize orthostatic hypotension and danger of syncope. This effect generally tends to disappear within a few days.

▷ 3 Limit the initial dose of prazosin to 1 mg, make dosage adjustments gradually, and add other antihypertensive medications cautiously to avoid excessive hypotensive reactions.

▶ NURSING CONSIDERATIONS

▷ 1 Be aware that maximum antihypertensive action of prazosin may require several weeks to develop.

▷ 2 Consider giving initial doses at bedtime to minimize orthostatic hypotension.

▷ 3 Inform patients that drowsiness, headache, and dizziness can occur during early stages of therapy, but will gradually disappear with continued therapy.

▷ 4 Note that tolerance may develop with continued use, and that drug may lose effectiveness within a few months.

▷ 5 Advise patients to avoid taking over-the-counter medications (*e.g.,* cough or cold remedies, nasal sprays, allergy medication) without consulting physician or pharmacist.

▶ propranolol

Inderal, Inderal LA

Propranolol is a beta-adrenergic blocking agent used in the treatment of several disease states, including hypertension. A complete discussion of propranolol and the other beta-blockers appears in Chapter 12, and only those aspects of its pharmacology relevant to its use as an antihypertensive drug will be discussed here.

Mechanism

Not completely established; reduces heart rate and force of contraction, suppresses renin release, and decreases outflow of sympathetic vasoconstrictor and cardio-accelerator fibers from brain stem vasomotor centers

Uses

1 Treatment of mild to moderate hypertension, usually combined with a diuretic or other antihypertensive drug

Dosage

Initially 40 mg twice a day (or 80-mg long-acting capsule once daily); increase gradually to gain optimal response; usual maintenance range is 160 mg to 480 mg/day in 2 to 3 divided doses or once daily with long-acting capsules; *not* indicated for hypertensive emergencies

▶ rauwolfia derivatives

Alseroxylon	Rescinnamine
Deserpidine	Reserpine
Rauwolfia whole root	

The rauwolfia derivatives are a group of products derived from the Rauwolfia family of plants, comprising whole root rauwolfia, an extraction of alkaloids (alseroxylon) and the refined alkaloids deserpidine, rescinnamine, and reserpine. Although individual alkaloids differ somewhat in their pharmacologic actions, they have similar indications and adverse reactions and are discussed together. Individual compounds are then listed in Table 31-3.

Mechanism

Deplete central and peripheral neuronal stores of biogenic amines (*i.e.,* norepinephrine, serotonin) by blocking amine uptake into vesicular storage sites within the nerve ending; decrease blood pressure, heart rate, and cardiac output; exert a CNS-depressant (sedating) action; do not markedly affect renal blood flow

Uses

1 Treatment of mild to moderate essential hypertension, either alone or combined with other antihypertensive medications
2 Management of psychotic behavior, primarily in pa-

Table 31-3. Rauwolfia Alkaloids

Drug	Preparations	Usual Dosage Range	Remarks
Alseroxylon (Rauwiloid)	Tablets—2 mg	Initially 2 mg to 4 mg/day Usual maintenance dose is 2 mg/day	Mixture of alkaloids derived from Rauwolfia; used for treatment of mild essential hypertension; serious mental depression can occur at high doses
Deserpidine (Harmonyl)	Tablets—0.1 mg, 0.25 mg	Hypertension—initially 0.75 mg to 1 mg/day; maintenance dose 0.25 mg/day Psychoses—initially 0.5 mg/day; usual range is 0.1 mg to 1 mg/day	An alkaloid derived from Rauwolfia; used for treatment of mild essential hypertension and for relief of symptoms in agitated psychotic states; do not make dosage adjustments more frequently than every 10 to 14 days because effects of the drug are slow to develop
Rauwolfia whole root (Raudixin and various other manufacturers)	Tablets—50 mg, 100 mg	Usual starting dose is 200 mg to 400 mg/day in divided doses Maintenance dose is 50 mg to 300 mg/day in a single or 2 divided doses	Powdered whole root of *Rauwolfia serpentina*, which contains several alkaloids, including reserpine; used in mild essential hypertension, and for relief of symptoms in agitated psychotic states; usually administered with food or milk to minimize GI upset; rarely used today
Rescinnamine (Moderil)	Tablets—0.25 mg, 0.5 mg	Initially 0.5 mg twice a day Usual maintenance dose is 0.25 mg to 0.5 mg daily	Alkaloid derived from the Rauwolfia plant; used in mild essential hypertension, and may be effective as an adjunct to other antihypertensive medications in more severe forms of hypertension; lower incidence of sedation and bradycardia reported with rescinnamine than with reserpine
Reserpine (Serpasil and various other manufacturers)	Tablets—0.1 mg, 0.25 mg, 0.5 mg, 1 mg Timed-release capsules—0.5 mg Injection—2.5 mg/ml	Oral: Hypertension—initially 0.5 mg/day; reduce slowly to 0.1 mg to 0.25 mg/day Psychiatric disorders—0.1 mg to 1 mg/day adjusted to patient's response IM: Hypertensive crises—initially 0.5 mg to 1 mg, followed by doses of 2 mg and 4 mg at 3-hour intervals Psychiatric emergencies—2.5 mg to 5 mg; administer a small test dose, if possible, to test sensitivity	An alkaloid derived from Rauwolfia; used orally for treating mild hypertension and for relief of symptoms of agitated psychotic states; IM administration is indicated for hypertensive emergencies (usually not drug of choice, however) and to quickly control symptoms of extreme agitation; oral doses higher than 0.25 mg/day may cause severe depression; combined with other antihypertensive drugs (*e.g.,* diuretics, hydralazine) for treatment of more severe forms of hypertension

tients intolerant of other antipsychotic drugs (except alseroxylon and rescinnamine)

Dosage
See Table 31-3.

Fate
Onset of action following oral administration is generally slow (several days); maximum antihypertensive effect requires several weeks to develop; effects persist for weeks following discontinuation of therapy; primarily excreted in the urine, mainly as metabolites; following IM injection, reserpine has an onset in approximately 1 hour to 2 hours with maximum effects occurring within 4 hours to 6 hours.

Common Side-Effects
Drowsiness, nasal congestion, diarrhea, and bradycardia

Significant Adverse Reactions
GI—nausea, vomiting, abdominal pain, hypersecretion, bleeding

CNS—nervousness, anxiety, nightmares, depression, extrapyramidal symptoms (large doses)

Cardiovascular—palpitations, arrhythmias, anginal-like symptoms, orthostatic hypotension, syncope, cutaneous vasodilation and flushing

Other—rash, pruritus, uveitis, blurred vision, dryness of mouth, epistaxis, headache, dysuria, impotence, breast engorgement, pseudolactation, gynecomastia, asthma, dyspnea, muscle aching, weight gain, menstrual irregularities

Contraindications

Mental depression, active peptic ulcer, ulcerative colitis, pheochromocytoma, patients receiving ECT, therapy with MAO inhibitors

Interactions

1 Enhanced hypotensive effects may be seen when rauwolfia derivatives are combined with anesthetics, barbiturates, diuretics and other antihypertensive drugs, methotrimeprazine, phenothiazines, quinidine, propranolol, and vasodilators.
2 Cardiac arrhythmias can occur if reserpine is given with digitalis or quinidine.
3 CNS-depressant effects of other agents (*e.g.,* alcohol, barbiturates, narcotics, antihistamines, phenothiazines) may be enhanced by reserpine.
4 Rauwolfia derivatives may decrease the effects of anticholinergics (antisecretory action), anticonvulsants, indirect-acting sympathomimetics (*e.g.,* ephedrine, amphetamine), levodopa, morphine, salicylates, vasopressors (*e.g.,* metaraminol, mephentermine).
5 If used with tricyclic antidepressants, rauwolfia derivatives can be antagonized and excitation and mania can occur.
6 Excitation and hypertension can initially result from combined use of rauwolfia drugs and MAO inhibitors, but prolonged therapy can lead to severe depression and markedly increased GI activity.

▶ NURSING ALERTS

▷ 1 Carefully observe patients with a history of or tendency toward depression during therapy. Discontinue drug at first sign of drug-induced depression (despondency, insomnia, anorexia, impotence), and be aware that depressive effects of these drugs can persist for months after withdrawal.
▷ 2 Use cautiously in patients with cardiac damage or arrhythmias, epilepsy, obesity, renal insufficiency, bronchitis, asthma, and gallstones, and in elderly, debilitated, pregnant, or nursing patients.

▶ NURSING CONSIDERATIONS

▷ 1 Advise patients to monitor weight regularly and report excessive or too-rapid weight gain.
▷ 2 Administer drug with food or milk to minimize GI distress.
▷ 3 Caution patients to show care in performing hazardous tasks (*e.g.,* driving, operating machinery) because drugs commonly cause drowsiness, especially during early stages of therapy.
▷ 4 Note that although orthostatic hypotension is uncommon, patients should be made aware of the possibility of dizziness and fainting occurring during drug treatment. Urge gradual position changes.
▷ 5 If a vasopressor is needed to treat excessive hypotension, use a direct-acting sympathomimetic (*e.g.,* levarterenol) rather than an indirect-acting drug (*e.g.,* ephedrine).

▷ 6 Recognize that therapeutic effects of these drugs may take several weeks to develop and may persist for up to 1 month following termination of therapy. Discontinue drugs several weeks prior to elective surgery, to avoid severe hypotension during anesthesia.
▷ 7 Advise patients that alcohol may increase both the hypotensive and CNS-depressant effects of the drugs.

▶ timolol

Blocadren, Timoptic

A nonselective beta-blocker, oral timolol (Blocadren) is indicated for treatment of hypertension and to reduce the risk of reinfarction in patients surviving the acute phase of a myocardial infarction. It is also used as eye drops (Timoptic) for management of chronic open-angle glaucoma. Timolol is very similar to propranolol, but is slightly longer-acting and does not possess significant myocardial depressant or local anesthetic action. Oral timolol is also available in combination with hydrochlorothiazide as Timolide.

The complete pharmacology of timolol is presented in Chapter 12; only its dosage for treating hypertension is given here.

Dosage

Hypertension

Initially 10 mg twice a day; increase gradually to obtain optimal control; usual maintenance range is 20 mg to 40 mg per day

Myocardial infarction
10 mg twice a day

▶ trimethaphan

Arfonad

Trimethaphan is a ganglionic blocking agent used parenterally for rapid blood pressure reduction. In addition to blocking ganglionic receptor sites, it may also exert a direct relaxant effect on peripheral vascular smooth muscle. Onset of action is rapid, and the effects persist for only a short time after the infusion is terminated. Trimethaphan is discussed with the other ganglionic blocking drug mecamylamine in Chapter 13.

Uses

1 Production of controlled hypotension during surgery
2 Short-term management of hypertensive emergencies, *e.g.,* dissection of the aorta
3 Emergency treatment of pulmonary edema in patients with pulmonary hypertension

Dosage

Dilute 10 ml of drug to 500 ml 5% Dextrose Injection; infuse initially at a rate of 3 ml to 4 ml/minute and adjust to desired blood pressure control; range is 0.3 ml to 6 ml/minute

Summary. Antihypertensive Drugs

Drug	Preparations	Usual Dosage Range
Atenolol (Tenormin)	Tablets—50 mg, 100 mg	Initially 50 mg/day in a single dose; increase to 100 mg/day in 2 weeks if response is inadequate
Captopril (Capoten)	Tablets—25 mg, 50 mg, 100 mg	Initially 25 mg 3 times/day; increase to 50 mg 3 times/day in 1 week to 2 weeks; may increase further in 50-mg increments with addition of a diuretic; Range is 25 mg to 150 mg 3 times/day
Clonidine (Catapres)	Tablets—0.1 mg, 0.2 mg, 0.3 mg	Initially 0.1 mg twice a day; increase by 0.1 mg to 0.2 mg/day to desired response (maximum 2.4 mg/day)
Diazoxide Parenteral (Hyperstat IV)	Injection—300 mg/20 ml	1 mg/kg to 3 mg/kg (maximum 150 mg) by IV push within 30 seconds; repeat at 5 minute to 15-minute intervals
Guanabenz (Wytensin)	Tablets—4 mg, 8 mg	Initially 4 mg twice a day; increase in increments of 4 mg to 8 mg every 1 week to 2 weeks; maximum dosage is 32 mg/day
Guanadrel (Hylorel)	Tablets—10 mg, 25 mg	Initially 10 mg/day; increase gradually until optimal effect is reached; usual dosage range is 20 mg to 75 mg daily in 2 divided doses
Guanethidine (Ismelin)	Tablets—10 mg, 25 mg	Ambulatory—10 mg/day initially; increase slowly every 5 to 7 days; usual dose is 25 mg to 50 mg/day. Hospital—10 mg to 50 mg initially; increase by 10 mg to 25 mg every 2 to 4 days
Hydralazine (Apresoline)	Tablets—10 mg, 25 mg, 50 mg, 100 mg; Injection—20 mg/ml	Oral—initially 10 mg 4 times/day for 2 to 4 days; increase to 25 mg 4 times/day for balance of first week, then to 50 mg 4 times/day if necessary. IM, IV—20 mg to 40 mg repeated as necessary
Mecamylamine (Inversine)	Tablets—2.5 mg, 10 mg	Initially 2.5 mg twice a day; increase by 2.5 mg every 2 days until desired response; average dose is 25 mg/day in 3 to 4 divided doses
Methyldopa (Aldomet)	Tablets—125 mg, 250 mg, 500 mg; Injection—250 mg methyldopate HCl/5 ml; Oral suspension—250 mg/5 ml	Oral: Adults—250 mg 3 to 4 times/day; adjust to desired response; usual dosage range is 500 mg to 2000 mg/day in 2 to 4 divided doses. Children—10 mg/kg/day in 2 to 4 divided doses (maximum 65 mg/kg/day or 3 g). IV infusion: Adults—250 mg to 500 mg at 6-hour intervals infused over 30 minutes to 60 minutes; maximum dose 1 g every 6 hours. Children—20 mg to 40 mg/kg in divided doses every 6 hours; maximum dose 3 g/day
Metoprolol (Lopressor)	Tablets—50 mg, 100 mg; Injection—1 mg/ml	Initially 100 mg/day in a single or divided doses; increase at weekly intervals; usual maintenance range 100 mg to 450 mg/day
Metyrosine (Demser)	Capsules—250 mg	Initially 250 mg 4 times/day; increase by 250 mg to 500 mg every day to a maximum of 4 g/day

(continued)

Summary. Antihypertensive Drugs *(continued)*

Drug	Preparations	Usual Dosage Range
Minoxidil (Loniten)	Tablets—2.5 mg, 10 mg	Adults—initially 5 mg/day; increase gradually until optimal control is attained (usual range 10 mg–40 mg/day)
		Children (under 12)—initially 0.2 mg/kg/day; increase in 50% to 100% increments (usual range is 0.25 mg/kg–1 mg/kg/day)
Nadolol (Corgard)	Tablets—40 mg, 80 mg, 120 mg, 160 mg	Initially 40 mg once daily; increase in 40-mg to 80-mg increments; usual dose is 80 mg to 320 mg/day
Nitroprusside (Nipride, Nitropress)	Injection—50 mg/5 ml	IV infusion *only*—3 mcg/kg/minute (range 0.5 mcg/kg–10 mcg/kg/min) of a 50 mg in 250 ml to 1000 ml 5% Dextrose in Water dilution
Pargyline (Eutonyl)	Tablets—10 mg, 25 mg, 50 mg	Initially 10 mg to 25 mg/day in a single dose; increase by 10 mg/wk until desired response is achieved; usual range is 50 mg to 75 mg/day
Phenoxybenzamine (Dibenzyline)	Capsules—10 mg	Initially 10 mg/day; increase by 10 mg/4 days until optimal effects are noted; usual range is 20 mg to 60 mg/day
Pindolol (Visken)	Tablets—5 mg, 10 mg	Initially 10 mg twice a day or 5 mg 3 times a day; adjust in increments of 10 mg/day at 2-week to 3-week intervals
Phenoxybenzamine (Dibenzyline)	Capsules—10 mg	Initially 10 mg/day; increase by 10 mg/4 days until optimal effects are noted; usual range is 20 mg to 60 mg/day
Phentolamine (Regitine)	Tablets—50 mg Injection—5 mg/ampule	Oral—25 mg to 50 mg 4 to 6 times/day
		IV, IM—5 mg (adults); 1 mg (children)
		Prevent necrosis—10 mg/liter of infusion solution
		Treat necrosis—5 mg to 10 mg/10 ml saline injected into area
Prazosin (Minipress)	Capsules—1 mg, 2 mg, 5 mg	Initially 1 mg 2 to 3 times/day; increase *slowly* to desired level, up to 20 mg/day
Propranolol (Inderal, Inderal LA)	Tablets—10 mg, 20 mg, 40 mg, 60 mg, 80 mg, 90 mg Long-acting capsules—80 mg, 120 mg, 160 mg Injection—1 mg/ml	Initially 40 mg twice a day or 80 mg once daily; increase gradually until optimal response is achieved; usual maintenance range is 160 mg to 480 mg/day in 2 to 3 divided doses, or once daily with long-acting capsule
Rauwolfia derivatives	See Table 31-3.	
Timolol (Blocadren)	Tablets—5 mg, 10 mg, 20 mg	Initially 10 mg twice a day; increase gradually; usual maintenance range is 20 mg to 40 mg/day
Trimethaphan (Arfonad)	Injection—50 mg/ml	Dilute 10 ml of drug solution to 500 ml with 5% Dextrose Injection
		Infuse at a rate of 3 ml to 4 ml/minute (range is 0.3 ml–6 ml/min)

Drugs that can improve blood flow through circulatory vessels by increasing their diameter are termed *vasodilators*. These agents are usually effective in reducing the incidence and severity of exertional pain in patients with coronary artery disease (*e.g.*, angina), but are generally of limited clinical usefulness for improving circulation in peripheral vascular diseases. The drugs discussed in this chapter are therefore divided into those principally used for the treatment of angina pectoris and those usually indicated for the treatment of peripheral and cerebrovascular insufficiency.

Antianginal Agents— Vasodilators

32

I Antianginal Agents

Angina pectoris is a condition characterized by intermittent substernal (chest) pain, often of a "crushing" nature, which may remain localized in the sternal region or may radiate to other areas of the body (*e.g.*, the left shoulder or left arm). The pain is the result of ischemia (reduced blood supply) in an area of the myocardium, leading to decreased cardiac oxygenation, especially during periods of exertion or stress. Acute anginal attacks are triggered when the oxygen demand of the heart exceeds the capacity of the coronary circulation to supply the needed oxygen. However, merely attempting to increase myocardial blood flow via coronary artery dilation, of itself, is not usually beneficial in the absence of a reduced workload on the heart. For example, although they dilate coronary arteries, catecholamines (*e.g.*, epinephrine) are of no value in treating angina because they increase the workload, and hence oxyen demand of the heart, to an even greater degree. Effective management of the anginal condition therefore requires the use of drugs that can increase overall myocardial oxygenation. In fact, the primary effect of the vasodilators used in the treatment of angina is reduction of *total* peripheral vascular resistance rather than selective dilation of coronary arteries. The resultant decrease in venous return to the heart reduces the oxygen requirement of the myocardium and the workload on the anginal heart.

Drug therapy of angina is twofold; namely, to provide relief of pain during an acute anginal attack, and to decrease the overall frequency and severity of attacks by improving the oxygen supply/demand ratio. Treatment of an acute anginal attack is usually accomplished by sublingual administration of one of the rapid-acting nitrites or nitrates (*e.g.*, nitroglycerin, isosorbide dinitrate), which are drugs that have a quick onset and a relatively short duration of action. Prophylaxis against anginal episodes can be conferred by use of longer acting, orally effective nitrates (*e.g.*, pentaerythritol, erythrityl), topical nitroglycerin, beta-adrenergic blockers, calcium channel blockers, and possibly dipyridamole.

While the efficacy of the rapid-acting agents in aborting an acute anginal attack is unquestioned, controversy surrounds the use of the long-acting nitrates as prophylactic drugs. Although clinical evidence suggests that these long-acting agents may improve exercise tolerance in some anginal patients, there are conflicting data on their efficacy in reducing the frequency and severity of recurring attacks. Long-acting nitrates are quickly transported to the liver following ingestion, being rapidly and almost completely metabolized in most cases before attaining significant plasma concentrations. Cross-tolerance has been noted between the long-acting and rapid-acting nitrates. This condition may prove hazardous if a rapid-acting drug is administered in a crisis situation, only to exhibit greatly reduced effectiveness because of the increased tolerance. Currently, use of the long-acting nitrates is rated as only "possibly effective" for the prophylaxis of angina, and their use remains largely a matter of physician preference.

Another method for administering chronic nitroglycerin is the transdermal infusion system (Nitrodisc, Nitro-Dur, Transderm-Nitro). A small adhesive bandage containing nitroglycerin in a specialized medium (*e.g.,* solid polymer, gel-like matrix) or encased in a semipermeable membrane is applied to a nonhairy skin area once a day, and provides for constant absorption of drug over a 24-hour period. Thus, maintenance of steady-state venous plasma levels is possible, improving clinical efficacy and reducing untoward reactions.

A chemically unique type of compound, the calcium channel blocker, has recently become available for *prophylaxis* of anginal attacks. The calcium channel blockers (*i.e.,* diltiazem, nifedipine, verapamil) act by impairing the influx of calcium through the so-called slow membrane channels, thus reducing the contractile activity of smooth muscle and cardiac muscle. They are effective in alleviating pain and improving exercise tolerance in a high percentage of anginal patients while exhibiting a fairly low incidence of side-effects. The calcium channel blockers are employed orally in chronic, stable angina as well as in the vasospastic (Prinzmetal's) variant form. In addition, verapamil reduces AV conduction and SA nodel automaticity and prevents abnormal impulse re-entry at the AV node, and is also used IV in the management of supraventricular tachyarrhythmias, a condition in which the drug is now considered by many to be the drug of choice. This latter indication is reviewed in detail in Chapter 30.

The nitrites and nitrates are discussed as a group because they exhibit qualitatively similar actions; individual drugs are then listed in Table 32-1. The calcium channel blockers are likewise considered together; the individual drugs are then detailed in Tables 32-2 and 32-3. Propranolol, nadolol, and dipyridamole, other drugs used chronically in angina, are then reviewed individually.

Nitrites/Nitrates

Amyl nitrite	Nitroglycerin
Erythrityl tetranitrate	Pentaerythritol tetranitrate
Isosorbide dinitrate	

Mechanism

Direct relaxing effect on vascular smooth muscle, resulting in generalized vasodilation, reduced venous return, and decreased cardiac output, thereby lowering myocardial oxygen demand; reduced venous return decreases left ventricular end-diastolic pressure, thereby improving blood flow to deeper (subendocardial) layers of the myocardium; relax most other nonvascular smooth muscles as well, possibly by interfering with enzyme systems necessary for maintenance of normal smooth muscle tone

Uses

1 Relief of pain of acute anginal attacks (rapid-acting drugs only)
2 Prevention of anginal episodes, and reduction in frequency and severity of acute attacks (long-acting nitrates, transdermal nitroglycerin, sustained-release forms of nitroglycerin)
3 Reduce cardiac work load in patients with myocardial infarction or congestive heart failure
4 Relief of smooth muscle spasm (*e.g.,* biliary, GI, urethral, bronchial) (infrequent use)

Dosage

See Table 32-1.

Fate

Onset with sublingual administration is 2 minutes to 5 minutes; duration ranges from 10 minutes to 15 minutes (nitroglycerin) to 2 hours (erythrityl); onset following oral ingestion is 15 minutes to 60 minutes, with a duration of 4 hours to 6 hours for regular tablets or capsules, and up to 12 hours with sustained-release dosage forms. Topical administration (ointment, transdermal patch) results in effects within 30 minutes to 60 minutes; duration of action with ointment is 4 hours to 6 hours, while effects with transdermal patch persist for at least 24 hours; drugs are rapidly metabolized in the liver to inactive metabolites, which are excreted in the urine.

Common Side-Effects

(Most frequent with rapid-acting drugs) Headache, flushing, dizziness, palpitation, and burning sensation in sublingual area

Significant Adverse Reactions

Orthostatic hypotension, tachycardia, vertigo, confusion, weakness, skin rash, and exfoliative dermatitis (rare)

Occasional hypersensitivity reaction, marked by vomiting, profound weakness, restlessness, tachycardia, incontinence, syncope, perspiration, pallor, pronounced hypotension, and collapse

Contraindications

Severe anemia, marked hypotension, increased intracranial pressure, cerebral hemorrhage, and acute stages of myocardial infarction

Interactions

1 Hypotensive effects of nitrites and nitrates may be enhanced by alcohol, beta-blockers, antihypertensives, narcotics, tricyclic antidepressants.
2 Nitrates can potentiate the effects of antihistamines,

tricyclic antidepressants, and other anticholinergic drugs.

3 Cross-tolerance can occur between all nitrites and nitrates.

4 Nitrites and nitrates can antagonize the pressor actions of sympathomimetic drugs.

▶ **NURSING ALERTS**

▷ 1 Inform patient that dizziness, weakness, syncope, and other signs of orthostatic hypotension can occur following administration, especially sublingually. Advise patient to sit or lie down when taking medication and to rest for 10 minutes to 15 minutes after taking tablet.

▷ 2 Instruct patient to take additional sublingual tablets (up to 3) at 5-minute intervals if necessary. If pain is not relieved after 15 minutes, a physician should be contacted immediately, or the patient should report to the hospital.

▷ 3 Advise patient to inform physician if blurring of vision, dry mouth, or severe headaches occur. Dosage may need to be adjusted.

▷ 4 Use cautiously in patients with glaucoma, because increased intraocular pressure can result from generalized vasodilation.

▷ 5 Warn patients of danger associated with alcohol consumption in conjunction with nitroglycerin therapy because a shock-like syndrome (flushing, pallor, weakness, hypotension, syncope) can occur.

▷ 6 Advise patients to be alert for development of tolerance to the rapid-acting drugs, marked by lack of adequate relief of pain following several tablets. Temporary discontinuation of the drug (several days) is usually sufficient to restore sensitivity. Tolerance can be minimized by using smallest effective dose.

▶ **NURSING CONSIDERATIONS**

▷ 1 Instruct patients to keep a record of the frequency of anginal attacks, number of tablets required for relief, and development of any side-effects.

▷ 2 Inform patients that headaches may occur following drug administration, but will usually disappear within 20 minutes to 30 minutes. Prolonged headache can be relieved with analgesics.

▷ 3 Dispense and store drugs (especially sublingual nitroglycerin) in original manufacturer's glass container. Tablets may lose potency rapidly in metal, plastic, or cardboard containers.

▷ 4 Suggest that patients discard unused sublingual tablets 6 months after original container is opened because potency is probably reduced. Note that the presence of a burning or stinging sensation under the tongue following administration is a good indication that potency is adequate.

▷ 5 Observe for appearance of skin rash, visual disturbances, or persistent headache in patients taking long-acting nitrates, and advise physician.

▷ 6 Suggest that patients learn to avoid situations that might precipitate anginal pain (*e.g.,* stress, heavy exercise, smoking, overeating); urge reduction in caloric intake

and development of a program of regular sensible exercise.

▷ 7 Suggest that patient use sublingual nitroglycerin in anticipation of situations in which acute anginal episodes have predictably occurred.

▷ 8 Instruct patients that sublingual tablets should be placed under the tongue, while long-acting tablets or capsules should be swallowed whole.

▷ 9 Recognize that the topical dosage forms of nitroglycerin are *not* intended for relief of acute attacks of angina, due to their slower onset of action.

▷ 10 Suggest patient apply new transdermal patch 30 minutes before removing old one to minimize fluctuations in plasma level of drug. At least 30 minutes are required for sufficient absorption from new patch to attain steady state plasma concentration.

▷ 11 Caution patients to check that patch hasn't loosened following showering, swimming, or heavy perspiration—these factors generally do *not* affect the drug response.

▷ *Dietary precautions*

▷ 1 Counsel patients on the danger of excessive consumption of coffee, sodas, tea, and other foods high in caffeine; increased anginal episodes can result.

Calcium Channel Blockers

Diltiazem	Verapamil
Nifedipine	

Calcium channel blockers are used orally for prophylaxis of angina. In addition, one of these agents, verapamil, is administered IV for treatment of supraventricular tachyarrhythmias; this latter application is considered in Chapter 30. The following discussion pertains to the oral use of these agents in angina. While all of the calcium blockers are effective in treatment of angina pectoris, significant differences exist among the drugs with regard to their pharmacologic effects on cardiovascular function. Table 32-2 outlines some of the more important differences in the actions of the various calcium channel blockers, while Table 32-3 presents dosage ranges and additional information.

Mechanism

Calcium channel blockers inhibit the influx of extracellular calcium ions into cardiac muscle and smooth muscle cells through specific "slow calcium channels." Antianginal effects include dilation of coronary arteries and arterioles and prevention of coronary artery spasm. Dilation of peripheral arterioles also occurs, reducing total resistance against which the heart must work; thus, there is a corresponding reduction in myocardial energy consumption and oxygen demand. Verapamil also markedly decreases calcium influx into cardiac contractile and conductile cells of the SA node and AV node. This latter action slows AV conduction, prolongs effective AV refractory period, and interrupts reentry

Table 32-1. Nitrites and Nitrates (see general discussion of drug class)

Drug	Preparations	Usual Dosage Range	Remarks
Amyl nitrite (Aspirols, Vaporole)	Inhalation ampules—0.18 ml, 0.3 ml	0.18 ml to 0.3 ml inhaled as required	Available as thin ampules in a woven fabric cover; ampule is wrapped in gauze or cloth, crushed between fingers, and contents inhaled; drug has a strong, fruity odor; volatile and highly flammable; tachycardia often occurs for a brief period following inhalation; has been employed to relieve renal and gallbladder colic, but infrequently used now due to odor, cost, and inconvenience; excessive doses may cause methemoglobinemia, an impaired oxygen-carrying capacity of red blood cells.
Erythrityl tetranitrate (Cardilate)	Tablets Oral—5 mg, 10 mg Chewable—10 mg Sublingual—5 mg, 10 mg	Sublingual—10 mg 3 times/day or prior to stressful episodes Oral—5 mg to 15 mg 3 times/day; additional dose at bedtime if nocturnal attacks are frequent	Comparable onset but longer duration (4 hr) of action than nitroglycerin; primarily used for prophylaxis in patients with frequent, recurrent anginal pain and reduced exercise tolerance; vascular headaches are common early in therapy; less frequent with oral than sublingual administration; GI disturbances are noted with high oral doses.
Isosorbide dinitrate (Isordil, Sorbitrate, and various other manufacturers)	Tablets Sublingual—2.5 mg, 5 mg, 10 mg Oral—5 mg, 10 mg, 20 mg, 30 mg, 40 mg Sustained release—40 mg Chewable—5 mg, 10 mg Capsules—40 mg Capsules (sustained release)—40 mg	Sublingual—2.5 mg to 10 mg as needed for relief of pain or every 2 hours to 6 hours Chewable—5 mg initially for relief of acute attack, or 5 mg every 2 hours to 3 hours for prophylaxis Tablets—10 mg to 20 mg 4 times a day for prophylaxis Sustained release—40 mg every 6 hours to 12 hours	Sublingual and chewable forms rated "probably effective" for treatment of acute anginal attacks and to prevent attacks in high-risk situations (e.g., stress); oral dosage forms rated "possibly effective" for prevention of anginal episodes; should be taken on an empty stomach, unless vascular headaches are severe; then drug may be taken with meals; duration following sublingual administration is 1 hour to 2 hours, and up to 6 hours with oral administration (12 hr with sustained-release forms).
Nitroglycerin, sublingual (Nitrostat and various other manufacturers)	Tablets—0.15 mg, 0.3 mg, 0.4 mg, 0.6 mg	0.3 mg to 0.6 mg under the tongue or in the buccal pouch at first indication of acute anginal attack; repeat as needed up to 3 tablets	Very effective in relieving pain of acute anginal episodes, and for preventing attacks when taken immediately prior to a stressful event; onset is almost immediate, and effects persist 10 minutes to 15 minutes; keep bottles tightly capped, store in cool and dry place, and, if possible, only a week's supply of tablets should be carried at any one time; remainder should be kept in stock bottle.
Nitroglycerin transmucosal (Susadrin)	Buccal tablets—1 mg, 2 mg, 3 mg	Initially 1 mg 3 times/day; titrate dosage upward as necessary in small increments	Tablets are placed between lip and gum above the upper incisors and adhere to the mucosa; drug is released over an extended period of time; dissolution time ranges from 3 hours to 5 hours; subsequent tablets should be placed in mouth within 1 hour of previous tablet's dissolution.

Table 32-1. Nitrites and Nitrates (see general discussion of drug class) (continued)

Drug	Preparations	Usual Dosage Range	Remarks
Nitroglycerin topical ointment (Nitro-Bid, Nitrol, Nitrong, Nitrostat)	Ointment—2%	Initially, half-inch strip of ointment every 4 hours to 8 hours; apply by spreading a thin, uniform layer on skin; do *not* rub in; increase by half-inch increments until optimal response is obtained	Effective prevention of anginal attacks, especially at night. Begin with half-inch of ointment/dose, and increase by half-inch every succeeding dose until vascular headache occurs, then decrease slightly; ointment is measured by squeezing a ribbon onto calibrated measuring tapes provided; rotate sites of application to prevent dermal inflammation and sensitization; area may be covered with plastic wrap to protect clothing; equally effective when applied to any skin area; *gradually* reduce dosage and frequency of application upon termination of drug, to prevent sudden withdrawal reaction; one inch ointment equals approximately 15 mg nitroglycerin.
Nitroglycerin sustained release (Nitro-Bid, Nitrospan, Nitrostat, and various other manufacturers)	Sustained-release tablets— 2.6 mg, 6.5 mg, 9.0 mg Sustained-release capsules— 2.5 mg, 6.5 mg, 9.0 mg	2.5 mg to 9.0 mg every 8 hours to 12 hours	Rated "possibly effective" for prophylaxis of anginal attacks. Drug should be taken on an empty stomach, and tablets or capsules should be swallowed whole.
Nitroglycerin transdermal systems (Nitrodisc, Nitro-Dur, Transderm-Nitro)	Adhesive Pads Nitrodisc—8 cm²—5 mg/24 hours; 16 cm²—10 mg/24 hours Nitro-Dur—5 cm²—2.5 mg/24 hours; 10 cm²—5 mg/24 hours; 15 cm²—7.5 mg/24 hours; 20 cm²—10 mg/24 hours; 30 cm²—15 mg/24 hours Transderm-Nitro—5 cm²—2.5 mg/24 hours; 10 cm²—5 mg/24 hours; 20 cm²—10 mg/24 hours; 30 cm²—15 mg/24 hours	Apply one patch to a nonhairy skin area once every 24 hours	Transdermal patch system provides a continuous source of drug absorbed at a constant rate over 24 hours; the larger the patch, the greater the content of drug in the reservoir and the larger the amount of drug absorbed over 24 hours. Dosage is stated in mg drug absorbed per 24 hours; rotate application sites; steady-state venous plasma levels are rapidly attained (30 min) and then maintained for 24 hours; new bandage should be applied 30 minutes before removing old one; dosage titration depends on clinical response, reduction in sublingual nitroglycerin usage, and degree of hypotension; most frequent side-effects are headache and flushing; terminate usage gradually over 4 weeks to 6 weeks to prevent sudden withdrawal reactions; not intended for treatment of acute anginal attacks
Nitroglycerin Injection (Nitrostat IV, Nitrol IV, Nitro-Bid IV, Tridil)	Injection—0.8 mg/ml, 5 mg/ml	Initially 5 mcg/minute by IV infusion; increase gradually in 5-mcg/minute increments every 3 minutes to 5 minutes up to 20 mcg/minute; if no response, further increases should be made in increments of 10 mcg/minute, then 20 mcg/minute until an effect is noted	Used to reduce the incidence of myocardial ischemic injury resulting from an acute myocardial infarction; to control hypertension associated with certain surgical procedures; to provide "controlled hypotension" during surgery; and to treat acute angina pectoris in patients not responding to other means of therapy

(continued)

Table 32-1. Nitrites and Nitrates (see general discussion of drug class) *(continued)*

Drug	Preparations	Usual Dosage Range	Remarks
Pentaerythritol tetranitrate (P.E.T.N., Peritrate, and various other manufacturers)	Tablets—10 mg, 20 mg, 40 mg, 80 mg Sustained-release tablets—80 mg Sustained-release capsules—30 mg, 45 mg, 60 mg, 80 mg	Initially 10 mg to 20 mg 3 to 4 times/day; increase gradually to a maximum 40 mg 4 times/day; maintenance 30 mg to 80 mg sustained-release forms every 12 hours	Rated "possibly effective" for prophylactic treatment of angina; observe for development of skin rash or persistent headaches and caution patient that prlonged use may reduce effectiveness of rapid-acting drugs; available in combination with nitroglycerin (10 mg P.E.T.N./0.3 mg nitroglycerin) for sublingual use, and combined with phenobarbital, meprobamate, hydroxyzine, or isosorbide for oral administration

of impulses at the AV node, thus restoring normal sinus rhythm.

Uses

1 Management of chronic, stable (effort-induced) angina in patients intolerant of or unresponsive to beta-blockers or nitrates
2 Management of vasospastic (Prinzmetal's variant) angina
3 Treatment of supraventricular tachyarrhythmias and control of rapid ventricular rate in atrial flutter or atrial fibrillation (IV verapamil—see Chap. 30)

Dosage

See Table 32-3.

Fate

(See Table 32-2.) All drugs are well absorbed orally, but diltiazem and verapamil undergo extensive first-pass hepatic metabolism; onset of action is within 30 minutes and effects persist for 4 hours to 6 hours. All drugs are highly protein bound. Hepatic metabolism is extensive and excretion proceeds largely via the kidney, with smaller amounts of metabolites appearing in the feces.

Common Side-Effects

(Most frequent with nifedipine and least frequent with diltiazem) Flushing, headache, weakness, dizziness, nausea, lightheadedness, peripheral edema; also, constipation with verapamil

Significant Adverse Reactions

Cardiovascular—palpitations, hypotension, bradycardia, myocardial infarction, heart failure; in addition, third-degree AV block with verapamil

Respiratory—dyspnea, cough, wheezing, chest congestion, pulmonary edema

GI—heartburn, diarrhea, cramping, flatulence, sore throat

CNS—fatigue, weakness, tremor, nervousness, confusion, mood changes, blurred vision, insomnia

Musculoskeletal—muscle cramping, joint stiffness, inflammation

Other—hair loss, menstrual irregularities, claudication, dermatitis, urticaria, fever, sweating, chills, impotence

Table 32-2. Pharmacokinetic and Pharmacologic Properties of Calcium Channel Blockers

	Diltiazem	Nifedipine	Verapamil
Pharmacokinetics			
Onset of action (min)	15–30	20	30 (2–5 IV)
Peak effect (hr)	0.5–1	1–2	2–4 (0.2 IV)
Half-life (hr)	4–8	2–4	2–5
Protein binding (%)	70–80	90–95	90
Pharmacologic effects			
Coronary vasodilation	↑↑↑	↑↑↑	↑↑↑
Peripheral vasodilation	↑	↑↑↑	↑↑
Heart rate	↓	↑ (reflex)	↑ or ↓
Contractility	0 (↓)	↓ or ↑ (reflex)	↓↓
AV nodal conduction	↓↓	0 (↓)	↓↓↓
SA nodal automaticity	↓	0	↓↓

↑↑↑ or ↓↓↓ = marked effect; ↑↑ or ↓↓ = moderate effect; ↑ or ↓ = minimal effect; 0 (↑) or 0 (↓) = variable effect; 0 = no effect

Table 32-3. Calcium Channel Blockers

Drug	Preparations	Usual Dosage Range	Remarks
Diltiazem (Cardizem)	Tablets—30 mg, 60 mg	Initially 30 mg 4 times/day; increase gradually at 1- to 2-day intervals to achieve optimal response; maximum dose is 240 mg/day in divided doses	Potent coronary vasodilator with little or no negative inotropic effect; weak peripheral vasodilation results in a modest fall in blood pressure; heart rate is slightly reduced; slows AV conduction, and may have additive bradycardic effects with beta-blockers or digitalis; incidence of adverse reactions is very low; nausea, headache and peripheral edema are occasionally reported.
Nifedipine (Procardia)	Capsules—10 mg	Initially 10 mg 3 times/day; increase slowly until optimal effect is noted; usual dosage range is 10 mg to 20 mg 3 times/day; maximum recommended dose is 180 mg/day	Orally effective calcium blocker used in chronic, stable angina as well as vasospastic angina; does not alter conduction system of the heart as does verapamil, thus is of no use in arrhythmias; marked reduction in peripheral resistance coupled with minimal increase in heart rate suggests possible use as an antihypertensive; discontinue drug gradually if necessary.
Verapamil (Calan, Isoptin)	Tablets—80 mg, 120 mg	Initially 80 mg 3 to 4 times/day; increase at daily or weekly intervals until optimal effect is attained; usual dosage range is 300 mg to 480 mg daily	Orally effective calcium blocker used in angina; also administered IV for treatment of supraventricular tachyarrhythmias (see Chap. 30); significantly reduces SA nodal automaticity and AV conduction and decreases force of contraction; high doses are necessary due to extensive first-pass metabolism; use with caution in patients with left-ventricular dysfunction.

Contraindications

(Verapamil and diltiazem) Severe left ventricular dysfunction, sick sinus syndrome, second- or third-degree heart block, cardiogenic shock, systolic pressure less than 90 mm Hg; in addition, do not give IV verapamil and IV beta-blockers concurrently (see Chap. 30)

Interactions

1 Calcium blockers and beta-blockers together may be beneficial in some patients with chronic, stable angina, but can also increase the likelihood of congestive heart failure or severe hypotension and may worsen existing angina, especially when given IV in patients with left ventricular dysfunction or conduction defects.
2 Verapamil can elevate serum levels of digoxin if used concurrently, possibly leading to digitalis toxicity.
3 Calcium blockers may have an additive antihypertensive effect if administered together with other antihypertensive drugs.
4 Actions of calcium blockers may be enhanced by concomitant use of other highly protein-bound drugs (*e.g.,* anticoagulants, anti-inflammatory agents, sulfonamides, barbiturates, etc.).

▶ **NURSING ALERTS**

▷ 1 Carefully monitor blood pressure during initial stages of therapy and whenever dosage alterations are made, because excessive hypotension can occur, especially in patients already receiving beta-blockers or other blood pressure lowering drugs.

▷ 2 Recognize that verapamil and to a lesser extent diltiazem (see Table 32-2) have significant negative inotropic effects and markedly slow AV conduction. Be alert for development of bradycardia, sometimes accompanied by nodal escape rhythms. First-degree AV block has also occurred during peaks of serum concentration. If above changes persist or worsen, reduce dose and be prepared to institute appropriate antidotal therapy if necessary.

▷ 3 Be alert for signs of developing congestive heart failure, which can occur especially in patients also receiving a beta-blocker. Discontinue drug and monitor patient closely.

▷ 4 Use drugs cautiously in patients with impaired hepatic or renal function, hypotension, congestive heart failure, pulmonary edema, and in pregnant women and nursing mothers.

▷ 5 Note that mild peripheral edema, usually of the lower extremities, can occur, especially with nifedipine, and may be treated with diuretics. Be careful to differentiate this edema from that resulting from the left ventricular dysfunction of congestive heart failure.

▶ **NURSING CONSIDERATIONS**
(See Table 32-3 for additional information)

▷ 1 Monitor liver enzymes periodically during therapy, because occasional elevations of transaminase and alkaline phosphatase have been reported. These elevations are usually not associated with clinical symptoms and their significance is unclear; nevertheless, the potential for hepatic injury does exist with these drugs.

▷ 2 Inform patients that sublingual nitroglycerin may be used as needed to control acute anginal attacks while taking a calcium channel blocker.

▷ 3 Establish optimal dosage by careful titration over a period of several days to several weeks if necessary. Excessive dosing frequently results in hypotension.

Dipyridamole (Persantine)

Dipyridamole is an orally effective vasodilator and inhibitor of platelet aggregation. It is widely employed to prevent reinfarction and to decrease the incidence of transient ischemic attacks due to platelet hyperaggregation, although these above indications are viewed solely as investigational. Dipyridamole is also indicated for the symptomatic management of chronic angina; however, it is only rated "possibly effective" for this application.

Mechanism

Lowers coronary vascular resistance, possibly by causing accumulation of adenosine and other vasodilatory nucleotides; inhibits phosphodiesterase enzyme, thus increasing functional levels of cyclic AMP, which dilates resistance vessels and reduces platelet adherence; stimulates production of vessel wall prostacyclin (PGI_2), a potent vasodilator and inhibitor of platelet aggregation

Uses

1 Long-term symptomatic therapy of chronic angina; "possibly effective" in reducing frequency of anginal episodes and in improving exercise tolerance; not useful in acute attacks
2 Prevention of thrombotic complications associated with cerebrovascular or ischemic heart diseases (investigational use only)

Dosage

25 mg to 75 mg 3 times/day

Fate

Well absorbed orally; clinical response may take several months to develop; metabolized in the liver, and excreted both as intact drug and metabolites largely through the feces

Common Side-Effects

GI distress

Significant Adverse Reactions

Headache, nausea, weakness, dizziness, syncope, and skin rash; occasionally, aggravation of angina pectoris

Contraindications

Acute myocardial infarction

Interactions

1 Dipyridamole can enhance the effects of oral anticoagulants and heparin.

▶ **NURSING ALERTS**
▷ 1 Use cautiously in patients with hypotension.

▶ **NURSING CONSIDERATIONS**
▷ 1 Administer 1 hour before meals.
▷ 2 Advise patients that headache or dizziness may occur, but that these effects are usually transient.

Beta-Blockers

▶ **propranolol**
Inderal, Inderal LA

A beta-adrenergic blocking agent employed in the treatment of several disease states, including angina, propranolol is reviewed in detail in Chapter 12, and only those aspects of its pharmacology that pertain to its use as an antianginal drug will be discussed here.

Mechanism

Competitive antagonism of beta-adrenergic receptor sites on the heart, resulting in a decreased heart rate, force of contraction, and cardiac output, which reduces myocardial oxygen demand; lowered systemic blood pressure may also reduce cardiac workload

Uses

1 Prophylactic management of moderate to severe angina not controlled by other drugs, usually in combination with nitroglycerin or isosorbide

Dosage

Initially 10 mg to 20 mg 3 to 4 times/day; increase gradually at weekly intervals until optimal response is obtained; usual maintenance dosage range is 80 mg to 160 mg/day in divided doses

▶ **NURSING ALERTS**
See Chapter 12. In addition:
▷ 1 Be aware that worsening of anginal symptoms and occasional myocardial infarction have occurred following abrupt discontinuation of therapy. Discontinue drug gradually over several weeks, and monitor patient during withdrawal.

▶ **NURSING CONSIDERATIONS**
See Chapter 12. In addition:
▷ 1 Re-evaluate patient periodically since dosage requirements may change as condition stabilizes or deteriorates.

▶ **nadolol**
Corgard

A nonspecific beta-adrenergic blocking agent indicated for the long-term management of patients with angina, its actions resemble those of propranolol, and both drugs are discussed in detail in Chapter 12. Unlike propranolol, however, nadolol does not appear to exert a direct depressant action on the myocardium. The long half-life of nadolol (20 hr–24 hr) permits once daily dosing.

Dosage

Initially 40 mg once daily; increase by 40 mg to 80 mg at 3- to 7-day intervals until optimal clinical response is observed, or until there is pronounced slowing of heart rate; usually maintenance dose is 80 mg to 240 mg/day

II Peripheral Vasodilators

Vasodilator drugs are capable of increasing blood flow through circulatory vessels by either a direct action (smooth muscle relaxing) or an indirect action (interference with sympathetic nerve supply). Although these agents may significantly enhance blood flow to limbs and body organs in the *normal* person, their efficacy in relieving the ischemia of peripheral vascular disease is severely limited. Reduced blood flow can result from either vasospasm or vascular occlusion, such as that caused by deposition of a fatty plaque on the vessel wall. Although vasospastic diseases (*e.g.,* Raynaud's disease) may in some cases be more amenable to treatment with direct-acting peripheral vasodilators than vaso-occlusive diseases (*e.g.,* arteriosclerosis obliterans), there is little evidence to indicate that *either* type of disease is significantly benefitted by any of the direct-acting peripheral vasodilators. Likewise, drugs that interfere with sympathetic activation of blood vessels (*e.g.,* reserpine, guanethidine) have also been reported to decrease persistent vasospasm in some cases of Raynaud's disease, although complete relief has rarely been obtained. These indirect-acting agents are not usually employed to treat peripheral vascular diseases, however, because of their many side-effects. Therefore, minimal therapeutic benefit should be expected from the treatment of peripheral vascular diseases with any of the currently available peripheral vasodilators.

▶ cyclandelate
Cyclan, Cyclospasmol, Cydel

Mechanism

Direct relaxation of vascular smooth muscle, with no significant action on sympathetic innervation of blood vessels

Uses

1 Adjunctive therapy of ischemic peripheral vascular diseases, *e.g.,* Raynaud's disease, intermittent claudication, and arteriosclerosis obliterans (Effectiveness has *not* been conclusively demonstrated.)

Dosage

Initially 400 mg 3 to 4 times/day; usual maintenance dose is 400 mg to 800 mg/day in 2 to 4 divided doses

Fate

Well absorbed orally; onset of action in 15 minutes to 30 minutes; duration of 3 hours to 4 hours.

Common Side-Effects

Flushing

Significant Adverse Reactions

Dizziness, sweating, headache, weakness, tachycardia, and GI distress

▶ **NURSING ALERTS**
▷ 1 Use cautiously in patients with obliterative coronary artery disease, cerebral vascular disease, active bleeding or bleeding tendencies, glaucoma, and during pregnancy or lactation.

▶ **NURSING CONSIDERATIONS**
▷ 1 Suggest taking drug with meals or milk to minimize GI upset.
▷ 2 Inform patients that flushing, headache, and tachycardia can occur during initial stages of therapy, but usually disappear with slight dosage reduction.
▷ 3 Make patients aware that clinical benefit may occur gradually and that adherence to dosage schedule is important to obtain maximal therapeutic benefit.
▷ 4 Stress the importance of good physical hygiene (*e.g.,* proper diet, rest, exercise, cessation of smoking) to the successful management of peripheral vascular disease.

▶ ergoloid mesylates
Hydergine and various other manufacturers

Ergoloid mesylates contain equal parts of three dihydrogenated ergotoxine alkaloids, namely dihydroergocornine, dihydroergocristine, and dihydroergocryptine. The compound is used to provide symptomatic relief of those signs and symptoms associated with a decline in mental acuity and capacity in the elderly, such as confusion, forgetfulness, lessened self-care, sociability, and appetite. Improvement in the above parameters are observed within 8 weeks to 12 weeks, and may be the result of improved cerebral circulation.

Mechanism

Not completely established; exerts an alpha-adrenergic blocking action, which may increase cerebral vasodilation, but also decreases blood pressure and can lead to orthostatic hypotension; increased metabolic activity in the brain has been postulated to also improve cerebral vascular flow

Uses

1 Symptomatic treatment of decreased mental capacity and function in elderly patients (*possibly* effective)

Dosage

Initially, 1 mg (orally or preferably sublingually) 3 times/day; adjust dosage gradually to obtain optimal effect

Fate

Erratically absorbed orally; undergoes extensive first-pass hepatic metabolism; probably less than one third of a dose reaches the systemic circulation following oral absorption; peak blood levels occur within 1 hour to 2 hours, probably earlier with sublingual administration; half-life is about 4 hours; metabolized in the liver; excretion pattern is not completely known.

Common Side-Effects

GI upset, transient nausea, and sublingual irritation

Significant Adverse Reactions

Orthostatic hypotension, lightheadedness, blurred vision, skin rash, nasal stuffiness, and bradycardia

Contraindications

Acute or chronic psychoses

▶ **NURSING ALERTS**

▷ 1 Note that drug efficacy is apparently greater following sublingual administration than with oral administration; however, sublingual usage may be more difficult in elderly or senile patients.

▷ 2 Use cautiously in patients susceptible to acute intermittent porphyria because acute attacks have been precipitated.

▶ **NURSING CONSIDERATIONS**

▷ 1 Inform patients that beneficial effects may not be observed for several weeks.

▷ 2 Caution patient to change position slowly, especially when rising from a recumbent position, because orthostatic hypotension can occur.

▷ 3 Instruct patients how to monitor heart rate, because sinus bradycardia can occur. Discontinue drug if heart rate is abnormally reduced.

▶ **ethaverine**

Circubid, Ethaquin, Ethatabs, Ethavex-100, Isovex-100

Mechanism

Direct relaxation of vascular smooth muscle (see papaverine—drug is a closely related analog)

Uses

1 Treatment of peripheral and cerebral vascular insufficiency associated with arterial spasm (*possibly* effective)

2 Relief of gastrointestinal and genitourinary spasms (*possibly* effective)

Dosage

100 mg to 200 mg 3 times/day; alternately, 150 mg to 300 mg sustained-release capsules every 12 hours

Fate

See Papaverine.

Common Side-Effects

Nausea, abdominal distress, and flushing

Significant Adverse Reactions

Anorexia, drowsiness, malaise, headache, sweating, constipation or diarrhea, hypotension, vertigo, skin rash, respiratory depression, cardiac depression, and arrhythmias

Contraindications

Serious arrhythmias, complete AV block, and liver disease

Interactions

See Papaverine.

▶ **NURSING ALERTS**

See Papaverine. In addition:

▷ 1 Administer cautiously to patients with pulmonary embolism because arrhythmias may develop. Have necessary equipment and drugs on hand to treat arrhythmia should it occur.

▶ **NURSING CONSIDERATIONS**

See Papaverine.

▶ **isoxsuprine**

Vasodilan, Voxsuprine

A direct-acting beta-adrenergic activator used in the treatment of peripheral vascular diseases, isoxsuprine is discussed in detail in Chapter 11 and is reviewed only briefly here.

Mechanism

Direct activation of beta-adrenergic receptor sites on vascular smooth muscle; however, vasodilator effects on muscle blood flow are *not* prevented by beta-blockers; may exert a *direct* relaxant effect on vascular smooth muscle and block alpha-adrenergic receptors; other effects include increased heart rate, contractility, and cardiac output, decreased blood pressure (possibly resulting in small *reductions* in cerebral blood flow), relaxation of uterine smooth muscle, and, in high doses, decreased platelet aggregation

Uses

(Clinical effectiveness has not been conclusively demonstrated.)

1 Relief of symptoms of peripheral and cerebral vascular insufficiency

2 Cessation of premature labor and prevention of threatened abortion (parenteral use only)

Dosage

Oral: 10 mg to 20 mg 3 to 4 times/day

IM: 5 mg to 10 mg 2 to 3 times/day in severe or acute conditions

▶ **nicotinyl alcohol**

Roniacol, Rontinol

Mechanism
Converted to nicotinic acid, which is responsible for much of its action; produces direct relaxation of vascular smooth muscle, particularly cutaneous vessels; no significant increase in muscle or cerebral blood flow

Uses
1 "Possibly effective" for symptomatic treatment of peripheral vascular disease, vascular spasm, varicose and decubital ulcers, Meniere's syndrome, and vertigo

Dosage
50 mg to 100 mg 3 times/day or 1 to 2 sustained-release tablets (150 mg) twice a day

Fate
Action is gradual in onset; long-acting tablets provide 10-hour to 12-hour action; converted to nicotinic acid, which exerts a vasodilating action of its own

Common Side-Effects
Flushing, GI upset

Significant Adverse Reactions
Skin rash, paresthesias, urticaria, angio-edema, dizziness, orthostatic hypotension

Interactions
1 Large doses of nicotinyl alcohol may antagonize the action of antidiabetics.
2 Nicotinyl alcohol may intensify the hypotensive effects of antihypertensive medications.

▶ NURSING CONSIDERATIONS
▷ 1 Inform patients that flushing and sensation of warmth can occur.
▷ 2 Administer drug with or shortly before meals to minimize GI upset.
▷ 3 Caution patients against excessive use of alcohol because increased vasodilation and dizziness can occur.

▶ nylidrin
Adrin, Arlidin

A beta-adrenergic activator, possessing actions similar to those of isoxsuprine, nylidrin is reviewed in detail in Chapter 11, and only a brief description of its actions is presented here.

Mechanism
Dilates peripheral arterioles and increases cerebral blood flow, probably by a beta-adrenergic activating action and a direct relaxant effect on vascular smooth muscle; increases heart rate and cardiac output, and reduces blood pressure, which may decrease cerebral blood flow

Uses
(Clinical effectiveness has not been conclusively demonstrated.)
1 Treatment of peripheral vascular diseases, such as Raynaud's disease, night leg cramps, diabetic vascular disease, and thromboangiitis obliterans
2 Relief of circulatory disturbances of the inner ear, *e.g.,* cochlear cell, macular or ampullar ischemia; labyrinthine artery spasm or obstruction

Dosage
3 mg to 12 mg 3 to 4 times/day

▶ papaverine
Cerespan, Pavabid, Paverolan, and various other manufacturers

Mechanism
Direct relaxation of vascular smooth muscle, independent of autonomic innervation, with predominant effects on coronary, cerebral, pulmonary, and systemic peripheral blood vessels; depresses myocardial conduction and irritability, and prolongs the refractory period; relaxes most other smooth muscles (*e.g.,* bronchioles, GI tract, biliary tract, ureters) by direct action on muscle fibers

Uses
(Clinical effectiveness has not been conclusively demonstrated.)
1 Relief of cerebral and peripheral ischemia associated with vascular spasm
2 Treatment of myocardial ischemia, complicated by arrhythmias
3 Relief of various smooth muscle spastic conditions, *e.g.,* biliary, ureteral, or GI colic

Dosage
Oral: 100 mg to 300 mg 3 to 5 times/day (sustained-released forms—150 mg every 8 hr–12 hr)
IM, IV: 30 mg to 120 mg every 3 hours

Fate
Well absorbed orally; undergoes extensive (60%–70%) first-pass hepatic metabolism; onset of action is 30 minutes to 60 minutes, with duration of 4 hours to 6 hours (10 hr–12 hr with sustained-release forms); highly bound (90%) to plasma proteins; metabolized by the liver, and excreted chiefly in the urine as metabolites

Common Side-Effects
(Infrequent with oral use) Nausea, abdominal distress, sweating, and flushing

Significant Adverse Reactions
Oral—vertigo, headache, drowsiness, anorexia, skin rash, constipation or diarrhea, tachycardia, increased respiration, hepatic hypersensitivity reactions (jaundice, eosinophilia), altered liver function tests

Parenteral—excessive sweating and flushing; increased blood pressure, respiratory rate, and heart rate; sedation

Contraindications
Complete AV block

Interactions
1 Papaverine may enhance the hypotensive effects of other blood pressure lowering agents.
2 Papaverine may reduce the efficacy of levodopa.
3 The smooth muscle relaxant action of papaverine can be antagonized by morphine and other opiates.

▶ **NURSING ALERTS**
▷ 1 In patients on prolonged therapy, perform periodic blood and liver function tests and be alert for early signs of developing hepatoxicity (*e.g.,* jaundice, eosinophilia). Withdrawal of drug will result in reversal of hepatotoxic effects.
▷ 2 Use cautiously in the presence of glaucoma, myocardial depression, or history of cardiac arrhythmias.
▷ 3 Monitor blood pressure, respiration, and heart rate frequently in patients receiving the drug parenterally.

▶ **NURSING CONSIDERATIONS**
▷ 1 Do not add parenteral form to lactated Ringer's solution, because precipitate can result.
▷ 2 Advise patients that dizziness has been reported following administration of papaverine; urge caution in driving and performing other hazardous tasks until effects of the drug have been established.

▷ 3 Administer drug IV slowly over 1 minute to 2 minutes. In treating cardiac extrasystoles, two doses may be given 10 minutes apart.

▶ **tolazoline**
Priscoline

A reversible alpha-adrenergic blocking agent and peripheral vasodilator that is employed parenterally to improve blood flow in spastic peripheral vascular disorders, tolazoline is discussed in detail in Chapter 12 and is only reviewed briefly here.

Mechanism
Reversible competitive antagonism of alpha-adrenergic receptor sites and direct relaxation of vascular smooth muscle; exhibits beta-adrenergic, cholinergic, and histaminergic activity as well, which may contribute to its vasodilatory action; cutaneous blood flow is most improved; produces cardiac and GI stimulation

Uses
1 "Possibly effective" for the treatment of peripheral vascular disorders, *e.g.,* acrocyanosis, arteriosclerosis obliterans, diabetic arteriosclerosis, and post-thrombotic complications

Dosage
IM, IV, SC: 10 mg to 50 mg 4 times/day
Intra-arterial: Initially 25 mg, followed by 50-mg to 75-mg/dose 2 to 3 times/week to sustain circulatory improvement (given only by trained personnel)

Summary. Antianginal Drugs—Vasodilators

Drug	Preparations	Usual Dosage Range
I. Antianginal Drugs		
Nitrites/nitrates see Table 32-1		
Calcium channel blockers See Table 32-3		
Dipyridamole (Persantine)	Tablets—25 mg, 50 mg, 75 mg	25 mg to 75 mg 3 times/day
Propranolol (Inderal)	Tablets—10 mg, 20 mg, 40 mg, 60 mg, 80 mg, 90 mg Long-acting capsules—80 mg, 120 mg, 160 mg	10 mg to 20 mg 3 to 4 times/day; increase gradually at 3- to 7-day intervals; usual range is 80 mg to 160 mg/day
Nadolol (Corgard)	Tablets—40 mg, 80 mg, 120 mg, 160 mg	Initially 40 mg once daily; increase by 40 mg to 80 mg every 3 to 5 days; usual range is 80 mg to 240 mg/day
II. Peripheral Vasodilators		
Cyclandelate (Cyclan, Cyclospasmol, Cydel)	Tablets—100 mg Capsules—200 mg, 400 mg	Initially 400 mg 3 to 4 times/day; usual maintenance dose is 400 mg to 800 mg/day in divided doses

Summary. Antianginal Drugs—Vasodilators *(continued)*

Drug	Preparations	Usual Dosage Range
Ergoloid mesylates (Hydergine and various other manufacturers)	Tablets (oral)—1 mg Tablets (sublingual)—0.5 mg, 1 mg Liquid—1 mg/ml Capsules—1 mg	Initially 1 mg 3 times/day; adjust upward gradually, depending upon response
Ethaverine (Circubid, Ethaquin, Ethatabs, Ethavex-100, Isovex-100)	Tablets—100 mg Capsules—100 mg Capsules (timed-release)—150 mg	100 mg to 200 mg 3 times/day; alternately, 150 mg to 300 mg every 12 hours
Isoxsuprine (Vasodilan, Voxsuprine)	Tablets—10 mg, 20 mg Injection—5 mg/ml	Oral—10 mg to 20 mg 3 to 4 times/day IM—5 mg to 10 mg 2 to 3 times/day
Nicotinyl Alcohol (Roniacol, Rontinol)	Tablets—50 mg Long-acting tablets—150 mg Elixir—50 mg/5 ml	50 mg to 100 mg 3 times a day, or 1 to 2 long-acting tablets (150 mg) twice a day
Nylidrin (Adrin, Arlidin)	Tablets—6 mg, 12 mg	3 mg to 12 mg 3 to 4 times/day
Papaverine (Cerespan, Pavabid, Paverolan, and various other manufacturers)	Tablets—30 mg, 60 mg, 100 mg, 200 mg, 300 mg Tablets (timed release)—200 mg Capsules (timed release)—150 mg, 300 mg Injection—30 mg/ml	Oral: 100 mg to 300 mg 3 to 5 times/day Oral (timed release): 150 mg every 8 hours to 12 hours IM, IV: 30 mg to 120 mg every 3 hours as required
Tolazoline (Priscoline)	Injection—25 mg/ml	IM, IV, SC: 10 mg to 50 mg 4 times/day Intrarterial: 25 mg initially, followed by 50-mg to 75-mg dose 2 to 3 times/week

33 Prophylaxis of Atherosclerosis— Hypolipemic Drugs

Atherosclerosis is a condition characterized by deposition of lipid (fatty) material within the walls of the arterial system, resulting in a gradual occlusion of blood flow. Clinical consequences of this lipid deposition include the development of ischemic heart disease, cerebrovascular disease (including stroke), peripheral ischemia, and renovascular hypertension. The presence of generalized atherosclerosis greatly increases the risk of mortality from one or more of these conditions.

Although the basic mechanism involved in the development of the atherosclerotic process is still somewhat uncertain, there appears to be a metabolic disturbance in the synthesis, transport, and utilization of lipids; this, in combination with damage to the vascular endothelial lining, results in the adherence and eventual buildup of fatty deposits within the lining of the vessel walls.

Lipids do not circulate freely in the blood stream, but rather are bound to plasma proteins (albumin, globulins). These complexes are termed *lipoproteins* and contain varying proportions of high-density proteins and low-density lipids. The four major types of lipoproteins, and a brief description of their characteristics, are listed below.

1 *Chylomicrons*—largest and lightest of the lipoproteins, formed in the intestine during absorption of dietary fat; composed mainly (80%–90%) of triglycerides, and impart a cloudiness to plasma; normally cleared rapidly from the blood, their presence in plasma taken from a fasting patient suggests an inability to handle dietary fats

2 *Very low density lipoproteins (VLDL)*—pre-beta lipoproteins containing large amounts (50%–60%) of triglycerides that were synthesized in the liver; major means by which endogenous triglycerides are carried from the liver to the plasma

3 *Low-density lipoproteins (LDL)*—beta lipoproteins derived partly from breakdown of VLDL, containing about 50% to 60% cholesterol, 25% protein, and very little triglycerides; most of the circulating serum cholesterol is transported in this form, and elevated plasma levels of LDL indicate excessive cholesterol levels and suggest that the patient is at high risk for developing atherosclerosis

4 *High-density lipoproteins (HDL)*—alpha lipoproteins, the smallest and most dense (heaviest) of the lipoproteins, containing approximately 50% protein, 25% cholesterol, and very small amounts of triglycerides; believed to play an important role in clearing cholesterol from body tissues, and may protect against development of atherosclerosis by blocking uptake of LDL cholesterol by vascular smooth muscle cells

Patients having defects in lipid transport or metabolism can be classified on the basis of the types of lipoproteins that are elevated in the plasma; this grouping allows precise diagnosis and treatment of each patient's condition. The term *hyperlipoproteinemia* is used to indicate an increase in one or more of the classes of lipoproteins. Table 33-1 lists the types of hyperlipoproteinemias that are currently recognized, with a brief description of each type and the most effective treatment of each subgroup.

It has not been conclusively established whether lowering serum lipids or cholesterol has a beneficial effect on the

Table 33-1. Classification of Hyperlipoproteinemias

Type	Descriptive Name	Characteristic Features	Treatment Diet	Drugs
I	Fat-induced (exogenous)	Relatively rare; increase in plasma chylomicrons containing large amounts of triglycerides of dietary origin; frequently seen in infancy, and marked by abdominal pain; does not lead to atherosclerosis	Low fat; no restrictions on proteins, carbohydrates, or cholesterol	None effective
IIa	Familial hypercholesterolemia	High levels of LDL; normal VLDL; slight elevation of triglycerides; fairly common, and a definite risk for development of atherosclerosis and coronary heart disease	Low cholesterol; low saturated fats; increased intake of polyunsaturated fats	Cholestyramine Colestipol Dextrothyroxine Probucol
IIb	Combined hyperlipoproteinemia	Elevated LDL and VLDL; presence of hypercholesterolemia and hypertriglyceridemia; lipid deposits occur on feet, elbows, knees	See IIa	Cholestyramine Colestipol Dextrothyroxine Nicotinic acid Probucol
III	Broad beta lipoproteinemia	Elevated LDL and VLDL; cholesterol and triglycerides are elevated; relatively uncommon but associated with atherosclerosis; recessively inherited disorder	Weight reduction; low cholesterol; low saturated fats; maintain high protein	Clofibrate Dextrothyroxine Nicotinic acid
IV	Carbohydrate-induced (endogenous)	Marked elevation of VLDL; triglycerides are increased, but LDL and cholesterol are normal or slightly elevated; most common type; definite risk for atherosclerosis and coronary heart disease	Weight reduction; low carbohydrate; low cholesterol; low alcohol; maintain protein intake	Clofibrate (?) Gemfibrozil Nicotinic acid
V	Mixed hyperlipemia	Elevated VLDL and triglycerides; chylomicrons are increased; relatively uncommon type not generally associated with atherosclerosis or heart disease	Low fat; high protein, low carbohydrate; low alcohol	Clofibrate (?) Gemfibrozil (?) Nicotinic acid

morbidity or mortality associated with atherosclerosis or coronary heart disease. Therefore, dietary and drug therapy for the prevention of atherosclerotic vascular disease remains a subject of controversy. Nevertheless, regulation of the diet and use of lipid-lowering drugs (hypolipemic agents) are widely employed in a significant percentage of the population with hyperlipoproteinemia. However, in view of the potential for many hypolipemic drugs to cause untoward reactions, dietary changes should always be undertaken initially before drug therapy is instituted. Only if diet alone is ineffective in controlling the plasma lipid picture should drugs be employed, and then only upon careful diagnosis of the type of hyperlipoproteinemia present. To date, drug therapy is entirely prophylactic—that is, hypolipemic agents can reduce the rate and extent of fatty deposition within arterial walls by lowering plasma lipid concentrations, but they do *not* dissolve or remove existing lipid deposits.

Finally, one must recognize that diet and drug therapy are only a part of the total therapeutic regimen for the prophylaxis of coronary heart disease and other vascular disorders. Attention to and modifications of other known risk factors such as obesity, physical inactivity, behavioral patterns, smoking, hypertension, and stress can greatly enhance the clinical response to hypolipemic drugs and may significantly reduce mortality.

Bile Acid Sequestering Resins

Cholestyramine   Colestipol

These two bile acid sequestering agents are anion-exchange resins that combine with bile acids in the intestines, preventing their reabsorption and therefore increasing their excretion in the feces. They are effective plasma cholesterol-lowering drugs, and cholestyramine is also used for relieving pruritus associated with partial biliary obstruction. They are discussed together, here, then listed individually in Table 33-2.

Mechanism

Form an insoluble complex with bile acids in the intestine, increasing their fecal excretion; this leads to increased oxidation of cholesterol to bile acids, decreased serum cholesterol levels, and reduced beta lipoprotein (LDL) levels; little effect on serum triglyceride levels; may interfere with absorption of calcium, fats, fat-soluble vitamins (A, D, E, K), and many other drugs (see Interactions)

Uses

1   Adjunctive treatment of primary type II hyperlipoproteinemia
2   Relief of pruritus associated with partial biliary obstruction (cholestyramine only)
3   Investigational uses for cholestyramine include treatment of antibiotic-induced pseudomembranous colitis and treatment of poisoning with the pesticide chlordecone (Kepone)

Dosage

See Table 33-2.

Table 33-2. Bile Acid Sequestering Resins

Drug	Preparations	Usual Dosage Range	Remarks
Cholestyramine (Questran)	Powder—4 g resin/9 g powder	Initially 4 g resin 2 to 3 times/day before meals, adjust to patient's needs (range 16 g–24 g/day)	Place drug on surface of 4 oz to 6 oz liquid; allow to stand 1 minute to 2 minutes without stirring, then gently twirl container or stir slowly to obtain a uniform suspension; rinse glass with fluid to assure taking entire dose; may also be mixed with soups or pulpy fruits (*e.g.,* applesauce); relief of pruritus may take 1 week to 2 weeks to become evident; decline in serum cholesterol is usually apparent by 1 month
Colestipol (Colestid)	Water-insoluble beads—5-g packets or 500-g bottles	15 g to 30 g/day in divided doses 2 to 4 times/day	Add prescribed amount of drug to at least 3 oz of liquid, and stir until completely mixed (does *not* dissolve); may also be added to cereals, soups, or pulpy fruits; does not have the disagreeable odor or taste of cholestyramine

Fate

Not absorbed from the GI tract, nor hydrolyzed by digestive enzymes; excreted in feces as insoluble bile acid complex

Common Side-Effects

Constipation (occasionally severe), abdominal discomfort, flatulence, belching, nausea, and anorexia.

Significant Adverse Reactions

Vomiting; steatorrhea; fecal impaction; vitamin-K deficiency with bleeding tendencies; vitamin A, D, and E deficiencies; rash and irritation of the skin, tongue, and perianal region; and osteoporosis

A wide variety of other adverse reactions have been reported in persons taking these drugs, but their relationship to the drugs themselves is unclear.

Contraindications

Complete biliary obstruction

Interactions

1 May interfere with oral absorption of anticoagulants, cephalexin, clindamycin, digitalis drugs, iron preparations, phenobarbital, phenylbutazone, thiazide diuretics, thyroid drugs, tetracyclines, trimethoprim, and vitamins A, D, E, and K

▶ NURSING ALERTS

▷ 1 Be alert for development of constipation, especially when dose is high or in elderly patients. Dosage may be lowered, or a stool softener or laxative may be used.

▷ 2 Observe patients for early symptoms of hypoprothrombinemia (vitamin K deficiency), such as petechiae, mucosal bleeding, and tarry stools. Parenteral vitamin K₁ is indicated. Recurrences can be prevented by oral administration of vitamin K (2.5 mg–10 mg).

▷ 3 Dissolve drugs as instructed before giving orally be-cause ingestion of powder itself is very irritating and may cause esophageal impaction.

▶ NURSING CONSIDERATIONS

▷ 1 Determine baseline serum cholesterol and triglyceride levels at start of therapy and at regular intervals during therapy.

▷ 2 Ensure that patients consume a high-bulk diet (fruit, raw vegetables) and maintain an adequate fluid intake to minimize constipation.

▷ 3 Mix powder in an appropriate vehicle (*e.g.,* flavored liquids, thin soups, juices) to disguise disagreeable taste (see Table 33-2).

▷ 4 Administer oral drugs at least 1 hour before or 4 hours following resin administration, if possible, to avoid interference with absorption.

▷ 5 Consider supplemental therapy with parenteral or water-miscible forms of vitamins A, D, E, and K in patients on prolonged resin therapy because vitamin deficiencies can occur.

▷ 6 Note that a dosage schedule has not been established for infants or children; if so used, initiate therapy with small doses and carefully observe patients, because hypochloremic acidosis has occurred in very young and very small patients.

▷ 7 Advise patients that GI side-effects usually subside with continued therapy.

▶ clofibrate

Atromid-S

Mechanism

Not definitively established; lowers elevated triglyceride and VLDL levels, possibly by increasing breakdown of free fatty acids in the liver via action of lipoprotein lipase; also, decreases release of VLDL from liver to plasma, and interferes with binding of free fatty acids to albumin; may slightly reduce plasma cholesterol and LDL, presumably by inhibiting cholesterol biosynthesis and increasing biliary and fecal excretion of cholesterol; reduces serum fibrinogen levels and platelet adhesiveness

Uses

1 Adjunctive therapy for reduction of elevated serum triglycerides and cholesterol in patients with type III hyperlipoproteinemia, and possibly in conjunction with bile sequestering resins in type II.b where serum triglyceride levels are elevated
2 Treatment of patients with xanthoma tuberosum (external nodules or lesions usually grouped about the joints, resulting from elevated blood lipids) associated with hyperlipidemia

Dosage

Adults: Initially 2 g/day in divided doses; adjust to desired response

Fate

Following administration, drug is hydrolyzed to p-chlorophenoxyisobutyric acid (CPIB), the active form of the drug, which is slowly but completely absorbed; peak CPIB plasma levels occur in 3 hours to 6 hours; plasma half-life ranges from 6 hours to 24 hours; much longer (up to 100 hr) in patients with renal impairment; highly protein bound (90%–95%); largely metabolized in the liver and excreted in the urine

Common Side-Effects

Nausea, dyspepsia, abdominal distress, and flatulence

Significant Adverse Reactions

GI—diarrhea, vomiting, gastritis, stomatitis, increased gallstones, hepatomegaly
Cardiovascular—arrhythmias, swelling, and phlebitis at site of xanthoma, angina, thromboembolic complications
Dermatologic—rash, urticaria, pruritus, alopecia, dry skin, dry hair
Hematologic—leukopenia, anemia, eosinophilia
Neurologic—drowsiness, weakness, dizziness, headache
Other—myalgia and "flu-like" symptoms, arthralgia, impotence, decreased libido, dysuria, hematuria, decreased urinary output, weight gain, polyphagia, abnormal liver function tests, hepatic tumors

Contraindications

Hepatic or renal dysfunction, primary biliary cirrhosis, pregnancy, and nursing mothers

Interactions

1 Clofibrate may enhance the effects of oral anticoagulants, antidiabetics, cholinesterase inhibitors, furosemide, and thyroxine.
2 Oral contraceptives and other estrogens can antagonize the action of clofibrate.
3 The effects of clofibrate may be enhanced by acidifying agents, neomycin, sitosterols, and thyroxine.

▶ NURSING ALERTS

Warning: Clofibrate has produced benign and malignant tumors in rats at 5 to 8 times the human dose. The drug has the potential to elicit hepatic tumors in humans, produce cholelithiasis (twice the risk of nonusers), and evoke a wide range of other untoward reactions. Due to these characteristics, coupled with the lack of substantial evidence for a beneficial effect for clofibrate on cardiovascular mortality, it should be reserved for those patients with *significant* hyperlipidemia and a high risk of coronary heart disease who have not responded adequately to diet, weight loss, and other less toxic drugs.

▷ 1 Urge strict birth-control measures by women of childbearing age taking clofibrate because fetal damage can occur. Withdraw drug several months prior to attempted conception.
▷ 2 Perform frequent liver function tests and blood counts during therapy, and withdraw drug if results are abnormal.
▷ 3 Use with caution in patients with a history of jaundice or hepatic disease, peptic ulcer, cardiac arrhythmias, gout, and in patients taking oral anticoagulants or hypoglycemic drugs.
▷ 4 Notify physician immediately if chest pain, dyspnea, irregular heartbeat, stomach pain, vomiting, fever, chills, sore throat, hematuria, oliguria, or swelling of the extremities occur.

▶ NURSING CONSIDERATIONS

▷ 1 Determine serum cholesterol and triglyceride levels before initiating therapy and at 2- to 4-week intervals during treatment.
▷ 2 Advise patients to report development of flu-like symptoms (muscle aching, weakness, soreness, cramping) because these may indicate a need for dosage reduction.
▷ 3 Observe patients for clinical response, and discontinue drug after 3 months if response is inadequate, except in treating xanthomas, in which case the drug may be continued for longer periods if there is a reduction in the number or size of lesions.
▷ 4 Note that a *rebound rise* in lipid levels my occur after 2 to 3 months of therapy, but that further decreases will then ensure.
▷ 5 Before initiating therapy, attempt to control serum lipids by diet, weight loss, and other nondrug measures. Stress importance of adherence to diet during therapy as well.

▶ dextrothyroxine

Choloxin

Mechanism

Synthetic d-isomer of thyroxine, possessing much less metabolic stimulating action than the naturally occurring l-isomer (l-thyroxine); reduces serum cholesterol and LDL levels but has no *consistent* effect on triglycerides or VLDL; accelerates breakdown of cholesterol in the liver resulting in increased biliary excretion

Uses

1 Adjunctive treatment for reduction of elevated cholesterol and LDL levels in type II (and possibly type III) euthyroid patients with no evidence of organic heart disease
2 Treatment of hypothyroidism in patients with cardiac disease who cannot tolerate other thyroid drugs

Dosage

Hypercholesterolemia

Adults: initially 1 mg to 2 mg/day; increase by 1-mg to 2-mg increments at monthly intervals to a maintenance range of 4 mg to 8 mg/day
Children: initially 0.05 mg/kg/day; increase by 0.05-mg/kg/month increments to desired level (usually 0.1 mg/kg/day)

Hypothyroidism

Initially, 1 mg; increase in 1-mg/month increments to optimal level (usually 4 mg/day)

Fate

Adequately absorbed from GI tract; metabolized by the liver and excreted in both the urine and feces

Common Side-Effects

Nervousness, sweating, flushing, palpitations, and dyspepsia

Significant Adverse Reactions

(Most frequent in hypothyroid patients or patients with organic heart disease)
Cardiovascular—angina, arrhythmias, myocardial damage, increased heart size
CNS—insomnia, tremors, headache, hyperthermia, dizziness, visual disturbances, tinnitus, paresthesia, psychic changes
GI—vomiting, diarrhea, anorexia
Other—hair loss, weight loss, diuresis, menstrual irregularities, altered libido, hoarseness, muscle pain, skin rash, gallstones, hyperglycemia, elevated PBI, worsening of peripheral vascular disease

Contraindications

Organic heart disease (angina, arrhythmias, myocardial infarction, congestive heart failure, rheumatic heart disease), hypertension (other than mild, labile forms), liver or kidney disease, pregnancy, and nursing mothers

Interactions

1 Dextrothyroxine may potentiate the effects of oral anticoagulants.
2 Toxic actions of digitalis preparations may be enhanced by dextrothyroxine.

3 Dextrothyroxine can antagonize the effects of oral hypoglycemics and insulin by increasing blood sugar levels.
4 Increased response to injections of epinephrine or norepinephrine (*e.g.*, episodes of coronary insufficiency) may occur in the presence of dextrothyroxine.

▶ NURSING ALERTS

▷ 1 Closely observe patients with previous or suspected cardiac disease for signs of increasing cardiac decompensation (*e.g.,* dyspnea, nocturnal coughing, pain on exertion, palpitations, edema), and advise physician immediately. Dose should be reduced or discontinued.
▷ 2 Advise patient to promptly report symptoms of iodism (excessive use of iodine-containing compounds) such as acneiform rash, itching, coryza, conjunctivitis); drug may have to be withdrawn.
▷ 3 Stress the necessity of adherence to birth-control measures in women of childbearing potential receiving dextrothyroxine because a risk of fetal damage exists.
▷ 4 In patients receiving digitalis therapy, do not exceed 4 mg dextrothyroxine per day because myocardial oxygen requirements may be dangerously elevated.

▶ NURSING CONSIDERATIONS

▷ 1 Note that increased serum PBI levels will occur in patients taking dextrothyroxine. Elevated levels indicate absorption and transport of the drug rather than a hypermetabolic state. Level in the range of 10 mcg% to 25 mcg% are common and do not necessitate dosage adjustment.
▷ 2 Observe diabetic patients carefully for loss of control (*e.g.,* glycosuria, polyuria, polydipsia) during dextrothyroxine therapy. Dosage adjustments may be needed (increase antidiabetic drugs or decrease dextrothyroxine).
▷ 3 Note that decreased cholesterol levels may not occur for several weeks after initiation of therapy and that maximal response may require 2 months to 3 months.
▷ 4 Discontinue drug at least 2 weeks prior to elective surgery to reduce danger of cardiac arrhythmias resulting from anesthesia or surgery.
▷ 5 Determine serum lipids prior to therapy and at monthly intervals thereafter during therapy.

▶ gemfibrozil

Lopid

Mechanism

Not completely established; lowers elevated serum triglycerides, primarily the VLDL fraction and less frequently the LDL fraction; may also increase the high-density lipoprotein fraction, an action also considered to be beneficial in atherosclerosis; biochemical mechanisms of action may include inhibition of peripheral lipolysis, reduction of liver triglyceride production, and impairment in the synthesis of VLDL carrier apoprotein; may also reduce incorporation of long-chain fatty acids into newly formed triglycerides and accelerate removal of cholesterol from the liver

Uses

1 Treatment of type IV hyperlipidemia in patients who do not respond to a dietary regimen, and who present a risk of abdominal pain and pancreatitis (*e.g.,* triglyceride levels in excess of 750 mg/dl)

Dosage

600 mg twice a day, 30 minutes before the morning and evening meal

Fate

Well absorbed from the GI tract; peak serum levels occur in 1 hour to 2 hours; plasma half-life is 1 hour to 2 hours; excreted in the urine largely as unchanged drug (70%) and some metabolites; small amounts are also eliminated in the feces

Common Side-Effects

Abdominal pain, diarrhea, and nausea

Significant Adverse Reactions

GI—vomiting, constipation, dry mouth, gas pain, anorexia
CNS—headache, dizziness, blurred vision, vertigo, insomnia, tinnitus, paresthesias
Musculoskeletal—arthralgia, back pain, myalgia, muscle cramping, swollen joints
Skin—rash, dermatitis, pruritus, urticaria
Hepatic—liver function abnormalities (increased SGOT, SGPT, LDH, CPK, alkaline phosphatase)
Other—anemia, eosinophilia, leukopenia, malaise, syncope, cholelithiasis

Contraindications

Hepatic or severe renal dysfunction, gallbladder disease

Interactions

1 Gemfibrozil may potentiate the effects of oral anticoagulants.

▶ NURSING ALERTS

Note: Due to pharmacologic similarities between gemfibrozil and clofibrate, the serious adverse effects reported in patients receiving clofibrate must be considered a possibility in patients receiving gemfibrozil as well. Refer to the discussion of clofibrate for details.

▷ 1 Perform periodic blood counts and liver function tests during therapy. If abnormalities persist for any length of time or worsen, discontinue the drug.
▷ 2 If signs and symptoms of gallbladder disease occur (*e.g.,* upper abdominal discomfort, bloating, belching, fried food intolerance), perform appropriate diagnostic studies and discontinue drug if gallstones are found.
▷ 3 Note that incidence of benign liver nodules and liver carcinomas was significantly increased in animals receiving 10 times the human dose. Administer the drug *only* to the patient population described under Uses.

▷ 4 Use with caution in patients with cardiac arrhythmias, in pregnant or nursing mothers, and in children.
▷ 5 Urge caution in performing hazardous tasks, especially in early stages of therapy, because drug may cause dizziness or blurred vision.

▶ NURSING CONSIDERATIONS

▷ 1 Stress the importance of adherence to prescribed diet and restriction of intake of sugars, cholesterol, saturated fats, and alcohol to the successful control of the hyperlipidemia.
▷ 2 Inform patients to advise physician if GI symptoms (abdominal pain, nausea, vomiting, diarrhea) persist or worsen. Dosage may have to be reduced or drug discontinued.
▷ 3 If lipid response is still inadequate after 3 months, as determined by laboratory serum lipid determinations, withdraw drug.

▶ nicotinic acid
Niacin

Nicotinic acid (vitamin B_3) is a water-soluble vitamin that is discussed in Chapter 75. In large doses, it can lower elevated plasma lipid levels and has been used as adjunctive therapy in certain types of hyperlipoproteinemias.

Mechanism

Not completely established; reduces lipolysis and release of free fatty acids from adipose tissue, and decreases hepatic synthesis of VLDL and triglycerides; LDL formation is also reduced; increases activity of lipoprotein lipase, and accelerates removal of chylomicron triglycerides; hepatic cholesterol synthesis may also be inhibited

Uses

1 Adjunctive therapy in treatment of hypercholesterolemia and hyperbetalipoproteinemia (types IIb, III, IV, and V) in patients who do not respond to diet and weight loss

Dosage

1 g to 2 g 3 times/day; increase slowly, first to 4.5 g, then to 6 g/day after several weeks if necessary

Fate

Readily absorbed orally; peak serum levels occur within 1 hour; elimination half-life is 45 minutes to 60 minutes; metabolized by the liver, and excreted as both metabolites and unchanged drug by the kidney

Common Side-Effects

GI distress, flushing, feeling of warmth, pruritus, and paresthesias

Significant Adverse Reactions

Headache, dizziness, palpitations, diarrhea, hypotension, hyperuricemia, gouty arthritis, skin rash, dermatoses, epigastric pain, jaundice, decreased glucose tolerance, activation of peptic ulcer, increased sebaceous gland activity, toxic amblyopia, and impaired liver function

Contraindications

Hepatic dysfunction, active peptic ulcer, severe hypotension, hemorrhaging, and gastritis

Interactions

1 Nicotinic acid may enhance the blood pressure lowering effects of antihypertensive medications.
2 Nicotinic acid may antagonize the effects of antidiabetic drugs by elevating blood glucose levels.

▶ NURSING ALERTS

▷ 1 Use cautiously in patients with allergic disorders, glaucoma, jaundice, gallbladder disease, diabetes, gout, and in pregnant or lactating women.
▷ 2 Perform frequent liver function tests and blood glucose determinations during early stages of therapy to determine if adverse effects are occurring.
▷ 3 Caution patients that hypotension with accompanying dizziness or weakness can occur following ingestion of nicotinic acid. Inform physician because dosage may need to be reduced.

▶ NURSING CONSIDERATIONS

▷ 1 Inform patients that drug should be taken with cold water, not hot beverages, to facilitate swallowing.
▷ 2 Note that reduction in serum lipids may be enhanced if tablets are chewed rather than swallowed whole, and ingested with large amounts of water.
▷ 3 Administer drug with food to minimize GI distress.

▶ probucol
Lorelco

Mechanism

Not determined; may inhibit hepatic synthesis of cholesterol at an early stage; does not affect later stages; increased excretion of fecal bile acids occurs, and absorption of dietary cholesterol may be impaired

Uses

1 Adjunctive therapy for the reduction of elevated serum cholesterol in type II hyperlipoproteinemia

Dosage

500 mg twice a day

Fate

Variable GI absorption; peak blood levels are higher and less variable when taken with food; accumulates in fatty tissues and very slowly eliminated

Common Side-Effects

Diarrhea, flatulence, abdominal pain, and nausea

Significant Adverse Reactions

Sweating, angio-edema, dizziness, palpitations, syncope, vomiting, chest pain, headache, paresthesias, eosinophilia, and reduced hemoglobin; abnormal liver function tests, and uric acid, blood urea nitrogen, and blood glucose levels have been reported.

Contraindications

Patients with cardiac arrhythmias or prolongation of the Q–T interval, pregnant or nursing mothers

▶ NURSING ALERTS

▷ 1 Advise women of childbearing potential to utilize birth-control measures during therapy and for several months thereafter because the possibility of drug-induced fetal damage exists.

▶ NURSING CONSIDERATIONS

▷ 1 Perform baseline serum cholesterol studies, and determine cholesterol levels frequently during initial months of therapy. Reductions should occur within first 2 months of therapy, and drug may be continued as long as a favorable trend continues.
▷ 2 Monitor serum triglycerides during probucol therapy; if levels are elevated and remain so, do not continue probucol therapy but switch to other drugs that reduce both cholesterol and triglycerides.
▷ 3 Administer drug with food to minimize GI upset and to provide more consistent blood levels.

Several other drugs have the capacity to lower elevated serum lipid levels, but are largely unsuitable for the treatment of hyperlipoproteinemia, primarily because of their high incidence of untoward reactions and the availability of more effective and less toxic agents. *Neomycin sulfate* reduces plasma cholesterol by blocking its gastric absorption, and lowers LDL levels as well, especially when given in combination with cholestyramine resin. However, neomycin is highly toxic (GI distress, ototoxicity, kidney damage) and is only employed in type II disease that is resistant to other forms of therapy.

Estrogens effectively lower cholesterol and LDL levels but may elevate triglycerides and VLDL. They are obviously unsuited for use in males because of their feminizing action, and they can result in thromboembolic disorders, abdominal pain, and pancreatitis in women. Administration of *norethindrone acetate,* a progestin, has decreased VLDL levels in some women with type V hyperlipoproteinemia. However, this agent has significant estrogenic activity and is therefore associated with many of the same adverse effects as the estrogens themselves.

Finally, although *heparin* can increase the conversion of triglycerides to free fatty acids, resulting in degradation of chylomicrons to soluble, dispersible complexes, heparin is of no clinical use as a hypolipemic drug because of its potential to cause hemorrhage and its need to be administered parenterally.

Summary. Hypolipemic Drugs

Drug	Preparations	Usual Dosage Range
Bile acid sequestering resins	See table 33-2.	
Clofibrate (Atromid-S)	Capsules—500 mg	2 g/day in divided doses; adjust to desired response
Dextrothyroxine (Choloxin)	Tablets—1 mg, 2 mg, 4 mg, 6 mg	Initially 1 mg to 2 mg/day; increase by 1-mg to 2-mg/month increments to desired response (usual range is 4 mg to 8 mg/day)
		Children—0.05 mg/kg/day increased by 0.05-mg/kg/month increments to desired level (usual dose is 0.1 mg/kg/day)
Gemfibrozil (Lopid)	Capsules—300 mg	600 mg twice a day, 30 minutes before the morning and evening meals
Nicotinic acid (Niacin)	Tablets—50 mg, 100 mg, 500 mg	1 g to 2 g 3 times/day, with or following meals; increase slowly to a maximum of 6 g/day
	Timed-release capsules—125 mg, 200 mg, 250 mg, 300 mg, 400 mg, 500 mg	
	Timed-release tablets—150 mg	
	Elixir—50 mg/5 ml	
	Injection—50 mg, 100 mg/ml	
Probucol (Lorelco)	Tablets—250 mg	500 mg twice a day

34 Antianemic Drugs

The term *anemia* describes a group of clinical conditions characterized by a reduction in the number of erythrocytes or in the hemoglobin concentration within erythrocytes, or both. Because oxygen is transported in the bloodstream primarily in combination with hemoglobin contained within the red blood cell, either condition will result in an impaired oxygen-carrying capacity of the blood and therefore inadequate tissue oxygenation.

Red cells are formed continually in the bone marrow, their synthesis requiring many nutrients, of which the most important are iron, folic acid, and vitamin B_{12} (cyanocobalamin). These substances are usually present in sufficient amounts in the diet; if they are adequately absorbed from the GI tract, erythrocyte formation and hemoglobin synthesis proceed normally. However, when the diet is deficient in any of these nutrients, or when their GI absorption is impaired, symptoms of anemia develop. Anemia may also result from extreme loss or destruction of red blood cells (*e.g.,* trauma, hemorrhage, excessive menstruation), thereby increasing the nutritional requirements above the level that can be supplied by diet alone.

Although anemias can occur in a number of ways (*e.g.,* deficiency or impaired availability of dietary factors, excessive destruction or loss of red blood cells, loss of bone marrow cells), most anemias are the result of inadequate amounts of iron, folic acid, or vitamin B_{12}, and so they are considered *deficiency* anemias. Correction of the deficiency has proven highly successful in treating these conditions, if an accurate diagnosis of the type of anemia as well as any underlying causative factor (*e.g.,* ulcers, malignancy) has been made.

Of the deficiency anemias, those that result from lack of iron are characterized by fewer than normal erythrocytes, which are frequently smaller (microcytic) and paler (hypochromic) than usual, because they contain less hemoglobin. These anemias are referred to as *microcytic* or *hypochromic*. Other hypochromic microcytic anemias result from failure to incorporate adequate iron into the developing cells, although an actual nutritional deficiency may not be present.

Anemias that occur because of insufficient levels of folic acid or vitamin B_{12} (*i.e.,* dietary deficiency, reduced absorption) are characterized by the presence of large, immature red cells (megaloblasts) in the bone marrow and blood, as well as enlarged erythrocytes (macrocytes) that may contain abnormally high levels of hemoglobin. These anemias are labeled *megaloblastic, macrocytic,* or *hyperchromic*. It should be noted that hypochromic and hyperchromic anemias seldom occur together, further underlining the importance of accurate diagnosis for proper replacement therapy. Likewise, carefully differentiating those anemias caused by nutritional iron deficiency from those caused by failure of iron incorporation into red blood cells is essential, because supplemental iron in the latter case is not only ineffective but can result in iron overload (hemochromatosis) and subsequent toxicity. The "shotgun" approach of combining many factors (*e.g.,* iron, B_{12}, folic acid) in treating anemias has no place in clinical medicine, and should never be used in lieu of careful diagnosis and *selective* replacement of the deficient factor, as well as correction of any underlying pathologic disorder.

The antianemic drugs to be discussed in this chapter include the iron preparations, folic acid, and vitamin B_{12}. In addition to these agents, therapy may also include other drugs and measures to correct any underlying abnormality that may be responsible for the anemia. Self-medication with any of the antianemic drugs should be strongly discouraged, because the apparent beneficial effects gained by treating oneself often may mask the symptoms of a more serious underlying disorder (*e.g.*, internal bleeding, neurologic dysfunction).

Oral Iron Preparations

Ferrous fumarate   Polysaccharide–iron complex
Ferrous gluconate   Soy protein–iron complex
Ferrous sulfate

The various types of preparations containing iron (capsules, tablets, liquids, injections) are used as replacement therapy in iron-deficiency anemias. The oral forms of therapy are preferred. Parenteral administration of iron is largely restricted to those persons who cannot tolerate oral iron because of its gastric irritative action, those who do not absorb sufficient iron from the GI tract, or those who are noncompliant. Oral iron is available in either the bivalent (ferrous) or trivalent (ferric) forms; bivalent iron is more widely used because it is better absorbed and somewhat less irritating than the trivalent form. An acid environment favors reduction of trivalent to bivalent iron, which increases absorption. GI distress can be reduced by using one of the iron complexes or sustained-release forms, but the absorption of elemental iron may be retarded with use of these specialized dosage forms, because much of their iron content may be released beyond the major iron absorptive sites in the duodenum and jejunum.

The oral iron preparations are essentially alike in terms of their pharmacologic action, because they all release elemental iron, and therefore are reviewed as a group. Individual salts and dosage forms are then listed in Table 34-1. The parenteral iron preparation, iron dextran, is then discussed in detail.

Mechanism

Provide replacement for insufficient iron, thereby correcting the hemoglobin and tissue iron deficiency; iron is

Table 34-1. Oral Iron Preparations

Drug	Preparations	Usual Dosage Range	Remarks
Ferrous fumarate (Feco-T, Feostat, Fumasorb, Fumerin, Hemocyte, Ircon, Palmiron, Toleron)	Tablets—195 mg, 200 mg, 300 mg, 324 mg, 325 mg Chewable tablets—100 mg Timed-release tablets—324 mg Suspension—100 mg/5 ml Drops—45 mg/0.6 ml	Adults—200 mg 1 to 4 times/day Children (under 6)—100 mg to 300 mg/day in divided doses	Contains 33% elemental iron; essentially similar to ferrous sulfate in most respects, with slightly lower incidence of some GI side-effects; available in combination with docusate as timed-release capsules (Ferocyl, Ferro-Sequels)
Ferrous gluconate (Fergon, Ferralet, Simron)	Tablets—300 mg, 320 mg, 325 mg Capsules—86 mg, 325 mg, 435 mg Elixir—300 mg, 325 mg/5 ml	Adults—300 mg to 640 mg 3 times/day Children (6 yr–12 yr)—300 mg 1 to 3 times/day Children (under 6)—100 mg to 300 mg/day in divided doses	Contains 11.6% elemental iron; somewhat better tolerated and better utilized than other forms of iron; lower incidence of GI distress; available in combination with polysorbate 20 as Simron
Ferrous sulfate (Feosol, Fer-In-Sol, Fer Iron, Ferralyn, Fero-Gradumet, Ferospace. Ferusal, Fumaral, Hematinic, Iromal, Mol-Iron, Slow FE)	Tablets—195 mg, 200 mg, 300 mg, 325 mg Capsules—190 mg Timed-release capsules—150 mg, 167 mg, 225 mg, 250 mg, 390 mg Timed-release tablets—160 mg, 324 mg, 525 mg Syrup—90 mg/5 ml Elixir—220 mg/5 ml Liquid—195 mg/4 ml Drops—75 mg/0.6 ml; 125 mg/ml	Adults—300 mg to 1200 mg/day in divided doses Children (6 yr–12 yr)—120 mg to 600 mg/day in divided doses Children (under 6 years)—300 mg/day in divided doses	Contains 20% elemental iron; most widely used form of oral iron; best absorbed and least expensive; high degree of GI irritation that can be minimized by using sustained-release forms; available in combination with magnesium–aluminum hydroxide as Fermalox
Polysaccharide–iron complex (Hytinic, Niferex, Nu-Iron)	Tablets—50 mg iron Capsules—150 mg iron Elixir—100 mg iron/5 ml	Adults—50 mg to 300 mg/day in divided doses as required Children—50 mg to 100 mg/day	Water-soluble complex of elemental iron and a low molecular weight polysaccharide; fewer GI side-effects than with other forms of iron, no teeth staining, and no metallic aftertaste; fairly expensive
Soy protein–iron Complex (Fe-Plus)	Tablets—50 mg iron	50 mg 3 times/day	Iron–protein complex made with specially isolated soy protein; should be taken with meals

an essential component of hemoglobin because transport of oxygen by hemoglobin requires molecular iron in the bivalent state; corrects the abnormal red blood cell picture

Uses

1 Prevention and treatment of iron-deficiency anemias
2 Prophylactic therapy during periods of increased iron requirements, *e.g.,* pregnancy, rapid growth, and sustained hemorrhaging

Dosage

See Table 34-1.

Fate

Absorption occurs at most levels of the GI tract, although it is very poor; only 5% to 10% of dose is absorbed in normal persons and up to 20% in iron-deficient patients; bivalent iron can pass directly into the bloodstream, where it is bound to transferrin; a fraction of absorbed bivalent iron is converted to the trivalent form in epithelial cells, and combined with the protein apoferritin to yield ferritin; iron in the plasma circulates bound to transferrin, a protein that is ordinarily 33% saturated with iron, although the percent can vary depending on the physiologic state of the patient; distributed to storage sites in bone marrow, liver, spleen, and hemoglobin; excretion occurs mainly in the feces through sloughing of iron-containing mucosal cells of the bowel; smaller amounts are found in the bile, urine, and sweat; readily crosses the placental barrier, and is also present in breast milk

Common Side-Effects

GI irritation, nausea, constipation

Significant Adverse Reactions

(Usually result of overdosage) Vomiting, diarrhea, allergic reactions, drowsiness, abdominal pain, stomach and intestinal erosion, hypotension, weak pulse, shock, convulsions, cardiovascular collapse, and liver necrosis

Contraindications

Peptic ulcer, ulcerative colitis, hemochromatosis, hemosiderosis, hemolytic anemia, and cirrhosis of the liver

Interactions

1 Absorption of iron may be impaired by antacids (especially those containing magnesium trisilicate), cholestyramine, pancreatic extracts, as well as by ingestion of eggs or milk.
2 Oral iron retards absorption of tetracyclines.
3 Effectiveness of iron may be impaired by vitamin E, hydroxyurea, and oral contraceptives.
4 Vitamin C may facilitate iron absorption.
5 Chloramphenicol can delay clearance of iron from the plasma.
6 Allopurinol may interfere with the action of an enzyme that controls iron absorption, leading to excessive absorption.

▶ NURSING ALERTS

▷ 1 Caution patients against self-medication with iron preparations because this may mask symptoms of a more severe underlying disease.

▶ NURSING CONSIDERATIONS

▷ 1 Inform patients that iron preparations can cause black or dark green stools, which are *not* usually a sign of GI bleeding.
▷ 2 Administer iron preparations with food, if necessary, to minimize GI irritation (absorption may be further impaired, however). Avoid giving milk or antacids, because they may also retard GI absorption of iron.
▷ 3 Instruct patients taking liquid forms of iron to use a straw for administration because preparation can stain teeth. Suggest immediate rinsing of mouth following drug ingestion to prevent tooth discoloration.
▷ 4 Perform blood counts and hemoglobin determination before prescribing iron. Assess dietary iron intake, if possible, and note other drugs that patient is taking that may contribute to the observed anemia (*e.g.,* quinidine, anti-inflammatory drugs, sulfonamides).
▷ 5 Monitor hemoglobin and reticulocyte values periodically during therapy. Improvement should be noted within 2 weeks to 4 weeks; if not, reassessment is warranted.
▷ 6 Inform patients that GI disturbances (irritation, cramping, constipation) are common in initial stages of therapy, but can usually be minimized by reducing dose, taking drug with food, or by changing the type of preparation being taken.
▷ 7 Note that oral iron preparations are available in combination with many other drugs (*e.g.,* B and C vitamins, folic acid, dessicated liver, antacids, and stool softeners).

▶ iron dextran

Feostat, Ferotran, Hematran, Hydextran, I.D.-50, Imferon, Irodex, K-Feron, Norferan, Proferdex

Iron dextran is a complex of ferric hydroxide with dextran in physiologic saline used either IV or IM for treating iron-deficiency anemias in patients intolerant of or resistant to oral iron preparations.

Mechanism

Hydrolysis of the iron–dextran complex by reticuloendothelial cells of liver, spleen, and bone marrow releases ferric iron, which combines with transferrin and is transported to the bone marrow to be used in the synthesis of hemoglobin.

Uses

1 Treatment of iron-deficiency anemias in patients where oral iron administration is ineffective or poorly tolerated

Dosage

(1 ml iron dextran complex equals 50 mg elemental iron)
To determine quantity of iron needed, the following formula
may be used:

$$0.3 \times \text{wt (lb)} \times \left(100 - \frac{\text{g\% Hb} \times 100}{14.8}\right) = \text{mg iron}$$

A more practical rule is 250 mg iron for each gram of hemoglobin below normal.

IM: test dose of 25 mg (*i.e.,* 0.5 ml) on first day to test
for allergic reactions; if no evidence of hypersensitivity
within 1 hour to 2 hours, the remainder of the first
day's dose can be given. Each day's dose should not
exceed 25 mg iron for infants under 10 lb, 50 mg iron
for children under 20 lb, 100 mg iron for patients
under 110 lb, and 250 mg iron for other patients until
the calculated total dose has been given.

IV: 0.5 ml first day; increase to 2 ml/day within 2 to 3
days, and continue until total calculated dose has been
given.

Oral iron should be discontinued prior to administration
of iron dextran, to prevent iron overload.

Fate

Slowly but well absorbed from IM injection sites (60%
within 2–3 days and 90% within 1 week–2 weeks); distributed
through the reticuloendothelial system; excreted in urine,
bile, and feces

Common Side-Effects

Paresthesias, nausea

Significant Adverse Reactions

Anaphylactic reactions, other hypersensitivity reactions
(rash, pruritus, urticaria, dyspnea, arthralgia, fever, chills,
sweating, myalgia), soreness and inflammation at injection
site, brown discoloration and sterile abscesses at IM injection
sites, headache, vomiting, shivering, hypotension, lymphadenopathy, peripheral flushing, local phlebitis (IV injection), chest pain, tachycardia, arrhythmias, and convulsions

Contraindications

Anemias other than iron-deficiency anemias, marked liver
impairment, and pregnancy

▶ NURSING ALERTS

▷ 1 Be aware that fatal anaphylactic-type reactions have
occurred with iron–dextran injection. Always administer initial small test dose to determine patient's sensitivity, and carefully observe for signs of hypersensitivity. Have epinephrine (1:1000) solution available
for treating acute hypersensitivity reactions

▷ 2 Use IV only in patients with insufficient muscle mass,
impaired IM absorptive capacity (*e.g.,* edema), and
uncontrolled bleeding, or in cases in which massive
or prolonged therapy is indicated.

▷ 3 Be aware that multiple dose vials contain a preservative
(phenol) and should not be used IV.

▷ 4 Use cautiously in patients with asthma or a history of
allergies, rheumatoid arthritis, liver impairment, ankylosing spondylitis, and in women of childbearing
potential.

▶ NURSING CONSIDERATIONS

▷ 1 Administer IM injections into upper, outer buttock
area using a large (19-gauge–20-gauge, 2-in-3-in)
needle. Use Z-track technique to avoid leakage into
and staining of overlying subcutaneous tissue (see
Chap. 1). Do not inject more than 5 ml at one IM
injection site.

▷ 2 Instruct patient receiving injection to bear weight on
leg opposite to injection site if standing, or position
patient in lateral position with injection site uppermost
if lying down.

▷ 3 Perform periodic determinations of hemoglobin, hematocrit, and reticulocytes during therapy, and initiate
oral iron therapy as soon as it is feasible.

▷ 4 Keep patient recumbent for 30 minutes to 60 minutes
following IV administration to minimize orthostatic
hypotension.

▷ 5 Note that iron–dextran administration may increase
pain and swelling associated with rheumatoid arthritis.

▷ 6 Do not mix other drugs in solution with iron–dextran.

▶ cyanocobalamin, crystalline

Betalin 12, Redisol, Rubramin PC, and various other manufacturers

Cyanocobalamin (vitamin B_{12}) is a cobalt-containing substance essential for normal growth, cell reproduction, hematopoiesis, and nucleoprotein synthesis. It is a biologically
potent compound, so only minute amounts (1 mcg–2 mcg)
are necessary in the daily diet to supply the normal body
needs. The most common cause of vitamin B_{12} deficiency
is insufficient GI absorption, due primarily to reduced availability of the intrinsic factor, a glycoprotein secreted by the
gastric mucosal cells that is necessary for adequate absorption
of B_{12}. This condition is referred to as pernicious anemia
and is characterized hematologically by megaloblasts in the
bone marrow and macrocytes in the plasma. The patient
feels fatigued, and frequently there are GI and neurologic
complications. Symptoms are usually readily reversed by
supplemental injections of cyanocobalamin crystalline.

Cyanocobalamin is available over-the-counter for oral use
as tablets and by prescription for IM or SC injection. Tablets
containing less than 500 mcg are *not* intended for treatment
of pernicious anemia, but should only be used as nutritional
supplements (see Chap. 75).

Mechanism

Provides needed vitamin B_{12} to reverse the deficiency
state resulting from inadequate GI absorption of dietary B_{12};
allows megaloblasts to mature into normal erythrocytes; improves GI function, relieves most neurologic symptoms (*e.g.,*
numbness, tingling, confusion, incoordination), and arrests
further neurologic damage

Uses

1 Treatment of vitamin B$_{12}$ deficiency states caused by impaired GI absorption (*e.g.,* pernicious anemia, GI dysfunction or surgery, tapeworm infestation, sprue)
2 Prevention of vitamin B$_{12}$ deficiency resulting from increased requirements (*e.g.,* pregnancy, hemorrhage, malignancy, thyroid, liver or renal disease) or inadequate dietary intake (*e.g.,* poverty, famine, alcoholism, vegetarian diet)
3 Performance of the Vitamin B$_{12}$ absorption test (Schilling test)

Dosage
(Variable depending on extent of vitamin B$_{12}$ deficiency)

Pernicious anemia
Adults:
Oral—1000 mcg/day (if GI absorption is impaired)
IM, SC—30 mcg/day for 5 to 10 days, then 100 mcg to 200 mcg/month
Children: 100 mcg/dose to a total of 1 mg to 5 mg over 2 weeks, then 60 mcg/month

Schilling test
1000 mcg IM 2 hours after an oral dose of radioactive cobalt-B$_{12}$ (0.5 mcg–1 mcg); urine collected for 24 hours and radioactivity is measured; impaired absorption indicated by less than 5% urinary excretion of vitamin B$_{12}$ (normal is 10%–30%)

Fate
GI absorption depends on presence of intrinsic factor, which binds vitamin B$_{12}$ to protect it from intestinal microorganisms; well absorbed from IM injection sites; small (less than 50 mcg) injected doses largely retained by the body; larger doses excreted rapidly (50%–90% within 48 hr; most within 8 hr) by the kidney

Common Side-Effects
(Usually with parenteral therapy) Transient diarrhea, itching, and flushing

Significant Adverse Reactions
Polycythemia vera, peripheral vascular thrombosis, exanthema, hypokalemia, pulmonary edema, congestive heart failure, and anaphylactic shock

Contraindications
Cobalt hypersensitivity, optic nerve damage

Interactions

1 GI absorption of cyanocobalamin may be impaired by alcohol, p-aminosalicylic acid, colchicine, neomycin, and potassium chloride.
2 Chloramphenicol may antagonize the beneficial therapeutic response to vitamin B$_{12}$.

▶ **NURSING ALERTS**
▷ 1 Administer vitamin B$_{12}$ parenterally in cases of pernicious anemia, because oral administration is unreliable, and prolonged oral therapy may therefore result in permanent neurologic complications.

▷ 2 Monitor serum potassium levels prior to treatment and regularly during initial days of therapy. Improvement of condition increases erythrocyte potassium requirements and may result in severe hypokalemia, possibly with a fatal outcome.
▷ 3 Be alert for symptoms of pulmonary edema (*e.g.,* dyspnea, night cough), which can occur early in therapy with vitamin B$_{12}$.
▷ 4 Determine if megaloblastic anemia is caused by folic acid or vitamin B$_{12}$ deficiency. Although folic acid may improve some symptoms of vitamin B$_{12}$ deficient anemias, exclusive use of folic acid could result in irreversible neurologic damage.

▶ **NURSING CONSIDERATIONS**
▷ 1 Obtain a dietary history in all patients taking vitamin B$_{12}$, and attempt to correct diet deficiencies. Because single vitamin B$_{12}$ deficiency is rare, multiple vitamin supplementation is often indicated.
▷ 2 Recognize that persons taking most antibiotics or methotrexate will not exhibit valid vitamin B$_{12}$ or folic acid blood assays.
▷ 3 Note that therapeutic response to drug therapy is generally rapid (within 48 hr) as measured by improved blood picture, lessening of GI and neurologic symptoms, and decreased fatigue. Reticulocyte counts rise in 3 to 4 days, peak in 7 to 8 days, then gradually decline as erythrocyte and hemoglobin rise.
▷ 4 Administer oral vitamin B$_{12}$ with meals to increase absorption (food stimulates production of intrinsic factor). Avoid mixing drug with citrus juices, because ascorbic acid may adversely affect the stability of vitamin B$_{12}$.
▷ 5 Advise patient to report the development of an infection, because decreased vitamin B$_{12}$ effectiveness can result. Dosage may have to be temporarily increased.
▷ 6 Stress the importance of *continual* vitamin B$_{12}$ therapy in patients with pernicious anemia. Interruption of treatment can result in progressive neurologic damage.
▷ 7 Recognize that doses of vitamin B$_{12}$ greater than 10 mcg/day may mask symptoms of folate deficiency. Check with physician before using multiple B vitamin preparations.

▷ *Dietary precautions*
▷ 1 Be aware that strict vegetarian diets can lead to vitamin B$_{12}$ deficiency. Good sources of vitamin B$_{12}$ are red meats, liver, egg yolk, dairy products, clams, oysters, and sardines.
▷ 2 Caution patients against excessive alcohol intake because malabsorption of vitamin B$_{12}$ can occur.

▶ **hydroxocobalamin, crystalline**
AlphaRedisol, Neo-Betalin 12 and various other manufacturers

Hydroxocobalamin is a source of vitamin B$_{12}$ similar in actions, indications, and untoward reactions to cyanocobalamin. It is more slowly absorbed than cyanocobalamin, resulting in a more sustained rise in serum cobalamin levels and less urinary excretion of cobalamin following each injection, and may be taken up by the liver in larger quantities than cyanocobalamin. Its therapeutic advantage over regular vitamin B_{12} injection is questionable, however. IM dosage is 30 mcg/day for 5 to 10 days, then 100 mcg/month as maintenance. Mild pain and irritation at injection site has been reported.

▶ folic acid
Folvite

Folic acid or folate (vitamin B_9) is a member of the B-complex vitamin group essential for synthesis of nucleoproteins and maintenance of normal erythrocyte production. Folic acid stimulates production of red and white blood cells as well as platelets in megaloblastic anemias. Dietary folate is converted in the body to a metabolite, tetrahydrofolic acid, which functions as a coenzyme in many reactions, especially the synthesis of purine and pyrimidine precursors of nucleic acids. Folate is available in many different foods (*e.g.,* vegetables, milk, eggs, liver), so deficiencies rarely occur. Most likely causes are malnutrition, greatly increased demands (*e.g.,* repeated pregnancy), and malabsorption syndromes such as sprue or celiac disease. Patients lacking sufficient folic acid usually develop a megaloblastic anemia similar to that observed in pernicious anemia, although the incidence of neurologic damage is much less than the damage observed in cases of vitamin B_{12} deficiency. Oral or parenteral administration of folic acid readily corrects the anemia, both symptomatically and hematologically, and improvement can be maintained by very small daily doses of folic acid.

Mechanism
Converted to tetrahydrofolic acid, which is essential for proper synthesis of purines and pyrimidines, and ultimately nucleic acids; deficiency of folic acid impairs production of bone marrow blood cell precursors.

Uses
1   Treatment of megaloblastic anemias caused by deficiency of folic acid, as seen in malnutrition, alcoholism, pregnancy, infancy, sprue or celiac disease

Dosage
Initially 0.25 mg to 1.0 mg daily; maintenance is 0.1 mg to 0.4 mg daily depending on age; 0.8 mg daily for pregnant or lactating women

Fate
Well absorbed from GI tract; maximum effect in 30 minutes to 60 minutes; highly bound to plasma proteins; metabolized in the liver, primarily to a biologically active form; excreted largely by the kidney

Common Side-Effects
(Rare) Flushing following IV injection

Significant Adverse Reactions
(Rare) Allergic reactions (rash, itching, bronchospasm), GI distress, irritability, confusion, and depression

Interactions
1   Effects of folic acid may be decreased by barbiturates, chloramphenicol, oral contraceptives, phenytoin, and primidone.
2   Folic acid may reduce phenytoin blood levels, requiring an increase in dosage.
3   Trimethoprim, triamterene, and pyrimethamine may interfere with utilization of folic acid.

▶ NURSING ALERTS
▷ 1   Be aware that use of folic acid may obscure some symptoms of pernicious anemia by improving hematologic picture. Irreversible neurologic damage could result.
▷ 2   Determine if a mixed megaloblastic anemia is present before administration, and replace vitamin B_{12} only if it is lacking.

▶ NURSING CONSIDERATIONS
▷ 1   Note that beneficial effects of folate therapy can appear within 24 hours (decreased malaise, improved outlook), while improvements in hematologic picture require 3 to 5 days.
▷ 2   Increase normal dosage levels in the presence of alcoholism, hemolytic anemia, chronic infection, and anticonvulsant therapy (especially with hydantoins).
▷ 3   Caution patients against self-medication with folic acid, because this may delay recognition of other types of anemias.
▷ 4   Use orally except in cases of known GI malabsorption. IM, IV, or SC administration can be employed in severe diseases or if GI absorption is impaired.

▷ *Dietary precautions*
▷ 1   Advise patients that foods high in folates include green vegetables, fruits, liver, and yeasts. Note that much of the folate content is destroyed by prolonged cooking or canning.

▶ leucovorin calcium
Folinic Acid

Leucovorin is the active metabolite of folic acid that is used IM to treat folate-deficient megaloblastic anemia when oral folic acid therapy is not feasible. The drug is also indicated for ''leucovorin rescue,'' that is, to minimize the cellular toxicity resulting from large doses of methotrexate used in certain neoplastic diseases. Leucovorin prevents severe methotrexate-induced toxicity by preferentially protecting or ''rescuing'' normal cells from the action of folic acid antagonists such as methotrexate without interfering with the desired oncolytic action of the drug. This cellular protective function is considered further in Chapter 74.

In treating megaloblastic anemia, leucovorin is administered IM in a dose of 1 mg/day. It should not be used in anemias secondary to a vitamin B_{12} deficiency, because the hematologic picture may improve, while the neurologic deficit continues to accrue. Allergic reactions represent the principal group of adverse reactions.

Summary. Antianemic Drugs

Drug	Preparations	Usual Dosage Range
Oral iron preparations	See Table 34-1	
Iron dextran (Feostat, Ferotran, Hematran, Hydextran, I.D.-50, Imferon, Irodex, K-Feron, Norferan, Proferdex)	Injection—ferric hydroxide and dextran equivalent to 50 mg iron/ml	See text
Cyanocobalamin, crystalline (Betalin 12, Redisol, Rubramin PC, and various other manufacturers)	Tablets—500 mcg, 1000 mcg Injection—30 mcg, 100 mcg, 120 mcg, 1000 mcg/ml (See also Chap. 75)	Adults: Oral—1000 mcg/day (if absorption is impaired) SC, IM—30 mcg/day for 5 to 10 days, then 100 mcg to 200 mcg/month Children: 100 mcg/dose to a total of 1 mg to 5 mg over 2 weeks, then 60 mcg/month
Hydroxocobalamin, crystalline (AlphaRedisol, Neo-Betalin 12, and various other manufacturers)	Injection—1000 mcg/ml	IM—30 mcg/day for 5 to 10 days, then 100 mcg/month
Folic acid (Folvite)	Tablets—0.1 mg, 0.4 mg, 0.8 mg, 1.0 mg Injection—5 mg/ml	Initially 0.25 mg to 1.0 mg/day Maintenance is 0.1 mg to 0.4 mg/day depending on age; 0.8 mg/day for pregnant women
Leucovorin calcium (Folinic acid)	Injection—3 mg, 10 mg/ml	Megaloblastic anemia—IM is 1 mg/day; Leucovorin Rescue—see Chap. 74

The process of blood clot formation, and subsequent clot resolution or lysis, is characterized by a chemically complex series of events that involves the interaction of a large number of substances (factors) present in blood plasma, blood cells (especially thrombocytes), and, to a lesser extent, body tissues. The overall reaction can be summarized as follows:

1 *Stage I*—formation of prothrombin activator either through an extrinsic (extravascular) or intrinsic (intravascular) mechanism
2 *Stage II*—conversion of prothrombin to thrombin
3 *Stage III*—conversion of fibrinogen to fibrin, and subsequent clot formation
4 *Stage IV*—dissolution of fibrin by fibrinolysin, and clot resolution or breakdown

Drugs capable of affecting the coagulation process generally act on one or more of the stages outlined above. Agents preventing the formation of new clots are termed *anticoagulants*. Drugs increasing the rate of resolution (or lysis) of preformed clots are referred to as *thrombolytic agents*. Compounds enhancing blood clot formation, thereby reducing bleeding, are characterized as *hemostatic drugs*.

Anticoagulant, Thrombolytic, and Hemostatic Drugs

35

I Anticoagulant Drugs

Therapy with anticoagulant drugs is directed primarily toward preventing development of intravascular thromboses, a major cause of death in the various kinds of thromboembolic disorders. Although these compounds are widely used, therapy with them is still largely empirical, and their efficacy in treating some conditions for which they are utilized has been questioned. Moreover, they are potentially dangerous drugs, capable of causing severe, possibly fatal hemorrhaging, and therefore must be carefully prescribed and closely monitored. *Long-term* therapy with anticoagulant drugs remains a controversial area; nevertheless, when judiciously selected and properly employed, the various anticoagulant agents have an important place in clinical therapy, and can markedly reduce the incidence of vascular clotting.

There are two classes of therapeutically useful anticoagulant drugs, the parenteral and oral agents. Heparin is the sole representative of the parenteral class, while the oral anticoagulant group encompasses several drugs, characterized as coumarin derivatives. Following a separate discussion of heparin, the oral anticoagulants are discussed as a group, followed by a listing of individual drugs. Mention is also made under this heading of both protamine sulfate, a heparin antagonist, and vitamin K and its derivatives, which are antagonists of the oral anticoagulant drugs.

Parenteral Anticoagulant

▶ **heparin sodium**
Lipo-Hepin, Liquaemin

▶ heparin calcium
Calciparine

Heparin is a mucopolysaccharide extracted from bovine lung or porcine intestinal tissue. Its potency is standardized by a biological assay and is expressed in units. The compound is a strong organic acid, possessing an electronegative charge that is essential for its anticoagulant activity. Blood clotting is inhibited *in vivo* as well as *in vitro,* and the effects of heparin are noted immediately upon administration. Heparin is usually given as the sodium salt but is also available as heparin calcium, which is equally effective.

Mechanism
Accelerates the rate at which antithrombin III, an alpha-2-globulin produced by the liver, inactivates factors IX, X, XI and XII, as well as thrombin; conversion of fibrinogen to fibrin is blocked, and activation of the fibrin-stabilizing factor (XIII) is also impaired; the rate-limiting step in the coagulation cascade is activation of factor X, which is inhibited by lower doses of heparin than those needed to neutralize thrombin, thus, prophylactic therapy is accomplished with much lower doses than those necessary once the coagulation process has begun; may also reduce platelet adhesiveness; no fibrinolytic activity but may exert a diuretic and hypolipemic action

Uses
1 Prophylaxis and treatment of venous thromboses, pulmonary embolism, and atrial fibrillation with embolization
2 Prevention of postoperative deep venous thrombosis and pulmonary embolism in patients undergoing major (abdominothoracic, cardiac, arterial) surgery (low-dose regimen)
3 Prevention of cerebral thrombosis in evolving stroke
4 Diagnosis and treatment of acute and chronic consumption coagulopathies (disseminated intravascular coagulation)
5 Prevention of peripheral venous thrombosis following acute myocardial infarction
6 Anticoagulant in blood transfusion, dialysis procedures, blood samples for laboratory procedures, and extracorporeal circulation

Dosage
The dosage depends upon the patient's coagulation tests. Dosage is adequate when whole blood clotting time is 2.5 to 3 times the control value *or* the partial thromboplastin time (PTT) is 1.5 to 2.5 times the control value.

Anticoagulation
SC: 10,000 to 20,000 units initially, then 8000 to 20,000 units every 8 hours to 12 hours
IV injection: 10,000 units initially, then 5000 to 10,000 units every 4 hours to 6 hours
IV infusion: 20,000 to 40,000 units/day in 1000 ml of isotonic sodium chloride solution, preceded by a 5000-unit IV loading dose

Postoperative prophylaxis
SC: 5000 units 2 hours before surgery and 5000 units every 8 hours to 12 hours for 7 days following surgery

Heart/blood vessel surgery
IV: 150 units/kg to 400 units/kg depending on length of surgery

Blood transfusion
7500 units/100 ml sterile Sodium Chloride Injection; 6 ml to 8 ml of dilution is added per 100 ml whole blood

Laboratory samples
70 to 150 units/10 ml to 20 ml whole blood sample

Fate
Not active orally; immediate onset IV, with peak effect in 5 minutes to 10 minutes and duration of 2 hours to 6 hours; gradually absorbed SC, with onset of 30 minutes to 60 minutes, and duration of 8 hours to 12 hours; highly bound to plasma proteins; metabolized by the liver, and slowly excreted in the urine; not found in appreciable amounts in the fetus or breast milk

Common Side-Effects
Spontaneous bleeding, local irritation at SC and IM injection sites

Significant Adverse Reactions
Hemorrhaging, hypersensitivity (chills, urticaria, fever, rhinitis, asthmatic-like reaction, lacrimation, diarrhea, anaphylactic reaction), vasospastic reaction, acute reversible thrombocytopenia, delayed (*i.e.,* 8–12 days) thrombocytopenia, alopecia, osteoporosis, and impaired renal function

Contraindications
Active bleeding or significant bleeding tendencies (*e.g.,* hemophilia, purpura, thrombocytopenia), presence of a drainage tube, and threatened abortion

Interactions
1 Increased risk of bleeding can occur if heparin is used in combination with oral anticoagulants, salicylates and other anti-inflammatory drugs, cancer chemotherapeutic agents, dextran, guaifenesin, dipyridamole, probenecid, or quinine.
2 Anticoagulant action of heparin may be partially antagonized by antihistamines, hydroxyzine, nicotine, digitalis, phenothiazines, tetracyclines, and vitamin C.
3 Heparin markedly elevates levels of free thyroxin, possibly resulting in arrhythmias.

▶ NURSING ALERTS
▷ 1 Use with extreme caution in any condition where there is increased risk of hemorrhage, *e.g.,* following surgery of the brain, eye, or spinal cord, shock, severe hypertension, jaundice, ulcerative lesions, and indwelling catheters.
▷ 2 Do not administer to any patient who cannot be kept under careful observation with periodic coagulation

tests, such as partial thromboplastin time (PTT). Careful titration of dosage based upon test results is critical for effective and safe therapy.

▷ 3 Observe patient carefully for signs of unusual bleeding (*e.g.,* discoloration of urine or feces, bruising) as well as low back pain which may indicate abdominal bleeding, and report these signs immediately.

▷ 4 Use cautiously in patients with a history of allergy (heparin is derived from animal tissue), renal or hepatic disease, alcoholism, during menstruation, pregnancy, or the immediate postpartum period, and when administering acid citrate dextrose (A.C.D.)-converted blood, because heparin activity persists for several weeks following conversion of such blood.

▷ 5 Be alert for early signs of an allergic reaction (chills, fever, itching, dyspnea), and advise physician immediately.

▷ 6 Perform platelet counts prior to beginning therapy and at regular intervals thereafter, and examine patient for bruises or petechiae, which are signs of possible thrombocytopenia. A delayed form of thrombocytopenia occurs 8 to 12 days after initiation of therapy, is often severe and may be associated with a significant risk of hemorrhage and paradoxical thromboembolism.

▷ 7 Avoid IM administration, because hematoma can occur.

▷ 8 Have available protamine sulfate, a specific heparin antagonist, as well as whole blood or plasma in case of heparin overdosage. Monitor vital signs during therapy.

▶ **NURSING CONSIDERATIONS**

▷ 1 Determine clotting time prior to each SC or IV injection, and at 4-hour intervals during early stages of IV infusion.

▷ 2 Give SC injection deep into fatty layers of abdomen or above iliac crest to minimize local irritation. Alternate injection sites and observe for hematoma. Do not aspirate syringe. Use the "bunching" technique or the Z-track method (see Chap. 1).

▷ 3 Be aware that resistance to heparin may be encountered in patients with infections, thrombophlebitis, thrombosis, myocardial infarction, and cancer, and in postoperative patients. Advise physician if fever or other symptoms of infection develop during heparin therapy.

▷ 4 When administering heparin with oral anticoagulants, allow at least 5 hours after the last IV dose and 24 hours after the last SC dose before drawing blood for a prothrombin time. Heparin may be withdrawn when prothrombin activity is in the desired range following oral anticoagulant therapy. Administration of oral anticoagulant usually overlaps heparin for 3 to 5 days.

▷ 5 Advise patients that diuresis can occur following heparin therapy. During prolonged treatment, suggest potassium supplementation (*e.g.,* orange juice, bananas).

▷ 6 Note that heparin is available as dilute solutions (10 units or 100 units/ml) in saline for use as an IV flush (Heparin Sodium Lock Flush Solution) to maintain the patency of indwelling IV catheters; these dilute solutions are *not* intended for therapeutic use.

▷ 7 Reassure patient that alopecia, if it occurs, is temporary.

▷ 8 Caution patients against indiscriminate use of alcohol or over-the-counter preparations containing aspirin or the cough suppressant guaifenesin because these may alter the response to heparin.

Heparin Antagonist

▶ **protamine sulfate**

Protamine sulfate is a mixture of proteins exhibiting a strongly positive charge that is capable of chemically combining with heparin, producing a stable salt, and thereby neutralizing the anticoagulant action of heparin. However, it may exert an anticoagulant effect when administered alone or when dosage exceeds that required to neutralize heparin.

Uses

1 Treatment of heparin overdosage

Dosage

Each mg of protamine sulfate neutralizes approximately 90 units of heparin activity derived from lung tissue and 115 units of heparin activity derived from intestinal mucosa.

Administer slowly IV over 1 minute to 3 minutes, not to exceed 50 mg in a 10-minute period.

Fate

Onset of action within 5 minutes; duration lasts 1 hour to 2 hours

Common Side-Effects

Flushing, feeling of warmth

Significant Adverse Reactions

Sudden hypotension, bradycardia, dyspnea, and allergic reactions

▶ **NURSING ALERTS**

▷ 1 Be aware that protamine itself has weak anticoagulant properties, and very large doses may lead to increased bleeding.

▷ 2 Do not administer protamine in cases of hemorrhage resulting from conditions other than heparin overdosage.

▷ 3 Use cautiously in patients with cardiovascular disease or fish allergies (protamine is derived from fish sources), and have facilities available to treat shock.

▷ 4 Inject slowly, because too-rapid administration can lead to sudden, severe hypotension.

▶ **NURSING CONSIDERATIONS**

▷ 1 Monitor vital signs during protamine infusion and at regular intervals for at least 3 hours to 4 hours following administration.

▷ 2 Perform appropriate blood coagulation studies (*e.g.,* heparin titration test, plasma thrombin time) to de-

termine necessity for repeat administrations of protamine.

Oral Anticoagulants

Coumarin derivatives	Indandione
Dicumarol	Phenindione
Phenprocoumon	
Warfarin	

Mechanism
Depress the hepatic synthesis of vitamin K-dependent
clotting factors II, VII, IX, and X by inhibiting vitamin K–
2, 3-epoxide reductase enzymes; factor VII is the first to be
depleted, followed sequentially by factors IX, X, and II.
Thus, initial prolongation of prothrombin time occurs within
8 hours to 12 hours, but maximal anticoagulant activity requires several days to develop. These drugs exert no effect
on established thrombus, but may prevent further extension
of the formed clot, thereby preventing secondary thromboembolic complications.

Uses
1 Prophylaxis and treatment of venous thrombosis and
   its extension
2 Treatment of atrial fibrillation with embolism
3 Prophylaxis and treatment of pulmonary embolism
4 Adjunctive treatment of coronary occlusion
5 Prophylaxis in patients with prosthetic valves

6 Reduce risk of recurrent myocardial infarction (investigational use)

Dosage
See Table 35-1.

Fate
(See Table 35-1 for individual drug properties) Most are
almost completely absorbed orally, although absorption rates
vary widely; peak activity usually occurs within 2 to 4 days
(1–2 days with phenindione); effects persist 2 to 7 days
following single doses of the coumarins and 1 to 3 days
with the indandiones; all drugs are highly but weakly bound
to plasma proteins; metabolized by hepatic microsomal enzymes, and excreted primarily in the urine as inactive metabolites

Common Side-Effects
Coumarins—hemorrhagic episodes
Indandiones—hemorrhagic episodes, hypersensitivity
   reactions

Significant Adverse Reactions
Coumarins—nausea, anorexia, severe bleeding, adrenal
   hemorrhage, vomiting, abdominal cramping, diarrhea,
   urticaria, dermatitis, alopecia, fever, agranulocytosis,
   leukopenia, mucosal ulceration, nephropathy

Contraindications
Hemorrhagic tendencies; hemophilia; thrombocytopenic
purpura; recent or contemplated surgery (especially eye or

Table 35-1. Oral Anticoagulants

Drug	Preparations	Usual Dosage Range	Remarks
Coumarins			
Dicumarol (Dicumarol)	Tablets—25 mg, 50 mg, 100 mg Capsules—25 mg, 50 mg	200 mg to 300 mg first day; 25 mg to 200 mg/day thereafter, depending on prothrombin time	Slowly and incompletely absorbed orally; peak effect in 3 to 5 days; be alert for accumulation toxicity (especially bleeding), because drug is long acting; poorly water soluble; half-life increases with increasing dose
Phenprocoumon (Liquamar)	Tablets—3 mg	Initially 24 mg; maintenance—0.75 mg to 6 mg/day based on prothrombin time	Long-acting derivative; peak activity in 2 to 3 days, and duration of 4 to 7 days; prolonged action increases danger of hemorrhage
Warfarin Sodium (Coufarin, Coumadin, Panwarfin)	Tablets—2 mg, 2.5 mg, 5 mg, 7.5 mg, 10 mg Injection—50 mg/vial with 2-ml diluent	Initially 10 mg to 15 mg/day (up to 60 mg/day) orally IM or IV—adjust based on prothrombin time Usual maintenance—2 mg to 10 mg/day	Well absorbed orally; peak effect in 1 to 2 days, and duration of 4 to 5 days; most widely used oral anticoagulant, giving most uniform response; reduce dose by one half in elderly or debilitated patients; do not use injectable solution if precipitate is present
Warfarin Potassium (Athrombin-K)	Tablets—5 mg	Initially 10 mg to 30 mg/day (up to 60 mg/day) Maintenance—2.5 mg to 10 mg/day	Similar to warfarin sodium in most respects; may be indicated in sodium-restricted patients

CNS surgery); active bleeding; ulcerative, traumatic, or surgical wounds; visceral carcinoma; diverticulitis; colitis; aneurysm; acute nephritis; suspicion of cerebrovascular hemorrhage; eclampsia or preeclampsia; threatened abortion; uncontrolled hypertension; hepatic insufficiency; polyarthritis; polycythemia vera; subacute bacterial endocarditis; ascorbic acid (vitamin C) deficiency; spinal puncture; continuous GI drainage; and regional block anesthesia

Interactions

1 The hypoprothrombinemic effect of oral anticoagulants may be enhanced by drugs that decrease vitamin K levels (antibiotics, cholestyramine, mineral oil); drugs that displace the anticoagulants from their protein binding sites (clofibrate, chloral hydrate, diazoxide, nalidixic acid, phenylbutazone, salicylates, sulfonamides, oral hypoglycemics); drugs that inhibit the metabolism of anticoagulants (alcohol, allopurinol, chloramphenicol, cimetidine, co-trimoxazole, disulfiram, methylphenidate, metronidazole, phenylbutazone, sulfinpyrazone, tricyclic antidepressants); and also by anabolic steroids, glucagon, sulindac, danazol, quinidine, and thyroid drugs.

2 Increased incidence of hemorrhage can occur with combined use of oral anticoagulants and inhibitors of platelet aggregation (dipyridamole, indomethacin, pyrazolones, salicylates), inhibitors of procoagulant factors (antimetabolites, alkylating agents, quinidine, salicylates), or ulcerogenic drugs (corticosteroids, indomethacin, pyrazolones, potassium salts, salicylates).

3 A decreased anticoagulant effect may be observed if oral anticoagulants are used in the presence of enzyme inducers (barbiturates, carbamazepine, ethchlorvynol, glutethimide, griseofulvin, phenytoin, rifampin); activators of procoagulant factors (estrogens, oral contraceptives, vitamin K); and drugs that can decrease GI absorption (cholestyramine, colestipol).

4 Oral anticoagulants may potentiate the action of phenytoin and the oral hypoglycemic drugs by inhibiting their liver metabolism.

▶ NURSING ALERTS

▷ 1 Stress the necessity of strict compliance to the prescribed dosage schedule. Obtain a careful drug history prior to initiation of therapy, and caution patients to avoid adding or discontinuing any other medication while taking oral anticoagulants.

▷ 2 Urge patients to observe carefully for signs of abnormal bleeding (*e.g.,* hematuria, tarry stools, hematemesis, petechiae, ecchymoses, bleeding gums, nosebleed, excessive menses), and advise physician immediately. Dosage adjustment is indicated.

▷ 3 Warn patients to note development of early signs of agranulocytosis (fever, chills, sore throat, malaise, mucosal ulceration) or hepatitis (itching, darkened urine, jaundice), and report at once. Discontinuation of medication is advisable.

▷ 4 Use with caution in the presence of congestive heart failure, mild liver or kidney dysfunction, alcoholism, tuberculosis, history of ulcerative disease, diabetes, allergic disorders, poor nutritional states, collagen disease, pancreatic disorders, vitamin K deficiency, hypothyroidism, x-ray therapy, edema, and hyperlipidemia.

▷ 5 Inform patients that minor overdosage, which is characterized by petechiae, oozing from cuts, or bleeding of gums after brushing, can be successfully treated by omitting one or more doses until prothrombin time returns to therapeutic range. Check with physician. More severe bleeding can be treated with oral (1 mg–10 mg) or parenteral (20 mg–40 mg) vitamin K, depending on severity. Occasionally, transfusions with fresh whole blood or fresh-frozen plasma may be indicated.

▷ 6 Be aware that compliance with the prescribed drug regimen is poorest in elderly, alcoholic, and emotionally unstable persons. Closely monitor their drug-taking practices.

▶ NURSING CONSIDERATIONS

▷ 1 Perform daily prothrombin determinations during initial stages of therapy and during periods of dosage adjustment or addition of other drugs. Prothrombin time should be maintained at 1.5 to 2 times the control value.

▷ 2 Note that onset of clinical effects with these agents is delayed several days. Be alert for signs of overdosage during early stages of therapy because of accumulation of drug.

▷ 3 During maintenance therapy, ensure that prothrombin time is determined at 1-week to 4-week intervals depending upon drug response. Periodic blood counts, urinalysis, and liver function tests should also be carried out.

▷ 4 Advise patients that many factors may affect anticoagulant response (*e.g.,* illness, diet, climate, presence of other drugs). Urge maintenance of a well-balanced diet, avoidance of excessive alcohol consumption, adherence to prescribed dosage schedule, and avoidance of any other drugs except when prescribed.

▷ 5 Urge patients to carry some form of identification at all times stating the type of medication they are taking and their physician's name.

▷ 6 Begin therapy at anticipated maintenance dosage level, and adjust daily dosage based upon prothrombin time. Excessive loading doses have been associated with increased bleeding complications. Heparin is preferred if rapid anticoagulation is desired.

▷ 7 Do not terminate therapy abruptly; withdraw gradually over 3 weeks to 4 weeks. Prothrombin activity returns to normal within 2 to 10 days following cessation of therapy.

▷ 8 Carefully weigh benefits *versus* risks when using oral anticoagulants in pregnant women. Fetal hemorrhage and congenital malformations have occurred with use of oral anticoagulants.

▷ *Dietary precautions*
▷ 1 Advise patients to avoid large amounts of green leafy vegetables, cabbage, cauliflower, fish, and liver because these are high in vitamin K and may reduce the effectiveness of the oral anticoagulants.

Oral Anticoagulant Antagonist

▶ vitamin K

Vitamin K is effective as an antidote to overdosage with the oral anticoagulant drugs. Three types of vitamin K preparations are available; (1) phytonadione (vitamin K_1), a fat-soluble derivative resembling naturally occurring vitamin K; (2) menadione (vitamin K_3), another synthetic fat-soluble derivative which is less effective than K_1 as an antidote to oral anticoagulants; and (3) menadiol (vitamin K_4), a synthetic water-soluble analog to menadione which is converted to menadione *in vivo* but is only about half as potent. Phytonadione is the preferred drug for treatment of anticoagulant-induced prothrombin deficiency because the other derivatives (K_3 and K_4) are less potent, less dependable, less rapid acting, and shorter acting than K_1.

The complete pharmacology of the various vitamin K preparations is reviewed in detail in Chapter 76. The present discussion is limited to the use of these preparations solely for the treatment of oral anticoagulant overdosage. Thus, only phytonadione (vitamin K_1), the preferred antidote, is reviewed at this time.

▶ phytonadione (K_1)

AquaMEPHYTON, Konakion, Mephyton

Mechanism
Promotes hepatic synthesis of blood clotting factors II, VII, IX, and X, thereby reversing oral anticoagulant-induced prothrombin depression; no antidotal effects against heparin

Uses
1 Treatment of anticoagulant-induced prothrombin deficiency (oral or parenteral K_1)
2 Treatment of hypoprothrombinemia secondary to antibacterial therapy, obstructive jaundice, biliary fistulas, or salicylate administration (oral or parenteral K_1)
3 Prophylaxis and therapy of newborn hemorrhagic disease (parenteral K_1)
4 Treatment of hypoprothrombinemia secondary to malabsorption or impaired synthesis of vitamin K such as can occur in ulcerative colitis, obstructive jaundice, celiac disease, intestinal resection, or regional enteritis (parenteral K_1)

Dosage
(Use smallest effective dose)
Anticoagulant overdosage:
Oral—2.5 mg to 10 mg (maximum 50 mg) initially; repeat in 12 hours to 24 hours as needed

SC, IM—0.5 mg to 10 mg (maximum 25 mg) initially; repeat in 6 hours to 8 hours as needed
IV (emergency only—see Significant Adverse Reactions)—0.5 mg to 10 mg at a rate of 1 mg/minute

Fate
Effects appear in 6 hours to 10 hours with oral use and 1 hour to 2 hours with parenteral use (15 min following IV injection); oral absorption requires presence of bile in the GI tract; normal prothrombin level usually is obtained within 12 hours to 16 hours.

Common Side-Effects
Flushing, GI upset

Significant Adverse Reactions

Warning: Severe anaphylactic reactions have occurred following IV injection of AquaMEPHYTON (an aqueous colloidal solution of K_1), resulting in shock, cardiac arrest, and respiratory arrest. Therefore, the IV route should be used only when other routes are not feasible and with full consideration of all risks.

Pain, swelling, and tenderness at injection site, allergic reactions (bronchospasm, dyspnea, anaphylaxis), cramping, chills, fever, weakness, dizziness, chest constriction, profuse sweating, erythema, cyanosis

▶ NURSING ALERTS
▷ 1 Be aware that several hours are required for vitamin K to enhance prothrombin synthesis. In cases of severe hemorrhage, whole blood or plasma transfusions are indicated.
▷ 2 Administer IV only when other routes of administration are not feasible. Dilute injection with sodium chloride or dextrose solution, and administer very slowly. Severe reactions (including fatal anaphylaxis) have occurred following IV injection—see above).
▷ 3 Use smallest dose that is effective in restoring normal prothrombin time. Be aware that overzealous use of phytonadione may promote return of thromboembolic complications and can interfere with action of oral anticoagulants for an extended period (2 wk–3 wk).

▶ NURSING CONSIDERATIONS
▷ 1 Perform frequent prothrombin times during therapy, to aid in determining dosage and frequency of administration.
▷ 2 Use IV dilution immediately upon preparation, and discard unused portion. Protect from light by wrapping container during use.
▷ 3 Note that patients who have received large doses of phytonadione may exhibit resistance to subsequent oral anticoagulant therapy. If anticoagulant effect is desired, larger than normal doses of the oral drugs or use of heparin may be required.

▷ 4 Inform patient that temporary pain or swelling, or both, may occur following SC or IM injection.
▷ 5 Avoid use of drugs that can interfere with vitamin K activity (*e.g.,* oral antibiotics, quinidine, salicylates) during phytonadione therapy.

▷ *Dietary precaution*
▷ 1 Advise patient to restrict intake of foods rich in vitamin K (*e.g.,* leafy vegetables, tomatoes, meats, egg yolks) during phytonadione treatment.

II Thrombolytic Drugs

Drugs possessing the ability to degrade blood clots directly, or to accelerate the endogenous dissolution process, are termed thrombolytic agents. These drugs are potentially dangerous agents, associated with a high risk of severe hemorrhage, which is often difficult to manage, and should be administered only by persons trained and experienced in their use. Their clinical effectiveness is subject to considerable doubt, and it is imperative that the potential benefit be carefully weighed against the considerable risk before prescribing these agents to treat thromboembolic conditions.

The currently available thrombolytic drugs are two enzymes, one derived from beta-hemolytic streptococci (streptokinase) and the other from human kidney cells (urokinase).

▶ streptokinase
Kabikinase, Streptase

Mechanism
Converts plasminogen to the proteolytic enzyme plasmin (fibrinolysin), which breaks down fibrin clots

Uses
1 Lysis of acute, massive pulmonary emboli
2 Lysis of acute, extensive deep vein thromboses
3 Clearance of occluded arteriovenous cannulae
4 Lysis of coronary artery thrombi associated with an evolving myocardial infarction, as an aid to reperfusion of the blocked vessel (conclusive evidence that treatment reduces mortality or salvages myocardial tissue is lacking)

Dosage
Venous thrombosis and pulmonary embolism
Initially, 250,000 units IV over 30-minute period, then 100,000 units/hour over 72 hours for venous thrombosis, or 100,000 units/hour over 24 hours to 72 hours for pulmonary embolism or arterial thrombosis
Reconstitute contents of each vial with 5 ml Sodium Chloride Injection, then dilute further to a total volume of 45 ml.

Arteriovenous cannula occlusion
Infuse by pump at a constant rate, 250,000 units/2 ml IV solution, into each occluded limb of cannula over a 30-minute period, then clamp off for 2 hours; aspirate contents of infusion cannula, flush with saline, and reconnect cannula.
Reconstitute contents of 250,000 units/vial with 2 ml Sodium Chloride Injection or 5% Dextrose Injection.

Myocardial infarction
Initially—250,000 units IV, followed by 100,000 units/hour for 24 hours; alternately, 500,000 units to 1,500,000 units in a single IV infusion over 1 hour.
  Intracoronary—10,000 units to 20,000 units initially, followed by 2000 units to 4000 units/minute until lysis occurs, then 2000 units/minute for 1 hour.

Common Side-Effects
Fever, bleeding episodes (*e.g.,* ecchymoses, gum bleeding, hematuria), urticaria, itching, flushing, nausea, headache, and muscle pain

Significant Adverse Reactions
Severe hemorrhage (cerebral, GI, retroperitoneal); allergic reactions (dyspnea, angio-edema, periorbital swelling, bronchospasm, anaphylactic reaction); blood pressure alterations, and phlebitis at site of IV injection

Contraindications
Active internal bleeding, intracranial or intraspinal surgery, intracranial neoplasm, and recent cerebrovascular accident

Interactions
1 Drugs that alter platelet function (*e.g.,* salicylates, dipyridamole, indomethacin, phenylbutazone) or coagulation (*e.g.,* heparin, warfarin) may increase the risk of hemorrhage with streptokinase.

▶ NURSING ALERTS
▷ 1 Discontinue drug in case of serious bleeding. If necessary, administer whole fresh blood, packed red cells, or fresh-frozen plasma. Aminocaproic acid may be given if hemorrhage is unresponsive to blood replacement.
▷ 2 Use with extreme caution in the following situations: recent or imminent surgery, ulcerative wounds, trauma with internal injuries, malignancies, urinary or GI lesions (*e.g.,* colitis, diverticulitis), severe hypertension, diabetic retinopathy, hepatic or renal disease, hemorrhagic disorders, chronic lung disease, rheumatic heart disease, subacute bacterial endocarditis, history of allergic reactions, pregnancy, immediate postpartum period, and in children.
▷ 3 If clinical signs of potentially serious bleeding occur (hematuria, ecchymoses, epistaxis, gum bleeding) or if thrombin time is less than half normal, discontinue drug. Re-institute therapy only if signs of bleeding cease.
▷ 4 Do not administer IM (danger of hematoma), and avoid arterial invasive procedures before and during treat-

ment. Perform venipuncture as carefully and infrequently as possible, and apply prolonged pressure to site following procedure.

▷ 5 Observe patients very carefully during first few hours of infusion for signs of serious allergic reactions (*e.g.,* asthmatic symptoms, blood pressure changes). Discontinue infusion and initiate symptomatic treatment (*e.g.,* epinephrine, antihistamines, corticosteroids) if allergic manifestations occur.

▷ 6 Note that streptokinase is not indicated for treatment of superficial thrombophlebitis.

▷ 7 Prior to instituting therapy, streptokinase resistance should be measured. If levels exceed 1,000,000 units, do not administer streptokinase.

▶ **NURSING CONSIDERATIONS**

▷ 1 Prior to initiating therapy, draw a blood sample to determine thrombin time and streptokinase resistance.

▷ 2 Have appropriate measures or drugs on hand to treat fever (*e.g.,* acetaminophen), allergic reactions (*e.g.,* corticosteroids, epinephrine, antihistamines), and excessive bleeding (*e.g.,* whole blood, dextran, aminocaproic acid).

▷ 3 Avoid unnecessary handling of patient because bruising can occur easily.

▷ 4 Avoid concurrent use of anticoagulants, and allow sufficient time for their effects to diminish before instituting streptokinase therapy.

▷ 5 Be aware that a recent streptococcal infection may require use of higher loading doses of streptokinase because of higher resistance levels.

▷ 6 Use dilution within 24 hours of reconstitution, and discard unused portion of solution.

▷ 7 Following termination of therapy, begin continuous IV heparin infusion, but not until the thrombin time has decreased to less than twice the normal control level. Discontinue heparin when prothrombin time reaches 2 to 3 times the normal control value.

▶ **urokinase**

Abbokinase

Mechanism

Converts plasminogen to plasmin (fibrinolysin), thereby degrading fibrin clots

Uses

1 Lysis of acute, massive pulmonary emboli
2 Lysis of acute thrombi obstructing coronary arteries associated with evolving myocardial infarction.
3 Clearance of IV catheters, including central venous catheters

Dosage

(IV infusion only) Initially 4400 units/kg of urokinase–saline mixture over a period of 10 minutes, followed by continuous infusion of 4400 units/kg/hr for 12 hours; ap-

proximately 3 hours to 4 hours following urokinase therapy, a continuous heparin IV infusion should be initiated.

Reconstitute urokinase solution by adding 5.2 ml Sterile Water for Injection to vial of urokinase, then dilute reconstituted urokinase solution with normal saline prior to IV infusion.

Common Side-Effects

See Streptokinase; also, lowered hematocrit

Significant Adverse Reactions

See Streptokinase; however, severe allergic reactions are infrequent with urokinase, because it is a protein of human origin.

Contraindications

See Streptokinase.

Interactions

See Streptokinase.

▶ **NURSING ALERTS**

See Streptokinase.

▶ **NURSING CONSIDERATIONS**

See Streptokinase. In addition:

▷ 1 Reconstitute urokinase solution *only* with Sterile Water for Injection. (Do not use bacteriostatic water.)

▷ 2 Do not reconstitute until immediately before using, because solution contains no preservatives. Discard unused portion.

III Hemostatic Drugs

Hemostatic drugs may be used to control bleeding in a variety of situations. Systemically administered agents are employed to elevate or replenish one or more coagulation factors that may be deficient because of a hereditary or acquired defect, and to treat excessive systemic bleeding resulting from surgical complications, hematologic disorders, or neoplastic disease. Topically applied hemostatics are primarily used to control continual oozing or mild bleeding from capillaries and other small blood vessels (*e.g.,* following surgery), or in the treatment of decubitus or chronic leg ulcers.

Systemic Hemostatics

▶ **aminocaproic acid**

Amicar

Mechanism

Inhibits profibrinolysin activators and exerts an antifibrinolysin action, thereby retarding clot breakdown

Uses

1 Treatment of severe bleeding resulting from systemic hyperfibrinolysis, such as that associated with heart surgery, hematologic disorders, abruptio placentae, cirrhosis of the liver, or neoplastic disorders
2 Treatment of urinary hyperfibrinolysis, such as that associated with severe trauma, shock, prostatectomy, nephrectomy, or renal malignancies
3 Treatment of overdosage with fibrinolytic drugs (*e.g.,* streptokinase, urokinase)
4 Prevent recurrence of subarachnoid hemorrhage, abort or prevent attacks of hereditary angioneurotic edema, and decrease need for platelet transfusion in cases of amegokaryocytic thrombocytopenia (investigational uses only)

Dosage

Oral: 5 g initially, followed by 1 g to 1.25 g/hour for 8 hours or until bleeding has ceased; maximum dose— 30 g/day

IV infusion: 4 g to 5 g in 250 ml diluent during first hour, followed by continuous infusion at a rate of 1 g/hour in 50 ml diluent for 8 hours or until bleeding ceases

Fate

Rapidly absorbed orally; peak plasma levels occur in 1 hour to 2 hours; widely distributed; rapidly excreted, largely in the form of unmetabolized drug

Common Side-Effects

Nausea, cramping

Significant Adverse Reactions

Diarrhea, dizziness, tinnitus, malaise, weakness, fatigue, pruritus, headache, hypotension, delirium, nasal congestion, skin rash, menstrual cramping, reversible acute renal failure, thrombophlebitis, and auditory and visual hallucinations

Contraindications

Active intravascular clotting, hematuria of upper urinary tract origin, and pregnancy

Interactions

1 Oral contraceptives may increase the danger of increased coagulation.
2 Serum potassium levels can be elevated by aminocaproic acid.

▶ NURSING ALERTS

▷ 1 Do not administer unless a definite diagnosis of hyperfibrinolysis has been made.
▷ 2 In life-threatening bleeding situations, be prepared to administer emergency treatment, *e.g.,* fresh whole blood transfusion, fibrinogen infusions.
▷ 3 Do not administer by rapid IV injection because bradycardia, arrhythmias, or marked hypotension can occur. Infuse slowly as outlined under Dosage, above.
▷ 4 Use cautiously in patients with hepatic, renal, or cardiac disease, and in children.

▷ 5 Be alert for signs of possible thromboembolic complications (*e.g.,* chest or leg pain, dyspnea), and advise physician.

▶ NURSING CONSIDERATIONS

▷ 1 Note that plasma levels should be .13 mg/ml or higher to inhibit systemic hyperfibrinolysis.

▶ antihemophilic factor, human

Factorate, Hemofil, Koāte, Profilate

Mechanism

A plasma protein (factor VIII) that is essential for the conversion of prothrombin to thrombin; replaces deficient endogenous factor VIII in cases of classic hemophilia, thereby decreasing bleeding tendency

Uses

1 Treatment of classic hemophilia A, to control bleeding episodes, or perform surgical procedures

Dosage

(Administered IV) Must be individualized to needs of each patient; dosage expressed in AHF units; one AHF unit equals the activity present in 1 ml of human plasma pooled from at least 10 donors and tested within 3 hours of collection.

Average dosage levels

Overt bleeding: 10 units/kg to 20 units/kg every 6 hours to 8 hours for 24 hours, then every 12 hours for 3 to 4 days

Massive wounds: give until bleeding stops, then 20 units/kg every 8 hours

Muscle hemorrhage: 10 units/kg to 20 units/kg initially, then 10 mg/kg every 8 hours to 12 hours for up to 48 hours

Surgery: 30 units/kg to 40 units/kg prior to surgery, then 20 units/kg every 8 hours after surgery

Prophylaxis of bleeding episodes: 250 units to 500 units/day, in the morning

Fate

Following IV administration, plasma half-life is 6 hours to 8 hours; rapidly inactivated in solution

Common Side-Effects

Mild allergic reactions, headache, and flushing

Significant Adverse Reactions

Nausea, vomiting, chills, erythema, hives, fever, tachycardia, hypotension, backache, visual disturbances, clouded consciousness; massive doses may cause hemolytic anemia, increased bleeding tendency, and hyperfibrinogenemia; viral hepatitis has been reported.

▶ NURSING ALERTS

▷ 1 Administer only after diagnosis of factor VIII deficiency has been made. Drug is of no benefit in other forms of bleeding disorders.

▷ 2 Note that a small percentage of patients (about 10%) develop inhibitors to factor VIII, necessitating use of much larger than normal doses or administration of anti-inhibitor coagulation complex (see following discussion).

▶ **NURSING CONSIDERATIONS**

▷ 1 Administer only by the IV route, using a plastic syringe.

▷ 2 Keep drug vials stored between 2°C and 8°C until reconstituted. Do *not* refrigerate after reconstitution, and avoid precipitation.

▷ 3 During reconstitution of drug solution, rotate vial gently but do not shake. Warm the concentrate and diluent to room temperature before mixing. Do not use if gel formation occurs.

▷ 4 Administer drug within 3 hours after reconstitution, to avoid possible untoward effects caused by bacterial contamination during mixing.

▷ 5 Do not administer at a rate greater than 10 ml/minute because vasomotor reactions can occur.

▶ **anti-inhibitor coagulant complex**

Autoplex

Mechanism

Concentrate of activated and precursor clotting factors and factors of the kinin generating system prepared from pooled human plasma; reduces level of factor VIII inhibitory activity in hemophilic patients, thus decreasing bleeding episodes

Uses

1 Treatment of symptoms of hemophilia in patients with significant levels of factor VIII inhibitors who are bleeding or about to undergo surgery

Dosage

(IV only) 25 to 100 factor VIII correctional units/kg depending on severity of bleeding at a rate of 2 ml infusion solution/minute; repeat in 6 hours if necessary (one unit of factor VIII correctional activity is that amount of activated prothrombin complex which, upon addition to an equal amount of factor VIII deficient plasma, will correct the clotting time to 35 sec)

Significant Adverse Reactions

Hypersensitivity reactions (fever, chills, alterations in blood pressure); headache, flushing, tachycardia, hypercoagulability (dyspnea, chest pain, cough, changes in pulse rate)

Contraindications

Fibrinolysis, disseminated intravascular coagulation (DIC)

▶ **NURSING ALERTS**

▷ 1 Recognize that a risk of transmission of viral hepatitis and possibly other diseases (*e.g.,* AIDS) exists with the use of the concentrated product. Use only when apparent clinical benefit outweighs potential risk.

▷ 2 Observe closely for indications of intravascular coagulation (*e.g.,* dyspnea, coughing, chest or leg pain) and terminate infusion.

▷ 3 Use with caution in patients with liver disease or a history of allergies, and in small children.

▶ **NURSING CONSIDERATIONS**

▷ 1 Have appropriate medications (*e.g.,* epinephrine, corticosteroids, antihistamines) available to manage any allergic reactions that may develop.

▷ 2 Avoid too-rapid infusion rates (*e.g.,* 5 ml/min–10 ml/min), because incidence of side-effects is much higher.

▷ 3 Monitor prothrombin time in all patients. Do not reinfuse drug unless *post*infusion prothrombin time is at least two thirds of the *pre*infusion value.

▷ 4 Store unreconstituted product under refrigeration. Use diluent provided to prepare infusion solution according to package directions. Each bottle is labeled with the units of factor VIII correctional activity that it contains.

▶ **factor IX complex, human**

Konȳne, Profilnine, Proplex

Mechanism

Concentrate of dried plasma fractions of human coagulation factors II, VII, IX, and X with small amounts of other plasma proteins; provides replacement therapy for a congenital or acquired deficiency of one or more factors that can result in increased bleeding tendencies

Uses

1 Treatment of deficiency states involving coagulation factors II, VII, IX, or X where prevention or cessation of bleeding is necessary

2 Treatment of hemorrhagic disease of the newborn with proven deficiency of factors II, VII, IX, and X

3 Treatment or prevention of bleeding in children or adults with acquired hepatic insufficiency having a proven deficiency of above-named factors

Dosage

Highly individualized depending on patient status, severity of bleeding, and degree of factor deficiency as determined by coagulation assays prior to treatment; dosage measured in units (1 unit is the activity present in 1 ml of normal plasma less than 1 hr old). Potency is adjusted based on factor IX, because the other factors (II, VII, X) are present in approximately the same amount.

Dosage guidelines

Factor IX deficiency: 2 units/kg yields an average increase of 3%

Factor VII deficiency: 2 units/kg yields an average increase of 4%

Refer to package instructions for complete dosage information.

Common Side-Effects

Flushing, tingling (especially with too-rapid infusion)

Significant Adverse Reactions

Chills, fever, headache, tachycardia, hypotension, viral hepatitis, and intravascular hemolysis

Contraindications

Liver disease with signs of intravascular coagulation or fibrinolysis, and patients undergoing elective surgery

▶ **NURSING ALERTS**

▷ 1   Be aware that the preparation may contain the causative agent of viral hepatitis and possibly other diseases such as AIDS. Use very cautiously in cases of suspected or confirmed liver impairment, and observe carefully for signs of hepatitis.

▷ 2   Monitor infusion rate constantly, and note development of symptoms (*e.g.,* cough, chest pain, respiratory distress, altered pulse and pressure) that signify increased intravascular coagulation. Stop infusion immediately. To minimize risk of intravascular coagulation, do not attempt to raise factor IX level to more than 50% of normal.

▷ 3   Do not administer unless a deficiency of one of the four factors (II, VII, IX, X) has been definitively established.

▶ **NURSING CONSIDERATIONS**

▷ 1   Perform coagulation assays prior to initiation of treatment and at regular intervals thereafter. Dosage is adjusted based upon assay results.

▷ 2   Infuse *slowly* IV. Rapid infusion (greater than 10 ml/min) can produce vasomotor symptoms (*e.g.,* tachycardia, hypotension).

▷ 3   Monitor levels of coagulation factors repeatedly during infusion because excessive levels increase the risk of intravascular coagulation.

▷ 4   Store products under normal refrigeration until reconstituted, but do not freeze. Warm to room temperature before mixing. Do not use if gel forms.

▷ 5   Administer drug within 3 hours following reconstitution, and do not refrigerate reconstituted solution because precipitation can occur.

▷ 6   Advise patient to report development of chills, fever, tingling, flushing, or headache during infusion; dosage reduction (slower infusion rate) is indicated.

Topical Hemostatics

▶ **gelatin film, absorbable**
Gelfilm

Mechanism

Nonantigenic, absorbable gelatin film with the consistency of cellophane; moistened and cut to desired size and shape, and applied to tissue to reduce bleeding; absorbed completely within one half to 3 months

Uses

1   Reduce local bleeding in thoracic, ocular, or neurosurgery

Dosage

Immerse in sterile saline, and allow to soak until pliable; cut to desired size and shape, and apply to surface of tissue.

▶ **NURSING CONSIDERATIONS**

▷ 1   Do not use in grossly contaminated or infected surgical wounds, because rate of absorption is markedly increased.

▷ 2   Use immediately after opening package envelope to minimize contamination.

▶ **gelatin sponge, absorbable**
Gelfoam

Mechanism

A pliable, nonantigenic sponge capable of absorbing many times its weight in whole blood; prepared from specially treated, purified gelatin solution; completely absorbed in 4 weeks to 6 weeks when implanted into tissues; presence of anticoagulants does not interfere with its effectiveness; liquefies within several days when applied to actively bleeding areas

Uses

1   Provide control of capillary and small blood vessel bleeding in many forms of surgery

2   Enhance wound healing by providing a framework for granulation tissue

Dosage

(Use sterile technique) Cut to desired size, and apply either dry or saturated with Sodium Chloride Injection or Thrombin Solution to desired area. Hold in place with moderate pressure for 10 seconds to 15 seconds, then allow to remain in contact with bleeding site. Wound may be closed over sponge.

Decubitus ulcers may be packed with sponge and a dressing applied.

Contraindications

Presence of infection, postpartum bleeding, menorrhagia, bleeding due to blood dyscrasias, and closure of skin incisions

▶ **NURSING CONSIDERATIONS**

▷ 1   Compress sponge before inserting into cavities or closed tissue spaces, to reduce expansion and possible disturbances of surrounding structures. Do *not* overpack a particular area, because sponge may expand excessively, interfering with function of surrounding structures.

▷ 2   Note that effectiveness can be enhanced by soaking in a thrombin solution.

▷ 3   Use sponges as soon as possible after opening package to minimize bacterial contamination.

▷ 4   Do not resterilize by heating (changes absorption time) or with ethylene oxide (irritating to tissues).

▶ **microfibrillar collagen hemostat**
Avitene

Mechanism

A dry, fibrous, water-insoluble preparation of purified bovine corium collagen; when applied to the source of bleeding, it attracts platelets, which adhere to the fibrils of the preparation, triggering further platelet aggregation into thrombi; stimulates a mild, chronic inflammatory response; response is not inhibited by heparin; does not interfere with bone regeneration or healing

Uses

1 Adjunct to hemostasis in surgical procedures when control of bleeding by conventional procedures (*e.g.,* ligation) is ineffective or impractical

Dosage

Compress surface to be treated with a dry sponge prior to applying dry hemostat preparation, then apply pressure over the hemostat for several minutes. The amount of product required depends on size of area and severity of bleeding. Remove excess material after several minutes. Do not handle with wet instruments or gloves.

Significant Adverse Reactions

Potentiation of infection, hematomas (sealing over of exit site for deeper hemorrhage), adhesion formation, and allergic reactions

Contraindications

Closure of skin incisions, use on bone surfaces to which prosthetic materials are to be attached

▶ NURSING ALERTS

▷ 1 Do not sterilize product, because it is inactivated by autoclaving. Avoid wetting product, because its hemostatic efficacy is impaired.
▷ 2 Avoid spilling product on nonbleeding surfaces (especially abdominal or thoracic viscera), because it will adhere to any moist surface, possibly resulting in adhesions.

▶ NURSING CONSIDERATIONS

▷ 1 Remove excess material after several minutes by gentle teasing or irrigation. If breakthrough bleeding occurs, apply additional hemostat.
▷ 2 Do not use gloved fingers to apply pressure; a dry sponge is preferred.

▶ negatol

Negatan

Mechanism

Highly acidic compound that coagulates protein substances and possesses a germicidal action

Uses

1 Astringent and hemostatic on skin and mucous membranes (*e.g.,* vagina, cervix, vulvae)

Dosage

Cleanse and dry area to be treated; apply either full strength (45%) or as a 1:10 dilution.
  Vaginal: soak gauze in 1:10 dilution and use as a pack; remove within 24 hours and douche
  Cervical: soak gauze in full strength solution, and insert into cervical canal

Significant Adverse Reactions

Skin irritation, burning, erythema, and superficial desquamation

▶ NURSING CONSIDERATIONS

▷ 1 Make initial application in vagina with 1:10 dilution, and observe for signs of hypersensitivity. Concentration can be increased if no untoward reactions are noted.
▷ 2 Advise patients to wear perineal pads to avoid soiling of clothing.

▶ oxidized cellulose

Novocell, Oxycel, Surgicel

Mechanism

Upon saturation of cellulose material with blood, it swells into a gelatinous tenacious mass that serves as a clot nucleus; slowly absorbed from sites of implantation with minimal tissue reaction; does not alter normal blood clotting mechanism

Uses

1 Adjunctive control of minor hemorrhage (capillary, venous, small arterial) in cases in which conventional methods (*e.g.,* ligation) are inappropriate
2 Production of hemostasis in oral and dental surgery

Dosage

Place desired size pad, strip, or pellet of material on bleeding site; usually removed following development of hemostasis by irrigation with sterile water or saline

Significant Adverse Reactions

Stinging, burning, headache, sneezing (nasal application), foreign body reactions, encapsulation of fluid, obstruction (*e.g.,* urinary, intestinal) caused by adhesion formation, necrosis of nasal membranes

Contraindications

Implantation in bone defects (*e.g.,* fractures), use as packing or wadding (must be removed following hemostasis), hemorrhage from large arteries, and control of nonhemorrhagic oozing

▶ NURSING ALERTS

▷ 1 Do not enclose oxidized cellulose in contaminated wounds without drainage.
▷ 2 *Always* remove following development of hemostasis in laminectomy procedures (may cause nerve damage), from foramina of bone, and from large open wounds.

▷ 3 Do not apply silver nitrate or other similar materials before using oxidized cellulose because absorption may be impaired.

▷ 4 Avoid wadding or packing the cellulose material, especially within rigid cavities, because swelling may cause obstruction or necrosis.

▷ 5 Ensure that none of the material is aspirated by the patient, as when it is used to control bleeding following tonsillectomy or to reduce epistaxis.

▶ **NURSING CONSIDERATIONS**

▷ 1 Avoid adding anti-infective agents, buffers, or other hemostatics to oxidized cellulose. The low *p*H of the product destroys these other additives.

▷ 2 Always irrigate before removal of oxidized cellulose, to avoid tearing of tissues and re-institution of bleeding.

▷ 3 Do not moisten prior to application, because hemostatic effect is greater when dry.

▷ 4 Do not resterilize, because autoclaving causes physical breakdown. Discard opened, unused product.

▷ 5 Use least amount necessary to produce hemostasis. Remove any excess before surgical closure.

▶ **thrombin, topical**

Thrombinar, Thrombostat

Mechanism

Catalyzes the conversion of fibronogen to fibrin

Uses

1 Reduce oozing and minor bleeding from capillaries and small venules (*e.g.,* laryngeal or nasal surgery, plastic surgery, bleeding from cancellous bone, dental extractions)

Dosage

Prepare solutions in sterile distilled water or saline; intended use determines concentration of solution, which may range from 100 unit to 2000 units/ml depending on extent and severity of bleeding.

Spray or flood area (using syringe and fine-gauge needle) with solution; alternately, dried powder from vial may be placed directly on area, or absorbable gelatin sponge may be soaked in thrombin solution and then placed on area of bleeding.

Significant Adverse Reactions

Allergic reactions, fever

▶ **NURSING ALERTS**

▷ 1 Never administer thrombin parenterally or allow it to enter large blood vessels because extensive intravascular clotting and death can result.

▶ **NURSING CONSIDERATIONS**

▷ 1 Use solutions the day they are prepared. Refrigerate solutions if several hours are to elapse between preparation and use.

▷ 2 Be aware that acids, alkalies, heat, and heavy metal salts reduce thrombin activity.

▷ 3 Do not sponge treated surfaces because clot may be dislodged.

▷ 4 Ensure that wound is relatively free from blood before application of drug.

Summary. Anticoagulant, Thrombolytic and Hemostatic Drugs

Drug	Preparations	Usual Dosage Range
Anticoagulants		
Parenteral Anticoagulant		
Heparin sodium (Lipo-Hepin, Liquaemin) Heparin calcium (Calciparine)	Injection—1000; 2500; 5000; 7500; 10,000; 12,500; 15,000; 20,000; 40,000 units per ml or per unit dose	Anticoagulant: SC—10,000 units to 20,000 units initially then 8000 to 20,000 units every 8 hours to 12 hours
		IV—10,000 units initially, then 5000 to 10,000 units every 4 hours to 6 hours
		IV infusion—20,000 to 40,000 units/day
		Postoperative: SC—5000 units 2 hours before surgery, then 5000 units every 8 hours to 12 hours for 7 days
Heparin Sodium in Saline (Hep-Lock, Liquaemin Lock Flush)	Injection—10 units, 100 units/ml	Use as IV flush in indwelling IV catheters

(continued)

Summary. Anticoagulant, Thrombolytic and Hemostatic Drugs *(continued)*

Drug	Preparations	Usual Dosage Range
Heparin Antagonist		
Protamine Sulfate	Injection—10 mg/ml Powder—50 mg, 250 mg/vial with 5 ml diluent	1 mg neutralizes 90 units to 120 units of heparin; administer slowly IV over 1 minute to 3 minutes; maximum dosage is 50 mg within 10-minute period
Oral Anticoagulants	See Table 35-1.	
Oral Anticoagulant Antagonist		
Phytonadione (AquaMEPHYTON, Konakion, Mephyton)	Tablets—5 mg Injection—2 mg, 10 mg/ml (Konakion for IM use only)	Oral—2.5 mg to 25 mg initially; may repeat in 12 hours to 24 hours SC, IM—0.5 mg to 10 mg initially; may repeat up to 25 mg in 6 hours to 8 hours IV—0.5 mg to 10 mg at a rate of 1 mg/minute
Thrombolytics		
Streptokinase (Kabikinase, Streptase)	Powder for reconstitution—250,000; 600,000; 750,000 units/vial	Initially 250,000 units IV over a 30-minute period, followed by 100,000 units/hour for 24 hours to 72 hours For AV cannula occlusion—250,000 units/2 ml IV solution infused into each cannula limb over a 30-minute period Myocardial infarction—250,000 units IV, followed by 100,000 units/hour for 24 hours or 10,000 to 20,000 units into blocked coronary artery, followed by 2000 to 4000 units/minute until lysis occurs, then 2000 units/minute for 1 hour
Urokinase (Abbokinase)	Powder for reconstitution—250,000 units/vial	4400 units/kg of urokinase–saline mixture over a period of 10 minutes by IV infusion, followed by continuous infusion of 4400 units/kg/hour for 12 hours
Hemostatics		
Systemic Hemostatics		
Aminocaproic Acid (Amicar)	Tablets—500 mg Syrup—250 mg/ml Injection—250 mg/ml	Oral—5 g initially then 1 g to 1.25 g/hour until bleeding stops (maximum is 30 g/day) IV infusion—4 g to 5 g initially, during first hour, then 1 g/hour thereafter
Antihemophilic Factor, Human (Factorate, Hemofil, Koate, Profilate)	Vials—10 ml, 20 ml, 25 ml, 30 ml, 40 ml, 50 ml and single dose containing a dried preparation of human antihemophilic factor (units indicated on vial) with diluent	Individualized depending on patient's weight, severity of bleeding, presence of factor VIII inhibitors Average dose range is 10 units to 20 units/kg every 6 hours to 12 hours; prior to surgery 30 units to 40 units/kg; prophylaxis 250 units to 500 units/day, in the morning

Summary. Anticoagulant, Thrombolytic and Hemostatic Drugs *(continued)*

Drug	Preparations	Usual Dosage Range
Anti-inhibitor Coagulant Complex (Autoplex)	Vials—30 ml containing a dried auto-inhibitor coagulant complex obtained from pooled human plasma (units of factor VIII correctional activity indicated on each vial) with diluent	25 to 100 factor VIII correctional units/kg at a rate of 2 ml infusion solution/minute; repeat in 6 hours if necessary
Factor IX Complex, Human (Konyne, Profilnine, Proplex)	Dried plasma fraction of factors II, VII, IX, and X in vials with diluent	Highly individualized; coagulation assays should be performed prior to treatment and at regular intervals during treatment, and dosage should be based upon assay results
Topical Hemostatics		
Gelatin Film, Absorbable (Gelfilm)	Strips—100 mm × 125 mm, and 25 mm × 50 mm	Soak in sterile saline until pliable, cut to desired size, and apply to tissue surface
Gelatin Sponge, Absorbable (Gelfoam)	Sponges, dental packs, and prostatectomy cones of various dimensions	Apply dry or saturated with saline injections or thrombin solution
Microfibrillar Collagen Hemostat (Avitene)	Jars—1 g, 5 g (fibrous form) Strips—70 mm × 70 mm and 70 mm × 35 mm	Place on area and apply pressure for several minutes; remove excess material after several minutes
Negatol (Negatan)	Solution—45%	Apply either full strength or as a 1:10 dilution; also used as a soak for gauze packing
Oxidized Cellulose (Novocell, Oxycel, Surgicel)	Pads, strips, and pledgets of various sizes Pellets for dental application	Place desired size pad, strip, or pellet onto bleeding area; remove following the development of hemostasis by irrigation
Thrombin, Topical (Thrombinar, Thrombostat)	Powder—1000-; 5000-; 10,000-; 20,000-unit vials	Topical—spray or flood area of bleeding with solution of thrombin in sterile water or saline; alternately, dry powder from vial may be placed on bleeding site

Drugs Acting on the Renal System

IV

The kidneys play a major role in the maintenance of homeostasis by regulating the volume and composition of the extracellular fluid that serves as the internal environment for each cell. In addition to controlling the water, electrolyte, and solute concentrations of the extracellular fluid, the kidneys selectively excrete drugs, hormones, and by-products of metabolism. The kidneys also participate in the maintenance of acid–base balance, renin and angiotensin production, and vitamin D metabolism.

Renal Physiology— A Review

36

Gross Anatomy of the Kidney

The kidneys are paired, bean-shaped organs located retroperitoneally on each side of the vertebral column at the level of the 12th thoracic to the third lumbar vertebrae. The right kidney is placed slightly lower than the left because of displacement by the liver.

Each kidney is invested with a fibrous capsule that is interrupted medially at the *hilus* for passage of blood vessels, lymphatics, nerves, and a ureter.

A frontal section of the kidney reveals an outer granular *cortex* located deep to the capsule and an inner *medulla* composed of several striated *pyramids* (Fig. 36-1). Interspersed among the pyramids are columns of cortical tissues known as the renal columns of Bertin.

The apex of each renal pyramid forms a *papilla,* which projects into a cup-like minor *calyx.* Several minor calyces unite to form major calyces, and the latter merge to form the *renal pelvis.* The renal pelvis is continuous with the *ureter,* which drains its contents into the *urinary bladder.*

Renal Blood Supply

Paired *renal arteries* arise from the abdominal aorta, branching as they enter the hilus. These branches divide into *interlobar arteries,* which pass between the medullary pyramids. At the corticomedullary junction the vessels form the *arcuate arteries,* which arch over the bases of the pyramids. Branching from the arcuate arteries are numerous *interlobular arteries,* which penetrate the cortical substance and give rise to *afferent arterioles* supplying individual nephron units.

Each afferent arteriole terminates in a tuft of capillaries, the *glomerulus,* which rejoin to form the *efferent arteriole.* Efferent arterioles terminate in *peritubular capillaries,* which surround the renal tubules. The peritubular capillaries eventually converge into venules that carry the blood into a series of veins corresponding in name and in course to the arteries described above.

A series of long, straight peritubular capillaries termed *vasa recta* course through the medulla, turning sharply at various levels. The vasa recta participate in countercurrent exchange of substances between the renal tubules and vascular bed as detailed later in this chapter.

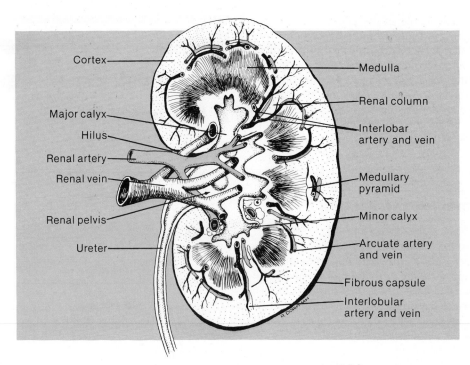

Figure 36-1 Frontal section of a human kidney.

Microscopic Anatomy of the Kidney

The basic anatomical and functional unit of the kidney is the *nephron* (Fig. 36-2). There are approximately 1 million nephrons in each human kidney. A nephron consists of a renal corpuscle and a long, often tortuously coiled renal tubule composed of the following anatomically modified and functionally distinct segments: the proximal convoluted tubule, the loop of Henle, and the distal convoluted tubule, which empties into a confluent collecting tubule.

Each nephron originates as a double-walled cup, the *Bowman's capsule,* which encloses the glomerular capillaries. Collectively, the Bowman's capsule and the glomerulus are termed the *renal (malpighian) corpuscle.* The epithelium of the Bowman's capsule is simple squamous, with the inner (visceral) layer containing modified cells called *podocytes.* The podocytes exhibit numerous foot-like extensions called *pedicels,* which contact the basement membrane of the glomerular capillaries.

The podocyte layer (visceral epithelium) of the Bowman's capsule together with the basement membrane and fenestrated endothelium of the glomerulus form a functional filtration membrane.

The outer (parietal) layer of the Bowman's capsule becomes continuous with the epithelium of the *proximal convoluted tubule.* The proximal convoluted tubule then straightens and plunges toward the medulla, forming the thick descending segment (pars recta) of the *loop of Henle.*

The loop of Henle is a U-shaped structure composed of a thick descending segment (pars recta), a thin segment, and a thick ascending segment. The thick ascending segment becomes continuous with the *distal convoluted tubule* at a modified site, the *macula densa,* where the tubular cells and their prominent nuclei are densely crowded.

The distal tubule coils in the area of the renal cortex before joining a collecting tubule. The latter descends into the medulla as part of a renal pyramid and empties through the papilla into a minor calyx.

Histologically, the proximal and distal segments of the tubule differ somewhat, reflecting differences in function.

The epithelium of the proximal segments (proximal convoluted tubule and pars recta) is characterized by a luminal "brush border" of extensive microvilli that greatly increase the free surface area available for reabsorption of filtered substances.

By contrast, the epithelia of the thick ascending limb of Henle's loop and the distal tubule are flatter with few microvilli. The epithelium of the thin segment of Henle's loop is simple squamous and lacks microvilli.

Juxtaglomerular Apparatus

At its origin the distal convoluted tubule lies close to the afferent and efferent arterioles. Here the distal tubular epithelium cells with their prominent nuclei are densely crowded, forming a discrete area termed the *macula densa.* Adjacent to the macula densa are modified afferent arteriolar cells called *juxtaglomerular cells,* which contain granules of the proteolytic enzyme *renin.* Collectively the juxtaglo-

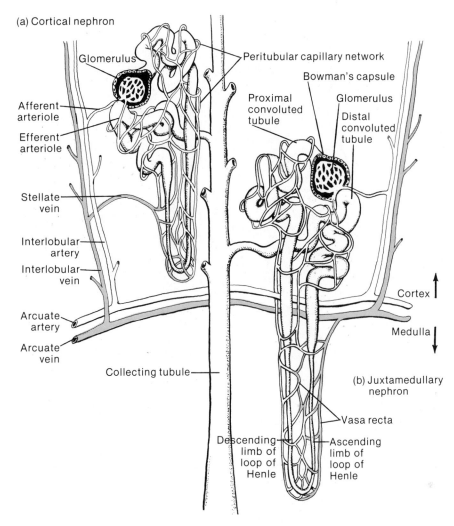

(a) Cortical nephron

Glomerulus

Afferent arteriole

Efferent arteriole

Stellate vein

Interlobular artery

Interlobular vein

Arcuate artery

Arcuate vein

Collecting tubule

Peritubular capillary network

Bowman's capsule

Proximal convoluted tubule

Glomerulus

Distal convoluted tubule

Cortex ↑

Medulla ↓

(b) Juxtamedullary nephron

Vasa recta

Descending limb of loop of Henle

Ascending limb of loop of Henle

Figure 36–2   Diagram of two nephrons and their blood supply. One nephron (*left*) has a short loop of Henle; the other nephron (*right*) has a long loop of Henle and a more extensive blood supply. (After Chaffee EE, Lytle IM: Basic Physiology and Anatomy, 4th ed. Philadelphia, JB Lippincott, 1980)

merular cells and the macula densa are termed the *juxtaglomerular apparatus* (Fig. 36-3).

The juxtaglomerular cells secrete renin in response to reduced renal perfusion (renal ischemia), hypotension, hyponatremia, hyperkalemia, and beta-adrenergic receptor stimulation.

By way of the macula densa, the nature of the tubular fluid in the distal tubule can also influence renin secretion by the juxtaglomerular cells.

Upon entering the blood, renin converts the plasma protein angiotensinogen into the decapeptide *angiotensin I.* Converting enzymes found largely in the lungs split a dipeptide from angiotensin I to form the physiologically active *angiotensin II.* Angiotensin II is a potent vasopressor substance that elevates blood pressure by promoting intense peripheral vasoconstriction and by stimulating secretion of the sodium-retaining hormone aldosterone, as outlined in Figure 28-4.

Control of Renal Blood Flow

Sympathetic vasoconstrictor nerve fibers arising from thoracolumbar segments of the spinal cord innervate the kidneys. In an average adult at rest the kidneys receive 20% to 25% of the cardiac output. Pain, cold, fright, strenuous exercise, hemorrhage, deep anesthesia, and other stressors reduce renal blood flow by activating sympathetic mechanisms for constriction of renal blood vessels.

Renal Physiology

The formation of urine by the nephrons involves three basic processes: glomerular filtration, renal tubular reabsorption, and renal tubular secretion.

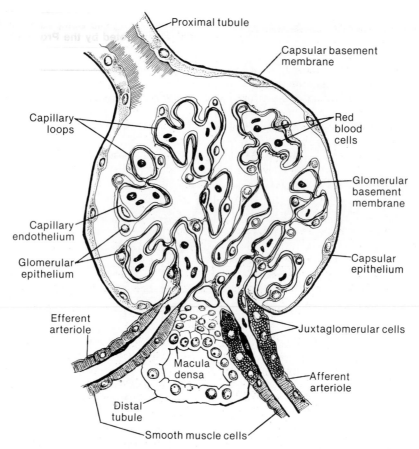

Figure 36–3 Semidiagrammatic drawing of a renal corpuscle. Note that the distal tubule appears to be attached to the afferent arteriole. Also depicted are the macula densa and the juxtaglomerular cells. The combined structure at the point of attachment is called the juxtaglomerular apparatus.

Glomerular Filtration

Glomerular filtration is a process whereby approximately one fifth of the plasma flowing through the glomerulus is passively transferred into the Bowman's capsule. The glomerular filtration membrane described earlier acts as a sieve, allowing passage of small molecules while restricting transfer of large molecular weight substances such as proteins.

The driving force for filtration is the hydrostatic pressure within the glomerular capillaries, which is ultimately derived from the work of the heart. The hydrostatic pressure in the glomerular capillaries is notably higher than that in other capillaries because the glomerulus is interposed between two arterioles.

Forces opposing filtration include the colloidal osmotic pressure of the plasma and the hydrostatic pressure of the Bowman's capsule. The colloidal osmotic pressure of the Bowman's capsule is close to zero because the glomerular filtrate is essentially protein-free.

The equation below shows how net filtration pressure can be calculated:

Net filtration pressure

  = Glomerular capillary hydrostatic pressure

    − [Plasma colloidal osmotic pressure

                         + Capsular hydrostatic pressure]

    (50 mm Hg) − (30 mm Hg + 10 mm Hg)

Therefore,

      Net filtration pressure = 10 mm Hg

Approximately 125 ml of filtrate are formed each minute. The glomerular filtration rate remains remarkably stable within a rather wide range of blood pressure variation due to an intrinsic mechanism of autoregulation. Glomerular filtration may be affected by changes in plasma colloidal osmotic presure, a force that opposes glomerular filtration. Decreases in plasma colloidal osmotic pressure will enhance filtration and *vice versa.*

The high rate of glomerular filtration (125 ml/min) yields a total of 180 liters of plasma filtered in 1 day. Yet the average volume of urine excreted in 1 day is less than 2 liters. Hence, over 99% of the glomerular filtrate is reabsorbed during passage through the renal tubules.

Renal Tubular Reabsorption and Secretion

Renal tubular reabsorption involves the transport of filtered substances across the renal tubular epithelium from the tubular lumen to the blood of the peritubular capillaries.

Renal tubular secretion, on the other hand, involves transtubular movement of substances from the blood of the peritubular capillaries to the tubular lumen.

Substances may be reabsorbed or secreted passively by diffusion along existing chemical, electrical, or osmotic gradients. They may also be actively transported against electrical or chemical gradients into or out of the tubular lumen by selective, carrier-mediated and energy-requiring transport systems. Each active renal transport system exhibits a *transport maximum* (T_m), which is the maximal rate at which a given substance can be carried across the renal tubular epithelium. For actively reabsorbed substances such as glucose, the plasma concentration of the substance that causes its transport maximum to be exceeded is termed the *renal threshold.*

Nutrients such as glucose and amino acids, and vitamins such as ascorbic acid are actively reabsorbed in the proximal tubule. Uric acid, an end product of purine metabolism, is actively reabsorbed and actively secreted in the proximal tubule. Urea, the major end product of nitrogen metabolism, is formed chiefly in the liver in accordance with the rate of protein catabolism. Filtered urea is passively reabsorbed by the renal tubules to an extent determined by the rate of urine flow and degree of water reabsorption.

Creatinine, a product of muscle metabolism, and histamine are actively secreted in the proximal tubule.

Many organic compounds of medical importance are also actively secreted in the proximal tubule. Among these are the drugs and diagnostic agents listed in Table 36-1. Because renal tubular secretion supplements glomerular filtration and enhances the removal of substances from the blood, impaired renal function may interfere with the excretion of therapeutic agents and may therefore require an adjustment (reduction) in drug dosage.

Renal Handling of Ions and Water

The amount of sodium excreted is normally equivalent to the amount ingested, over a wide range of dietary sodium intake. Renal handling of sodium is of singular importance to the maintenance of extracellular fluid volume, because renal tubular reabsorption of sodium is the major driving force for the passive reabsorption of water. Also linked to the active reabsorption of sodium are the secretion of hydrogen and potassium and the reabsorption of chloride and bicarbonate in certain tubular segments. Chloride and bicarbonate reabsorption are reciprocally related. If chloride reabsorption increases, bicarbonate reabsorption decreases, and *vice versa,* so that total anion concentration of the plasma remains constant.

Table 36-1. Organic Compounds of Medical Importance Actively Secreted by the Proximal Tubule

Compound	Medical Use
Drugs	
Acetazolamide (Diamox)	Carbonic anhydrase (CA) inhibitor
Chlorothiazide (Diuril)	Diuretic
Penicillin	Antibiotic
Probenecid (Benemid)	Uricosuric agent
Salicylates	Analgesic and anti-inflammatory agents
Tolazoline (Priscoline)	Alpha-adrenergic blocking agent
Diagnostic Agents	
Iodopyract (Diodrast)	Urologic contrast medium
Para-aminohippuric acid (PAH)	Measurement of renal plasma flow and tubular secretion
Phenolsulfonphthalein (Phenol red or PSP)	Measurement of renal plasma flow

The bulk (approximately 70%) of sodium reabsorption takes place actively in the proximal tubule. Chloride and bicarbonate passively follow the sodium out of the proximal tubule, accompanied by an osmotic equivalent of water so that tubular fluid osmolarity in this segment equals that of plasma. The reabsorption of water in this tubular segment is therefore termed *obligatory.*

In the loop of Henle, chloride is actively pumped out of the thick ascending limb, followed passively by sodium. The water impermeability of the ascending limb of Henle's loop leads to a net loss of salt (sodium chloride) and thus hypoosmolarity of the tubular fluid entering the distal tubule.

Active reabsorption of sodium resumes in the distal tubule and continues in the collecting tubules. Much of the reabsorbed sodium is accompanied by anion (chloride or bicarbonate). Other reabsorbed sodium ions are exchanged for secreted cations (hydrogen and potassium).

Sodium–potassium exchange in the renal tubules is controlled by the adrenal cortical hormone aldosterone, which favors sodium reabsorption and potassium secretion.

The passive reabsorption of water from the distal and collecting tubules is under the control of antidiuretic hormone (ADH). In the absence of ADH the epithelium of the distal and collecting tubules is essentially impermeable to water. The tubular fluid remains hypotonic and urinary volume is high. In the presence of ADH the epithelium of these tubular segments becomes highly permeable to water, permitting the *facultative* reabsorption of water according to osmotic gradients established in the loop of Henle through the countercurrent mechanism.

Countercurrent Mechanism

The conservation of water and concentration of urine by the kidneys is made possible by the operation of a countercurrent mechanism. Within this mechanism the loops of Henle act as countercurrent multipliers that establish an osmotic gradient in the renal medulla, while the vasa recta serve as countercurrent exchangers to maintain this gradient.

In the water-impermeable thick ascending limb of Henle's loop, chloride is actively transported out of the tubular fluid, followed passively by sodium, thus creating a *hyper*osmolarity in the medullary interstitium. The permeability of the epithelium in the descending limb of Henle's loop permits diffusion of water from the tubular fluid into the hyperosmolar medullary interstitium, and diffusion of sodium chloride and urea into the tubular fluid. Thus, a gradually increasing osmolarity of the tubular fluid and medullary interstitium is created as the turn in the loop of Henle is approached. ADH controls the final volume of urine available for excretion by promoting the facultative reabsorption of water from the collecting tubules passing through the medullary pyramids according to the osmotic gradient established by the countercurrent mechanism.

Renal Function in Acid–Base Regulation

The renal tubular epithelium participates in acid–base regulation by reabsorbing sodium bicarbonate and secreting hydrogen ions and ammonia. The hydrogen ions are derived from the dissociation of carbonic acid (H_2CO_3), which forms when carbon dioxide and water combined in the presence of the enzyme catalyst *carbonic anhydrase*. Hydrogen ions thus secreted into the tubular lumen combine chemically with phosphate buffers present in the tubular fluid to form monosodium phosphate (NaH_2PO_4).

Secreted hydrogen ions may also combine with the ammonia produced by the renal tubular epithelium from the deamination of amino acids such as glutamine. The secreted hydrogen ions and ammonia combine to form the ammonium ion (NH_4^+), which is excreted together with tubular anions such as chloride (Cl^-).

A diuretic is an agent capable of increasing the volume of urine and promoting a net loss of body water. The principal aim of diuretic therapy is to reduce the extracellular fluid volume, thus relieving or preventing edema, that is, excessive fluid accumulation in tissues. The retention of excess fluid by the body depends in large measure on the retention of *sodium.* Therefore, the effectiveness of a diuretic is primarily related to its ability to increase the excretion of sodium, which is accomplished in most cases by interfering with the reabsorption of sodium ions in the tubules of the kidney. Loss of sodium is accompanied by excretion of an osmotically equivalent quantity of water, which is derived from body fluids removed from the tissues.

The handling of electrolytes by the kidney involves a complex series of interrelated mechanisms. Drugs such as diuretics that affect the handling of one electrolyte (*e.g.,* sodium) almost invariably alter the handling of other electrolytes as well (such as chloride, potassium, hydrogen, bicarbonate). Depending on the mechanism of action of the individual diuretic drugs, therefore, various electrolyte or acid–base balance disturbances, or both, can develop during diuretic therapy. These electrolyte imbalances are often responsible for many of the disturbing and occasionally serious side-effects resulting from diuretic administration, and an understanding of the sites and mechanisms of action of the diuretics can aid in predicting the types of electrolyte changes expected with any one drug. The overall drug regimen can then be tailored to produce an optimal diuretic action with a minimal degree of electrolyte-induced side-effects (*e.g.,* combining a drug that produces potassium loss with a potassium-sparing drug).

It should be noted that the effectiveness and safety of diuretics are greatly compromised in the presence of kidney disease. Most diuretics are of little value in patients with significantly impaired renal function, and in many instances they can be quite hazardous. These drugs should be prescribed to patients with known or suspected kidney impairment only after consideration of the potential risks.

A large number of chemically dissimilar compounds have a diuretic action, and the diuretic drugs are usually classified on the basis of their predominant sites and mechanisms of action. The major categories of diuretics reviewed in this chapter are listed in Table 37-1, along with their principal sites of action in the kidney and the major electrolyte disturbances associated with each group. Refer to Chapter 36 for a discussion of the renal handling of the various ions present in the kidney; reference to Chapter 36 will also aid in understanding the sites and mechanisms outlined for each class of diuretics in the subsequent discussion.

Diuretics

37

I Carbonic Anhydrase Inhibitors

Acetazolamide   Methazolamide
Dichlorphenamide

Compounds in the group of carbonic anhydrase inhibitors are sulfonamide derivatives that interfere with the activity

Table 37-1. Diuretic Drugs: Sites of Action and Electrolyte Disturbances

Classes of Diuretics	Major Sites of Action	Electrolyte Disturbances
I. Carbonic anhydrase inhibitors (*e.g.,* acetazolamide)	Proximal tubule and distal tubule	Hyponatremic acidosis Hyperchloremic acidosis Hypokalemia
II. Indolines (*e.g.,* Indapamide)	Distal tubule and cortical ascending loop of Henle	Hypokalemia Hypochloremia Hyponatremia
III. Loop (high-ceiling) diuretics (*e.g.,* furosemide)	Thick ascending loop of Henle and proximal and distal tubules	Hypokalemia Hypochloremic alkalosis Hyponatremia (excessive diuresis) Hypocalcemia
IV. Mercurials (*e.g.,* mersalyl)	Thick ascending loop of Henle and possibly proximal and distal tubule sites	Hypochloremic alkalosis Hypokalemia (mild) Hyponatremia (excessive diuresis)
V. Osmotics (*e.g.,* mannitol)	Proximal tubule, descending loop of Henle, and collecting tubule	Minimal
VI. Potassium-sparing diuretics (*e.g.,* triamterene)	Distal tubule and collecting duct	Hyperkalemia
VII. Thiazides/sulfonamides (*e.g.,* hydrochlorothiazide, chlorthalidone)	Distal tubule and possibly *cortical* ascending loop of Henle	Hypokalemia Hypochloremic alkalosis Hyponatremia Hypercalcemia

of the enzyme carbonic anhydrase (CA), thus blocking the hydration of carbon dioxide (CO_2) to carbonic acid (H_2CO_3) and subsequent ionization to yield hydrogen (H^+) and bicarbonate (HCO_3^-) ions. In addition to their mild diuretic action, these agents also reduce aqueous humor production and are occasionally used in the treatment of glaucoma. They are also used adjunctively in treating some forms of epilepsy (see Chap. 25). The CA inhibitors are reviewed as a group, followed by a listing of individual drugs in Table 37-2.

Mechanism
Reduce formation of H^+ and HCO_3^- in renal tubules, thus decreasing HCO_3^- reabsorption in the proximal convoluted tubule and also decreasing the amount of H^+ available for $Na^+ - H^+$ exchange in the distal tubule and collecting duct. Increased urinary excretion of Na^+, HCO_3^-, K^+, and water ensues although diuresis is limited. Extended therapy leads to metabolic acidosis (loss of extracellular Na^+ and HCO_3^-), and tolerance to the diuretic action of the drugs.

Uses
1 *Adjunctive* treatment of drug-induced edema or edema due to congestive heart failure refractory to single drug therapy (not indicated alone in edema)
2 *Adjunctive* treatment of glaucoma (open-angle, secondary glaucoma, preoperative in narrow angle) to lower intraocular pressure
3 Adjunctive treatment of certain forms of epilepsy, especially *petit mal*
4 Prophylaxis of acute mountain sickness (*e.g.,* weakness, dizziness, nausea) at high altitudes (investigational use for acetazolamide–500 mg/day)

Dosage
See Table 37-2.

Fate
Readily absorbed from GI tract; onset of action following oral administration is 30 minutes to 60 minutes (longer with methazolamide); peak plasma levels occur in 2 hours to 4 hours (except sustained-release forms, which peak in 8 hr–12 hr); largely excreted within 24 hours, either as unchanged drug or *N*-dealkylated metabolites, some of which are active

Common Side-Effects
Paresthesias, drowsiness

Significant Adverse Reactions
CNS—confusion, myopia, tinnitus, malaise, vertigo, headache, xerostomia, depression, nervousness, weakness, flaccid paralysis, convulsions, tremor, ataxia
Dermatologic—skin eruptions, urticaria, pruritus, melena, photosensitivity
Hepatic/renal—hepatic insufficiency, pancreatitis, polyuria, dysuria, glycosuria, hematuria, urinary frequency, ureteral colic
Electrolyte—hypokalemia, hyponatremia
Other—aplastic anemia, diarrhea, vomiting, anorexia, loss of taste and smell
Note: Drugs are sulfonamide derivatives. See Chapter 57 for other potential adverse reactions.

Contraindications
Marked liver or kidney disease, chronic pulmonary disease, adrenocortical insufficiency, hyperchloremic acidosis,

Table 37-2. Carbonic Anhydrase Inhibitors

Drug	Preparations	Usual Dosage Range	Remarks
Acetazolamide (Ak-Zol, Dazamide, Diamox)	Tablets—125 mg, 250 mg Sustained-release capsules—500 mg Injection—500 mg/vial (sodium salt)	Glaucoma—250 mg orally, 1 to 4 times/day depending on response Edema—250 mg to 375 mg orally, once daily in the morning for 1 day to 2 days; then skip a day IV—500 mg initially; then 125 mg to 250 mg every 4 hours as needed in acute situations (500 mg/5 ml Sterile Water for Injection) Children—5 mg/kg/day Epilepsy—Adults and children: 8 mg to 30 mg/kg/day	Used for edema of congestive heart failure, minor and motor epilepsies, chronic open-angle glaucoma, and preoperatively in narrow-angle glaucoma; doses in excess of 1000 mg do not usually produce an increased effect. Sustained release form may be used on a twice-daily basis. Reconstituted injection solution should be used within 24 hours. Avoid IM administration if possible because alkaline solution is very painful upon injection.
Dichlorphenamide (Daranide)	Tablets—50 mg	100 mg to 200 mg initially, followed by 100 mg every 12 hours until desired response is achieved, maintenance 25 mg to 50 mg 1 to 3 times/day	Indicated as adjunctive treatment for open-angle glaucoma and preoperatively in narrow-angle glaucoma, together with miotics and osmotic diuretics
Methazolamide (Neptazane)	Tablets—50 mg	50 mg to 100 mg 2 to 3 times/day	Adjunctive therapy for both open-angle and narrow-angle glaucoma, with miotics and osmotic diuretics; contraindicated in *severe* or *absolute* glaucoma, hemorrhagic glaucoma, or that due to peripheral anterior synechiae; higher incidence of drowsiness than with other CA inhibitors

electrolyte imbalances, sensitivity to sulfonamides, pregnancy, and chronic noncongestive angle closure glaucoma

Interactions

1 CA inhibitors make the urine alkaline and thus may enhance the action of amphetamines, catecholamines, procainamide, quinidine, tricyclic antidepressants, and any other basic drug by increasing their reabsorption.
2 CA inhibitors can decrease the effects of lithium, barbiturates, nitrofurantoin, salicylates, and other acidic substances by reducing their renal tubular reabsorption.
3 A reduced hypoglycemic response to insulin and oral antidiabetics has been reported with CA inhibitors.
4 Increased hypokalemia can result with combinations of CA inhibitors and other diuretics, corticosteroids, and amphotericin B.
5 CA-induced hypokalemia may augment digitalis toxicity.

▶ NURSING ALERTS

▷ 1 Use cautiously in patients with respiratory acidosis, diabetes, and gout.
▷ 2 Counsel patients to note and report early signs of hypokalemia (palpitations, muscle weakness or cramping, fatigue, respiratory difficulty, orthostatic hypotension) and metabolic acidosis (nausea, vomiting, malaise, abdominal pain, hyperpnea, tinnitus, disorientation, dysuria, numbness in extremities). If signs occur, stop drug temporarily and reduce dosage upon resumption.
▷ 3 Be alert for signs of hypersensitivity (rash, fever) and possible blood dyscrasias (sore throat, bruising, mucosal ulceration) because drugs are sulfonamide derivatives. Advise physician immediately. Periodic (4 mo–6 mo) blood cell counts are recommended during prolonged therapy.
▷ 4 Do not interchange brands of carbonic anhydrase inhibitors in a patient stabilized on one product, because therapeutic equivalence among the different available products is not always realized.

▶ NURSING CONSIDERATIONS

▷ 1 Administer drugs on an alternate-day regimen (see Usual Dosage Range, Table 37-2) to minimize development of tolerance and loss of diuretic potency.
▷ 2 Monitor intake and output continually during acute drug therapy for edema. If diuretic effect decreases, *reducing* dose or frequency of administration often restores effectiveness.
▷ 3 Recognize that these drugs may increase antidiabetic drug requirements by increasing blood glucose levels. An adjustment in antidiabetic drug dosage may be necessary.
▷ 4 Administer drugs in the morning to provide most diuretic action during the day while patient is awake.
▷ 5 Caution patients against prolonged exposure to sunlight, because photosensitivity can occur.

▷ *Dietary precaution*
▷ 1 Encourage patient to consume foods high in potassium as part of his diet to minimize hypokalemia. Potassium-rich foods include orange and other fruit juices, bananas, fish, fowl, dates, prunes, raisins, cereal, and cola beverages.

II Indolines

▶ indapamide

Lozol

Indapamide is an indoline diuretic/antihypertensive drug structurally unrelated to the other classes of diuretics, but exhibiting many of the same pharmacologic and toxicologic actions as the thiazides.

Mechanism

Similar to that of the thiazide/sulfonamide diuretics (see discussion later in the chapter), with the addition of a possible direct vascular smooth muscle relaxant action, perhaps due to alterations in membrane calcium ion transfer; no significant effect on heart rate, force of contraction, cardiac output, glomerular filtration rate, or renal blood flow. Electrolyte and metabolic disturbances include hypokalemia, hypochloremia, hyponatremia, and hyperuricemia.

Uses

1 Treatment of hypertension, either alone in milder forms or in combination with other drugs in more severe forms
2 Treatment of edema associated with congestive heart failure

Dosage

Initially 2.5 mg as a single daily dose; increase to 5 mg/day after 1 week to 4 weeks if response is inadequate, or combine with other antihypertensive drugs.

Fate

Completely absorbed orally; peak blood levels are attained within 2 hours; approximately 70% to 80% protein-bound; extensively metabolized and excreted, primarily (70%) by the kidneys, with smaller amounts (20%–50%) by the GI tract. Plasma half-life is 12 hours to 15 hours.

Common Side-Effects

Headache, fatigue, weakness, and malaise

Significant Adverse, Reactions

CNS—dizziness, nervousness, irritability, anxiety, numbness of the extremities, vertigo, insomnia, depression, and blurred vision

GI—constipation, nausea, diarrhea, gastric irritation, abdominal cramping, and anorexia
Cardiovascular—palpitations, orthostatic hypotension, and irregular heart beats
Allergic—rash, urticaria, pruritus, and vasculitis
Miscellaneous—urinary frequency, nocturia, polyuria, impotence, flushing, dry mouth, paresthesias, rhinorrhea, hypokalemia, hyperuricemia, hyperglycemia, glycosuria, and increased serum creatinine and BUN

Contraindications

Anuria, sulfonamide hypersensitivity

Interactions

See Thiazides/Sulfonamides.

▶ NURSING ALERTS

See Thiazides/Sulfonamides.

▶ NURSING CONSIDERATIONS

See Thiazides/Sulfonamides. In addition:
▷ 1 Note that doses greater than 5 mg/day do not provide additional effects on blood pressure or edema, but are associated with a greater degree of hypokalemia

III Loop (High-Ceiling) Diuretics

Bumetanide   Furosemide
Ethacrynic acid

Several diuretic drugs are classified as "high-ceiling" agents, inasmuch as their peak diuretic effect is much greater than that observed with other clinically available oral diuretic drugs. Moreover, they exhibit a prompt onset of action when given orally, their action is independent of acid–base disturbances, and they are effective in patients with impaired renal function. The term *loop* derives from the fact that their site of action includes the thick ascending loop of Henle, as well as the proximal and distal tubules. The multiple sites of action of these drugs are responsible not only for their extreme potency, but also for the high incidence of fluid and electrolyte disturbances associated with their use. Careful medical supervision is, therefore, essential whenever these drugs are employed, and the dose must be critically adjusted for each patient. The drugs in this category are reviewed together; information pertaining to each individual drug is then presented in Table 37-3.

Mechanism

Inhibit active tubular reabsorption of sodium and chloride in the thick ascending loop of Henle, as well as other segments of the proximal and distal tubules, resulting in excretion of sodium, chloride, potassium, hydrogen, other electrolytes, and large quantities of water; renal blood flow is usually unaffected, and drugs have little effect on carbonic anhydrase or aldosterone. See Thiazides/Sulfonamides for other pharmacologic actions.

Table 37-3. Loop (High-ceiling) Diuretics

Drug	Preparations	Usual Dosage Range	Remarks
Bumetanide (Bumex)	Tablets—0.5 mg, 1 mg Injection—0.25 mg/ml	Oral—0.5 mg to 2 mg/day, as a single dose; maximum oral dose is 10 mg/day IV, IM—0.5 mg to 1 mg; repeat at 2-hour to 3-hour intervals to a maximum of 10 mg as needed	Drug is more chloruretic than natriuretic; does not appear to have a significant effect on the distal tubule; hypokalemia may be less severe than with furosemide; cross-sensitivity with furosemide is rare; use an intermittent dosage schedule for prolonged therapy; use parenteral solutions within 24 hours; safety and efficacy in children under 18 has not been established.
Ethacrynic acid (Edecrin)	Tablets—25 mg, 50 mg Injection—50 mg/vial (sodium salt)	Oral: Adults—initially 50 mg to 100 mg daily; maintenance dose 50 mg to 200 mg/day on an intermittent schedule Children—initially 25 mg/day; adjust dosage in 25-mg increments to achieve optimal response IV 0.5 mg/kg to 1 mg/kg (usual adult dose 50 mg); a second dose of 50 mg at a different site may be required (maximum 100 mg/dose)	Reconstitute IV solution by adding 50 ml 5% Dextrose Injection or Sodium Chloride Injection to vial; do *not* inject SC or IM, because pain and irritation may occur; direct IV injection should be made over several minutes; do not use solution if cloudy; discard within 24 hours after preparation; when used IV, be alert for presence of pain in calf, chest, or pelvic area, possible signs of thromboembolic complications; safety and efficacy of ethacrynic acid in treating hypertension has not been established; hypoproteinemia may reduce response to ethacrynic acid; discontinue drug if diarrhea occurs.
Furosemide (Lasix, SK-Furosemide)	Tablets—20 mg, 40 mg, 80 mg Oral solution—10 mg/ml Injection—10 mg/ml	Oral: Adults Diuresis—20 mg to 80 mg as a single dose; may increase by 20-mg to 40-mg increments to a maximum of 600 mg/day Hypertension—40 mg twice a day; adjust according to response; usual maintenance dose 40 mg to 80 mg/day in a single or two divided doses Children Initially 2 mg/kg as a single dose; may increase by 1-mg/kg to 2-mg/kg increments to a maximum of 6 mg/kg/day Parenteral: Adults 20 mg to 40 mg IV or IM as a single dose; may increase by 20-mg increments every 2 hours to 3 hours until desired response is obtained Acute Pulmonary Edema—40 mg IV over 1 minute to 2 minutes; may increase to 80 mg IV after 1 hour Children 1 mg/kg IV or IM; may increase by 1 mg/kg no sooner than 2 hours after previous dose; maximum 6 mg/kg	Oral doses should be given on an intermittent schedule (*e.g.*, 2 to 4 days/wk); parenteral therapy is indicated for emergency situations only, and should be replaced by oral therapy as soon as possible; do not mix parenteral solutions with highly acidic preparations; use mixture within 24 hours of preparation and do not use if solution is yellow; use cautiously in patients allergic to sulfonamides, because cross-reactions can occur; when adding drug to an existing antihypertensive regimen, reduce dose of other drugs by ½ to avoid excessive drop in blood pressure and titrate furosemide dosage to obtain optimal hypotensive effect; in patients with impaired renal function, use controlled IV infusion (4 mg/min) to minimize danger of azotemia or oliguria; drug can stimulate renal synthesis of prostaglandin E_2, which can complicate the neonatal respiratory distress syndrome.

Uses

1 Treatment of severe edema associated with congestive heart failure, hepatic cirrhosis, and renal disease
2 Relief of acute pulmonary edema (IV administration)
3 Adjunctive treatment of hypertension (furosemide)
4 Management of ascites due to malignancy, idiopathic edema, and lymphedema (ethacrynic acid)
5 Short-term management of pediatric patients with congenital heart disease or the nephrotic syndrome (ethacrynic acid)

Dosage
See Table 37-3.

Fate
Onset of diuresis following oral administration is 30 minutes to 60 minutes; peak effect occurs in 1 hour to 2 hours, and duration is 6 hours to 8 hours, except for bumetanide (4 hr). IV injection produces a diuretic response within 5 minutes to 10 minutes, which then peaks within 15 minutes to 30 minutes and persists for 2 hours. Drugs are highly bound to plasma proteins (94%–98%) and are rapidly excreted in the urine, both as metabolites and unchanged drug. Approximately one third of the dose is eliminated by way of the bile in the feces.

Common Side-Effects
Bumetanide: abdominal discomfort, orthostatic hypotension
Ethacrynic acid: anorexia, abdominal discomfort
Furosemide: orthostatic hypotension (initial period of therapy)

Significant Adverse Reactions
All drugs
GI—vomiting, diarrhea, dysphagia, acute pancreatitis, jaundice
CNS—headache, blurred vision, tinnitus, hearing loss, weakness, vertigo
Electrolyte—hypokalemia, hyponatremia, hypochloremic alkalosis, hypomagnesemia, hypocalcemia
Other—rash, pruritis, hyperglycemia, hyperuricemia, azotemia, increased serum creatinine, agranulocytosis, thrombocytopenia

Bumetanide
Dry mouth, arthritic pain, muscle cramping, hives, premature ejaculation, ECG changes, chest pain, hyperventilation, breast tenderness

Ethacrynic acid
GI bleeding, *profuse* watery diarrhea, fever, chills, hematuria, neutropenia, confusion, fatigue, hypovolemia, hypocalcemia, orthostatic hypotension, muscle cramping, and nystagmus

Furosemide
GI irritation, constipation, paresthesias, leukopenia, anemia, urticaria, photosensitivity, erythema multiforme, exfoliative dermatitis, necrotizing angiitis, weakness, urinary frequency, urinary bladder spasm, and thrombophlebitis

Contraindications
Anuria, hepatic coma, dehydration, severe electrolyte depletion, early pregnancy, and in infants

Interactions
▷ 1 Loop diuretics may potentiate the action of antihypertensive medications.
▷ 2 Loop diuretics may increase the toxicity of aminoglycoside antibiotics (ototoxicity), cephalosporins (nephrotoxicity), salicylates, lithium, and cardiac glycosides.
▷ 3 Increased orthostatic hypotension can occur with combinations of loop diuretics and alcohol, narcotics, or barbiturates.
▷ 4 Increased potassium loss may occur when corticosteroids are given with loop diuretics.
▷ 5 Loop diuretics may reduce the effectiveness of uricosuric drugs by elevating serum uric acid levels.
▷ 6 Probenecid may reduce the diuretic effectiveness of bumetanide and furosemide.
▷ 7 Phenytoin, indomethacin, and possibly other nonsteroidal anti-inflammatory drugs may impair the action of loop diuretics.
▷ 8 Loop diuretics can potentiate the muscle relaxing effects of the antidepolarizing neuromuscular-blocking drugs (*e.g.,* tubocurare, gallamine).
▷ 9 Increased requirements for oral antidiabetic drugs or insulin may occur in persons taking loop diuretics, which can elevate blood glucose levels.
▷ 10 Furosemide (and possibly bumetanide) can potentiate the pharmacologic effects of theophylline.
▷ 11 Ethacrynic acid may displace oral anticoagulants from their protein-binding sites.

▶ NURSING ALERTS
▷ 1 Be aware that these drugs can cause profound dehydration and electrolyte depletion (especially in the elderly or debilitated), possibly leading to circulatory collapse. Initiate therapy with small doses and adjust dosage carefully based on serum electrolyte levels as well as clinical response.
▷ 2 Perform periodic CO_2, BUN, WBC, and liver function studies as well as electrolyte determinations during prolonged drug therapy.
▷ 3 Observe for signs of electrolyte imbalance (anorexia, thirst, dry mouth, tachycardia, GI disturbances, restlessness, dizziness, weakness, fatigue, muscle cramps), and advise physician. Dosage should be adjusted or supplemental medications (*e.g.,* potassium or sodium) should be considered.
▷ 4 Caution patient to make positional changes slowly, because orthostatic hypotension can result in dizziness and fainting.
▷ 5 Discontinue drug if profound hypotension, hypovolemia, hematuria, or profuse diarrhea occurs. Inform physician.
▷ 6 Do not initiate diuretic therapy in persons in hepatic coma or in states of electrolyte deficiency. Correct underlying condition first.
▷ 7 Alert patient to report immediately any indication of impaired hearing (often preceded by vertigo and tinnitus). Dosage should be reevaluated, because danger of permanent hearing loss exists with prolonged high-dose therapy.
▷ 8 Monitor IV administration closely. Rapid or excessive diuresis can lead to hypovolemia, hypotension, and vascular collapse. Check blood pressure frequently and avoid extravasation of drug, because pain and irritation are common.

▷ 9 Perform periodic determinations of blood and urine glucose in known and suspected diabetics. Be alert for increases in blood glucose and altered glucose tolerance, and advise physician if they occur.

▷ 10 Use cautiously in patients with hepatic cirrhosis, diabetes, gout, or cardiogenic shock, in persons receiving digitalis drugs or potassium-depleting steroids, and in elderly patients.

▶ **NURSING CONSIDERATIONS**

▷ 1 Administer drug in the morning and early afternoon, if necessary, to avoid nocturia and interruption of sleep. Stress the importance of taking the drugs regularly as prescribed.

▷ 2 Determine baseline (predrug) body weight; weigh patient daily during therapy. Weight loss of 1 to 2 pounds/day during initial stages of therapy is desirable. Caution patient to report any *weight gain*.

▷ 3 Monitor infusion rate when drug is given IV. Rate should not exceed 4 mg/minute.

▷ 4 Watch for signs of joint swelling, tenderness, or pain, because these may signify onset of gout. Discontinue drug and advise physician.

▷ 5 Note that GI side-effects occur most frequently after 1 month to 2 months of therapy. Advise patients to report development of diarrhea or abdominal pain because dosage adjustment may be warranted.

▷ 6 Administer drugs with meals or food if necessary to reduce GI irritation.

▷ 7 Use intermittent dosage schedule where possible (*i.e.,* 3 days–4 days/wk, interspersed with rest period) to allow for stabilization of electrolyte and acid–base balance.

▷ 8 To minimize loss of potassium, provide potassium supplements or administer a potassium-sparing diuretic, especially in cirrhotic or nephrotic patients.

▷ *Dietary precautions*

▷ 1 To minimize excessive potassium loss, advise patients to consume potassium supplements or potassium-rich foods (*e.g.,* orange juice or other citrus fruits, cola beverages, bananas, raisins, beef, chicken, fresh fish, milk, prunes, raw carrots).

▷ 2 Advise patient to avoid licorice, because it contains glycyrrhizic acid, which can cause severe hypokalemia if ingested in large amounts.

IV Mercurial Diuretics

The use of mercurial diuretics has declined dramatically in recent years with the availability of equally effective and safer diuretic drugs. Currently, only one mercurial diuretic, mersalyl, is available, and it is very infrequently used. Mercurial diuretics are so named because they are complex organic compounds containing mercury in the divalent (mercuric) state. Mersalyl produces prompt and copious diuresis and is primarily indicated in severe edematous states secondary to other conditions such as congestive heart failure, renal disease, or cirrhosis. Its principal disadvantage is that it must be administered IM for optimal effect and thus is of limited usefulness for ambulatory or out-of-hospital patients.

Mersalyl elicits a lower degree of hypokalemia than most other potent diuretics and thus may prove useful in patients in whom excess potassium loss might be harmful. The preparation contains theophylline, which increases the absorption of the mercurial from the injection site and also assists in the removal of the potentially toxic mercury ions by the kidneys, reducing the danger of cumulation and possible nephrotoxicity.

▶ **mersalyl with theophylline**
Mercutheolin, Theo-Syl-R

Mechanism

In an acid environment, free mercuric ions (Hg^{++}) are liberated, which inhibit enzymes that supply energy for active tubular reabsorption of sodium and chloride; sodium and chloride reabsorption is decreased, primarily in the medullary segment of the ascending loop of Henle, leading to excretion of electrolytes and water. Hyperuricemia is rare. Tolerance develops in time, and patients become refractory due to development of hypokalemic, hypochloremic alkalosis. Responsiveness can be restored by administration of ammonium chloride (6 g–10 g/day) or by lengthening the time interval between injections.

Use

1 Treatment of severe edema secondary to congestive heart failure, hepatic cirrhosis, nephrotic syndrome, nephrotic stage of glomerulonephritis, or portal obstruction in the hospitalized patient

Dosage

(Injection contains 100 mg mersalyl and 50 mg theophylline per ml)
   Adults: 1 ml to 2 ml daily or every other day IM or by slow IV injection (diluted with 5 ml to 10 ml Sterile Water for Injection)
   Children: 0.5 ml to 1 ml
(Initial test dose to determine susceptibility is 0.5 ml in adults and 0.25 ml in children.)

Fate

Rapidly absorbed from injection site; diuretic response is seen within 1 hour to 2 hours, peaks in 4 hours to 8 hours, and persists for 12 hours to 24 hours; rapidly excreted (approximately one half dose within 3 hr)

Common Side-Effects

Flushing, pruritus

Significant Adverse Reactions

GI—vomiting, diarrhea, abdominal pain
Allergic—urticaria, fever, rash, anaphylactic reactions

Hematologic—thrombocytopenia, leukopenia, agranulocytosis

Electrolyte—hyponatremia, hypochloremic alkalosis, hypokalemia, hypomagnesemia

Other—ecchymoses, azotemia, transient urinary retention, vertigo, headache, hyperuricemia, mercurialism (stomatitis, gingivitis, metallic taste, salivation, gastric pain, diarrhea, proteinuria)

Contraindications

Acute or subacute nephritis, ulcerative colitis, severe liver or kidney disease, dehydration, and hypersensitivity to mercury

Interactions

1 Diuretic effects may be enhanced by other diuretics, chloride ion, and urinary acidifying agents (*e.g.,* ammonium chloride, l-lysine monochloride) and can be reduced by alkalinizing agents (*e.g.,* sodium bicarbonate).

2 Mersalyl may increase the risk of ventricular arrhythmias from catecholamines.

3 Diuretic-induced hypokalemia may increase digitalis toxicity and interfere with the hypoglycemic action of insulin and oral antidiabetics.

▶ NURSING ALERTS

▷ 1 If possible, administer a small initial test dose of the drug to ascertain if hypersensitivity exists. (It may be manifested as chills, fever, rash, or vomiting.)

▷ 2 Monitor intake–output ratio and vital signs at least daily during initial stages of therapy. Note lack of diuretic response or excessive diuresis, and advise physician. Too vigorous therapy can induce dehydration, hypovolemia, hypotension, and vascular thromboses.

▷ 3 In patients receiving repeated injections, perform electrolyte, CO_2, and BUN determinations and monitor urine for albumin, blood cells, and casts, possible indications of renal toxicity.

▷ 4 Instruct patients to watch for early signs of electrolyte imbalance (muscle cramping, paresthesias, thirst, nausea, abdominal pain, weakness, faintness, confusion), and advise physician immediately.

▷ 5 Use cautiously in patients with recent myocardial infarction, arrhythmias, benign prostatic hypertrophy, and in patients with a BUN above 60 mg/100 ml, in patients receiving digitalis drugs, and in pregnant or lactating women.

▷ 6 Discontinue drug if albuminuria, hematuria, or oliguria appears.

▷ 7 Have dimercaprol (BAL) on hand as antidote to prevent toxic effects in case of overdosage.

▶ NURSING CONSIDERATIONS

▷ 1 Administer drug in the morning to avoid nocturnal diuresis.

▷ 2 Select a nonedematous area for injection. The IM route (gluteus maximus, deltoid) is preferable for obese or emaciated patients, but drug may be given by deep

SC injection if necessary although a painful local reaction can result. Mersalyl may also be used by slow IV injection (diluted in 5 ml to 10 ml of Sterile Water for Injection) in the presence of marked edema.

▷ 3 Record daily weight loss of patient (2 lb–4 lb/day is the optimal rate). Report sudden, extreme weight changes.

▷ 4 Note that diuresis can be potentiated if desired by oral administration of 2 g to 3 g ammonium chloride 3 to 4 times a day for 2 days, before injection. Theophylline preparations and bed rest may also increase diuresis.

▷ 5 Caution patient against excessively reducing salt intake, especially in hot weather, because hypochloremic alkalosis and subsequent loss of drug responsiveness can occur. Dietary sodium should be reduced but *not* severely restricted (muscle cramps often signal sodium deficiency).

V Osmotic Diuretics

The term *osmotic diuretic* refers to any solute that is readily filtered by the kidney but poorly reabsorbed in the renal tubules. Consequently, the large amount of nonreabsorbed material increases the osmotic pressure of the tubular fluid, causing an osmotically equivalent amount of water to be carried through the tubule with it, eventually to be excreted. Sodium excretion is not significantly increased, however, by normal therapeutic doses of the osmotic diuretics. For this reason, as well as the fact that most of these diuretics must be administered IV in large doses, they are infrequently used for routine treatment of edema, and are primarily indicated for the prevention of acute renal failure associated with a sharply reduced glomerular filtration rate.

Their osmotic effects are not confined to the kidney, but extend to the bloodstream as well, where the presence of the drug in the circulation draws fluid from tissue spaces *into* the blood. This effect underlies their application in reducing elevated intraocular and intracranial pressures, actions important in treating cranial injuries and acute congestive glaucoma, and as an aid to neurosurgery.

▶ glycerin

Glyrol, Osmoglyn

Mechanism

Elevates plasma osmotic pressure, thus drawing fluid from extravascular spaces; decreases intraocular and intracranial pressure

Uses

1 Preoperative reduction in intraocular pressure as an aid to ophthalmic surgery (*e.g.,* for glaucoma, cataracts)

2 Lower intracranial pressure (investigational use for IV administration)

Dosage

Orally 1 g/kg to 1.5 g/kg of a 50% or 75% solution 1 hour to 1½ hours before surgery

Fate

Rapidly absorbed when taken orally; intraocular pressure is reduced within 15 minutes, maximal effect occurring in 1 hour; action persists 4 hours to 6 hours; metabolized in the liver

Significant Adverse Reactions

Nausea, vomiting, diarrhea, headache, disorientation, confusion, arrhythmias, dehydration, and hyperglycemia

▶ NURSING ALERT

▷ 1 Use cautiously in patients with diabetes, congestive heart disease, severe dehydration, hypervolemia, or confused mental states, and in elderly or senile persons.

▶ NURSING CONSIDERATIONS

▷ 1 Suggest that patients lie down during drug administration to minimize degree of headache from cerebral dehydration.

▷ 2 Note that glycerin is for oral administration *only;* do not inject. The 50% solution is lime flavored. Unflavored solutions may be made more palatable by addition of lemon juice or other flavoring agent.

▶ isosorbide

Ismotic

Mechanism

Increases plasma osmotic pressure, thereby reducing elevated intraocular pressure by promoting redistribution of fluid toward the circulatory vessels

Uses

1 Short-term reduction of elevated intraocular pressure prior to and following surgery for glaucoma or cataract
2 Interrupt an acute attack of glaucoma

Dosage

Initially, 1.5 g/kg orally 2 to 4 times a day; usual range is 1 g/kg to 3 g/kg 2 to 4 times a day.

Fate

Rapidly absorbed orally; onset of action is within 30 minutes; peak effect occurs in 1 hour to 1½ hours and duration lasts 5 hours to 6 hours.

Significant Adverse Reactions

Nausea, vomiting, diarrhea, thirst, headache, dizziness, lightheadedness, lethargy, irritability, rash, hiccoughs, and hypernatremia

Contraindications

Anuria due to severe renal disease, severe dehydration, acute pulmonary edema, and hemorrhagic glaucoma

▶ NURSING ALERTS

▷ 1 Maintain proper fluid and electrolyte balance during prolonged administration.

▷ 2 Monitor urinary output and discontinue drug if output continues to decrease, because extracellular fluid overload can occur.

▶ NURSING CONSIDERATION

▷ 1 Pour medication over cracked ice and sip to improve palatability.

▶ mannitol

Osmitrol

Mechanism

Not appreciably metabolized following IV injection, rapidly excreted by the kidneys; not reabsorbed in the renal tubules; hence raises the osmotic pressure of tubular fluid, which reduces reabsorption of water and increases urine flow; may increase electrolyte excretion when used in large doses; decreases elevated intracranial and intraocular pressure by raising plasma osmotic pressure

Uses

1 Prevention and treatment of the oliguric phase of acute renal failure before irreversible renal failure occurs
2 Treatment of cerebral edema and elevated intracranial pressure (*e.g.,* resulting from head injury or surgery)
3 Reduction of elevated intraocular pressure in acute congestive glaucoma
4 Treatment of acute chemical poisoning, by enhancing renal excretion of toxic substances
5 Measurement of glomerular filtration rate

Dosage

(IV infusion *only*)

Acute renal failure—50 g to 100 g as a 5% to 25% solution
Reduction of intracranial pressure—1.5 g–2 g/kg as a 15% to 25% solution over 30 minutes to 60 minutes
Reduction of intraocular pressure—1.5 g/kg to 2 g/kg as a 15% to 25% solution over 30 minutes
Acute chemical poisoning—100 g to 200 g depending on fluid requirement and urinary output
Measurement of glomerular filtration rate—100 ml of 20% solution diluted with 180 ml of Sodium Chloride Injection infused at a rate of 20 ml/minute
Test dose (patients with marked oliguria)—0.2 g/kg infused over 3 minutes to 5 minutes to produce a urine flow of at least 30 ml to 50 ml/hour

Fate

Confined to extracellular space; only slightly metabolized and rapidly excreted by the kidneys (80% of a dose appears in the urine within 3 hr); less than 10% is reabsorbed by the kidneys; diuresis occurs in 1 hour to 2 hours, and elevated cranial and ocular pressures are reduced within 30 minutes

Significant Adverse Reactions

(Infrequent) Dry mouth, thirst, headache, blurred vision, nausea, vomiting, rhinitis, diarrhea, marked diuresis, electrolyte imbalance, acidosis, fever, chills, dizziness, hypotension, dehydration, tachycardia, and angina-like pain

Contraindications

Anuria, severe pulmonary edema or congestive heart failure, intracranial bleeding, severe dehydration, progressive renal disease after initiating mannitol therapy, and in children under 12 years of age

Interactions

1 Edetate (EDTA, Versenate) may increase the absorption rate of mannitol.
2 The combination of mannitol and kanamycin has been reported to cause deafness.

▶ NURSING ALERTS

▷ 1 Monitor urine output continually and terminate therapy if output declines during infusion. Accumulation of mannitol can result in expanded extracellular fluid volume and congestive heart failure.
▷ 2 With prolonged administration, perform plasma electrolyte measurements and adjust infusion to prevent electrolyte imbalance.
▷ 3 Do not administer concurrently with whole blood unless at least 20 mEq of sodium chloride is added to mannitol solution to prevent pseudoagglutination.
▷ 4 Carefully evaluate patient's cardiovascular status before administering mannitol solution IV, because sudden expansion of extracellular fluid volume may aggravate or precipitate congestive heart failure.
▷ 5 In patients with severe renal impairment, use a test dose to determine effectiveness of drug. A second test dose may be given if an inadequate response (urine flow less than 30 ml/hr) occurred to the first.
▷ 6 Use cautiously in patients with marked cardiopulmonary or renal dysfunction and in pregnant women.

▶ NURSING CONSIDERATIONS

▷ 1 Avoid extravasation of solution and observe infusion site for inflammation and edema.
▷ 2 Adjust infusion rate to maintain a urine flow of at least 30 ml to 50 ml/hour.
▷ 3 Consult physician about allowable fluid intake.
▷ 4 If solution is crystallized (exposed to low temperatures), warm in hot water bath, then cool to body temperature before injecting. Do not administer if crystals are present.

▶ urea

Ureaphil

Mechanism

Filtered but not reabsorbed by the kidney; increased osmotic pressure in tubular fluid prevents water reabsorption and increases rate and volume of urine flow; elevates osmotic pressure of blood, thus increasing movement of fluid from body tissues to blood stream

Uses

1 Reduction of intracranial and intraocular pressure
2 Prevention of acute renal failure (*mannitol* is the preferred drug)
3 Induction of abortion (intra-amniotic injection)—*investigational use*

Dosage

(IV infusion *only*)
Maximum infusion rate 4 ml/min; maximum dose 120 g/day
Adults: 1 g/kg–1.5 g/kg
Children: 0.5 g/kg–1.5 g/kg
Infants: 0.1 g/kg–0.5 g/kg

Fate

Onset of diuretic effect is 4 hours to 8 hours; intracranial-intraocular pressure is reduced within 1 hour to 2 hours; widely distributed by the bloodstream and excreted by the kidney essentially unchanged

Common Side-Effects

Headache, nausea

Significant Adverse Reactions

Syncope, disorientation, confusion, agitation, pain, irritation, phlebitis and thrombosis at site of infusion, electrolyte imbalances, tachycardia, and hypotension

Contraindications

Severely impaired renal function, marked dehydration, intracranial bleeding, and frank liver failure

Interactions

1 Urea may potentiate the action of anticoagulants.
2 Urea can reduce the effectiveness of lithium by increasing its excretion.

▶ NURSING ALERTS

▷ 1 Closely monitor intake *and* output during urea infusion. If diuresis does not occur within 6 hours to 12 hours after injection, or if BUN exceeds 75 mg/100 ml, discontinue drug and reevaluate renal function.
▷ 2 Use extreme care to avoid extravasation of solution, because irritation, thrombosis, and tissue necrosis can occur.
▷ 3 Do not infuse into veins of lower extremities in elderly patients because thrombosis and phlebitis of deep veins may result.
▷ 4 Use cautiously in patients with liver impairment or kidney disease, and in pregnant or lactating women.

▶ NURSING CONSIDERATIONS

▷ 1 Do not infuse through the administration set used for blood infusion. Keep infusion rate below 4 ml/minute to avoid hemolysis.
▷ 2 Ensure that comatose patients receiving urea have an indwelling catheter for bladder emptying.
▷ 3 Prepare solution by reconstituting it with 5% or 10%

dextrose injection or 10% invert sugar in water. Use solution within a few hours if stored at room temperature (within 48 hr if stored at 2°C–8°C). Discard unused portion.

VI Potassium-Sparing Diuretics

Unlike most other major classes of diuretic drugs, the potassium-sparing diuretics do not cause a loss of potassium *via* the kidney. The potassium-sparing action is due to their inhibition of the sodium–potassium exchange mechanism in the distal segments of the renal tubule. These agents are not potent diuretic drugs when used alone and their use as single agents can result in significant hyperkalemia. Their principal application, therefore, is in combination with other oral diuretics (*e.g.,* thiazides, high-ceiling drugs) both to increase the excretion of sodium and water and, more importantly, to minimize the potassium loss normally induced by the more potent drugs. Because several important differences exist among the available potassium-sparing diuretics, they are reviewed individually.

▶ amiloride
Midamor

Mechanism
Acts on the distal segments of the renal tubules to reduce loss of potassium; does not function as an aldosterone antagonist; possesses weak diuretic and antihypertensive activity and only slightly enhances sodium excretion; little effect on renal blood flow or glomerular filtration rate

Use
1 Adjunctive treatment with potassium-depleting diuretics (*e.g.,* thiazides, high-ceiling drugs) to minimize potassium loss or restore normal serum potassium levels (rarely used alone)

Dosage
Initially 5 mg/day orally as a single dose added to the diuretic regimen; increase if necessary to 10 mg/day. Maximum recommended dose is 20 mg/day for severe, persistent hypokalemia.

Fate
Onset of action with oral administration is 2 hours; peak effects occur between 6 hours and 10 hours; duration is 24 hours; plasma half-life is 6 hours to 9 hours; not metabolized, but excreted unchanged in both the urine and feces in approximately equivalent amounts

Common Side-Effects
Nausea, anorexia, diarrhea, headache, flatulence, skin rash, hyperkalemia (paresthesias, muscle weakness, fatigue, bradycardia)

Significant Adverse Reactions
GI—vomiting, abdominal pain, dyspepsia, constipation, GI bleeding
CNS—dizziness, encephalopathy
Respiratory—dyspnea, coughing
Musculoskeletal—muscle cramping
Other—impotence, photosensitivity
A variety of other untoward reactions have occurred during amiloride therapy, but the causal relationship is uncertain.

Contraindications
Hyperkalemia, impaired renal function, and concomitant use with other potassium-sparing diuretics or potassium supplements

Interactions
1 Amiloride may increase lithium toxicity by reducing its renal clearance.
2 Hyperkalemia may be augmented by concomitant use of other potassium-sparing drugs (*e.g.,* spironolactone, triamterene) or potassium supplements.
3 Amiloride can reduce the clinical effectiveness of digitalis drugs, but also reduces the risk of toxicity resulting from hypokalemia.

▶ NURSING ALERTS
▷ 1 Be alert for early signs of hyperkalemia (see Common Side-Effects) and advise physician immediately. Monitor serum potassium levels regularly, particularly in the initial stages of therapy.
▷ 2 Use cautiously in patients with diabetes, renal impairment, cardiopulmonary disease, in pregnant women or nursing mothers, in children, and in elderly, debilitated, or severely ill patients.
▷ 3 Caution patients to avoid potassium supplementation or excessive consumption of potassium-rich foods (*e.g.,* orange juice, bananas, raisins, fresh fish, dates, raw carrots) during therapy with amiloride, because serum potassium levels may rise significantly.
▷ 4 Urge care while driving or operating other machinery, because drug may cause dizziness, headache, or visual disturbances.

▶ NURSING CONSIDERATIONS
▷ 1 Administer drug with food to minimize GI upset.
▷ 2 Monitor serum electrolytes and BUN frequently during extended therapy, and advise physician in the event of electrolyte imbalance or change in renal function.
▷ 3 Note that amiloride (5 mg) is available in fixed combination with hydrochlorothiazide (50 mg) as Moduretic.

▶ spironolactone
Aldactone, Spiractone

Mechanism
Competitive antagonism of the naturally occurring hormone aldosterone at renal tubular sites involved in the ex-

change of sodium for potassium; aldosterone normally stimulates enzymes that supply energy for the active ion-exchange process; inhibition of aldosterone thus impairs sodium–potassium exchange, resulting in excretion of sodium and retention of potassium; spironolactone does not appear to elevate serum uric acid or alter carbohydrate metabolism; interferes with testosterone synthesis, leading to increased estrogenic/androgenic activity ratio

Uses

1 Management of edema associated with congestive heart failure, primary hyperaldosteronism, cirrhosis of the liver, and nephrotic syndrome
2 Treatment of essential hypertension, usually combined with other diuretics or antihypertensive drugs
3 Adjunctive therapy with other potent diuretics to minimize potassium loss
4 Diagnosis and treatment of primary hyperaldosteronism

Dosage

(Oral administration only)
Edema—adults, 25 mg to 200 mg/day in a single dose or divided doses; children, 3.3 mg/kg in a single dose or divided doses
Hypertension—50 mg to 100 mg daily in a single dose or divided doses; maximum 200 mg/day
Diagnosis of hyperaldosteronism—400 mg/day for 4 days; if serum potassium increases during this time, then falls when drug is stopped, a presumptive diagnosis of primary hyperaldosteronism may be considered.
Treatment of hyperaldosteronism—100 mg to 400 mg/day
Hypokalemia—25 mg to 100 mg/day to prevent diuretic-induced potassium loss

Fate

Peak plasma levels occur in 3 hours to 4 hours following a single dose; maximal diuretic action is seen in 2 days to 3 days and may persist for several days after therapy is discontinued; highly bound to plasma proteins; rapidly and extensively metabolized and excreted primarily in the urine, with small amounts in the bile

Common Side-Effects

Gynecomastia and breast tenderness (in men and women), GI upset, and lethargy

Significant Adverse Reactions

Warning: Spironolactone has been shown to be a tumorigen in chronic toxicity studies in rats at significantly higher than recommended doses. Its use should be restricted to those indications outlined above for which other diuretic drugs are ineffective or inappropriate.

Cramping, diarrhea, vomiting, cutaneous eruptions, urticaria, fever, ataxia, drowsiness, confusion, impotence, hirsutism, irregular menses, voice deepening, postmenopausal bleeding, fluid and electrolyte disturbances (especially hyperkalemia and hyponatremia), mild acidosis, and elevated BUN

Contraindications

Anuria, acute renal insufficiency or significantly impaired renal function, and hyperkalemia

Interactions

1 Spironolactone potentiates the effects of other diuretics and antihypertensive drugs.
2 Salicylates may reverse the effects of spironolactone.
3 Spironolactone may reduce the clinical effectiveness of digitalis drugs but also reduces the likelihood of digitalis-induced arrhythmias occurring as a result of hypokalemia.
4 The renal clearance of lithium may be reduced by spironolactone.
5 The effects of oral anticoagulants may be reduced due to hemoconcentration of clotting factors resulting from diuretic action.
6 Ammonium chloride and other acidifying agents can induce systemic acidosis when given in combination with spironolactone.
7 Hyperkalemia may result if potassium supplements are used together with spironolactone, or if patients consume a potassium-rich diet.

▶ NURSING ALERTS

▷ 1 Be aware that spironolactone has been shown to induce malignant tumors in rats following chronic therapy with 25 to 250 times the usual human dose. Restrict use of the drug to those persons in whom other diuretic drugs are either ineffective or inappropriate.
▷ 2 Monitor serum potassium levels daily during early stages of therapy. Hyperkalemia may lead to cardiac irregularities. Advise patients to report early any signs of hyperkalemia (weakness, confusion, paresthesias, heaviness in the legs).
▷ 3 Avoid potassium supplementation during spironolactone therapy and caution patients against excessive intake of potassium-rich foods (*e.g.,* bananas, orange juice, citrus fruits, dates).

▶ NURSING CONSIDERATIONS

▷ 1 Monitor intake–output ratio, blood pressure, and body weight regularly during therapy. Report any marked changes in blood pressure or alterations in body weight.
▷ 2 Inform patients that swelling and tenderness of the breasts may occur, most often with prolonged therapy, but that this effect is usually reversible upon cessation of therapy.
▷ 3 Instruct patients to be alert for signs of hyponatremia (lethargy, thirst, dryness of the mouth, drowsiness) and advise physician.
▷ 4 Note that spironolactone is available in two fixed dosage combination with hydrochlorothiazide as Alazide, Aldactazide, Spiractazide, Spironazide, and Spirozide.

▶ triamterene

Dyrenium

Mechanism

Inhibits the exchange of sodium for potassium and hydrogen in the distal segment of the renal tubule; does *not* interfere with aldosterone but appears to act directly on the distal tubule

Uses

1 Treatment of edema associated with congestive heart failure, cirrhosis of the liver, or the nephrotic syndrome, and in steroid-induced or idiopathic edema
2 Adjunctive therapy of hypertension, in combination with other diuretics, for its added diuretic effect as well as its potassium-conserving effect

Dosage

When used alone 100 mg twice a day (maximum 300 mg/day); dose should be reduced when given in combination with other diuretics.

Fate

Erratically absorbed from the GI tract; onset of action is 2 hours to 4 hours; maximal diuretic effect occurs within 2 days to 3 days; duration of action is 6 hours to 9 hours after a single dose; significantly bound to plasma proteins; metabolized primarily in the liver and excreted by the kidneys

Common Side-Effects

GI upset, nausea, and leg cramps

Significant Adverse Reactions

Headache, weakness, metallic taste, dryness of the mouth, skin rash, photosensitivity, elevated BUN, hyperuricemia, hyperkalemia, hypotension, and blood dyscrasias (rare)

Contraindications

Anuria, severe hepatic disease, hyperkalemia, and severe or progressive kidney dysfunction (except nephrosis)

Interactions

See Spironolactone. In addition:
1 Serum levels of digitalis glycosides may be increased by triamterene.
2 Acute renal failure has been reported when indomethacin was given with triamterene.

▶ NURSING ALERTS

▷ 1 Use cautiously in patients with impaired renal or hepatic function, diabetes, or a history of gouty arthritis, and in elderly patients. Observe carefully for signs of electrolyte imbalances (*e.g.,* confusion, weakness, paresthesias, drowsiness, abdominal cramps, dry mouth, thirst), and advise physician immediately.
▷ 2 Perform periodic BUN and serum creatinine determinations during extended therapy especially in patients with kidney dysfunction as well as in elderly and diabetic patients. Note possible early signs of renal insufficiency (*e.g.,* fatigue, vomiting, stomatitis, confusion, bad taste in mouth).
▷ 3 Counsel patients to report immediately the development of fever, sore throat, mucosal ulceration, extreme fatigue, or weakness. These symptoms may indicate a blood dyscrasia, and blood counts should be performed.
▷ 4 Avoid potassium supplementation and excessive ingestion of potassium-rich foods during triamterene therapy. Severe hyperkalemia can occur, resulting in cardiac irregularities.

▶ NURSING CONSIDERATIONS

▷ 1 Administer drug with meals to minimize nausea. Be aware that nausea and vomiting may also be a sign of electrolyte imbalance and should be reported immediately.
▷ 2 Monitor intake–output ratio, blood pressure, and body weight regularly during prolonged therapy. Advise physician of any unusual or excessive changes.
▷ 3 Closely monitor diabetic patients for hyperglycemia during triamterene therapy, because drug can elevate blood glucose level.
▷ 4 Withdraw drug *gradually* over several days to prevent excessive rebound potassium excretion.
▷ 5 Note that triamterene is available in combination with 25 mg of hydrochlorothiazide as Dyazide.

VII Thiazides/Sulfonamides

Bendroflumethiazide	Hydroflumethiazide
Benzthiazide	Methyclothiazide
Chlorothiazide	Metolazone
Chlorthalidone	Polythiazide
Cyclothiazide	Quinethazone
Hydrochlorothiazide	Trichlormethiazide

The largest group of orally effective diuretic drugs, thiazides/sulfonamides are structurally related to the sulfonamide antibacterial drugs; however, they possess no anti-infective properties. Most of these sulfonamide diuretics are derived from a benzothiadiazine nucleus, and hence are commonly referred to as thiazide diuretics. A few other sulfonamide diuretics differ slightly in their chemical structure from the thiazides, although their pharmacologic and toxicologic properties are essentially similar, and these compounds are referred to as sulfonamide or thiazide-like diuretics. Structural differences notwithstanding, all of these drugs possess parallel dose-response curves, that is, there is essentially no difference among them in their clinical efficacy, and all drugs in this category possess similar sites and mechanisms of diuretic action.

The thiazide/sulfonamide diuretics are the most widely used drugs for the treatment of edematous states and for the control of mild to moderate hypertension. Because of the similarity of action among the various drugs in this class,

Table 37-4. Thiazide/Sulfonamide Diuretics

Drug	Preparations	Usual Dosage Range	Remarks
Bendroflumethiazide (Naturetin)	Tablets—2.5 mg, 5 mg, 10 mg	Edema—initially 5 mg to 20 mg/day; maintenance 2.5 mg to 5 mg/day Hypertension—initially, 5 mg to 20 mg/day; maintenance 2.5 mg to 15 mg/day	Long-acting preparation (18 hr–24 hr); low doses do not appreciably alter serum electrolyte levels; available in fixed combinations with potassium chloride (Naturetin-K), rauwolfia (Rauzide), and potassium plus rauwolfia (Rautrax-N)
Benzthiazide (Aquatag, Exna, Hydrex, Marazide, Proaqua)	Tablets—25 mg, 50 mg	Edema—initially 50 mg to 200 mg/day; maintenance 50 mg to 150 mg/day Hypertension—initially 50 mg to 100 mg/day; maintenance 50 mg 2 to 4 times/day	Maximal effect in 4 hours to 6 hours, with a duration of 12 hours to 18 hours
Chlorothiazide (Diachlor, Diuril, SK-Chlorothiazide)	Tablets—250 mg, 500 mg Suspension—250 mg/5 ml Injection—500 mg/20 ml	Edema Adults—0.5 g to 1 g 1 to 2 times a day, 3 to 5 days/week Children—22 mg/kg/day in 2 doses Hypertension—0.5 to 1 g/day, adjusted to optimal response	Following oral administration, onset within 2 hours and duration of 6 hours to 12 hours; IV solution prepared by adding 18 ml Sterile Water to vial; do not administer with plasma or whole blood, nor give SC or IM; use IV *only* in emergency situations and avoid extravasation; IV injections are not recommended in children; solutions may be stored up to 24 hours at room temperature; available with reserpine (Diupres) and methyldopa (Aldoclor) in oral form
Chlorthalidone (Hygroton, Hylidone, Thalitone)	Tablets—25 mg, 50 mg, 100 mg	Edema—50 mg to 100 mg/day or 100 mg/day 3 times a week on alternate days Hypertension—initially 25 mg to 50 mg; adjust to optimal response; maximum 100 mg/day Children—3 mg/kg/day, 3 times/week	Sulfonamide diuretic; onset 2 hours to 3 hours and duration 48 hours to 72 hours; given by single daily dosage in the morning; effective hypotensive agent, often used as initial therapy in mild hypertension; may elevate plasma levels of cholesterol, triglycerides, and LDL; available with clonidine (Combipres) and reserpine (Regroton, Demi-Regroton)
Cyclothiazide (Anhydron, Fluidil)	Tablets—2 mg	Edema—1 mg to 2 mg/day; reduce to 1 mg to 2 mg 2 to 3 times a week as necessary Hypertension—2 mg once a day (maximum 6 mg once a day) Children—0.02 mg to 0.04 mg/kg/day in divided doses	Slow onset (4 hr–6 hr) and prolonged duration of action (18 hr–24 hr); given in early morning to minimize sleep disturbance
Hydrochlorothiazide (Esidrix, Hydrodiuril, and various other manufacturers)	Tablets—25 mg, 50 mg, 100 mg	Edema—initially 25 mg to 200 mg/day; maintenance 25 mg to 100 mg/day, usually on an intermittent schedule Hypertension—initially 50 mg to 100 mg/day; adjust to desired response; usual range 25 mg to 100 mg/day Children—2.2 mg/kg/day	Most widely used thiazide diuretic; onset 1 hour to 2 hours and duration 6 hours to 12 hours; available in fixed combination with many other antihypertensive drugs; oral absorption may be improved if taken with food
Hydroflumethiazide (Diucardin, Saluron)	Tablets—50 mg	Edema—initially 50 mg to 100 mg/day; usual maintenance dose 25 mg to 200 mg/day on an intermittent schedule Hypertension—50 mg twice a day; adjusted to desired response	Rapid onset (1 hr–2 hr) and short duration (6 hr–12 hr); do not exceed 200 mg/day; available with reserpine (Salutensin)
Methyclothiazide (Aquatensen, Enduron, Ethon)	Tablets—2.5 mg, 5 mg	Edema—2.5 mg to 10 mg daily Hypertension—2.5 mg to 5 mg daily	Onset in 2 hours and duration lasts about 24 hours; do not exceed 10 mg/day; available with reserpine (Diutensen-R), deserpidine (Enduronyl), pargyline (Eutron), and cryptenamine (Diutensen)

Table 37-4. Thiazide/Sulfonamide Diuretics (continued)

Drug	Preparations	Usual Dosage Range	Remarks
Metolazone (Diulo, Zaroxolyn)	Tablets—2.5 mg, 5 mg, 10 mg	Edema—5 mg to 20 mg once daily Hypertension—2.5 mg to 5 mg once daily	Sulfonamide derivative with rapid onset (1 hr) and moderate duration (12 hr–24 hr) of action; dosage should be in upper end of range in patients with congestive heart failure to ensure diuretic effect for full 24 hours; not recommended in children; profound volume and electrolyte depletion can occur in combination with furosemide
Polythiazide (Renese)	Tablets—1 mg, 2 mg, 4 mg	Edema—1 mg to 4 mg/day Hypertension—2 mg to 4 mg/day Children—0.02 mg to 0.08 mg/kg/day	Onset 1 hour to 2 hours and duration 24 hours to 36 hours; available with reserpine (Renese-R) and prazosin (Minizide)
Quinethazone (Hydromox)	Tablets—50 mg	50 mg to 100 mg in a single daily morning dose; maximum 200 mg/day	Sulfonamide diuretic with an onset of 2 hours and a duration of 18 hours to 24 hours; available with reserpine as Hydromox-R
Trichlormethiazide (Diurese, Metahydrin, Mono-Press, Naqua, Niazide, Trichlorex)	Tablets—2 mg, 4 mg	Edema—1 mg to 4 mg/day Hypertension—2 mg to 4 mg/day Children—0.07 mg/kg/day	Onset 2 hours and duration 24 hours or longer; available with reserpine (Metatensin, Naquival)

they are reviewed as a group. Individual drugs are then listed in Table 37-4.

Mechanism

Diuretic

Impair active sodium and chloride reabsorption in the early portion of the distal segment of the renal tubule and possibly also in the cortical thick ascending loop of Henle, resulting in excretion of these ions with an osmotically equivalent volume of water; possess weak carbonic anhydrase inhibitory activity, although the importance of this action to their diuretic effect is probably minimal. Bicarbonate excretion is slightly increased, whereas calcium excretion is reduced. Potassium is lost *via* exchange with sodium in the more distal portions of the tubule.

Antihypertensive

May be due to (1) reduction of plasma volume and sodium levels, (2) direct relaxation of arteriolar smooth muscle, and (3) decreased reactivity of vascular smooth muscle to endogenous pressor substances, possibly the result of alterations in sodium content within the muscle fibers

Other

Interfere with insulin release, possibly a result of hypokalemia, and compete with uric acid for renal tubular secretory sites, thus elevating serum uric acid levels; exert a paradoxical *anti*diuretic effect in diabetes insipidus, possibly by enhancing the action of antidiuretic hormone (ADH) as consequence of sodium depletion

Uses

1 Treatment of edema associated with congestive heart failure, hepatic cirrhosis, renal dysfunction, and steroid or estrogen therapy
2 Management of all forms of hypertension, either alone (mild cases) or in combination with other antihypertensive drugs (moderate to severe cases)
3 Symptomatic treatment of diabetes insipidus to reduce polyuria
4 Prevent formation and recurrence of calcium stones in hypercalciuria, either alone or with amiloride or allopurinol (investigational use)

Dosage

See Table 37-4.

Fate

Well absorbed orally; onset of diuresis is usually 1 hour to 2 hours after oral administration (except cyclothiazide 4 hr–6 hr); peak diuretic effect generally occurs in 4 hours to 6 hours, and duration ranges from 6 hours to 72 hours (average duration is 12 hr–18 hr); several days are necessary for development of the antihypertensive action, and peak antihypertensive effects generally occur after 2 weeks to 4 weeks; many drugs are highly bound to plasma proteins; excreted in the urine, both as unchanged drug and metabolites

Common Side-Effects

Lightheadedness, hypokalemia (muscle weakness, dizziness, paresthesias, cramping), especially if potassium supplements are not employed

Significant Adverse Reactions

GI—nausea, GI irritation, vomiting, anorexia, dry mouth, diarrhea, cramping, bloating, jaundice, pancreatitis, sialadenitis, hepatitis
Cardiovascular—orthostatic hypotension, palpitation, angina-like pain, hemoconcentration
CNS—headache, vertigo, blurred vision, syncope, fatigue, drowsiness

Hypersensitivity—rash, photosensitivity, fever, purpura, urticaria, vasculitis, Stevens–Johnson syndrome, dyspnea, pneumonitis, anaphylactic reactions

Hematologic—blood dyscrasias (rare)

Other—muscle spasm, chills, impotence, hyperglycemia, hyperuricemia, elevated BUN, hypercalcemia

Contraindications

Sulfonamide hypersensitivity, anuria, renal decompensation, IV administration in infants and children; metolazone is also contraindicated in patients with hepatic coma or precoma.

Interactions

1 Thiazides potentiate the hypotensive action of other antihypertensive drugs, and may increase the incidence of orthostatic hypotension due to alcohol, narcotics, barbiturates and other CNS depressants, phenothiazines, and tricyclic antidepressants.

2 The effects of oral anticoagulants, vasopressors, hypouricemic drugs, and oral antidiabetics may be antagonized by thiazide diuretics.

3 Hypokalemia may be intensified if thiazides are combined with corticosteroids.

4 Thiazide-induced hypokalemia may increase digitalis toxicity.

5 Indomethacin and the pyrazolones may reduce the diuretic efficacy of the thiazides.

6 Hypercalcemia can occur if thiazides are given with calcium carbonate or other calcium-containing products.

7 Thiazides can potentiate amphetamines, quinidine, and lithium by decreasing their excretion.

8 Prolonged relaxation of skeletal muscle (including respiratory) may occur if thiazides are given together with nondepolarizing muscle relaxants (*e.g.,* curare, gallamine, pancuronium, atracurium).

▶ NURSING ALERTS

▷ 1 Use with caution in patients with renal or hepatic disease, bronchial asthma, diabetes, gout, history of allergies, lupus erythematosus, advanced arteriosclerosis, or advanced heart disease, and in elderly or debilitated persons and pregnant women or nursing mothers.

▷ 2 Monitor intake–output ratio and be alert for development of excessive diuresis, which can lead to severe electrolyte imbalance.

▷ 3 Inform patients that physician should be advised at

first sign of possible electrolyte imbalance (*e.g.,* thirst, dryness of mouth, anorexia, weakness, fatigue, muscle pain, oliguria, GI disturbances, tachycardia, paresthesias, confusion, irritability). Imbalances are more likely in elderly or debilitated patients or after excessive loss of fluid (*e.g.,* brisk diuresis, vomiting, diarrhea).

▷ 4 Advise patients to make positional changes slowly to minimize danger of orthostatic hypotension (dizziness, ataxia, fainting).

▶ NURSING CONSIDERATIONS

▷ 1 Perform baseline and periodic determinations of serum electrolytes, BUN, CO_2, uric acid, blood sugar, blood counts, body weight, and blood pressure.

▷ 2 Closely observe patients taking digitalis drugs, hypouricemic agents, and oral antidiabetics for loss of effectiveness or development of toxic reactions during thiazide therapy. Dosage adjustments may be necessary.

▷ 3 Discontinue thiazides 48 hours before surgery, because they may enhance the action of muscle relaxants and reduce the effectiveness of pressor amines.

▷ 4 Stress the importance of adjunctive measures (*e.g.,* proper diet, cessation of smoking, decreased caffeine and sodium intake) in the overall control of hypertension with thiazide diuretics.

▷ 5 When adding thiazides to an existing antihypertensive regimen, reduce the dose of each by one half to avoid excessive hypotension. Dosage may then be slowly titrated to obtain maximal benefit.

▷ 6 Discontinue thiazides for several days before performing parathyroid function tests because drugs may decrease calcium excretion.

▷ 7 If possible, give drug in the morning to avoid nocturia. Administer with food to minimize gastric irritation.

▷ 8 Use an intermittent dosing schedule whenever possible to minimize excessive diuresis and undesirable electrolyte imbalances.

▷ *Dietary precautions*

▷ 1. Suggest that patient's daily diet contain high-potassium foods (*e.g.,* citrus fruits, bananas, cola drinks, potatoes, prunes, dates) to decrease possibility of hypokalemia.

▷ 2 Urge patient to avoid high-sodium foods (*e.g.,* lunch meats, smoked meats, Chinese food, processed cheeses, snack foods) and not to add any table salt to other foods.

▷ 3 Caution patient to avoid licorice, because hypokalemia may be worsened if it is consumed in large amounts.

Summary. Diuretics

Drug	Preparations	Usual Dosage Range
Carbonic Anhydrase (CA) Inhibitors		
See Table 37-2.		
Indolines		
Indapamide (Lozol)	Tablets—2.5 mg	Initially 2.5 mg/day; increase to 5 mg/day as needed

Summary. Diuretics *(continued)*

Drug	Preparations	Usual Dosage Range
Loop (High-Ceiling) Diuretics		
See Table 37-3.		
Mercurials		
Mersalyl with Theophylline (Mercutheolin, Theo-Syl-R)	Injection—100 mg mersalyl and 50 mg theophylline per ml	IM—1 ml to 2 ml daily or every other day until desired weight is attained; then individualize
		Children—0.5 ml to 1 ml
		IV—1 ml to 2 ml as needed—(dilute injection with 5 ml to 10 ml Sterile Water for Injection and administer slowly)
		(Test dose 0.5 ml IM in adults and 0.25 ml in children)
Osmotic Diuretics		
Glycerin (Glyrol, Osmoglyn)	Oral solution—50%, 75%	1 g/kg to 1.5 g/kg, 1 hour to 1½ hour before ocular surgery
Isosorbide (Ismotic)	Oral solution—100 g/220 ml	1 g/kg to 3 g/kg 2 to 4 times a day
Mannitol (Osmitrol)	Injection—5%, 10%, 15%, 20%, 25%	50 g to 200 g/24 hours by IV infusion
		Rate adjusted to maintain a urine flow of 30 ml to 50 ml/hour
Urea (Ureaphil)	Injection—40 g/150 ml	Adults—1 g/kg to 1.5 g/kg
		Children—0.5 g/kg to 1.5 g/kg
		Infants—0.1 g/kg to 0.5 g/kg
		(Maximum dose 120 g/day)
Potassium-Sparing Diuretics		
Amiloride (Midamor)	Tablets—5 mg	5 mg to 10 mg/day added to the diuretic regimen; maximum dose is 20 mg/day
Spironolactone (Aldactone, Spiractone)	Tablets—25 mg, 100 mg	Edema—25 mg to 200 mg/day in divided doses
		Children—3.3 mg/kg/day in divided doses
		Hypertension—50 mg to 100 mg/day in divided doses
		Hyperaldosteronism—100 mg to 400 mg/day prior to surgery
Triamterene (Dyrenium)	Capsules—50 mg, 100 mg	100 mg twice a day (maximum 300 mg/day)
Thiazides/Sulfonamides		
See Table 37-4.		

Drugs Acting on the Endocrine Glands

The endocrine system functions in close harmony with the nervous system in regulating, coordinating, and integrating the wide range of metabolic and physiologic activities essential to the maintenance of homeostasis in an everchanging environment.

The anatomically distinct and functionally diverse organs of the endocrine system participate in the regulation of the following basic activities: (1) energy metabolism, (2) electrolyte and water metabolism, (3) reproduction, (4) growth and development, and (5) response to stress.

The products of endocrine glands, the *hormones,* are characteristically produced in small amounts by specialized glandular cells and are secreted directly into the bloodstream, whereby they are transported to specific target tissues upon which they exert regulatory control.

Chemically, hormones may be

1 Polypeptides or proteins (*e.g.,* insulin and growth hormone)
2 Steroids (*e.g.,* aldosterone and cortisol)
3 Amines (*e.g.,* epinephrine and thyroxine)

The Endocrine Glands— A Review

38

Transport and Metabolism of Hormones

Most hormones are transported through the blood bound to plasma proteins. Because only free (unbound) hormone is physiologically active and subject to biodegradation (metabolic transformation), protein binding affords a mechanism for readily available reserve hormone. Hormones may be inactivated by the liver, kidneys, or, more rarely, by the target tissues themselves. Because of the great importance of the liver and kidneys in the metabolism and excretion of hormones, the state of hepatic and renal function should be established during the course of diagnosing specific endocrine dysfunction.

Mechanisms of Hormone Action

The mechanisms whereby hormones exert their specific effects on target tissues vary. Steroid hormones such as aldosterone bind to intracellular receptors and affect DNA transcription, ultimately modifying protein synthesis. Several hormones, including epinephrine and glucagon, act through a second messenger to activate specific enzymes, while others, such as insulin and antidiuretic hormone (ADH), alter permeability characteristics of selected cell membranes to certain substrates.

Second Messenger Mechanism

Several hormones have been shown to exert their effects by way of a "second messenger." The hormone, acting as the

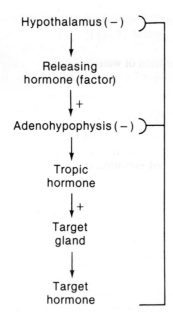

Figure 38-1 Negative feedback mechanism regulating endocrine hormone secretion.

first messenger, binds to specific receptors at the outer surface of a target cell membrane. The hormone–receptor interaction leads to the activation of the enzyme *adenyl cyclase,* which then converts cytoplasmic adenosine triphosphate (ATP) into cyclic adenosine monophosphate (*cyclic AMP*).

Before being inactivated by phosphodiesterase enzymes, the cyclic AMP acts as the second messenger to bring about a specific cellular action (*e.g.,* enzyme activation or change in membrane permeability to a given substrate).

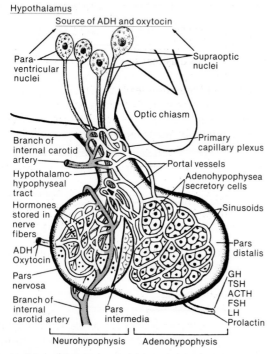

Figure 38-2 The pituitary gland (hypophysis) and its relationship with the hypothalamus.

Regulation of Hormone Secretion

Secretion of certain hormones is under the direct control of the nervous system. Other hormones are controlled by the blood level of an electrolyte (*e.g.,* calcium) or a metabolite (*e.g.,* glucose). Most, however, are controlled by a negative feedback mechanism (Fig. 38-1) whereby an elevation in the plasma concentration of a given hormone inhibits its production by the endocrine gland.

Pituitary Gland

The pituitary gland, sometimes called the "master gland," secretes several polypeptide hormones that directly or indirectly regulate a wide variety of metabolic and physiologic processes essential to normal growth and development as well as to the maintenance of homeostasis. Many of the hormones secreted by the pituitary gland are critical to the activity of target glands, including the thyroid, adrenals, and gonads.

Anatomy

The pituitary gland (*hypophysis cerebri*) is located at the base of the brain, resting within the sella turcica of the sphenoid bone. The pituitary gland maintains elaborate neural and vascular connections with the hypothalamus of the brain, which plays a central role in the integration of neuroendocrine activity (Fig. 38-2).

The pituitary gland has two major divisions: the *neurohypophysis* and the *adenohypophysis.*

Neurohypophysis

The *neurohypophysis,* which is connected directly to the hypothalamus by the *infundibular* (pituitary) *stalk,* is rich in nerve fibers of hypothalamic origin (the *hypothalamohypophyseal tract*).

Neurosecretory cells in the *supraoptic* and *paraventricular nuclei* of the hypothalamus produce two hormones: *antidiuretic hormone* (ADH or vasopressin) and *oxytocin.* These hormones are then transported along the axons of the hypothalamohypophyseal tract to the *pars nervosa* (posterior lobe) of the pituitary gland for storage and ultimate release.

Adenohypophysis

The *adenohypophysis* is served by an elaborate vascular system, including the *hypothalamohypophyseal portal system,* which transports hypothalamic regulating hormones (factors) to the glandular cells of the adenohypophysis.

The largest portion of the adenohypophysis is the *pars distalis* (anterior lobe). Its secretory chromophilic cells include the following:

1 *Acidophils* (alpha cells), which constitute 40% of the cellular population, and which secrete *growth hormone* (GH; somatotropin; STH) and *prolactin* (luteotropic hormone; LTH)

2 *Basophils* (beta cells), which represent 10% of the glandular cells, and which secrete four hormones: *thyroid-stimulating hormone* (TSH; thyrotropin); *adrenocorticotropic hormone* (ACTH; corticotropin); *follicle-stimulating hormone* (FSH), and *luteinizing hormone* (LH)

The remaining 50% of the cells in the adenohypophysis, the *chromophobes,* are believed to be undifferentiated precursors of the chromophils. Nevertheless, chromophobe tumors have been associated with excessive secretion of ACTH and GH.

The *pars intermedia* (intermediate lobe) of the adenohypophysis contains basophilic (beta) cells, which secrete *melanocyte-stimulating hormone* (MSH or intermedin).

A third region, the *pars tuberalis,* forms an incomplete sheath around the infundibular stalk. To date, no specific hormones have been associated with the pars tuberalis.

Hormones of the Neurohypophysis

Antidiuretic Hormone (ADH; Vasopressin)

Control of Secretion

Antidiuretic hormone (ADH) is a polypeptide hormone of hypothalamic origin (supraoptic nuclei) that is stored in and released from the neurohypophysis in response to a variety of stimuli. Included among these are increased plasma osmolality, reduced extracellular fluid (ECF) volume, pain, emotional stress, and pharmacologic agents such as morphine, nicotine, ether, and the barbiturates.

Decreased plasma osmolality, increased ECF volume, and alcohol inhibit ADH secretion.

Osmoreceptors found in the anterior hypothalamus monitor changes in plasma osmolality, while ECF volume changes are detected by volume ("stretch") receptors located in the wall of the left atrium. The osmoreceptors and volume receptors work in concert to exert precise control over ADH secretion, thus forming a delicate homeostatic feedback mechanism for the regulation of ECF volume and concentration.

Actions

The principal physiologic role of ADH is to regulate extracellular fluid volume and osmolality by controlling the final volume and concentration of urine.

ADH, acting through the second messenger cyclic AMP, increases the permeability of the distal nephron (distal convoluted tubules and collecting tubules) to water. The enhanced reabsorption of water from the renal tubules results in the production of a concentrated urine that is reduced in volume.

Pharmacologic amounts of ADH produce a *pressor* (hypertensive) effect that results from a direct constrictor action of the hormone on vascular smooth muscle.

The early observations that posterior pituitary extracts produce a marked elevation of arterial blood pressure led to the initial naming of this hormone as *vasopressin.*

Clinical States

Diabetes Insipidus

Inadequate ADH secretion results in the excretion of large volumes of dilute urine (polyuria). Intense thirst and consumption of large amounts of liquid (polydipsia) are also characteristic of diabetes insipidus.

This disorder may be idiopathic, or it may follow trauma or cranial injury, central nervous system disease, infection, or emotional shock. The deficit may be related to the supraoptic nuclei, the hypothalamohypophyseal tract, or the neurohypophysis.

A rare ADH-resistant or *nephrogenic* diabetes also exists. In this inherited disorder, ADH secretion is normal; however, the renal tubules are unresponsive to the hormone. Treatment of diabetes insipidus is discussed in Chapter 39.

Inappropriate ADH Syndrome

The inappropriate ADH syndrome, a clinical state characterized by hypersecretion of ADH, may result from generalized infection, mediastinal tumors, metastatic tumors to the brain, pathologic CNS changes, or intracranial surgery.

Abnormal fluid retention leads to dilution of plasma sodium (dilutional hyponatremia), and urine becomes inappropriately concentrated. Fluid intake must be stringently restricted to minimize water intoxication.

Oxytocin

Control of Secretion and Actions

The two major physiologic actions of oxytocin are exerted upon female reproductive structures.

Galactokinetic Action

The ejection of milk from a primed, lactating mammary gland follows a neuroendocrine reflex in which oxytocin serves as the efferent limb. The reflex is normally initiated by suckling, which stimulates cutaneous receptors in the areola of the breast. Afferent nerve impulses travel to the paraventricular nuclei of the hypothalamus to effect the release of oxytocin from the neurohypophysis. Oxytocin is carried by the blood to the mammary gland, where it causes contraction of *myoepithelial cells* surrounding the alveoli and lactiferous ducts to bring about the ejection of milk (milk let-down).

In lactating women, tactile stimulation of the breast areola, emotional stimuli, and genital stimulation may also lead to oxytocin release.

Oxytocic Action

Oxytocin acts directly upon uterine smooth muscle to elicit strong, rhythmic contractions of the myometrium. Uterine sensitivity to oxytocin varies with its physiologic state and with hormonal balance. The gravid (pregnant) uterus is highly sensitive to oxytocin, particularly in the late stages of gestation. Uterine sensitivity to oxytocin is greatly enhanced by estrogen and inhibited by progesterone.

Oxytocin release appears to follow a neuroendocrine reflex initiated by genital stimulation.

There is some evidence that oxytocin may affect sperm transport through the female genital tract.

Hormones of the Adenohypophysis

The secretion of hormones by the adenohypophysis (pars distalis and pars intermedia) is controlled by hypothalamic regulatory hormones (factors) that are transported to the pituitary gland by the hypothalamohypophyseal portal system illustrated in Figure 38-2.

There appear to be 10 such regulatory (hypophysiotropic) hormones produced by the hypothalmus:

1 Thyrotropin-releasing hormone (TRH)
2 Corticotropin-releasing hormone (CRH)
3 Growth hormone-releasing hormone (GRH)
4 Growth hormone-inhibiting hormone (GIH) or *somatostatin*
5 Follicle stimulating hormone-releasing hormone (FRH)
6 Luteinizing hormone-releasing hormone (LRH)
7 Prolactin-inhibiting hormone (PIH)
8 Prolactin-releasing hormone (PRH)
9 Melanotropin-releasing hormone (MRH)
10 Melanotropin-inhibiting hormone (MIH)

The secretion of hypothalamic regulatory hormones is controlled by neurotransmitters, many of which have been specifically identified.

Growth Hormone (GH; Somatotropin; STH)

Control of Secretion

Factors Promoting GH Secretion
GRH
Hypoglycemia and fasting
Elevated plasma levels of amino acids (*e.g.,* arginine)
Stress
Exercise
Levodopa
Glucagon

Factors Inhibiting GH Secretion
GIH
Hyperglycemia
Elevated plasma levels of free fatty acids
Cortisol
Alpha-adrenergic blocking agents
GH (negative feedback mechanism)
    GH secretion in response to hypoglycemia, fasting, and exercise appears to be reduced by obesity.

Actions

Effects on Growth

GH accelerates overall body growth by increasing the mass of both skeletal and soft body tissues through hyperplasia (increased cell number) and hypertrophy (increased cell size).

The effects of GH are particularly evident in hard tissues where chondrogenesis (cartilage formation) and osteogenesis (bone formation) are enhanced, leading to an increase in linear growth and stature before epiphyseal closure and in bone thickness following closure of the epiphyses.

GH stimulates certain tissues, notably the liver and kidneys, to produce *somatomedins* (formerly termed *sulfation factor*). Somatomedins are low molecular weight peptides that mediate certain effects of GH, including the stimulation of collagen synthesis, chondrogenesis, and incorporation of sulfate into cartilage.

Metabolic Effects

1 *Protein metabolism*—GH increases protein synthesis and nitrogen retention by enhancing the incorporation of amino acids into protein. The protein anabolic action results from (1) accelerated entry of amino acids into cells and (2) increased ribonucleic acid (RNA) synthesis.
2 *Lipid metabolism*—GH stimulates the mobilization and utilization of fats, enabling the body to use stored fats as an energy source. The elevation of plasma levels of free fatty acids resulting from the hydrolysis of triglycerides (stored neutral fats) is potentially ketogenic.
3 *Carbohydrate metabolism*—GH causes hyperglycemia by increasing the hepatic output of glucose and impairing glucose transport into muscle ("anti-insulin" action on muscle).
    Excessive secretion of GH may precipitate or increase the severity of clinical diabetes mellitus ("diabetogenic" effect).
4 *Electrolyte metabolism*—GH enhances gastrointestinal absorption of calcium and phosphorus, and reduces renal excretion of sodium and potassium.

Prolactin (Lactogenic Hormone;

Mammotropin; Luteotropic Hormone; LTH)

Control of Secretion

Prolactin secretion is controlled by the hypothalamus, with PIH normally dominating. Tactile stimulation of the breast may initiate neuronal activity leading to the release of PRH from the hypothalamus, thus promoting prolactin secretion from the alpha cells of the adenohypophysis. Levodopa inhibits prolactin secretion by liberating PIH from the hypothalamus.

Actions

Prolactin initiates and maintains milk secretion from breasts primed for lactation by other hormones such as estrogens, progesterone, and insulin.

Prolactin also appears to act synergistically with estrogen to stimulate growth of the mammary glands.

Prolactin and GH are very closely related structurally and may, therefore, exert some overlapping functions.

Follicle Stimulating Hormone (FSH)

Control of Secretion

FSH secretion is controlled by the hypothalamus by way of the releasing hormone, FRH. Circulating levels of androgens (testosterone) and estrogens participate in this control by inhibiting FRH secretion by the hypothalamus. Surgical stress usually inhibits FSH secretion. The pineal gland has also been implicated in the control of gonadotropin secretion.

Actions

FSH directly stimulates the germinal epithelium of testicular seminiferous tubules, thereby promoting spermatogenesis in the male. In the female, FSH stimulates follicular growth and development within the ovaries.

Luteinizing Hormone (LH; Interstitial Cell

Stimulating Hormone; ICSH)

Control of Secretion

LH secretion is controlled by the hypothalamus through LRH.

The release of LH is inhibited by testosterone and by estrogens, except for a brief priming effect exerted by estrogen to allow a surge of LH needed to effect ovulation.

Actions

In the male, this hormone stimulates testosterone production by testicular interstitial cells (of Leydig); hence the name, interstitial cell stimulating hormone.

In the female, LH stimulates ripening of the ovarian follicles, controls ovulation, and promotes the formation and maintenance of the corpus luteum.

In many animals, LH elicits the behavioral manifestations of estrus (heat).

Thyrotropin (Thyroid Stimulating

Hormone; TSH)

Control of Secretion

TRH and cold promote secretion of TSH by the beta cells of the adenohypophysis. Elevated plasma levels of free thyroid hormones inhibit thyrotropin secretion as outlined in Figure 38-3.

Actions

TSH stimulates growth (hypertrophy) of the thyroid gland and promotes the synthesis and release of thyroid hormones thyroxine and triiodothyronine. The actions of TSH upon the thyroid gland are mediated by cyclic AMP, and they are detailed in the section on the thyroid gland.

TSH may also act directly on the ocular orbital tissue to cause exophthalmos (protrusion of the eyeballs).

Corticotropin (Adrenocorticotropic

Hormone; ACTH)

Control of Secretion

ACTH secretion is regulated by neural factors and a hormonal negative feedback mechanism. ACTH is secreted in response to CRH and to various forms of stress, including fear, pain, cold, trauma, and hypoglycemia.

Elevated plasma glucocorticoid (cortisol) levels inhibit CRH and ACTH secretion.

Actions

ACTH exerts its tropic effects upon the adrenal glands, promoting growth and steroidogenesis in the adrenal cortex.

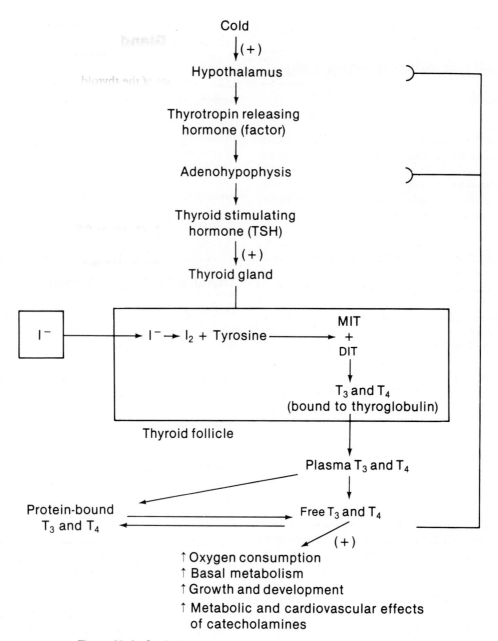

Figure 38–3 Synthesis, storage, release, and action of thyroid hormones.

The stimulation of corticosteroid production (steroidogenesis) in response to ACTH is mediated by the second messenger, cyclic AMP.

Melanotropin (Melanocyte-Stimulating Hormone; MSH; Intermedin)

Control of Secretion

MSH secretion by the pars intermedia is controlled by hypothalamic inhibiting and releasing hormones.

Actions

MSH acts upon the skin of fish, reptiles, and amphibians to disperse melanophore granules leading to changes in skin coloration.

Mammals, including humans, do not possess melanophores, but rather melanin-containing cells called melanocytes. Thus there appears to be no major physiologic role for MSH in humans. Some neurotropic effects of MSH have been observed; however, the physiologic significance of these remains unclear.

Abnormally large amounts of MSH (such as with functional pituitary tumors) may produce hyperpigmentation of skin in humans.

ACTH and MSH are structurally similar, so that hyperpigmentation associated with certain pathologic states may result from ACTH or MSH hypersecretion, or both.

Disorders of the Adenohypophysis

Hypofunctional States

Hypopituitarism (Pituitary Insufficiency)

In the adult, hypopituitarism may be manifested in a variety of forms, such as panhypopituitarism, Simmond's disease (pituitary cachexia), or Sheehan's syndrome.

Pituitary insufficiency may result from hypothalamic lesions, cysts or tumors affecting the pituitary, surgical hypophysectomy, infiltrative granulomatous disease, vascular collapse, or thrombosis.

The deficiency in the production of tropic hormones leads to functional deficiency and atrophy of target glands such as the adrenal cortex, thyroid, and gonads. Symptoms of pituitary insufficiency may include weakness; decreased resistance to stress, cold, and infection; sexual dysfunction (*e.g.*, infertility, amenorrhea, decreased secondary sex characteristics); sallow, dry, wrinkled skin; and hypotension.

Pituitary Dwarfism

The hallmark of hypopituitarism in children is growth retardation or dwarfism. Despite the small stature, the pituitary dwarf has normal body proportions. Hypoglycemia, hypogonadism, and hypothyroidism may also occur.

Hyperfunctional States

Gigantism and Acromegaly

Excessive secretion of GH is usually caused by acidophilic adenomas. Hypersecretion of GH occurring before closure of the epiphyses leads to proportional but immense growth. An individual may grow to 7 or 8 feet in height; hence the term *gigantism*.

Excessive secretion of GH following epiphyseal closure results in *acromegaly*. Because the bones can no longer increase in length, overall height (stature) is not affected. However, the bones thicken considerably, an effect particularly noticeable in the face, hands, and feet. Overgrowth of the mandible results in prognathism (jaw protrusion) and separation of the lower teeth. The skeletal changes predispose to joint disorders such as osteoarthritis.

Increased sweating, thickening of the skin, and increased body hair (in women) are common. Hyperglycemia and glucose intolerance may be noted. Headaches and visual disturbances may result from pressure by the tumor.

Thyroid Gland

The hormones of the thyroid gland exert a wide spectrum of metabolic and physiologic actions that affect virtually every tissue in the body.

Anatomy

The thyroid gland is a bilobed organ overlying the trachea anteriorly. The thyroid gland is composed of numerous closely packed spheres or *follicles.*

Each follicle consists of a simple cuboidal epithelium (*follicular cells*) enclosing a lumen or cavity containing a viscous hyaline substance termed *colloid*. The chief constituent of the colloid is the iodinated glycoprotein *thyroglobulin.*

Interspersed among the follicles are small clusters of *parafollicular* (C) cells, which secrete *calcitonin* (thyrocalcitonin), a hormone affecting calcium metabolism.

Thyroid Hormones

The follicular cells of the thyroid gland secrete two hormones, *thyroxine* (tetraiodothyronine or T$_4$) and *triiodothyronine* (T$_3$). The plasma levels of these hormones are regulated by the hypothalamopituitary axis as outlined in Figure 38-3. Intrinsic (intrathyroidal) mechanisms, as well as bioavailability of iodine, influence thyroid hormone production.

Biosynthesis of Thyroid Hormones

1 *Iodide uptake*—Ingested iodine is readily absorbed from the GI tract in the reduced iodide state. Iodide ions are actively transported from the blood into the thyroid follicles by an energy-requiring "trapping" mechanism often termed the *iodide pump.* The normal thyroid/serum ratio of iodide is 25:1. The uptake of iodide is enhanced by TSH and may be blocked by anions such as perchlorate and thiocyanate.

2 *Oxidation to iodine*—Upon entering the colloid, iodide is rapidly oxidized to iodine in the presence of peroxidase enzymes. Thiouracil appears to inhibit peroxidase activity.

3 *Iodination of tyrosine*—Free molecular iodine spontaneously combines with tyrosine residues on the thyroglobulin to form 3-monoiodotyrosine (MIT) and 3,5-diiodotyrosine (DIT). This organic iodination is enhanced by TSH and blocked by agents such as propylthiouracil and methimazole. Goitrogens found in cabbage, kale, and turnips, as well as cobalt and phenylbutazone, also block organification of iodine.

4   *Coupling reaction*—Two iodinated tyrosines combine to form either T_3 or T_4. The coupling occurs within the thyroglobulin molecule, and the reaction appears to be promoted by TSH.

5   *Storage and release of thyroid hormones*—T_4 and T_3 remain stored within the colloid bound to thyroglobulin until released by protease enzymes that free the hormones, allowing them to diffuse out of the colloid, through the follicular cells into the plasma.

TSH, acting through cyclic AMP, increases the production of thyroid hormones by promoting various steps in the biosynthetic mechanism, including the release of the hormones from storage in thyroglobulin.

Transport

Circulating thyroid hormones bind specifically with *thyroxine-binding globulin* and *thyroxine-binding prealbumin,* and nonspecifically with serum albumin. The extent of plasma protein binding can be measured as protein-bound iodine (PBI).

Only a small fraction of circulating thyroid hormones is in the free (unbound), biologically active form.

Several drugs, including phenytoin and the salicylates, compete for plasma protein binding sites, thus lowering the PBI and increasing the percentage of free, active hormones. High levels of estrogen, such as those occurring in pregnancy or oral contraceptive therapy, elevate plasma protein levels, thereby increasing PBI levels.

Fate

Thyroid hormones are inactivated by deiodination, deamination, decarboxylation, or conjugation with glucuronic acid or sulfate. Much of the iodine released during biodegradation is recycled and reutilized for synthesis of new hormones. The remainder is excreted in the urine. Metabolism occurs chiefly in the liver, and excretion is mainly through the kidneys. The conjugated hormones are excreted through the bile and eliminated in the feces.

Actions

The thyroid hormones increase the rate of metabolism, total heat production, and oxygen consumption in most body tissues. They also promote normal physical and mental development and growth, and they potentiate the cardiovascular and metabolic actions of the catecholamines (epinephrine and norepinephrine).

At the cellular level, the thyroid hormones increase mitochondrial permeability, accelerate protein synthesis, and uncouple oxidative phosphorylation. Although T_4 is quantitatively the major hormone produced by the thyroid follicles, it appears that T_3 is biologically more potent. It is likely that T_4 is converted peripherally into the more active T_3 form.

The pharmacologic uses of the thyroid hormones are discussed in Chapter 40.

Disorders of the Thyroid

Simple Goiter

Goiter, an enlargement of the thyroid gland, most commonly results from an insufficient dietary intake of iodine. The gland becomes hyperplastic and filled with colloid lacking in iodine. TSH levels are usually high because plasma levels of free thyroid hormones are insufficient to suppress TSH production by the adenohypophysis. More rarely, goiter may result from excessive intake of goitrogens (such as cabbage) or may be due to congenital lack of biosynthetic enzymes.

Transient simple goiter may occur during pregnancy or at the onset of puberty, when the demand for the hormones increases.

Hypothyroidism

Hypothyroidism may result from primary disease of the thyroid gland itself, or it may be secondary to a deficiency of pituitary TSH or hypothalamic TRH.

Because thyroid hormones affect a wide range of physiologic and metabolic processes including growth and development, the time of onset of a deficiency state is most important.

Cretinism (Congenital or Neonatal Hypothyroidism)

Cretinism results from fetal or neonatal thyroid hormone deficiency, which may be due to anatomical dysgenesis of the thyroid, iodine deficiency, or inborn errors of iodine metabolism.

Cretinism is characterized by mental retardation and dwarfism due to delayed skeletal maturation. Other signs of this disorder include the presence of thick, dry skin, large protruding tongue, and umbilical hernia. The child appears apathetic or lethargic and has a low body temperature. TSH and serum cholesterol levels are elevated.

Myxedema (Adult Hypothyroidism)

Primary myxedema may follow thyroidectomy, eradication of the thyroid by radioactive iodine, ingestion of goitrogens, or chronic thyroiditis. Idiopathic atrophy, possibly involving autoimmune mechanisms, may also lead to hypothyroidism.

Early symptoms of myxedema include cold intolerance, weakness, fatigue, dryness of the skin, thinning hair, and thin brittle nails. Among later signs are weight gain, pallor, dyspnea, peripheral edema, anginal pain, bradycardia, and slow speech. Cardiac enlargement may result from pericardial effusion, and macrocytic anemia may occur.

The low turnover of protein leads to the accumulation

of a protein-rich fluid under the skin, lending a puffiness and thickness to the skin.

Manifestations of personality changes and organic psychoses ("myxedema madness") may occur.

It is noteworthy that myxedematous patients are unusually sensitive to opiates, and may die from average doses of these agents.

Hyperthyroidism (Thyrotoxicosis)

Hyperthyroid states are characterized by some degree of glandular hyperplasia and excessive thyroid hormone production. Nervousness, excessive sweating, heat intolerance, warm moist skin, weight loss despite increased appetite, restlessness, and tremor are common signs of hyperthyroidism. Tachycardia, high pulse pressure, and systolic hypertension frequently occur.

When associated with toxic diffuse goiter, elevated metabolic rate and exophthalmos, hyperthyroidism is termed *Graves' disease.* Long-acting thyroid stimulator (LATS) is an immunoglobulin (antibody) with TSH-like activity that has been isolated from the serum of patients with Graves' disease.

The treatment of thyroid disorders is detailed in Chapter 40.

Calcitonin

Calcitonin (thyrocalcitonin) is a polypeptide hormone secreted by the cells of the thyroid gland in response to *hypercalcemia* (elevated blood calcium).

Calcitonin lowers serum calcium primarily by inhibiting the rate of calcium release from bone.

In addition to inhibiting bone resorption, calcitonin appears to accelerate bone formation and mineral deposition. Calcitonin may also inhibit the renal calcium reabsorptive action of *parathyroid hormone* (PTH).

In addition to the parafollicular cells of the thyroid, calcitonin-secreting cells have been found in the parathyroid and thymus glands. Because calcitonin is not the principal calcium-regulating hormone, there are no clinical syndromes associated with abnormal rates of calcitonin secretion.

Parathyroid Glands

The parathyroid glands, usually four in number, are embedded in the dorsal surface of the thyroid gland.

In response to *hypocalcemia* (low serum calcium), the chief cells of the parathyroid glands secrete a single polypeptide hormone known as *parathyroid hormone* (PTH or parathormone).

PTH regulates serum calcium levels by exerting its effects on the following three target tissues:

1 *Bone*—PTH stimulates bone resorption by activating the bone-destroying osteoclasts. The demineralization of bone elevates serum calcium and phosphate levels.

2 *Kidneys*—PTH promotes renal tubular reabsorption of calcium, and increases renal excretion of phosphate by blocking its reabsorption.

3 *GI tract*—PTH enhances calcium and phosphate absorption from the small intestine in the presence of adequate amounts of vitamin D.

The major actions of PTH are mediated by cyclic AMP. Calcium metabolism and the clinical uses of PTH and calcitonin are discussed in Chapter 41.

Disorders of the Parathyroid Glands

Hypoparathyroidism

Hypoparathyroidism is not common. When it occurs, usually following accidental removal of or damage to the parathyroid glands during thyroidectomy, signs of *hypocalcemia* ensue. Among these are neuromuscular hyperexcitability (related in severity to the degree of hypocalcemia), tetany, and mental disturbances. Respiratory difficulties mimicking asthma may occur.

Hyperparathyroidism

Primary hyperparathyroidism may result from adenoma, carcinoma, or primary hyperplasia of the parathyroid glands. It may also be associated with ectopic production of PTH by carcinomas elsewhere in the body.

Signs and symptoms characteristic of hyperparathyroidism include *hypercalcemia,* anorexia, vomiting, thirst, polyuria, and renal calculi (kidney stones). Skeletal manifestations may range from simple joint or back pain to pathologic fractures and cystic bone lesions throughout the skeleton (*osteitis fibrosa cystica*). The skeletal abnormalities result from the excessive demineralization of bone, while the occurrence of kidney stones is related to excessive renal excretion of minerals (calcium and phosphate).

Pancreas

The endocrine functions of the pancreas are performed by the *islets of Langerhans,* small, highly vascularized masses of cells scattered throughout the pancreas and representing only 1% to 3% of the entire organ.

The islets of Langerhans contain three types of secretory cells, as follows:

1 *Alpha* (A) cells that secrete *glucagon*

2 *Beta* (B) cells that secrete *insulin*

3 *Delta* (D) cells that secrete *somatostatin*

Insulin-secreting beta cells are the most numerous, making up 70% to 80% of the islet cell population.

The physiologic roles of glucagon and insulin in the regulation of intermediary metabolism are well established. The exact physiologic role of pancreatic somatostatin remains unclear. Because somatostatin inhibits the release of both glucagon and insulin from the pancreatic islets, it may function, at least in part, as a hormone-regulating pancreatic secretion.

Glucagon

Glucagon is a 29 amino-acid polypeptide hormone secreted by the alpha cells of the pancreatic islets primarily in response to *hypoglycemia*. Glucagon is essentially a catabolic hormone that decreases carbohydrate and lipid energy stores, and increases the amount of glucose and fatty acids available for oxidation.

Extrapancreatic glucagon ("gut glucagon") is secreted by certain cells of the stomach and duodenum. Both pancreatic glucagon and gut glucagon stimulate secretion of insulin from the beta cells of the pancreatic islets.

Control of Secretion

The plasma glucose concentration is the major physiologic regulator of glucagon secretion. In addition to hypoglycemia and fasting, the following factors promote glucagon secretion: ingestion of a high protein meal (amino acids), exercise, stress, gastrin, pancreozymin, and beta-adrenergic stimulation. The rate of glucagon secretion is inhibited by elevated blood levels of glucose and free fatty acids, by somatostatin, phenytoin, and alpha-adrenergic stimulation.

Major Actions

1 *Carbohydrate metabolism*—Glucagon stimulates hepatic glycogenolysis, thereby promoting the release of glucose from liver glycogen stores. This action is mediated by cyclic AMP, which stimulates protein kinase activity leading to the activation of phosphorylase, the glycogenolytic enzyme. In addition to stimulating hepatic glycogenolysis, glucagon inhibits glycogenesis and increases the rate of hepatic gluconeogenesis. The net effect is an elevation of blood glucose (hyperglycemia).

2 *Lipid metabolism*—Glucagon stimulates lipolysis, thereby increasing the release of free fatty acids and glycerol from adipose tissue. Glucagon also promotes the uptake and oxidation of fatty acids by liver and muscle.

3 *Protein metabolism*—Glucagon exerts a catabolic action on proteins, and inhibits the incorporation of amino acids into hepatic protein.

4 *Cardiac effects*—Large amounts of exogenous glucagon produce a positive inotropic effect on the heart by increasing myocardial levels of cyclic AMP. A direct chronotropic effect has also been reported. The net effect is an increase in cardiac output resulting from an increased force of myocardial contraction and increased heart rate.

All the major actions of glucagon—hepatic glycogenolysis, lipolysis, stimulation of insulin release, and the inotropic effect on the heart—are mediated by cyclic AMP.

Insulin

Structure, Biosynthesis, and Secretion

Insulin is a polypeptide hormone composed of 51 amino acids arranged in two chains (A and B), linked by disulfide bridges.

Insulin is derived from a large, polypeptide precursor—*proinsulin*—which is synthesized in the endoplasmic reticulum of beta cells and packaged into membrane-bounded granules within the Golgi complex.

A connecting (C) peptide is removed from the proinsulin molecule by proteolytic cleavage before the secretion of insulin in its biologically active form.

Insulin secretion occurs through exocytosis (emiocytosis), a calcium-dependent process that is enhanced by cyclic AMP and potassium. Upon entering the circulation, insulin is transported largely in free molecular form, not bound to plasma proteins.

Control of Secretion

The secretion of insulin is controlled primarily by the blood glucose level, with an elevation of blood glucose (hyperglycemia) increasing both production and release of insulin. Ingested glucose effects a far greater secretion of insulin than an equivalent amount of intravenously administered glucose because several gastrointestinal hormones, including gastrin, secretin, pancreozymin, and glucagon, stimulate insulin secretion.

Insulin secretion is also increased by mannose, fructose, certain amino acids, vagal stimulation (acetylcholine), cyclic AMP, potassium, and oral hypoglycemic drugs such as tolbutamide. Hyperglycemia, somatostatin, alpha-adrenergic stimulation, thiazide diuretics, phenytoin, and diazoxide inhibit insulin secretion.

Major Actions

1 *Cellular membrane permeability*—Insulin facilitates the transport of glucose across selected cell membranes, thereby accelerating the entry of glucose into muscle, adipose tissue, fibroblasts, leukocytes, mammary glands, and the anterior pituitary. The transport

of glucose into the liver, brain, renal tubules, intestinal mucosa, and erythrocytes is *independent* of insulin. Exercise and hypoxia mimic the effect of insulin upon cellular permeability to glucose in skeletal muscle. The insulin requirements of diabetics engaging in strenuous exercise may be reduced substantially, and therefore must be monitored carefully to avoid hypoglycemia. Insulin also increases cellular permeability to amino acids, fatty acids, and potassium, particularly in muscle and adipose tissue.

2 *Carbohydrate metabolism*—Insulin effectively lowers the level of blood glucose by enhancing the transport and peripheral utilization of glucose. Insulin increases muscle and liver glycogen stores by activating enzymes involved in glycogenesis, while inhibiting those that produce glycogenolysis. Glycolytic enzymes are also activated by insulin, while several enzymes involved in gluconeogenesis are inhibited.

3 *Protein metabolism*—Insulin is strongly anabolic, increasing protein synthesis and inhibiting protein catabolism. Insulin increases the incorporation of amino acids into protein by accelerating the entry of amino acids into the cell and possibly by increasing RNA synthesis.

4 *Lipid metabolism*—Insulin stimulates formation of triglycerides (*lipogenesis*) and inhibits their breakdown (*lipolysis*). Insulin accelerates fatty acid and glycerol phosphate synthesis, and enhances cellular permeability to fatty acids, leading to increased deposition of triglycerides in adipose tissue.

Somatostatin (Growth Hormone

Inhibiting Hormone)

Somatostatin is a tetradecapeptide that has been isolated from the hypothalamus, the pancreas, and the upper gastrointestinal tract. Within the pancreatic islets, the somatostatin secreting delta (D) cells are located between the glucagon-secreting alpha (A) cells and the central mass of insulin-secreting beta (B) cells. Such an arrangement could permit the product of the D cells—somatostatin—to directly influence the secretion of glucagon and insulin by the A and B cells, respectively.

Actions

Although the precise role or roles of somatostatin remain unclear, several endocrine and nonendocrine activities have been attributed to this hormone. These biological actions include the following:

Endocrine
Inhibition of secretion of:
GH
TSH
Glucagon
Insulin
Gastrin
Secretin
Renin

Nonendocrine
Inhibition of:
Gastric acid secretion and gastric emptying
Pancreatic bicarbonate and enzyme release
Gallbladder contraction
Xylose absorption
Splanchnic blood flow
Platelet aggregation
Electrical activity of CNS neurons
Acetylcholine release from peripheral nerves

Disorders of Glucose Metabolism

Hypoglycemia

Hypoglycemic states are characterized by the presence of an abnormally low blood glucose level. This represents a threat to the brain, which depends upon glucose as its source of energy.

Normally, when the blood glucose falls below a critical level, insulin secretion is inhibited and release of glucagon, epinephrine, GH, and glucocorticoids is increased. Only the release of the catecholamine epinephrine leads to observable symptoms, such as sweating, palpitation, anxiety, and weakness.

Impairment of brain function, confusion, amnesia, bizarre behavior, or blurred vision may occur if the blood glucose falls below a level of 40 mg/100 ml. Severe hypoglycemia may ultimately lead to hypothermia, convulsions, and coma. Hypoglycemic disorders may be divided into two types: *fasting* (food-deprived) and *postprandial* (food-stimulated or reactive).

Possible causes of fasting hypoglycemia are listed below:

1 *Hyperinsulinism*—insulinomas (insulin-secreting tumors of the pancreas), overdosage with exogenous insulin or sulfonylurea drugs (oral hypoglycemic agents)

2 *Endocrine disorders*—Addison's disease (adrenocortical insufficiency), hypopituitarism (*e.g.,* Simmonds' disease), myxedema

3 *Liver disease*—hepatic necrosis, malignancy, or advanced cirrhosis, which may lead to impairment of glycogenesis and gluconeogenesis, thereby reducing liver glycogen stores and hepatic output of glucose

4 *Acute alcoholism*

5 *Extrapancreatic tumors*

The possible causes of *postprandial* (*reactive*) hypoglycemia include early or alimentary hypoglycemia, which may follow gastric intestinal surgery or result from increased vagal tone, and late hypoglycemia (early or occult diabetes mellitus).

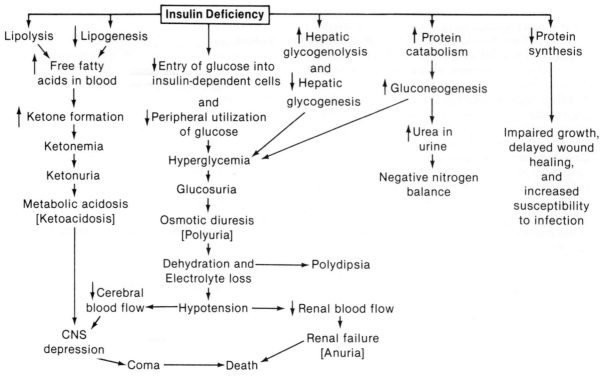

Figure 38-4   Metabolic consequences of severe insulin deficiency.

Diabetes Mellitus

Diabetes mellitus is a chronic disorder of metabolism characterized by carbohydrate intolerance and inappropriate hyperglycemia resulting from a deficiency of insulin secretion or a reduction in its biological efficacy ("relative" insulin deficiency).

The insulin deficiency, be it absolute or relative, triggers a series of biochemical changes in the metabolism of carbohydrates, lipids, and proteins, as outlined in Figure 38-4. These metabolic abnormalities lead to the classic symptoms of diabetes mellitus—*polyuria* (frequent urination), *polydipsia* (excessive thirst), *polyphagia* (hunger), and fatigue.

Long-term, serious complications of diabetes mellitus include gangrene, visual impairment resulting from proliferative retinopathy, myocardial infarction, polyneuropathy, and uremia. Pathologic changes in the blood vessels, particularly in the microcirculation (microangiopathy), appear to underlie the majority of these complications.

Diabetes mellitus is a disorder of heterogenous etiology. Predisposition to diabetes is inherited, although the genetic factors are complex. There are two generally recognized types of diabetes mellitus: (1) *insulin dependent* (type I or *juvenile onset*) and (2) *noninsulin dependent* (type II or *maturity onset*).

Insulin-Dependent (Type I) Diabetes

Generally occurs in nonobese persons before the age of 30, most commonly in adolescence. Circulating insulin is virtually absent, and the beta pancreatic cells fail to respond to all normal stimuli for insulin secretion. The islet beta cell reserve is markedly reduced or totally absent, and ketosis usually develops in the course of the disease. Patients respond to exogenous insulin, which is required to reverse the hyperglycemia and the general catabolic state and to prevent ketosis.

Immunopathologic mechanisms have been strongly implicated in this type of diabetes. Specific histocompatibility (HLA) antigens have been linked to this disorder, and circulating antibodies to islet cells have been detected in some patients early in the course of the disease.

Viruses such as mumps, coxsackie B4 virus, and rubella have been associated epidemiologically with the onset of juvenile-onset diabetes. It is possible that an underlying genetic defect of the immune system may predispose an individual to beta cell destruction following these viral infections.

Noninsulin-Dependent (Type II) Diabetes

Usually has its onset after the age of 40, although it may occur at any age. Obesity is a major risk factor to the development of this disease, beta cell mass may be only moderately reduced, and autoimmunity is not demonstrable. There is no correlation with HLA antigens; however, there is a strong genetic component. Ketosis rarely occurs.

In at least some cases of noninsulin-dependent diabetes, a defect in insulin binding to cellular receptors is likely. Insulin apparently exerts a negative feedback control over its own receptors. In the presence of obesity, certain tissues (such as muscle and adipose tissue) display insensitivity to insulin. Perhaps the hyperinsulinism that results from chronic excessive caloric intake and sustained beta cell stimulation actually reduces the number of available insulin receptors and leads to glucose intolerance.

In addition to obesity and excessive carbohydrate intake, diabetes mellitus may be precipitated by pancreatitis, pregnancy, and endocrine disorders associated with overproduction of GH, glucocorticoids, or catecholamines.

Almost all forms of clinical and experimental diabetes mellitus are associated with increased secretion of glucagon, a potent hyperglycemic hormone whose glycogenolytic, gluconeogenic, lipolytic, and ketogenic actions are intensified by insulin deficiency.

Adrenal Glands

The *adrenal* (suprarenal) glands are paired, yellowish masses of tissue situated at the superior pole of each kidney. Each gland consists of two distinct entities—an outer *adrenal cortex* and an inner *adrenal medulla*—that differ in embryologic origin, character, and function.

Adrenal Medulla

The *adrenal medulla* develops from the embryonic ectoderm. It remains functionally associated with the sympathetic nervous system, being essentially a modified sympathetic ganglion whose postganglionic neurons have lost their axons and become secretory.

Histologically, the adrenal medulla contains large, ovoid cells arranged in clumps or irregular cords around numerous blood vessels. The medullary cells, often termed *chromaffin* cells because their granules possess affinity for chromium salts, secrete the catecholamine hormones *epinephrine* (adrenalin) and *norepinephrine* (noradrenalin). The principal secretory product is epinephrine, with norepinephrine normally accounting for only 20% of the total secretion.

Adrenal medullary secretion of the catecholamines is physiologically controlled by the posterior hypothalamus. The hormones are stored in cellular granules, bound to adenosine triphosphate (ATP) and protein, and are released in response to the following stimuli: sympathetic nervous system activation, hypoglycemia, pain, hypoxia, hypotension, cold, emotional stress, acetylcholine, histamine, and nicotine.

Epinephrine and norepinephrine are rapidly metabolized to inactive products, principally by the liver and kidneys. Major products of biodegradation include metanephrine, normetanephrine, and vanillylmandelic acid (VMA). These appear in the urine and may be assayed during the course of clinical diagnosis.

Actions of Adrenal Medullary Hormones

Epinephrine and norepinephrine mimic the effects of sympathetic nerve discharge, producing the following effects:

1 Direct increase in cardiac rate and myocardial force of contraction
2 Elevation of blood pressure
3 Dilation of coronary and skeletal muscle blood vessels
4 Constriction of the cutaneous and visceral vasculature
5 Relaxation of respiratory smooth muscle
6 Inhibition of GI motility
7 Pupillary dilation (mydriasis)
8 Glycogenolysis in liver and muscle
9 Lipolysis

The cardiac excitatory effects and the metabolic actions of lipolysis and glycogenolysis are mediated by cyclic AMP, the latter involving the activation of phosphorylase enzyme by protein kinase.

The catecholamines also elevate the metabolic rate (calorigenic action), stimulate the central nervous system, increase alertness, and stimulate respiration.

Clinical Disorders

Adrenal medullary function is not essential to life; therefore, hyposecretion of adrenal medullary hormones does not constitute a recognized clinical entity.

Pheochromocytoma

Pheochromocytoma is a chromaffin-cell tumor of the sympathoadrenal system, most commonly involving one of the adrenal glands or both. It is characterized by hypersecretion of the catecholamines epinephrine and norepinephrine, the latter usually dominating. Clinical manifestations of pheochromocytoma include paroxysmal or persistent hypertension, severe headaches, tachycardia, profuse sweating, epigastric pain, nausea, irritability, and dyspnea. Metabolic signs of this disorder include hyperglycemia, increased basal metabolic rate, weight loss, and elevated levels of urinary catecholamines or their metabolites.

Adrenal Cortex

The *adrenal cortex* develops from the mesoderm during embryonic life. The cells of the adrenal cortex, which are arranged in continuous cords separated by capillaries, are characterized by an abundance of mitochondria, endoplasmic reticulum, and accumulation of lipid.

Adrenal cortical tissue is structurally arranged into three concentric regions or zones: a thin outer *zona glomerulosa,* a thick middle *zona fasciculata,* and an inner *zona reticularis* bordering on the adrenal medulla.

Chemically, the steroid hormones of the adrenal cortex, the *adrenocorticoids,* are all derivatives of cholesterol. The adrenocorticoid hormones are usually divided into three functional groups: the *mineralocorticoids,* such as aldosterone, which regulate electrolyte and water balance; the *glucocorticoids,* such as cortisol, which affect carbohydrate, protein, and fat metabolism; and the *adrenogenital steroids* or *sex hormones.*

The adrenogenital steroids are of three types: *androgens* (such as dehydroepiandrosterone), *estrogens* (such as estradiol), and *progestins* (such as progesterone).

Under normal physiologic conditions the adrenogenital steroids are secreted (under ACTH control) in minute amounts and, therefore, they exert minimal effects on reproductive functions. Excessive secretion of adrenal androgens results in precocious pseudopuberty in boys, and causes masculinization of females (*adrenogenital syndrome*).

Mineralocorticoids

Control of Secretion and Actions

Aldosterone is the principal physiologic mineralocorticoid secreted by the zona glomerulosa. Its secretion is regulated primarily by the renin–angiotensin mechanism described in Chapter 36. The plasma concentrations of sodium and potassium are central factors in the control of aldosterone secretion, for low sodium or elevated potassium levels stimulate the zona glomerulosa both directly and indirectly (by way of the renin–angiotensin system). Other factors contributing to the control of aldosterone secretion include blood volume and ACTH, the latter exerting a limited, nonselective stimulatory effect.

Aldosterone plays a major physiologic role in the maintenance of electrolyte and fluid balance by promoting the renal tubular reabsorption of sodium and the secretion of potassium and hydrogen. Aldosterone binds to nuclear receptors and stimulates DNA-directed RNA synthesis leading to increased formation of specific proteins involved in sodium transport.

A similar sodium-retaining, potassium-excreting action is exerted on other target tissues, including salivary glands and sweat glands.

Glucocorticoids

Control of Secretion and Actions

Glucocorticoid secretion, which occurs primarily in the zona fasciculata, is controlled by ACTH. A variety of stressful stimuli including anxiety, fear, hypoglycemia, hypotension, and hemorrhage increase secretion of corticotropin releasing hormone (CRH) from the hypothalamus. CRH promotes ACTH secretion by the adenohypophysis, and ACTH stimulates adrenal cortical secretory activity, thereby elevating blood levels of cortisol (the principal physiologic glucocorticoid). Elevated blood levels of free cortisol normally exert a negative feedback control over further secretion of CRH and ACTH. Prolonged ACTH secretion results in hypertrophy and hyperplasia of the adrenal cortex and excessive secretion of all adrenocorticoid hormones. The metabolic and physiologic actions of the glucocorticoids are summarized below. The pharmacologic actions and clinical uses of these hormones are discussed in Chapter 43.

1 *Carbohydrate metabolism*—Glucocorticoids stimulate hepatic gluconeogenesis and inhibit peripheral uptake and utilization of glucose, thereby promoting hyperglycemia. Hepatic glycogenesis is also enhanced.

2 *Protein metabolism*—Glucocorticoids exert protein catabolic and antianabolic actions, promoting the breakdown of existing proteins while inhibiting the incorporation of amino acids into new proteins, except in the liver, where protein synthesis is stimulated.

3 *Lipid metabolism*—Glucocorticoids inhibit lipogenesis and favor mobilization of fats from adipose tissues. When present in large amounts, these hormones favor redistribution of adipose stores by promoting loss of fat from the extremities, and accumulation of fat depots in central body regions (*e.g.,* "moon face" and "buffalo hump" formation).

4 *Blood and immunologic effects*—Glucocorticoids inhibit the immune response, cause involution of lymphoid tissue, and reduce blood levels of lymphocytes, eosinophils, and basophils. These hormones also stimulate erythropoiesis and elevate circulating levels of platelets and neutrophils.

5 *GI tract effects*—Glucocorticoid hormones stimulate gastric acid and pepsin secretion and inhibit the production of protective mucus, thereby favoring development of gastric ulcers.

Disorders of the Adrenal Cortex

Addison's Disease

Addison's disease (chronic adrenocortical insufficiency) may result from idiopathic adrenocortical atrophy, adrenocortical destruction by disease (*e.g.,* tuberculosis or cancer), or deficiency of ACTH or CRH secretion.

Weakness and fatigability are early signs of the disease, and weight loss, dehydration, and hypotension are characteristic. Emotional changes and GI disturbances (such as anorexia, nausea, vomiting, diarrhea) frequently occur. Hyperpigmentation is a major characteristic of primary adrenocortical insufficiency, with increased pigmentation being prominent on skin folds, pressure points (bony prominences), extensor surfaces, nipples, perineum, tongue, and buccal mucosa.

In Addison's disease, aldosterone (mineralocorticoid) deficiency results in increased excretion of sodium and retention of potassium. The salt and water depletion causes severe dehydration, reduced circulatory volume, hypotension, and eventual circulatory collapse.

Glucocorticoid (cortisol) deficiency leads to reduced gluconeogenesis, hypoglycemia, diminished hepatic glycogen, and extreme insulin sensitivity. The inability to withstand stress (such as infection, trauma, surgery) may result in acute adrenal insufficiency (adrenal crisis).

Cushing's Syndrome

Cushing's syndrome is a clinical state characterized by glucocorticoid excess resulting from adrenocortical tumors, hypersecretion of ACTH, or from the administration of large amounts of exogenous corticosteroids or ACTH.

Clinical manifestations of this syndrome include truncal obesity, moon face, and buffalo hump, resulting from the characteristic redistribution of fat from the extremities to central body regions (abdomen, face, and upper back). The increased central subcutaneous fat depots stretch the skin, rupturing the subdermal tissue and causing formation of purple striae.

Excessive protein catabolism results in protein depletion and causes thin skin, muscular wasting, easy bruising, and poor wound healing. Osteoporosis develops, predisposing the patient to fractures and skeletal deformities.

Increased gluconeogenesis and decreased peripheral utilization of glucose result in hyperglycemia and glucose intolerance, and frank diabetes mellitus may develop in genetically predisposed individuals.

Hypertension and renal calculi frequently occur, and psychiatric disturbances are common.

Primary Hyperaldosteronism (Conn's Syndrome)

Conn's syndrome, a clinical state resulting from excessive production of the mineralocorticoid aldosterone, is generally characterized by potassium depletion, sodium retention, hypertension, polyuria, fatigue, and muscular weakness. Hypokalemic alkalosis and tetany may also be observed.

Gonadal Hormones

The physiologic and metabolic actions of the gonadal hormones, together with their clinical uses, are reviewed in Chapter 44 (Estrogens and Progestins) and Chapter 46 (Androgens and Anabolic Steroids). The menstrual (endometrial) cycle is presented schematically in Chapter 45, Figure 45-1.

39 Hypophysial Hormones

The hypophysis, or pituitary gland, is composed of two major divisions, the adenohypophysis (anterior lobe), which contains at least six hormones, and the neurohypophysis (posterior lobe), which contains two hormones. No bodily function is exempt from the influence of at least one of these eight hypophysial hormones, and collectively they serve to regulate and integrate the physiologic processes necessary for the maintenance of homeostasis.

Hormones of the Adenohypophysis

Of the six principal hormones of the adenohypophysis, growth hormone (GH), adrenocorticotropic hormone (ACTH), and thyroid stimulating hormone (TSH) are available clinically as purified preparations. However, because they must be extracted from pituitary glands of animals (ACTH, TSH) or humans (GH), they are in limited supply and thus quite expensive. These three hormones are peptides, and hence they must be administered parenterally because they would be rapidly digested if taken by mouth. Furthermore, because of their protein nature, they may stimulate antibody production and lead to allergic reactions. Should synthetic derivatives of these pituitary hormones become available in the future, it is possible that they may enjoy a wider application as well as significantly reduced side-effects and allergic reactions. GH, ACTH, and TSH are reviewed in this chapter.

The two adenohypophysial gonadotropins, follicle stimulating hormone (FSH) and luteinizing hormone (LH), are extracted from the urine of pregnant and postmenopausal women. The commercial preparation, human menopausal gonadotropin (HMG), is used in the treatment of infertility and cryptorchidism (undescended testes) and is discussed in Chapter 45. The remaining adenohypophysial hormone, prolactin (luteotropic hormone, LTH), is as yet unavailable for therapeutic use.

All adenohypophysial hormones except GH exert their effects on selective target organs, such as the adrenal cortex, thyroid gland, or gonads. Replacement therapy in cases of hormonal deficiency states is usually best accomplished by supplying the individual target gland hormones (thyroxine, hydrocortisone, estrogen, progesterone) instead of the pituitary hormones for many of the reasons mentioned above. In the case of the gonadal hormones, moreover, the individual purified hypophysial hormones are not clinically available. Deficiency of GH, on the other hand, can be rectified only by replacement therapy with GH itself, and because of the high degree of species specificity that exists among the various types of GH, only *human* GH possesses significant biological activity in humans. The extremely limited supply makes this a very expensive form of therapy.

▶ **adrenocorticotropic hormone**

▶ **corticotropin injection**
ACTH, Acthar

▶ **corticotropin repository**

ACTH Gel, Cortigel, Cortrophin Gel, Cotropic Gel, H.P. Acthar Gel

▶ **corticotropin zinc**

Cortrophin-Zinc

A polypeptide containing 39 amino acids, extracted from the pituitary glands of various animals, ACTH is commercially available either as a stable aqueous solution for injection, an aqueous solution containing gelatin to delay absorption and prolong the action, or a zinc hydroxide complex to prevent tissue destruction, which also prolongs the effect. A synthetic subunit (*i.e.,* 24 amino acids) of ACTH is available as cosyntropin, and is used to test for adrenocortical insufficiency. Cosyntropin is reviewed in Chapter 78. A second diagnostic agent, metyrapone, can also be employed to ascertain whether pituitary secretion of ACTH is adequate, and is likewise considered in Chapter 78.

Mechanism

Stimulates the adrenal cortex to produce and secrete all of its products and activates adenyl cyclase in adrenal cortical tissue, thus increasing cyclic adenosine monophosphate (AMP) levels, which enhance the synthesis of adrenal steroids, principally cortisone and hydrocortisone

Uses

1. Diagnostic testing of adrenocortical function
2. Management of severe myasthenia gravis and acute exacerbations of multiple sclerosis
3. Treatment of nonsuppurative thyroiditis, tuberculous meningitis (with appropriate antibacterial therapy), trichinosis with neurologic or myocardial involvement, and hypercalcemia associated with cancer; also may be used for many of the indications of systemic glucocorticoids (see Chap. 43), such as rheumatic, hematologic, respiratory, and neoplastic diseases

Dosage

Adrenal responsiveness must first be verified.
Diagnosis—10 U to 25 U/500 ml 5% Dextrose by IV infusion over 8 hours
Treatment of deficiency states—regular injection: 20 U four times a day IM or SC
Repository injection—40 U to 80 U every 1 to 3 days IM or SC
Myasthenia—100 U/day to a total of 1000 U to 2000 U
Multiple sclerosis—80 U to 120 U/day for 2 weeks to 3 weeks IM

Fate

Readily absorbed from injection sites; effects are rapid following IM or IV injection and persist for 4 hours to 6 hours. Duration with repository injection is 24 hours to 48 hours. Half-life following IV injection is 20 minutes to 30 minutes; binds to plasma proteins; excreted partly by the kidney

Significant Adverse Reactions

(Usually observed with prolonged use)
GI—ulceration and hemorrhage (cause and effect relationship not established), pancreatitis, abdominal distention
Musculoskeletal—weakness, osteoporosis, steroid myopathy, loss of muscle mass, vertebral compression fractures
Dermatologic—erythema, petechiae, ecchymoses, delayed wound healing, sweating, hyperpigmentation, acneiform reactions, thinning skin
CNS—convulsions, vertigo, headache, insomnia, depression, mood swings, euphoria, personality alterations
Endocrine—menstrual irregularities, hirsutism, diabetes, decreased carbohydrate tolerance, growth suppression
Electrolyte—hypernatremia, hypokalemia, hypocalcemia, fluid retention
Cardiovascular—hypertension, necrotizing angiitis
Other—subcapsular cataracts, increased intraocular pressure, exophthalmos, negative nitrogen balance, allergic reactions

Contraindications

Osteoporosis, scleroderma, systemic fungal infections, ocular herpes simplex, recent surgery, congestive heart failure, hypertension, IV use (except diagnostic testing), alone in active tuberculosis, and sensitivity to proteins of porcine origin

Interactions

1. Increased requirements for antidiabetic drugs may occur with use of ACTH, due to the hyperglycemic action of corticosteroids.
2. ACTH may enhance the hypoprothrombinemic action of aspirin.
3. Marked hypokalemia may result if ACTH is given with diuretics that cause potassium loss.
4. ACTH may antagonize oral anticoagulants.
5. The adverse effects of vaccines may be enhanced by ACTH.

▶ NURSING ALERTS

▷ 1. Do not administer in full therapeutic doses until adrenal responsiveness has been verified by a rise in plasma or urinary corticosteroid values following an IM or SC test injection.
▷ 2. Perform a skin sensitivity test in all patients with suspected sensitivity to proteins of porcine origin. Observe patients closely for sensitivity reactions during IV infusion or immediately following IM or SC injection.
▷ 3. Use cautiously in patients with diabetes, hypothyroidism, cirrhosis, abscess, infections, diverticulitis, renal insufficiency, myasthenia gravis, in pregnant and lactating women, and in emotionally unstable individuals.
▷ 4. Do not discontinue ACTH therapy abruptly, but gradually reduce dose to minimize the relative adrenal cortical insufficiency that can result from prolonged ACTH therapy. Reinstitute full dose treatment if periods of stress occur during steroid withdrawal.
▷ 5. Observe patients for signs of electrolyte imbalances (*e.g.,* thirst, weakness, muscle cramping), sodium or water retention, or psychic changes (*e.g.,* mood swings, insomnia, depression, euphoria), and advise physician.

▷ 6 Undertake immunization procedures with extreme caution during ACTH therapy because lack of antibody response and neurologic complications have been reported. Do not vaccinate against smallpox during treatment with ACTH.

▷ 7 Urge patients to notify physician if illness or infection develops, because ACTH can produce immuno-suppression and impair the ability of the body to fight infections.

▶ NURSING CONSIDERATIONS

▷ 1 Make dosage adjustments gradually and only after full effects of the drug have become apparent.

▷ 2 Do not administer repository forms of ACTH IV; inject deeply IM. The zinc repository form should not be given SC.

▷ 3 Ensure that proper anti-infective therapy is administered in the presence of an infection, because resistance and ability to localize infections may be impaired by ACTH.

▷ 4 Advise patients to report any weight gain or signs of edema and monitor blood pressure regularly during ACTH treatment.

▷ 5 Recognize that maximal therapeutic effect with ACTH may take several days to develop. Use more rapid acting steroids when an immediate effect is desired.

▷ 6 Reconstitute prepared powder with Sterile Water for Injection or Sterile Saline Solution. Refrigerate and discard unused portion after 24 hours.

▶ growth hormone
GH

▶ somatotropin
Asellacrin, Crescormon

GH (Somatropin, Somatotropin) is a purified polypeptide hormone extracted from human pituitary glands at necropsy. Because of the limited supply, GH is available only to physicians who submit to the suppliers documented clinical and laboratory evidence of GH deficiency in their patients.

Mechanism
An anabolic agent that stimulates linear growth in patients with pituitary growth hormone deficiency; anabolic effects are mediated by another group of peptide hormones, termed *somatomedins,* whose hepatic synthesis is stimulated by growth hormone; promotes intracellular transport of amino acids, cellular protein synthesis, net retention of nitrogen, phosphorus, and potassium, and urinary excretion of calcium; may stimulate DNA duplication, facilitate synthesis of messenger RNA, and activate cyclic AMP, resulting in subsequent coupling of amino acids to their respective transfer RNAs

Elevates serum concentrations of phosphorus and alkaline phosphatase and augments synthesis of chondroitin sulfate and collagen; stimulates lipolysis, increases plasma free fatty acids, and enhances oxidation of fatty acids; inhibits intra-cellular glucose metabolism; may exert a diabetogenic action in large doses by increasing blood glucose levels, decreasing glucose tolerance, and reducing sensitivity to exogenous insulin

Use
1 Treatment of growth failure due to a deficiency of pituitary growth hormone (hypopituitary dwarfism)

Dosage
Initially 2 International Units (IU) three times a week IM, with 48 hours between injections; if growth rate does not exceed 2.5 cm in a 6-month period, dose may be doubled for next 6 months. If there is still no satisfactory response, discontinue drug.

Fate
Short half-life in plasma (15 min–60 min) but effects persist for several days; largely metabolized in the liver and excreted in the kidney

Common Side-Effects
Increased calcium excretion

Significant Adverse Reactions
Myalgia, pain and swelling at injection site, hyperglycemia, ketosis

Contraindications
Patients with closed epiphyses, progressive intracranial lesions or tumors

Interactions
1 Accelerated epiphyseal closure (fusion of ends of long bones) can occur if GH is combined with androgens or thyroid hormones.
2 Hydrocortisone and other anti-inflammatory steroids may inhibit the response to GH.
3 GH may decrease responsiveness to insulin or to oral antidiabetic drugs by increasing blood glucose levels.

▶ NURSING ALERTS

▷ 1 Use cautiously in patients with diabetes or a family history of diabetes, because drug induces hyperglycemia and ketosis. Regular urine testing for glycosuria should be employed.

▷ 2 Before initiating treatment, document growth hormone deficiency by failure of serum growth hormone concentration to rise above 5 mg to 7 mg/ml in response to at least two standard stimuli, *e.g.,* insulin-induced hypoglycemia, IV arginine (see Chap. 78), oral levodopa, or IM glucagon.

▷ 3 Perform annual bone age assessments in all patients, especially those receiving thyroid or androgen therapy concurrently, because premature epiphyseal closure can occur.

▷ 4 Be alert for possible development of hypotension, tachycardia, or atrial arrhythmias.

▶ **NURSING CONSIDERATIONS**

▷ 1 Do not inject SC, because lipoatrophy or lipodystrophy can occur. SC injection also increases the chance of developing neutralizing antibodies. Administer IM and rotate injection sites.

▷ 2 Be alert for signs of hypercalciuria (*e.g.,* flank pain, renal colic, chills, fever, urinary frequency, hematuria) especially during first 2 months to 3 months of therapy.

▷ 3 Discontinue injections when satisfactory height has been achieved, epiphyses have fused, or patient fails to exhibit proper growth response.

▷ 4 Perform periodic thyroid function tests and initiate thyroid hormone therapy if hypothyroidism occurs.

▷ 5 Reconstitute each vial with 5 ml of Bacteriostatic Water for Injection. Do *not* shake vial vigorously. Store in refrigerator and discard after 1 month.

▶ **thyroid-stimulating hormone**

▶ **thyrotropin**

Thytropar

A purified extract of TSH isolated from bovine pituitary glands, this preparation is devoid of significant amounts of other pituitary hormones.

Mechanism

Increases uptake of iodide by the thyroid gland, enhances formation of thyroid hormones, and increases release of thyroid hormones from the thyroid gland; in large doses, produces hyperplasia of thyroid glandular tissue, which is readily reversible upon termination of the drug

Uses

1 Determination of subclinical hypothyroidism or low thyroid reserve

2 Differentiation between primary and secondary hypothyroidism

3 Differentiation of primary hypothyroidism from euthyroidism (normal thyroid function) following thyroid suppression by thyroid replacement therapy

4 Aid in the detection of metastases of thyroid carcinoma

5 Adjunct in the management of certain types of thyroid carcinoma and resulting metastases, in combination with ^{131}I to enhance isotope uptake by the thyroid

Dosage

10 IU (contents of 1 vial) IM or SC daily for 1 to 8 days depending on condition

Fate

Short acting and rapidly excreted by the kidney; half-life is 30 minutes to 40 minutes with normal thyroid function, longer in hypothyroidism and shorter in hyperthyroidism

Common Side-Effects

Transient hypotension, thyroid swelling (especially from large doses)

Significant Adverse Reactions

Vomiting, fever, headache, urticaria, menstrual irregularities, tachycardia, atrial fibrillation, anaphylactic reactions, angina (large doses), and congestive heart failure (large doses)

Contraindications

Coronary thrombosis, untreated Addison's disease

▶ **NURSING ALERT**

▷ 1 Use cautiously in patients with angina pectoris, cardiac failure, hypopituitarism, adrenal cortical insufficiency.

▶ **NURSING CONSIDERATION**

▷ 1 Prepare solution by adding 2 ml sterile physiologic saline solution to vial containing 10 IU thyrotropic activity. Solution may be kept for up to 2 weeks if refrigerated.

Hormones of the Neurohypophysis

The neurohypophysis or posterior lobe of the pituitary contains two hormones, oxytocin and vasopressin, both of which are available for clinical use. In addition, a posterior pituitary preparation, an extract of pituitary glands possessing the activity of both oxytocin and vasopressin, is used both by injection and by inhalation for certain therapeutic indications.

Oxytocin exerts two principal actions in the body: contraction of uterine smooth muscle (oxytocic effect) and contraction of the myoepithelial cells surrounding the ducts of the mammary gland, resulting in ejection of milk (galactokinetic effect). The sensitivity of the uterus to the effects of oxytocin is dependent both on the stage of gestation (maximal at term and immediately postpartum) as well as on the existing balance of female sex hormones (increased in the presence of estrogen and reduced in the presence of progesterone). Natural oxytocin is no longer available for clinical use, and has been replaced by a synthetic derivative. It is most frequently employed to enhance uterine contractions during labor. Although not derived from pituitary sources, two other drugs used for their oxytocic effects, ergonovine and methylergonovine, are also considered in this chapter.

Vasopressin is frequently referred to also as the antidiuretic hormone (ADH), because it promotes reabsorption of water from the distal tubules and collecting ducts of the kidney. Its other pharmacologic effects include contraction of vascular smooth muscle, especially of the portal and splanchnic (visceral) vessels, and a direct spasmogenic effect on gastrointestinal smooth muscle. Available preparations of vasopressin include a synthetic derivative of the naturally occurring hormone possessing marked pressor and antidiuretic activity and two structural analogs, desmopressin and lypressin, which exhibit relatively selective antidiuretic activity with minimal pressor effects. These drugs are reviewed individually in this chapter.

▶ posterior pituitary injection
Pituitrin-S

Posterior pituitary injection is a sterile aqueous extract of pituitary glands containing the equivalent of either 10 United States Pharmacopeia (USP) posterior pituitary U/ml (Pituitrin) for obstetric use or 20 USP U/ml (Pituitrin-S) for hemostasis in surgery.

Mechanism
Possesses oxytocic, vasopressor, smooth muscle spasmogenic, and antidiuretic activity

Uses
1 Control of postoperative ileus and to facilitate expulsion of gas before pyelography
2 Aid to achieving hemostasis in surgical procedures
3 Assistance in uterine involution and control of postpartum hemorrhage following placental expulsion, supplemented with ergot alkaloids

Dosage
SC, IM, 5 U to 20 U (average 10 U)

Common Side-Effects
Facial pallor, uterine cramping, GI spasms

Significant Adverse Reactions
Tinnitus, mydriasis, anxiety, diarrhea, urticaria, albuminuria, angioedema, eclamptic episodes, loss of consciousness, and anaphylaxis

Contraindications
Toxemia of pregnancy, cardiac disease, hypertension, epilepsy, and advanced arteriosclerosis

Interactions
1 Increased incidence of cardiac arrhythmias and coronary insufficiency can occur if Pituitrin is combined with barbiturates or general anesthetics.
2 Antidiuretic effects can be potentiated by chlorpropamide, clofibrate, and carbamazepine.

▶ NURSING ALERTS
▷ 1 Be aware that the drug is not recommended to assist labor, because its action is rather short-lived and there is a high risk of fetal distress or asphyxia and uterine rupture.
▷ 2 Do not use for treatment of surgical shock, because the vasoconstriction and increased peripheral resistance are accompanied by decreased coronary blood flow and cardiac output, further aggravating the conditions that may have been responsible for shock.

▶ posterior pituitary, intranasal
Posterior Pituitary

An intranasal dosage form of posterior pituitary extract is available for the control of symptoms of diabetes insipidus due to an endogenous deficiency of ADH. The drug is supplied as capsules containing 40 mg of posterior pituitary powder, which is administered 3 to 4 times a day using an Armour Powder Inhalator. Nasal irritation, rhinorrhea, and nasal mucosal ulceration have occurred, and inadvertent inhalation into the bronchioles has resulted in dyspnea and coughing. Intranasal posterior pituitary should be used cautiously in patients with coronary artery disease, because vasoconstriction can occur if appreciable amounts are absorbed systemically. Use of the product in pregnant women may induce abortion.

▶ vasopressin
Pitressin Synthetic

▶ vasopressin tannate
Pitressin Tannate In Oil

A synthetic compound structurally identical to naturally occurring vasopressin possessing vasopressor and antidiuretic activity, vasopressin injection is available as an aqueous solution containing 20 pressor U per milliliter. Vasopressin tannate injection is a water-insoluble tannate salt of vasopressin suspended in peanut oil, containing 5 pressor units per milliliter and having a prolonged (36 hr–72 hr) duration of action.

The principal indication for these agents is the treatment of diabetes insipidus, a condition characterized by excretion of excessive quantities of dilute urine (polyuria) and extreme thirst (polydipsia). Insufficient ADH secretion from the neurohypophysis is often the cause of this condition, and vasopressin provides replacement therapy to correct the symptoms. Occasionally, however, the problem is unresponsiveness of the renal tubules to the action of vasopressin and, in these cases, vasopressin is ineffective in treating the condition. Successful therapy of this latter type of diabetes insipidus is difficult, but clinical benefit has been reported with use of thiazide diuretics and chlorpropamide. Vasopressin is also used to reduce excessive bleeding based upon its ability to strongly contract vascular smooth muscle.

Mechanism
Increases distal tubular reabsorption of water by increasing the permeability of the tubular epithelium via activation of cyclic AMP in cells of the renal collecting ducts; enhances contraction of vascular and nonvascular smooth muscle, resulting in decreased peripheral blood flow and GI, urinary, and uterine smooth muscle spasm; constriction of coronary arteries may precipitate or worsen existing angina

Uses
1 Treatment of diabetes insipidus of central (hypophysial) origin
2 Prevention and treatment of postoperative abdominal distention
3 Dispersion of gas shadows to aid abdominal roentgenography
4 Control of bleeding esophageal varices and hemorrhage due to abdominal surgery (experimental use)

Dosage

Vasopressin injection

Diabetes insipidus—5 U to 10 U 2 to 3 times a day IM, SC, or intranasally on cotton pledgets

Abdominal distention—5 U IM initially; increase to 10 U every 3 hours to 4 hours as necessary

Abdominal roentgenography—10 U IM 2 hours and ½ hour before films are exposed

Bleeding episodes—20 U by IV infusion over 5 minutes to 10 minutes or occasionally intra-arterially

Vasopressin tannate in oil

0.3 ml to 1 ml (1.5 U–5 U) IM; repeat as needed every 36 hours to 72 hours

Fate

Duration of action with aqueous injection is 2 hours to 8 hours; effects of tannate injection persist 36 hours to 96 hours, primarily due to slow, cumulative absorption from IM injection site; rapidly removed from the plasma (half-life 15 min); inactivated by the liver and kidneys and excreted in the urine as metabolites and unchanged drug

Common Side-Effects

Facial pallor, nausea, GI disturbances, and uterine cramping

Significant Adverse Reactions

Vertigo, sweating, headache, vomiting, urticaria, bronchoconstriction, hypersensitivity reactions, anaphylactic reaction, and anginal pain

Following nasal insufflation: congestion, irritation, rhinorrhea, headache, conjunctivitis, and mucosal ulceration

Contraindications

Chronic nephritis, advanced arteriosclerosis, and severe coronary artery disease

Interactions

1 Action of vasopressin may be potentiated by antidiabetics, acetaminophen, fludrocortisone, ganglionic blocking agents, neostigmine, and general anesthetics.

2 Antidiuretic activity can be increased by chlorpropamide, clofibrate, or carbamazepine.

3 Antidiuretic action of vasopressin may be reduced by alcohol, epinephrine, cyclophosphamide, heparin, and lithium.

▶ NURSING ALERTS

▷ 1 Do not use in patients with disease of the coronary arteries, except with extreme caution. Anginal attacks and myocardial infarction can occur. Appropriate treatment (*e.g.,* nitroglycerin, oxygen, antiarrhythmics) should be available.

▷ 2 Do not inject vasopressin tannate IV.

▷ 3 Be alert for early signs of water intoxication (nausea, vomiting, drowsiness, listlessness, headaches, confusion), because convulsions and coma can occur. Withdraw drug and restrict fluid intake until specific

gravity of urine is at least 1.015 and polyuria occurs. Diuretics may be used with caution.

▷ 4 Use cautiously in patients with epilepsy, asthma, migraine, heart failure, angina, renal disease, goiter, and in elderly, very young, or pregnant patients.

▶ NURSING CONSIDERATIONS

▷ 1 Administer 1 or 2 glassfuls of water with a large dose of vasopressin to reduce side-effects such as cramping, skin blanching, and nausea.

▷ 2 Before therapy, determine baseline values for blood pressure, body weight, and intake–output ratio. Monitor values regularly (daily if possible) during therapy and report any sudden changes.

▷ 3 When vasopressin is used to relieve abdominal distention, observe patients for appearance of peristaltic sounds, passage of flatus, and return of normal pattern of bowel movements. Abdominal measurements should be done prior to and during treatment.

▷ 4 Note that the polyuria and thirst of diabetes insipidus are controlled for 36 hours to 72 hours following a single dose of the tannate salt. Do not administer more frequently than every 36 hours to 48 hours.

▷ 5 Note the tannate injection is indicated *only* for treatment of diabetes insipidus.

▷ 6 Inform patients that tannate injection may be painful. Be alert for development of allergic reactions, to both the vasopressin and the vehicle.

▷ 7 Injections should be warmed to body temperature before administration. Shake the tannate suspension vigorously to ensure uniform dispersion.

▶ desmopressin acetate

DDAVP, Stimate

A synthetic analog of vasopressin, desmopressin acetate is used as an intranasal spray, or by injection, and possesses prolonged, potent antidiuretic activity with no vasopressor or oxytocic effects at normal doses.

Mechanism

Provides replacement therapy for antidiuretic hormone in treating polyuria and polydipsia

Uses

1 Treatment of diabetes insipidus of central (hypophysial) origin

2 Treatment of polyuria and polydipsia associated with trauma or surgery of the pituitary gland

3 Treatment of hemophilia A and certain forms of von Willebrand's disease (injectable form)

Dosage

Inhalation

Drug is supplied with a flexible calibrated plastic tube (rhinyle); desired quantity of solution is drawn into tube, one end is inserted into nostril, and patient blows on other end to deposit drug deep into nasal cavity; infants and young children require assistance (*e.g.*, air-filled syringe attached to tube).

> Adults: 0.1 ml to 0.4 ml/day, either as a single dose or in 2 or 3 divided doses
>
> Children (under 12): 0.05 ml to 0.3 ml/day in a single or 2 divided doses

IV

Diabetes insipidus—0.5 ml to 1.0 ml daily in 2 divided doses

Hemophilia A/von Willebrand's Disease—0.3 mcg/kg by slow IV infusion over 15 minutes to 30 minutes. In adults use 50 ml of sterile saline diluent; in children less than 10 kg, use 10 ml diluent.

Fate

Onset in 1 hour to 2 hours; provides control of symptoms for 8 hours to 20 hours; metabolized by liver and kidney and excreted in the urine

Common Side-Effects

Nasal irritation and congestion

Significant Adverse Reactions

(Usually with high doses only) Headache, nausea, flushing, rhinitis, abdominal cramping, vulval pain, and hypertension

▶ NURSING ALERT

▷ 1 Use cautiously in patients with coronary artery disease, and hypertension, and in very young or elderly patients.

▶ NURSING CONSIDERATIONS

▷ 1 Decrease fluid intake as necessary to decrease possibility of water intoxication and hyponatremia.

▷ 2 Administer a diuretic as needed if excessive fluid retention occurs.

▷ 3 Provide complete instructions for administering medication (see Dosage) and ensure that patients understand how to use the calibrated plastic tube (rhinyle).

▶ lypressin

Diapid

A synthetic vasopressin, lypressin possesses little or no vasopressor or oxytocic activity. It is stable in aqueous solution and administered in the form of a nasal spray containing 50 USP Posterior Pituitary Pressor U/ml.

Mechanism

Provides replacement therapy for antidiuretic hormone; useful in patients who are unresponsive to or intolerant of other forms of replacement therapy, or who experience allergic reactions or other adverse reactions with systemically administered vasopressin

Use

1 Management of the symptoms of diabetes insipidus of central (hypophysial) origin

Dosage

One or two sprays in each nostril 4 times a day, with an additional dose at bedtime to eliminate nocturia if needed (one spray provides approximately 2 USP Posterior Pituitary Pressor U).

Fate

Rapidly absorbed from the nasal mucosa; maximal effects occur in 1 hour to 2 hours and persist 3 hours to 4 hours; metabolized in the liver and kidney and excreted in the urine

Common Side-Effects

(Infrequent) Irritation and congestion of the nasal mucosa

Significant Adverse Reactions

Headache, rhinorrhea, conjunctivitis, nasal ulceration, abdominal cramping, and increased bowel movements

Inadvertent inhalation may cause coughing, chest tightness, and dyspnea

▶ NURSING ALERTS

▷ 1 Warn patient not to inhale while spraying and to avoid use of excessive doses (sprays), because systemic effects may be increased.

▷ 2 Use cautiously in patients with coronary artery disease or hypertension and in pregnant women, because some residual vasopressor or oxytocic effects can occur.

▶ NURSING CONSIDERATIONS

▷ 1 Note that effectiveness may be impaired in patients with nasal congestion, allergic rhinitis, upper respiratory infections, and colds. Dosage adjustment may be required.

▷ 2 Be aware that more than 2 or 3 sprays in each nostril usually results in wastage, the unabsorbed excess draining into the digestive tract to be inactivated. If increased dosage is indicated, increase frequency of usage rather than number of sprays with each use.

▷ 3 Instruct patient to clear nasal passages before administering, hold bottle upright when spraying, and keep head in an upright position.

▶ oxytocin

Pitocin, Syntocinon

Oxytocin is a synthetic peptide possessing the pharmacologic effects of the endogenous hormone. It is available as an injection for IM or IV use containing 10 U/ml, and as a nasal spray containing 40 U/ml.

Mechanism

Direct spasmogenic effect on uterine smooth muscle; increases permeability of the cell membranes of myofibrils to sodium ions, thereby augmenting contractile activity; also contracts myoepithelial cells surrounding the ducts and alveoli of the mammary gland, facilitating ejection of milk from the properly primed gland; large doses may exhibit antidiuretic activity.

Uses

1. Initiation or augmentation of uterine contractions to assist in delivery of the fetus for *valid fetal or maternal reasons only*, such as the following:
   a. Maternal diabetes
   b. Rh problems
   c. Uterine inertia
   d. Premature rupture of membranes
   e. Preeclampsia or eclampsia
2. Control of postpartum hemorrhage
3. Facilitation of uterine involution
4. Management of inevitable, incomplete, or missed abortion
5. Aid in milk let-down during breast-feeding or relief of postpartum breast engorgement (only indication for the nasal spray)

Dosage

Injection

Induction or enhancement of labor—0.001 U to 0.002 U/minute (0.1 ml–0.2 ml/min of a 1:1000 dilution; see below) by IV infusion; increase gradually in 0.001-U to 0.002-U/min increments at 15-minute to 30-minute intervals until a desirable contraction pattern has been established; adjust rate according to uterine response

Dilution—1-ml ampul (10 U) added to 1000 ml of 0.9% aqueous sodium chloride or other suitable IV fluid; use constant infusion pump to accurately control dose

Postpartum uterine bleeding: IV—10 U to 40 U/1000-ml diluent infused at a rate to control bleeding; IM—10 U after delivery of the placenta

Incomplete abortion—10 U/500 ml diluent infused IV at a rate of 0.020 U to 0.040 U/minute

Nasal spray

One spray into one nostril or both nostrils 2 minutes to 3 minutes before nursing or pumping of breasts

Fate

Onset of effect is within 1 minute with IV infusion, 3 minutes to 7 minutes with IM injection, and 5 minutes to 10 minutes with nasal spray; although nasal absorption is erratic, short plasma half-life (several minutes); rapidly cleared from the plasma by the liver, kidney, and mammary gland; primarily excreted as metabolites by the kidney, with small amounts as active drug

Significant Adverse Reactions

Fetus

Bradycardia, arrhythmias, neonatal jaundice, hypoxia, and trauma from too rapid expulsion

Mother

Arrhythmias, nausea, vomiting, pelvic hematoma, afibrinogenemia, uterine hypertonicity or spasm, uterine rupture, anaphylactic reaction, subarachnoid hemorrhage, hypertension, water intoxication, convulsions, and postpartum hemorrhage

Contraindications

Unfavorable fetal position, significant cephalopelvic disproportion, fetal distress where delivery is not imminent, hypertonic uterine patterns, undilated cervix, prolonged use in uterine inertia or severe toxemia, conditions in which vaginal delivery is contraindicated (*e.g.,* prolapsed cord, total placenta praevia, vasa praevia), previous cervical or uterine surgery, invasive cervical carcinoma, dead fetus, and abruptio placentae

Interactions

1. Severe persistent hypertension can occur if oxytocin is given in the presence of other vasopressor drugs, *e.g.,* epinephrine, ephedrine, methoxamine, or metaraminol.
2. Estrogens may augment and progestins may decrease the uterine spasmogenic action of oxytocin.
3. Oxytocin can be potentiated by cyclophosphamide.

▶ NURSING ALERTS

▷ 1 Recognize that oxytocin is indicated for medical rather than elective induction of labor and should be used only in the best interests of the mother and fetus.

▷ 2 Ensure that oxytocin used for induction of labor be given only by IV infusion, and administered by trained personnel. A physician should be readily available at all times to manage complications.

▷ 3 Do not administer by more than one route simultaneously for any indication.

▷ 4 Except in unusual circumstances, do not use in the following conditions: prematurity, partial placenta praevia, previous surgery on the cervix or uterus, overdistention of the uterus, grand multiparity, or history of uterine sepsis.

▷ 5 Carefully regulate flow rate of infusion to obtain optimal contractions. Monitor uterine contractions, fetal heart rate, and maternal blood pressure and pulse regularly during infusion, and report any significant changes immediately.

▷ 6 During prolonged infusion, be alert for signs of water intoxication due to ADH effect of oxytocin. Early signs are confusion, headache, and drowsiness. Intake–output ratio should be checked during labor, and edema and anuria should be promptly noted.

▷ 7 Stop infusion if contractions are frequent (less than 2-min intervals), prolonged, or excessive (*i.e.,* greater than 50 mm Hg) to prevent fetal anoxia. Place patient on her side and be prepared to administer oxygen. Effects will decrease rapidly, because oxytocin is short acting.

▷ 8 If local anesthetics containing epinephrine are used durign labor in patients receiving oxytocin, be alert for development of excessive blood pressure elevations. Symptoms may include throbbing headache, palpitations, sweating, fever, vomiting, stiff neck, photophobia, chest pain.

▷ 9 Do not administer *undiluted* solution IV, nor give oxytocin by more than one route of administration at any one time.

▶ NURSING CONSIDERATIONS

▷ 1 Begin IV infusion with non-oxytocin-containing solution (*e.g.,* physiologic electrolyte solution). Oxytocin solution is then added to the system using a constant infusion pump to accurately regulate the rate of infusion. Flow rate should not exceed 2 ml/minute.

▷ 2 Instruct patients using nasal spray to hold bottle upright and maintain a sitting or standing position. Nasal passages should be cleared before spraying.

▷ 3 When oxytocin is given IM (deep deltoid injection), have magnesium sulfate solution available to relax myometrium if necessary.

▶ ergonovine
Ergotrate

An alkaloid obtained from ergot, a fungus that grows on the rye plant, ergonovine exerts a more prolonged oxytocic action than oxytocin itself and elicits fewer side-effects.

Mechanism
Direct stimulating effect on smooth muscle of the uterus; small doses increase force and frequency of uterine contractions, but normal relaxant phase follows; larger doses produce sustained, forceful contractions, with markedly elevated resting tone; cerebral vasoconstriction is moderate, although less than that observed with ergotamine, a related alkaloid used in migraine (see Chap. 14)

Uses
1 Prevention and treatment of postpartum or post-abortion hemorrhage due to uterine atony
2 Investigational uses, including alternate therapy of migraine (especially when use of ergotamine causes paresthesias) and diagnosis of Prinzmetal's variant angina during coronary arteriography

Dosage
Oral—0.2 mg to 0.4 mg 2 to 4 times a day until danger of atony has passed (usually 48 hr)
IM—0.2 mg following placental delivery; may repeat in 2 hours to 4 hours as needed
IV—0.2 mg for excessive uterine bleeding

Fate
Rapidly absorbed orally and parenterally; onset of action is usually within 10 minutes by any route of administration; duration of action is 2 hours to 4 hours; metabolized largely by the liver

Significant Adverse Reactions
(Most frequent with IV administration) Nausea, vomiting, weak and rapid pulse, paresthesias, allergic reactions (including shock), hypertension, tinnitus, headache, dyspnea, cramping, dizziness, confusion, decreased lactation, and muscle weakness

Contraindications
For induction of labor, threatened spontaneous abortion

Interactions
1 Blood pressure may be further elevated if ergonovine is combined with vasopressors or other oxytocics.
2 Oxytocic action may be antagonized by hypocalcemia.

▶ NURSING ALERTS

▷ 1 Use with extreme caution before delivery of the placenta, and only in the presence of a staff member well versed in the use of ergonovine, because very high uterine tone may be produced.

▷ 2 Use IV only in extreme emergencies, because danger of hypertension and severe nausea and vomiting is increased.

▷ 3 Monitor blood pressure, pulse, vaginal blood flow, and uterine response following injection until condition has stabilized, and report marked changes in pulse or pressure.

▷ 4 Use cautiously in patients with heart disease, hypertension, mitral valve stenosis, renal or hepatic impairment, obliterative vascular disease, or sepsis.

▶ NURSING CONSIDERATIONS

▷ 1 To avoid development of ergotism (ergot poisoning) do not use for prolonged periods of time. Early symptoms include vomiting, cramping, headache, and confusion.

▷ 2 If uterus is not responding to ergonovine, patient may be hypocalcemic. Determine serum calcium levels and, if they are deficient, consider cautious administration of IV calcium gluconate (10 ml–30 ml of a 10% solution). Do not use calcium gluconate in patients taking digitalis.

▷ 3 Store injection in a cool place and do not use solution over 60 days old.

▷ 4 Note that cramping is usually an indication of drug effectiveness, but persistent or severe cramping may indicate a need for dosage reduction.

▶ methylergonovine
Methergine

A synthetic ergot alkaloid, methylergonovine is similar in most respects to ergonovine.

Mechanism
Direct spasmogenic action on uterine smooth muscle; weak cerebral vasoconstrictive action

Uses
1 Management of postpartum atony, hemorrhage, or subinvolution of the uterus following delivery of the placenta
2 Facilitation of labor (given in the second stage following delivery of the anterior shoulder)

Dosage
Oral—0.2 mg 3 or 4 times a day for a maximum of 1 week
IM, IV—0.2 mg after delivery of the anterior shoulder,

after delivery of placenta, or during the puerperium; may repeat as required at 2-hour to 4-hour intervals

Fate

Well absorbed orally or parenterally; onset of action is 5 minutes to 10 minutes orally and IM and almost immediate with IV injection

Significant Adverse Reactions

Nausea, vomiting, hypertension, dizziness, tinnitus, sweating, palpitation, chest pain, and dyspnea

Contraindications

Hypertension, toxemia, and pregnancy

Interactions

1 Pressor effects may be enhanced by concurrent use of vasopressors or other oxytocics.

▶ NURSING ALERTS

▷ 1 Do not use routinely IV, because risk of hypertension and cerebral vascular accident is increased. When used IV, administer slowly and closely monitor blood pressure.

▷ 2 Use cautiously in patients with sepsis, obliterative vascular disease, and hepatic or renal dysfunction.

▶ NURSING CONSIDERATION

▷ 1 Do not use solution if discolored. Store in a cool place and protect from light.

Summary. Hypophysial Hormones

Drug	Preparations	Usual Dosage Range
Adenohypophysis		
Corticotropin injection (ACTH, Acthar)	Powder for injection—25 U/ml, 40 U/ml, 80 U/ml	20 U 4 times/day SC or IM 10 U to 25 U/500 ml 5% Dextrose infused IV over 8 hours
Corticotropin repository (ACTH Gel, Cortigel, Cortrophin Gel, Cortropic Gel, H.P. Acthar Gel)	Injection—40 U/ml, 80 U/ml	40 U to 80 U IM or SC every 1 to 3 days
Corticotropin zinc (Cortrophin-Zinc)	Injection—40 U/ml	40 U to 80 U IM (only) every 1 to 3 days
Somatotropin (GH) (Asellacrin, Crescormon)	Injection—2 U/vial, 4 U/vial, 10 U/vial	Initially, 2 IU IM 3 times/week, 48 hours apart; if growth rate does not exceed 2.5 cm in a 6-month period, double the dose for next 6 months
Thyrotropin (TSH) (Thytropar)	Powder for injection—10 U/vial with diluent	10 U IM or SC daily for 1 to 8 days depending on condition
Neurohypophysis		
Posterior pituitary injection (Pituitrin-S)	Injection—10 U/ml (Pituitrin) 20 U/ml (Pituitrin-S)	5 U to 20 U (average 10 U) IM or SC
Posterior pituitary, intranasal (Posterior Pituitary)	Capsules for inhalation—40 mg posterior pituitary hormone	Administer using an Armour Powder Inhalator 3 to 4 times a day according to package directions
Vasopressin (ADH) (Pitressin Synthetic)	Injection—20 U/ml	Diabetes insipidus—5 U to 10 U 2 to 3 times/day IM, SC, or intranasally on cotton pledgets Abdominal distention—5 U IM, increased to 10 U every 3 hours to 4 hours as needed Roentgenography—10 U IM 2 hours and ½ hour before film
Vasopressin tannate (Pitressin Tannate in Oil)	Injection—5 U/ml	Diabetes insipidus—0.3 ml to 1 ml (1.5 U–5 U) IM only every 36 hours to 48 hours as needed
Desmopressin acetate (DDAVP, Stimate)	Nasal solution—0.1 mg/ml Injection—4 mcg/ml	Inhalation—Adults: 0.1 ml to 0.4 ml/day either a single dose or in 2 to 3 divided doses Children (under 12): 0.05 ml to 0.3 ml/day in 2 divided doses

(continued)

Summary. Hypophysial Hormones *(continued)*

Drug	Preparations	Usual Dosage Range
		IV: Diabetes insipidus—0.5 ml to 1.0 ml daily in 2 divided doses Hemophilia A/von willebrand's Disease—0.3 mcg/kg by slow infusion (15 minutes to 30 minutes) in sterile saline diluent (adults—50 ml; children—10 ml)
Lypressin (Diapid)	Nasal spray—0.185 mg/ml	1 to 2 sprays in each nostril 4 times/day with an additional dose at bedtime if needed to control nocturia
Oxytocin (Pitocin, Syntocinon)	Injection—10 U/ml	Induction of labor—0.001 U to 0.002 U/minute by slow IV infusion; increase gradually until optimal effect is noted
		Postpartum uterine bleeding—10 U to 40 U/1000 ml by constant IV infusion or 10 U IM after delivery of placenta
		Incomplete Abortion—10 U/500 ml infused IV at a rate of 0.020 U to 0.040 U/minute
Oxytocin, synthetic nasal (Syntocinon)	Nasal spray—40 U/ml	1 spray into one nostril or both 2 minutes to 3 minutes before nursing or pumping of breast
Nonhypophysial Oxytocics		
Ergonovine (Ergotrate)	Tablets—0.2 mg Injection—0.2 mg/ml	0.2 mg to 0.4 mg orally 2 to 4 times/day until danger of atony has passed 0.2 mg IM or IV
Methylergonovine (Methergine)	Tablets—0.2 mg Injection—0.2 mg/ml	0.2 mg orally 3 to 4 times/day 0.2 mg IM or IV, repeat every 2 hours to 4 hours as required

The endogenous thyroid hormones thyroxine (T_4) and triiodothyronine (T_3) play an important role in normal physical and mental growth and development, and in regulating the metabolic activity of essentially every cell of the body. They affect a wide range of physiologic activities including central nervous system, cardiovascular, and gastrointestinal function; carbohydrate, lipid, and protein metabolism; temperature regulation; muscle activity; water and electrolyte balance; and reproduction. Unlike many other hormones, however, they do not act upon discrete target organs but exert a diffuse effect throughout the body. Their onset of action is slow and their activity prolonged; thus, they generally provide long-term regulation of bodily functions rather than moment-to-moment control.

The synthesis, storage, and release of the thyroid hormones by the thyroid gland are regulated in large part by the thyroid stimulating hormone (TSH) of the adenohypophysis; this schema is discussed in the review of endocrine function in Chapter 38. The principal clinical application of the thyroid hormones is in the treatment of *hypo*thyroidism. This disease, characterized by reduced or absent secretion of endogenous thyroid hormones, can be clinically subdivided into cretinism (fetal or neonatal hypothyroidism) and myxedema (adult hypothyroidism), and each of these conditions is reviewed in Chapter 38. It should be noted that use of thyroid hormones in hypothyroidism merely constitutes replacement therapy and does not effect a cure. Because normal thyroid function is usually not reestablished of its own, clinical benefit is attained only as long as thyroid hormones are supplied.

Several types of thyroid hormone preparations are available, both natural extracts of animal thyroid glands and synthetic derivatives. Although the natural animal extracts exhibit more variation in potency than the synthetic derivatives, the pharmacologic effects of all the thyroid hormone preparations are essentially identical. Principal differences occur in onset and duration of action.

The available thyroid preparations are the following:

1 *Desiccated thyroid*—powdered, dried thyroid glands of domesticated animals, standardized on the basis of iodine content
2 *Thyroglobulin*—purified extract of porcine thyroid gland, standardized by iodine content and bioassayed for metabolic activity
3 *Levothyroxine sodium*—sodium salt of the synthetic l-isomer of T_4
4 *Liothyronine sodium*—sodium salt of the synthetic l-isomer of T_3
5 *Liotrix*—combination of levothyroxine sodium (T_4) and liothyronine sodium (T_3) in a 4:1 ratio, on a weight basis

The pharmacology of the thyroid hormones is discussed as a group, because their overall effects are similar. Individual drugs are then listed in Table 40-1.

Secretion of excessive amonts of thyroid hormones reflects a *hyper*thyroid state, the most common cause of which is overstimulation of the gland by circulating immunoglobulins synthesized by B-lymphocytes. One such antibody is thyroid stimulating immunoglobulin (TSI), which interacts

Thyroid Hormones and Antithyroid Drugs

40

Table 40-1. Thyroid Hormones

Drug	Preparations	Usual Dosage Range	Remarks
Thyroid, desiccated (Armour Thyroid, S-P-T, Thyrar, Thyro-Teric, Westhroid)	Tablets—16 mg, 32 mg, 65 mg, 98 mg, 130 mg, 195 mg, 260 mg, 325 mg Coated tablets—32 mg, 65 mg, 130 mg, 195 mg Capsules (timed release)—65 mg, 130 mg, 195 mg, 325 mg	Adults: Myxedema—16 mg/day for 2 weeks; 32 mg/day for 2 weeks; then 65 mg/day; increase daily dosage at monthly or greater intervals based on laboratory tests (usual range 65 mg–195 mg/day) Hypothyroidism without myxedema—65 mg/day increased by 65 mg every 30 days until desired response Children: Dosage regimen same as adults, with increments made at 2-week intervals; maintenance doses may be higher in growing child than in adult	Desiccated animal thyroid glands containing active thyroid hormones (T_3 and T_4) in their natural state and ratio; potency can vary significantly from lot to lot; clinical effects develop slowly and are very prolonged; caution in transferring patient from thyroid to T_3 alone; discontinue thyroid, begin T_3 at very low doses and gradually increase dosage levels; drug should be stored in dark, moisture-free bottles
Thyroglobulin (Proloid)	Tablets—32 mg, 65 mg, 100 mg, 130 mg, 200 mg	Initially 32 mg/day; increase at 1-week to 2-week intervals until optimal response is attained; usual maintenance dosage range 32 mg/day to 200 mg/day	Purified extract of hog thyroid containing T_4 and T_3 in an approximate 2.5:1 ratio; biologically assayed and standardized in animals; action is similar to that of desiccated thyroid with comparable onset and duration
Levothyroxine sodium—T_4 (l-thyroxine, Levothroid, Noroxine, Synthroid)	Tablets—0.025 mg, 0.05 mg, 0.075 mg, 0.1 mg, 0.125 mg, 0.15 mg, 0.175 mg, 0.2 mg, 0.3 mg Injection—100 mcg/ml	Oral: Adults—0.1 mg/day initially; increased by 0.05-mg to 0.1-mg increments every 1 week to 3 weeks until desired response is obtained; in elderly, myxedematous, or cardiovascular patients, initial dose 0.025 mg with 0.025-mg to 0.05-mg increments as needed; usual range 0.1 mg to 0.2 mg/day Children—0.05 mg initially, with increments of 0.025-mg to 0.05-mg/day at 1-week to 3-week intervals until desired response is obtained; usual range 0.2 mg to 0.4 mg/day Parenteral: Myxedematous coma—0.2 mg to 0.5 mg IV first day; 0.1 mg to 0.3 mg second day if necessary; daily injections maintained until patient can accept a daily oral dose	Synthetic monosodium salt of the naturally occurring l-isomer of thyroxine; 0.1 mg is equivalent to 65 mg of desiccated thyroid; used orally for hypothyroid replacement therapy and IV for treatment of myxedema coma or stupor demanding immediate replacement; may be given IM when oral route is not feasible; slower onset and longer duration than synthetic T_3; discontinue T_4 before switching to T_3; conversely, begin T_4 several days before stopping T_3; parenteral solution is prepared with Sodium Chloride Injection and shaken until clear, use immediately; administer IV very cautiously to patients with heart disease; inject slowly in small doses, and carefully observe patient
Liothyronine Sodium— T_3 (Cytomel)	Tablets—5 mcg, 25 mcg, 50 mcg	Adults and children over 3 years: Mild hypothyroidism—25 mcg/day initially; increase by 12.5 mcg/day to 25 mcg/day every 1 week to 2 weeks; usual maintenance is 25 mcg to 75 mcg/day in divided doses Myxedema—5 mcg/day initially; increased by 5 mcg to 10 mcg/day every 1 week to 2 weeks; usual maintenance is 50 mcg to 100 mcg/day Simple nontoxic goiter—see Myxedema	Synthetic form of the naturally occurring l-triiodothyronine (T_3); 25 mcg is equivalent to 65 mg of desiccated thyroid; possesses similar actions and uses of other thyroid hormones, but has a more rapid onset of maximal effect and shorter duration (half-life 1–2 days), allowing quicker dosage adjustments; serum TSH levels are most reliable laboratory index for monitoring T_3 replacement; also used in T_3 suppression test to differentiate borderline hyperthyroid from euthyroid

Table 40-1. Thyroid Hormones (continued)

Drug	Preparations	Usual Dosage Range	Remarks
		T_3 supression test—75 mcg to 100 mcg/day for 7 days; then repeat ^{131}I uptake test; in hyperthyroid patient, uptake is not affected; in normal patient, uptake will fall to less than 20%	(normal); useful in patients allergic to naturally extracted derivatives; be alert for possible additive effects due to residual action of longer acting thyroid drugs when T_3 is substituted for them
		Children under 3 years: Cretinism—initially 5 mcg/day; increase by 5 mcg every 3 to 4 days until desired response is achieved; infants a few months old require about 20 mcg/day; at 1 year, 50 mcg/day is required	
Liotrix (Euthroid, Thyrolar)	Tablets containing T_4 and T_3 in a fixed 4:1 ratio | T_4 (mcg)	T_3 (mcg)	Thyroid equivalent (mg)
---	---	---
12.5	3.1	15
25	6.25	30
30	7.5	30
50	12.5	60
60	15	60
100	25	120
120	30	120
150	37.5	180
180	45	180
250	62.5	300		Dosage given in thyroid equivalents Initially 15 mg to 30 mg/day; increased gradually every 1 week to 2 weeks until desired response is obtained Replacement therapy for other thyroid products is based on the equivalency: 60 mg liotrix = 65 mg desiccated thyroid or thyroglobulin = 0.1 mg T_4 = 25 mcg T_3	A constant mixture of synthetic T_4 and T_3 in a fixed 4:1 ratio by weight; although the product is claimed to more closely approximate the endogenous ratio of T_4:T_3, when differences in potency, absorption, binding, peripheral conversion of T_4 to T_3, and metabolism are considered, the fixed ratio offers *no* apparent advantage over other thyroid hormones used at optimal doses (except in those few intolerant persons); tablets have a shelf life of 2 years

with receptor sites in the thyroid cell to stimulate hormonal output.

Therapy of hyperthyroidism includes surgical removal of a part of the gland (subtotal thyroidectomy), use of radioactive iodide (^{131}I) to destroy thyroid tissue, or administration of antithyroid drugs that interfere with synthesis and release of thyroid hormones. The antithyroid drugs methimazole and propylthiouracil are reviewed in this chapter and listed in Table 40-2, and a discussion of ^{131}I is also presented.

Certain types of thyroid disorders can also be effectively treated with elemental iodine preparations, and these products are considered at the end of the chapter. A final thyroid related drug is Protirelin, a synthetic thyrotropin-releasing hormone used for diagnosis of thyroid dysfunction. This drug is reviewed in Chapter 78 along with various other diagnostic drugs.

Effective treatment of thyroid disorders depends upon accurate assessment of the thyroid state. Several laboratory parameters used to ascertain thyroid functioning are listed below, with average (normal) values given beside each test.

Table 40-2. Antithyroid Drugs

Drug	Preparations	Usual Dosage Range	Remarks
Methimazole (Tapazole)	Tablets—5 mg, 10 mg	Adults—15 mg to 60 mg initially depending on degree of hyperthyroidism in 3 daily doses at 8-hour intervals; maintenance is 5 mg to 15 mg/day Children—0.4 mg/kg initially in 3 divided doses at 8-hour intervals; maintenance is ½ initial dose	More potent than propylthiouracil, longer duration of action, and somewhat more toxic; skin rash is an indication for discontinuing drug
Propylthiouracil (Propacil, PTU)	Tablets—50 mg	Adults—100 mg initially 3 times/day every 8 hours; maintenance is 100 mg to 150 mg/day Children (over 10 yr)—50 mg to 100 mg 3 times/day every 8 hours Children (6 yr–10 yr)—50 mg to 150 mg/day in divided doses	Least toxic antithyroid drug; administer with meals to reduce GI distress; monitor prothrombin time regularly during therapy, because drug can cause hypoprothrombinemia

Commonly Used

1 *Free thyroxine index:* 1.4 ng/100 ml to 4.2 ng/100 ml
2 *Resin uptake of radioactive T$_3$ in vitro:* 27% to 37% uptake of T$_3$
3 *TSH levels:* up to 10 μU/ml

Infrequently Used

1 *Basal metabolic rate (BMR):* ±10%
2 *Protein-bound iodine (PBI):* 4 mcg/100 ml to 8 mcg/100 ml serum
3 *Radioactive iodine uptake:* 5% to 10% at 2 hours; 10% to 20% at 6 hours; 20% to 40% at 24 hours
4 *Radioimmunoassays for T$_3$ and T$_4$:*
   T$_3$—80 ng/100 ml to 180 ng/100 ml (adults)
   T$_4$—5 mcg/100 ml to 12 mcg/100 ml (adults)
5 *Thyroxine-binding globulin levels:* 10 mcg/100 ml to 26 mcg/100 ml
6 *Free T$_3$ index:* 20 ng/100 ml to 60 ng/100 ml

Because of the possibility of false increases or decreases in the readings of any one of these tests as a result of other medications taken by the patient (*e.g.,* barbiturates, corticosteroids, diazepam, heparin, hormones, lithium, nitroprusside, oral contraceptives, phenytoin, propranolol, pyrazolones, thiazide diuretics), or the presence of certain disease states (*e.g.,* hepatitis, nephrosis), *several* tests should be performed before a diagnosis is made, and the results should be used only in combination with a thorough clinical assessment of the patient.

Thyroid Hormones

▶ **levothyroxine**

▶ **liothyronine**

▶ **liotrix**

▶ **thyroglobulin**

▶ **thyroid, dessicated**

Mechanism

Incompletely understood, but multiple sites and mechanisms are probably involved; probably bind to receptors on cellular surfaces, increasing uptake of glucose and amino acids; may also diffuse into cells, and interact with receptors on mitochondria and chromatin material; increased mRNA synthesis can occur, resulting in accelerated protein synthesis; cellular utilization of oxygen is increased, and sodium–potassium transport is facilitated.

Clinical effects include increases in heart rate, cardiac output, body temperature, respiration, carbohydrate, fat and protein metabolism, and enzymatic activity; growth and maturation of tissues is also stimulated; T$_3$ is approximately 4 times more potent than T$_4$ and the ratio of T$_4$/T$_3$ released by the gland is about 20:1 (see Fate below).

Uses

1 Replacement or substitution therapy of primary hypothyroidism (*e.g.,* cretinism, myxedema, nontoxic goiter, hypothyroid state of childhood, pregnancy, or old age) or secondary hypothyroidism (*e.g.,* surgery, radiation, drug-induced)
2 Adjuncts to thyroid-inhibiting agents when they are used to reduce release of thyrotropic hormones in treatment of thyrotoxicosis (Thyroid drugs prevent development of goiter and hypothyroidism.)
3 Differentiation of hyperthyroidism from euthyroidism (T$_3$ only—T$_3$ suppression test)

Dosage

See Table 40-1.

Fate

Oral absorption is variable, T$_3$ being absorbed to a greater extent (95% within 4 hr) than T$_4$ (50%–75%). Onset of action is within 6 hours to 8 hours for T$_3$, but much slower with T$_4$ (2 to 3 days). Peak effects may require up to 8 to 10 days to develop, however. Plasma half-lives are 1 to 2 days for T$_3$ and 6 to 7 days for T$_4$. Both hormones are highly bound (99%–100%) to plasma proteins (thyroxine-binding globulin, thyroxine-binding prealbumin, and albumin). Approximately 35% of T$_4$ is deiodinated in the periphery to T$_3$. Drugs are metabolized by the liver and excreted in the urine (70%–80%) or bile (20%–30%) both as free drug and conjugated metabolites.

Common Side-Effects

(If dosage is excessive) Palpitations, nervousness, and tachycardia

Significant Adverse Reactions

(Usually result of overdosage or too-rapid increase in dosage) Headache, diarrhea, sweating, arrhythmias, anginal pain, tremors, insomnia, menstrual irregularities, heat intolerance, allergic skin reactions, congestive heart failure, and shock

Contraindications

Thyrotoxicosis, nephrosis, hypogonadism, hyperthyroidism, hypoadrenalism, and cardiovascular diseases uncomplicated by hypothyroidism

Interactions

1 Thyroid hormones enhance the cardiovascular effects of catecholamines, possibly resulting in angina or arrhythmias.
2 Effects of thyroid hormones may be increased by phenytoin and tricyclic antidepressants.

3 Thyroid hormones can potentiate the pharmacologic effects of anticoagulants, digitalis glycosides, ketamine, and indomethacin.

4 Cholestyramine (decreased absorption) and estrogens (increased protein binding) may impair the action of thyroid hormones.

5 Thyroid hormones may increase blood sugar levels, thus increasing requirements for insulin and oral hypoglycemic drugs.

▶ NURSING ALERTS

▷ 1 Use very cautiously in patients with cardiovascular diseases, including hypertension. Begin therapy with small doses, and advise physician at onset of chest pain, dyspnea, or other signs of possible cardiovascular complications.

▷ 2 In patients with severe or prolonged hypothyroidism, use supplemental adrenocortical steroids with thyroid hormone replacement to prevent development of adrenocortical insufficiency.

▷ 3 Do not use thyroid preparations for treatment of obesity, depression, or reproductive disorders, because they are ineffective and potentially dangerous.

▷ 4 Perform regular testing of urine of diabetics during thyroid hormone therapy, because drugs may increase dosage requirements of antidiabetic drugs.

▷ 5 Be alert for development of signs of thyroid hormone overdosage, such as irritability, nervousness, sweating, tachycardia, increased bowel motility, menstrual irregularities. Drug should be stopped for several days, then reinstituted at a lower dosage.

▶ NURSING CONSIDERATIONS

▷ 1 Begin therapy at small doses in hypothyroid individuals, because they are extremely sensitive to thyroid hormones, and make dosage changes gradually. Earliest clinical responses in adult hypothyroid patients are usually diuresis, increased appetite, and increased pulse rate.

▷ 2 Be aware that the action of oral anticoagulants can be enhanced by thyroid hormones, necessitating a dosage reduction.

▷ 3 Instruct parents of juveniles taking thyroid hormones to monitor growth regularly. Too-rapid increases in height can result in premature closure of epiphyses and resultant skeletal deformities.

▷ 4 Stress the importance of taking the drug regularly even though patient may feel well. Thyroid hormone replacement therapy is generally a life-long requirement.

▷ 5 Recognize that maintenance dosage may be higher in an actively growing child than in an adult. The sleeping pulse and basal morning temperature are important guides to treatment.

▷ 6 Monitor pulse rate and rhythm during periods of dosage adjustment, and notify physician if rate exceeds 100 or if there is a marked change in rate or rhythm, because drug may need to be withheld.

▷ 7 Note that effects, both pharmacologic and toxicologic, may persist for 10 days to 14 days after withdrawal of T_3, and for 4 weeks to 6 weeks after withdrawal of T_4.

▷ 8 Warn juvenile hypothyroid patients and their parents that initial response to thyroid hormone therapy may be dramatic (excessive hair loss, rapid growth, assertiveness). These reactions tend to lessen with continued therapy.

▷ 9 Note that drugs are administered once a day, and should preferably be given in the morning to minimize the possibility of sleep disturbances.

Antithyroid Drugs (Thioamides)

▶ methimazole

▶ propylthiouracil

The antithyroid drugs impair the synthesis of the thyroid hormones T_3 and T_4 in the thyroid gland, and are used in the treatment of hyperthyroid states. Unlike other means of hyperthyroid therapy, such as subtotal thyroidectomy, or ^{131}I, antithyroid drugs do not tend to damage thyroid tissue beyond repair and thus are usually the initial treatment of choice. Long-term therapy may produce remission of the disease in some cases, but relapse is not uncommon. Patients who fail to respond fully to drug therapy or who show evidence of relapse should be considered as candidates for either surgery or radioisotope therapy.

Because the antithyroid drugs do not interfere with the release or activity of previously formed thyroid hormones, their clinical effects are delayed for several weeks, until body stores of preformed T_4 and T_3 are exhausted. Likewise, the action of exogenously administered thyroid hormones is unimpaired by antithyroid drugs.

Several kinds of compounds are capable of exerting an antithyroid effect. Large amounts of the iodide ion (6 mg–10 mg/day) can suppress release of thyroid hormones from the gland, and are thus occasionally used for treating some forms of hyperthyroidism and for reducing the size and vascularity of the gland before thyroidectomy. Certain monovalent inorganic anions (*e.g.,* perchlorate, thiocyanate, periodate) block uptake of iodide by the gland and can exert an antithyroid action. They are rarely used clinically, however, because of the availability of more effective and less toxic drugs. The principal antithyroid agents are the thioamide derivatives methimazole and propylthiouracil and they are discussed below, then summarized in Table 40-2.

Mechanism

Inhibit the biosynthesis of thyroid hormones possibly by inhibiting the enzyme system that catalyzes the conversion of iodine to iodide and by reducing the concentration of free iodine available for reaction with tyrosine; may also block oxidative coupling of mono- and diiodotyrosine to form T_3 and T_4 (see Chap. 38) and can partially inhibit conversion of T_4 to T_3 in the periphery; do not inactivate existing T_3 and T_4, nor interfere with the action of exogenous thyroid hormones

Drug-induced depression of circulating hormone levels results in compensatory increase in TSH release from adenohypophysis. Excess TSH increases size and vascularity of thyroid gland (goitrogenic action).

Uses

1 Treatment of hyperthyroidism (most effective in milder cases in which thyroid gland is not excessively enlarged)
2 Preparation for subtotal thyroidectomy (to reduce hyperthyroidism and to lessen surgical risks)

Dosage

See Table 40-2.

Fate

Well absorbed orally and oral bioavailability is high; concentrated in the thyroid gland; effects are noted within 30 minutes–60 minutes, and persist for 2 hours to 4 hours. Plasma half-lives are relatively short (2 hr–3 hr), but do *not* reflect duration of antithyroid effect, which is due to action within the thyroid gland. Propylthiouracil is excreted more quickly than methimazole, and thus requires more frequent dosing.

Common Side-Effects

Skin rash, itching, nausea, and epigastric distress

Significant Adverse Reactions

Paresthesias, arthralgia, myalgia, loss of taste, loss of hair, dizziness, drowsiness, neuritis, edema, skin pigmentation, lymphadenopathy, sialadenopathy, and jaundice

Less commonly: agranulocytosis, granulopenia, thrombocytopenia, drug fever, lupus-like reaction, hepatitis, periarteritis, hypoprothrombinemia, and bleeding

Goitrogenic action is indicated by enlarged thyroid, periorbital edema, fatigue, paresthesias, muscle cramps, cool skin, sensitivity to cold, and bradycardia.

Contraindications

Nursing mothers

Interactions

1 Antithyroid drugs can magnify the effects of oral anticoagulants by causing hypoprothrombinemia.
2 Use cautiously in the presence of other drugs known to cause agranulocytosis, *e.g.*, antidepressants, carbamazepine, clofibrate, indomethacin, methyldopa, meprobamate, phenothiazines, phenylbutazone, procainamide, quinidine, tetracyclines, and tolbutamide.

▶ NURSING ALERTS

▷ 1 Warn patient to report development of sore throat, rash, fever, headache, or malaise immediately, because these may be early indication of developing blood dyscrasia. Discontinue drug and perform hematologic studies.

▷ 2 Monitor prothrombin time regularly during therapy and advise patient to report appearance of petechiae, ecchymoses, or any other unexplained bleeding, because drugs can cause hypoprothrombinemia.

▷ 3 Note that these drugs readily cross the placental barrier and may produce goiter and cretinism in the developing fetus. Use smallest effective dose during pregnancy and discontinue drug if possible 2 weeks to 3 weeks before delivery. Thyroid hormones are often given concurrently with antithyroid drugs during pregnancy to prevent hypothyroidism in mother and fetus. Advise mothers not to nurse infants if taking antithyroid drugs.

▶ NURSING CONSIDERATIONS

▷ 1 Note that when the euthyroid state is attained, thyroid hormones may be added to the regimen to prevent goiter.

▷ 2 In patients receiving antithyroid drugs, administer iodine (*e.g.*, Lugol's solution, Potassium Iodide Solution) for 7 days to 10 days before thyroidectomy to reduce the size and vascularity of the gland.

▷ 3 Be alert for symptoms of excessive dosage (*e.g.*, depression, nonpitting edema, or cold intolerance), and advise physician.

▷ 4 Caution patients against use of over-the-counter preparations that contain iodide (*e.g.*, cough syrups, asthma preparations) because they may interfere with effectiveness of antithyroid drugs.

▷ 5 Stress the importance of rigid adherence to the prescribed dosage regimen. Teach patients how to monitor pulse rate and advise them to report increased pulse rate, anxiety, weight loss, or tremor, possible indications of inadequate clinical response.

▷ 6 Be aware that therapy usually lasts 1 year to 2 years, whereupon remission is attained in about 50% of patients. Instruct patients in remission to continue monitoring pulse rate and weight and to report any significant changes.

Radioactive Iodide

▶ radioactive sodium iodide—^{131}I

Iodotope

Of the several radioactive isotopes of iodine, ^{131}I is the most widely used clinically. Although its major indication is the treatment of certain types of hyperthyroidism, it has also been successfully employed for therapy of thyroid carcinoma and as a diagnostic tool for measuring thyroid function.

Mechanism

Rapidly and efficiently taken up by the thyroid gland, incorporated into T_3 and T_4 and stored in the follicle of the gland; emits both beta radiation, which penetrates only 1 mm to 2 mm and thus remains localized in the thyroid gland, and small amounts of longer wave length gamma radiation, which can be detected and measured externally; large quantities of released beta radiation destroy thyroid tissue.

Uses

1 Treatment of hyperthyroidism, especially in patients over 30 years of age who do not respond to other antithyroid medications
2 Treatment of thyroid carcinoma and metastases (effectiveness is questionable in all cases because some thyroid neoplasms, *e.g.,* giant cell, spindle cell, and amyloid solid carcinomas, do *not* concentrate sufficient iodide ion)
3 Diagnosis of thyroid disorders, based on uptake of isotope by gland (infrequently used)

Dosage

Dose is measured in millicuries (mCi) and varies depending on indication, size of the thyroid, uptake of a small initial tracer dose, and rate of release of radioactive iodine from the gland.

Average doses are as follows:

Hyperthyroidism: 4 mCi to 10 mCi as a single dose or two divided doses 6 weeks to 8 weeks apart

Thyroid carcinoma: 50 mCi to 150 mCi

Usually administered orally in a glass of water (colorless and tasteless) or as capsules

Treatment may be repeated every 3 months to 4 months until euthyroid state is attained.

Fate

Rapidly absorbed when taken orally, and quickly and efficiently concentrated by the thyroid gland as well as by the stomach and salivary glands; radioactivity can be detected in the thyroid within minutes. Half-life of ^{131}I isotope is 8 days. Thyroid function begins to decrease within 2 weeks; maximum effects are observed in 8 weeks to 12 weeks; excreted mainly by the kidneys

Common Side-Effects

Hypothyroidism (see Nursing Alerts, No. 2), soreness over the thyroid area, nausea, dysphagia, cough, and thinning of the hair

Significant Adverse Reactions

Glandular swelling, thyroiditis, sialadenitis, gastritis, bone marrow depression, blood dyscrasias, acute leukemia, alopecia, petechiae, and angioedema

Contraindications

Pregnant and nursing women, very young children, preexisting vomiting and diarrhea, and persons with recent myocardial infarction

Interaction

1 Uptake of ^{131}I by thyroid gland can be impaired by recent intake of iodine in any form (*e.g.,* x-ray contrast media; see Chap. 78).

▶ **NURSING ALERTS**

▷ 1 Observe proper procedures for handling and administering radioactive materials.
▷ 2 Provide necessary thyroid hormone replacement therapy following radioactive iodide to minimize the incidence and severity of hypothyroidism. Recognize that hypothyroidism is often insidious in development but probably occurs in *almost everyone* receiving this treatment but may take years to become manifest. Stress the need for continual replacement therapy for as long as necessary should hypothyroidism develop.
▷ 3 Use with caution in women of childbearing age. If use is necessary, administer drug during first few days of menses.

▶ **NURSING CONSIDERATIONS**

▷ 1 Perform periodic thyroid function studies on patients receiving radioactive iodide to detect possible development of hypothyroidism.
▷ 2 Note that solution may darken upon standing but this does not affect potency.
▷ 3 Be aware that adequate control of hyperthyroidism may require several treatments with radioactive iodide over many months. If therapy is inadequate, it is apparent usually within 2 months to 3 months, that is, patient remains hyperthyroid.
▷ 4 Discontinue antithyroid drug therapy for 3 days to 4 days before administration of radioiodide.
▷ 5 Reassure patients that when usual doses are used, no special precautions are necessary and that the radioactivity hazard is minimal.

Iodine/Iodide Compounds

▶ **potassium iodide**

▶ **saturated solution potassium iodide**

▶ **sodium iodide**

▶ **strong iodine solution**

At one time, iodine and iodide were the only available treatment for hyperthyroidism. In spite of the rapid beneficial action, effects were short-lived, and within a few weeks symptoms usually returned and in many instances were intensified. Largely for this reason, these drugs have only a limited therapeutic application today, and are primarily used to suppress hyperthyroidism and reduce the size and vascularity of the thyroid gland *before thyroidectomy.* The available compounds include strong iodine solution (5%

iodine and 10% potassium iodide), sodium iodide injection, saturated solution of potassium iodide (SSKI) and tablets containing potassium iodide and niacinamide (Iodo-Niacin). The pharmacology of these agents is discussed in general terms and individual drugs are then listed in Table 40-3. In addition, certain iodide-containing products useful as expectorants are detailed in Chapter 54.

Mechanism

Not completely established; may suppress release of thyroid hormones from thyroglobulin, and interfere with synthesis of thyroid hormones; improvement in symptoms is rapid, hence they are of value in treating thyroid storm; reduce size and vascularity of the thyroid gland and increase quantity of bound iodine within the gland

Uses

1 Preparation for thyroidectomy, by decreasing size, vascularity, and friability of the thyroid gland
2 Temporary suppression of hyperthyroid states
3 Treatment of thyroid storm (IV Sodium Iodide)

Dosage

See Table 40-3.

Fate

Well absorbed when taken orally; effects usually noted within 24 hours to 48 hours and maximal effect occurs within 10 days to 14 days; cleared from plasma by either renal excretion or thyroid uptake; eliminated in either urine or feces by way of the bile

Common Side-Effects

Unpleasant metallic taste, GI distress

Significant Adverse Reactions

Gum soreness, mucosal ulceration, salivary gland enlargement, excessive salivation, rhinitis, fever, joint pain, dyspnea, edema, skin rash, vomiting, headache, and goiter

IV administration can result in acute iodide poisoning, characterized by edema (bronchial, laryngeal); mucosal hemorrhaging; serum sickness; acneiform, maculopapular, vesicular or bullous eruptions; and generalized inflammation.

Contraindications

Potassium iodide is contraindicated in hyperkalemia; sodium iodide is contraindicated in pulmonary tuberculosis.

Interactions

1 Lithium may enhance the hypothyroid action of potassium iodide.
2 Estrogens and progestins can increase protein-bound iodine.

▶ **NURSING ALERTS**

▷ 1 Be alert for development or exacerbation of hyperthyroidism if radioactive iodide is given following iodine solution, because release of large amounts of

---

Table 40-3. Iodine/Iodide Compounds

Drug	Preparations	Usual Dosage Range	Remarks
Potassium iodide (various brands)	Liquid—325 mg 500 mg/ 15 ml Tablets—650 mg Enteric-coated tablets— 300 mg	Adults—300 mg to 650 mg every 4 hours to 6 hours Children—250 mg to 1000 mg daily in divided doses	Useful for hyperthyroidism, thyrotoxic crisis (with antithyroid drugs), preoperatively for thyroidectomy, and to facilitate bronchial drainage and cough in chronic pulmonary diseases; discontinue if skin rash appears; see also Chapter 54
Saturated solution potassium iodide (SSKI)	Solution—1 g/ml	0.3 ml to 0.6 ml 4 to 12 times/day diluted in water, juice, or milk	Used presurgically for reducing size and fragility of thyroid gland; do not allow to stand uncovered for prolonged periods of time because solution may evaporate; slight discoloration of solution does not affect potency
Sodium iodide (various manufacturers)	Injection—10%, 20%	Thyroid crisis—2 g/day by IV infusion	Primarily used for acute treatment of thyroid crisis; be alert for development of acute iodism (e.g., metallic taste, stomatitis, sneezing, vomiting, swollen salivary glands), and pulmonary edema
Strong iodine solution (Lugol's solution)	Solution—5% iodine and 10% potassium iodide	0.1 ml to 0.3 ml (approximately 2 to 6 drops) 3 times/day (usually for 10 days–14 days before thyroidectomy)	Principally used to prepare thyroid gland for surgery; also used with an antithyroid drug for treating thyrotoxic crisis; discontinue if signs of iodism appear (see above); administer solution diluted in juice, milk, or water, preferably after meals

stored hormone can occur if gland is destroyed by radiation.

▷ 2 Administer cautiously during pregnancy, because compounds can induce goiter in the newborn.

▶ **NURSING CONSIDERATIONS**

▷ 1 Continually observe patients receiving these drugs for development of goiter. Withdrawal of iodide or administration of thyroid hormones will correct the condition, although the mechanism is incompletely understood.

▷ 2 Be aware that a patient recently treated with iodine/iodides cannot be given radioactive iodide, because the gland will be saturated and cannot take up the radioiodide.

▷ 3 Caution patients against indiscriminate use of over-the-counter drugs containing iodides (*e.g.,* cough preparations, asthma medications, salt substitutes) because these may increase the response to iodide therapy.

▷ 4 Urge strict adherence to prescribed dosage regimen when drugs are used before thyroidectomy to avoid possibility of loss of iodide effectiveness and gland enlargement.

▷ *Dietary precaution*

▷ 1 Check with physician concerning the need for restricting iodine-rich foods (*e.g.,* seafoods, vegetables) or iodized salt.

Summary. Thyroid Hormones and Antithyroid Drugs

Drug	Preparations	Usual Dosage Range
Thyroid hormones T$_3$ and T$_4$	See Table 40-1.	
Antithyroid drugs Methimazole Propylthiouracil	See Table 40-2.	
Radioactive iodide ^{131}I (Iodotope)	Solution or capsules containing a known amount of ^{131}I in mCi suitable for oral or IV administration	Highly variable Average doses: Hyperthyroidism—4 mCi to 10 mCi 6 weeks to 8 weeks apart Carcinoma—50 mCi to 150 mCi
Iodine/Iodide Products	See Table 40-3.	

---

41 Parathyroid Drugs, Calcitonin, and Calcium

Calcium, the most abundant cation in the body, plays an important role in many vital physiologic processes, such as bone formation, blood coagulation, muscle contraction, nerve conduction, hormone secretion, and enzyme activity. The level of free calcium and phosphate in the blood is dependent on a complex series of interactions among several substances, most important of which are parathyroid hormone (PTH) and vitamin D. PTH is a polypeptide synthesized by the parathyroid glands and is secreted in response to reductions in serum calcium. PTH elevates plasma calcium levels by increasing resorption of calcium ions from bone, by promoting renal tubular reabsorption of calcium, and by enhancing calcium absorption from the GI tract (see Chap. 38). *Vitamin D* is the term commonly applied to two biologically similar substances, ergocalciferol (D_2) and cholecalciferol (D_3). Its major actions on calcium metabolism are essentially identical to those of PTH, namely, increased resorption from bone and enhanced GI absorption. A third endogenous substance, *calcitonin,* can also influence calcium and phosphate metabolism. Calcitonin is a polypeptide secreted by the parafollicular (C) cells of the *thyroid* gland in response to a rise in serum calcium levels. It lowers serum calcium by inhibiting bone resorption, and promotes renal excretion of calcium, probably by interfering with renal tubular reabsorption of the ion.

Serum levels of calcium are normally maintained within a narrow range (10 ± 1 mg/100 ml), and deviation from this level results in the appearance of symptoms of either *hyper*calcemia or *hypo*calcemia. *Hyper*calcemia may result from hyperparathyroidism, excessive vitamin D intake, malignant tumors, or hyperthyroidism, and is characterized by vomiting, constipation, muscle weakness, electrocardiographic abnormalities, and deposition of calcium in soft tissues such as the kidney. Significant elevations in serum calcium can lead to progressive loss of sensation and eventually coma. Principal causes of *hypo*calcemia are hypoparathyroidism, inadequate vitamin D levels, and dietary calcium deficiency. Symptoms include muscle twitching, tetanic spasms, and convulsions.

Drugs discussed in this chapter are used to regulate body calcium stores, provide replacement for inadequate calcium, and to treat Paget's disease, a decalcification of bone leading to skeletal deformities, joint impairment, and development of vascular fibrous tissue in marrow spaces. Although once used clinically, bovine extracts of parathyroid hormone are no longer available, because tolerance usually developed quickly, and allergic reactions were noted in a number of patients. Synthetic calcitonin and a nonhormonal substance, etidronate, two drugs used in moderate to severe forms of Paget's disease, are reviewed individually below. Mention is also made of mithramycin, an antibiotic used to treat hypercalcemia and hypercalciuria in patients not responsive to conventional treatment. Mithramycin is also used to treat testicular tumors, and that aspect of its pharmacology is reviewed in Chapter 74. Oral calcium salts, employed as dietary supplements for calcium deficiency states, are also considered in this chapter. Preparations with vitamin D-like activity (calcifediol, calcitriol, dihydrotachysterol) can be used to control hypocalcemic states resulting from a number of conditions, and these agents are discussed with the other fat-soluble vitamins in Chapter 76.

▶ calcitonin, salmon
Calcimar

Salmon calcitonin is a synthetic preparation of the hormone secreted by the C cells of the thyroid gland. The amino acid sequence of salmon calcitonin results in a more potent and more stable (longer duration) preparation than that of human calcitonin.

Mechanism
Decreases serum calcium levels by directly inhibiting osteoclastic bone resorption (effects become less intense with prolonged administration—possibly due to development of neutralizing antibodies); increases renal excretion of calcium and phosphorus by blocking their tubular reabsorption; transiently but markedly reduces output of gastric and pancreatic secretions, such as hydrochloric acid, gastrin, trypsin, and amylase

Uses
1 Treatment of moderate to severe Paget's disease (osteitis deformans), characterized by polyostotic involvement, and elevated serum alkaline phosphatase and urinary hydroxyproline excretion
2 Treatment of hypercalcemia, especially hypercalcemic emergencies

Dosage
Expressed in Medical Research Council (MRC) units. One MRC unit is equivalent to approximately 4 μg of pure porcine calcitonin.
Paget's disease: initially 100 MRC U/day SC (preferred) or IM; maintenance 50 MRC U-100 MRC U daily or on alternate days
Hypercalcemia: initially 4 MRC U/kg/12 hours SC or IM; may increase to 8 MRC U/kg/12 hours after 1 day to 2 days, then to a maximum of 8 MRC U/kg/6 hours if response is still unsatisfactory

Fate
Onset of action is usually within 30 minutes to 60 minutes; peak effect occurs in 4 hours to 6 hours, and duration is 12 hours to 24 hours; salmon calcitonin is rapidly metabolized by the kidney to smaller, inactive fragments and excreted in the urine.

Common Side-Effects
Nausea, vomiting, local inflammatory reaction at injection site, facial flushing, paresthesias

Significant Adverse Reactions
Diuresis, urticaria, skin rash, diarrhea, hypocalcemic tetany; antibodies may form to calcitonin upon repeated usage, reducing its efficacy.

Contraindications
Young children, pregnancy, and nursing mothers

Interactions
1 Calcitonin may antagonize the hypercalcemic action of PTH, dihydrotachysterol, and vitamin D.
2 The effects of calcitonin can be augmented by androgens.

▶ NURSING ALERTS
▷ 1 In patients with suspected sensitivity to calcitonin, perform a skin test before administration. Presence of more than mild erythema or slight wheal formation within 15 minutes of intracutaneous injection is a positive sign of hypersensitivity.
▷ 2 Ensure that proper provisions (*e.g.,* epinephrine, antihistamines, oxygen) are available to treat allergic reactions should they develop.
▷ 3 Have parenteral calcium available to treat possible hypocalcemic tetany that may develop, especially during the initial stages of therapy.
▷ 4 Use with caution in osteoporosis, renal impairment, and pernicious anemia.

▶ NURSING CONSIDERATIONS
▷ 1 Assess drug effect by periodic measurement of serum alkaline phosphatase and 24-hour urinary hydroxyproline levels as well as observation for symptoms. Biochemical abnormalities and bone pain should decrease during first few months of therapy.
▷ 2 Test for antibody titer in patients who evidence relapse after an initial good response. Following overnight fast, serum calcium is measured and 100 MRC U calcitonin are then given IM. Blood samples are withdrawn at 3 hours and 6 hours after injection. A decrease in serum calcium of 0.3 mg/100 ml or less suggests antibody presence, and drug should be withdrawn.
▷ 3 Stress the importance of continued therapy even though clinical symptoms have abated.
▷ 4 Note that increases in dosage beyond 100 MRC U/day do not result in a greater clinical response.
▷ 5 Instruct patient in the proper technique for handling and injecting drug at home.
▷ 6 Reassure patients that should nausea and vomiting occur during the initial stages of therapy, these symptoms will disappear as treatment continues.

▶ etidronate
Didronel

A nonhormonal substance, etidronate acts primarily to reduce the rate of bone turnover. It is principally used for symptomatic treatment of Paget's disease.

Mechanism
Absorbs onto calcium hydroxyapatite crystals, disrupting both crystal growth and resorption, depending on concentration of drug; decreases urinary hydroxyproline excretion

and serum alkaline phosphatase; also reported to reduce vascularity of Pagetic bone, and decrease elevated cardiac output associated with active Paget's disease.

Uses

1 Treatment of moderate to severe Paget's disease (osteitis deformans); symptomatic improvement occurs in approximately three out of five patients.
2 Reduction of heterotopic bone ossification due to spinal cord injury or that complicating total hip replacement

Dosage

Paget's disease: initially 5 mg/kg/day for up to 6 months (maximum dose 20 mg/kg/day); retreatment may be initiated after at least a 3-month drug-free period if reactivation of the disease has occurred.

Heterotopic ossification due to spinal cord injury: 20 mg/kg/day for 2 weeks, followed by 10 mg/kg/day for 10 weeks

Heterotopic ossification complicating total hip replacement: 20 mg/kg/day for 1 month preoperatively; then 20 mg/kg/day for 3 months postoperatively.

Fate

Very poorly absorbed if taken orally (1% at 5 mg/kg); cleared from the blood within 6 hours; one half of absorbed dose is excreted in the urine within 24 hours, the remainder being adsorbed onto bone and very slowly eliminated. Unabsorbed drug is eliminated in the feces. Clinical response is evident only after 1 month–3 months of treatment.

Common Side-Effects

Loose stools, nausea

Significant Adverse Reactions

Increased bone pain at previously asymptomatic sites, demineralization of bone leading to fractures

▶ NURSING ALERTS

▷ 1 Adhere to the recommended dose regimen to avoid overdosage. Incidence of untoward reactions (*e.g.,* GI distress, bone pain, fractures) rises dramatically at elevated doses.

▷ 2 If fracture occurs, discontinue drug and do not resume until fracture is completely healed.

▷ 3 Use with caution in patients with renal impairment, enterocolitis, multiple long bone fractures, in pregnant or nursing women, and in children.

▷ 4 Recognize that response to therapy is gradual and continues for months after drug is stopped. Dosage increases should be made cautiously, treatment should not be resumed until clear evidence of disease recurrence is present, and therapy should never be reinstituted before at least a 3-month drug-free period.

▶ NURSING CONSIDERATIONS

▷ 1 Ensure that patients maintain an adequate intake of calcium and vitamin D during treatment, through either dietary sources, calcium supplementation, or both.

▷ 2 Administer drug on an empty stomach, 2 hours before meals, unless GI distress is extreme, because food impairs absorption.

▷ 3 Monitor urinary hydroxyproline and serum alkaline phosphatase levels periodically during therapy. Usually, the first evidence of clinical benefit is reduced urinary hydroxyproline excretion. Serum alkaline phosphatase is also lowered by 30% in most patients.

▷ 4 Note that no evidence exists to support the prophylactic use of etidronate in asymptomatic patients. Most patients with mild symptoms can be effectively treated with analgesics.

▶ mithramycin
Mithracin

Mithramycin (also known as plicamycin) is an antibiotic produced by *Streptomyces plicatus.* It is employed by IV infusion to treat hypercalcemia and hypercalciuria in patients not responsive to conventional therapy, such as those with advanced neoplasms. Due to its potential to elicit serious toxicity (thromocytopenia, hemorrhage, liver or kidney dysfunction), however, the potential benefit from the drug must be carefully weighed against the risk. Mithramycin is contraindicated in patients with thrombocytopenia, coagulation disorders, increased susceptibility to bleeding, and bone marrow depression. Platelet counts, prothrombin time, and bleeding time must be determined frequently during therapy and for several days following the last dose. Epistaxis or hematemesis may be early indications of a developing hemorrhagic syndrome and should be reported immediately. GI symptoms (nausea, diarrhea, anorexia, stomatitis) represent the most frequent side-effects. The recommended dose is 25 mcg/kg/day by IV infusion over 4 hours to 6 hours for 3 or 4 days. If the desired degree of reversal of hypercalcemia is not attained, the dosage may be repeated at intervals of one week or more. Normal calcium balance can often be maintained with single weekly doses or 2 to 3 doses/week. Rapid IV injections should be avoided, because the incidence of GI disturbances is much greater with this method. Extravasation of the solution should be avoided, because local irritation, cellulitis, and possibly thrombophlebitis can occur. Moderate heat applied to the site of extravasation may help disperse the compound and minimize discomfort.

Mithramycin is also employed in the treatment of testicular neoplasms, and that application is considered in detail in Chapter 74.

Oral Calcium Salts

▶ calcium carbonate

▶ calcium glubionate

▶ **calcium gluconate**

▶ **calcium lactate**

▶ **dibasic calcium phosphate**

Adequate intake of calcium is essential for normal homeostasis, and is particularly critical during periods of active bone growth; for example, during childhood, adolescence, pregnancy, or lactation. In addition, sufficient calcium intake is necessary for the prevention and treatment of disease-induced calcium deficiency states such as hypoparathyroidism, postmenopausal osteoporosis, and tetany of the newborn. The use of oral calcium supplements, particularly as they apply to the adjunctive treatment of calcium deficiency states resulting from hypoparathyroidism, is discussed here. Parenteral therapy with calcium, on the other hand, is indicated for treatment of hypocalcemic states requiring a *prompt* elevation in plasma calcium, for example, neonatal tetany, severe vitamin D deficiency, and systemic alkalosis. Parenteral calcium therapy is reviewed along with other parenteral electrolytes in Chapter 77. The pharmacology of the oral calcium preparations is detailed for the group, then individual drugs are listed in Table 41-1.

Mechanism
Replace deficient calcium stores in the body; presence of sufficient calcium is essential for bone development, blood coagulation, muscle contraction, cardiac functioning, and many other physiologic processes.

Use
1 Prevention or treatment of calcium deficiency states, such as those associated with hypoparathyroidism, osteoporosis, rickets, and osteomalacia

Dosage
See Table 41-1.

Fate
Absorption is good when taken orally in the presence of adequate levels of vitamin D and PTH. Metabolism of calcium is likewise controlled by vitamin D and PTH. It is excreted largely in urine.

Common Side-Effects
Occasional GI distress

Significant Adverse Reactions
Hypercalcemia (nausea, vomiting, abdominal pain, constipation, polyuria, fatigue, muscle weakness, bradycardia, arrhythmias, confusion), and hypercalciuria

Contraindications
Renal calculi, hypercalcemia

Interactions
1 GI absorption of calcium can be enhanced by vitamin D and impaired by corticosteroids, phosphorus (*e.g.,* milk, dairy products), oxalic acid (*e.g.,* spinach, rhubarb), and phytic acid (*e.g.,* bran cereals).
2 Calcium may reduce the muscle-relaxing effects of neuromuscular-blocking agents.
3 Elevated serum calcium levels may increase digitalis toxicity.

Table 41-1. Oral Calcium Salts

Drug	Preparations	Usual Dosage Range	Remarks
Calcium carbonate (BioCal, Caltrate 600, Os-Cal 500)	Tablets—600 mg, 650 mg, 1.25 g	1 g to 1.5 g 3 times/day (maximum 8 g/day)	Contains 40% calcium; very potent antacid (see Chap. 48); high incidence of constipation; tablet should be chewed before swallowing or dissolved in mouth and followed by water
Calcium glubionate (Neo-Calglucon)	Syrup—1.8 g/5 ml	Adults—15 ml 3 times/day Pregnancy—15 ml 4 times/day Children—10 ml 3 times/day Infants—5 ml 5 times/day	Contains 6% calcium; GI disturbances are rare; administer before meals to enhance absorption
Calcium gluconate	Tablets—500 mg, 650 mg, 1 g Injection—10%	1 g to 2 g orally 3 to 4 times/day Children—500 mg/kg/day in divided doses	Contains 9% calcium; can be given IV (see Chap. 77); GI irritation is minimal, but may be constipating
Calcium lactate	Tablets—325 mg, 650 mg	325 mg to 1.3 g 3 times/day	Contains 13% calcium; similar to calcium gluconate; tablets may be dissolved in hot water, then cool water added to taste; absorption may be enhanced by lactose; administer with meals
Dibasic calcium phosphate dihydrate (Dicalcium phosphate)	Tablets—500 mg	500 mg to 1500 mg 2 to 3 times/day	Contains 23% calcium; Administer with meals

4   Calcium can inhibit the GI absorption of tetracyclines. Do not give within 1 hour of each other.

▶ **NURSING ALERT**

▷ 1   Administer cautiously to patients receiving digitalis glycosides and to persons with renal insufficiency or a history of renal stones.

▶ **NURSING CONSIDERATIONS**

▷ 1   Give oral calcium ½ hour before meals or 1 hour to 1½ hours after meals to increase utilization.

▷ 2   Make frequent determinations of plasma and urinary calcium levels during prolonged therapy to avoid hypercalcemia and hypercalciuria.

Summary. Parathyroid Drugs, Calcitonin and Calcium

Drug	Preparations	Usual Dosage Range
Parathyroid hormone (PTH)	Injection—100 U/ml	Hypoparathyroidism—20 U to 40 U IM, SC, or IV every 12 hours
		Diagnosis—200 U IV
Calcitonin-salmon (Calcimar)	Injection—200 MRC U/ml	Initially 100 MRC U/day SC (preferred) or IM
		Maintenance—50 MRC U to 100 MRC U daily or on alternate days
Etidronate (Didronel)	Tablets—200 mg	Paget's disease—initially 5 mg/kg/day for up to 6 months; retreatment after a 3-month drug-free period if symptoms return
		Heterotopic ossification (spinal injury)—20 mg/kg/day for 2 weeks then 10 mg/kg/day for 10 weeks
		Heterotopic ossification (hip replacement)—20 mg/kg/day for 1 month before and 3 months following surgery
Mithramycin (Mithracin)	Injection—2.5 mg/vial	Hypercalcemia—0.025 mg/kg/day for 3 days to 4 days; repeat at 1-week intervals as necessary
		Testicular carcinoma—0.025 mg to 0.03 mg/kg/day for 8 days to 10 days *or* 0.025 mg to 0.05 mg/kg/day on alternate days for 3 to 8 doses
Oral calcium salts	See Table 41-1.	

Alterations in blood glucose levels occur with a wide variety of drugs; in most cases these changes represent undesired side-effects of the compounds. A few drugs, however, are employed specifically for their ability to lower or raise blood glucose levels and thus are termed *hypoglycemic* and *hyperglycemic agents,* respectively.

Hypoglycemic drugs produce a decline in blood and urinary levels of glucose, and are used primarily in the treatment of diabetes mellitus, a chronic metabolic disorder resulting from a deficiency of functional endogenous insulin and characterized by elevated levels of glucose in the blood (hyperglycemia) and urine (glycosuria). The etiology and types of diabetes mellitus and the associated metabolic disturbances are reviewed in Chapter 38. Drug therapy of diabetes mellitus may be undertaken by either providing replacement insulin obtained from bovine or porcine sources or synthesized *in vitro* or by oral administration of synthetic, sulfonamide-related hypoglycemic drugs (sulfonylureas), which increase release of endogenous insulin and increase the number and affinity of insulin receptors on body cells.

The antidiabetic drugs considered in this chapter include the various kinds of insulin preparations, which are indicated in absolute insulin-deficient forms of diabetes (type I, insulin-dependent diabetes or juvenile-onset diabetes; see Chap. 38) and the *oral hypoglycemic drugs,* which are used primarily in milder diabetes, frequently associated with obesity, in which insulin levels are near normal but the hormone is relatively ineffective (type II, non-insulin-dependent diabetes or maturity-onset diabetes; see Chap. 38).

Successful treatment of diabetes mellitus, however, requires more than mere drug therapy. Among the many adjunctive measures that should be considered in properly managing the diabetic state are (1) weight reduction, (2) regulation of the diet, (3) proper amounts of exercise, (4) maintenance of good hygiene, and (5) education of the patient about proper monitoring procedures to avoid untoward effects. In fact, milder forms of maturity-onset diabetes (see Chap. 38) can be adequately controlled in many instances without resorting to drugs, simply by weight loss and careful regulation of the diet. Drug treatment of diabetes mellitus, when necessary, is a highly individualized matter and requires accurate diagnosis, continual monitoring of the patient, and proper drug dosage modifications as necessitated by changes in patient status.

On the other hand, drugs that elevate blood glucose levels can be employed to reverse hypoglycemia resulting from diseases (such as pancreatic carcinoma, hormonal imbalances, liver and kidney dysfunction) or antidiabetic drug overdosage. Parenteral glucose is the most effective agent for elevating blood glucose levels and should be employed in acute situations whenever feasible. Other effective hyperglycemic drugs include glucagon, a purified peptide extracted from pancreatic alpha (A) cells and diazoxide, a thiazide derivative that blocks insulin release. These compounds are also reviewed in this chapter.

Antidiabetic and Hyperglycemic Agents

42

Insulins

▶ **insulin injection**

▶ **insulin zinc suspension**

▶ **insulin zinc suspension, extended**

▶ **insulin zinc suspension, prompt**

▶ **isophane insulin suspension**

▶ **protamine zinc insulin suspension**

Endogenous insulin is a 51 amino acid polypeptide hormone secreted by the beta (B) cells of the islets of Langerhans of the pancreas. The clinically available insulin preparations include purified extracts from beef or pork pancreas that possess biological effects qualitatively identical to those of human insulin, differing from human insulin by only three (beef) or one (pork) amino acid in the sequence. In addition, *human* insulin (*i.e., exact* amino acid sequence of endogenous insulin) is now available, and is derived by either recombinant DNA techniques utilizing strains of *E. coli* or chemical modification of animal-extracted pork insulin to replace the lone amino acid that is different from that of human insulin.

All commercially available insulins are termed *single-peak* insulins, and due to improved purification procedures, are less likely to produce allergic reactions and lipodystrophy at the injection site than the previously available United States Pharmacopeia (USP) insulin. Moreover, the various purification techniques used to remove allergenic contaminants (*e.g.,* proinsulin, an insulin precursor, and the other islet cell hormones such as glucagon, somatostatin, and vasoactive intestinal peptide) have been refined to the point that a new class of further purified single-peak insulins is now available. These products, indicated by the term *purified insulin* on the label, contain less than 10 parts per million (ppm) of proinsulin and elicit even fewer allergic reactions in hypersensitive patients than conventional single-peak insulins.

Most diabetics can be managed equally well on conventional single-peak insulin or purified insulin. Generally, candidates for the purified insulins are those patients who exhibit local or systemic allergic reactions or severe lipodystrophy with conventional insulin preparations. A few patients may require dosage adjustments when switched from conventional to highly purified insulins, because the highly purified preparations are less bound by insulin antibodies and therefore may be slightly more potent. All stabilized diabetics being switched to a purified insulin preparation should be monitored closely to determine if a dosage modification is required. The possible advantages of human insulin over purified porcine insulin are still subject to debate, and absolute indications for human insulin preparations are rare.

Several types of insulin preparations are available. In addition to regular insulin, modified forms of insulin have been formulated that display important differences in onset, peak, and duration of action, thereby allowing the physician to carefully control the response in each patient. The time course of action of the different insulins is largely dependent on the physical properties of the various preparations, such as the presence of conjugating metals or proteins (*e.g.,* zinc, globin, protamine), types of buffers, and the *p*H of the medium. Thus, insulin preparations can conveniently be divided into three groups based upon their onset and duration of action. This classification is outlined in Table 42-1, where several characteristics of the different insulins are listed. All available insulin preparations are presented in Table 42-2, where specific indications and other pertinent information are given for each individual drug.

Insulin preparations are standardized on the basis of their hypoglycemic action in fasted rabbits, and doses are measured in units. One insulin unit possesses the activity of 1/24 mg of Zinc Insulin Crystals Reference Standard. Insulin is marketed in 10-ml vials containing 40 U/ml or 100 U/ml as well as a 20-ml concentrated solution containing 500 U/ml. The U100 insulins have virtually replaced the older U40 insulins today.

Mechanism
Facilitates uptake of glucose by cells of striated muscle and adipose tissue, probably by activating a carrier system for transport of glucose across the cell membrane; stimulates glycogen synthesis in muscle and liver by increasing enzyme activity, and suppresses gluconeogenesis; enhances formation of triglycerides and retards release of free fatty acids from adipose tissue; facilitates incorporation of amino acids into muscle protein and may thus promote protein synthesis; restoration of efficient glucose utilization decreases hyperglycemia, reduces glucosuria, and prevents diabetic acidosis and coma.

Uses
1   Treatment of diabetes mellitus, especially the insulin-dependent type and complicated forms of non-insulin-dependent (*i.e.,* maturity-onset) diabetes not adequately controlled by diet
2   Emergency treatment of severe ketoacidosis or diabetic coma
3   Induction of hypoglycemic shock for therapy of certain psychiatric states

Dosage
Must be individualized based on blood glucose, urinary glucose, and ketone determinations

Table 42-1. Characteristics of Insulin Preparations

Drug	Synonym	Onset	Peak Action	Duration
Rapid Acting				
Insulin injection	Regular insulin	½ hour to 1 hour	2 hours to 4 hours	6 hours to 8 hours
Insulin zinc suspension, prompt	Semilente insulin	½ hour to 1 hour	4 hours to 8 hours	12 hours to 16 hours
Intermediate Acting				
Insulin zinc suspension	Lente insulin	1 hour to 2 hours	8 hours to 14 hours	18 hours to 24 hours
Isophane insulin suspension	NPH insulin	1 hour to 1½ hours	8 hours to 12 hours	18 hours to 24 hours
Long Acting				
Insulin zinc suspension, extended	Ultralente insulin	4 hours to 8 hours	12 hours to 24 hours	30 hours to 36 hours
Protamine zinc insulin suspension	Protamine zinc insulin (PZI)	4 hours to 8 hours	14 hours to 20 hours	30 hours to 36 hours

Fate

Inactivated when taken orally; absorbed at varying rates from SC injection sites (see Table 42-1 for onset, peak action, and duration of effect); metabolized by both the liver and kidney and excreted in the feces and to a small extent in the urine.

Common Side-Effects

Mild hypoglycemia (fatigue, headache, drowsiness, nausea, mild tremor), local allergic reactions at injection site (itching, swelling, erythema)

Significant Adverse Reactions

Marked hypoglycemia (sweating, tremor, hypothermia, weakness, hunger, palpitations, nervousness, paresthesias, irritability, blurred vision, numbness in mouth, confusion, delirium, convulsions, and loss of consciousness)

Systemic allergic reactions (urticaria, angioedema, anaphylactic episodes), lipodystrophy at injection sites, insulin resistance, and visual disturbances

Contraindications

Hypersensitivity to specific animal proteins (*e.g.*, bovine, porcine)

Interactions

1 Hypoglycemia may be augmented by alcohol, anabolic steroids, anticoagulants, oral antidiabetics, antineoplastics, monoamine oxidase (MAO) inhibitors, methamphetamine, pyrazolones, propranolol and other nonselective beta-blockers, salicylates, and sulfonamides

2 The hypoglycemic effects of insulin can be antagonized by corticosteroids, diuretics, diazoxide, epinephrine, estrogens, glucagon, lithium, oral contraceptives, phenothiazines, phenytoin, and thyroid preparations.

3 Insulin may lower serum potassium levels, and can increase the toxicity of digitalis glycosides.

▶ NURSING ALERTS

▷ 1 Ensure that the patient always administers insulin with a syringe that coordinates with the strength of the insulin to avoid improper dosage. Vial labeling and syringe calibrations are color coded red (U40) and black (U100).

▷ 2 Note early signs of hypoglycemia (see Common Side-Effects), which may occur with excess insulin, reduced food intake, increased exercise, or emotional upset.

▷ 3 Upon development of hypoglycemic symptoms, advise patient to take 4 oz sweetened orange juice or other beverage, 2 tsp of sugar, honey, or corn syrup, or several candies. A solution of glucose (40%) is also available for oral use. If symptoms do not abate within 30 minutes, more vigorous therapy is indicated. Consult physician.

▷ 4 To treat severe hypoglycemia, obtain a blood sample for measurement of glucose level and administer 10% to 50% intravenous glucose. Begin oral carbohydrate supplements as soon as patient is conscious, and closely monitor blood glucose until stable.

▷ 5 Be aware that ketoacidosis can be precipitated in diabetics (especially juvenile) by rapid growth, illness, emotional upset, infection, surgery, or other stressors. Advise patients and their parents of signs and symptoms of ketoacidosis (see Significant Adverse Reactions) and stress the importance of immediate reporting to physician.

▷ 6 Treat ketoacidosis with IV insulin (regular insulin injection *only*). If necessary 1 g dextrose per unit of insulin being administered may be added. Monitor blood sugar, check blood pressure, intake–output, and urinary ketone levels, and observe other vital signs

Table 42-2. Insulins

Drug	Preparations	Remarks
Rapid Acting		
Insulin injection (Insulin, Regular Iletin I)	Injection—40 U/ml, 100 U/ml (pork, beef and pork)	Short acting; solution is clear; may be administered SC 15 minutes to 30 minutes before meals for control of diabetes, or IV (only insulin suitable for IV use) for severe ketoacidosis or diabetic coma; give 1 g dextrose/U insulin when administered IV, and monitor blood sugar, blood pressure, and intake–output ratio every hour until stable; be alert for development of rapid hypoglycemia and insulin shock
Purified (Actrapid, Regular Iletin II, Velosulin)	Purified injection—100 U/ml (beef, pork)	
Human (Actrapid Human, Humulin R)	Human—100 U/ml	
Insulin injection, concentrated		
Purified (Regular Concentrated Iletin II)	Purified injection—500 U/ml (pork)	Indicated for control of diabetes in patients with marked insulin resistance; may be administered SC or IM; concentrated from pork pancreas, solution is clear and colorless; accuracy in dosage is essential due to potency; marked hypoglycemia can occur
Insulin zinc suspension, prompt (Semilente Iletin I, Semilente Insulin)	Injection—40 U/ml, 100 U/ml (beef, beef and pork)	Suspension of small particles of insulin and zinc chloride; solution is cloudy; administered SC 30 minutes before meals, usually breakfast; may only be mixed with other lente insulins; mix thoroughly by rolling vial and inverting end to end; do *not* shake; if suspension is granular or clumped, discard vial
Purified (Semitard)	Purified injection—100 U/ml (pork)	
Intermediate Acting		
Insulin zinc suspension (Lente Iletin I, Lente Insulin)	Injection—40 U/ml, 100 U/ml (beef, beef and pork)	Cloudy suspension containing a mixture of 30% prompt zinc suspension and 70% extended zinc suspension; contains no proteins, thus allergic reactions are rare; administered SC 30 minutes to 60 minutes before breakfast; action closely approximates that of NPH insulin, although duration of action may be slightly longer; see Insulin zinc suspension, prompt for mixing instructions and compatibilities
Purified (Lentard, Lente Iletin II, Monotard)	Purified injection—100 U/ml (beef, pork, beef and pork)	
Human (Monotard Human)	Human—100 U/ml	
Isophane insulin suspension (Isophane Insulin NPH, NPH Iletin I)	Injection—40 U/ml, 100 U/ml (beef, beef and pork)	Suspension of protamine zinc insulin crystals; administered SC 30 minutes before breakfast; a second injection in the evening may be required; see Insulin zinc suspension, prompt for mixing instructions; it may be mixed with regular insulin injection, but not lente forms; available in fixed combination with purified regular pork insulin as Mixtard
Purified (Insulatard NPH, NPH Iletin II, Protaphane NPH)	Purified injection—100 U/ml (beef, pork)	
Human (Humulin N)	Human—100 U/ml	
Long Acting		
Insulin zinc suspension, extended (Ultralente Iletin I, Ultralente Insulin)	Injection—40 U/ml, 100 U/ml (beef, beef and pork)	Cloudy suspension of large particles of zinc insulin, which delay absorption and prolong effects; no protein, and low incidence of allergic reactions; administered SC 30 minutes to 90 minutes before breakfast; may be mixed with other lente preparations
Purified (Ultratard)	Purified injection—100 U/ml (beef)	
Protamine zinc insulin suspension (Protamine, Zinc and Iletin I, Protamine Zinc Insulin)	Injection—40 U/ml; 100 U/ml (beef, beef and pork)	Cloudy suspension of fine particles of protamine zinc insulin; administered 30 minutes to 60 minutes before breakfast; duration of action may exceed 36 hours; balanced diet and regular meals are essential; may be mixed with regular insulin only; clinical effects may be delayed several days, supplemental doses of regular insulin may be needed during that time; hypoglycemia may be gradual in onset and often unnoticed
Purified (Protamine, Zinc and Iletin II)	Purified injection—100 U/ml (beef, pork)	

frequently until stable. Monitor serum potassium levels and be prepared to provide supplemental potassium as blood glucose falls.

▷ 7 Alert patient to the importance of advising physician of any illness or other change in normal living pattern (*e.g.,* pregnancy, injury) that might alter insulin or diet requirements. In case of sudden illness, bed rest and liberal amounts of fluids should be instituted immediately and the physician advised.

▷ 8 In *acute* situations (*e.g.,* severe hyperglycemia, acidosis) regular insulin is the drug of choice. Longer acting derivatives should never be used.

▶ **NURSING CONSIDERATIONS**

▷ 1 Educate diabetic patients about the nature of their disease, the techniques involved in insulin administration and urine testing, the importance of adherence to diet schedules, and the necessity of recognizing early symptoms of blood sugar abnormalities.

▷ 2 Do not use outdated, discolored, clumped, or cloudy solutions or partially used vials that have been open for several weeks.

▷ 3 To ensure proper dispersion of suspension preparations, rotate vial and invert end to end several times just before withdrawal of each dose. Do *not* shake strongly, because frothing may occur, resulting in inadequate dosage withdrawal. Note that regular and globin insulins do not contain precipitates.

▷ 4 Store vials in a cool place (refrigeration is no longer necessary, but is desirable). Avoid freezing or high temperatures and protect from strong light. Avoid injecting cold insulin, however, because lipodystrophy and reduced absorption can result. Inject SC into areas with substantial fatty layers. Do not inject IM.

▷ 5 Aspirate needle before injection, because inadvertent intravascular injection can result in immediate and marked hypoglycemic response.

▷ 6 Rotate injection sites systematically to minimize trauma and tissue hypertrophy in any one area.

▷ 7 Alert patients to the fact that visual disturbances may occur during early stages of therapy. Eyeglass lenses should not be altered for at least several weeks after therapy has been initiated.

▷ 8 Observe for development of local allergic reaction at injection site. Symptoms usually disappear with continued use, but an antihistamine may be used to alleviate local discomfort. Allergic reactions can also be minimized by switching from pork to beef insulin (or *vice versa*) or use of the corresponding *purified* insulin.

▷ 9 Suggest that patients always carry candy or sugar lumps for use should symptoms of hypoglycemia occur. Some form of medical identification should likewise be carried at all times, stating condition, drugs, dosage used, and physician's name and location.

▷ 10 Counsel patients to carry a sufficient supply of syringes and needles when traveling, and to store the vial of insulin in a cool place if refrigeration is not available.

▷ 11 Urge maintenance of good personal hygiene to prevent infections and vascular complications in the diabetic patient.

▷ 12 Administer insulin 15 minutes to 60 minutes before a meal, depending on type of insulin used (see Table 42-2 for individual dosages). If a dose of insulin is unavailable for any reason, food intake should be decreased temporarily and fluids increased.

▷ 13 Caution patients against use of any other medications unless advised by the physician.

▷ 14 If an insulin mixture is required, note that regular insulin may be mixed with crystalline PZI insulin in any proportion. Lente, semilente, and ultralente may likewise be combined in any ratio. Mixtures of regular insulin with NPH or lente insulins may not be stable beyond 10 minutes to 15 minutes and should be used immediately.

▷ 15 Take care not to contaminate vials of insulin that do not contain protein (*e.g.,* regular insulin) with protein-containing insulin (*e.g.,* NPH, protamine zinc). Withdraw appropriate volume from regular insulin vial *before withdrawing protamine-containing insulin from its vial.*

▷ 16 Recognize that insulin can be adsorbed onto the surface of plastic IV infusion sets, perhaps removing 25% to 50% of the dose. Closely monitor patients receiving insulin in this manner to ensure the proper response.

▷ *Dietary precautions*

▷ 1 Carefully outline required diet to patients and impress upon them the necessity of maintaining a regular meal schedule.

▷ 2 Caution against excessive alcohol consumption, because enhanced hypoglycemia may result.

Oral Antidiabetic Drugs

▶ **acetohexamide**

▶ **chlorpropamide**

▶ **glipizide**

▶ **glyburide**

▶ **tolazamide**

▶ **tolbutamide**

The orally effective hypoglycemic agents are sulfonamide derivatives classified as sulfonylureas. The clinically useful oral antidiabetics have similar mechanisms of action, that is, release of endogenous insulin from functional beta cells in the pancreas and enhanced sensitivity of insulin receptor sites on cellular membranes. However, they display significant differences in the duration of their hypoglycemic action. These differences are detailed in Table 42-3, which lists the available drugs, dosages, and other pertinent characteristics.

The principal indication for the oral hypoglycemic agents is management of mild, stable, non-insulin-dependent, maturity-onset diabetes that cannot be adequately controlled by diet alone. They are of no value in diabetes complicated

Table 42-3. Oral Antidiabetic Drugs

Drug	Preparations	Usual Dosage Range	Remarks
Acetohexamide (Dymelor)	Tablets—250 mg, 500 mg	250 mg to 1500 mg/day in a single dose or 2 divided doses if over 1000 mg/day	Intermediate acting drug (duration 12 hr–24 hr); possesses significant uricosuric activity at therapeutic doses; metabolized to active intermediate by the liver (2½ times as potent as parent compound); use with caution in renal insufficiency
Chlorpropamide (Diabinese)	Tablets—100 mg, 250 mg	Initially 250 mg/day (100 mg to 125 mg/day in older patients); maintenance 100 mg to 500 mg/day (usual 250 mg/day) depending on condition	Longest acting oral antidiabetic drug (duration up to 60 hr); more potent and generally more toxic than other oral drugs; also indicated for treatment of polyuria of diabetes *insipidus;* may enhance effects of ADH; give as a single morning dose, with food, to minimize GI upset; if hypoglycemia occurs, give frequent feedings or glucose for at least 3 days to 5 days, as drug is very long acting, and observe patient closely during this time
Glipizide (Glucotrol)	Tablets—5 mg, 10 mg	Initially, 5 mg before breakfast; increase in 2.5 mg to 5 mg increments every 7 days until optimal response; maximum daily dose is 40 mg	Peak plasma concentrations occur in 1 hr–3 hr. Elimination half-life is 2 hr–4 hr, but blood sugar control persists for up to 24 hr. Liver metabolism is rapid and extensive. Daily doses greater than 15 mg should be divided and given before meals. Reduce dosage in elderly, debilitated, or malnourished persons, and in the presence of impaired renal or hepatic function
Glyburide (Diabeta, Micronase)	Tablets—1.25 mg, 2.5 mg, 5 mg	Initially, 2.5 mg to 5 mg before breakfast; usual maintenance dose is 5 mg to 20 mg daily in a single dose or two divided doses; maximum daily dose is 20 mg	Peak plasma levels are attained within 4 hr, and effects persist for at least 24 hr. Elimination half-life is approximately 10 hr. Excreted in the bile and urine, 50% by each route; thus, can be used in patients with renal impairment with greater safety than other oral antidiabetics
Tolazamide (Tolinase)	Tablets—100 mg, 250 mg, 500 mg	Initially 100 mg to 250 mg/day in a single dose depending on fasting blood sugar; maintenance 100 mg to 500 mg/day	Intermediate-acting drug (duration 10 hr–14 hr); may be effective in patients who do not respond to other sulfonylureas or in some patients with a history of ketoacidosis or coma; close observation of these patients is required; converted to several weakly active metabolites by the liver
Tolbutamide (Orinase, SK-Tolbutamide)	Tablets—250 mg, 500 mg Vials—1 g with diluent	Initially 1 g to 2 g/day orally; Maintenance 0.25 g to 2 g/day, usually in divided doses 1 g IV	Short-acting drug (duration 6 hr–12 hr); mildly goitrogenic at high doses and may reduce radioactive iodide uptake after prolonged administration without producing clinical hypothyroidism; rapidly metabolized to inactive metabolites; useful in patients with kidney disease; Orinase IV is used to diagnose islet cell adenoma (see Chap. 78); in presence of tumor, there is a rapid, marked drop in blood glucose that persists for up to 3 hours; IV injection may produce local irritation or thrombophlebitis

by acidosis or coma, and there is no justification for and significant hazard in their use in labile, insulin-dependent forms of diabetes.

In fact, considerable support exists for the view that initial control of most if not all non-insulin-dependent diabetes should be attempted by diet and weight reduction alone, together with small amounts of insulin in selected cases as necessary. Oral antidiabetic drugs are primarily used in those patients not stabilized by diet and weight loss *and* who are unwilling or unable to take insulin for any reason (*e.g.,* allergies, physical disabilities, fear of injections). Thus, the current status of oral hypoglycemic drugs is uncertain and their use is largely a matter of physician preference and experience.

Mechanism

Stimulate release of preformed endogenous insulin from functional beta cells in the pancreas; also appear to increase the number and sensitivity of insulin receptor sites on tissues, thus increasing the utilization of available insulin; may inhibit hepatic glucose production and reduce serum glucagon concentrations

Uses

1 Treatment of stable, nonketotic, or nonacidotic maturity-onset (non-insulin-dependent) diabetes mellitus not adequately controlled by diet and weight reduction
2 Adjunct to insulin in certain types of *insulin-dependent* diabetes (allows reduced insulin dosage)
3 Diagnosis of pancreatic insulinoma (tolbutamide)
4 Adjunctive treatment of diabetes insipidus (chlorpropamide *only*)

Dosage

See Table 42-3.

Fate

Well absorbed when taken orally; onset of action is 1 hour to 2 hours, but duration varies widely among different drugs (see Table 42-3); most are metabolized in the liver to active as well as inactive metabolites and excreted in the urine; highly bound to plasma proteins

Common Side-Effects

Mild hypoglycemia (fatigue, drowsiness, headache, weakness, hunger, nervousness), GI distress (anorexia, nausea, abdominal cramps, heartburn)

Significant Adverse Reactions

Severe hypoglycemia (tachycardia, vomiting, diarrhea, sweating, blurred vision, irritability, delirium, convulsions), dizziness, edema, and hyponatremia

  Dermatologic—urticaria, pruritus, photosensitivity, morbilliform or maculopapular rash, erythema multiforme, exfoliative dermatitis
  Hepatic—cholestatic jaundice, altered liver function tests, hepatic porphyria
  Hematologic (rare)—thrombocytopenia, leukopenia, mild anemia, eosinophilia, agranulocytosis

Contraindications

Insulin-dependent diabetes, hepatic or renal dysfunction, uremia, ketosis, acidosis, coma, pregnancy, *severe* cases of stress, fever, infection, or trauma, and before surgery

Interactions

1 Effects of oral hypoglycemic drugs may be prolonged or enhanced by oral anticoagulants, alcohol, allopurinol, anti-inflammatory drugs, chloramphenicol, insulin, MAO inhibitors, probenecid, phenytoin, salicylates, sulfonamides, and other highly protein-bound drugs.
2 Thiazide diuretics and beta-blocking agents can reduce the response to oral antidiabetic drugs.
3 Alcohol may elicit a "disulfiram-like" toxic reaction in patients taking oral hypoglycemics (see Chap. 80), and may also produce photosensitivity reactions.
4 Chlorpropamide and possibly other sulfonylureas may prolong the effects of barbiturates.
5 Oral hypoglycemics may increase the metabolism of digitoxin.
6 Oral hypoglycemic requirements can be increased by corticosteroids, estrogens, and thyroid hormones.

▶ NURSING ALERTS

(See Nursing Alerts for Insulin, because many apply to oral antidiabetic drugs as well. Specific alerts associated with the oral drugs are given below.)

▷ 1 Recognize that the sulfonylureas are *not* insulin substitutes and should never be employed alone in juvenile-onset diabetes, or in any form of diabetes complicated by ketoacidosis.
▷ 2 Caution patient that control of diabetes with oral hypoglycemic drugs may be insufficient during periods of stress, illness, and following surgery. Supplemental insulin therapy is indicated on these occasions, and the physician should immediately be apprised of any change in the patient's health state.
▷ 3 Transfer patients from insulin to oral antidiabetic drugs gradually unless patient has been receiving 20 U/day or less of insulin, in which case insulin may be discontinued abruptly. Urine should be tested frequently during transitional period. No transitional period is required when switching between different oral hypoglycemic drugs.
▷ 4 Stress the importance of rigid adherence to prescribed diet, dosage schedules, exercise program, and hygiene to the overall successful management of the disease.
▷ 5 Use very cautiously in patients with cardiac impairment or adrenal or thyroid dysfunction, in women of childbearing age, in elderly or debilitated patients, and in alcoholics.
▷ 6 Carefully weigh benefit *versus* risk in prescribing oral antidiabetic drugs to patients with cardiovascular disease. An older study revealed a higher mortality rate from cardiovascular disease in patients receiving oral antidiabetic drugs than in those treated with diet alone or diet plus insulin. Although these results have not been replicated and are subject to some controversy due to flaws in patient selection processes and experimental design, oral antidiabetic drugs should be used with caution, and patients should be closely monitored.
▷ 7 Urge patient to immediately report any indications of hypersensitivity or hepatic dysfunction (*e.g.,* itching, rash, fever, sore throat, dark urine, light-colored stools, diarrhea, vomiting).

▶ NURSING CONSIDERATIONS

▷ 1 Counsel patient on the early signs of hypoglycemia (see Common Side-Effects) and the importance of eating meals and taking drug on a *regular* schedule to minimize significant fluctuations in blood glucose.
▷ 2 Suggest that patient always carry or have access to some form of soluble glucose (*e.g.,* candy, soda, sweetened juices) in the event a hypoglycemic reaction occurs. If symptoms do not subside within 30 minutes after glucose ingestion, advise physician.
▷ 3 Caution patient against alcohol consumption with oral antidiabetic drugs, because a disulfiram-like reaction may occur, resulting in symptoms of severe illness (*e.g.,* vomiting, tachycardia, headache, hypertension, sweating). Alcohol may also intensify and prolong the hypoglycemic response to oral hypoglycemic drugs.

▷ 4 Instruct all patients taking oral hypoglycemic drugs in the proper use of insulin, should it become necessary to administer it in an emergency.

▷ 5 During initial weeks of therapy, perform necessary laboratory tests and physical examinations on a weekly basis. If insulin is being withdrawn at the same time, observe patient closely and avoid precipitating ketosis, acidosis, or coma by too-rapid dosage adjustments.

▷ 6 Be alert for lack of adequate control with oral drugs, manifested by signs of hyperglycemia (thirst, polyuria, flushing, fatigue, weight loss, hypotension, fruity odor on breath, diarrhea, blurred vision, irritability, abdominal cramping). Report development of symptoms promptly.

▷ 7 Administer drugs in the morning whenever possible to minimize nocturnal hypoglycemia. Give drugs with food to decrease gastric upset.

▷ 8 Caution patients beginning therapy to avoid excessive sunlight, because photosensitivity reactions can occur. Urge gradual exposure to sun until effects of the drug are known.

▷ 9 Begin therapy in elderly patients at low dosage levels, because hyperresponsiveness has been reported. Check blood and urinary sugar daily and adjust dosage accordingly.

▷ 10 Recognize that patients should be under continuous medical supervision, because drug requirements can change frequently. Patient compliance is essential for optimal control of the diabetic state.

▷ *Dietary precaution*

▷ 1 Emphasize the importance of maintaining regular dietary habits and of consuming proper amounts of carbohydrates. Weight control should be attempted, but *not* at the expense of sharply reduced food intake.

Hyperglycemic Agents

Although the most effective means of elevating the blood sugar level in cases of marked hypoglycemia is direct IV injection of glucose, this method is not always available or feasible. Alternatives include the oral administration of glucose gel, or *diazoxide,* a thiazide-like drug that inhibits release of insulin from the pancreas and is used in the management of hypoglycemia due to hyperinsulinism. Also, the parenteral use of *glucagon,* a polypeptide produced by pancreatic alpha cells, can increase conversion of glycogen to glucose.

Most drug-induced hypoglycemic episodes are mild and generally can be reversed by oral ingestion of some form of glucose (such as candy, soda, sweetened orange juice). Only in those instances in which the hypoglycemic response is severe (*e.g.,* insulin shock) or prolonged (when symptoms persist longer than 30 min after oral consumption of glucose) is the use of IV glucose or glucagon indicated.

▶ glucose

Glutose, Insta-Glucose, Monojel

Although glucose (dextrose) is commonly administered by IV infusion (see Chap. 77), mild hypoglycemic reactions can be controlled by the oral use of a 40% glucose gel. This product is squeezed into the buccal cavity; unconscious patients then usually swallow the gel by a reflex action. Blood glucose levels are quickly elevated because the drug is rapidly absorbed from the GI tract. Glucose is not absorbed from the buccal cavity and must be swallowed to be effective. Thus, whenever possible, other drugs should be employed to treat hypoglycemia in the unconscious patient, because the swallowing reflex does not always occur, and the absence of the normal gag reflex can lead to aspiration as well. The usual dose is one third of a bottle (approximately 10 g glucose). The dose may be repeated in 10 minutes if consciousness is not regained.

▶ glucagon

Mechanism

Accelerates synthesis of cyclic AMP, thus increasing phosphorylase activity resulting in glycogenolysis and increased blood glucose levels; inhibits glycogen synthetase, promotes uptake of amino acids into liver, and stimulates hepatic gluconeogenesis; exerts effects on heart similar to catecholamines, that is, increased rate and force of contraction

Use

1 Treatment of severe drug-induced hypoglycemic reactions in diabetic patients or persons undergoing insulin shock therapy (minimal effectiveness in states of starvation, adrenal insufficiency, or chronic hypoglycemia)

2 Production of GI hypotonia as a diagnostic aid for radiologic examination of stomach, duodenum, small intestine, and colon

Dosage

Hypoglycemia: 0.5 mg to 1 mg SC, IM, or IV; repeat once or twice at 20-minute intervals if no response has occurred

Insulin shock therapy: 0.5 mg to 1 mg SC, IM, or IV after 1 hour of coma; if no response within 15 minutes to 25 minutes, repeat

Diagnostic aid: 0.25 mg to 2 mg IV or IM

Fate

Blood glucose begins to increase in 5 minutes to 20 minutes; duration of action is approximately 1 hour to 2 hours; metabolized by the liver

Significant Adverse Reactions

(Rare) Nausea, vomiting, and hypersensitivity reactions

Interaction

1 Glucagon may potentiate the action of oral anticoagulants.

▶ NURSING ALERTS

▷ 1 Note that glucagon is of little benefit in states of starvation, adrenal insufficiency, chronic hypoglycemia, or other conditions in which liver glycogen is unavailable. IV Glucose should be available and must be used if patient is in a deep coma or fails to respond to glucagon.

▷ 2 Begin oral carbohydrates as soon as possible after patient regains consciousness in order to restore liver glycogen and prevent secondary hypoglycemia.

▷ 3 Use cautiously in patients with a history of insulinoma (increased *hypo*glycemia can occur) and pheochromocytoma (increased blood pressure can occur).

▷ 4 Be aware that insulin-dependent diabetics usually do not respond to glucagon with as large an increase in blood glucose as noninsulin-dependent diabetics and supplemental carbohydrates may also be necessary.

▶ **NURSING CONSIDERATIONS**

▷ 1 Be alert for possibility of a hypersensitivity reaction to glucagon injection, because the drug is a protein substance.

▷ 2 Do not mix glucagon solution with solutions containing sodium, potassium, or calcium chlorides, because precipitation will occur. Glucagon does not precipitate in Dextrose Solution.

▷ 3 Inform physician of the occurrence of hypoglycemic episodes, because dosage of insulin or oral antidiabetic drugs may have to be adjusted.

▶ **diazoxide, oral**

Proglycem

Mechanism

Inhibits secretion of insulin from the pancreas and may increase glycogen synthesis; effect on insulin release is antagonized by alpha-adrenergic blocking agents; other pharmacologic actions include hyperuricemia, decreased sodium and water excretion, tachycardia, and increased serum free fatty acid levels; drug is used IV (Hyperstat, see Chap. 31) as an antihypertensive agent, because it directly relaxes vascular smooth muscle; effects on blood pressure are minimal when it is used orally in therapeutic doses.

Use

1 Management of hypoglycemia due to hyperinsulinism (*e.g.*, islet cell proliferation, hyperplasia, or carcinoma; extrapancreatic malignancy; leucine sensitivity) where other medical or surgical treatment is ineffective or inappropriate

Dosage

Initially 3 mg/kg/day in three divided doses every 8 hours
Maintenance 3 mg/kg to 8 mg/kg/day in divided doses; (Infants) 8 mg/kg to 15 mg/kg/day in 2 or 3 equal doses every 8 hours to 12 hours.

Fate

Onset of hyperglycemia is 1 hour; duration is 6 hours to 8 hours; highly bound to plasma albumin; plasma half-life is 10 hours to 24 hours in children and 24 hours to 36 hours in adults; excreted in the urine

Common Side-Effects

Sodium and fluid retention, hirsutism, GI distress (nausea, diarrhea, abdominal pain, loss of taste), palpitations, tachycardia, hyperuricemia, skin rash, headache, and weakness

Significant Adverse Reactions

Cardiovascular—hypotension, chest pain
CNS—anxiety, dizziness, insomnia, extrapyramidal symptoms
Hematologic—thrombocytopenia, neutropenia, eosinophilia, excessive bleeding, decreased hemoglobin
Ocular—transient cataracts, subconjunctival bleeding, blurred vision, scotoma, lacrimation
Hepatic/renal—azotemia, hematuria, proteinuria, decreased urinary output, nephrotic syndrome, increased alkaline phosphatase and SGOT
Other—fever, lymphadenopathy, pancreatitis, galactorrhea, gout, dermatitis, pruritus, herpes, loss of scalp hair, paresthesias, hyperglycemia, glycosuria, ketoacidosis

Contraindications

Functional hypoglycemia, hypersensitivity to sulfonamides or thiazides

Interactions

1 Hypotensive effects of diazoxide may be intensified by antihypertensives and diuretics.
2 Thiazides may potentiate the hyperglycemic and hyperuricemic action of diazoxide.
3 Effects of diazoxide may be enhanced by other protein-bound drugs (*e.g.*, anti-inflammatory agents, anticoagulants, barbiturates, phenytoin, sulfonamides).
4 Chlorpromazine can strongly potentiate the hyperglycemic effect of diazoxide.

▶ **NURSING ALERTS**

▷ 1 Closely monitor intake–output ratio and check frequently for appearance of edema. Drug can cause significant fluid retention and be hazardous in the cardiac patient. Conventional diuretic therapy is usually sufficient to overcome fluid retention.

▷ 2 Be alert for development of ketoacidosis in cases of overdosage, which may lead to coma. Overdosage responds promptly to insulin and restoration of fluid and electrolyte balance. Observe patients closely for at least 7 days following suspected overdosage because diazoxide is long acting.

▷ 3 Use in pregnancy only when potential benefit outweighs the risk of fetal damage that has been reported in experimental animal studies.

▷ 4 Use cautiously in patients with diabetes, renal dysfunction, impaired cerebral or cardiac circulation, or history of gout, in children, and in persons taking corticosteroids.

▶ **NURSING CONSIDERATIONS**

▷ 1 Monitor urine regularly for sugar and ketones and immediately report abnormalities to physician.

▷ 2 Caution patients to report any changes in vision during diazoxide therapy. Transient cataracts have occurred.

▷ 3 Be alert for signs of hirsutism (mainly on forehead, back, and limbs), especially in children and women. Condition is reversible upon drug withdrawal.

▷ 4 Note that some individuals show higher diazoxide blood levels with the liquid than with the capsule formulation. Use caution in changing formulations

▷ 5 Reduce dosage in patients with impaired renal functions and monitor serum electrolytes closely.

▷ 6 Monitor clinical response and blood glucose levels frequently until condition has stabilized. Drugs should be discontinued if satisfactory response is not obtained within 2 weeks to 3 weeks.

Summary. Antidiabetic and Hyperglycemic Drugs

Drug	Preparations	Usual Dosage Range
Insulins	See Table 42-2.	
Oral antidiabetics	See Table 42-3.	
Glucagon (Glucagon)	Powder for injection—1 mg, 10 mg (1 mg = 1 U)	0.5 mg to 1 mg SC, IM, or IV; may repeat in 15 minutes to 25 minutes if no response is noted
Glucose (Glutose, Insta-Glucose, Monojel)	Gel—40%	⅓ bottle squeezed into the buccal cavity, then swallowed; repeat in 10 minutes if necessary
Diazoxide, oral (Proglycem)	Capsules—50 mg Suspension—50 mg/ml	Adults—3 mg/kg to 8 mg/kg/day in 2 to 3 divided doses every 8 hours to 12 hours Infants—8 mg/kg to 15 mg/kg/day in 2 to 3 divided doses

The adrenal cortex secretes a large number of steroidal compounds possessing a variety of physiologic actions. These substances are termed *adrenocorticoids,* or simply *corticoids.* According to their predominant action in the body, they may be divided into one of the three following categories:

I. Mineralocorticoids (*e.g.,* aldosterone)
II. Glucocorticoids (*e.g.,* hydrocortisone)
III. Adrenogenital corticoids (*e.g.,* dehydroepiandrosterone)

The mineralocorticoids, of which aldosterone is the major endogenous representative, exert their principal action on electrolyte and water metabolism, especially in the kidney; there they facilitate the reabsorption of sodium and water from the urine by the ionic exchange mechanisms in the distal segments of the tubule. Aldosterone itself is not available for therapeutic use, and those mineralocorticoids employed clinically are the synthetic derivatives desoxycorticosterone and fludrocortisone.

The glucocorticoids are those compounds that primarily influence carbohydrate, fat, and protein metabolism and thus can elicit varied effects in the body and alter the body's immune response to diverse stimuli. Hydrocortisone and cortisone are the major endogenous glucocorticoids. Metabolic actions of the glucocorticoids include gluconeogenesis, hyperglycemia, increased protein catabolism, decreased utilization of amino acids, impaired lipogenesis, and increased lipolysis. In addition, they can suppress the inflammatory process, and this action is responsible for their major clinical application, the control of symptoms of inflammation. Both naturally occurring glucocorticoids (such as cortisone, hydrocortisone) as well as synthetic glucocorticoids (*e.g.,* betamethasone, prednisone) are available for therapeutic use, and they differ primarily in potency and degree of side-effects.

The adrenogenital corticoids are male and female sex hormones (such as estrogen, progesterone, testosterone) found in very small amounts in the adrenal cortex. Other than dehydroepiandrosterone, a precursor of both testosterone and the estrogens, the adrenogenital corticoids are present in the adrenal cortex in amounts too small to be of clinical significance. The sex hormones are discussed in Chapters 44 to 46.

Although the classification of the major adrenal corticoids into mineralocorticoids and glucocorticoids is convenient for discussion purposes, it represents an oversimplification from a functional standpoint. With the exception of a few potent synthetic glucocorticoids, *complete* separation of mineralocorticoid from glucocorticoid activity has not been achieved and considerable overlapping of activity exists with most compounds, especially when employed in large doses. This overlapping is responsible for many of the side-effects associated with adrenal corticosteroid therapy, although in some cases it may represent a desirable extension of the clinical activity of a particular drug. For example, in the treatment of primary adrenal cortical hypofunction (Addison's disease), the mineralocorticoid action (salt and water retention) of glucocorticoid compounds such as hydrocortisone is desirable from a therapeutic point of view. In fact, mineralocorticoid supplementation is often provided with

Adrenal Cortical Steroids

43

glucocorticoid therapy in the treatment of Addison's disease. On the other hand, a mineralocorticoid action might prove undesirable in the cardiac patient, because salt and water retention may aggravate the already compromised cardiac function.

Regulation of adrenal corticosteroid secretion is reviewed in Chapter 38. Synthesis of adrenal corticoids is controlled primarily by ACTH (corticotropin) released from the adenohypophysis. ACTH itself is used in certain clinical situations and is discussed in Chapter 39; the remaining adrenal cortical drugs are reviewed in this chapter. In addition, aminoglutethimide, a drug used in the treatment of adrenal cortical *hyper*function (Cushing's syndrome) will be considered at the end of the chapter.

I Mineralocorticoids

The clinically useful mineralocorticoids possess actions qualitatively similar to those of the major endogenous agent aldosterone, that is, they facilitate the reabsorption of sodium and water from the distal segment of the nephron by the ionic exchange mechanisms involving potassium and hydrogen. They are indicated as partial replacement therapy for adrenocortical insufficiency and for treatment of salt-losing adrenogenital syndrome. The clinically available drugs include desoxycorticosterone (DOC), a synthetic intermediate in the synthesis of aldosterone and fludrocortisone, the most potent and most frequently employed synthetic mineralocorticoid.

▶ desoxycorticosterone acetate
DOCA, Percorten Acetate

▶ desoxycorticosterone pivalate
Percorten Pivalate

A synthetic form of 11-desoxycorticosterone, the drug is available as an aqueous injection (acetate), a repository (long-acting) injection (pivalate), and implantation pellets (acetate).

Mechanism
Promotes sodium and water retention and potassium and hydrogen excretion by facilitating renal distal tubular ionic exchange mechanisms; increases sodium retention in sweat glands, salivary glands, and gastrointestinal mucosa; does *not* exhibit glucocorticoid activity and has no antiinflammatory activity

Uses
1 Partial replacement therapy for primary and secondary adrenocortical insufficiency (in combination with glucocorticoids, fluids, electrolytes, and other adjunctive measures)
2 Treatment of salt-losing adrenogenital syndrome (with adequate glucocorticoid therapy)

Dosage
Injection: 2 mg to 5 mg/day IM
Repository injection: 25 mg to 100 mg every 4 weeks depending on daily requirement of regular injection (25 mg pivalate for 1 mg acetate)
Pellets: 1 pellet for each 0.5 mg of acetate required daily, implanted SC every 8 months to 12 months.

Fate
Not absorbed dependably from GI tract; duration of action is 24 hours to 48 hours with regular injection, 4 weeks to 6 weeks with repository injection, and 8 months to 12 months with pellets; excreted primarily in urine

Common Side-Effects
Hypokalemia (muscle weakness, paresthesias, fatigue), and edema

Significant Adverse Reactions
Hypertension, pulmonary congestion, cardiac arrhythmias, headaches, arthralgia, muscle paralysis, hypersensitivity reactions, and pain and irritation at site of pellet implantation

Contraindications
Hypertension, congestive heart failure, or other cardiac disease

Interactions
See Glucocorticoids for *potential* drug interactions, although the incidence with desoxycorticosterone is lower.

▶ **NURSING ALERTS**

▷ 1 Observe for signs of edema, weight gain, or hypertension, and report immediately. Edema may be relieved by restricting dietary sodium.

▷ 2 Do not administer repository injection more often than once a month or pellets more often than every 8 months to 10 months. Determine dosage of the preparations based on daily requirements of regular injection.

▷ 3 Advise patients to notify physician of infection, trauma, or other stressful situation, because supplemental therapy may be required (*e.g.,* anti-infectives, glucocorticoids, salt replacement).

▶ **NURSING CONSIDERATIONS**

▷ 1 Determine baseline weight, blood pressure, and electrolyte levels. Perform periodic determinations of these parameters during extended therapy and advise physician of any significant changes.

▷ 2 Be alert for signs of excessive hypokalemia (*e.g.,* muscle cramping or weakness, paresthesias, palpitations, fatigue, nausea, polyuria) or drug overdosage (*e.g.,* weight gain, hypertension, pulmonary congestion, insomnia). Supplemental potassium may be indicated.

▷ 3 Inform patients receiving pellet implantation to note signs that drug effect is decreasing (*e.g.,* weight loss, hypotension, fatigue, loss of appetite), and report immediately. Daily injections of acetate are then resumed until a new maintenance requirement is established (usually 2 wk–4 wk). Do *not* reimplant pellets until a *new* maintenance level is determined.

▷ 4 Inject IM into upper outer quadrant of the buttock with a 20-gauge (pivalate dosage form) or 22- to 23-gauge (acetate dosage form) needle, because pivalate is more viscous. Pellets are implanted aseptically SC through an incision, usually in the infrascapular region.

▷ 5 Stress the importance of controlling salt intake for optimal drug effects. Excess salt intake increases sodium retention and potassium excretion, reducing drug efficacy and necessitating potassium supplementation.

▶ fludrocortisone acetate

Florinef

An orally effective, potent mineralocorticoid, fludrocortisone also has marked glucocorticoid activity, and is the most commonly used mineralocorticoid.

Mechanism

Possesses both sodium-retaining and water-retaining properties (see Desoxycorticosterone) and has effects on carbohydrate, fat, and protein metabolism (see Glucocorticoids); small doses produce marked sodium retention and potassium excretion and elevate blood pressure. Large doses can induce a negative nitrogen balance unless protein intake is adequate.

Uses

1 Partial replacement therapy for primary and secondary adrenocortical insufficiency in Addison's disease
2 Treatment of salt-losing adrenogenital syndrome
3 Management of idiopathic or neurologic orthostatic hypotension (Shy-Drager syndrome)

Dosage

Orally 0.1 mg/day; range is 0.1 mg 3 times a week to 0.2 mg/day.

Fate

Adequately absorbed orally; metabolized in the liver and excreted primarily in the urine

Significant Adverse Reactions

See Desoxycorticosterone and Glucocorticoids.

Contraindications

Treatment of conditions other than those specifically indicated (see Uses), hypertension, cardiac disease, and systemic fungal infections

Interactions

See Glucocorticoids.

▶ NURSING ALERTS

(Because fludrocortisone possesses significant mineralocorticoid as well as glucocorticoid activity, refer to the Nursing Alerts listed under these headings for those applicable to the oral use of fludrocortisone.)

▶ NURSING CONSIDERATIONS

See Nursing Alerts statement above. In addition,

▷ 1 Monitor blood pressure regularly during therapy. If transient hypertension develops, reduce dose to 0.05 mg/day.

▷ 2 Note that drug is usually administered in conjunction with cortisone (10 mg–37.5 mg/day in divided doses) or hydrocortisone (10 mg–30 mg/day in divided doses) when used in the treatment of Addison's disease.

▷ 3 Stress the need for maintaining a diet adequate in protein.

II Glucocorticoids

Amcinonide	Fluocinonide
Beclomethasone	Fluorometholone
Betamethasone	Flurandrenolide
Clocortolone	Halcinonide
Cortisone	Hydrocortisone
Desonide	Medrysone
Desoximetasone	Methylprednisolone
Dexamethasone	Paramethasone
Diflorasone	Prednisolone
Flumethasone	Prednisone
Flunisolide	Triamcinolone
Fluocinolone	

The glucocorticoids encompass a large number of naturally occurring and synthetic steroids, possessing similar pharmacologic actions, but differing widely in potency and the type and severity of side-effects. The principal naturally occurring adrenal cortical steroids are cortisone and hydrocortisone, and they exhibit both mineralocorticoid (salt-retaining) as well as glucocorticoid (anti-inflammatory) effects. As such, they are primarily used as replacement therapy for adrenocortical deficiency states.

Synthetic glucocorticoids are characterized by their greater glucocorticoid potency compared to natural adrenal cortical steroids and by their reduced (and in some cases complete absence of) mineralocorticoid action. The synthetic drugs are used principally for their potent anti-inflammatory action and are available in many different dosage forms. The relative potencies of the various systemically employed glucocorticoids are listed in Table 43-1, which compares their oral effectiveness, anti-inflammatory activity, and mineralocorticoid potency.

It is important to recognize that the majority of adverse reactions associated with glucocorticoid use occur following the systemic use of these compounds. When a local effect is desired, the drug may be applied topically in various dosage forms (*e.g.,* ointment, cream, lotion, aerosol, nasal spray, ophthalmic drops) or administered by an intralesional or intra-articular injection. A number of different corticosteroids are used topically, and the relative potency of topical steroids is dependent on several factors, including the concentration of drug applied, the basic characteristics of the

Table 43-1. Comparative Activities of Systemic Glucocorticoids

Drug	Equivalent Oral Doses (mg)	Relative Anti-Inflammatory Activity	Relative Mineralocorticoid Potency
Short Acting			
Cortisone	25	0.8	++
Hydrocortisone	20	1	++
Intermediate Acting			
Prednisone	5	3–4	+
Prednisolone	5	4	+
Methylprednisolone	4	5	0
Triamcinolone	4	5	0
Long Acting			
Paramethasone	2	10	0
Dexamethasone	0.75	25–30	0
Betamethasone	0.6	25–30	0

drug molecule, and the type of vehicle used. For example, fluorinated derivatives (*e.g.,* betamethasone, fluocinonide, halcinonide) are more potent than nonfluorinated agents (*e.g.,* hydrocortisone, desonide) but may have a higher incidence of local adverse effects. A relative potency ranking of the various topical steroid preparations is presented in Table 43-2.

The discussion of glucocorticoids below focuses mainly on their systemic pharmacology. Following this general review of glucocorticoids, individual drugs, both systemic and local, are listed in Table 43-3; the available dosage forms are given along with recommended dose levels for each dosage form, and specific remarks pertaining to each drug are presented.

Mechanism

Mechanism of anti-inflammatory action is not completely established, but may include one or more of the following actions: (1) stabilization of lysosomal membranes, reducing release of tissue-destructive enzymes; (2) inhibition of capillary dilation and permeability; (3) interference with the biosynthesis, storage, or release of allergic substances (*e.g.,* bradykinin, histamine); (4) suppression of leukocyte migration and phagocytosis; (5) inhibition of fibroblast formation and collagen deposition; and (6) reduction of antibody formation by lymphocytes and plasma cells. Drugs may also enhance the responsiveness of the cardiovascular system to circulating catecholamines, thus increasing cardiac output as well as local perfusion pressure. Derivatives possessing mineralocorticoid activity exert effects on fluid and electrolyte balance as well (see Mechanism for Desoxycorticosterone).

Uses

1. Replacement therapy in primary or secondary adrenal cortical insufficiency (hydrocortisone is drug of choice)
2. Treatment of congenital adrenal hyperplasia
3. Symptomatic treatment of various inflammatory,

allergic, or immunoreactive disorders including the following:
   a. *Rheumatic*—rheumatoid arthritis, bursitis, osteoarthritis, acute gouty arthritis, tenosynovitis, synovitis, ankylosing spondylitis
   b. *Collagen*—acute rheumatic carditis, systemic lupus erythematosus
   c. *Allergic*—allergic rhinitis, bronchial asthma, status asthmaticus, dermatitis, serum sickness, drug hypersensitivity
   d. *Dermatologic*—erythema multiforme (Stevens–Johnson syndrome) exfoliative dermatitis, severe psoriasis, angioedema, urticaria, chronic eczema
   e. *Ophthalmic*—conjunctivitis, keratitis, iritis, uveitis, acute optic neuritis, chorioretinitis, allergic corneal marginal ulcers
   f. *Gastrointestinal*—ulcerative colitis, regional enteritis
   g. *Hematologic/neoplastic*—thrombocytopenic purpura, hemolytic anemia (autoimmune), erythroblastopenia, leukemias, Hodgkin's disease, multiple myeloma
   h. *Other*—nephrotic syndrome, gout, hypercalcemia, multiple sclerosis, acute myasthenic episodes, anaphylactic shock, tuberculous meningitis, nonsuppurative thyroiditis
4. Testing of adrenal cortical hyperfunction (dexamethasone only)
5. Treatment of pulmonary emphysema with bronchospasm and edema (triamcinolone)
6. Investigational uses include prevention of cisplatin-induced vomiting (dexamethasone), prevention of respiratory distress syndrome in premature neonates (betamethasone), treatment of septic shock (methylprednisolone IV), and diagnosis of depression (dexamethasone)

Dosage
See Table 43-3.

Table 43-2. Relative Potencies of Topically Applied Corticosteroids*

Generic Name	Trade Name	Dosage form/Strength	
Group I			
Amcinonide	Cyclocort	Ointment	0.1%
Betamethasone dipropionate	Diprolene, Diprosone	Ointment	0.05%
Desoximetasone	Topicort	Cream	0.25%
Diflorasone	Florone, Maxiflor	Ointment	0.05%
Fluocinonide	Lidex	Cream	0.05%
	Lidex	Ointment	0.05%
	Topsyn	Gel	0.05%
Group II			
Betamethasone benzoate	Benisone, Uticort	Gel	0.025%
Betamethasone dipropionate	Diprosone	Cream	0.05%
Betamethasone valerate	Betatrex, Valisone	Ointment	0.1%
Triamcinolone	Aristocort	Cream	0.5%
Group III			
Betamethasone valerate	Betatrex, Valisone	Lotion	0.1%
Fluocinolone	Synalar	Ointment	0.025%
	Synalar-HP	Cream	0.2%
Flurandrenolide	Cordran	Ointment	0.05%
Triamcinolone	Aristocort, Kenalog	Ointment	0.1%
Group IV			
Betamethasone valerate	Betatrex, Valisone	Cream	0.1%
Clocortolone	Cloderm	Cream	0.1%
Fluocinolone	Fluonid, Synalar, Synemol	Cream	0.025%
Fluoromethalone	Oxylone	Cream	0.025%
Flurandrenolide	Cordran	Cream	0.05%
Hydrocortisone valerate	Westcort	Cream	0.2%
Triamcinolone	Aristocort, Kenalog	Cream	0.1%
	Kenalog	Lotion	0.025%
Group V			
Desonide	Tridesilon	Cream	0.05%
Dexamethasone	Hexadrol	Cream	0.04%
Flumethasone	Locorten	Cream	0.03%
Hydrocortisone	Alphaderm, Hytone	Cream	1.0%
	Cortril, Hytone	Ointment	1.0%
	Cort-Dome, Hytone	Lotion	1.0%
Methylprednisolone	Medrol	Ointment	1.0%
Prednisolone	Meti-Derm	Cream	0.5%

* Group I drugs are the most potent; group V drugs are the least potent. Drugs in each group are listed alphabetically; there is no significant difference among agents in each group.

Fate

Most drugs are well absorbed from the GI tract and circulate in the blood partially bound to plasma proteins; duration of action varies among derivatives (see Table 43-1); metabolized in the liver and excreted largely by the kidney in conjugated form; induction of hepatic enzymes will increase the metabolic clearance of glucocorticoids; renal clearance is accelerated when plasma levels are increased. (See Table 43-3 for specific data for individual drugs.)

Common Side-Effects

Salt and water retention, sweating, increased appetite

Significant Adverse Reactions

GI—vomiting, peptic ulcer, pancreatitis, abdominal distention, ulcerative esophagitis

Cardiovascular—hypertension, arrhythmias, congestive heart failure, shock, thrombophlebitis, fat embolism

Dermatologic—petechiae, ecchymoses, purpura, hirsutism, acne, thinning of skin, striae, fatty redistribution in subcutaneous layers, impaired wound healing, abnormal pigmentation

Musculoskeletal—osteoporosis, muscle weakness, tendon rupture, vertebral compression fractures, spontaneous fractures, steroid myopathy

Neurologic—vertigo, headache, syncope, personality changes, irritability, insomnia, convulsions, catatonia

Fluid/Electrolyte—hypokalemia, hypocalcemia, alkalosis

Endocrine—menstrual irregularities, growth retardation, decreased carbohydrate tolerance, steroid diabetes

Ophthalmic—posterior subcapsular cataracts, glaucoma exophthalmos

Table 43-3. Glucocorticoids

Drug	Preparations	Usual Dosage Range	Remarks
Amcinonide (Cyclocort)	Cream—0.1%	Apply 2 to 3 times/day	Effective against steroid-responsive dermatoses; drug is formulated in nonsensitizing hydrophilic base
Beclomethasone (Beclovent, Beconase, Vancenase, Vanceril)	Aerosol for oral inhalation—42 mcg/dose Aerosol for intranasal inhalation—42 mcg/dose	Oral inhalation: Adults—2 inhalations 3 to 4 times a day (maximum 20/day) Children—1 or 2 inhalations 3 to 4 times a day (maximum 10/day) Nasal inhalation: 1 inhalation 2 to 4 times a day	Synthetic corticosteroid related to prednisolone; used by oral inhalation for chronic management of bronchial asthma not controlled by bronchodilators and other nonsteroidal drugs; dry mouth, hoarseness, and localized fungal infections of mouth and pharynx can occur; danger of adrenal insufficiency if patients are transferred from oral to inhaled steroids too quickly or during periods of stress; oral steroids should be available at all times; *not* indicated for relief of acute asthmatic attack; intranasal solution is used for relief of symptoms of seasonal or perennial rhinitis, minimal systemic effects; do not use in children under 12; nasal irritation and dryness are most common side-effects; effects are evident only with several days use; patients with blocked nasal passages should use a decongestant (see Chap. 11) prior to administration; do not use longer than 3 weeks if no effect
Betamethasone (Celestone) Phosphate (Celestone Phosphate, Cel-U-Jec, Selestoject) Benzoate (Benisone, Uticort) Diproprionate (Diprolene, Diprosone) Valerate (Betatrex, Valisone)	Tablets—0.6 mg Syrup—0.6 mg/5 ml Injection—4 mg/ml Repository injection—3 mg acetate and 3 mg phosphate/ml Cream—0.01%, 0.025%, 0.05%, 0.1%, 0.2% Ointment—0.025%, 0.05%, 0.1% Lotion—0.025%, 0.05%, 0.1% Gel—0.025% Aerosol 0.1%, 0.15%	Oral—0.6 mg to 7.2 mg/day IM, IV (phosphate only)—up to 9 mg/day IM (repository)—0.5 mg to 9.0 mg/day Intra-articular—2 mg to 8 mg (0.25 ml–2 ml) depending on joint size and disease Topical—1 to 3 times/day	Long-acting agent with no mineralocorticoid activity; phosphate salt has a prompt onset of action and is given IV or IM, may be combined with acetate salt (prolonged action) for repository IM injections, given every 3 to 10 days into joints, lesions, or bursae; up to 2 ml may be injected into very large joints; *not used* in Addison's disease where salt- and water-retaining action is desirable; used topically for dermatoses, pruritus, and psoriatic lesions; use aerosol cautiously because systemic absorption may be substantial, resulting in increased adverse effects. Dipropionate is available in a specially formulated waxy vehicle that enhances drug absorption (Diprolene)
Clocortolone (Cloderm)	Cream—0.1%	Apply 1 to 3 times/day	Indicated for relief of inflammatory manifestations of corticosteroid responsive dermatoses
Cortisone (Cortone)	Tablets—5 mg, 10 mg, 25 mg Injection—25 mg/ml, 50 mg/ml	Oral, IM—20 mg to 300 mg/day; reduce to lowest effective dosage	Short-acting glucocorticoid with prominent mineralocorticoid activity; it is largely converted to hydrocortisone, which is responsible for most of its pharmacologic action
Desonide (Tridesilon)	Cream—0.05% Ointment—0.05%	Apply 2 to 3 times/day	Possesses anti-inflammatory, antipruritic, and vasoconstrictive activity; discontinue if irritation develops; less potent than most other topical steroids

Table 43-3. Glucocorticoids (continued)

Drug	Preparations	Usual Dosage Range	Remarks
Desoximetasone (Topicort)	Cream—0.05%, 0.25% Gel—0.05%	Apply 1 to 2 times/day	Higher strength (0.25%) cream is very potent; weaker strength cream (Topicort LP) and gel are of moderate potency
Dexamethasone (Decadron, Hexadrol, various other manufacturers	Tablets—0.25 mg, 0.5 mg, 0.75 mg, 1.0 mg, 1.5 mg, 2 mg, 4 mg, 6 mg Oral solution—1 mg/ml Elixir—0.5 mg/5 ml Injection—4 mg/ml, 10 mg/ml, 20 mg/ml, 24 mg/ml Repository injection—(acetate salt) 2 mg/ml, 8 mg/ml, 10 mg/ml Ophthalmic solution—0.1% Ophthalmic suspension—0.1% Ophthalmic ointment—0.05% Cream—0.04%, 0.1% Gel—0.1% Aerosol—0.01% Aerosol (Respihaler)—12.6 g (84 mcg/dose) Aerosol (Turbinaire)—12.6 g (84 mcg/dose)	Oral—0.75 to 9 mg/day Children—0.2 mg/kg/day Parenteral—⅓ to ½ oral dose every 12 hours (usual range 0.5–5 mg/day) Repository injection—8 mg to 16 mg IM every 1 week to 3 weeks Intra-articular, intralesion, or soft-tissue injection—0.4 mg to 6 mg depending on area Ophthalmic—1 to 2 drops or thin film of ointment 3 to 4 times/day Topical—2 to 4 times/day as needed Respihaler—2 to 3 inhalations 3 to 4 times/day Turbinaire—2 sprays in nostril 2 to 3 times/day	Widely used, potent corticosteroid; long-acting, and not recommended for alternate-day dosing; phosphate salt is freely soluble and is given IM or IV; prompt onset of action; acetate salt is highly insoluble and has a prolonged effect when given IM; aerosol therapy may result in nasal or bronchial irritation, drying of mucosa, rebound congestion, asthmatic-like reaction, and other systemic effects; Turbinaire aerosol is used for nasal inflammation, whereas Respihaler aerosol is indicated for bronchial asthma; available with lidocaine for soft-tissue injection (*e.g.*, bursitis, tenosynovitis); systemic adverse effects may follow long-term or high-dose topical intralesional, or inhalation therapy; protect eyes from topical spray in the face area; discontinue ophthalmic use if eye irritation develops
Diflorasone (Florone, Maxiflor)	Ointment—0.05% Cream—0.05%	Apply 2 to 3 times/day	Used in steroid-responsive dermatoses; cream is in an emulsified hydrophilic base
Flumethasone (Locorten)	Cream—0.03%	Apply 3 to 4 times/day	Treatment should be continued for several days after clearing of lesions; drug has fairly weak anti-inflammatory, antipruritic, and vasoconstrictive action
Fluocinolone (Fluonid, Flurosyn, Synalar, Synemol)	Ointment—0.025% Cream—0.01%, 0.025%, 0.2% Solution—0.01%	Apply 2 to 4 times/day in a thin layer	Possesses moderate anti-inflammatory and antipruritic activity; high potency cream (0.2%) should be used for short periods of time only
Fluocinonide (Lidex, Topsyn)	Ointment—0.05% Cream—0.05% Gel—0.05% Solution—0.05%	Apply 3 to 4 times/day	Used for anti-inflammatory action in steroid responsive dermatoses; one of the more potent topical corticosteroids; available in several different vehicles
Fluorometholone (FML Liquifilm)	Ophthalmic suspension—0.1%	Ophthalmic—1 to 2 drops 3 to 4 times/day	Be alert for ocular irritation with drops and discontinue drug
Flurandrenolide (Cordran)	Ointment—0.025%, 0.05% Cream—0.025%, 0.05% Lotion—0.05% Tape—4 mcg/cm²	Apply 2 to 3 times/day Tape—Cut tape to size of area; apply to clean dry skin and replace every 12 hours	Good anti-inflammatory, antipruritic, and vasoconstrictive activity; ointment is slightly more effective than cream; both preparations are available with neomycin (Cordran-N); for use in dermatoses complicated by bacterial infections; tape is usually removed every 12 hours but may be left in place for 24 hours if well tolerated; if irritation or infection develops, remove tape and advise physician

(continued)

Table 43-3. Glucocorticoids *(continued)*

Drug	Preparations	Usual Dosage Range	Remarks
Halcinonide (Halog, Halog E)	Ointment—0.1% Cream—0.025%, 0.1% Solution—0.1%	Apply 2 to 3 times/day in a thin film	Similar to most other topical corticosteroids; ointment is formulated in a polyethylene and mineral oil gel base; cream (0.1%) is available in a vanishing base (Halog E)
Hydrocortisone (Cort-Dome, Cortef, and several other manufacturers)	Tablets—5 mg, 10 mg, 20 mg Oral suspension—10 mg/5 ml Injection—25 mg/ml, 50 mg/ml; 100 mg/vial, 250 mg/vial, 500 mg/vial, 1,000 mg/vial Respository injection (acetate)—25 mg/ml, 50 mg/ml Enema—100 mg/60 ml Rectal foam aerosol—90 mg/application Ophthalmic ointment—1.5% Ointment—0.5%, 1%, 2.5% Cream—0.1%, 0.125%, 0.2%, 0.25%, 0.5%, 1%, 2.5% Lotion—0.125%, 0.25%, 0.5%, 1%, 2.5% Gel—1% Aerosol spray—0.5% Topical aerosol foam—1%	Oral—20 mg to 240 mg/day in divided doses Parenteral—⅓ to ½ oral dose every 12 hours Enema—100 mg/night for 21 days Intralesional, intra-articular, or soft-tissue injection—10 mg to 50 mg depending on area Ophthalmic—A thin film of ointment 3 to 4 times/day Topical—A thin film or spray onto area 2 to 4 times/day	Short-acting corticosteroid possessing mineralocorticoid activity; similar in action but less potent than many other synthetic derivatives; local injection as acetate provides long lasting effect due to low solubility; phosphate and succinate salts are water soluble and may be given IV; topical hydrocortisone preparations of 0.5% or weaker are available over-the-counter
Medrysone (HMS Liquifilm)	Ophthalmic suspension—1%	1 to 2 drops 2 to 4 times/day as needed	Used for steroid-responsive inflammatory conditions of the eye; discontinue drug if irritation develops; prolonged use has resulted in cataract formation; shake suspension well before using
Methylprednisolone (Medrol, various other manufacturers)	Tablets—2 mg, 4 mg, 8 mg, 16 mg, 24 mg, 32 mg Injection—40 mg/ml, 125 mg/2 ml, 500 mg/8 ml, 1000 mg/16 ml Repository injection (acetate)—20 mg/ml, 40 mg/ml, 80 mg/ml Enema—40 mg Ointment—0.25%, 1%	Oral—4 mg to 48 mg/day in divided doses Injection—4 mg to 48 mg/day IM or IV Children—0.5 mg/kg or less every 24 hours Repository injection—40 mg to 120 mg IM every 1 week to 4 weeks depending on condition Enema—40 mg 3 to 7 times a week for 2 or more weeks Topical—2 to 3 times/day	Available as base (tablets), sodium succinate (rapid acting injection) or acetate (repository injection, topical ointment); use alternate-day regimen when administered over extended periods of time; do not inject acetate salt IV
Paramethasone (Haldrone)	Tablets—1 mg, 2 mg	2 mg to 24 mg/day in divided doses depending on severity of condition	Approximately 10 times more potent than hydrocortisone, with minimal mineralocorticoid activity; hypocalcemia is common with prolonged high doses
Prednisolone (various manufacturers)	Tablets—1 mg, 5 mg Injection—20 mg/ml, 25 mg/ml, 50 mg/ml, 100 mg/ml Repository injection—25 mg/ml, 50 mg/ml, 100 mg/ml Ophthalmic drops—0.12%, 0.125%, 0.25%, 0.5%, 1%	Oral—5 mg to 60 mg/day Injection (IM, IV)—4 mg to 60 mg/day Repository injection (IM only)—4 mg to 60 mg/day Intralesional, intra-articular, or soft-tissue injection—4 mg to 30 mg (regular injection)	Synthetic derivative of hydrocortisone, approximately 5 times more potent; administer orally with meals to minimize GI irritation; sodium and water retention is minimal with normal doses; alternate-day therapy is advisable with prolonged use to reduce incidence of adverse

Table 43-3. Glucocorticoids (continued)

Drug	Preparations	Usual Dosage Range	Remarks
		or 5 mg to 100 mg (respository injection) Ophthalmic—1 to 2 drops into conjunctival sac every 4 hours	effects; ophthalmic use may increase intraocular pressure; frequent ocular examinations are advisable during extended therapy; injections are available as phosphate (rapid onset; short duration), acetate (prolonged action), tebutate (prolonged action) and a combination of acetate and phosphate (prompt onset and prolonged effect)
Prednisone (various manufacturers)	Tablets—1 mg, 2.5 mg, 5 mg, 10 mg, 20 mg, 25 mg, 50 mg Syrup—5 mg/5 ml	5 mg to 60 mg/day in divided doses Children—0.1 to 0.15 mg/kg/day divided every 12 hours	Synthetic derivative of hydrocortisone; therapeutic action is due to metabolism to prednisolone; use with caution in patients with liver disease; may produce sodium and water retention and potassium loss, especially at high doses; administer on alternate days during prolonged therapy; frequently combined with antineoplastic drugs in certain forms of carcinoma (See Chap. 74)
Triamcinolone (Aristocort, Azmacort, Kenalog, and various other manufacturers)	Tablets—1 mg, 2 mg, 4 mg, 8 mg, 16 mg Syrup—2 mg/5 ml, 4 mg/5 ml Injection—25 mg/ml, 40 mg/ml Repository injection—5 mg/ml, 10 mg/ml, 20 mg/ml, 40 mg/ml Ointment—0.025%, 0.1%, 0.5% Cream—0.025%, 0.1%, 0.5% Lotion—0.025%, 0.1% Gel—0.1% Spray—50 g, 150 g Oral inhaler—approximately 100 mcg are delivered with each activation	Oral—4 mg to 60 mg/day depending on condition Repository injection (IM)—40 mg once a week Intralesional, intra-articular injection: Diacetate—5 mg to 40 mg Acetonide—2.5 mg to 15 mg Hexacetonide—2 mg to 20 mg Topical—2 to 4 times/day as needed Inhalation—2 inhalations 3 to 4 times/day	Synthetic corticosteroid approximately 5 times more potent than hydrocortisone; no significant mineralocorticoid activity at normal doses; diacetate has an intermediate onset and moderate duration of action; acetonide and hexacetonide derivatives possess a slow onset and prolonged duration of action. Do not use in children. Injections should be made IM; do not administer IV. Oral inhalation is used in steroid-responsive bronchial asthma.

Other—increased susceptibility to or masking of infections, fatty embolism, negative nitrogen balance, hypersensitivity and anaphylactic reactions, renal stones, leukocytosis

Contraindications

Systemic fungal infections, active peptic ulcer, active tuberculosis, acute glomerulonephritis, and thrombocytopenic purpura (IM use)

Interactions

1 The pharmacologic effects of corticosteroids may be reduced by barbiturates, phenytoin, ephedrine, and rifampin, drugs that enhance the metabolic clearance of steroids.

2 Corticosteroids may increase the dosage requirements for insulin and oral antidiabetic agents, isoniazid, salicylates, and oral anticoagulants.

3 Increased intraocular pressure can result from combinations of corticosteroids and anticholinergics, tricyclic antidepressants, or adrenergics.

4 Excessive hypokalemia has resulted from concomitant use of corticosteroids and potassium-depleting diuretics or amphotericin.

5 Corticosteroids can increase digitalis toxicity as a result of potassium loss.

6 The anti-inflammatory action of corticosteroids may be enhanced by estrogens, indomethacin, nicotine, salicylates, and pyrazolones.

7 GI absorption of corticosteroids can be impaired by cholestyramine and colestipol.

8 Corticosteroids may increase the pharmacologic effects of theophylline.

▶ **NURSING ALERTS**

▷ 1 Warn patients to avoid infections and to report immediately if one is suspected (*e.g.,* slow wound healing, prolonged inflammation, persistent fever, or sore throat). Corticosteroids may mask some signs of infection, encourage their spread, and decrease the patients' resistance. Appropriate antibiotic therapy is essential.

▷ 2 Do not immunize patients undergoing high-dose corticosteroid therapy because of impaired antibody response and danger of neurologic complications.

▷ 3 Advise patients to report any visual disturbances immediately, because prolonged glucocorticoid therapy may produce cataracts, glaucoma, or optic nerve damage. Periodic ophthalmic examinations should be performed during chronic steroid treatment.

▷ 4 Observe patients closely for signs of mental changes (*e.g.,* euphoria, insomnia, depression, mood swings), because psychic derangements have occurred during glucocorticoid therapy. Use cautiously in persons with a history of emotional instability or psychotic tendencies.

▷ 5 Be alert for possibility of hypersensitivity reactions with parenteral use of these drugs. Severe anaphylactic reactions have been reported.

▷ 6 Withdraw drug gradually following extended therapy in order to minimize the danger of adrenal suppression. Note symptoms of adrenal insufficiency (*e.g.,* nausea, dyspnea, fever, hypotension, myalgia, hypoglycemia) and provide supplementary steroids as needed to reverse the symptoms. An alternate-day dosing regimen may reduce the incidence and severity of adrenal suppression.

▷ 7 Use glucocorticoids cautiously in patients with hypothyroidism, ulcerative colitis, diverticulitis, cirrhosis, peptic ulcer, diabetes mellitus, nephritis, hypertension, osteoporosis, renal insufficiency, thrombophlebitis, myasthenia gravis, convulsive disorders, pyogenic infections, Cushing's syndrome, varicella, and glaucoma, and in pregnant or nursing women.

▷ 8 Counsel patients that glucocorticoid requirements may be increased during periods of stress. Supplementary doses of a rapid-acting corticosteroid should be administered during these stressful periods.

▷ 9 Do not inject a steroid into a joint suspected of being infected or unstable. Recognize that frequent intraarticular injections can result in damage to joint.

▶ **NURSING CONSIDERATIONS**

▷ 1 Determine baseline values for blood pressure, body weight, intake–output ratio, blood glucose, and serum potassium before instituting glucocorticoid treatment and then at regular intervals thereafter.

▷ 2 Individualize dosage in each patient based upon disease state being treated and clinical response. Initial dosage should be adjusted and then maintained until a satisfactory response is evident. Dosage may then be gradually reduced to the lowest effective dose. Alternate-day therapy is generally preferred where feasible to minimize adrenal suppression.

▷ 3 Note that alternate-day therapy is usually accomplished by administering twice the daily maintenance dose every other morning. Provide patient with a schedule of doses to be taken each day to effect the changeover from daily to alternate-day dosing. Do *not* employ long-acting glucocorticoids on alternate-day therapy.

▷ 4 Administer drugs with food or milk in a single daily morning dose, preferably before 9:00 AM. Corticosteroids suppress adrenal function least when given at the time of maximal adrenocortical activity, which is early morning.

▷ 5 Inform patients to notify physician if excessive weight gain, edema, hypertension, muscle weakness, bone pain, sore throat, fever, cold, or infection occurs.

▷ 6 Alert women to the possibility that menstrual irregularities may develop during glucocorticoid therapy.

▷ 7 Caution patients against overusing a joint following cessation of pain, because inflammatory focus may still be present, and further deterioration can occur with excessive movement.

▷ 8 Urge patients to use a firm mattress and bedboard and to report persistent backache or chest pain, because these may indicate presence of spontaneous vertebral or rib fractures (see Significant Adverse Reactions).

▷ 9 Monitor weight and height of children receiving corticosteroids, because drugs can suppress normal growth pattern.

▷ 10 Observe diabetics closely during glucocorticoid therapy, because hyperglycemia and loss of control can occur.

▷ 11 Reassure patients that sudden worsening of condition during periods of dosage adjustments is temporary.

▷ 12 Urge patients to advise physician if gastric distress is severe or persistent, because drugs can cause gastric ulceration. Supplemental antacids may alleviate the distress.

▷ 13 Suggest that patients always carry information describing their condition, and the drug and dosage being taken.

▷ 14 If signs and symptoms of corticosteroid toxicity occur without obvious cause, question the patient as to possible history of excessive over-the-counter hydrocortisone application.

▷ *Dietary precautions*

▷ 1 Advise patients to restrict intake of excessive salt.

▷ 2 Encourage regular consumption of potassium-rich foods (*e.g.,* fruit juices, bananas, leafy vegetables) especially if patient is taking a glucocorticoid with significant mineralocorticoid activity (see Table 43-1).

▷ 3 Urge patients to avoid licorice, because hypokalemia may be intensified.

III Adrenal Steroid Inhibitor

An inhibitor of the synthesis of adrenal steroids is available for treating selected cases of Cushing's syndrome (*i.e.,* adrenal corticol hyperfunction).

▶ aminoglutethimide

Cytadren

Mechanism

Inhibits the conversion of cholesterol to delta-5-pregnenolone, thus impairing normal synthesis of adrenal steroids; probably acts by binding to cytochrome P-450

Uses

1 Suppression of adrenal function in selected patients with adrenocortical hyperfunction (Cushing's syndrome). Usually given only until more definitive therapy (*i.e.,* surgery) can be undertaken.
2 Investigational uses include treatment of advanced mammary carcinoma in postmenopausal women and metastatic prostatic carcinoma.

Dosage

Initially 250 mg 4 times a day; may increase in increments of 250 mg/day at intervals of 1 week to 2 weeks to a total daily dose of 2 g; may be necessary to provide mineralocorticoid replacement therapy (*e.g.,* 25 mg–30 mg hydrocortisone, orally, daily in the morning)

Common Side-Effects

Drowsiness, skin rash, nausea, anorexia, headache, dizziness

Significant Adverse Reactions

Hematologic—Neutropenia, transient leukopenia, pancytopenia, thrombocytopenia
Cardiovascular—orthostatic hypotension, tachycardia
GI—vomiting
Dermatologic—pruritus, urticaria
Other—adrenal insufficiency, hypothyroidism, hirsuitism, fever, myalgia, altered liver function tests, cholestatic jaundice

Contraindications

Sensitivity to glutethimide (Doriden), pregnancy

Interactions

1 Aminoglutethimide can accelerate the metabolism of dexamethasone.

▶ NURSING ALERTS

▷ 1 Be aware that the drug can produce adrenal cortical hypofunction, especially under conditions of stress, trauma, surgery, or acute illness. Monitor patients closely and provide hydrocortisone and fludrocortisone as needed (see Dosage).
▷ 2 Monitor blood pressure in all patients receiving the drug, and alert patients to the possibility of orthostatic hypotension (dizziness, faintness, ataxia, weakness). Urge caution in performing hazardous tasks and advise patient to rise *slowly* from a supine or seated position.
▷ 3 Perform thyroid function tests at regular intervals, and observe for clinical signs of hypothyroidism (fatigue, hypotension, weakness). Supplementary thyroid drugs may be required.
▷ 4 Perform baseline hematologic studies, and repeat at regular intervals during therapy.

▶ NURSING CONSIDERATIONS

▷ 1 Perform periodic liver function tests during therapy as well as regular determinations of serum electrolytes. Advise physician of any abnormality.
▷ 2 Advise patients that nausea and loss of appetite can occur during first few weeks of therapy. Consult physician if these effects are pronounced or prolonged.
▷ 3 Reduce dosage or temporarily discontinue drug if adverse reactions become too severe (*e.g.,* skin rash, drowsiness). If skin rash persists longer than 1 week, drug should be stopped.

Summary. Adrenal Cortical Steroids

Drug	Preparations	Usual Dosage Range
Desoxycorticosterone *Acetate* (DOCA, Percorten, Acetate) *Pivalate* (Percorten Pivalate)	Injection—5 mg/ml Repository Injection— 25 mg/ml Pellets—125 mg	Injection—2 mg to 5 mg a day IM Repository injection—25 mg to 100 mg IM every 4 weeks Pellets—1 pellet SC for each 0.5 mg acetate injection required for daily maintenance
Fludrocortisone (Florinef)	Tablets—0.1 mg	0.1 mg a day (Range 0.1 mg 3 times a week to 0.2 mg a day)
Glucocorticoids	See Table 43-3.	
Aminoglutethimide (Cytadren)	Tablets—250 mg	Initially 250 mg 4 times/day; increase in increments of 250 mg/day at 1-week to 2-week intervals; maximum 2 g/day

44 Estrogens and Progestins

The female hormones may be categorized into two types—estrogens and progestins. Both groups are made up of steroidal compounds secreted by the ovaries, beginning around the time of puberty, as well as by the placenta during pregnancy, and in much lesser amounts by the adrenal cortex. The female sex hormones play a major role in the development and maintenance of the reproductive system and also affect the functioning of many other physiologic systems.

Estrogens

Chlorotrianisene	Estradiol
Combined estrogens	Estrone
Conjugated estrogens	Estropipate
Dienestrol	Ethinyl estradiol
Diethylstilbestrol	Polyestradiol phosphate
Esterified estrogens	Quinestrol

The estrogens are a group of both naturally occurring and synthetic derivatives that exhibit similar pharmacologic and toxicologic effects, differing primarily in suitability for a particular route of administration, potency, and therapeutic indications. One useful classification for the estrogens divides them into the following categories:

1 *Natural (endogenous) estrogens* (*e.g.,* estradiol, estriol, estrone)
2 *Esters and conjugates of natural estrogens* (*e.g.,* estradiol valerate, estropipate, polyestradiol phosphate, conjugated estrogens
3 *Semisynthetic and synthetic estrogens* (*e.g.,* ethinyl estradiol, chlorotrianisene, dienestrol, diethylstilbestrol)

The naturally occurring estrogens are synthesized principally in the ovary and are secreted during the early phase of the menstrual cycle through the synergistic action of follicle-stimulating hormone (FSH) and luteinizing hormone (LH) on the maturing ovarian follicle. The endogenous hormone is composed of several related substances, the principal one being estradiol, which is the most potent. Estradiol is rapidly converted to estrone, which is approximately one half as potent. Estrone in turn is metabolized to estriol, the weakest of the three. These endogenous estrogens promote the growth and development of the endometrium and exert a wide range of effects on other body structures (see Mechanism).

Naturally occurring estrogens are poorly absorbed when administered orally, are rapidly inactivated, and are quickly eliminated, and thus are largely unsuited for oral therapy. Estradiol is available for injection as either the cypionate or valerate salt in an oily vehicle (long acting), whereas estrone is available in either an aqueous suspension (short acting) or oily vehicle (long acting). Crystalline estrone sulfate stabilized with piperazine (estropipate) can be used as a vaginal cream, as can dienestrol, a synthetic estrogen. Orally effective estrogens include micronized estradiol, estropipate, conjugated and esterified estrogenic substances, and a number of semisynthetic and synthetic derivatives. Two very potent, orally effective semisynthetic estrogens, ethinyl estradiol and mestranol, are the only estrogens found in the combination oral contraceptive formulations, and these products are reviewed in Chapter 45.

Principal indications for use of estrogens include relief of the symptoms of menopause, symptomatic management of atrophic vaginitis, treatment of primary female hypogonadism and ovarian failure, palliation of certain types of carcinoma, suppression of lactation, relief of postpartum breast engorgement, and control of abnormal uterine bleeding due to hormonal imbalance. In addition, certain estrogens are used in combination with progestins for contraception. Of these uses, the treatment of menopause has been the most controversial application for estrogens, and much division of opinion still exists on the safety and efficacy of oral estrogen replacement therapy for menopausal symptomatology. There is fairly general agreement that *low-dose* oral estrogen therapy can reduce the incidence and severity of vasomotor symptoms associated with the menopause (such as sweating, flushing, "hot flashes") and that topical application is effective in retarding the atrophic changes in the vaginal epithelium (as in senile vaginitis). Conversely, there is no evidence to support the use of estrogenic substances for the control of the mental and emotional changes that often accompany the onset of menopause. Similarly, estrogens are regarded as only "probably effective" in retarding progression of the osteoporotic changes in the bony structure associated with the menopause, and there is no evidence that estrogen therapy thickens or further strengthens bone. The use of estrogens in menopausal women must be undertaken cautiously, minimal effective doses must be used, and cyclic administration should be employed (*e.g.,* 3 weeks on, 1 week off). Therapy should be re-evaluated at 3-month to 6-month intervals and the dosage reduced or the drug terminated when possible. Appropriate tests and physical examinations should be performed frequently because of the possibility of significant adverse effects, including thromboembolic complications, gallbladder disease, and most especially endometrial carcinoma, the risk of which is 5 times to 12 times greater in users than in nonusers, depending on dosage and duration of therapy.

The discussion of the estrogens considers the agents together as a group. Individual drugs and dosages are listed in Table 44-1 along with comments pertaining to each individual drug.

Mechanism

Produce thickening and increase development of blood vessels and glands of the endometrium; increase volume and acidity of cervical and vaginal secretions; promote growth and cornification of vaginal epithelium and enhance glycogen deposition; accelerate uterine motility; assist growth and development of the duct system of the mammary glands; metabolic actions include a protein anabolic action, accelerated closure of the epiphyses, decreased bone resorption rate, increased serum triglycerides, decreased serum cholesterol and low-density lipoproteins, and enhanced sodium and water retention; reduce platelet adhesiveness and increase levels of vitamin K-dependent clotting factors; *large doses* reduce release of FSH and prolactin from the anterior pituitary by negative feedback, thus inhibiting follicular maturation and lactation; appear to increase release of LH, assisting ovulation

Uses

(See Table 44-1 for specific indications for each drug.)
1 Relief of vasomotor, atrophic, and possibly osteoporotic symptoms of the menopause
2 Treatment of atrophic vaginitis and kraurosis vulvae (dryness and pruritus of genitalia)
3 Replacement therapy in female hypogonadism, female castration, and primary ovarian failure
4 Palliative treatment of advanced prostatic carcinoma, and mammary carcinoma in women who are at least 5 years postmenopausal (see Chap. 74)
5 Relief of postpartum breast engorgement (benefit *versus* risk must be critically weighed)
6 Control of abnormal uterine bleeding due to lack of estrogen secretion
7 Relief of severe acne resistant to more conventional therapy (in female patients only)
8 Postcoital contraception (investigational use only)

Dosage

See Table 44-1.

Fate

Estradiol is metabolized to estrone and further to estriol *in vivo,* then is conjugated and excreted in the urine. Natural estrogens are rapidly inactivated in the GI tract. Esterification of natural estrogens delays metabolism and prolongs action. Aqueous solution of estrogens provides rapid onset and relatively short duration of action. Suspensions or solutions in oil allow slower absorption from IM injection sites, delayed onset, and prolonged duration of action. Oral absorption of synthetic estrogens is good, and they are less rapidly inactivated than natural derivatives. They circulate in both free and conjugated forms, which are 50% to 75% protein-bound.

Common Side-Effects

Nausea, fluid retention, "breakthrough" (mid-cycle) menstrual bleeding, change in menstrual flow, and breast fullness or tenderness

Significant Adverse Reactions

(See also Chap. 45, Oral Contraceptives.)
GI—vomiting, abdominal cramps, bloating, diarrhea, anorexia, cholestatic jaundice, colitis
Dermatologic—skin rash, pruritus, hirsutism, chloasma, melasma, erythema multiforme, erythema nodosum, alopecia, acne
CNS—irritability, depression, headache, migraine attacks, dizziness, insomnia, paresthesias
Genitourinary—dysmenorrhea, amenorrhea, vaginal candidiasis, increased cervical secretions, cystitis-like reaction, endometrial hyperplasia, increase in size of uterine fibromyomata; in males, feminization of genitalia, testicular atrophy, impotence
Other—endometrial carcinoma, gallbladder disease, thromboembolic complications, hepatic adenoma,

(*Text continues on p. 436.*)

Table 44-1. Estrogens

Drug	Preparations	Usual Dosage Range	Remarks
Chlorotrianisene (Tace)	Capsules—12 mg, 25 mg, 72 mg	Menopause—12 mg to 25 mg/day cyclically for 30 days Breast engorgement—12 mg 4 times/day for 7 days or 50 mg every 6 hours for 6 doses or 72 mg twice a day for 2 days Hypogonadism—12 mg to 25 mg/day cyclically for 21 days, followed by 100 mg progesterone IM Prostatic carcinoma—12 mg to 25 mg/day	Synthetic estrogen with delayed onset and prolonged duration of action; stored in adipose tissue; 72-mg cap is used only for postpartum breast engorgement in non-nursing mothers; first dose should be given within 8 hours of delivery; drug is not recommended for mammary carcinoma, because it induces uterine bleeding and endometrial hyperplasia (see Chap. 74)
Combined estrogens, aqueous (Gynogen R.P.)	Injection—2.0 mg estrone and 0.1 mg estradiol/ml	Replacement for estrogen deficiency—0.1 mg to 1 mg estrone weekly, IM Abnormal uterine bleeding—2 mg to 5 mg estrone for several days Prostatic carcinoma—2 mg to 4 mg estrone 2 to 3 times/week Breast carcinoma—5 mg 3 or more times/week	Combination of estrone and estradiol providing rapid onset and moderate duration of action; administer IM only
Conjugated estrogens (Estrocon, Evestrone, Premarin)	Tablets—0.3 mg, 0.625 mg, 0.9 mg, 1.25 mg, 2.5 mg Injection—25 mg/vial with 5 ml diluent Vaginal cream—0.625 mg/g	Menopause—0.3 mg to 0.9 mg/day cyclically Hypogonadism, ovarian failure—2.5 mg to 7.5 mg/day in divided doses for 20 days; oral progestin during last 5 days Prostatic carcinoma—1.25 mg to 2.5 mg 3 times/day for several weeks (maintenance ½ initial dose) Breast cancer—10 mg 3 times/day for 2 months to 5 months as needed to obtain desired response Vaginitis, kraurosis vulvae—Insert vaginal cream 1 to 2 times/day Abnormal uterine bleeding—25 mg IV or IM; repeat in 6 hours to 12 hours if necessary	Water-soluble mixture of conjugated estrogens (sodium estrone sulfate, 50%–65%, and sodium equilin sulfate, 20%–35%) obtained from the urine of pregnant mares; commonly used orally, although vaginal cream is employed for atrophic vaginitis and pruritus vulvae and injection can be used to control abnormal uterine bleeding due to hormonal imbalance; perform IV injection slowly to minimize flushing; do not use if solution is darkened or a precipitate is noted; solution is incompatible with other solutions having an acid pH; it is also available in combination with meprobamate (Milprem and PMB); (see Chap. 74)
Dienestrol (DV, Estraguard, Ortho Dienestrol)	Vaginal cream—0.01% Vaginal suppositories—0.7 mg	Atrophic vaginitis, kraurosis vulvae—1 to 2 applicators of cream or 1 to 2 suppositories daily for 1 week to 2 weeks	Synthetic estrogen employed vaginally; systemic absorption may be significant during prolonged use; it is available with sulfanilamide, aminacrine, and allantoin (AVC/Dienestrol vaginal cream and suppositories)
Diethylstilbestrol (Stilbestrol)	Tablets—0.1 mg, 0.25 mg, 0.5 mg, 1 mg, 5 mg Enteric-coated tablets—0.1 mg, 0.25 mg, 0.5 mg, 1 mg, 5 mg Vaginal suppositories—0.1 mg, 0.5 mg	Menopause—0.2 mg to 0.5 mg/day cyclically Hypogonadism—0.2 mg to 0.5 mg/day cyclically Breast cancer—15 mg/day Prostatic carcinoma—1 mg to 3 mg/day Vaginitis—1 to 2 suppositories/day Postcoital contraception—25 mg twice a day for 5 days (investigational)	Potent synthetic estrogen, usually given orally; frequently produces nausea, vomiting, and headache; should be administered cyclically when given for prolonged periods; contraindicated during pregnancy, because drug has been implicated in causing vaginal and cervical cancer in offspring of women receiving the drug during first trimester

Table 44-1. Estrogens (continued)

Drug	Preparations	Usual Dosage Range	Remarks
Diethylstilbestrol diphosphate (Stilphostrol)	Tablets—50 mg Injection—0.25 g/5 ml	Advanced prostatic carcinoma—50 mg to 200 mg orally 3 times/day or 0.5 g by IV infusion first day, then 1 g/day on subsequent 5 days; maintenance 0.25 g to 0.5 g 1 to 2 times/week	High-dose diethylstilbestrol used for treatment of prostatic carcinoma unresponsive to other estrogens; be alert for early signs of thrombotic complications; for IV administration, dissolve 0.5 g to 1 g of drug in 300 ml saline or dextrose and infuse slowly (20 drops–30 drops a min) during first 10 minutes to 15 minutes; adjust rate thereafter so that entire amount is given over 1 hour (see Chap. 74.)
Esterified estrogen (Estratab, Evex, Menest)	Tablets—0.3 mg, 0.625 mg, 1.25 mg, 2.5 mg	Menopause—0.3 mg to 1.25 mg/day Hypogonadism, ovarian failure—2.5 mg to 7.5 mg/day in divided doses for 20 days, then stop for 10 days Breast cancer—10 mg 3 times/day for 3 months Prostatic carcinoma—1.25 mg to 2.5 mg 3 times/day; maintenance—reduce by ½ after several weeks	Mixture of sodium estrone sulfate (75%–85%) and sodium equilin sulfate (6%–15%); action is similar to conjugated estrogens
Estradiol (Estrace)	Tablets—1 mg, 2 mg	Menopause—1 mg to 2 mg/day orally for 3 weeks; then 1 week off Prostatic carcinoma—1 mg to 2 mg 3 times/day Breast cancer—10 mg 3 times/day for 3 months	Estrogenic hormone derived from estrone, but more potent; readily absorbed orally; available in salt form for injection (see below) providing slow onset and more prolonged duration of action
Estradiol cypionate (Depo-Estradiol, Cypionate and various other manufacturers)	Injection—1 mg/ml, 5 mg/ml	Menopause—1 mg to 5 mg IM every 3 weeks to 4 weeks Hypogonadism—1.5 mg to 2 mg once a month	Salt of estradiol in cottonseed oil providing a depot effect; duration of action 3 weeks to 6 weeks; administered IM only (see Chap. 74)
Estradiol valerate (Delestrogen and various other manufacturers)	Injection—10 mg/ml, 20 mg/ml, 40 mg/ml	Menopause—10 mg to 20 mg IM every 4 weeks Hypogonadism, ovarian failure—10 mg to 20 mg IM every 4 weeks Prostatic carcinoma—30 mg every 1 week to 2 weeks	Salt of estradiol in sesame or castor oil provides 2 weeks to 3 weeks of estrogenic activity following a single IM dose (see Chap. 74)
Estrone (Theelin Aqueous and various other manufacturers)	Injection: Aqueous suspension—2 mg/ml, 5 mg/ml Oil—2 mg/ml	Menopause—0.1 mg to 0.5 mg IM 2 to 3 times/week Hypogonadism, ovarian failure—0.1 mg to 2 mg/week IM in single or divided doses Prostatic carcinoma—2 mg to 4 mg IM 2 to 3 times/week	Estrogenic hormone derived from both natural and synthetic sources; oil base injections may become cloudy upon chilling, warm before injecting; response to therapy for prostatic carcinoma should become apparent within 3 months; if response occurs, continue drug until disease again becomes progressive (see Chap. 74)
Estropipate (Ogen)	Tablets—0.75 mg, 1.5 mg, 3 mg, 6 mg Vaginal cream—1.5 mg/g	Menopause—0.625 mg to 5 mg/day cyclically each month Hypogonadism, ovarian failure—1.25 mg to 7.5 mg/day for 3 weeks, followed by 8-day to 10-day rest period; repeated as needed Atrophic vaginitis—1 g to 2 g vaginal cream daily	Crystalline form of estrone solubilized as sulfate and stabilized with piperazine, making preparation orally effective; tablets contain 83% sodium estrone sulfate equivalent; formerly known as piperazine estrone sulfate

(continued)

Table 44-1. Estrogens *(continued)*

Drug	Preparations	Usual Dosage Range	Remarks
Ethinyl estradiol (Estinyl, Feminone)	Tablets—0.02 mg, 0.05 mg, 0.5 mg	Menopause—0.02 mg to 0.05 mg/day for 21 days cyclically each month Hypogonadism—0.05 mg 1 to 3 times/day for 2 weeks, followed by an oral progestin for 2 weeks Breast cancer—1 mg 3 times/day Prostatic carcinoma—0.15 mg to 2 mg/day	Potent, orally effective synthetic estrogen is found in many oral contraceptives (see Chap. 45); also used for menopausal symptoms, female hypogonadism, and certain carcinomas (see Chap. 74)
Polyestradiol phosphate (Estradurin)	Injection—40 mg/vial with 2 ml diluent	Advanced prostatic carcinoma—40 mg IM every 2 weeks to 4 weeks up to 80 mg	Provides a stable level of active estrogen over a prolonged period; quickly cleared from blood (24 hr) and passively stored in reticuloendothelial system; estradiol levels are maintained constant by continuous replacement from storage sites; increasing the dose prolongs the duration of action but does not significantly enhance the response; may produce temporary burning at IM injection site; clinical response should be evident within 3 months; continue drug until disease becomes progressive (see Chap. 74)
Quinestrol (Estrovis)	Tablets—100 mcg	Menopause, hypogonadism, ovarian failure, kraurosis vulvae, atrophic vaginitis—100 mcg once daily for 7 days, then 100 mcg to 200 mcg once a week thereafter	A derivative of ethinyl estradiol that is stored in body fat and slowly released, thus providing a prolonged duration of action; once-weekly administration is as effective as cyclic therapy with shorter acting estrogens, and may improve patient compliance

hypertension, hypercalcemia, decreased carbohydrate tolerance, aggravation of porphyria, changes in libido, pain at injection site, sterile abscess, fetal damage

Contraindications

Pregnancy, known or suspected breast cancer in premenopausal women, estrogen-dependent neoplasia, undiagnosed genital bleeding, a history of or active thromboembolic disease, incomplete bone growth, or epiphyseal closure

Interactions

1 Estrogens can enhance the effects of corticosteroids, folic acid antagonists, meperidine, and oxytocin.
2 Effects of oral anticoagulants, anticonvulsants, antidiabetic drugs, and cholesterol-lowering agents may be impaired by estrogens.
3 Phenothiazines, phenylbutazone, barbiturates, and other hypnotic drugs can reduce the effects of estrogens by increasing their hepatic metabolism.

▶ NURSING ALERTS

▷ 1 Obtain a comprehensive patient history and perform a physical examination before instituting estrogen therapy and repeat at regular intervals during prolonged therapy. Administer estrogens very cautiously

to persons with a family history of breast cancer or thromboembolic or other cardiovascular disorders.
▷ 2 Stress the importance of regular physician's visits during estrogen treatment, because the potential for adverse reactions is considerable and early detection is important.
▷ 3 Be alert for signs of embolic disorders (*e.g.,* severe headache, chest pains, dyspnea, calf pains, leg swelling, visual disturbances) and discontinue drug if they occur.
▷ 4 Use lowest effective doses to control menopausal symptoms and administer on a cyclic schedule. During extended therapy, perform periodic "Pap" smears, and investigate any vaginal bleeding immediately.
▷ 5 Avoid use of estrogens during pregnancy, because fetal abnormalities have occurred. Caution women receiving estrogens to advise physician immediately if pregnancy is suspected.
▷ 6 Observe patients for behavioral changes or signs of depression and advise physician. Drug should be discontinued unless absolutely necessary to avoid further mental deterioration.
▷ 7 Use with caution in persons with cerebrovascular or coronary artery disease, severe hypertension, epilepsy, migraine, renal or hepatic dysfunction, diabetes mel-

litus, depression or other emotional disturbances, gallbladder disease, metabolic bone disease associated with hypercalcemia, thyroid dysfunction, endometriosis, and in patients with a history of jaundice or a family history of breast or genital cancer.

▷ 8 Advise patients to report symptoms of abdominal distress, because gallbladder disease and benign hepatic adenomas have been reported during estrogen therapy.

▷ 9 Instruct patients to be alert for signs of developing jaundice (yellow skin or sclera, itching, darkened urine, light-colored stools), and discontinue drug.

▷ 10 Urge patients to curtail smoking during estrogen therapy, because the risk of cardiovascular complications is significantly higher in smokers.

▶ **NURSING CONSIDERATIONS**

▷ 1 Reassure patients that the nausea that frequently occurs early in therapy will disappear within 1 week to 2 weeks.

▷ 2 Be alert for excess fluid retention and weight gain. Advise physician should this occur, because dose may have to be adjusted.

▷ 3 Inform diabetic patients that estrogens may increase antidiabetic drug requirement by decreasing glucose tolerance.

▷ 4 Administer drugs on a cyclic schedule (*e.g.*, 3 wk on, 1 wk off) whenever possible, to minimize untoward reactions.

▷ 5 Advise postmenopausal women taking estrogens *cyclically* that withdrawal bleeding is normal and is not indicative of return of fertility.

▷ 6 Note appearance of symptoms of vaginal candidiasis (thick, whitish vaginal secretion, local inflammation), and administer appropriate antifungal agent.

▷ 7 Reassure male patients receiving estrogens that the signs of feminization and impotence that may occur during therapy are reversible upon cessation of drug.

▷ 8 Provide necessary emotional support to menopausal patients and be prepared to discuss their fears concerning use of estrogens and their possible adverse effects, including carcinoma and thromboembolic complications.

▷ 9 Be aware that use of estrogens can alter many laboratory values; for example, increased prothrombin, thyroid binding globulin, serum triglyceride, phospholipid, sulfobromophthalein retention and norepinephrine-induced platelet aggregability and decreased serum folate, glucose tolerance, pregnanediol excretion, antithrombin 3, and triiodothyronine (T_3) uptake; in addition, estrogens may cause an impaired response to the metyrapone test.

PROGESTINS

Hydroxyprogesterone	Norethindrone
Medroxyprogesterone	Norgestrel
Megestrol	Progesterone

The term *progestins* refers to a group of naturally occurring and synthetic steroids having the physiologic effects of progesterone, the principal endogenous progestational hormone. Progesterone is normally secreted by the corpus luteum and also by the placenta during pregnancy, and elicits a variety of actions in the body, which are reviewed under Mechanism. Due to its rapid inactivation following oral ingestion, progesterone is administered intramuscularly only, either in an aqueous or oily vehicle. A group of synthetic progestational steroids is also available, which exhibit effects qualitatively similar to progesterone itself, but which differ from the endogenous progestin in that they possess greater potency, longer duration of action, and in some cases, oral or sublingual effectiveness.

Primary indications for the various progestins are amenorrhea, abnormal uterine bleeding, endometriosis, and endometrial carcinoma. In addition, several of the orally effective synthetic derivatives are used either alone or in fixed combinations with estrogen for the prevention of conception. A discussion of the oral contraceptive agents is presented in Chapter 45.

A previous use for progestational drugs is no longer considered a valid indication for these compounds. Progestins have been employed during the first trimester of pregnancy in an attempt to prevent habitual abortion or to treat threatened abortion. There is no conclusive evidence that such treatment is effective, however, and several reports have suggested that fetal damage (*i.e.*, congenital heart or limb reduction defects) and delayed spontaneous abortion of defective ova can result from use of progestational agents during early pregnancy. If exposed to progestins during the initial stages of pregnancy, patients should be apprised of the potential risks to the fetus.

The discussion of the progestational drugs treats them as a group, inasmuch as their pharmacology is similar. Individual drugs are listed in Table 44-2.

Mechanism
Induce biochemical changes in the endometrium in preparation for implantation of the fertilized egg; inhibit secretion of pituitary gonadotropins (primarily LH), preventing maturation of the follicle and ovulation; stimulate cervical mucus secretion, relax uterine smooth muscle, and induce secretory changes in the endometrium; aid in development of secretory apparatus of the breast; possess some estrogenic and androgenic activity

Uses
(See Table 44-2 for specific indications for each drug.)
1 Treatment of primary and secondary amenorrhea and dysmenorrhea
2 Control of abnormal uterine bleeding due to hormonal imbalance, in the absence of organic pathology
3 Treatment of endometriosis
4 Palliative and adjunctive treatment of advanced, inoperable, or metastatic breast or endometrial carcinoma
5 Prevention of conception (alone or combined with estrogens)

Dosage
See Table 44-2.

Table 44-2. Progestins

Drug	Preparations	Usual Dosage Range	Remarks
Hydroxyprogesterone caproate (Delalutin, Deprolutin-250, Duralutin, Gesterol L.A., Hylutin, Hyprogest 250, Hyproval P.A., Pro-Depo)	Injection—125 mg/ml, 250 mg/ml	Amenorrhea, uterine bleeding—375 mg IM; if no bleeding after 21 days, begin cyclic therapy with estradiol and repeat every 4 weeks for 4 cycles Uterine adenocarcinoma—1 g or more IM initially; repeat 1 or more times each week (maximum 7 g a wk); stop when relapse occurs or after 12 weeks with no response Test for endogenous estrogen production—250 mg IM; repeat in 4 weeks; bleeding 7 days to 14 days after injection indicates endogenous estrogen	Long-acting synthetic progestin, available in either sesame oil or castor oil; duration of action is approximately 10 days to 17 days; devoid of estrogenic or androgenic activity and does not prevent conception; may produce dyspnea, coughing, constriction of the chest, and allergic-like reactions, especially at high doses; solution should be protected from light and stored at room temperature (see also Chap. 74)
Medroxyprogesterone acetate (Amen, Curretab, Depo-Provera, Provera)	Tablets—2.5 mg, 10 mg Injection (Depo-Provera)—100 mg/ml, 400 mg/ml	Amenorrhea—5 mg to 10 mg a day orally for 5 days to 10 days Uterine bleeding—5 mg to 10 mg a day for 5 days to 10 days beginning on 16th or 21st day of cycle Endometrial or renal carcinoma—400 mg to 1000 mg a week IM; maintenance therapy following improvement 400 mg a month	Synthetic progestin used orally for inducing secretory changes in the estrogen-primed endometrium and IM in a depot injectable form for adjunctive therapy of inoperable, recurrent, or metastatic endometrial or renal carcinoma; also has been used orally to stimulate respiration in the obesity–hypoventilation syndrome; has produced malignant mammary nodules in dogs, the human significance of this finding is not established (see also Chap. 74)
Megestrol acetate (Megace, Palace)	Tablets—20 mg, 40 mg	Breast or endometrial carcinoma—40 mg to 80 mg 4 times a day for at least 2 months	Orally effective synthetic progestin indicated for palliative treatment of advanced breast or endometrial carcinoma; malignant breast tumors have occurred in megestrol-treated dogs; no serious side-effects have been reported in humans in doses as high as 800 mg a day (see also Chap. 74)
Norethindrone (Micronor, Norlutin, Nor-Q.D.)	Tablets—0.35 mg, 5 mg	Amenorrhea, uterine bleeding—5 mg to 20 mg a day from days 5 to 25 of cycle Endometriosis—10 mg a day for 2 weeks, then increase by 5 mg a day every 2 weeks to 30 mg a day Contraception—0.35 mg daily	Synthetic progestin possessing androgenic, anabolic, and antiestrogenic properties, especially in high doses; component of several oral contraceptive products and used alone (0.35 mg) as well as a progestin-only contraceptive (see Chap. 45)
Norethindrone acetate (Aygestin, Norlutate)	Tablets—5 mg	Amenorrhea, uterine bleeding—2.5 mg to 10 mg a day from days 5 to 25 of cycle Endometriosis—5 mg a day for 2 weeks; then increase by 2.5 mg a day every 2 weeks to 15 mg a day	Potent synthetic progestin possessing androgenic, anabolic, and *anti*estrogenic activity; component of several oral contraceptive drugs (see Chap. 45)
Norgestrel (Ovrette)	Tablets—0.075 mg	Contraception—0.075 mg a day	Potent progestational hormone used as a progestin-only oral contraceptive ("mini-pill") (see Chap. 45)

Table 44-2. Progestins (continued)

Drug	Preparations	Usual Dosage Range	Remarks
Progesterone (Femotrone, Progelan)	Injection: Aqueous—25 mg/ml, 50 mg/ml, 100 mg/ml Oil—25 mg/ml, 50 mg/ml, 100 mg/ml	Amenorrhea—5 mg to 10 mg IM for 6 to 8 consecutive days Uterine bleeding—5 mg to 10 mg a day IM for 6 days	Endogenous progestin possessing *anti*estrogenic activity; large doses may have a catabolic action and produce loss of sodium and chloride; warm solution before injecting to assure dissolution of all particles; should not be used for diagnosis of pregnancy

Fate

Progesterone is quickly inactivated orally. Other derivatives are rapidly absorbed following oral administration or aqueous IM injection; metabolized by the liver and excreted both in the urine and feces

Common Side-Effects

(Usually seen with large doses) Fluid retention, breakthrough bleeding

Significant Adverse Reactions

(Usually seen with prolonged use or high doses) Menstrual flow irregularities, amenorrhea, cervical erosion, changes in cervical secretion, altered libido, masculinization of the female fetus, edema, weight gain, breast tenderness, hirsutism, alopecia, rash, melasma, decreased glucose tolerance, photosensitivity, cholestatic jaundice, pruritus, diarrhea, depression, nervousness, migraine, coughing, dyspnea, allergic reactions, and retinal vascular lesions

See also Oral Contraceptives (Chap. 45).

Contraindications

Thromboembolic disorders, markedly impaired liver function, known or suspected genital or breast malignancy, undiagnosed vaginal bleeding, missed abortion, and cerebral apoplexy

Interactions

1 Progestins can impair the action of sympathomimetic drugs by enhancing their metabolism and can reduce the effectiveness of antidiabetic drugs by decreasing glucose tolerance.
2 The effects of progestins may be reduced by antihistamines, barbiturates, or phenylbutazone.
3 Phenothiazines can be potentiated by progesterone.

▶ NURSING ALERTS

▷ 1 Apprise patients of the danger to the fetus if progestins are taken during the initial months of pregnancy. Urge patients using progestins to advise physician immediately if pregnancy is suspected.
▷ 2 Be alert to the early manifestations of thromboembolic complications (*e.g.,* chest or calf pain, dyspnea,

numbness in arm or leg, edema, dizziness, visual disturbances), and discontinue drug.
▷ 3 Caution patients to note occurrence of any visual changes, diplopia, ptosis, or headache, and to advise physician. If ophthalmic examination reveals retinal vascular lesions or papilledema, discontinue drug.
▷ 4 Warn patients to observe for symptoms of jaundice (dark urine, pruritus, yellowish skin, or sclera) and to report these symptoms immediately.
▷ 5 Use cautiously in patients with diabetes, migraine, epilepsy, cardiac or renal disease, asthma, and psychoses.
▷ 6 Counsel patients about the difference between normal withdrawal bleeding (3 days–4 days following discontinuation of drug) and breakthrough bleeding or spotting (during course of drug therapy). The latter type of bleeding should be reported, because dosage adjustment may be necessary.

▶ NURSING CONSIDERATIONS

▷ 1 Perform pretreatment and periodic follow-up examinations of the breast and pelvic region, including a Pap smear. Teach female patients how to examine their own breasts.
▷ 2 Observe diabetic patients closely for loss of control because progestins may decrease glucose tolerance. Monitor urine sugar carefully and report any changes.
▷ 3 During progestin therapy closely observe patients with a history of psychic depression. Be alert for any mood changes or signs of recurring depression.
▷ 4 Advise patients to note occurrence of vaginal itching or burning, possible indications of a local candidal infection. Administer appropriate antifungal medication (see Chap. 72).
▷ 5 Be aware that progestins may alter the results of various laboratory tests for hepatic or endocrine function.
▷ 6 Instruct patients to monitor their weight regularly and to observe for signs of edema. Significant weight variations should be reported.
▷ 7 Administer oral progestins with food to minimize GI distress.
▷ 8 Alert patients receiving IM injections that pain or local allergic reactions can occur, but that they are generally transient.

45 Drugs Used in Fertility Control

Several different kinds of pharmacologic agents are employed to control female fertility. They may be grouped according to their action as the following:

I. *Steroid contraceptives* (*e.g.,* estrogen–progestin combinations)
II. *Ovulation stimulants* (*e.g.,* clomiphene, menotropins)
III. *Abortifacients* (*e.g.,* prostaglandins, sodium chloride 20%)

Fertility control is widely practiced and is highly successful in most instances. However, serious and occasionally fatal adverse effects have occurred in some women taking these drugs. Proper dosing of fertility control drugs is essential for their safe and effective use, and these drugs should always be prescribed and monitored by persons aware of their pharmacologic actions and toxicologic potential as well as the pituitary hormone–ovarian relationship. A graphic representation of the menstrual (endometrial) cycle and the various hormonal influences upon ovarian function and endometrial growth and development is presented in Figure 45-1. In addition, patient education is a vital component of a safe and successful contraceptive regimen, and all persons receiving contraceptives for the first time should be given the literature included in the package.

I Steroid Contraceptives

The widest application for estrogens and progestins is in the prevention of pregnancy. Combinations of estrogens and progestins, commonly referred to as oral contraceptives or "the pill," are the most frequently employed and most effective means for preventing pregnancy in fertile women. The many fixed-combination products differ both in the amount and potency of the two components and in the relative estrogen–progestin activity ratio. One of only two estrogens, ethinyl estradiol or mestranol, are found in all of the oral contraceptives, although the amounts vary among the different products. The progestin component of these preparations, however, may be comprised of one of five different compounds, which vary not only in potency, but also in degree of estrogenic, antiestrogenic, and androgenic activity. Although contraceptive efficacy varies little among the currently available oral contraceptive combinations, frequency and severity of side-effects are often related to the relative strength of the estrogen or progestin component. Achieving the proper hormonal balance of estrogen–progestin activity in each individual can often significantly reduce the degree of untoward effects and thus maximize patient compliance. Table 45-1 presents the important side-effects resulting from either estrogen or progestin excess and provides a listing of currently available oral contraceptives grouped according to their relative estrogen–progestin ratio.

While the fixed estrogen–progestin combination products are generally recognized as being the most effective nonsurgical means of contraception, other types of steroidal and nonsteroidal products are used to prevent conception. Progestin-only oral contraceptives (the "mini-pill") are claimed to elicit fewer adverse effects than the combination products,

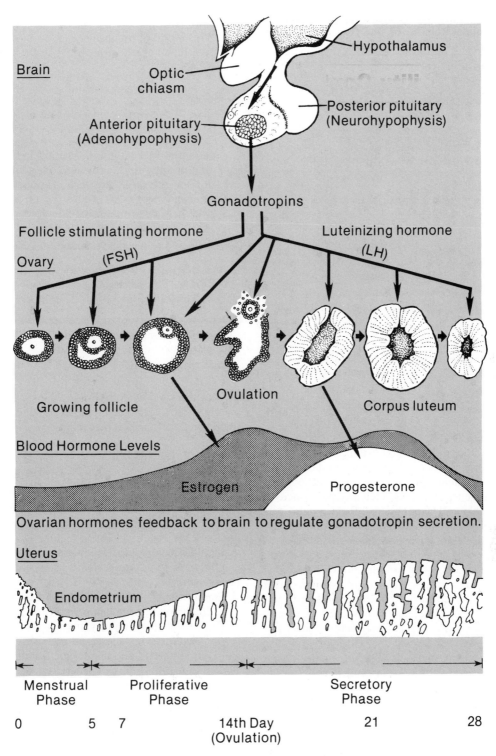

Figure 45–1 The menstrual (endometrial) cycle.

but are also somewhat less effective, having approximately a threefold higher incidence of pregnancy than the estrogen–progestin combinations.

Another steroidal preparation is the intrauterine progesterone contraceptive system, a T-shaped device containing a reservoir of progesterone that is continuously released in small amounts into the uterine cavity following implantation.

The unit is effective for up to 1 year and must be replaced at 1-year intervals. Contraceptive efficacy is equivalent to that of progestin-only drugs.

Diethylstilbestrol (DES), a synthetic estrogen, has been effective as a postcoital contraceptive in large doses (25 mg twice a day for 5 days), provided the drug is given within 72 hours after intercourse. At these doses, DES apparently

Table 45-1. Hormonal Balance of Oral Contraceptives and Relation to Adverse Effects

I. Hormonal Balance

Estrogen dominant

Enovid-E, Norinyl 2 mg, Ortho-Novum 2 mg, Ovulen

Intermediate

Brevicon; Demulen; Enovid-5 mg; Modicon; Norinyl 1+35, 1+50, and 1+80; Norlestrin 1/50 and 2.5/50; Ortho-Novum 1/35, 1/50, 1/80, 10/11, and 7/7/7; Ovcon-35 and -50, Tri-Norinyl

Progestin dominant

Demulen 1/35, Loestrin 1.5/30, Lo/Ovral, Nordette, Ovral

II. Adverse Effects

Estrogen excess

Cervical mucorrhea, edema, nausea, bloating, breast tenderness, migraine, hypertension, chloasma

Estrogen deficiency

Early or mid-cycle breakthrough bleeding, spotting, nervousness, hypomenorrhea

Progestin excess

Acne, depression, hirsutism, fatigue, increased appetite, weight gain, monilial vaginitis, oily skin, pruritus, hypomenorrhea

Progestin deficiency

Late-cycle bleeding, dysmenorrhea, delayed withdrawal bleeding

---

blocks implantation of the fertilized ovum. Because of the hazards of such large doses of DES, this method of contraception is not recommended for routine use, but should be restricted to emergency situations, such as rape or incest.

Many other chemical (spermicidal foams, gels, and creams) and mechanical (diaphragm, intrauterine device, condom) methods of contraception are available, and although usually somewhat less reliable than steroidal drugs, do not present as great a risk of serious untoward reactions as does the use of steroid drugs. Choice of a contraceptive method is a highly personal one, and the advantages and disadvantages of the available methods should be clearly understood by both prescriber and user before a decision is reached.

The oral contraceptives are discussed as a group, inasmuch as they are essentially alike in their pharmacologic action. A complete list of available products is given in Table 45-2, along with their respective estrogen and progestin content. A review of the intrauterine progestin system is also presented.

Mechanism

Interfere with follicular maturation (estrogen decreases release of FSH) and inhibit ovulation (progestin suppresses release of LH); (see Fig. 45-1); induce structural and biochemical changes in the endometrium making it unfavorable for implantation of the fertilized ovum; progestins reduce the amount and increase the viscosity of cervical mucus, thus interfering with motility of sperm cells; may also impair the ciliary and peristaltic activity of the fallopian tubes, impeding movement of the ova

Uses

1 Prevention of pregnancy
2 Treatment of menstrual irregularities (see Progestins, Chap. 44)

Dosage

Estrogen–progestin combinations: 1 tablet daily for 20 days or 21 days beginning on cycle day 5 (day 1 is first day of bleeding); some products are supplied as 28-tablet packs, the last 7 tablets being inert or containing only iron, allowing continuous daily dosage for the entire 28-day cycle; resume next course of therapy 7 days after cessation of previous course, whether or not menstrual flow has occurred.

Note: Due to the association between the dose of estrogen and the risk of thromboembolism, new patients should be given a preparation containing *50 mcg or less* of estrogen.

Progestin-only products: 1 tablet daily without interruption

Fate

Well absorbed when taken orally; metabolized predominantly by the liver and excreted in both the urine and feces; small amounts found in breast milk

Common Side-Effects

(Depends to a large extent on the estrogen–progestin ratio—see Table 45-1) Nausea, vomiting, headache, fluid retention, weight gain, dizziness, breast tenderness, breakthrough bleeding, and leg cramps

Significant Adverse Reactions

(Depends to a large extent on the estrogen–progestin ratio—see Table 45-1)

Cardiovascular—thromboembolic disorders, myocardial infarction, hypertension, and cerebral hemorrhage

GI/hepatic—abdominal cramping, diarrhea, gallbladder disease, benign adenomas and other hepatic lesions, cholelithiasis, and cholestatic jaundice

Genitourinary—dysmenorrhea, amenorrhea, infertility after discontinuation, change in cervical secretions, increased urinary tract and vaginal infections

Ophthalmic—neuro-ocular lesions (*e.g.,* retinal thrombosis, optic neuritis), papilledema, change in corneal curvature, intolerance to contact lenses

CNS—migraine, depression, menstrual tension, fatigue

Other—rash, chloasma, reduced lactation, impaired carbohydrate tolerance, altered laboratory values (*e.g.,* liver function, thyroid function, serum triglycerides, blood glucose)

Contraindications

Thromboembolic disorders, coronary artery or cerebrovascular disease, myocardial infarction or previous history of these disorders, known or suspected breast or other es-

Table 45-2. Oral Contraceptives

Trade Name	Estrogen	Progestin
Estrogen dominant		
Enovid-E	Mestranol 100 mcg	Norethynodrel 2.5 mg
Norinyl 2 mg	Mestranol 100 mcg	Norethindrone 2 mg
Ortho-Novum 2 mg	Mestranol 100 mcg	Norethindrone 2 mg
Ovulen	Mestranol 100 mcg	Ethynodiol diacetate 1 mg
Intermediate		
Brevicon	Ethinyl estradiol 35 mcg	Norethindrone 0.5 mg
Demulen	Ethinyl estradiol 50 mcg	Ethynodiol diacetate 1 mg
Enovid 5 mg	Mestranol 75 mcg	Norethynodrel 5 mg
Modicon	Ethinyl estradiol 35 mcg	Norethindrone 0.5 mg
Norinyl 1+80	Mestranol 80 mcg	Norethindrone 1 mg
Norinyl 1+50	Mestranol 50 mcg	Norethindrone 1 mg
Norinyl 1+35	Ethinyl estradiol 35 mcg	Norethindrone 1 mg
Norlestrin 2.5/50	Ethinyl estradiol 50 mcg	Norethindrone 2.5 mg
Norlestrin 1/50	Ethinyl estradiol 50 mcg	Norethindrone 1 mg
Ortho-Novum 1/80	Mestranol 80 mcg	Norethindrone 1 mg
Ortho-Novum 1/50	Mestranol 50 mcg	Norethindrone 1 mg
Ortho-Novum 1/35	Ethinyl estradiol 35 mcg	Norethindrone 1 mg
Ortho-Novum 10/11	Ethinyl estradiol 35 mcg	Norethindrone 0.5 mg (10 tablets)/1.0 mg (11 tablets)
Ortho-Novum 7/7/7	Ethinyl estradiol 35 mcg	Norethindrone 0.5 mg (7 tablets)/0.75 mg (7 tablets)/ 1.0 mg (7 tablets)
Ovcon-50	Ethinyl estradiol 50 mcg	Norethindrone 1 mg
Ovcon-35	Ethinyl estradiol 35 mcg	Norethindrone 0.4 mg
Tri-Norinyl	Ethinyl estradiol 35 mcg	Norethindrone 0.5 mg (7 tablets)/1.0 mg (9 tablets)/0.5 mg (5 tablets)
Progestin dominant		
Demulen 1/35	Ethinyl estradiol 35 mcg	Ethynodiol diacetate 1 mg
Loestrin 1.5/30	Ethinyl estradiol 30 mcg	Norethindrone 1.5 mg
Loestrin 1/20	Ethinyl estradiol 20 mcg	Norethindrone 1 mg
Lo/Ovral	Ethinyl estradiol 30 mcg	Norgestrel 0.3 mg
Nordette	Ethinyl estradiol 30 mcg	Levonorgestrel 0.15 mg
Ovral	Ethinyl estradiol 50 mcg	Norgestrel 0.5 mg
Progestin only		
Micronor		Norethindrone 0.35 mg
Nor-Q.D.		Norethindrone 0.35 mg
Ovrette		Norgestrel 0.075 mg

trogen-dependent carcinoma, undiagnosed vaginal bleeding, known or suspected pregnancy, severe liver disease, or liver tumors

Interactions

See Estrogens and Progestins, Chapter 44. In addition:

1 Increased incidence of breakthrough bleeding may occur with barbiturates, penicillin, ampicillin, chloramphenicol, sulfonamides, primidone, phenytoin, carbamazepine, rifampin, isoniazid, phenylbutazone, or nitrofurantoin.

2 Oral contraceptives may impair the effectiveness of anticonvulsants, anticoagulants, antihypertensives, tricyclic antidepressants, antidiabetics, and certain vitamins (folic acid, D₃).

3 Oral contraceptive effectiveness may be reduced by barbiturates, meprobamate and other sedatives, phenytoin, phenylbutazone, antihistamines and other drugs that are liver microsomal enzyme inducers (see Chap. 7), as well as by broad-spectrum antibiotics, especially tetracyclines.

4 Oral contraceptives may reduce elimination of corticosteroids, caffeine, chlordiazepoxide, clomipramine, diazepam, imipramine, metoprolol, phenytoin, phenylbutazone, and propranolol.

▶ NURSING ALERTS

See Nursing Alerts for Estrogens and Progestins, Chapter 44. In addition:

▷ 1 Advise women that cigarette smoking markedly increases the risk of cardiovascular complications from oral contraceptive use. The risk increases with age and with heavy smoking. Urge cessation of smoking in women using these drugs.

▷ 2 Use combination with the lowest estrogen content that is effective and tolerated by the patient. A positive correlation exists between dose of estrogen and risk of both thromboembolism and endometrial carcinoma.

▷ 3 Alert patients to observe for signs and symptoms of possible thromboembolism (*e.g.,* calf pain, redness, swelling) and to advise physician immediately should these occur.

▷ 4 Rule out pregnancy before initiating or continuing an oral contraceptive regimen, because use of female sex hormones during early pregnancy may seriously damage the fetus. Pregnancy should always be considered if withdrawal bleeding does not occur following each course of therapy.

▷ 5 Advise patient who misses 3 consecutive days of therapy to begin a new compact of tablets 7 days after last tablet was taken and to use alternate method of contraception for the next 14 days. If one tablet is missed, patient should take two tablets the next day. If two tablets are missed, she should take two tablets daily for the next 2 consecutive days.

▷ 6 Advise patient to report any abnormal vaginal bleeding immediately. If it is sparse (*e.g.,* spotting), medication may be continued uninterrupted but physician should be notified if spotting continues past the second month. If flow is heavy (*e.g.,* menstrual-like flow) patient should discontinue medication and begin a new package of tablets on the fifth day after the start of new bleeding.

▷ 7 When pregnancy is desired, advise patient to terminate oral contraceptives and use alternative means of birth control for an additional 3 months to minimize risk of congenital abnormalities from residual effects of steroidal hormones.

▶ **NURSING CONSIDERATIONS**

See Nursing Considerations for Estrogens and Progestins, Chapter 44. In addition:

▷ 1 Provide users with patient information contained in each package and urge them to read brochure carefully.

▷ 2 Suggest patient use another method of contraception during the first week of administration in the initial cycle of therapy.

▷ 3 Note that after several months of therapy, menstrual flow may be greatly reduced.

▷ 4 Consider changing to another oral contraceptive formulation if a certain pattern of side-effects persists. See Table 45-1.

▷ 5 Be aware that breakthrough bleeding and altered menstrual pattern are more likely to occur with progestin-only products than with combinations.

▷ 6 Perform a physical examination before instituting therapy and at yearly intervals thereafter.

▷ 7 Avoid use of oral contraceptives in adolescents until at least 2 years after establishment of regular menstrual cycles.

▷ 8 Do not administer oral contraceptives to nursing mothers until infant has been weaned.

▷ 9 Suggest patients take medication at the same time every day to minimize the possibility of missing a dose.

▶ **intrauterine progesterone contraceptive system**
Progestasert

The intrauterine progesterone contraceptive system is a T-shaped intrauterine device (IUD) containing 38 mg progesterone dispersed in silicone oil. Following insertion of the unit into the uterine cavity, progesterone is continuously released at an average rate of 65 mcg/day. The contraceptive effectiveness approximates that of progestin-only tablets and is retained for a period of 1 year, after which the system must be replaced.

Mechanism

Suppresses proliferation of endometrial tissue, creating an environment unfavorable for implantation; may decrease sperm survival time, possibly by altering cervical mucus; does not appear to prevent ovulation

Uses

1 Prevention of pregnancy

Dosage

Insert system into the uterine cavity following manufacturer's instructions; replace after 1 year.

Common Side-Effects

(Usually soon after insertion) Bleeding, cramping

Significant Adverse Reactions

Dysmenorrhea, amenorrhea, cervical erosion, pelvic infection, vaginitis, endometritis, spotting, prolonged menstrual flow, delayed menses, dyspareunia, septicemia, septic abortion, cervical or uterine perforation, ectopic pregnancy, pain, and bradycardia or syncope upon insertion

Contraindications

Pregnancy or suspicion of pregnancy, previous ectopic pregnancy, pelvic inflammatory disease, venereal disease, previous pelvic surgery, uterine abnormalities, uterine or cervical malignancy, vaginal bleeding of undetermined origin, and acute cervicitis

Interactions

1 Excessive bleeding may occur in patients receiving anticoagulants.

▶ **NURSING ALERTS**

▷ 1 If pregnancy occurs with system in place, remove it by the thread if possible. Consider termination of pregnancy if system cannot be removed, because risk of spontaneous abortion and sepsis is considerable.

▷ 2 Note that incidence of ectopic pregnancies is higher in patients with an IUD in place. Be alert for delayed menses, unilateral pelvic pain and falling hematocrit, possible indications of an ectopic fetus.

▷ 3 Use cautiously in patients with anemia, hypermenorrhea, valvular heart disease, or a history of thromboembolic disorders.

▶ **NURSING CONSIDERATIONS**
▷ 1 Perform insertion during or shortly following menstruation to ensure that undetermined pregnancy has not occurred.
▷ 2 Caution patients not to pull on threads or to attempt to move unit once inserted.
▷ 3 Re-examine patient within 3 months of insertion to ensure unit is in place.
▷ 4 Teach patients to recognize symptoms of pelvic inflammatory disease (abdominal pain, fever, nausea, vomiting, malaise, purulent vaginal discharge) because risk is increased in IUD users.

II Ovulation Stimulants

Although an infrequent cause of infertility, anovulation, when it occurs, has responded to the use of ovulation-stimulating drugs, and conception has been made possible in previously anovulatory women. Because therapy with these agents is expensive, often tedious, and potentially hazardous, selection of patients with a reasonable expectation for success is important. Thus, women with primary ovarian failure, uterine abnormalities, fallopian tube obstruction, or endometrial carcinoma should be excluded as potential candidates. Likewise, impaired or absent sperm production in the partner should be ruled out. When careful patient selection is observed, 25% to 50% of those persons completing a course of therapy can be expected to conceive. However, treatment with ovulation-inducing drugs is not without its hazards, such as ovarian enlargement, often accompanied by pain and ascites. The incidence of early abortion is increased with use of these drugs, and the occurrence of multiple pregnancies with recommended dosage schedules has been estimated as high as 20%.

Ovulation-inducing agents include clomiphene, a drug capable of increasing release of FSH and LH from the adenohypophysis, and human menopausal gonadotropins (HMG, menotropins), a purified extract of FSH and LH. Clomiphene is used alone, while HMG therapy is followed by an injection of human chorionic gonadotropin (HCG) to induce ovulation. These drugs are reviewed individually.

▶ **clomiphene**
Clomid, Serophene

A nonsteroidal, synthetic estrogen possessing weak estrogenic as well as antiestrogenic activity, clomiphene stimulates release of FSH and LH from the adenohypophysis, and thus requires both a functioning pituitary and a responsive ovary for its therapeutic effect. A single ovulation is induced by each 5-day course of treatment, and the majority of patients who are going to respond will do so with the first course of therapy. A second and third course may be tried if conception has not occurred, but treatment beyond three courses in patients exhibiting no evidence of ovulation or who fail to conceive is not recommended. Approximately 30% to 40% of women with ovulatory dysfunction conceive with a course of clomiphene therapy.

Mechanism
Not completely established; increases release of FSH and LH from the adenohypophysis, enhancing maturation of the ovum and eliciting ovulation (see Fig. 45-1); gonadotropin release may result from removal of negative feedback on gonadotropin release from the adenohypophysis by virtue of the drug's decreasing the number of available estrogenic receptors (*i.e.,* antiestrogenic action); this is interpreted by the pituitary as a signal that estrogen levels are low, and secretion of FSH and LH is increased; may also increase biosynthesis of ovarian hormones

Uses
1 Treatment of ovulatory failure in properly selected patients desiring pregnancy, whose partners are fertile
2 Treatment of male infertility (investigational use)

Dosage
Female infertility: beginning on the fifth day of the cycle, 50 mg/day for 5 days (therapy may be started anytime in amenorrheic women); if ovulation does not occur, a second and third course of therapy (at 100 mg/day for 5 days) may be tried, with a minimum 30-day interval between treatment courses. Treatment beyond three courses of therapy is *not* recommended.
Male infertility: 25 mg/day for 25 days or 100 mg 3 times/week (Mon, Wed, and Fri)

Fate
Well absorbed when taken orally; metabolized in the liver and excreted largely in the feces, both as metabolites and unchanged drug

Common Side-Effects
Ovarian enlargement, abdominal discomfort, vasomotor symptoms (*e.g.,* hot flashes, flushing)

Significant Adverse Reactions
Nausea, vomiting, diarrhea, visual disturbances (*e.g.,* blurring, photophobia, diplopia, scotomata), headache, nervousness, lightheadedness, vertigo, insomnia, depression, abnormal uterine bleeding, breast tenderness, ovarian hemorrhage, urinary frequency, rash, dermatitis, fluid retention, weight gain; increased incidence of early abortion and multiple births.

Contraindications
Pregnancy, liver dysfunction or history of liver disease, ovarian cysts, thrombophlebitis, and abnormal uterine or vaginal bleeding

▶ **NURSING ALERTS**
▷ 1 Perform a complete pelvic examination, an endometrial biopsy, and liver function tests before therapy

and determine cause of any abnormal bleeding before giving the drug.

▷ 2 Advise patients to report development of any visual disturbances. If they occur, discontinue treatment, and perform a complete ophthalmologic examination.

▷ 3 Inform patients that drug may produce blurred vision, dizziness and lightheadedness, and caution against engaging in hazardous activities.

▷ 4 Urge patients to report development of pelvic or abdominal pain; examine them for ovarian enlargement.

▷ 5 Note that birth defects have occurred with clomiphene therapy, although a direct causal relationship is not firmly established.

▶ **NURSING CONSIDERATIONS**

▷ 1 Do not increase dosage beyond 100 mg/day for 5 days, because effectiveness is not enhanced but incidence of untoward reactions and danger of multiple births is increased.

▷ 2 Teach patients how to use a basal thermometer to ascertain time of ovulation.

▷ 3 Stress the importance of properly timed intercourse for conception.

▷ 4 Note that clomiphene may increase levels of serum thyroxine and thyroxine-binding globulin.

▶ **menotropins (human menopausal gonadotropins—HMG)**

Pergonal

A purified preparation of gonadotropins extracted from the urine of postmenopausal women, menotropins is biologically standardized for FSH and LH activity. It is frequently referred to as human menopausal gonadotropins or HMG and provides an exogenous source of pituitary gonadotropins and thus, unlike clomiphene, does not require the presence of functional hypophysial gonadotropins for its activity. Treatment with menotropins usually results only in follicular growth and maturation; subsequent ovulation is effected by sequential administration of HCG (see Chorionic Gonadotropin, below) when sufficient follicular maturation has occurred.

Mechanism

Provides a source of FSH and LH, thus promoting growth of ovarian follicles in women who do not have primary ovarian failure (see Fig. 45-1); does not usually elicit ovulation, which must be induced by injection of HCG, a polypeptide possessing significant LH activity

Uses

1 Treatment of infertility in women with primary or secondary amenorrhea (with or without galactorrhea), polycystic ovary syndrome, anovulatory cycles, or irregular menses (*not* effective in primary ovarian failure)

2 Stimulation of spermatogenesis in men who have primary or secondary hypogonadotropic hypogonadism

Dosage

Women (must be individualized): usually, 1 ampule/day (75 U each of FSH and LH) IM for 9 days to 12 days, followed by HCG, 10,000 U IM 1 day after the last dose of HMG; if ovulation occurs without pregnancy, may repeat course of therapy twice with same dosage levels at monthly intervals. If ovulation does not occur, repeat treatment with 2 ampules/day (150 U each of FSH and LH) for 3 days to 12 days, followed by 10,000 U HCG IM. Do not exceed 2 ampules/day.

Men (to increase spermatogenesis): HCG alone (5000 IU three times/week for 4–6 mo); then, 1 ampule menotropins IM 3 times/week and HCG, 2000 IU, twice a week for 4 months

Common Side-Effects

Mild uncomplicated ovarian enlargement, with or without abdominal pain (20% incidence)

Significant Adverse Reactions

(Usually with larger doses) Ovarian hyperstimulation syndrome (*e.g.,* abdominal pain, ascites, pleural effusion, sudden ovarian enlargement), fever, nausea, vomiting, diarrhea, hemoperitoneum, arterial thromboembolism (rare), and ovarian cysts

Multiple births have occurred with HMG–HCG treatment; occasional gynecomastia in men

Contraindications

Primary ovarian failure, pregnancy, ovarian cysts or enlargement *not* due to polycystic ovary syndrome, thyroid or adrenal dysfunction, intracranial lesion, abnormal bleeding of unknown origin, and infertility due to factors other than anovulation

In men, primary testicular failure and infertility *not* due to hypogonadotropic hypogonadism

▶ **NURSING ALERTS**

▷ 1 Perform a thorough gynecologic examination and endocrinologic evaluation before initiating therapy. Pregnancy and primary ovarian failure must be ruled out and the cause of any abnormal vaginal bleeding determined. Evaluation of the male partner is likewise essential.

▷ 2 Advise patient to be alert for signs of ovarian hyperstimulation (abdominal distention and pain, vaginal bleeding, dyspnea), and, if they occur, to refrain from intercourse and advise physician. Mild ovarian enlargement generally regresses within 2 weeks to 3 weeks.

▷ 3 Do *not* administer HCG if ovaries are abnormally enlarged or if estrogen excretion is greater than 100 mcg/24 hours on the last day of menotropins therapy, because risk of excessive ovarian stimulation is greatly increased.

▶ **NURSING CONSIDERATIONS**

▷ 1 Note that administration of HMG–HCG should only be undertaken by persons trained in their use, knowledgeable in the necessary estrogen and progesterone assays required to monitor the patient's status, and thoroughly familiar with treating female infertility.

▷ 2 Encourage the couple to have intercourse daily beginning the day before HCG administration until ovulation has occurred, as indicated by increased progesterone production.

▷ 3 Examine patients every other day during HMG–HCG treatment and for at least 2 weeks post-treatment for signs of excessive ovarian stimulation. Most ovarian hyperstimulation is noted 7 days to 10 days after ovulation.

▷ 4 In men with reduced or absent spermatogenesis, determine that the cause is lack of pituitary function before initiating therapy with menotropins.

▶ human chorionic gonadotropin
Android-HCG, A.P.L. Secules, Chorex, Corgonject-5, Follutein, Glukor, Gonic, Libigen, Pregnyl, Profasi HP

A purified polypeptide hormone, HCG is produced by the human placenta and extracted from the urine of women during the first trimester of pregnancy. The effect of HCG is due primarily to its LH-like activity, although it exhibits a slight degree of FSH-like activity as well.

Mechanism
Human chorionic gonadotropin stimulates the corpus luteum of the ovaries to produce progesterone, and triggers ovulation from FSH-primed follicles (see Fig. 45-1). In males, it stimulates the interstitial cells of the testes to produce androgens, thus promoting development of secondary sex characteristics and descent of the testicles.

Uses
1 Induction of ovulation in the anovulatory female who has been properly pretreated with HMG
2 Treatment of cryptorchidism (undescended testes) in instances *not* due to anatomical obstruction; therapy is usually instituted between ages 4 years and 9 years
3 Treatment of male hypogonadism secondary to a pituitary deficiency

Dosage
(Highly individualized; IM only; dosage measured in USP units)

Induction of ovulation
5000 U to 10,000 U 1 day following last dose of HMG

Cryptorchidism
1 4000 U three times a week for 3 weeks
2 5000 U every other day for four injections
3 15 injections of 500 U to 1000 U over 6 weeks
4 500 U to 1000 U three times a week for 4 weeks to 6 weeks

Hypogonadism
1 500 U to 1000 U three times a week for 3 weeks, then twice a week for 3 weeks
2 4000 U three times a week for 6 months to 9 months, then 2000 U three times a week for 3 months

Common Side-Effects
Headache, restlessness

Significant Adverse Reactions
Depression, fatigue, edema, gynecomastia, pain at injection site, and sexual precocity in prepubertal patients

Contraindications
Androgen-dependent neoplasms, precocious puberty

▶ NURSING ALERTS
▷ 1 Discontinue drug if signs of precocious puberty are noted in patients being treated for cryptorchidism.
▷ 2 Use cautiously in patients with cardiac or renal disease, asthma, migraine, or epilepsy.
▷ 3 Recognize that excessive treatment with HCG may damage a mechanically obstructed undescended testis. Cryptorchidism failing to respond to HCG within a reasonable period of time (6 wk–12 wk) usually requires surgical intervention.

▶ NURSING CONSIDERATIONS
▷ 1 Note that although HCG has been used in the treatment of obesity, there is no substantial evidence that the drug alters fat mobilization or distribution, retards appetite, or reduces hunger associated with low-calorie diets. Its use as an antiobesity drug should be avoided.
▷ 2 Be alert for signs of edema and advise patient to notify physician if needed. Dosage reduction usually eliminates fluid retention.

III Abortifacients

▶ carboprost tromethamine
Prostin/15 M

▶ dinoprost tromethamine
Prostin F$_2$ alpha

▶ dinoprostone
Prostin E$_2$

Termination of pregnancy can be accomplished by both mechanical and pharmacologic methods. During the early weeks of pregnancy, there is no safe and reliable method for pharmacologically inducing fetal expulsion, and suction curettage is the commonly performed procedure. Beginning at about the start of the second trimester, however, pharmacologic methods are usually employed; these consist of injections of either hypertonic saline solution or prostaglandins (F$_2$ alpha) into the amniotic sac, IM administration of a prostaglandin salt, or use of a prostaglandin (E$_2$) vaginal

Table 45-3. Prostaglandin Abortifacients

Drug	Preparations	Usual Dosage Range	Remarks
Carboprost tromethamine (Prostin/15 M)	Injection—250 mcg/ml	Initially 250 mcg IM; repeat at 1½-hour to 3½-hour intervals; may increase to 500 mcg per dose if necessary; maximum dose 12 mg	Administer deeply IM; abortion is incomplete in about 20% of cases; may produce transient elevation in body temperature (1°–3°F), which persists only as long as drug is being given; forced fluids are recommended during hyperpyrexia; an optional test dose of 100 mcg (0.4 ml) may be given initially to ascertain hypersensitivity to drug
Dinoprost tromethamine (Prostin F2 alpha)	Injection—5 mg/ml	Inject 40 mg *slowly* into the amniotic sac; may repeat in 24 hours with 10 mg to 40 mg if abortion is not established or complete	A transabdominal tap of the amniotic sac should be performed before drug injection and at least 1 ml of fluid withdrawn; do *not* inject drug if tap is bloody; if abortion is incomplete, other measures should be taken to ensure complete fetal expulsion, *e.g.*, hypertonic sodium chloride
Dinoprostone (Prostin E2)	Vaginal suppository—20 mg	Insert 1 suppository high into vagina; repeat at 3-hour to 5-hour intervals until abortion occurs	Keep patient supine for at least 10 minutes following insertion; vomiting occurs in about two thirds of all patients, and diarrhea in approximately half, provide assistance as needed; nausea, headache, chills, and hypotension (20 mm Hg to 30 mm Hg) have also been noted frequently

suppository. Certain prostaglandins (PGE_2, $PGF_{2\alpha}$) have been detected in amniotic fluid during labor or spontaneous abortion and appear to play a role in fetal expulsion by facilitating myometrial contractions. These observations have led to the development of several prostaglandin preparations indicated for the induction of second trimester elective abortion. Currently available drugs can be used by intra-amniotic or IM injections or insertion of a vaginal suppository. These agents are preferable to intra-amniotic injection of hypertonic sodium chloride (see below) because they have a more rapid onset of action and a lower incidence of side-effects. The prostaglandins used as abortifacients are reviewed as a group, followed by a listing of individual drugs and dosages in Table 45-3.

Mechanism
Elicit contractions of the gravid uterus, probably by a direct stimulation of the myometrium; may produce a regression of corpus luteum function; also increase contractile activity of the GI tract and other smooth muscle, especially following systemic injection

Uses
1 Termination of pregnancy from the 12th gestational week through the second trimester
2 Production of uterine evacuation in cases of missed abortion or fetal death up to 28 weeks gestational age (dinoprostone only)
3 Management of hydatidiform mole, that is, nonmeta-

static gestational trophoblastic disease (dinoprostone only)

Dosage
See Table 45-3.

Fate
Drugs are widely distributed in both fetal and maternal bodies; half-life in amniotic fluid is several hours, but much shorter in plasma; metabolized by maternal liver and excreted largely in the urine

Common Side-Effects
Vomiting (especially with IM injection), diarrhea, nausea, headache, shivering, chills, slight hyperthermia, flushing, and abdominal cramps

Significant Adverse Reactions
(Not all are clearly drug related) Chest pain, backache, leg or shoulder pain, breast tenderness, coughing, dyspnea, bronchospasm, wheezing, hyperventilation, hiccup, blurred vision, eye pain, diplopia, paresthesias, hot flashes, dizziness, sweating, fainting, muscle weakness, chest constriction, rash, dehydration, dysuria, hematuria, urine retention, anxiety, vasomotor symptoms, tremor, convulsions, arrhythmias, endometritis, vaginitis, and cervical perforation during abortion

Contraindications
Acute pelvic inflammatory disease; active cardiac, pulmonary, hepatic, or renal disease

Interaction

1 Aspirin and other anti-inflammatory drugs may prolong the time required for fetal expulsion with prostaglandins.

▶ **NURSING ALERTS**

▷ 1 Administer drugs only in a hospital or other health care facility where trained personnel, intensive care, and acute surgical facilities are available.

▷ 2 Recognize that prostaglandins, unlike hypertonic saline, are not usually lethal to the fetus, and the possibility of a liveborn fetus exists, especially if the drugs are given near the end of the second trimester.

▷ 3 Note that prostaglandins have the potential to damage the fetus. Thus, any failed pregnancy termination using these drugs should be completed by other means (*e.g.,* hypertonic sodium chloride; see below).

▷ 4 Use cautiously in patients with asthma, hypertension, heart disease, diabetes, glaucoma, epilepsy, renal or hepatic impairment, anemia, jaundice, vaginitis, and cervicitis.

▷ 5 Be alert for the possibility of cervical perforation during induced abortion, especially in primigravid patients or if oxytocin is used concurrently. Examine patient postabortion for cervical trauma.

▶ **NURSING CONSIDERATIONS**

▷ 1 Perform a transabdominal tap before intra-amniotic injection, and withdraw at least 1 ml of fluid. If no blood is present, injection may be started.

▷ 2 Inject the first milliliter of intra-amniotic solution slowly to determine possible sensitivity. Give remainder of dose over the next 5 minutes to 10 minutes. If abortion has not occurred within 24 hours, drug may be readministered.

▷ 3 Perform a vaginal examination before injection to ensure that intra-amniotic injection catheter has not prolapsed into vagina.

▷ 4 Be aware that transient pyrexia can occur with IM injections of carboprost. Temperature elevations greater than 2°F have been noted in approximately one eighth of the patients receiving the drug. Supplemental fluids

are recommended in cases of drug-induced fever, but other modes of treatment are generally unnecessary, because temperature reverts to normal shortly after therapy is discontinued.

▷ 5 Consider pretreating patients with antiemetic and antidiarrheal medication to minimize the incidence and severity of prostaglandin-induced nausea, vomiting, and diarrhea.

▷ 6 Note that drug-induced abortion is not always complete. If incomplete, other measures should be taken to ensure complete expulsion (*e.g.,* hypertonic sodium chloride; see below).

▷ 7 Monitor uterine activity and other vital signs following drug administration. Observe for any symptoms of vasomotor disturbance (*e.g.,* bradycardia, pallor, rapid fall in blood pressure) and report immediately.

▶ **sodium chloride**
20% Sodium Chloride Solution

Intra-amniotic injection of hypertonic sodium chloride can be used for second trimester abortion, but has been largely replaced by the prostaglandins, which are both safer and more effective. The principal indication for sodium chloride injection is in the patient desiring abortion who has not responded successfully or completely to one of the prostaglandins. When prostaglandin-induced abortion is incomplete, however, injection of hypertonic saline should be delayed until the uterus is no longer contracting. The volume of solution instilled should not exceed the volume of amniotic fluid removed. Injection should be performed at a relatively slow rate and fluid samples taken at regular intervals to ensure that the needle remains in the amniotic cavity. The maximum dose is considered to be 250 ml. Inadvertent intravascular injection should be avoided, because sudden, severe hypernatremia may result, possibly leading to cardiovascular shock, extensive hemolysis, and renal necrosis. The drug should be administered only in a medical unit with intensive care facilities readily available. If labor has not begun within 48 hours after instillation, a re-evaluation of the patient status is indicated.

Summary. Drugs Used in Fertility Control

Drug	Preparations	Usual Dosage Range
Oral contraceptives	See Table 45-2.	
Intrauterine progesterone contraceptive system (Progestasert)	T-shaped IUD—containing 38 mg progesterone; releases 65 mcg/day	Insert system into uterine cavity; replace after 1 year.
Clomiphene (Clomid, Serophene)	Tablets—50 mg	50 mg a day for 5 days; if no response, 100 mg a day for 5 days the second and third months
Menotropins (human menopausal gonadotropins—HMG) (Pergonal)	Injection—containing 75 units FSH activity and 75 units LH activity per ampule	2 ml a day IM for 9 days to 12 days, followed by 10,000 U HCG 1 day after last dose of HMG; may repeat twice at

(continued)

Summary. Drugs Used in Fertility Control *(continued)*

Drug	Preparations	Usual Dosage Range
		monthly intervals if ovulation has occurred
Human chorionic gonadotropin (HCG) (various manufacturers)	Powder for injection—200 U/ml; 5000-U, 10,000-U, and 20,000-U/vial with 10 ml diluent	Induction of ovulation—5,000 U to 10,000 U IM 1 day following last dose of HMG
		Cryptorchidism—highly individualized; see text
		Hypogonadism—500 U to 1000 U 3 times a week for 6 weeks *or* 4000 U 3 times a week for 6 months to 9 months, then 2000 U 3 times a week for 3 months (also highly individualized)
Prostaglandin abortifacients	See Table 45-3.	
Sodium chloride (20% Sodium Chloride Solution)	Injection—20%	Instill at a slow rate into the amniotic cavity, replacing amniotic fluid in equal amounts; maximum dose 250 ml

The term *androgen* refers to a number of naturally occurring or synthetic steroidal compounds exhibiting the masculinizing and tissue-building (anabolic) actions of testosterone, the principal endogenous physiologic androgenic hormone. Testosterone is produced in and secreted by the interstitial (Leydig) cells of the testes under the stimulus of interstitial cell-stimulating hormone (ICSH), which is identical to the luteinizing hormone (LH) of the female.

Testosterone is responsible for the development and support of the male sex organs and the appearance of the secondary sex characteristics (*e.g.,* deep voice, body hair), at the time of puberty. In addition, testosterone exerts a protein anabolic action, thus stimulating growth of skeletal muscle tissue, reduces excretion of sodium, potassium, chloride, nitrogen, and phosphorus, and enhances growth of long bones in prepubertal males. However, it also accelerates the ossification (hardening) process at the ends of long bones, eventually resulting in a conversion of cartilage into bone in the active growth areas (epiphyses) and cessation of further bone growth. For this reason, use of large amounts of androgens in young boys may actually result in a *reduction* of full potential growth due to a premature closing of the epiphyses after an initial spurt in growth. Likewise, androgenic therapy in young males can result in precocious puberty, that is, premature development of the male sex organs and secondary sex characteristics, with possible attendant psychological trauma.

Testosterone itself, although adequately absorbed from the GI tract, is not administered orally because it is rapidly inactivated by the liver. Thus, very large oral doses (*e.g.,* 400 mg/day) are needed to provide clinically effective blood levels. Testosterone may be given by IM injection (aqueous suspension); however, it is relatively short acting when administered by this route, again due to rapid metabolism. Several esters of testosterone (propionate, cypionate, enanthate) exhibit greater stability and slower metabolism and, when injected IM in an oily vehicle, display a prolonged duration of action. Other structural modifications of testosterone (*e.g.,* methyltestosterone, fluoxymesterone) can increase potency and confer resistance to hepatic metabolism, thus permitting use by the oral or buccal route.

A group of synthetic steroids structurally related to testosterone have been developed that display some separation of anabolic from androgenic activity, although the degree of separation is incomplete and variable. These compounds are termed *anabolic steroids* and have been used for a variety of conditions in which an anabolic activity is desired, such as retarded growth and development in children; senile, postmenopausal, or corticosteroid-induced osteoporosis; debilitation resulting from trauma, surgery, or illness; and certain types of anemia (*e.g.,* aplastic). Of course, sufficient caloric and protein intake must be maintained during drug therapy in order to achieve and maintain a positive nitrogen balance. While these compounds exhibit a higher anabolic–androgenic ratio than testosterone or methyltestosterone, excessive dosage or prolonged administration is associated with most of the same untoward effects as seen with testosterone itself. Moreover, anabolic steroids have *not* been proven to enhance athletic prowess to the extent that their use justifies the potential health hazards that can result from

Androgens and
Anabolic Steroids 46

their use. Thus, use of anabolic steroids, especially in women and children, should be closely supervised and restricted to those valid medications listed below.

Other steroids that bear structural resemblance to testosterone but exhibit reduced androgenic activity are used in the treatment of advanced or metastatic breast cancer in postmenopausal women. These drugs, dromostanolone and testolactone, are reviewed in Chapter 74. The rest of the androgenic and anabolic steroids are discussed here as a group, and then are listed in Table 46-1 with their specific indications and recommended doses. Finally, danazol, a synthetic androgen possessing antigonadotropic and androgenic activity that is used in the treatment of endometriosis, is reviewed at the end of this chapter.

Androgens and Anabolic Steroids

Ethylestrenol	Nandrolone
Fluoxymesterone	Oxandrolone
Methandriol	Oxymetholone
Methandrostenolone	Stanozolol
Methyltestosterone	Testosterone

Mechanism
Increase synthesis of RNA and cellular protein; testosterone itself is converted to its active metabolite dihydrotestosterone, other derivatives may enhance RNA and protein synthesis directly; stimulate growth of muscle, bone, skin, and hair and accelerate closure of epiphyses at ends of long bones; increase production of red blood cells; decrease excretion of nitrogen, phosphorus, sodium, and probably also calcium and potassium; temporarily arrest progression of estrogen-dependent carcinomas; *large doses* can suppress pituitary gonadotropin secretion, and decrease spermatogenesis through feedback inhibition of FSH.

Uses
(See Table 46-1 for specific indications.)
1 Replacement therapy in androgen deficiency states, such as testicular hypofunction, pituitary dysfunction, eunuchism (complete testicular failure), eunuchoidism (partial testicular failure), cryptorchidism, castration, or male climacteric
2 Treatment of low sperm count or impotence due to androgen deficiency (low doses only)
3 Palliative therapy of androgen-responsive inoperable breast cancer in 1-year to 5-year postmenopausal women
4 Production of a positive nitrogen balance in those conditions in which an anabolic action is desired, for example, retarded growth and physical development in children, osteoporosis, anemia, corticosteroid-induced catabolism, and debilitation resulting from injury, trauma, illness, and other causes
5 Relief of postpartum breast engorgement (*rarely* used)

Dosage
See Table 46-1.

Fate
Testosterone is rapidly inactivated when given orally or by IM injection. Pellet implantation provides a sustained release of medication for 3 months to 4 months. Esterification of testosterone increases stability, and thus prolongs the duration of action. Most other androgens are well absorbed when taken orally. They are metabolized in the liver and excreted primarily in the urine, with small amounts in the feces.

Common Side-Effects
Female virilization (*e.g.,* hirsutism, voice changes, clitoral enlargement), amenorrhea, changes in libido, flushing, nausea with oral preparations

Significant Adverse Reactions
Males
Prepubertal: phallic enlargement, increased erections, premature closing of epiphyses.

Postpubertal: impotence, testicular atrophy, bladder irritability, decreased sperm count, epididymitis, chronic priapism, gynecomastia

Females
Male pattern baldness, menstrual irregularities, suppression of ovulation or lactation

Both sexes
Acne; oily skin; excitation; insomnia; anxiety; depression; headache; paresthesia; chills; leukopenia; polycythemia; hypercalcemia; pain; swelling, urticaria, and irritation at injection sites; jaundice; hepatic necrosis; sodium and water retention; increased serum cholesterol; in addition, *oral* preparations may cause vomiting and ulcer symptoms; alterations can occur in many clinical laboratory tests.

Contraindications
Pregnancy, lactation, known or suspected prostatic or breast cancer in males; in addition, anabolic hormones are also contraindicated in prostatic hypertrophy, pituitary insufficiency, history of myocardial infarction, hepatic dysfunction, nephrosis, hypercalcemia, and in elderly asthenic males who may react adversely to overstimulation

Interactions
1 Androgens may potentiate the action of oral anticoagulants, phenylbutazone, and oxyphenbutazone.
2 Barbiturates and other hypnotics, phenytoin, and phenylbutazone may decrease the action of androgens by accelerating their metabolic breakdown.
3 Androgens can antagonize the action of calcitonin and parathyroid hormone.
4 Corticosteroids may increase the severity of androgen-induced edema.
5 Anabolic steroids may decrease blood glucose in diabetics, reducing insulin or oral hypoglycemic drug requirements.

Table 46-1. Androgens and Anabolic Steroids

Drug	Preparations	Usual Dosage Range	Remarks
Androgens			
Fluoxymesterone (Android-F, Halotestin, Ora-Testryl)	Tablets—2 mg, 5 mg, 10 mg	Hypogonadism, impotence—2 mg to 10 mg a day Delayed puberty—2 mg a day initially; increase gradually as necessary Breast cancer—15 mg to 30 mg a day in divided doses Postpartum breast engorgement—2.5 mg when active labor begins, thereafter, 5 mg to 10 mg a day in divided doses for 4 days to 5 days	Potent, orally effective, short-acting derivative of testosterone, approximately five times more active than testosterone itself; minimal sodium and water retention, but frequent GI distress (administer drug with food); be alert for symptoms suggestive of peptic ulcer; confirmatory tests should be performed (see also Chap. 74)
Methyltestosterone (Android, Metandren, Oreton, Testred, Virilon)	Tablets: Oral—10 mg, 25 mg Buccal—5 mg, 10 mg Capsules—10 mg	Male hypogonadism, impotence, male climacteric—10 mg to 40 mg a day (oral) or 5 mg to 20 mg a day (buccal) Cryptorchism—30 mg a day (oral) or 15 mg a day (buccal) Postpartum breast pain and engorgement—80 mg a day (oral) or 40 mg a day (buccal) for 3 days to 5 days Breast cancer—200 mg a day (oral) or 100 mg a day (buccal)	Orally effective, short-acting androgen somewhat less effective than testosterone esters; does not produce full sexual maturation in prepubertal testicular failure unless patient has been pretreated with testosterone; creatinuria is a common finding, although its significance is not known; buccal tablets should be placed between cheek and gum and allowed to dissolve; do not chew or swallow, and avoid eating, drinking, or smoking for at least 1 hour after ingestion; advise patient to report any inflammation or pain in oral cavity following drug usage; good oral hygiene should be stressed to reduce infection or irritation (see also Chap. 74)
Testosterone (Android-T, Andro 100, Histerone, Testaqua, Testoject)	Injection (aqueous)—25 mg, 50 mg, 100 mg/ml	Male hypogonadism, impotence, male climacteric—10 mg to 25 mg IM 2 to 3 times a week Postpartum breast engorgement—25 mg to 50 mg a day for 3 days to 4 days Breast carcinoma—100 mg 3 times a week	Male sex hormone used as replacement therapy in deficiency states, for relief of breast engorgement and treatment of mammary carcinoma in women; inject IM only deep into gluteal muscle; if crystals are present in the vial, warming and shaking will disperse them; absorption is slow and effects persist for several days; do not administer more frequently than recommended; regression of mammary tumors should be apparent within 3 months; occasionally, acceleration of tumor growth is encountered, in which case discontinue immediately; in some of these cases, estrogens will then cause regression (see also Chap. 74)
Testosterone propionate (Testex)	Injection (in oil)—25 mg, 50 mg, 100 mg/ml	IM—see Testosterone	Ester of testosterone formulated in an oily vehicle; absorption may be somewhat slower than testosterone aqueous, but duration of action is comparable
Testosterone cypionate (Andro-Cyp, Andronate, depAndro, Depo-Testosterone, Depotest,	Injection (in oil)—50 mg, 100 mg, 200 mg/ml	Hypogonadism, male climacteric—200 mg to 400 mg IM every 4 weeks Oligospermia—100 mg to 200	Long-acting esters of testosterone providing a therapeutic effect for approximately 4 weeks with a single injection; not recommended

(continued)

Table 46-1. Androgens and Anabolic Steroids (continued)

Drug	Preparations	Usual Dosage Range	Remarks
Duratest, Testa-C, Testoject-LA, Testionate, T-Ionate P.A.)		mg every 4 weeks to 6 weeks	for use in treating metastatic breast carcinoma; inject *deep* into gluteal muscle; Enanthate (200 mg/ml) is available in combination with propionate (25 mg/ml) as Testoject-E.P. (see also Chap. 74)
Testosterone enanthate (Android-T, Andro-L.A., Andryl, Anthatest, Delatestryl, Everone, Testate, Testone L.A., Testostroval P.A.)			
Anabolic Steroids			
Ethylestrenol (Maxibolin)	Tablets—2 mg Elixir—2 mg/5 ml	Weight gain, osteoporosis, anemias: Adults—4 mg a day up to 8 mg a day initially if needed Children—2 mg a day (range 1 mg–3 mg a day)	Anabolic steroid given for a 6-week period, then stopped for 4 weeks; if indication for its use is still evident, it may be resumed for additional 6-week period; in children, x-rays should be taken before reinstating therapy to determine stage of bone maturation
Methandriol (Andriol, Durabolic, Methydiol)	Injection: Aqueous—50 mg/ml Dipropionate in oil—50 mg/ml	Senile and postmenopausal osteoporosis: Adults—IM 10 mg to 40 mg a day (aqueous) or 50 mg to 100 mg 1 to 2 times a week (oil) Children—IM 5 mg to 10 mg a day	Anabolic steroid with approximately twice as much anabolic as androgenic activity; rated as only *possibly* effective and infrequently used
Nandrolone decanoate (Analone, Anabolin L.A., Androlone-D, Deca-Durabolin, Hybolin)	Injection (in oil)—50 mg, 100 mg, 200 mg/ml	Osteoporosis, tissue building, anemia: Adults—50 mg to 100 mg IM every 3 weeks to 4 weeks Children—25 mg to 50 mg every 3 weeks to 4 weeks Metastatic breast cancer: 100 mg to 200 mg a week	Long-acting ester of nandrolone (duration 3 wk to 4 wk); rated *probably* effective for adjunctive therapy of senile or postmenopausal osteoporosis and *possibly* effective for increasing tissue building activity postsurgically, for control of metastatic breast carcinoma, and in certain types of refractory anemia
Nandrolone phenproprionate (Anabolin I.M., Androlone, Durabolin, Hybolin Improved, Nandrobolic, Nandrolin)	Injection (in oil)—25 mg, 50 mg/ml	Metastatic breast cancer: 25 mg to 100 mg/week IM Osteoporosis, anemia, tissue building: Adults—25 mg to 50 mg a week Children—12.5 mg to 25 mg every 2 weeks to 4 weeks	Synthetic androgen with high anabolic–androgenic ratio; effects persist 1 week to 3 weeks; injection should be made deeply into gluteal muscle in adults; intermittent therapy is recommended, with 4-week to 8-week rest periods every 4 months (see Chap. 74)
Oxandrolone (Anavar)	Tablets—2.5 mg	Osteoporosis, tissue building: Adults—2.5 mg 2 to 4 times a day (up to 20 mg a day) for 2 weeks to 4 weeks; repeat after a rest period if desired Children—0.25 mg/kg a day	Synthetic anabolic steroid with low androgenic activity; used frequently to help promote weight gain following trauma, severe illness, major surgery, or prolonged corticosteroid administration; do not administer longer than 3 months
Oxymetholone (Anadrol-50)	Tablets—50 mg	Anemias—(adults and children) 1 mg to 2 mg/kg/day to a maximum of 5 mg/kg/day (highly individualized)	Synthetic anabolic steroid used primarily for anemias due to deficient red cell production, congenital or acquired aplastic anemia, and anemias resulting from administration of myelotoxic drugs; a minimum of 3 months to

Table 46-1. Androgens and Anabolic Steroids (continued)

Drug	Preparations	Usual Dosage Range	Remarks
			6 months should be allowed, because response is often slow; following remission, some patients may be able to stop drug, while others may require a minimum daily dosage
Stanozolol (Winstrol)	Tablets—2 mg	Osteoporosis, anemias, tissue building: Adults—initially 2 mg 2 to 3 times a day Children—1 mg to 2 mg 2 to 3 times a day	Anabolic steroid with minimal androgenic effects at normal doses; administer with meals to minimize GI distress; primarily used for aplastic anemia and senile or postmenopausal osteoporosis

▶ **NURSING ALERTS**

▷ 1 Observe female patients receiving androgens closely for signs of virilization (see Common Side-Effects) and decide if therapy should be continued. Some changes (e.g., voice deepening, hirsutism) may be irreversible even when drug is discontinued.

▷ 2 Test regularly for development of hypercalcemia, which occurs mainly in bedridden, immobilized patients or in persons with metastatic breast cancer. In the latter patients, elevated calcium levels usually indicate bone metastases. Discontinue medication if symptomatic hypercalcemia occurs (e.g., vomiting, constipation, loss of muscle tone, polyuria, lethargy), provide copious fluids to prevent renal calculi, and treat symptoms with appropriate medications.

▷ 3 Stop drug administration if liver tests are abnormal, if signs of excessive sexual stimulation occur (e.g., priapism), or if vaginal bleeding develops. Observe for signs of jaundice (yellow skin or sclera, itching) or for excessive stimulation in elderly patients.

▷ 4 Use cautiously in patients with a history of coronary artery disease or myocardial infarction and in prepubertal males.

▷ 5 When anabolic steroids are given to prepubertal males, carefully observe for signs of premature sexual development. Rate of bone growth and maturation should be periodically checked radiologically to minimize danger of premature fusion of epiphyses.

▶ **NURSING CONSIDERATIONS**

▷ 1 Instruct diabetic patients to be alert for signs of hypoglycemia (sweating, tremor, anxiety, vertigo) and to adjust antidiabetic drug dosage accordingly.

▷ 2 Perform periodic liver function tests, serum cholesterol determinations, and tests for serum calcium levels during therapy.

▷ 3 Advise male patients to notify physician if priapism, reduced ejaculatory volume, impotence, or gynecomastia occurs. These symptoms may be controlled by dosage reduction or temporary cessation of therapy.

▷ 4 Encourage bedridden patients to perform exercises regularly to minimize development of hypercalcemia.

▷ 5 Instruct patients on prolonged therapy to note signs of development of excessive fluid retention (e.g., edema, weight gain). Drug should be temporarily withdrawn or a diuretic administered.

▷ 6 Advise taking oral tablets with food to minimize GI distress. Buccal tablets should be allowed to dissolve between gum and cheek, or under the tongue, but should not be swallowed. Caution against eating, drinking, or smoking while tablet is in place.

▷ 7 Observe patients taking anticoagulants for signs of bleeding (e.g., petechiae, ecchymoses), because dosage of anticoagulant drug may have to be reduced during androgen therapy.

▷ 8 Recognize that anabolic steroids do not significantly enhance athletic ability and should not be used to improve performance or stamina, because the risk far outweighs the potential benefit.

▷ 9 Do not administer anabolic steroids for longer than 90 days without careful patient reassessment.

▷ 10 Be aware that androgens may alter the following clinical laboratory tests: liver function, thyroid function, glucose tolerance, blood coagulation, creatinine excretion, serum cholesterol, and the metyrapone test.

▶ **danazol**
Danocrine

A synthetic derivative of 17-alpha-ethinyl testosterone, danazol inhibits the release of gonadotropins from the pituitary gland and exhibits a weak androgenic effect. No estrogenic or progestational activity has been demonstrated. Danazol provides alternative therapy for endometriosis in those women who cannot tolerate or who fail to respond to other forms of treatment, and may also be employed in severe fibrocystic breast disease and hereditary angioedema.

Mechanism
Suppresses release of FSH and LH from the adenohypophysis, thus inhibiting ovarian function, resulting in anovulation and associated amenorrhea; consequently, complete resolution of endometrial lesions occurs in the majority of cases.

Uses

1 Treatment of endometriosis in those patients who cannot tolerate or who fail to respond to other means of therapy (not indicated in cases in which surgery is the treatment of choice)
2 Symptomatic treatment of severe fibrocystic breast disease
3 Prevention of attacks of all types (*e.g.,* cutaneous, laryngeal, abdominal) of hereditary angioedema
4 Treatment of gynecomastia, infertility, and menorrhagia (investigational use only)

Dosage

Endometriosis

400 mg twice a day for 6 months to 9 months; may reinstitute therapy if symptoms recur

Fibrocystic breast disease

100 mg to 400 mg/day in two divided doses for 3 months to 6 months

Angioedema

Initially, 200 mg two to three times/day; reduce dosage at 1-month to 3-month intervals if clinical response is favorable.

Common Side-Effects

Flushing, sweating

Significant Adverse Reactions

Virilization (acne, oily skin, hirsutism, deepening of the voice, decrease in breast size, clitoral hypertrophy), vaginitis, vaginal bleeding, edema, weight gain, nervousness; other effects for which a direct causal relationship has not been established are loss of hair, changes in libido, pelvic pain, muscle cramps, back, neck, or leg pain, skin rash, nasal congestion, nausea, vomiting, gastroenteritis, dizziness, headache, tremor, paresthesias, and visual disturbances

Contraindications

Pregnancy, lactation, undiagnosed vaginal bleeding, and markedly impaired cardiac, hepatic, or renal function

▶ NURSING ALERTS

▷ 1 Use cautiously in patients with cardiac or renal impairment, migraine, and epilepsy.
▷ 2 Begin therapy during menstruation, if possible, to ensure that patient is not pregnant. Otherwise, perform pregnancy test before initiating therapy if possibility of pregnancy exists.
▷ 3 Rule out carcinoma of the breast before initiating therapy for fibrocystic breast disease. If any nodule persists or enlarges during therapy, discontinue drug and perform appropriate tests.

▶ NURSING CONSIDERATIONS

▷ 1 Reassure patients that drug-induced anovulation and amenorrhea are reversible within 60 days to 90 days after termination of therapy.
▷ 2 Observe patients for development of signs of virilization and advise physician. Some of these symptoms may be irreversible.

Summary. Androgens and Anabolic Steroids

Drug	Preparations	Usual Dosage Range
Androgens and anabolic steroids	See Table 46-1.	
Danazol (Danocrine)	Capsules—50 mg, 100 mg, 200 mg	Endometriosis—400 mg twice a day for 6 months to 9 months
		Fibrocystic breast disease—100 mg to 400 mg a day in two divided doses for 3 months to 6 months
		Angioedema—200 mg initially, two to three times/day; reduce dosage at 1-month to 3-month intervals if clinical response is favorable

Drugs Acting on Gastrointestinal Function

VI

The digestive system functions to provide body cells with water, electrolytes, vitamins, and nutritive substances. During passage through the GI tract, ingested carbohydrates, fats, and proteins are converted into smaller, absorbable units by the action of digestive enzymes, aided by specialized secretions such as bile and hydrochloric acid.

The luminal contents of the digestive tract are transported and effectively mixed with digestive secretions and mucus by specialized muscular movements. GI motility and secretion are affected by a complex interaction of intrinsic and extrinsic neural influences and by several peptide hormones. This chapter briefly reviews the important anatomical features of the GI tract, then explores in detail the principal physiologic functions of the digestive system.

Gastrointestinal Physiology—A Review

47

I Organization of the Digestive System

A Gastrointestinal Tract

The GI tract (digestive tract or alimentary canal) is a continuous muscular tube lined with mucous membrane, extending from the mouth to the anus, with regional anatomical and functional modifications as outlined in Tables 47-1 and 47-2. The digestive tract includes the mouth, pharynx, esophagus, stomach, and the small and large intestines.

B Accessory Organs of Digestion

The salivary glands, pancreas, liver, and gallbladder contribute exocrine secretions essential to the chemical breakdown of food. Digestion is also aided mechanically by the teeth, tongue, and cheeks.

II General Histology of the Gastrointestinal Tract

The walls of the organs making up the digestive tract contain four basic layers (tunics) of tissue. From the lumen outward they are as follows:

A Tunica Mucosa

The tunica mucosa or mucous membrane consists of a lining *epithelium,* which is in direct contact with the luminal contents. The epithelium may be protective, secretory, or ab-

Table 47-1. Anatomical and Histologic Features of the Major Organs of the Digestive Tract

Organ	Gross Anatomical Features	Histologic Features
Esophagus	Muscular tube continuous with the pharynx	Mucosal epithelium is nonkeratinizing *stratified squamous*. Composition of the tunica muscularis: upper one third—striated muscle; middle one third—striated and smooth muscle; and lower one third—smooth muscle. Outer layer—adventitia
Stomach	Fundus—rounded upper portion lying above the entrance of the esophagus Body—dilated (major) central region Pyloric antrum—tapering distal portion terminating at the pyloric sphincter Greater curvature—Large convex curvature on the lateral border Lesser curvature—smaller, concave curvature on the medial border The empty (contracted) stomach exhibits longitudinal folds of mucosa termed *rugae*	Mucosal epithelium is *simple columnar*. Tunica muscularis contains three layers of smooth muscle: an inner *oblique*, a middle *circular*, and an outer *longitudinal*. Outer layer is a *serosa* formed by the visceral peritoneum, which reflects from the greater and lesser curvatures as the greater and lesser omenta.
Small Intestine	Duodenum—first 25 cm, which receives the common bile duct and the pancreatic duct Jejunum—middle segment representing about two fifths of the small intestine Ileum—remaining three fifths, rich in lymphatic aggregates (Peyer's patches)	Mucosal epithelium is *simple columnar*. Submucosa contains Brunner's glands. Outer layer is a *serosa*. Absorptive surface area is increased by the following structural features: 1. *Plicae circulares* (valves of Kerckring)—circular folds of the mucosa and submucosa projecting into the lumen 2. *Villi*—finger-like projections of mucous membrane containing a blood capillary and a lacteal (lymphatic) 3. *Microvilli*—microscopic projections of the free surfaces of lining epithelial cells
Large Intestine	Cecum—blind pouch from which the vermiform appendix is suspended Colon (ascending, transverse, descending and sigmoid) Rectum Anal canal	Mucosal epithelium is *simple columnar*. Outer layer is a *serosa* except for the rectum and anal canal, which are covered by adventitia. Prominent morphologic features include: 1. *Taeniae coli*—three strap-like bands of longitudinal smooth muscle 2. *Haustra*—sacculations or pouches giving the colon a scalloped appearance 3. *Epiploic appendages*—fat-filled tabs suspended from the colon

sorptive. Histologically, the epithelium is stratified squamous in the mouth, pharynx (except for the nasopharynx), esophagus, and anal canal, while it is simple columnar in the stomach and intestines.

A loose connective tissue, the *lamina propria,* supports the epithelium and binds it to the two underlying thin layers of smooth muscle, the *muscularis mucosa.*

B Tunica Submucosa

This loose connective tissue layer contains blood vessels, lymphatic tissue, and the nerve *plexus of Meissner* (submucosal plexus).

C Tunica Muscularis (Muscularis Externa)

Characteristically, the tunica muscularis is composed of two layers of smooth muscle, an inner, somewhat thicker circular layer and an outer longitudinal layer. Between these lies the *plexus of Auerbach* (myenteric plexus) which contains autonomic nerve fibers and ganglia.

D Tunica Serosa or Adventitia

Generally, the outermost tunic is a serous membrane or *serosa* (visceral peritoneum) composed of loose connective tissue covered by a layer of squamous mesothelial cells. In certain parts of the digestive tract (such as the esophagus and rectum) where the connective tissue is not covered by mesothelial cells, the outer tunic is termed the *adventitia*.

III Functional Overview

The principal activities of the digestive system include (1) motility, (2) secretion, (3) digestion, and (4) absorption.

A Motility

Muscular movements propel materials through the digestive tract, aid in the mechanical breakdown of food, promote mixing of luminal contents with mucus and digestive secretions, and facilitate absorption by renewing the absorptive surface.

The motor functions of the alimentary canal are of two basic types: *mixing* and *propulsive.* These movements are subject to intrinsic and extrinsic neural influences as well as to hormonal regulation.

The alimentary canal is extensively innervated by autonomic nerve fibers belonging to both the sympathetic and parasympathetic divisions. Autonomic elements are represented in the intrinsic nerve supply, the submucosal plexus (of Meissner) and more extensively in the myenteric plexus (of Auerbach). The nerves maintain muscle tone and regulate the force and velocity of muscular contractions.

GI motility is generally increased by parasympathetic (vagal and sacral nerve) stimulation and inhibited by sympathetic activation. Only the sphincters respond in an opposite manner, being relaxed by parasympathetic stimulation and contracted by sympathetic stimulation.

The motor functions of individual digestive organs are summarized in Table 47-2.

B Secretion

The major secretions of the digestive system are saliva, gastric juice, intestinal juice, pancreatic juice, and bile. These are produced by specialized exocrine glands associated with specific components of the digestive tract. Basically, each secretion consists of water, electrolytes, and one or more active organic constituents. Mucin, the active constituent of mucus, is produced by all segments of the digestive tract. Mucus serves to lubricate and protect each region of the alimentary canal from chemical and mechanical irritation.

Digestive secretions are produced in response to both mechanical and chemical stimulation. Nervous and humoral (hormonal) mechanisms control the rate and, in some instances, the relative composition of secretions. Generally, parasympathetic activity promotes GI secretion.

The major digestive secretions are characterized in Table 47-2.

1 Control of Gastric Secretion

Gastric secretion, which occurs in three phases, *cephalic, gastric,* and *intestinal,* is controlled by neural and humoral mechanisms.

The *cephalic phase,* which occurs before food enters the stomach, may be initiated by the thought, sight, smell, or taste of food. This phase, which is mediated by the vagus (X) nerve (and may therefore be abolished by vagotomy), elicits secretion of gastric juice high in acid and pepsin content.

The *gastric phase* of secretion, which is mediated by the hormone *gastrin,* takes place while food is present in the stomach. Gastrin is released from the pyloric antrum in response to mechanical distention or chemical stimulation (protein digestion products, alcohol, caffeine, others). Gastrin release is the major stimulus to acid secretion. Other actions of gastrin are listed in Table 47-3.

During the *intestinal phase,* the arrival of chyme in the duodenum causes the stomach to secrete small amounts of gastric juice. This stimulation is hormonally mediated by an intestinal gastrin.

2 Inhibition of Gastric Secretion

Contact of the duodenal mucosa with substances such as protein digestion products, fats, and acid inhibits gastric secretion. Further distention of the duodenum initiates the enterogastric reflex, which also inhibits gastric secretion and gastric motility (emptying).

Table 47-2. Major Activities of the Digestive Tract

Organ	Motor Activity	Secretion	Digestion	Absorption
Mouth	Chewing (mastication)—ingested food is subdivided into small particles by the teeth and mixed with saliva to form a bolus. Swallowing (deglutition)—oral phase of swallowing is initiated voluntarily as the tongue forces the bolus toward the oropharynx.	Saliva is secreted by buccal and salivary glands (parotid, submaxillary, and sublingual) in response to the sight, smell, or taste of food. Saliva moistens the mucous membranes, cleanses the mouth and teeth, lubricates the food to facilitate chewing and swallowing, and enhances the taste of food.	Digestion of complex carbohydrates (starches) is initiated by salivary amylase (ptyalin).	Certain drugs (e.g., nitroglycerin) are absorbed sublingually.
Pharynx	Swallowing (pharyngeal phase)—swallowing proceeds reflexly as the bolus enters the oropharynx and continues through the laryngopharynx into the esophagus.			
Esophagus	Swallowing (esophageal phase)—swallowing continues reflexly, coordinated by a swallowing center in the medulla. Bolus passes along the esophagus into the stomach through peristalsis.	Esophageal glands secrete mucus to facilitate passage of bolus and protect the mucosa.		
Stomach	Receptive relaxation—stomach adapts to increased volume without an increase in intragastric pressure Reservoir function—stomach stores contents ingested in a meal and allows partial digestion and gradual emptying into the intestine. Mixing function—mixing waves, aided by peristaltic waves, macerate the bolus, mix it with gastric juice, and reduce it into chyme. Propulsive function—peristaltic waves force the chyme through the pyloric sphincter into the duodenum. Gastric emptying—chyme leaves the stomach at a rate consistent with the most effective rates of digestion and absorption by the small intestine. The rate of gastric emptying is influenced by the physical and chemical composition of chyme (e.g., volume, viscosity, acidity, osmotic pressure). Hormonal and neural factors, including emotional state, can affect the gastric emptying rate.	Gastric juice contains: *Mucus* (secreted by mucous cells); protects the stomach wall from autodigestion *Hydrochloric acid* (secreted by parietal cells); converts pepsinogen into active pepsin; provides optimal *p*H for pepsin activity; inactivates ptyalin; bacteriostatic action *Rennin*—the milk curdling enzyme which acts upon the milk protein; of little importance in humans *Pepsinogen* (secreted by chief or zymogenic cells); inactive form of the proteolytic enzyme pepsin *Intrinsic factor* (secreted by parietal cells); forms a complex with vitamin B_{12} to allow intestinal absorption of cyanocobalamin	Protein digestion—pepsin begins the digestion of proteins by attacking certain amino-acid linkages and reducing proteins into proteoses and peptones. Fat digestion—gastric lipase acts principally on tributyrin and is not considered to contribute significantly to the digestion of fats.	Certain drugs (e.g., alcohol, aspirin), some water, and a few electrolytes are absorbed from the stomach.
Small Intestine	Segmentation—these fairly regular localized contractions of the circular smooth	*Succus entericus* (intestinal juice)—intestinal glands secrete	Fats are emulsified by bile and are digested principally by	Water, electrolytes, vitamins, and nutrients (products of

Table 47-2. Major Activities of the Digestive Tract (continued)

Organ	Motor Activity	Secretion	Digestion	Absorption
	muscle mix the chyme with pancreatic, intestinal, and hepatobiliary secretions. Pendular movements—these mixing contractions involve the longitudinal muscles of the tunica muscularis. Peristalsis—peristaltic waves propel the intestinal contents onward at a rate suitable for optimal absorption. Villus contractions—independent, asynchronous contractions of individual villi (stimulated by the putative hormone villikinin) renew the surface area for absorption.	a slightly alkaline fluid containing water, mucus, and enzymes that complete the digestion of carbohydrates, fats, and proteins. *Bile* (produced by the liver and concentrated by the gallbladder) and *pancreatic juice* are delivered to the duodenum by the common bile duct and pancreatic ducts, respectively.	Pancreatic lipase. Carbohydrates are digested by pancreatic amylase and by intestinal disaccharidases. Proteolytic enzymes produced by the pancreas and the small intestine digest proteins (as detailed in Table 47-4). Enterokinase converts pancreatic trypsinogen into active trypsin. Nucleic acids are broken down by pancreatic and intestinal nucleases.	carbohydrates, fat, and protein digestion) are absorbed readily from the small intestine (particularly the duodenum and jejunum), as are most orally administered drugs. Bile salts and vitamin B_{12} are absorbed from the ileum.
Large Intestine	Haustral churning—haustral (segmenting) contractions promote water and electrolyte absorption. Peristalsis—peristalic waves move the contents along the length of the large intestine. Mass peristalsis—strong propulsive contractions drive the luminal contents into the sigmoid colon and rectum. Defecation—reflex evacuation of the bowel initiated by distention of the rectum; reflex is integrated by the sacral segments of the spinal cord.	*Mucus* is secreted to protect the mucosa from chemical and mechanical trauma, and to lubricate the colonic contents, thereby facilitating passage of feces.		Water is absorbed, thereby reducing the contents from a semifluid to a semisolid mass. Some electrolytes and certain vitamins (B and K) synthesized in the colon are absorbed. Organic products of bacterial action (*e.g.,* indole and skatole) are absorbed and transported to the liver for biotransformation to less toxic substances. Rectally administered drugs are absorbed from the rectum.

C Digestion

Most substances ingested in the diet are structurally complex carbohydrates, fats, or proteins, which cannot be absorbed and utilized by the body in their natural states. During the process of digestion these complex organic constituents are chemically broken down into molecules that can be absorbed readily into body fluids. Specific digestive enzymes from the salivary glands, stomach, small intestine, and pancreas hydrolyze (1) complex carbohydrates into simple sugars; (2) fats into monoglycerides, fatty acids, and glycerol; and (3) proteins into amino acids.

The digestion of carbohydrates is initiated in the mouth by salivary amylase and is completed in the small intestine by pancreatic amylase and intestinal disaccharidases. Proteins are broken down by the combined actions of gastric, pancreatic, and intestinal proteolytic enzymes. Fats are emulsified by bile and are hydrolyzed mainly by pancreatic lipase.

The major digestive enzymes are presented in Table 47-4.

D Absorption

Absorption involves the transport of substances (water, electrolytes, vitamins, and products of digestion) across the wall of the digestive tract into the blood or lymph. Mechanisms of transport include diffusion, osmosis, active transport, and pinocytosis.

The proximal small intestine is the major site of absorption of vitamins, water, electrolytes, and nutrients. With the exception of vitamin B_{12} and the bile salts, which are absorbed mainly from the terminal ileum, most substrates are absorbed from the duodenum and upper jejunum. Intestinal villi, richly endowed with blood capillaries and lymphatic vessels (lacteals), provide an extensive surface area that greatly facilitates absorption. Epithelial cells lining the small intestine exhibit

Table 47-3. Major Hormones of the Digestive Tract

Hormone	Source	Stimulus for Secretion	Hormone Action
Gastrin	Gastric mucosa of pyloric antrum	Products of protein digestion Ingested Ca^{++} Acetylcholine Vagal stimulation Alcohol Caffeine	Stimulates gastric acid and pepsinogen secretion by the gastric mucosa; increases flow of hepatic bile; stimulates pancreatic enzyme secretion; promotes GI motility and gallbladder contraction
Intestinal gastrin	Duodenal mucosa	Entry of chyme into the duodenum	Stimulates secretion of gastric juice by the gastric glands
Enterogastrone*	Duodenal mucosa	Fats	Inhibits gastric acid secretion and motility
Secretin	Duodenal mucosa	Acid	Stimulates secretion of a watery, alkaline (bicarbonate-rich) pancreatic juice; promotes bile secretion
Enterocrinin*	Duodenal mucosa	Acid chyme	Stimulates secretion of intestinal juice (succus entericus)
Cholecystokinin (CCK) or Pancreozymin (PZ)	Duodenal and jejunal mucosa	Long-chain fatty acids Amino acids (tryptophan and phenylalanine) Acid Ca^{++}	Stimulates gallbladder contraction and relaxes the sphincter of Oddi to promote bile flow into the duodenum Stimulates secretion of an enzyme-rich pancreatic juice

* *Putative hormones*—Existence not conclusively established; other putative hormones affecting GI function include villikinin, gastric inhibitory peptide (GIP), vasoactive intestinal peptide (VIP), motilin, and chymodenin

Table 47-4. Major Digestive Enzymes

Source	Enzyme	Activator	Substrate	Action
Salivary glands	Salivary amylase (ptyalin)		Starch, glycogen	Initiates digestion of carbohydrates, converting starch into dextrins and disaccharides
Gastric glands	Pepsin (pepsinogen*)	HCl	Proteins, polypeptides	Converts proteins and polypeptides into smaller polypeptides (proteoses and peptones)
Exocrine pancreas	Trypsin (trypsinogen*)	Enterokinase	Proteins, polypeptides	Converts proteins and polypeptides into smaller peptides and amino acids
	Chymotrypsin (chymotrypsinogen*)	Trypsin	Proteins, polypeptides	Converts proteins and polypeptides into smaller peptides and amino acids
	Carboxypeptidase (procarboxypeptidase*)	Trypsin	Polypeptides	Converts polypeptides into smaller peptides and amino acids
	Pancreatic amylase (amylopsin)	Chloride ion	Starch, glycogen, dextrins	Converts complex carbohydrates into disaccharides
	Pancreatic lipase (steapsin)	Emulsifying agents	Triglycerides	Converts fats into fatty acids and glycerol
	Ribonuclease		RNA	Converts RNA into nucleotides
	Deoxyribonuclease		DNA	Converts DNA into nucleotides
Intestinal mucosa	Enterokinase		Trypsinogen	Converts trypsinogen into the active proteolytic enzyme trypsin
	Aminopeptidase		Polypeptides	Converts polypeptides into smaller units
	Dipeptidase		Dipeptides	Complete protein digestion by converting dipeptides into absorbable amino acids
	Disaccharidase		Disaccharides	Convert disaccharides into absorbable monosaccharides
	Sucrase		Sucrose	Converts sucrose into glucose and fructose
	Lactase		Lactose	Converts lactose into glucose and galactose
	Maltase		Maltose	Converts maltose into glucose
	Intestinal lipase		Monoglycerides	Converts fats into fatty acids and glycerol
	Nuclease (nucleotidase)		Nucleotides	Convert nucleotides into nucleosides and phosphates

* Inactive form of the enzyme

microvilli that further increase the absorptive surface. Finally, the epithelium of the small intestine contains a variety of specialized transport systems for certain substrates (such as amino acids and glucose).

Absorption through the gastric mucosa is very limited. Aspirin and alcohol are, however, rapidly absorbed from the stomach.

1 Absorption of Carbohydrates

Carbohydrates are absorbed mainly in the form of monosaccharides (pentoses or hexoses), principally from the duodenum and upper jejunum. Glucose and galactose are absorbed by an active carrier system intimately linked to the sodium transport mechanism. Fructose is transported by facilitated diffusion, while the remaining monosaccharides are transported by simple passive diffusion.

2 Absorption of Fats (Lipids)

The products of fat digestion—fatty acids, glycerol, and monoglycerides—are absorbed mainly in the duodenum. Fatty acids containing fewer than 12 carbons are transported directly into the portal blood. Those containing more than 12 carbons are transported into the lymphatics (lacteals) in the form of chylomicrons.

Glycerol may pass into the liver to be used for glycogen synthesis; it may be oxidized by the intestinal mucosal cells, or it may be utilized for intracellular resynthesis of triglycerides.

Certain essential fat-soluble substances and vitamins A, D, E, and K require bile for their absorption. Water-soluble aggregates containing fatty acids, monoglycerides, and bile salts are called micelles.

3 Absorption of Proteins

Ingested proteins are absorbed mainly as amino acids from the duodenum and jejunum. Three active, carrier-mediated transport systems for amino acids have been characterized. Some dipeptides and tripeptides are also actively transported.

Occasionally, whole proteins may be absorbed from the intestine through pinocytosis. For example, gamma globulins (antibodies) ingested by a suckling infant are absorbed intact in this manner.

4 Absorption of Water

The net absorption of water from the intestines is variable, being greatly affected by the osmotic pressure and electrolyte composition of the intestinal contents. The transport of water occurs mainly through osmosis, with the driving force for water absorption being generated by the active transport of various solutes (such as glucose, amino acids, and electrolytes). Pinocytotic vacuoles have also been proposed as bulk carriers of water together with certain solutes. Water is absorbed principally in the upper small intestine and to a limited extent in the colon.

5 Absorption of Electrolytes

The electrolytes absorbed from the intestine include minerals ingested in the diet and electrolyte constituents of various digestive juices.

Monovalent ions, such as potassium and chloride, are absorbed more readily than divalent ions, such as calcium and magnesium. Sodium, calcium, and iron are absorbed actively, while potassium, magnesium, and bicarbonate are transported passively.

Calcium and iron are absorbed by special mechanisms largely in accordance with the body's needs. The rate of calcium absorption from the duodenum is greatly enhanced by vitamin D. Iron can be absorbed only in the reduced, ferrous (Fe^{+2}) state, and its absorption is increased when the body's iron stores are low and erythrocyte production is increased.

6 Absorption of Vitamins

The water-soluble vitamins (B and C) are readily absorbed in the upper portions of the small intestine. Vitamin B_{12} (cyanocobalamin), however, requires a special mechanism for absorption. Vitamin B_{12} forms a complex with *intrinsic factor,* a mucoprotein produced by the gastric parietal cells. The vitamin B_{12}–intrinsic factor complex is taken up by the mucosal cells through pinocytosis, and then the vitamin B_{12} is liberated for uptake into the blood. Failure to elaborate intrinsic factor impairs absorption of vitamin B_{12} and results in pernicious anemia.

The fat-soluble vitamins (A, D, E, and K) require bile for proper absorption. Lack of bile or pancreatic lipase may impair adequate absorption of these fat-soluble vitamins.

Vomiting (Emesis)

Vomiting is the reflex expulsion of the gastric contents through the mouth. Vomiting involves a complex sequence of visceral and somatic events coordinated by a *vomiting center* in the medulla.

The medullary vomiting center may be stimulated through five pathways:

1   Chemoreceptor Trigger Zone (CTZ)

Located in the floor of the fourth ventricle of the brain near the vomiting center, the CTZ may be stimulated by the following:

a. Drugs, chemicals, and toxins (*e.g.,* cardiac glycosides and apomorphine)
b. Pathologic states (*e.g.,* uremia and diabetic ketoacidosis)
c. Variations in gonadotropin and progesterone levels (*e.g.,* pregnancy)
d. Radiation

The CTZ exerts a tonic influence on the vomiting center, maintaining a state of excitability to other incoming vestibular impulses (see below).

Drug-, chemical- or toxin-induced neuronal excitation of the CTZ is probably mediated by the release of dopamine from surrounding cells (*e.g.,* astrocytes) that form synaptic connections with the neurons of the CTZ.

2   Cortical Stimulation

Emesis may follow cortical stimulation induced by *psychic factors,* such as unpleasant scenes or disagreeable odors, or *increased intracranial pressure,* for example, hydrocephalus, brain tumors, or inflammation.

3   Disturbances of the Inner Ear (Labyrinth)

Motion (through mechanical stimulation of receptors in the labyrinths of the ear) and disorders affecting the vestibular apparatus may produce emesis. Impulses are carried by the vestibulocochlear (VIII) nerve and are transmitted through the cerebellum and CTZ to the vomiting center. Acetylcholine is thought to be the neurotransmitter involved with impulse transmission along the labyrinthine pathway to the vomiting center.

4   Visceral Stimulation

Afferent impulses from the abdominal viscera may be generated by *visceral distention* or *visceral irritation,* and these impulses can *directly* stimulate the vomiting center. Destruction of the CTZ abolishes vomiting of labyrinthine origin (suggesting a modulatory role for the CTZ in vestibular activation of the vomiting center) but does not alter the emetic effect of visceral stimulation.

5   Nodose Ganglion

Certain drugs may produce vomiting by stimulating the nodose ganglion of the vagus (X cranial) nerve.

Following stimulation of the vomiting center, the esophagus, gastroesophageal sphincter, and the body of the stomach relax, while the pyloric antrum and duodenum contract. Forced inspiration follows, and sudden, powerful contraction of the diaphragm and abdominal muscles generates increased intragastric pressure that propels the gastric contents through the esophagus and pharynx into the mouth. Reflex elevation of the soft palate prevents the vomitus from entering the nasopharynx, and closure of the glottis prevents pulmonary aspiration.

Emesis is often preceded by nausea and profuse salivary secretion. Severe nausea may be accompanied by sweating, pallor of the skin, and dizziness.

The drugs reviewed in this chapter, antacids and antiflatulents, represent the most widely used group of medications for the treatment of upper GI disorders, ranging from mild indigestion and heartburn to peptic ulcer.

The principal action of antacids is to neutralize acidity, thus raising gastric *p*H. Increasing the *p*H results in progressive inhibition of the proteolytic activity of pepsin, thereby reducing its digestive action on the gastric mucosa. Consequently, antacids can reduce pain resulting from activation of mucosal nerve endings by excessive gastric acid as well as promote healing of damaged or ulcerated mucosa by protecting it from the destructive effects of pepsin.

The efficacy of antacids depends on many factors, most importantly their acid-neutralizing capacity, formulation, and dosage schedule. Among the various commercially available antacid preparations, there is nearly a 20-fold difference in acid-neutralizing capacity. Sodium bicarbonate and calcium carbonate possess the greatest neutralizing capacity, whereas aluminum phosphate and magnesium trisilicate are considerably weaker.

It is important to recognize, however, that the most potent preparation may not always be the most suitable in terms of potential toxicity (*e.g.,* diarrhea, constipation, hypercalcemia, systemic alkalosis), patient acceptance (*e.g.,* taste, consistency), sodium content (danger in cardiovascular conditions), or cost. For example, persons with conditions such as edema, hypertension, or congestive heart failure that require low salt intake should be given antacid preparations containing little or no sodium, such as Riopan Plus. Magnesium-containing antacids, on the other hand, may cause central nervous system (CNS) toxicity in patients with renal failure and may intensify chronic diarrhea, and thus should be avoided in these conditions. Antacids containing aluminum require cautious use in the presence of constipation or gastric outlet obstruction because they may further reduce gastric emptying. Preparations containing calcium carbonate or sodium bicarbonate are only indicated for short-term therapy, because their side-effects (*e.g.,* systemic alkalosis, rebound hyperacidity, milk–alkali syndrome) are significantly enhanced during prolonged treatment.

Aluminum-containing antacids bind phosphate ions in the intestine, resulting in accelerated elimination and the possible danger of hypophosphatemia. However, clinical advantage is taken of this property in the use of aluminum carbonate gel for prevention of phosphatic urinary stones or in the management of hyperphosphatemia associated with advanced renal failure.

Product formulation (suspension, tablet, powder) may also be a determining factor in the effectiveness and acceptance of antacids—liquid suspensions generally providing the best neutralizing action and greatest palatability. Dosage schedules should be based upon the type and severity of the condition being treated; both the frequency and duration of therapy should be sufficient to provide maximum therapeutic benefit with minimal untoward reactions.

Antacid failure is frequently a result of poor selection, inadequate dosage, or improper administration, and can be eliminated in most cases by judicious choice of an agent appropriate for both the patient and the condition. Selection of an appropriate antacid regimen requires consideration of

Antacids and
Antiflatulents

48

many factors, and persons should be cautioned against indiscriminate use of these widely available and easily obtainable products.

Antacids are usually administered as one of the many available combination products, inasmuch as these products generally provide good acid-neutralizing activity with a reduced incidence of side-effects when compared to the individual components themselves. A popular pairing of antacids is aluminum hydroxide and magnesium hydroxide, a mixture that significantly reduces the occurrence of the constipation and diarrhea frequently observed with aluminum (constipation) and magnesium (diarrhea) alone.

It is inevitable that comparisons are made between the effectiveness of antacid regimens and that of the histamine H₂ blockers, cimetidine and rantidine, in the treatment of gastric and duodenal ulcers (see Chap. 14). Although the efficacy of the H₂ blockers in relieving pain and promoting healing of duodenal ulcers is unquestioned, comparative studies with large-dose antacid regimens have demonstrated a nearly comparable level of effectiveness for the antacid products when used on a sufficiently frequent basis. Increasingly, clinicians are prescribing both H₂ blockers and supplemental antacids, when necessary; it appears as if such a combination provides, in most cases of gastric and duodenal ulcers, optimal therapeutic benefit with minimal untoward reactions. On the other hand, less serious gastric disorders such as heartburn, acid indigestion, and gastritis generally respond quite well to antacid therapy alone and do not require H₂ blockers unless the antacids do not provide sufficient relief.

Antacid drugs are discussed as a group, then listed individually in Table 48-1, in which the major uses and characteristics (including acid-neutralizing capacity [ANC], where established) of each drug are presented. Because most antacid preparations are combination products, the composition of the most commonly used combination products, including sodium content and ANC, is given in Table 48-2. Another antiulcer drug discussed in this chapter is sucralfate, a sulfated sucrose–aluminum hydroxide complex that appears to form a protective barrier over the ulcerated area. Finally, a review of simethicone, an antiflatulent drug used to relieve symptoms associated with excessive production of gas in the digestive tract, and charcoal, an adsorbent, are presented at the end of the chapter.

Several other classes of drugs are used for the relief of symptoms of upper GI distress and have been discussed in previous chapters: for example, anticholinergics (see Chap. 10) and histamine H₂ receptor antagonists, such as cimetidine and ranitidine (see Chap. 14). Still other drugs are in various stages of preclinical and clinical evaluation and include structural analogues of prostaglandin E, which is a cytoprotective agent in the GI tract, colloidal bismuth compounds, and pepsin antagonists (*e.g.,* amylopectin).

Antacids

Aluminum carbonate gel	Aluminum phosphate
Aluminum hydroxide	Calcium carbonate
Dihydroxyaluminum sodium carbonate	Magnesium hydroxide
Magaldrate	Magnesium oxide
Magnesium carbonate	Magnesium trisilicate
	Sodium bicarbonate

Mechanism
Neutralize gastric acidity and usually elevate gastric *p*H above 3 to 4; proteolytic activity of pepsin on gastric mucosa is suppressed above *p*H 4 and totally abolished above *p*H 7 to 8; elevated *p*H also induces the pyloric antrum to release gastrin; acid neutralization may increase lower esophageal sphincter tone; antacids do not appear to "coat" the mucosal barrier but can bind bile acids (especially the aluminum products), although the contribution of this latter action to the therapeutic effects of the drugs is unclear.

Uses
1 Symptomatic treatment of GI symptoms associated with hyperacidity (*e.g.,* heartburn, acid indigestion)
2 Treatment of hyperacidity associated with gastritis, peptic ulcer, hiatal hernia, esophagitis

Dosage
See Table 48-1.

Fate
Most preparations (except sodium bicarbonate) are not appreciably absorbed from the GI tract and are excreted largely in the feces. Calcium and magnesium products can form chloride salts by reaction with hydrochloric acid, which may be partly absorbed and require elimination by the kidneys.

Common Side-Effects
Diarrhea (magnesium products); constipation (aluminum and calcium products)

Significant Adverse Reactions
Aluminum—intestinal impaction, phosphate depletion (anorexia, weakness, impaired reflexes, depression, tremors, bone pain, osteomalacia)

Magnesium—profound diarrhea, dehydration, hypermagnesemia (nausea, vomiting, impaired reflexes, hypotension, respiratory depression—high risk in patients with impaired renal function), bradyarrhythmias, renal stones (magnesium trisilicate)

Calcium carbonate—rebound hyperacidity, milk–alkali syndrome (metabolic alkalosis, hypercalcemia, vomiting, confusion, headache, renal insufficiency), renal calculi, neurologic impairment, GI hemorrhage, fecal impaction

Sodium bicarbonate—systemic alkalosis, sodium overload, milk–alkali syndrome, rebound hypersecretion

Contraindications
Depend on individual product (see Table 48-1)

Interactions

Note: Due to the absorptive capacity of most antacids and their ability to alter gastric *pH*, other drugs should not be administered within 1 hour to 2 hours of antacid ingestion, if possible.

1 Antacids can impair the absorption of tetracyclines, digoxin, digitoxin, phenothiazines, indomethacin, phenylbutazone, isoniazid, and possibly also phenytoin, oral anticoagulants, quinidine, oral iron products, propranolol, other antibiotics, barbiturates, and salicylates.
2 Antacids can increase the effects of pseudoephedrine, levodopa, and meperidine by *facilitating* their intestinal absorption, and can enhance the effects of amphetamines by decreasing urinary excretion.

▶ NURSING ALERTS
(See Table 48-1 for specific information on each drug.)
▷ 1 Monitor the number and consistency of stools in patients taking antacids because dehydration from excessive diarrhea or fecal impaction from excessive constipation can occur.
▷ 2 Use a low sodium preparation in patients on restricted or low-sodium diets (*e.g.,* hypertension, congestive heart failure, edema, pregnancy).
▷ 3 Do not administer magnesium- or calcium-containing products to patients with significant renal impairment, because hypermagnesemia and hypercalcemia can occur. See Significant Adverse Reactions for symptoms.
▷ 4 Caution patient to report GI pain that persists longer than 72 hours or the presence of tarry stools, because these symptoms may indicate ulcer perforation, gastric hemorrhage, or other serious complications.

▶ NURSING CONSIDERATIONS
(See Table 48-1 for specific information on each drug.)
▷ 1 Administer antacid in liquid form if possible, because efficacy is significantly greater than with tablet or capsule formulations.
▷ 2 If given in a tablet form, instruct patient to chew *thoroughly* before swallowing and follow with a small amount of water.
▷ 3 Note that food acts as a buffer to gastric acid for approximately 60 minutes and that the presence of food can enhance the action of antacids. Thus, antacids taken on an empty stomach have a duration of action of 30 minutes, whereas if they are taken 1 hour after meals, their duration is approximately 3 hours.
▷ 4 During chronic therapy administer antacids 1 hour and 3 hours after meals and at bedtime for optimal clinical effect.

▷ *Dietary precautions*
▷ 1 Recognize that milk has no antacid properties and may increase acid production.
▷ 2 Caution the ulcer patient to avoid coffee, other caffeine-containing beverages, and alcohol. Note that the value of bland diets, other than during the acute symptomatic period, is unproven; a closely followed *reasonable* diet is far more acceptable to most patients than a bland diet, and thus compliance is better.
▷ 3 Suggest that small, frequent meals or snacks may be better tolerated by the ulcer patient than larger meals consumed twice a day and result in less gastric acid secretion.

▶ sucralfate
Carafate

Sucralfate is a complex of sulfated sucrose and aluminum hydroxide used orally for the short-term treatment of duodenal ulcers. Because it is not absorbed from the GI tract, it is virtually free of systemic side-effects. It requires an acidic environment for optimal activity, so it should not be administered simultaneously with antacids or H₂ antagonists, because its effectiveness may be somewhat reduced.

Mechanism
Not completely established; possible actions include formation of an ulcer-adherent complex with exudative material at the ulcer site, thus protecting the ulcerated area from further attack by acid, pepsin, and bile salts; may also inhibit activity of pepsin and absorb bile salts; does not appear to neutralize gastric acid

Use
1 Short-term (*i.e.,* up to 8 weeks) treatment of duodenal ulcers

Dosage
1 g (1 tablet) four times a day on an empty stomach

Fate
Minimally absorbed from GI tract; absorbed fraction is excreted principally in the urine

Common Side-Effect
Constipation

Significant Adverse Reactions
(Rare) Diarrhea, nausea, GI distress, indigestion, dry mouth, rash, pruritus, dizziness, vertigo, and sleepiness

Interaction
1 Sucralfate may reduce GI absorption of tetracyclines.

▶ NURSING CONSIDERATIONS
▷ 1 Administer antacids as needed to control pain but do not give within ½ hour of sucralfate.
▷ 2 Inform patients that sucralfate tablets should be taken at least 1 hour before meals and at bedtime to obtain maximal benefit.

▶ simethicone
Gas-X, Mylicon, Silain

Table 48-1. Antacids

Drug	Preparations	Sodium Content	Acid Neutralizing Capacity (mEq)	Usual Dosage Range	Remarks
Aluminum carbonate gel, basic (Basaljel)	Suspension (equivalent to 400 mg of aluminum hydroxide per 5 ml)	0.48 mg/ml	14	Antacid—2 capsules or tablets, 2 tsp of regular suspension or 1 tsp extra-strength suspension 4 to 8 times a day	Used as an antacid and for preventing development of urinary phosphate stones; exhibits strong phosphate-binding capacity, increasing fecal and decreasing urinary phosphate excretion; periodic determinations of serum electrolytes, especially calcium and phosphate, should be performed; low-phosphate diet is recommended; excessive doses can lead to phosphate depletion (weakness, tremors, bone pain, demineralization); be alert for signs of urinary infection (fever, chills, dysuria); high fluid intake should be maintained
	Extra-strength suspension (equivalent to 1000 mg of aluminum hydroxide per 5 ml)	4.6 mg/ml	11	Prevention of phosphate stones—2 to 6 capsules or tablets 1 hour after meals and at bedtime or 1 to 2 tbsp suspension in water or juice 1 hour after meals and at bedtime	
	Capsules and swallow tablets (equivalant to 500 mg of aluminum hydroxide)	2.8 mg/capsule	13		
		2.1 mg/tablet	14		
Aluminum hydroxide gel (ALternaGEL, Alu-Cap, Alu-Tab, Amphojel, Dialume)	Suspension—320 mg/5 ml	0.5 mg/ml	6–7	600 mg 3 to 4 times a day between meals and at bedtime	Antacid with moderate acid-neutralizing capacity; does not produce acid rebound or alkalosis; possesses phosphate-binding capacity although to a lesser degree than aluminum carbonate; constipation is a frequent side-effect; do not use for prolonged periods in patients with low serum phosphate or those on a low-sodium diet
	Concentrated suspension—600 mg/5 ml		12		
	Capsules—475 mg, 500 mg	1 mg/capsule	10		
	Tablets—300 mg, 600 mg		9		
	Chewable tablets—487.5 mg		18		
Aluminum phosphate gel (Phosphaljel)	Suspension—233 mg/5 ml	2.5 mg/ml	1–2	15 ml to 30 ml every 2 hours between meals and at bedtime	Less effective than aluminum hydroxide in acid-neutralizing ability; does not alter phosphate excretion, hence is preferred when high-phosphorus diet cannot be maintained, or in patients with diarrhea or pancreatitis
Calcium carbonate (Alka-2, Amitone, Chooz, Dicarbosil, Equilet, Mallamint, Tums, Tums E-X)	Tablets—650 mg	Less than 5 mg/750-mg tablet	8–10	0.5 g to 2 g 3 to 6 times a day as needed	Very effective antacid, possessing high neutralizing capacity, rapid onset, and relatively prolonged duration of action; does not cause systemic alkalosis, but is constipating and may elicit acid rebound and gastric hypersecretion; converted to calcium chloride by gastric acid, which may be absorbed in sufficient quantities to produce hypercalcemia with prolonged treatment; chronic use with foods high in vitamin D (e.g., milk) may lead to milk–alkali syndrome (see Significant Adverse Reactions)
	Chewable tablets—350 mg, 420 mg, 500 mg, 750 mg	2.7 mg–3.2 mg/500-mg tablet; 0.32 mg/350-mg tablet			

Table 48-1. Antacids (continued)

Drug	Preparations	Sodium Content	Acid Neutralizing Capacity (mEq)	Usual Dosage Range	Remarks
Dihydroxyaluminum sodium carbonate (Rolaids)	Chewable tablets— 334 mg	53 mg/tablet	7–8	1 to 2 tablets 3 to 6 times a day as needed	Converted to aluminum hydroxide in the presence of gastric acid, releasing carbon dioxide; gives rapid but transient neutralizing effect; because of high sodium content, use with caution in sodium-restricted patients
Magaldrate (Riopan)	Suspension—400 mg/ 5 ml Tablets—400 mg Chewable tablets— 400 mg	0.06 mg–0.14 mg/ml 0.3 mg–0.7 mg/tablet	13–14 13–14	400 mg to 800 mg 3 to 6 times a day between meals and at bedtime	A *chemical* combination of magnesium and aluminum hydroxides equivalent to 28% to 39% magnesium oxide and 17% to 25% aluminum oxide; has somewhat lower neutralizing capacity than a physical mixture of the two ingredients; does not elicit acid rebound or systemic acidosis; has a low incidence of diarrhea and constipation, and very low sodium content; available with simethicone as Riopan Plus
Magnesium carbonate (various manufacturers)	Powder	NA		0.5 g to 2 g between meals with a full glass of water	Infrequently used antacid due to poor patient acceptance; high incidence of diarrhea, and may produce hypermagnesemia
Magnesium hydroxide (Milk of Magnesia)	Tablets—325 mg, 650 mg Liquid—390 mg/5 ml	0.8 mg/ml		Antacid—5 ml to 10 ml or 650 mg tablet 4 times a day Cathartic: Adults—15 ml to 30 ml Children—5 ml to 30 ml	Used as an antacid in small doses or as a cathartic in slightly higher doses. Elicits prompt and sustained neutralization of gastric acid without marked acid rebound or systemic alkalosis. However, laxative action is commonly observed at higher doses; therefore drug is often combined with aluminum or calcium antacids. Also available as an emulsion containing mineral oil (Haley's MO). Laxative dose should be given at bedtime, followed by a full glass of water. See Chap. 50.
Magnesium oxide (Mag-Ox 400, Maox, Par-Mag, Uro-Mag)	Tablets—400 mg, 420 mg, 500 mg, 650 mg Capsules—140 mg, 400 mg Powder	NA		250 mg to 1.5 g with water or milk 4 times a day	Slow-acting antacid with prolonged effects; high neutralizing capacity, but frequently elicits nausea and diarrhea; in large doses has been used as a cathartic; frequently used in powder form; available as light and heavy magnesium oxide; *light* is 5 times bulkier than *heavy*, but possesses greater neutralizing power due to larger surface area
Magnesium trisilicate (various manufacturers)	Tablets—488 mg Powder	NA		1 g to 4 g 4 times a day with water or milk	Combination of magnesium oxide and silicon dioxide with water; potent antacid with slow onset and prolonged duration of action; provides adsorptive as well as neutralizing action; frequently combined with aluminum hydroxide to yield a long-acting antacid relatively free from constipating side-effects
Sodium bicarbonate (Bell/ans, Soda Mint)	Tablets—325 mg, 487.5 mg, 520 mg, 650 mg Powder	27% sodium		0.3 g to 2 g as needed 1 to 4 times a day	Systemic, absorbable antacid, with a short duration of action; its use should be discouraged, because it frequently elicits acid rebound, belching (due to liberated carbon dioxide), and gastric distention, and may result in systemic alkalosis; high sodium content precludes its use in patients with hypertension, or cardiac or renal disease; large doses may cause phosphaturia

NA = Sodium content is not available.

Table 48-2. Antacid Combinations

Trade Name	Dosage Form	Aluminum Hydroxide	Calcium Carbonate	Magnesium Oxide or Hydroxide	Simethicone	Other	Sodium Content	Acid Neutralizing Capacity (mEq)
Alka-Seltzer	Tablet					Sodium bicarbonate 1 g; citric acid 800 mg; potassium bicarbonate 300 mg	296 mg/tablet	10
Alkets	Tablet		780 mg	65 mg		Magnesium carbonate 130 mg	NA	
Aludrox	Tablet	233 mg		83 mg			1.6 mg/tablet	11–12
	Liquid	61.4 mg/ml		20.6 mg/ml			0.22 mg/ml	14
Bisodol	Tablet		194 mg	178 mg			0.036 mg/tablet	
	Powder					Sodium bicarbonate 129 mg/g; magnesium carbonate 95 mg/g	31 mg/g	
Camalox	Tablet	225 mg	250 mg	200 mg			1.5 mg/tablet	18
	Liquid	45 mg/ml	50 mg/ml	40 mg/ml			0.5 mg/ml	18
Citrocarbonate	Effervescent powder					Sodium citrate 1.82 g and sodium bicarbonate 0.78 g per 3.9-g dose	700 mg/dose	
Creamalin	Tablet	248 mg		75 mg			Less than 41 mg/tablet	
Delcid	Liquid	120 mg/ml		133 mg/ml			3 mg/ml	
Di-Gel	Tablet	282 mg (co-dried with magnesium carbonate)		85 mg	25 mg		10.6 mg/tablet	42
ENO	Liquid	56.4 mg/ml		17.4 mg/ml	5 mg/ml		1.7 mg/ml	10–11
	Powder					Sodium tartrate 2.16 g and sodium citrate 495 mg	780 mg/dose	
Estomul-M	Tablet	500 mg (co-dried with magnesium carbonate)		45 mg			16 mg/tablet	8
	Liquid	61 mg/ml (co-dried with magnesium carbonate)					2.34 mg/ml	
Gaviscon	Tablet	80 mg				Magnesium trisilicate 20 mg	18 mg	
Gaviscon-2	Tablet	160 mg				Magnesium trisilicate 40 mg	37 mg	

Table 48-2. Antacid Combinations (continued)

Trade Name	Dosage Form	Aluminum Hydroxide	Calcium Carbonate	Magnesium Oxide or Hydroxide	Simethicone	Other	Sodium Content	Acid Neutralizing Capacity (mEq)
Gaviscon	Liquid	6.3 mg/ml				Magnesium carbonate 27.5 mg/ml	8 mg/ml	
Gelusil	Tablet	200 mg		200 mg	25 mg		0.8 mg/tablet	11
Gelusil	Liquid	40 mg/ml		40 mg/ml	5 mg/ml		0.14 mg/ml	12
Gelusil-II	Tablet	400 mg		400 mg	30 mg		2.1 mg/tablet	21
Gelusil-II	Liquid	80 mg/ml		80 mg/ml	6 mg/ml		0.26 mg/ml	24
Gelusil-M	Tablet	300 mg		200 mg	25 mg		1.3 mg/tablet	12–13
Gelusil-M	Liquid	60 mg/ml		40 mg/ml	5 mg/ml		0.24 mg/ml	15
Kolantyl	Wafer	180 mg		170 mg			NA	10–11
Kolantyl	Liquid	30 mg/ml		30 mg/ml			0.44 mg/ml	10–11
Lo-Sal	Tablet	585 mg		120 mg			0.12 mg	
Maalox	Liquid	45 mg/ml		40 mg/ml			0.27 mg/ml	13–14
Maalox Concentrate	Liquid	120 mg/ml		60 mg/ml			0.16 mg/ml	28
Maalox No. 1	Tablet	200 mg		200 mg			0.84 mg/tablet	8–9
Maalox No. 2	Tablet	400 mg		400 mg			1.8 mg/tablet	18
Maalox Plus	Tablet	200 mg		200 mg	25 mg		1.0 mg/tablet	8–9
Maalox Plus	Liquid	45 mg/ml		40 mg/ml	5 mg/ml		0.26 mg/ml	13–14
Magnatril	Tablet	260 mg		130 mg		Magnesium trisilicate 455 mg	NA	
Magnatril	Liquid	52 mg/ml		26 mg/ml		Magnesium trisilicate 52 mg/ml	NA	
Mylanta	Tablet	200 mg		200 mg	20 mg		0.77 mg/tablet	11–12
Mylanta	Liquid	40 mg/ml		40 mg/ml	4 mg/ml		0.14 mg/ml	12–13
Mylanta-II	Tablet	400 mg		400 mg	30 mg		1.3 mg/tablet	23
Mylanta-II	Liquid	80 mg/ml		80 mg/ml	6 mg/ml		0.23 mg/ml	25–26
Riopan Plus	Tablet				20 mg	Magaldrate 480 mg	0.3 mg/tablet	13–14
Riopan Plus	Liquid				4 mg/ml	Magaldrate 108 mg/ml	0.06 mg/ml	13–14
Silain-Gel	Liquid	56.4 mg/ml		57 mg/ml	5 mg/ml		0.96 mg/ml	15
Tempo	Tablet	133 mg	414 mg	81 mg	20 mg			
Titralac	Tablet		420 mg			Glycine 180 mg	0.3 mg/tablet	7–8
Titralac	Liquid		200 mg/ml			Glycine 60 mg/ml	2.2 mg/ml	
WinGel	Tablet	180 mg		160 mg			2.5 mg/tablet	12
WinGel	Liquid	36 mg/ml		32 mg/ml			0.5 mg/ml	

NA = Sodium content is not available.

A silicone derivative possessing an antifoaming action, simethicone is claimed to relieve flatulence by dispersing gas trapped in the GI tract.

Mechanism
Alters the surface tension of gas bubbles, causing coalescence of the gas, thereby facilitating its elimination by belching or flatus

Uses
1 Adjunctive treatment of conditions associated with retention of excessive gas (*e.g.,* dyspepsia, peptic ulcer, spastic colon, diverticulitis, or postoperative gaseous retention)

Dosage
Tablets: 40 mg to 80 mg four times a day
Drops: 40 mg four times a day

▶ NURSING CONSIDERATIONS
▷ 1 Counsel patients to consult physician if symptoms are not relieved within several days, because continual passage of gas may indicate a more serious underlying condition.
▷ 2 Administer after each meal and at bedtime, and advise patients to chew tablets thoroughly, because complete particle dispersion facilitates the antiflatulent action.

▷ 3 Note that simethicone is widely available in combination with various antacids (see Table 48-2).

▶ charcoal

Mechanism
Adsorbs toxins and gas onto surface of particles, thereby relieving cramping, diarrhea, and flatulence

Uses
1 Temporary relief of indigestion, bloating, cramping, and flatulence
2 Prevention of nonspecific pruritus associated with kidney dialysis treatment

Dosage
975 mg to 3.9 g three to four times a day, followed by a small amount of water

▶ NURSING CONSIDERATIONS
▷ 1 Do not administer for more than 3 days, and use only when condition is acute. Drug can absorb nutrients, digestive enzymes, and other essential substances.
▷ 2 Chew or dissolve tablets in the mouth before swallowing.
▷ 3 Administer to children under 3 years of age only if directed by physician.

Summary. Antacids and Antiflatulents

Drug	Preparations	Usual Dosage Range
Antacids	See Table 48-1.	
Antacid combinations	See Table 48-2.	
Sucralfate (Carafate)	Tablets—1 g	1 g four times a day on an empty stomach for 4 weeks to 8 weeks
Simethicone (Gas-X, Mylicon, Silain)	Tablets—50 mg Chewable tablets—40 mg, 80 mg Drops—40 mg/0.6 ml	Tablets—40 mg to 80 mg four times a day Drops—40 mg four times a day
Charcoal	Tablets—325 mg, 650 mg Capsules—260 mg	975 mg to 3.9 g three to four times a day

Digestants are those substances that assist the physiologic process of food digestion in the gastrointestinal (GI) tract. The usefulness of most enzymes (*e.g.,* amylase, lipase, protease, cellulose) as exogenous digestive aids is probably greatly overstated, inasmuch as symptoms of GI distress can rarely be attributed to an actual deficiency of endogenous digestive chemicals. Nevertheless, certain digestive substances, especially the pancreatic enzymes, pancreatin and pancrelipase, have proven valuable as replacement therapy in elderly or debilitated persons or in persons with conditions such as GI surgery, achlorhydria, chronic pancreatitis or gastric carcinoma, in whom there exists a definite lack of one or more of these digestive substances. In such cases, however, the deficient chemicals must be replaced in sufficient amounts to restore digestive activity, and it should be recognized that many commercially available products contain amounts *too small* to provide the required quantity of digestant. Thus, empiric use of combination or "shotgun" digestive products has no place in rational pharmacotherapy. Moreover, the inclusion of anticholinergics, barbiturates, or antacids in these formulations merely increases the likelihood of untoward reactions.

The digestive aids most frequently employed clinically may be grouped as follows:

1 Gastric acidifiers, *e.g.,* glutamic acid HCl
2 Digestive enzymes, *e.g.,* pepsin, pancreatin, pancrelipase
3 Bile salts and bile acids, *e.g.,* dehydrocholic acid, ox bile extract

Gastric hydrochloric acid deficiency (achlorhydria) can occur in association with various pathologic conditions such as pernicious anemia or gastric carcinoma, as well as in the absence of observable disease. Dilute solutions (10%) of hydrochloric acid were previously used to aid digestion in patients with achlorhydria and to relieve complaints such as belching, nausea, and epigastric distress. Today, glutamic acid hydrochloride is used as a source of hydrochloric acid, because it is available in capsule and tablet form and offers a safer and more convenient mode of therapy. However, glutamic acid does not yield as much free acid as did hydrochloric acid.

Pepsin is a proteolytic enzyme activated by gastric acid, and thus is sometimes administered with glutamic acid to stimulate digestion. It is of doubtful benefit in most instances, because absolute lack of pepsin is relatively rare, except perhaps in gastric carcinoma and occasionally in pernicious anemia, and the acid deficiency is usually of far greater consequence. On the other hand, deficiency of pancreatic enzymes is a frequent occurrence, especially in cases of pancreatitis and duct obstruction, and of course following pancreatectomy. In these instances, replacement therapy with either pancreatin, a powdered concentrate of hog pancreas containing amylase, lipase, and protease activity, or pancrelipase, a more concentrated mixture of pancreatic enzymes of porcine origin, is indicated.

Natural bile contains a series of organic acids secreted as sodium salts, which lower the surface tension of fat globules, breaking them into small droplets. Bile further aids fat digestion by stimulation of pancreatic secretions and activation of pancreatic lipase. Exogenous bile salts (*e.g.,* ox

Digestants

49

bile extract) have occasionally been used as replacement therapy in patients with partial biliary obstruction or following removal of the gallbladder (cholecystectomy), but their effectiveness in this regard is subject to dispute. Bile salts also exhibit a choleretic action, that is, they stimulate the outflow of bile. Certain bile salts, especially the synthetic derivative dehydrocholic acid, markedly increase the output of a thin, watery bile, and are termed *hydrocholeretics.* Dehydrocholic acid is used to facilitate flushing and drainage of partially obstructed bile ducts, thereby minimizing infections and preventing biliary calculi from lodging in the duct.

In addition to the bile salts, a naturally occurring human bile acid, chenodeoxycholic acid, is available for treating selected patients with gallstones. Chenodeoxycholic acid (Chenodiol) retards hepatic synthesis of cholesterol and cholic acid, resulting in gradual dissolution of cholesterol gallstones in some patients. Chenodeoxycholic acid is discussed in detail below.

It should be re-emphasized that the majority of clinically available digestive products are multiple formulations containing digestive enzymes, bile extracts, or hydrochloric acid derivatives, frequently combined with anticholinergics, antiflatulents, antacids, or barbiturates. Not only is the content of these products often insufficient to provide the needed replacement in cases of deficiency states, but the digestants included in these formulations are frequently unnecessary and usually ineffective for the symptomatic treatment of simple digestive dysfunction, inasmuch as lack of endogenous digestive substances is only rarely the cause of GI distress.

Bile Salts

▶ **ox bile extract**
  ox bile extract with iron
  Bilron

Bile salts are the dried extract of bile from cattle, the bile salt content approximating that of human bile. When combined with iron (Bilron), the complex is insoluble in an acid medium (*e.g.,* stomach). As the complex enters the small intestine, the iron dissociates and the bile salts become soluble and active.

Mechanism
Lower the surface tension of fat globules, breaking them into smaller, more easily digestible particles by exposing a greater surface area to the enzymatic action of pancreatic lipases; exhibit a mild stimulating effect on GI smooth muscle; exert a choleretic action (*i.e.,* increased flow of bile) following absorption

Uses
1 Symptomatic treatment of uncomplicated constipation
2 Replacement therapy in bile deficiency states (*e.g.,* partial biliary obstruction, cholecystectomy)

Note: Because their therapeutic effectiveness has not been conclusively established, *bile salts are rarely used.*

Dosage
150 mg to 600 mg during or after meals

Significant Adverse Reactions
Loose stools, nausea, cramping

Contraindications
Complete biliary obstruction, severe jaundice

Interactions
1 Bile salts may enhance the absorption of fat-soluble vitamins (A, D, E, K).

▶ **NURSING ALERT**
▷ 1 Use cautiously in the presence of marked hepatic insufficiency (*e.g.,* viral hepatitis, advanced cirrhosis), and when symptoms of appendicitis are present (*e.g.,* abdominal pain, nausea, vomiting).

Bile Acids

▶ **chenodeoxycholic acid**
  Chenodiol

When cholesterol is present in bile in concentrations that exceed the capacity of bile acids and lecithin to solubilize it, crystals can precipitate, and eventually coalesce into gallstones. Oral administration of chenodeoxycholic acid, a primary bile acid, can decrease the concentration of cholesterol in bile by inhibiting its hepatic synthesis. Thus, chronic treatment with chenodeoxycholic acid can, in some patients, result in gradual dissolution of noncalcified, radiolucent cholesterol gallstones. The drug is potentially hepatotoxic, and is not appropriate therapy for all patients with gallstones. Careful selection and close monitoring of patients, therefore, is essential to minimize complications and to offer the greatest chance for successful therapy.

Mechanism
Blocks hepatic synthesis of cholesterol and cholic acid, resulting in reduction of biliary cholesterol levels and gradual dissolution of radiolucent cholesterol gallstones; small, floatable gallstones are more likely to respond to drug treatment than pigmented or partially calcified stones.

Use
1 Treatment of patients with radiolucent gallstones in well opacified gallbladders, in whom surgery is not feasible due to age or presence of systemic disease

Dosage
Initially 250 mg twice a day for 2 weeks; increase by 250 mg/day each week thereafter until the recommended

dose (*i.e.,* 13 mg/kg to 16 mg/kg/day) or the maximally tolerated dose is attained.

Doses less than 10 mg/kg/day are usually ineffective and may be associated with an *increased* risk of cholecystectomy.

Fate

Well absorbed orally but undergoes extensive first-pass hepatic clearance (see Chap. 2); converted in the colon to lithocholic acid, which is excreted largely (80%) in the feces; the remainder is absorbed, and metabolized in the liver; in patients unable to form hepatic sulfate conjugates of lithocholic acid, liver toxicity can occur.

Common Side-Effects

Diarrhea, elevated serum aminotransferase

Significant Adverse Reactions

Abdominal cramping, nausea, vomiting, anorexia, dyspepsia, flatulence, elevated serum cholesterol and HDL, and decreased white cell count

Contraindications

Intrahepatic cholestasis, primary biliary cirrhosis, sclerosing cholangitis, radiopaque bile pigment stones, acute cholecystitis, gallstone pancreatitis, biliary GI fistula, and pregnancy

Interactions

1 Bile acid sequestering agents (cholestyramine, colestipol) and aluminum-based antacids may reduce absorption of chenodeoxycholic acid.
2 Estrogens, oral contraceptives, clofibrate and other lipid lowering drugs may decrease the effectiveness of chenodeoxycholic acid by increasing biliary cholesterol secretion.

▶ NURSING ALERTS

▷ 1 Be aware that lithocholic acid, a metabolite of chenodeoxycholic acid formed in the colon, may be partially absorbed and subsequently transported to the liver, where it may be hepatotoxic in certain persons who fail to adequately metabolize it to a sulfated conjugate.

▷ 2 Closely monitor serum aminotransferase during therapy. If SGPT levels rise to over 3 times the upper limit of normal, discontinue the drug. Enzyme levels return to normal following drug discontinuation. If levels increase to 1.5 to 3 times the limit, temporarily stop drug and carefully resume only after levels return to normal.

▷ 3 Recognize that doses below 10 mg/kg are usually not effective, and may actually result in an *increased* risk of cholecystectomy.

▷ 4 Note that chenodeoxycholic acid is a potential teratogen. Do not use in women who are or may become pregnant. Alert women to the possibility of fetal damage should they become pregnant while taking the drug.

▶ NURSING CONSIDERATIONS

▷ 1 Following stone dissolution, discontinue treatment and monitor serial cholecystograms for recurrence, which occurs in approximately 50% of patients within 5 years.

▷ 2 Urge patients to maintain low cholesterol and carbohydrate diets following dissolution of stones and to reduce weight to minimize stone recurrence.

▷ 3 Be aware that a prophylactic dose is not established; stones have recurred on doses as high as 500 mg/day.

▷ 4 If partial stone dissolution is not evident within 9 months to 12 months, the likelihood of successful therapy is greatly reduced. Discontinue treatment if there is no response by 15 months to 18 months.

▷ 5 Monitor serum cholesterol at 4-month to 6-month intervals. Drug should be discontinued if cholesterol levels rise above the age-adjusted limit for a given patient.

▷ 6 Should diarrhea become persistent or severe, consider a temporary dosage reduction to alleviate the condition.

Gastric Acidifiers

▶ glutamic acid HCl
Acidulin

Glutamic acid hydrochloride is a source of hydrochloric acid that aids digestion in conditions associated with reduced (hypoacidity) or absent (achlorhydria) gastric acid. It is used as a hydrochloride salt of glutamic acid in tablet or capsule form that releases hydrochloric acid in the stomach, thus minimizing oral mucosal irritation and damage to dental enamel. Some preparations also contain pepsin or pancreatin enzyme concentrate to further assist digestive action.

Mechanism

Facilitates conversion of pepsinogen to pepsin, and provides optimal *p*H for action of pepsin; may stimulate pancreatic secretions and neutralize bicarbonates in gastrointestinal fluid, maintaining electrolyte balance

Uses

1 Replacement therapy to assist digestion in hydrochloric acid deficiency states (*e.g.,* chronic gastritis, pernicious anemia, gastric carcinoma, primary achlorhydria, gastric resection)
2 Prevent growth of putrefactive microorganisms in ingested food

Dosage

1 to 3 tablets or capsules (325 mg–1000 mg) 3 times/day before each meal

Significant Adverse Reactions

Overdosage may lead to systemic acidosis.

Contraindications
Gastric hyperacidity, peptic ulcer

Interactions
1 Glutamic acid may antagonize the antineoplastic action of vinblastine.

▶ **NURSING CONSIDERATIONS**
▷ 1 Prevent tablets or capsules from becoming wet, because HCl is released upon contact with water.
▷ 2 Periodically determine acid–base status in patients on long-term or high-dose therapy.
▷ 3 Note that glutamic acid is available in combination with pepsin as Muripsin and with betaine HCl (hydrolyzed to release HCl), pepsin and pancreatic enzyme concentrate as Milco-Zyme.

Hydrocholeretics

▶ **dehydrocholic acid**
Cholan-DH, Decholin, Hepahydrin, Neocholan

Dehydrocholic acid, a semisynthetic derivative of cholic acid, is termed a *hydrocholeretic agent* because its principal pharmacologic action is to increase the volume of dilute bile output without markedly altering the amount of solid bile constituents. Its major use is to facilitate biliary tract drainage. Hydrocholeretics are much less effective than natural bile salts or choleretics (such as ox bile extract) in emulsifying GI fats and in promoting fat absorption.

Mechanism
Increases the volume of low-viscosity bile flow, but does not change the amount of bile constituents

Uses
1 Adjunctive treatment of chronic or recurrent biliary tract disorders (*e.g.,* biliary dyskinesia, chronic partial biliary obstruction, noncalculous cholecystitis) to provide a flushing action
2 Assist prolonged drainage from biliary fistulas or T tubes
3 Postoperative management following cholecystectomy or surgery on the biliary tract to prevent occlusion or infection of the common bile duct (rarely used)
4 Temporary relief of constipation

Dosage
250 mg to 500 mg three times a day after meals

Fate
Absorbed from upper intestines, passes through the liver and is recycled in the intestinal tract by the bile ducts; excreted in the feces

Significant Adverse Reactions
None at recommended oral doses

Contraindications
Jaundice, severe hepatitis, advanced cirrhosis, cholelithiasis, abdominal pain, vomiting, complete obstruction of the common or hepatic bile ducts or GI or urinary tract

▶ **NURSING ALERTS**
▷ 1 Use cautiously in patients with prostatic hypertrophy, acute hepatitis, acute yellow atrophy of the liver, partial obstruction of the GI or urinary tracts, history of asthma or allergies, and in children under 6 or in elderly persons.
▷ 2 Do not use hydrocholeretics as diuretics or as adjuncts to diuretics, or when abdominal pain, nausea, or vomiting are present.

▶ **NURSING CONSIDERATIONS**
▷ 1 Consider simultaneous administration of bile salts with hydrocholeretics during prolonged administration or when bile is draining away from the intestinal tract to ensure adequate digestion and absorption of nutrients.
▷ 2 Note that dehydrocholic acid is available in combination with homatropine plus phenobarbital (Cholan HMB, G.B.S.); however, use of combination products is rarely warranted.

Pancreatic Enzymes

▶ **pancreatin**
Viokase

▶ **pancrelipase**
Cotazym, Ilozyme, Ku-Zyme HP, Pancrease

Pancreatic enzyme concentrates of bovine or porcine origin containing lipase, protease, and amylase activity; aid in digestion and absorption of fats and carbohydrates. Pancrelipase has greater lipase activity than does pancreatin, and can be used in lower doses to control steatorrhea (see uses below).

Mechanism
Provide enzymatic activity necessary to assist in the digestion of carbohydrates, fats, and proteins; exert their primary effects in the duodenum and upper jejunum

Uses
1 Replacement therapy in pancreatic enzyme deficiency states, such as chronic pancreatitis or pancreatic insufficiency, steatorrhea of malabsorption syndrome, cystic fibrosis, postgastrectomy or postpancreatectomy

Dosage
(Tablets, capsules and powder packets of different manufacturers contain varying amounts of lipase, protease and amylase)

Pancreatin: 325 mg to 1000 mg (1 to 3 tablets) or 0.75 g of powder with meals or snacks; each milligram contains not less than 25 U amylase activity, 2 U lipase activity, and 25 U protease activity.

Pancrelipase: 1 to 3 tablets or capsules, or 1 or 2 powder packets before or with meals or snacks; each milligram contains not less than 100 U amylase activity, 24 U lipase activity, and 100 U protease activity.

Significant Adverse Reactions

(Usually with high doses) Nausea, diarrhea, vomiting, anorexia, hypersensitivity reactions (sneezing, rash, lacrimation)

Contraindications

Hypersensitivity to beef or pork

Interactions

1 Pancreatic enzymes may retard the absorption of oral iron.
2 Availability of pancreatin in the duodenum may be enhanced by cimetidine or ranitidine.
3 Antacids containing magnesium hydroxide or calcium carbonate may reduce the effects of the enzymes.

▶ NURSING CONSIDERATIONS

▷ 1 Ensure a balanced intake of starch, protein, and fat during therapy to minimize indigestion.
▷ 2 Consider use of supplemental antacids to control refractive steatorrhea; however, do not give antacids within 1 hour of pancreatic medication.
▷ 3 Administer drugs with meals. Enteric-coated tablets should be swallowed whole. Powder or granules may be added to milk or water, or sprinkled on food.
▷ 4 Evaluate patient's response to drug by noting appearance of stools, monitoring weight, and periodically determining fecal fat and nitrogen.
▷ 5 Note that pancreatin is available as either bovine or porcine origin. Determine any previous hypersensitivity to beef or pork products before prescribing.

A large number of combination products containing various proportions of digestive enzymes, bile extracts, hydrocholeretics, acidifiers as well as a myriad of other types of agents (*e.g.,* anticholinergics, antacids, charcoal, barbiturates, simethicone) are available for symptomatic treatment of digestive disorders and for other GI dysfunctions. These combination products are rarely of clinical benefit, inasmuch as a GI disorder is seldom the result of an overall deficiency of several substances at one time. Specific deficiency states are more appropriately treated with the actual substance that is lacking rather than by employing a "shot-gun" approach to therapy. Moreover, inclusion of many different drugs, especially barbiturates and anticholinergics in a single preparation, only serves to increase the likelihood of untoward reactions. Commercially available digestive combinations include Accelerase, Donnazyme, Entozyme, Festal, Festalan, Kanulase, and Phazyme.

Summary. Digestants

Drug	Preparations	Usual Dosage Range
Bile Salts		
Ox bile extract	Enteric-coated tablets— 325 mg	150 mg to 600 mg during or following each meal
Ox bile extract with iron (Bilron)	Capsules—150 mg, 300 mg with iron	
Gastric Acidifiers		
Glutamic acid, HCl (Acidulin)	Tablets—325 mg Capsules—340 mg	1 to 2 tablets or capsules 3 times a day with meals
Hydrocholeretics		
Dehydrocholic acid (Cholan-DH, Decholin, Hepahydrin, Neocholan)	Tablets—244 mg, 250 mg	250 mg to 500 mg 3 times a day after meals
Pancreatic Enzymes		
Pancreatin (Viokase)	Tablets Powder containing various amounts of lipase, amylase, and protease	1 to 3 tablets or 0.75 g powder with meals
Pancrelipase (Cotazym, Ilozyme Ku-Zyme HP, Pancrease)	Tablets Capsules Powder packets containing various amounts of lipase, amylase, and protease	1 to 3 tablets or capsules, or 1 to 2 powder packets before meals or snacks

50 Laxatives

A laxative is an agent that facilitates evacuation of the bowel. The valid indications for use of such drugs are few, and laxatives are frequently misused and abused by a large number of persons suffering from constipation, a condition characterized by a reduced frequency of fecal elimination. Diagnosis of constipation is made difficult by the realization that there is a tremendous variation in the frequency of "normal" bowel movements, estimated to range from as low as three per week to as high as three per day. Given this inherent variability, constipation cannot be characterized strictly in terms of bowel frequency, but must be viewed in relation to previous bowel habits, presence of disease states, or to other drug therapy, diet, and other conditions.

Chronic simple constipation can be relieved frequently by proper diet, adequate fluid intake, and sufficient exercise, and does not usually require drug therapy. When indicated, laxative therapy should be short term (that is, 1 wk–2 wk) and should be discontinued once bowel regularity has returned. Prolonged use of laxative drugs should be strongly discouraged because regular use of most laxatives can lead to dependence on the drug to achieve bowel movements rather than on the natural defecation reflex. Persistent constipation is most often a result of improper diet, chronic disease states, prolonged laxative use, or a mental outlook or behavioral pattern adversely affecting bowel function. As such, drug therapy is usually ineffective and frequently harmful and should never be employed in lieu of determining and correcting the underlying cause of the dysfunction.

Acute constipation, on the other hand, is often amenable to drug therapy, especially in those individuals who do not have a history of bowel irregularities. Certain laxative products (*e.g.,* stimulants, saline, or osmotics) are also indicated for rapid lower bowel evacuation in preparation for radiographic or endoscopic examination of the intestinal tract or in cases of poisoning with toxic substances.

There are a variety of laxative products available that function by a number of different mechanisms. The choice of a laxative product is dependent on many factors, including speed and intensity of evacuation desired (*e.g.,* chronic, mild constipation *versus* preradiologic intestinal flushing), presence of other disease states (*e.g.,* cardiac impairment, anorectal disorders), or need for sodium restriction.

A classification of laxatives based upon their respective mechanisms of action is presented in Table 50-1. In general, bulk producing agents (*e.g.,* methylcellulose) are considered the safest and most "physiologic" type of laxative and are the preferred agents for short-term treatment of most types of mild constipation. Emollients or fecal softeners are likewise relatively safe and are widely used in conditions in which hard or dry stools might prove painful or dangerous, such as after rectal or anal surgery, or in the presence of hemorrhoids and other conditions in which straining is undesirable (*e.g.,* heart disease, hernias).

The various laxative products are discussed as a group, and are followed by a tabular listing of each product with specific comments. It should be noted that in addition to the products reviewed here, several of the bile salts (see Chap. 49) have also been employed for the symptomatic treatment of mild, uncomplicated constipation, although their efficacy has been questioned.

Laxatives

Bisacodyl	Magnesium sulfate
Cascara sagrada	Methylcellulose
Castor oil	Mineral oil
Danthron	Nondiastatic barley malt
Dioctyl calcium sulfosuccinate	Phenolphthalein
Dioctyl potassium sulfosuccinate	Poloxamer 188
	Polycarbophil
Dioctyl sodium sulfosuccinate	Psyllium
Glycerin	Senna
Lactulose	Sodium biphosphate
Magnesium citrate	Sodium phosphate
Magnesium hydroxide	

Mechanism
See Table 50-1.

Uses
1 Short-term treatment of constipation
2 Evacuation of the lower intestinal tract in preparation for surgery or endoscopic or radiologic examination
3 Removal of toxic substances from the lower intestinal tract
4 Prevention of straining where such action is painful or hazardous (*e.g.,* anorectal disorders, hernia, cardiac disease)

Dosage
See Table 50-2.

Fate
(See Table 50-2 for specific information.) Administered orally or rectally; systemic absorption is minimal in most cases; onset of action varies from 5 minutes to 10 minutes with many suppositories or rectal enemas to 24 hours to 72 hours with some bulk-forming products; excreted largely unchanged in the feces, although a number of drugs may be partially metabolized upon systemic absorption and eliminated by the kidney, often producing a colored urine

Common Side-Effects
(Incidence varies among different preparations) Excessive bowel activity, nausea, and unpleasant taste

Significant Adverse Reactions
(Not associated with all drugs and usually observed with excessive or prolonged use) Vomiting, profound diarrhea, perianal irritation, electrolyte imbalance (especially with saline/osmotic laxatives, resulting in weakness, fainting, dizziness, palpitations, and sweating), hypersensitivity reactions (especially with phenolphthalein), esophageal, in-

Table 50-1. Classification of Laxatives

Bulk Forming (*e.g.,* methylcellulose, psyllium)

Cellulose derivatives that swell in intestinal fluid, stimulating peristalsis by retaining water in the stool; considered the safest and most physiologic type of laxative; each dose should be taken with sufficient water to minimize risk of intestinal or esophageal obstruction; onset of action is usually 12 hours to 24 hours

Emollient/Fecal Softeners (*e.g.,* dioctyl sodium sulfosuccinate)

Anionic surfactants, which increase the wetting efficiency of intestinal water, thus softening the fecal mass by facilitating mixture of aqueous and fatty substances; most useful in conditions in which straining is hazardous (*e.g.,* heart disease, perianal disease, hypertension, hernia, rectal surgery); may require several days before an effect is seen

Lubricant (*e.g.,* mineral oil)

Softens fecal matter by lubricating the intestinal mucosa, facilitating passage of the stool; may prevent absorption of fat-soluble vitamins and nutrients and delay gastric emptying; do not administer with meals; effects usually occur within 6 hours to 8 hours

Saline/Osmotic (*e.g.,* magnesium citrate, sodium phosphate, lactulose)

Nonabsorbable cations (magnesium), anions (phosphate), or sugars (lactulose) that retain water in the intestinal lumen, thus mechanically stimulating peristalsis and altering stool consistency; action is rapid (0.5 hr–2 hr) and should be used only for acute bowel evacuation, except for lactulose which may be administered in chronic constipation

Stimulants (*e.g.,* bisacodyl, castor oil, phenolphthalein)

Increase intestinal propulsion by either a direct irritant effect on the mucosa or an activation of sensory nerve endings in intestinal smooth muscle; may produce excessive catharsis, leading to fluid and electrolyte disturbances; prolonged use can result in habituation and laxative dependency; onset of action is generally 6 hours to 8 hours orally

testinal, or rectal obstruction (particularly with bulk laxatives), discoloration of urine or rectal muscosa, laxative dependence

Contraindications
Presence of abdominal pain, nausea, vomiting, or other signs of acute appendicitis, diverticulitis, colitis, or regional enteritis; acute surgical abdomen, fecal impaction, intestinal obstruction, or perforation, acute hepatitis, or late pregnancy

In addition, use of magnesium or potassium salts in patients with renal dysfunction, use of sodium salts in patients requiring sodium restriction, and use of emollients and mineral oil together

Interactions
1 Systemic absorption of mineral oil can be enhanced by emollient (*i.e.,* fecal softening) laxatives.
2 Mineral oil may impair the GI absorption of fat-soluble vitamins (A, D, E, K) or nutrients.
3 Laxatives (particularly bulk forming) may decrease absorption of other drugs present in the GI tract, either

(*Text continues on p. 488.*)

Table 50-2. Laxatives

Drug	Preparations	Usual Dosage Range	Remarks
Bulk Forming			
Methylcellulose (Cologel)	Liquid–450 mg/5 ml	Adults—5 ml to 20 ml 2 to 3 times a day with water Children—5 ml to 10 ml 1 to 2 times a day	Used orally for constipation; also available in ophthalmic drops for relief of dry, irritated eyes and as an ocular lubricant for artificial eyes and contact lenses; oral doses should be taken with 1 or more glasses of water for each dose, and additional fluids are indicated throughout the day to prevent fecal impaction; sodium carboxymethylcellulose is available in capsule form with dioctyl sodium sulfosuccinate (Disoplex)
Nondiastatic barley malt extract (Maltsupex)	Tablets—750 mg Liquid Powder	Tablets: Adults only—4 tablets with meals and at bedtime 4 times/day with liquid Powder/liquid: Adults—2 tbsp twice a day for 3 to 4 days; then 1 to 2 tbsp at bedtime Children—1 tbsp to 2 tbsp in milk 1 to 2 times a day	Useful in treating functional constipation in infants and children, as well as in adults, including those with laxative dependence; also may provide relief from itching in pruritus ani; use with caution in diabetics, because preparations contain 14 g carbohydrates per tbsp and 0.6 g per tablet; mixes more easily with cold liquids when first stirred with a little hot water; available in combination with powdered psyllium seed as Syllamalt
Polycarbophil calcium (Mitrolan)	Chewable tablets—(equivalent to 500 mg polycarbophil)	Adults—2 tablets 4 times a day Children (6 yr–12 yr)—1 tablet 3 times a day Children (3 yr–6 yr)—1 tablet twice a day	A hydrophilic agent that is used for treating both diarrhea and constipation; claimed to restore a more normal moisture level and to provide bulk in the GI tract; as a laxative, retains free water in the lumen of the intestine; a full glass of water or other liquid should be taken with each dose; discontinue use after 1 week if desired effects are not noted; also used for controlling simple diarrhea (see Chap. 51)
Psyllium hemicellulose (Mucilose, Perdiem Plain)	Flakes–100% Granules–50% (with 50% dextrose), 100%	1 tsp to 2 tsp twice a day in a full glass of liquid	Natural products derived from the blond psyllium seed (*Plantago ovata*); available in several dosage forms, many containing dextrose as a dispersing agent; contact with water in GI tract produces a bland, nonirritating bulk that aids peristalsis; sodium content is negligible, except in effervescent mixes containing sodium bicarbonate; drug should be taken with adequate water to prevent esophageal, gastric, intestinal, or rectal obstruction; each dose should be followed by a second full glass of water; do not attempt to swallow dry; available in combination with barley malt extract (Syllamalt) or senna (Perdiem, Prompt)
Psyllium hydrocolloid (Effersyllium)	Powder–3-g to 7-g packet or rounded teaspoon	Adults—1 tsp or 1 packet 1 to 3 times a day in water Children—½ tsp or ½ packet in ½ glass water at bedtime	
Psyllium hydrophilic muciloid (Hydrocil, Metamucil, Modane Bulk, Regacilium, Reguloid, Syllact, V-Lax)	Powder–50% muciloid with 50% dextrose Powder–100% Powder packets–3-g to 5-g/ packet with citric acid and sodium bicarbonate	1 tsp in a glass of liquid 1 to 3 times a day; follow with a second glass of liquid 1 packet in water 1 to 3 times a day	

Table 50-2. Laxatives (continued)

Drug	Preparations	Usual Dosage Range	Remarks
Psyllium seed husks (Siblin)	Powder–3 g to 5 g/tsp with an equal amount of dextrose Granules–2.5 g/tsp with 2.4 g sucrose	1 tsp in a full glass of liquid 1 to 3 times a day Children—½ adult dose with same quantity of fluid	
Emollient			
Dioctyl calcium sulfosuccinate—Docusate calcium (Surfak, Pro-Cal-Sof)	Capsules—50 mg, 240 mg	Adults—240 mg/day Children—50 mg to 150 mg/ day	Similar in action to dioctyl *sodium* sulfosuccinate, but does not contain sodium, which may be hazardous in patients with hypertension, congestive heart failure, edema, impaired renal function, or in persons on sodium-restricted diets; do not use in combination with mineral oil, because drug may enhance systemic absorption of the oil. (See dioctyl sodium sulfosuccinate) combined with danthron as Doxidan capsules
Dioctyl sodium sulfosuccinate—Docusate sodium (Colace, Disonate, Doxinate, D-S-S, Modane Soft, and various other manufacturers)	Capsules—50 mg, 60 mg, 100 mg, 120 mg, 240 mg, 250 mg, 300 mg Tablets—50 mg, 60 mg, 100 mg, 240 mg, 300 mg Solution—10 mg/ml, 50 mg/ ml Syrup—17 mg/5 ml, 20 mg/5 ml Suppositories—100 mg	Adults—50 mg to 240 mg Children (6 yr–12 yr)—40 mg to 120 mg Children (3 yr–6 yr)—20 mg to 60 mg Children (under 3 yr)—10 mg to 40 mg Larger doses may be given initially, then adjusted to optimal response	A surface-wetting agent that increases the wetting efficiency of intestinal water, thus facilitating the mixing of aqueous and fatty substances to soften the fecal mass for easier passage; effect on stools is apparent 1 day to 3 days after first dose; does not exert a laxative action itself, but is mainly used as adjunctive treatment in constipation associated with hard, dry stools or in patients who should avoid straining (*e.g.,* with cardiac disease, hernia, anorectal disorders); combined with casanthranol (*e.g.,* Peri-Colace), danthron (*e.g.,* Dorbantyl)—caution; this combination may produce liver damage with chronic administration), senna concentrate (*e.g.,* Senokot S, Senokap DSS), phenolphthalein (*e.g.,* Correctol), sodium carboxymethylcellulose (*e.g.,* Dialose), and various other laxatives; should not be used regularly by patients who must restrict sodium intake; May increase systemic absorption of mineral oil if given in combination
Dioctyl potassium sulfosuccinate—Docusate potassium (Dialose, Kasof)	Capsules—100 mg, 240 mg	100 mg to 240 mg/day with a full glass of water	See dioctyl sodium sulfosuccinate; may be used where sodium restriction is necessary; available in enema form with benzocaine and soft soap (Therevac) and in capsules combined with casanthranol (Dialose Plus)
Poloxamer 188 (Alaxin)	Capsules—240 mg	Adults—2 capsules at bedtime with a glass of water for a maximum of 1 week	Fecal softener similar to dioctyl sodium sulfosuccinate, but is a *nonionic* surfactant, thus is

(continued)

Table 50-2. Laxatives (continued)

Drug	Preparations	Usual Dosage Range	Remarks
		Children—1 to 2 capsules at bedtime with water	compatible with electrolytes; may also be used where sodium restriction is necessary
Lubricants			
Mineral oil (Agoral Plain, Fleet Mineral Oil Enema, Kondremul Plain, Neo-Cultol, Nujol, Petrogalar Plain, Zymenol)	Liquid Jelly Suspension—65% Emulsion—50%, 55% Enema	Oral: Adults—5 ml to 30 ml at bedtime Children—5 ml to 10 ml at bedtime Rectal: Adults—60 ml to 120 ml Children—30 ml to 60 ml	Useful to maintain soft stools to avoid straining, coats fecal contents, preventing colonic absorption of water; probably not as effective or safe as emollients; may interfere with absorption of fat-soluble vitamins and nutrients; therefore administer on an empty stomach; do not use during pregnancy or with emollients; enema may avoid interference with nutrient absorption, but oil seepage from rectum can stain clothing; use cautiously in the very old or debilitated or very young (under 2 yr), because danger of aspiration and possible development of lipid pneumonia is increased; emulsified preparations mask the objectionable consistency of plain oil and may be slightly more effective, but tend to increase systemic absorption of oil and are significantly more expensive; avoid prolonged or excessive use; available in combination with dioctyl sodium sulfosuccinate, phenolphthalein (Agoral, Petrogalar with Phenolphthalein), cascara extract (Kondremul with Cascara), and magnesium hydroxide (Haley's M-O)
Saline/Osmotic			
Lactulose (Cephulac, Chronulac)	Syrup—10 g/15 ml with several other sugars	Laxative (Chronulac)—15 ml to 30 ml/day to a maximum of 60 ml/day Portal–systemic encephalopathy (Cephulac)—30 ml to 45 ml 3 to 4 times a day	A complex sugar that is not hydrolyzed in the GI tract, but enters the colon unchanged, where it is broken down primarily to lactic acid by colonic bacteria; this elevates the osmotic pressure, increasing stool water content and softening the fecal matter; may require 24 hours to 48 hours to produce a bowel movement; use cautiously in pregnant or nursing women, in elderly or debilitated patients, and in diabetics; initial doses may produce flatulence and cramping; may be mixed with fruit juice or milk to improve palatability; reduces blood ammonia levels by 25% to 50% and hence is also used for prevention and treatment of portal–systemic encephalopathy, including the stages of hepatic precoma and coma; may be administered

Table 50-2. Laxatives (continued)

Drug	Preparations	Usual Dosage Range	Remarks
			chronically for this indication, dosage is usually adjusted to produce 2 to 3 soft stools a day
Magnesium citrate (Citroma, Citro-Nesia)	Liquid	200 ml to 250 ml (1 glassful) at bedtime	Chilling liquid improves the taste; do not use in patients with renal impairment; observe for signs of magnesium toxicity (thirst, drowsiness, dizziness); availabe in several bowel evacuation kits (Evac-Q-Kit, Evac-Q-Kwik, Tridrate Bowel Evacuant Kit)
Magnesium hydroxide (Milk of Magnesia)	Liquid—78 mg/ml, 233 mg/ml Tablets—325 mg	Adults—15 ml to 30 ml of regular liquid or 10 ml to 20 ml of concentrated liquid at bedtime Children—0.5 ml/kg/dose of regular liquid	Recommended for short-term use only, because accumulation of magnesium ions can result in serious toxicity (CNS or neuromuscular depression, fluid and electrolyte imbalances); tablets are less effective than liquid as a laxative; concentrated liquid (233 mg/ml) is lemon flavored to improve palatability; do not use in patients with renal impairment; also used as an antacid (see Chap. 48); available in emulsion form containing mineral oil (Haley's M-O)
Magnesium sulfate (Epsom Salt)	Powder	Adults—15 g in a glass of water or fruit juice Children—0.25 g/kg/dose	Administer in a flavored vehicle if necessary to mask the salty taste; effects are noted within several hours; infrequently used laxative
Sodium phosphate	Powder	4 g dissolved in water	Somewhat less effective than magnesium salts; not recommended where sodium must be restricted
Sodium phosphate and sodium biphosphate (Fleet Enema, Phospho-Soda)	Solution—1.8 g sodium phosphate and 4.8 g, sodium biphosphate per 10 ml Enema—6 g sodium phosphate and 16 g sodium biphosphate per 100 ml	Oral: 20 ml to 40 ml in ½ glass of water (Children—5 ml–15 ml) Rectal: Adults—120 ml Children—60 ml	Indicated only for acute evacuation of the bowel, e.g., prior to rectal or bowel examinations; high sodium content (555 mg/5 ml); available in packaged forms with bisacodyl tablets, suppositories, or enema (Fleet Barium Enema Prep Kits)
Stimulants			
Bisacodyl (Bisco-Lax, Deficol, Dulcolax, Fleet Bisacodyl, Theralax)	Tablets—5 mg Suppositories—10 mg Enema—10 mg/30 ml	Oral: Adults—10 mg to 15 mg Children—5 mg to 10 mg Rectal (suppository): Adults—10 mg following each bowel movement Children—5 mg Rectal enema: 1 container (37.5 ml)	Increases peristalsis, probably by a direct effect on sensory nerve endings in colonic mucosa; used to relieve constipation and to evacuate the bowel before examination; onset of action is 6 hours to 8 hours orally and 15 minutes to 60 minutes after insertion of suppository; tablets should not be crushed or chewed, and milk or antacids should not be consumed within 1 hour of the drug because they may prematurely dissolve the enteric coating on the tablet;

(continued)

Table 50-2. Laxatives (continued)

Drug	Preparations	Usual Dosage Range	Remarks
			rectal burning and itching may follow use of suppositories; no untoward systemic effects have been observed with either oral or rectal use; habituation can occur, with gradual loss of effectiveness
Bisacodyl Tannex (Clysodrast)	Powder packets—1.5 mg bisacodyl and 2.5 g tannic acid per packet	Cleansing enema—2.5 g in 1 liter warm water Barium enema—2.5 g to 5 g in 1 liter barium suspension (maximum 4 packets in 72 hr)	A nonabsorbable complex of bisacodyl and tannic acid used as a colonic evacuant; tannic acid is claimed to reduce intestinal secretions and when used with barium suspension, to improve the adherence of barium to intestinal walls; contraindicated in pregnant women and in children under 10 years, tannic acid may be hepatotoxic if sufficient quantities are absorbed; use cautiously where multiple enemas are being administered and in elderly or debilitated patients
Cascara sagrada	Tablets—325 mg Fluid extract Aromatic fluid extract	1 to 2 tablets, 1 ml fluid extract, or 5 ml aromatic fluid extract at bedtime	Direct chemical irritant that increases propulsive movements in the colon; onset of action is 6 hours to 10 hours; fluid extract is most effective preparation but taste is objectionable to some; aromatic fluid extract is less effective but more palatable; urine may be colored reddish to yellow brown, and rectal mucosa may become discolored; prolonged use should be avoided because habituation can result
Castor oil (Alphamul, Emulsoil, Neoloid, Purge)	Liquid or emulsion in various strengths	Adults—15 ml to 60 ml Children (over 2 yr)—5 ml to 15 ml Children (under 2 yr)—1 ml to 5 ml (depending on strength of emulsion)	Natural product that is broken down in small intestine to glycerol and ricinoleic acid, a local irritant; stimulates intestinal activity, resulting in production of liquid stools; primarily used for prompt evacuation of bowel before radiologic examination or in cases of poisoning; onset is 2 hours to 6 hours; do not use in pregnant women or to treat infestation with fat-soluble vermifuge, because systemic absorption may be increased
Danthron (Dorbane, Modane)	Tablets—37.5 mg, 75 mg Liquid—37.5 mg/5 ml	37.5 mg to 150 mg	Synthetic irritant laxative that stimulates peristalsis in the large intestine; onset of action is approximately 10 hours to 12 hours; administer in the evening for morning evacuation; do not use in nursing mothers (drug is excreted in breast milk); pink to brown discoloration of urine may occur; prolonged use may discolor rectal mucosa and

Table 50-2. Laxatives *(continued)*

Drug	Preparations	Usual Dosage Range	Remarks
			produce liver damage; combined with dioctyl sodium sulfosuccinate (*e.g.,* Dorbantyl, Doxan) or dioctyl calcium sulfosuccinate (Doxidan); this latter combination can produce liver damage with prolonged use
Phenolphthalein (Alophen, Espotabs, Evac-U-Lax, Evac-U-Gen, Ex-Lax, Feen-A-Mint, Phenolax, Prulet)	Tablets—60 mg, 90 mg, 97.2 mg Chewable tablets—30 mg, 60 mg, 90 mg, 97.2 mg Wafers—64.8 mg, 80 mg Gum tablets—97.5 mg Powder	30 mg to 200 mg at bedtime	Stimulant laxative similar to bisacodyl in most respects; onset of action is 6 hours to 8 hours; may color urine red to yellow brown; effects may be prolonged for several days due to enterohepatic circulation; allergic skin reactions can occur; drug should be discontinued at first sign of rash; some preparations are fruit or chocolate flavored; keep out of reach of children, because serious toxicity can result if large quantities are consumed; Available in combination with dioctyl sodium sulfosuccinate (*e.g.,* Correctol, Disolan) mineral oil (*e.g.,* Agoral, Kondremul w/ Phenolphthalein, Petrogalar w/ Phenolphthalein), and cascara (*e.g.,* Caroid w/ Phenolphthalein)
Senna concentrate (Senexon, Senokot, X-Prep)	Tablets—187 mg Granules—326 mg/tsp Suppositories—652 mg Powder paks—22.5 g	Constipation: Adults—2 tablets, 1 tsp granules, or 1 suppository at bedtime Children—½ adult dose Preradiographic bowel evacuation—1 container (22.5 g) taken between 2 PM and 4 PM on day before examination	Natural product prepared from species of *Cassia,* having a similar but more potent laxative action than cascara; concentrate may provide a more uniform effect than other preparations, with less colic; onset of action is usually 6 hours to 12 hours, but may require 24 hours in some cases; may impart a yellow brown to red color to the urine or feces
Senna equivalent (Black-Draught)	Tablets—600 mg Granules—1.65 g/0.5 tsp	Adults—2 tablets or ¼ tsp to ½ tsp granules with water	
Senna extract (Senokot, Senolax, X-Prep)	Tablets—217 mg Syrup—44 mg/ml, 100 mg/ml Liquid—75 ml single dose bottle Powder	Constipation: Adults—2 tablets or 5 ml to 15 ml syrup at bedtime Children—1.25 ml to 10 ml syrup at bedtime depending on age and weight Preradiographic bowel evacuation—75 ml taken between 2 PM and 4 PM on day before examination	
Hyperosmolar			
Glycerin (Fleet Babylax)	Suppositories Liquid	1 suppository or 4 ml of liquid inserted high into the rectum	Produces dehydration of exposed mucosal tissue, leading to irritation and subsequent evacuation; laxative effect occurs within 15 minutes to 30 minutes

by chemically combining with them or by hastening their passage through the intestinal tract.

4 Antacids, other alkaline substances, or histamine H₂ antagonists may prematurely dissolve the enteric coating on bisacodyl tablets, decreasing the laxative action, and leading to gastric or duodenal stimulation.

▶ **NURSING ALERTS**

▷ 1 Advise physician immediately if rectal bleeding, severe abdominal pain, or a sudden change in bowel function occurs during laxative therapy.

▷ 2 Do not use laxatives for more than 1 week to 2 weeks without consulting a physician, and avoid increasing the dosage if the product is ineffective. Laxative dependence or electrolyte imbalance can develop.

▷ 3 Monitor electrolytes regularly during prolonged therapy and urge patients to report signs of electrolyte imbalances, such as muscle cramping, weakness, or dizziness.

▷ 4 Do not use products containing magnesium, phosphate, or potassium salts in patients with renal dysfunction.

▶ **NURSING CONSIDERATIONS**

(See Table 50-2 for specific information on each drug.)

▷ 1 Suggest that patients experiencing occasional constipation include sufficient roughage in the diet, maintain an adequate fluid intake (6–10 glasses/day), and undergo a normal exercise routine instead of relying on laxative drugs.

▷ 2 Attempt to ascertain and relieve the cause of constipation rather than simply to treat it symptomatically.

▷ 3 Administer laxative products to provide maximal effect at a time most convenient to patient (*e.g.,* give a drug with a 6-hour to 8-hour onset at bedtime for evacuation in the morning).

▷ 4 Do not administer stimulant cathartics or laxative enemas to children under 2 years of age.

▷ 5 Inform patient that use of certain laxatives (*e.g.,* cascara, danthron, phenolphthalein, senna) may color urine pink to red to yellow–brown, and can discolor rectal mucosa as well.

▷ 6 Administer bulk laxatives in a large glass of water followed by a second glass of water to prevent esophageal impaction. Advise patient never to swallow powder dry.

▷ 7 Check sodium content of laxative product before administering to patients who must restrict salt intake. Use only those products containing little or no sodium.

▷ 8 Adjust dosage of laxative to provide sufficient but not excessive bowel activity. Discontinue drug when bowel regularity is achieved.

▷ 9 Advise patients taking laxative products before endoscopic or radiologic examinations to carefully follow instructions concerning timing of doses to achieve maximal bowel evacuation.

▷ *Dietary precautions*

▷ 1 Stress the importance of adequate bulk and roughage in the diet to minimize the occurrence and severity of constipation. Desirable foods include whole grain bread and cereal, raw and cooked vegetables, plums, and prunes. Adequate fluid intake (6–10 glasses/day) is likewise important.

Diarrhea, the passage of excessive, watery stools, is generally viewed as a *symptom* of an underlying pathologic condition rather than as a disease entity in itself. Distinction must be made, however, between acute and chronic diarrhea, because significant differences exist between the two conditions with respect to etiology, potential danger to the patient, and preferred treatment. *Acute* diarrhea, characterized by sudden onset of frequent, watery stools, often accompanied by fever, pain, vomiting, and weakness, may have several causes, including viral or bacterial infection, food or drug poisoning, or radiation exposure. The major danger of severe acute diarrhea is that it can quickly lead to dehydration and electrolyte imbalances, especially in pediatric patients. Fortunately, most episodes of acute diarrhea are self-limiting, that is, once the offending organisms, foods, or medications are removed, the symptoms soon subside.

Chronic diarrhea likewise has many possible causative factors, such as secondary disease states (*e.g.,* ulcerative colitis, diverticulitis, irritable colon, hyperthyroidism, gastric carcinoma), surgery (such as subtotal gastrectomy, vagotomy, ileal resection), or presence of excessive amounts of hormones, bile acids, or other substances in the GI tract. Chronic diarrhea may also be of psychogenic origin, a most difficult type to treat.

Whatever the type of diarrhea, every effort should be made to determine and remove the underlying cause of the distress. For example, diarrhea resulting from the presence of an infectious organism may best be treated by use of an appropriate antibiotic. Likewise, drug-induced diarrhea can often be corrected by simply discontinuing the offending drug. Successful treatment of secondary disease states associated with diarrhea usually reduces or eliminates the accompanying episodes of diarrhea. In those instances in which the cause of the diarrhea is not readily apparent or cannot be successfully eliminated by other means, use of antidiarrheal drugs for symptomatic relief should be considered on a short-term basis. In no instance, however, should antidiarrheal agents be employed in lieu of attempts to eradicate the cause of the condition, nor should these drugs be administered over prolonged periods of time except in unusual circumstances, because many of the more effective antidiarrheals have the potential to elicit a wide range of side-effects in addition to becoming habituating.

The most effective antidiarrheal medications are the opiates (such as paregoric) and related opiate derivatives (*e.g.,* diphenoxylate, loperamide), systemically acting agents that reduce intestinal hypermotility and slow peristalsis. Anticholinergics have also been used to reduce GI motility by impairing parasympathetic nerve stimulation to intestinal smooth muscle. Although they are possibly effective in some forms of diarrhea, the doses of anticholinergic drugs required to effectively slow peristalsis are quite high, and usually result in a wide range of unacceptable side-effects. Anticholinergic drugs are reviewed in detail in Chapter 10, and are not discussed here.

Various locally acting drugs have been employed for the symptomatic relief of diarrhea, frequently in combination form. Among the pharmacologic products used in this way are adsorbents (kaolin, pectin), astringents (zinc phenolsulfonate), antacids (aluminum hydroxide, bismuth salts),

Antidiarrheal Drugs

51

and bacterial cultures (*lactobacillus acidophilus*). These substances are relatively safe for normal use, but there is insufficient clinical evidence to establish their effectiveness for the intended purpose. Nevertheless, they are available without prescription and are widely used by the general public. A warning appearing on every product states that they should not be used for longer than 2 days, nor in the presence of high fever, and they should only be given to children under 3 years upon physicians' orders.

Treatment of most types of diarrhea, with the possible exception of severe acute diarrhea in infants and children, is usually best carried out conservatively. One of the locally acting drug combinations (such as kaolin and pectin) is usually satisfactory for the symptomatic management of mild, episodic diarrhea. More intense acute diarrhea may require addition of one of the opiate derivatives plus the ingestion of large amounts of fluids or possibly electrolyte solutions (*e.g.,* Lytren, Pedialyte—see Table 77-1) to prevent dehydration and electrolyte depletion. Persistent or recurrent diarrhea generally signifies an underlying pathologic condition that should be identified and corrected. Routine use of antidiarrheal drugs for extended periods should be confined to certain conditions (such as chronic inflammatory bowel disease, GI carcinoma, intestinal surgery, radiation therapy), only undertaken following careful examination, and closely supervised by a physician. Continuous self-use of antidiarrheal drug formulations by persons with mild, intermittent, or episodic diarrhea should be strongly discouraged, because the drug may not only elicit untoward reactions, but can mask the symptoms of a more severe underlying disease.

The potent systemically active antidiarrheal drugs are reviewed individually, followed by a brief, general discussion of the principal locally acting antidiarrheal agents, and a listing of commonly used antidiarrheal combination products.

Systemic Antidiarrheals

The systemic antidiarrheals comprise the opiates, principally camphorated tincture of opium (paregoric), anticholinergics, which are discussed in Chapter 10, and two opiate (meperidine) derivatives, diphenoxylate and loperamide, that are claimed to have a lower incidence of CNS effects and reduced addiction liability than other opiates.

▶ diphenoxylate HCl with atropine sulfate

Diphenatol, Enoxa, Lomotil, and various other manufacturers

Diphenoxylate is a structural analog of meperidine with a rather low risk of dependence at normal doses although typical opiate effects (such as euphoria) may occur with high doses. Prolonged ingestion can lead to habituation. Diphenoxylate is combined with a subtherapeutic amount of atropine to discourage deliberate abuse; excessive doses result in development of a variety of atropine-induced adverse effects that are distinctly unpleasant (see Significant Adverse Reactions).

Mechanism
Slows intestinal motility, probably by a direct inhibitory action on circular and longitudinal GI smooth muscle; may exert an antisecretory action as well; prolongs intestinal transit time, increases viscosity and density of intestinal contents, and reduces daily fecal volume; little or no analgesic effect

Use
1 Adjunctive treatment of diarrhea

Dosage
Adults: 5 mg four times a day; reduce when symptoms are controlled
Children: Initially 0.3 mg to 0.4 mg/kg/day in divided doses
   Average daily doses:
   2 yr–5 yr: 4 ml (2 mg) three times a day
   5 yr–8 yr: 4 ml (2 mg) four times a day
   8 yr–12 yr: 4 ml (2 mg) five times a day

Fate
Well absorbed when taken orally; onset of action is 30 minutes to 60 minutes; quickly and extensively metabolized to difenoxin, the major active circulating metabolite; peak plasma levels occur in 2 hours to 3 hours; elimination half-life is 12 hours to 15 hours; excreted primarily in the feces, with small amounts in the urine

Common Side-Effects
Dry mouth, drowsiness, and nausea

Significant Adverse Reactions
(Usually with large doses) Abdominal discomfort, vomiting, anorexia, headache, dizziness, restlessness, depression, malaise, numbness of extremities, pruritus, urticaria, angioneurotic edema, paralytic ileus, toxic megacolon, and respiratory depression

Atropine side-effects are more common in children and include flushing, diminished secretions, hyperthermia, tachycardia, urinary retention, hypotonia, miosis, nystagmus, and blurred vision

Contraindications
Obstructive jaundice, pseudomembranous colitis, severe dehydration, and in children under 2 years of age

Interactions
(See also Anticholinergics, Chap. 10.)
1 Diphenoxylate may potentiate the depressant effects of barbiturates, alcohol, narcotics and other tranquilizers, and sedatives.
2 Concurrent use with MAO inhibitors may precipitate a hypertensive crisis.

▶ **NURSING ALERTS**

▷ 1 Use with extreme caution in young children, because they exhibit a much reduced safety margin and a greater variability in response. If severe dehydration and electrolyte imbalance occur, withhold the drug until appropriate corrective measures have been taken.

▷ 2 Discontinue administration for acute diarrhea if clinical improvement is not noted within 48 hours.

▷ 3 Do not use in acute diarrhea associated with organisms that penetrate the intestinal mucosa (*e.g.*, salmonellae, shigellae) or in pseudomembranous colitis associated with broad-spectrum antibiotics (*e.g.*, lincomycin, clindamycin), because diarrhea may be intensified or prolonged.

▷ 4 Administer cautiously to patients with cirrhosis or other advanced liver disease, ulcerative colitis, glaucoma, to addiction-prone persons, and to pregnant or lactating women.

▷ 5 Observe patients for occurrence of abdominal distention or pain, possible indications of developing toxic megacolon due to delayed intestinal transit. Drug should be discontinued.

▷ 6 Caution patients not to exceed recommended dosage because incidence of adverse effects (*e.g.*, drowsiness, dizziness, tachycardia, blurred vision) greatly increases at high doses, and the danger of habituation is enhanced.

▷ 7 Be alert for respiratory depression in cases of overdosage. Naloxone (Narcan) is the drug of choice for reversing diphenoxylate-induced respiratory depression. Early signs of overdosage include flushing, drying of the skin or mucosa, tachycardia, hyperthermia, extreme miosis, and hypotonic reflexes.

▶ **NURSING CONSIDERATIONS**

▷ 1 Advise patients to avoid alcohol or other CNS depressants during therapy with diphenoxylate, because an additive depressant effect can result.

▷ 2 Continue to observe patients for at least 48 hours after last dose has been administered, because respiratory depression may not occur for some time after overdosage.

▷ 3 Be alert for signs of atropine overdosage (*e.g.*, dry mouth, blurred vision, flushing, tachycardia, urinary retention), especially in young children. Advise physician, because dose should be reduced or drug discontinued.

▷ 4 When administering the liquid preparation, use only the calibrated dropper provided with the bottle.

▷ 5 Note that drug is a Schedule V substance. Follow proper procedures for handling (see Appendix).

▶ **loperamide**

Imodium

A structural analog of meperidine with a reduced risk of dependence at recommend doses, loperamide is similar to diphenoxylate in action, but does not contain atropine;

therefore, anticholinergic side-effects are reduced. It is claimed to have slightly less abuse potential than diphenoxylate for chronic therapy, but caution is required during prolonged use, especially in patients with a history of drug abuse.

Mechanism

Slows intestinal motility and inhibits peristalsis by a direct depressant effect on intestinal smooth muscle; minimal action on the CNS at recommended dose levels

Uses

1 Control of acute nonspecific diarrhea and chronic diarrhea associated with inflammatory bowel disease

2 Reduction of volume of discharge from ileostomies

Dosage

Adults only

Acute diarrhea: initially 4 mg, followed by 2 mg after each loose stool; maximum dose 16 mg/day

Chronic diarrhea: as above for acute diarrhea, then reduce to an effective maintenance dose; usual dose range 4 mg to 8 mg/day

Fate

Well absorbed when taken orally; onset is 30 minutes to 60 minutes, and duration is 4 hours to 5 hours; elimination half-life is about 10 hours to 12 hours; metabolized by the liver and excreted mainly in the feces as both unchanged drug and metabolites with small amounts in the urine

Common Side-Effects

(With prolonged therapy) Abdominal discomfort, drowsiness

Significant Adverse Reactions

Abdominal distention, constipation, dizziness, nausea, vomiting, skin rash, and CNS depression

Contraindications

Patients in whom constipation should be avoided (*e.g.*, severe cardiac disease, intestinal obstruction)

Interactions

1 Loperamide may enhance the sedative effects of other CNS depressants (*e.g.*, barbiturates, alcohol, narcotics, hypnotics).

▶ **NURSING ALERTS**

See Diphenoxylate. In addition:

▷ 1 Use with caution in children under 2 years because safety and effectiveness have not been established in this group.

▶ **NURSING CONSIDERATIONS**

See Diphenoxylate. In addition:

▷ 1 Note that if clinical benefit is not obtained at a dose of 16 mg/day for 10 days, further administration is unlikely to be effective. However, drug may be con-

Table 51-1. Antidiarrheal Combination Products

Trade Name	Dosage Form	Opiate Derivative	Adsorbents Astringents	Anticholinergics	Other Ingredients
Amogel PG	Suspension	Powdered opium	Kaolin, pectin	Hyoscyamine, atropine, hyoscine	
Bacid	Capsules				*Lactobacillus acidophilus,* sodium carboxymethylcellulose
B.P.P.-Lemmon	Tablets	Powdered opium	Kaolin, pectin, bismuth subgallate, zinc phenolsulfonate		
Corrective Mixture	Suspension		Bismuth subsalicylate, zinc sulfocarbolate, phenyl salicylate		Pepsin
Corrective Mixture with Paregoric	Suspension	Paregoric	Bismuth subsalicylate, zinc sulfocarbolate, phenyl salicylate		Pepsin
Devrom	Chewable tablets		Bismuth subgallate		
Diabismul	Tablets	Powdered opium	Bismuth subcarbonate, calcium carbonate		
Diabismul	Suspension	Opium	Kaolin, pectin		
Dia-Eze	Suspension		Kaolin, bismuth subgallate		
Diar-Aid	Tablets		Activated attapulgite, pectin		
Dia-Quel	Suspension	Opium tincture	Pectin	Homatropine	
Diarkote	Tablets		Activated attapulgite, pectin	Belladonna alkaloids	
DoFus	Tablets				*Lactobacillus acidophilus*
Donnagel	Suspension		Kaolin, pectin	Hyoscyamine, atropine, hyoscine	
Donnagel-PG	Suspension	Powdered opium	Kaolin, pectin	Hyoscyamine, atropine, hyoscine	
Infantol Pink	Liquid	Opium	Pectin, bismuth subsalicylate, zinc phenolsulfonate		Extract Irish moss
Kaodene with Codeine	Suspension	Codeine phosphate	Kaolin, pectin, bismuth subsalicylate, sodium carboxymethylcellulose		
Kaodene with Paregoric	Suspension	Anhydrous morphine	Kaolin, pectin, bismuth subsalicylate, sodium carboxymethylcellulose		
Kaodene Non-Narcotic	Suspension		Kaolin, pectin, bismuth subsalicylate, sodium carboxymethylcellulose		
Kaodonna PG	Suspension	Powdered opium	Kaolin, pectin	Hyoscyamine, atropine, hyoscine	
Kaopectate	Suspension		Kaolin, pectin		
Kapectolin PG	Suspension	Powdered opium	Kaolin, pectin	Hyoscyamine, atropine, hyoscine	
KBP/O	Capsules	Powdered opium	Kaolin, pectin, bismuth, subcarbonate		
K-C	Suspension		Kaolin, pectin, bismuth subcarbonate		

Table 51-1. Antidiarrheal Combination Products (continued)

Trade Name	Dosage Form	Opiate Derivative	Adsorbents Astringents	Anticholinergics	Other Ingredients
K-P	Suspension		Kaolin, pectin		
K-Pec	Suspension		Kaolin, pectin		
Lactinex	Granules Tablets				*Lactobacillus bulgaricus, Lactobacillus acidophilus*
Mitrolan	Chewable tablets				Calcium polycarbophil
Parelixir	Suspension	Opium tincture	Pectin		
Parepectolin	Suspension	Opium	Kaolin, pectin		
Pektamalt	Suspension		Kaolin, pectin		Potassium gluconate, sodium citrate
Pepto-Bismol	Suspension Chewable tablets		Bismuth subsalicylate		
Polymagma Plain	Tablets		Activated attapulgite, pectin		
Rheaban	Liquid Tablets		Colloidal activated attapulgite		

tinued as a supplement to diet or specific treatment (*e.g.,* antibiotics).

▶ opium tincture, camphorated
Paregoric

Opium tincture is a mixture containing 0.04% anhydrous morphine, alcohol, benzoic acid, camphor, and anise oil. Its antidiarrheal effectiveness is due to its morphine content. Opium tincture, camphorated, should not be confused with *opium tincture, deodorized,* which contains 25 times the morphine equivalency, and should not be used routinely for treating diarrhea (refer to the discussion of narcotics in Chap. 18).

Mechanism
Decreases GI motility and peristalsis, reduces digestive secretions, and increases intestinal smooth muscle tone, thus slowing passage of intestinal contents

Use
1 Treatment of acute diarrhea

Dosage
Adults: 5 ml to 10 ml (2 mg–4 mg morphine equivalent) after loose bowel movements, up to four times a day
Children: 0.25 ml to 0.5 ml/kg up to four times a day

Common Side-Effects
Drowsiness, lightheadedness

Significant Adverse Reactions
Allergic reactions (*e.g.,* rash, urticaria, pruritus), vomiting, dizziness, sweating, constipation, and habituation
In addition, because the drug is a narcotic, large doses or prolonged administration can result in symptoms of narcotic overdosage (see Chap. 18 for other possible untoward reactions).

Interactions
1 Paregoric can enhance the depressive effects of alcohol, barbiturates, tranquilizers, and other CNS depressants.

▶ NURSING ALERT
▷ 1 Discontinue drug as soon as symptoms of diarrhea are controlled. Physician should be advised if diarrhea persists longer than 48 hours or if fever or abdominal pain develops during treatment with paregoric.

▶ NURSING CONSIDERATIONS
▷ 1 Administer drug with water to facilitate its passage through the GI tract.
▷ 2 Urge patients to adhere closely to recommended dosage. Prolonged use or excessive doses may lead to habituation and dependence.
▷ 3 Ensure that adequate fluid replacement is provided during periods of diarrhea to prevent dehydration and electrolyte imbalances.
▷ 4 Observe proper procedures for storing and handling paregoric, because it is a Schedule III drug (see Appendix). Note that small amounts of paregoric or powdered opium equivalent are contained in several over-

the-counter antidiarrheal preparations (*e.g.,* Parepectolin, Dia-Quel, Donnagel-PG; see Table 51-1). These are either Schedule III or Schedule V drug combinations. Paregoric alone is available only by prescription.

Locally Acting Antidiarrheals

A large number of compounds exhibiting diverse pharmacologic effects have been employed in the treatment of diarrhea. Other than those drugs previously discussed in this chapter, most other frequently used antidiarrheal agents are locally acting drugs; that is, they are primarily nonabsorbable chemicals that act within the lumen of the GI tract by a variety of mechanisms. The most commonly employed classes of locally acting antidiarrheal drugs are the adsorbents, antiseptics, and bacterial cultures, although astringents, antacids, bulk laxatives, digestive enzymes, and electrolytes have all been tried in the treatment of diarrhea. These locally acting agents, while essentially safe in recommended doses, have not been conclusively demonstrated to be clinically effective. Nevertheless, they are widely available over-the-counter, usually as combination products containing several different locally acting ingredients, and frequently including small doses of paregoric or other opium equivalents. Because they are readily available and relatively safe, they are most often the initial agents tried in cases of occasional, uncomplicated diarrhea, and in many instances provide sufficient relief. The warning that appears on every product should be heeded, however, and these agents should not be used for longer than 2 days to 3 days, or when high fever is present. Further, children under 3 years should be given these drugs only by prescription from a physician.

A general review of the pharmacology of the most frequently used locally acting antidiarrheals is presented here, followed by a listing of the ingredients of the commonly employed combination products in Table 51-1.

Adsorbents

The adsorbents are the antidiarrheal products most frequently used for the treatment of mild diarrhea. Commercial products usually contain two or more adsorbents, frequently combined with small amounts of opium derivatives or anticholinergics, or both. The extent to which the adsorbents contribute to the overall antidiarrheal efficacy of such mixtures is a subject of controversy, however. These compounds have the ability to bind to their particle surface toxins, bacteria, and other irritants that may be present in the GI tract; in addition, some adsorbents (*e.g.,* pectin) may also exert a soothing demulcent action on the mucosal surface of the irritated bowel. The adsorptive activity of these compounds is not selective for irritants or toxins, however, and they may also adsorb other drugs found in the intestinal tract at the same time. Thus, adsorbents can potentially interfere with the normal GI absorption of many drugs, and this possibility

should be noted whenever an adsorbent substance is given to a patient receiving medications for other conditions.

The most frequently encountered adsorbents in commercial preparations are kaolin, pectin, activated attapulgite, and certain bismuth salts (*e.g.,* subgallate, subsalicylate). Cholestyramine, an anion-exchange resin discussed in Chapter 33, has also been employed in some cases of severe diarrhea. It is thought to complex with bacterial toxins in the GI tract. Anion-exchange resins are not approved as antidiarrheal drugs, and their use in this manner is strictly experimental.

Antiseptics/Astringents

Drugs such as zinc phenolsulfonate, phenyl salicylate, and zinc sulfocarbolate are included in several proprietary antidiarrheal mixtures based on their astringent and reputed antiseptic action. It is doubtful whether inclusion of these substances significantly improves the antidiarrheal activity of the mixture.

Bacterial Cultures

Cultures of viable strains of *Lactobacillus acidophilus* and *Lactobacillus bulgaricus* have been used in the treatment of diarrhea resulting from a disruption of normal intestinal microorganism balance. Seeding the bowel with bacterial cultures is believed to re-establish the normal intestinal flora and suppress the growth of undesired microorganisms, thus improving those GI disturbances, including diarrhea, resulting from an altered intestinal flora. While possibly effective in those cases of diarrhea induced by treatment with antibiotics that can upset the normal bacterial population of the GI tract, lactobacillus preparations are not recommended for most episodes of diarrhea, inasmuch as they are somewhat more costly than other locally acting drugs, and there is no conclusive evidence that modification of intestinal flora has a beneficial effect in acute diarrhea.

Other

Among the other types of locally acting products that have been used in the treatment of diarrhea are the bulk-producing laxatives or hydrophilic colloids (*e.g.,* carboxymethylcellulose, polycarbophil, psyllium seed). The rationale behind this apparently paradoxical action is that these substances have the ability to absorb excess fecal fluid as they swell in the intestinal tract, thus aiding in the production of formed stools. Their suitability for most forms of diarrhea, however, remains speculative.

An important facet of the adjunctive treatment of persistent or severe, acute diarrhea is replenishment of fluid and electrolyte loss, especially in infants and young children. The various parenteral fluids and electrolyte solutions available for this purpose are reviewed in Chapter 77.

Summary. Antidiarrheal Drugs

Drug	Preparations	Usual Dosage Range
Diphenoxylate HCl with atropine sulfate (Diphenatol, Enoxa, Lomotil, and various manufacturers)	Tablets—2.5 mg with 0.025 mg atropine sulfate Liquid—2.5 mg/5 ml with 0.025 mg atropine/5 ml	Adults—5 mg 4 times a day Children—0.3 mg to 0.4 mg/kg a day in divided doses 2 yr to 5 yr—4 ml (2 mg) 3 times a day 5 yr to 8 yr—4 ml (2 mg) 4 times a day 8 yr to 12 yr—4 ml (2 mg) 5 times a day
Loperamide (Imodium)	Capsules—2 mg	Adults and children over 12—Initially 4 mg, followed by 2 mg after each loose stool to a maximum of 16 mg/day (usual maintenance dose 4 mg–8 mg a day)
Opium tincture, camphorated (Paregoric)	Liquid—2 mg morphine equivalent per 5 ml	Adults—5 ml to 10 ml (2 mg–4 mg morphine equivalent) after each loose stool to a maximum of 4 times a day Children—0.25 ml to 0.5 ml/kg

Locally Acting Antidiarrheals

See Table 51-1

52 Emetics and Antiemetics

Drugs having the ability to enhance vomiting reflex mechanisms, either through a peripheral (*i.e.,* local gastric mucosal irritation) or central (*i.e.,* stimulation of the medullary chemoreceptor trigger zone) action are termed *emetics*. They are used primarily to induce vomiting in cases of drug overdosage or poisoning with other types of chemicals or toxins.

Antiemetics are those agents that reduce the hyperreactive vomiting reflex, largely by a central action, either at the level of the vomiting center or chemoreceptor trigger zone (CTZ), or on the vestibular apparatus in the inner ear. The various mechanisms that may be involved in eliciting the vomiting reflex are reviewed in Chapter 47.

Emetics

Vomiting is an efficient means of removing unabsorbed drugs or toxins from the stomach; thus, emetics are frequently used in instances of drug overdosage or accidental ingestion of toxic chemicals or other substances. Prompt administration is essential in order to remove as much of the toxin as possible before significant amounts are absorbed into the system. Emetics generally should not be used, however, in certain types of poisoning, for example, with corrosive or caustic agents or petroleum products, because the expulsion of these substances by vomiting can severely irritate or damage the epithelium of the upper digestive tract. Likewise, patients who are comatose or semiconscious or who demonstrate hyperactive or convulsive activity should not receive emetics. Whenever possible, adjunctive drugs and other measures (*e.g.,* materials for gastric lavage or suction, oxygen, specific antidotes to the common poisons) should be available and employed when necessary. Drug overdosage or chemical poisoning is a potentially serious problem, and everyone, especially parents, should have ready access to a poisoning chart giving explicit instructions for handling poisoning emergencies. The phone number of the closest poison prevention center should be on hand, because speed of recognition and treatment is very often a critical factor for successful recovery.

▶ apomorphine

A synthetic derivative of morphine with a potent stimulant action on the CTZ, apomorphine can, like other narcotics, depress several areas of the CNS, including the respiratory and vasomotor centers, but its analgesic effects are greatly diminished compared to that of most other opiates. The degree of CNS depression is dose-dependent.

Mechanism
Stimulates the CTZ, thus increasing activation of the medullary vomiting center, resulting in emesis; exhibits dopamine receptor-stimulating action, thus may reduce secretion of prolactin and alter central motor regulatory function (*e.g.,* reduce akinesia or rigidity)

Use
1 Production of vomiting

Dosage
Adults: 5 mg SC (usual range 2 mg–10 mg)
Children: 0.05 mg/kg to 0.1 mg/kg SC
Do not repeat.

Fate
Onset of emesis is usually within 10 minutes to 15 minutes; metabolized by the liver and excreted chiefly in the urine.

Common Side-Effects
Sedation, nausea

Significant Adverse Reactions
Respiratory depression, orthostatic hypotension, dizziness, weakness, salivation, restlessness, tremors, and euphoria
Overdosage may cause violent vomiting, irregular respiration, cardiac depression, and vascular collapse.

Contraindications
Impending shock, poisoning with corrosives or petroleum products, overdosage with opiates, barbiturates, alcohol, or other CNS depressants

Interactions
1 Apomorphine may enhance the effects of levodopa.

▶ NURSING ALERTS
▷ 1 Recognize that use of apomorphine in cases of overdosage with CNS-depressant drugs (*e.g.,* narcotics, hypnotics, alcohol) may lead to profound depression, coma, and possibly death.
▷ 2 Have available naloxone (for apomorphine overdose) and atropine (for cardiac depression), as well as equipment for gastric lavage, suction, and respiratory assistance.
▷ 3 Use cautiously in patients with cardiac decompensation, in children, and in elderly or debilitated persons.

▶ NURSING CONSIDERATIONS
▷ 1 Administer 200 ml to 300 ml water or other liquid (smaller volumes in children) immediately before injection to elicit a more efficient vomiting reaction.
▷ 2 Position patients on their side to prevent aspiration of vomitus.
▷ 3 Do not use solutions that are discolored or that contain a precipitate.
▷ 4 Note that drug is available as soluble tablets, which should be dissolved in an appropriate parenteral vehicle before administration. Protect solution from light and air.
▷ 5 Monitor vital signs of patient for at least several hours after injection, because respiratory depression may be slow in developing.

▶ ipecac syrup

An alkaloidal mixture containing principally emetine and cephaline, ipecac exerts its emetic effect by a direct irritant action on the GI tract as well as a central action on the CTZ. Ipecac syrup is available in quantities up to 30 ml over the counter; larger sizes require a prescription. The syrup must not be confused with *ipecac fluid extract,* which is 14 times more potent, and can be fatal if given in the same dosage as the syrup.

Mechanism
Elicits emesis by a direct irritative action on the gastric mucosa and an activation of the CTZ; possesses an expectorant action, possibly by increasing bronchial secretions

Use
1 Induction of vomiting, primarily to remove unabsorbed drugs and poisons

Dosage
Adults and children (over 1 yr): 15 ml syrup followed by one or two glasses of water; may repeat in 20 minutes–30 minutes if vomiting has not occurred
Children (under 1 yr): 5 ml to 10 ml followed by one half to one glass of water

Fate
Vomiting occurs within 15 minutes to 30 minutes, and effects may persist for another 20 minutes to 30 minutes.

Significant Adverse Reactions
(Result of overdosage) Bloody diarrhea, arrhythmias, cardiotoxicity, shock, and convulsions

Contraindications
Semiconscious, unconscious or convulsing patients, shock, poisoning with corrosive or caustic substances

Interactions
1 Activated charcoal may absorb ipecac syrup, nullifying its emetic effect.

▶ NURSING ALERTS
▷ 1 Be aware that if vomiting does not occur, ipecac may be absorbed to a sufficient degree to have cardiotoxic effects.
▷ 2 Do not confuse ipecac syrup with ipecac fluid extract. The latter is 14 times stronger and can be fatal if ingested in the same amounts as the syrup.
▷ 3 If vomiting does not occur within 20 minutes after the second dose, contact a physician or emergency room immediately.

▶ NURSING CONSIDERATIONS
▷ 1 Do not administer milk or carbonated beverages with ipecac syrup.
▷ 2 Follow ipecac administration with 200 ml to 300 ml water.

Table 52-1. Antiemetic Drugs

I. Phenothiazines (e.g., chlorpromazine, perphenazine, prochlorperazine)

Potent antiemetic drugs acting by inhibition of CTZ via a dopaminergic blocking action; primarily effective for drug-induced emesis and nausea and vomiting associated with surgery, anesthesia, radiation, carcinoma, and severe infections; little usefulness in motion sickness, because drugs do not affect the vestibular apparatus; possibility of numerous side-effects (some serious); thus recommended for short-term use only (see Chap. 22)

II. Antihistamines (e.g., cyclizine, dimenhydrinate, meclizine, promethazine)

Act by decreasing sensitivity of vestibular apparatus of inner ear; thus most effective in treating nausea and vomiting of motion sickness, Meniere's disease, or labyrinthitis; all elicit varying degrees of drowsiness and may have significant anticholinergic activity (see Chap. 14)

III. Anticholinergics (e.g., scopolamine)

Depress the vestibular apparatus and inhibit cholinergic activation of the vomiting center; very effective in preventing motion sickness; high incidence of side-effects limits oral usefulness, but scopolamine is also available as Transderm-Scop in the form of a circular, flat disk that adheres to the skin behind the ear and provides for a continuous steady rate of drug release over 3 days (5 mcg/hr) with minimal side-effects (see Chap. 10)

IV. Sedatives (e.g., barbiturates)

Decrease anxiety and possibly reduce excess stimulation of the vomiting center; largely ineffective and associated with a high incidence of drowsiness (see Chap. 20)

V. Miscellaneous (e.g., benzquinamide, diphenidol, thiethylperazine, trimethobenzamide)

Predominantly centrally acting antiemetics possessing various mechanisms of action; individual drugs are discussed below

Antiemetics

The mechanisms involved in the vomiting reflex can involve several pathways and are outlined in detail in Chapter 47. To briefly review, the vomiting center in the medulla may be stimulated by the CTZ, also in the medulla, by the vestibular nuclei via the labyrinthine apparatus in the inner ear, and also directly by GI irritation. Dopamine appears to be the major neurotransmitter in the CTZ, whereas acetylcholine is believed to mediate the functioning of the vomiting center.

A variety of drugs have been successfully employed for the prophylaxis and treatment of vomiting of diverse etiology. Although vomiting may have many causes, for example, drug or chemical poisoning, motion sickness, radiation exposure, bacterial or viral infection, pregnancy, endocrine disorders, neurological or psychic disturbances, most successful antiemetic drugs act primarily by inhibition of the CTZ in the medulla or depression of vestibular apparatus sensitivity in the inner ear. The major groups of drugs used to control nausea and vomiting are the phenothiazines, anticholiner-

gics, antihistamines, and sedatives, along with a group of miscellaneous drugs, most of which also exhibit a central mechanism of action. These agents are listed in Table 52-1, with brief descriptions of their pharmacologic effects. In addition, a variety of other drugs, predominately local acting, have been used in the treatment of nausea and vomiting, and include antacids, adsorbents, antiflatulents, demulcents, and local anesthetics. The efficacy of most of these regionally acting antiemetic drugs is subject to considerable debate; nevertheless, the placebo effect of such medications cannot always be discounted, and their occasional use to settle an "upset stomach" is probably not harmful in the otherwise healthy patient.

The majority of clinically useful antiemetic drugs are considered elsewhere in the text. Thus, the phenothiazines, which are potent dopamine blocking agents and therefore very effective against drug-induced emesis at the level of the CTZ, are discussed in Chapter 22. Antihistamines, which are primarily useful in preventing the nausea and vomiting of motion sickness, because they apparently reduce vestibular activation of the vomiting center, are reviewed in Chapter 14. Scopolamine, a highly effective antinauseant for motion sickness, is now frequently used as a transdermal patch, which provides a prolonged action (i.e., 3 days) and greatly reduces the side-effects previously associated with oral administration of the drug. Scopolamine is considered in Chapter 10. A number of other drugs exhibiting an antiemetic action do not fall into one of the above categories and therefore are reviewed individually in this chapter.

▶ **benzquinamide**
Emete-Con

Mechanism
Not established; believed to depress the CTZ, and reduce activation of the vomiting center; possesses antihistaminic, anticholinergic, antiserotonin, and sedative action

Use
1 Prevention and treatment of nausea and vomiting associated with anesthesia or surgery

Dosage
IM: initially 0.5 mg/kg to 1 mg/kg at least 15 minutes before emergence from anesthesia; may repeat in 1 hour; then at 3-hour to 4-hour intervals as needed
IV: 0.2 mg/kg to 0.4 mg/kg as a single dose administered at a rate of 1 ml/minute; subsequent doses should be given IM

Fate
Rapidly absorbed from IM sites; onset of action within 15 minutes; duration is 2 hours to 4 hours; approximately one half of blood level is protein-bound; metabolized by the liver (plasma half-life is 45 min) and excreted in urine and feces, largely as metabolites

Common Side-Effects
Drowsiness, dry mouth

Significant Adverse Reactions

Autonomic—flushing, shivering, sweating, salivation, increased temperature, blurred vision, hiccups

Cardiovascular—hypotension, dizziness, atrial fibrillation, premature ventricular contractions (Sudden *hyper*tension may follow IV injection.)

CNS—restlessness, headache, excitement, fatigue, insomnia, weakness, tremors

GI—anorexia, nausea

Other—allergic reactions (rash, chills, fever, urticaria)

Contraindications

Pregnant women and young children, IV injection in cardiac patients.

Interactions

1 Markedly increased blood pressure may result from use of benzquinamide with other pressor agents.
2 Benzquinamide may enhance the effects of other CNS depressants.

▶ NURSING ALERTS

▷ 1 Do not administer IV to patients with cardiovascular disease, because the danger of sudden hypertension or arrhythmias is increased.

▷ 2 Note that the drug may mask signs of overdosage with other drugs or prevent accurate diagnosis of conditions associated with nausea and vomiting (*e.g.,* intestinal obstruction, carcinoma, brain tumors).

▶ NURSING CONSIDERATIONS

▷ 1 Administer drug at least 15 minutes before expected awakening from anesthesia when used to control postoperative nausea and vomiting.

▷ 2 Inject deeply IM into a large muscle. Aspirate to avoid accidental IV injection.

▷ 3 Administer cautiously to elderly or debilitated patients, and use lower range of recommended dosage.

▷ 4 Reconstitute powder for injection with 2.2 ml Sterile Water for Injection. This yields 2 ml of a solution containing 25 mg drug/ml and is stable for 14 days at room temperature.

▶ diphenidol
Vontrol

Mechanism

Depresses excitability of vestibular apparatus and CTZ; exhibits relatively weak antihistaminic, anticholinergic, and CNS depressant activity

Uses

1 Control of nausea and vomiting due to surgery, vestibular disturbances, infectious diseases, neoplasms, and radiation therapy
2 Treatment of vertigo due to Meniere's disease, labyrinthitis, or middle or inner ear surgery

Dosage

Adults: 25 mg to 50 mg every 4 hours orally

Children: 0.4 mg/lb (0.88 mg/kg) every 4 hours orally; maximum 2.5 mg/lb/day

Fate

Rapidly absorbed orally; onset of action is 30 minutes to 60 minutes; metabolized in the liver and excreted largely by the kidney

Common Side-Effects

Drowsiness, indigestion, and dry mouth

Significant Adverse Reactions

Auditory and visual hallucinations (see Nursing Alerts), confusion, disorientation, malaise, depression, insomnia, dizziness, headache, skin rash, slight hypotension, and mild jaundice

Contraindications

Anuria, IV administration in patients with sinus tachycardia, infants under 6 months or 25 lb, and pregnancy

Interactions

1 Additive CNS-depressant effects can occur in combination with other sedative or hypnotic drugs.

▶ NURSING ALERTS

▷ 1 Use only in hospitalized patients or in those under close continuous medical supervision, because drug has caused auditory and visual hallucinations, disorientation, and confusion. Discontinue drug if such reactions occur (incidence about 0.5%; onset usually within 3 days after starting therapy; symptoms subside within several days after discontinuation of therapy).

▷ 2 Because drug is a weak anticholinergic, use cautiously in patients with obstructive GI or urinary lesions, glaucoma, peptic ulcer, and hepatic disease.

▷ 3 Be aware the drug may mask signs of drug overdosage or underlying pathology.

▶ NURSING CONSIDERATIONS

▷ 1 Provide needed mouth care if patient is unable to take fluids for relief of dry mouth.

▷ 2 Warn patients that drowsiness can occur and may interfere with performance of tasks.

▷ 3 Do not administer to children less than 6 months of age; drug is not indicated for control of vertigo in children.

▶ phosphorated carbohydrate solution
Calm-X, Eazol, Emetrol, Especol, Nausetrol

These products are hyperosmolar solutions of various carbohydrates (*e.g.,* sucrose, dextrose, levulose) with phosphoric acid. The phosphorated carbohydrate solutions are locally acting antiemetics available over-the-counter.

Mechanism
Not established; probably exert a direct action on the wall of the GI tract, reducing smooth muscle contraction

Use
1 Symptomatic relief of nausea and vomiting

Dosage
Acute vomiting: adults—15 ml to 30 ml; children—5 ml to 10 ml (may be taken at 15-min intervals until vomiting ceases)
Regurgitation in infants: 5 ml to 10 ml, 10 minutes to 15 minutes before each feeding
Morning sickness: 15 ml to 30 ml on arising and every 3 hours as needed
Motion sickness: 15 ml as needed

Contraindications
Diabetes, hereditary fructose intolerance

▶ **NURSING CONSIDERATIONS**
▷ 1 Note that drug is quite safe when taken as directed, virtually free of side-effects, and will not mask symptoms of underlying pathology.
▷ 2 Do not dilute or take oral fluids immediately before or for at least 15 minutes after administration.
▷ 3 Advise patients to consult physician if symptoms are not relieved or recur following drug treatment.

▶ **thiethylperazine**
Torecan

A phenothiazine derivative used exclusively as an antiemetic–antivertigo agent, thiethylperazine is claimed to have less tranquilizing action than other phenothiazines.

Mechanism
Not definitively established; probably exerts a direct depressant action on both the CTZ and vomiting center

Use
1 Symptomatic relief of nausea and vomiting

Dosage
Oral, rectal, IM: 10 mg to 30 mg/day in divided doses

Fate
Onset of action is 30 minutes to 60 minutes with oral or rectal administration and 15 minutes to 30 minutes following IM injection; metabolized in the liver and excreted both in the urine and feces

Common Side-Effects
Drowsiness

Significant Adverse Reactions
Headache, dizziness, blurred vision, restlessness, fever, altered taste perception, orthostatic hypotension, and cholestatic jaundice
See also Phenothiazines, Chapter 22, for other possible adverse reactions.

Contraindications
Severe CNS depression, comatose states, IV administration, pregnancy, and children under 12 years of age

Interactions
See Phenothiazines, Chapter 22.

▶ **NURSING ALERTS**
▷ 1 Urge caution in driving or performing hazardous tasks, because drug can cause drowsiness, dizziness, and blurred vision.
▷ 2 Administer IM with patient recumbent, and keep patient in bed for at least 1 hour following injection to minimize orthostatic hypotension.
▷ 3 Be alert for appearance of extrapyramidal reactions (eye movements, difficulty in speaking, unusual body movements, gait disturbances) and advise physician. Dosage should be reduced or drug discontinued.
▷ 4 Use cautiously in patients with renal or hepatic disease, in nursing mothers, and following intracardiac or intracranial surgery.

▶ **NURSING CONSIDERATIONS**
▷ 1 Administer IM deeply into a large muscle mass. Aspirate carefully to avoid inadvertent IV injection. Never inject directly IV, because severe hypotension can occur.
▷ 2 Be alert for development of restlessness, agitation, or depression in patients recovering from anesthesia who were given the drug preoperatively.
▷ 3 If a vasopressor agent is needed to treat drug-induced hypotension, use norepinephrine or phenylephrine. Epinephrine is contraindicated, because it may cause a further drop in pressure.

▶ **trimethobenzamide**
Tegamide, Tigan

Mechanism
Not established; may directly depress the CTZ and interfere with vestibular activation of the CTZ or the vomiting center; does not appear to block *direct* activation of the vomiting center; possesses weak antihistamine activity

Use
1 Symptomatic control of nausea and vomiting (combined with other antiemetics if vomiting is severe)

Dosage
Oral: adults—250 mg three or four times a day; children—100 mg to 200 mg three or four times a day
Rectal: adults—200 mg three or four times a day; children—100 mg to 200 mg three or four times a day
IM: adults only—200 mg three or four times a day

Fate
Onset of action following oral or rectal administration is 15 minutes to 45 minutes, with duration of 3 hours to 4 hours; following IM injection, onset is 15 minutes and du-

ration is 2 hours to 3 hours; metabolized in liver and excreted primarily in the urine

Significant Adverse Reactions

Hypersensitivity reactions, hypotension (especially with IM use), blurred vision, depression, diarrhea, dizziness, drowsiness, jaundice, muscle cramping, and blood dyscrasias

In addition, during acute fever, gastroenteritis, dehydration, or electrolyte imbalance, drug has produced CNS reactions such as opisthotonos (tetanic spasm of back muscles), convulsions, extrapyramidal symptoms (rigidity, akathesia, tremor), and coma.

Following IM injection, redness, irritation, stinging, swelling, or burning at injection site

Contraindications

Parenteral use in children; rectal administration in newborns, premature infants, or persons hypersensitive to benzocaine or other local anesthetics; pregnancy; and nursing mothers

Interactions

1 Additive depressant effects can occur with other CNS-depressant drugs (e.g., narcotics, alcohol, barbiturates).
2 Extrapyramidal reactions, convulsions, and other CNS disturbances may be enhanced if trimethobenzamide is given together with phenothiazines or barbiturates.

▶ NURSING ALERTS

▷ 1 Caution patients to report development of rash, itching, or other signs of hypersensitivity. Drug should be discontinued.
▷ 2 Be alert for indications of CNS toxicity (e.g., disorientation, lethargy, tremors) and discontinue drug.

Recognize that the extrapyramidal reactions that occasionally occur with this drug can be confused with symptoms of certain CNS disorders that may be responsible for the vomiting, for example, encephalopathy, Reye's syndrome.

▷ 3 Administer with extreme caution to patients receiving other centrally acting drugs such as phenothiazines, barbiturates, or anticholinergics.
▷ 4 Urge caution in performing hazardous tasks (driving, operating machinery), because drug may produce drowsiness, dizziness, and loss of orientation.
▷ 5 Observe for abrupt onset of vomiting, confusion, lethargy, or irrational behavior, possible signs of Reye's syndrome, a potentially fatal condition terminating in convulsions, liver degeneration, encephalopathy, coma, and death (see Salicylates, Chap. 19). Although trimethobenzamide and other antiemetic drugs have not been *definitely* linked to Reye's syndrome, it has been associated with their use during acute febrile periods. Immediate medical attention is imperative if the above symptoms occur.

▶ NURSING CONSIDERATIONS

▷ 1 Monitor blood pressure following parenteral administration, because hypotension can occur.
▷ 2 Recognize that use of antiemetic drugs can mask symptoms of a more serious underlying disorder or impair diagnosis of a pathologic condition (e.g., appendicitis).
▷ 3 Do not administer IM in children of any age and do not use rectal suppositories in premature or newborn infants.
▷ 4 To minimize irritation and pain with IM injection, inject deeply into upper outer quadrant of gluteal region and avoid escape of solution along the injection route.

Summary. Emetics and Antiemetics

Drug	Preparations	Usual Dosage Range
Emetics		
Apomorphine	Soluble tablets—6 mg	Adults—5 mg SC (range 2 mg–10 mg)
		Children—0.05 mg/kg to 0.1 mg/kg
		Do not repeat
Ipecac syrup	Syrup	Adults—15 ml followed by 200 ml to 300 ml water
		Children (under 1 yr)—5 ml to 10 ml followed by 20 ml water
Antiemetics		
Benzquinamide (Emete-Con)	Injection—50 mg/vial	IM—initially 0.4 mg/kg to 1 mg/kg; repeat in 1 hour, then at 3-hour to 4-hour intervals as needed
		IV—0.2 mg/kg to 0.4 mg/kg at a rate of 1 ml/minute; do not readminister IV

(continued)

Summary. Emetics and Antiemetics *(continued)*

Drug	Preparations	Usual Dosage Range
Diphenidol (Vontrol)	Tablets—25 mg	Adults: Oral—25 mg to 50 mg every 4 hours Children: Oral—0.4 mg/lb every 4 hours
Phosphorated carbohydrate solution (Calm-X, Eazol, Emetrol, Especol, Nausetrol)	Syrup Solution	Adults—15 ml to 30 ml Children—5 ml to 10 ml; repeat at 15-minute intervals until vomiting ceases
Thiethylperazine (Torecan)	Tablets—10 mg Suppositories—10 mg Injection—5 mg/ml	10 mg to 30 mg a day in divided doses
Trimethobenzamide (Tegamide, Tigan)	Capsules—100 mg, 250 mg Suppositories—200 mg Pediatric suppositories— 100 mg Injection—100 mg/ml	Oral: Adults—250 mg 3 to 4 times a day Children—100 mg to 200 mg 3 to 4 times a day Rectal: Adults—200 mg 3 to 4 times a day Children—100 mg to 200 mg 3 to 4 times a day IM: Adults only—200 mg 3 to 4 times a day

Drugs Acting on Respiratory Function

VII

Normal metabolism requires the continual supply of oxygen (O_2) and removal of carbon dioxide (CO_2). The respiratory system functions in concert with the cardiovascular system to supply all body tissues with O_2 for cellular oxidative metabolism, and to remove CO_2, a major metabolic waste product.

The respiratory system also plays a critical role in the regulation of acid–base balance, adjusting its activities rapidly to maintain a constant pH of the internal environment.

Respiration, which may be broadly defined as the exchange of gases (O_2 and CO_2) between a living organism and its external environment, consists of five interrelated phases that operate continuously:

1 *Pulmonary ventilation*—the periodic flow of air into and out of the lungs
2 *Pulmonary exchange of gases*—the diffusion of O_2 from the alveoli into the pulmonary capillaries and the diffusion of CO_2 out of the blood into the alveoli
3 *Transport of gases*—the transport of O_2 by the blood from the lungs for distribution to all body tissues and the return of CO_2 from the tissues to the lungs for expiration
4 *Blood–tissue exchange of gases*—the exchange of gases at the tissue level with O_2 diffusing from the blood into the tissue cells and CO_2 diffusing from the cells into the blood
5 *Cellular respiration*—the cellular utilization of O_2 for oxidative metabolism with the production of CO_2.

Respiratory Physiology— A Review

53

Anatomy—Histology Overview

The respiratory system has two major functional divisions: the *conducting division* and the *respiratory division*.

Conducting Division

The components of the conducting division serve primarily as air conduits to the gas-exchanging areas of the lungs. During its passage through the upper segments of the conducting division, the air is filtered, warmed, and humidified. Components of the conducting division are the nose, pharynx, larynx, trachea, bronchi, bronchioles, and terminal bronchioles.

Respiratory Division

The respiratory bronchioles, alveolar ducts, alveolar sacs, and alveoli form the respiratory division of the lungs wherein the oxygen-rich, water-saturated air is exposed to the blood for gaseous exchange.

The Respiratory Tree

During inspiration the air passes through the nose (or mouth), pharynx, and larynx before entering the trachea. The trachea is structurally characterized by the presence of 16 to 20 C-shaped rings of hyaline cartilage (completed posteriorly by smooth muscle and connective tissue), which support the trachea and keep it patent. The tissue lining the trachea is pseudostratified cilated epithelium with goblet cells. The trachea terminates in the thorax by dividing into two primary bronchi that pass to the roots of the lungs. The right bronchus is shorter, wider, and more vertical than the left.

Within the lungs, the primary bronchi undergo successive branching to form a tree-like arrangement of smaller bronchi and bronchioles, often called the *bronchial tree*. The successive branching within the bronchial tree results in the formation of successively narrower tubes that collectively offer a greater total cross-sectional area of the lumina than the parent tubes.

The following histologic modifications occur with progressive branching:

1 The rings of cartilage are replaced by irregular plates of cartilage that gradually become smaller and finally disappear in the bronchioles.

2 As the amount of cartilage decreases the amount of smooth muscle progressively increases. The smooth muscle layer plays a major role in determining the airway resistance because it governs the caliber of the bronchioles (which no longer have cartilage rings to maintain tubular patency).

3 The pseudostratified ciliated epithelium loses its goblet cells and then the cilia and is eventually replaced by simple cuboidal epithelium in the terminal bronchioles.

Arising from the terminal bronchioles are the first components of the respiratory division—the *respiratory bronchioles*—whose free terminations open into *alveolar ducts*. The alveolar ducts communicate with spaces called *alveolar sacs*, which in turn open into a number of pocket-like expansions, the *alveoli*.

Histologically, the smooth muscle prominent in the latter segments of the conducting division is replaced by elastic connective tissue within the respiratory division.

The respiratory epithelium loses its cilia and thins out to a single squamous configuration, thus allowing gaseous exchange to occur. Increasing vascularity and a greater cross-sectional surface area further promote efficient exchange of gases. It has been estimated that human lungs contain approximately 300 million alveoli and provide a total surface area of 70 m² for gaseous exchange.

The Lungs

All the components of the respiratory tract beyond the primary bronchi are contained within the lungs. The lungs are cone-shaped, paired structures located in the thoracic cavity, surrounded by a cage-like framework composed of the sternum, costal cartilage, ribs, and vertebrae. The muscular, dome-shaped diaphragm serves as the floor of the thoracic cage.

Blood vessels, lymphatics, nerves, and the bronchi enter the lungs at the *hilus,* and form the root of the lung. The *parietal pleura,* which lines the thoracic cavity, and the *visceral pleura,* which covers the lung surface, are continuous serous membranes that reflect upon each other at the root of each lung. The potential space between these two membranes (the *pleural cavity*) contains a thin film of lubricating fluid that minimizes friction during respiratory movements.

The right lung contains three lobes and the left lung has two lobes, each of which is supplied by a *secondary* (or lobar) *bronchus.* Each lung is further subdivided into *bronchopulmonary segments* supplied by *tertiary* (or segmental) *bronchi.*

Each bronchopulmonary segment contains smaller anatomical units called *lobules,* supplied by a terminal bronchiole, arteriole, venule, and lymphatic vessel.

Blood Supply

The pulmonary artery and its branches carry blood from the right ventricle of the heart to the respiratory tissue of the lung for oxygenation and removal of CO_2. Venules, arising from the vast network of pulmonary capillaries that surround the alveoli, collect oxygenated blood, which is then returned to the left atrium of the heart by the *pulmonary veins.*

Oxygenated blood reaches the visceral pleura and other portions of the lung through the *bronchial arteries* and their branches. Some *bronchial veins* empty into the superior vena cava through the azygos system, while others drain into the pulmonary veins.

In contrast to the systemic circulation, the pulmonary circulation is a low-pressure, low-resistance circuit.

Nerve Supply

The bronchial tree is innervated by fibers from both divisions of the autonomic nervous system. Activation of parasympathetic (vagal) nerve fibers causes contraction of respiratory smooth muscle, whereas sympathetic stimulation brings about relaxation.

Autonomic nerves also supply pulmonary and bronchial blood vessels.

Respiratory Defense Mechanisms

Large particulate matter inhaled through the nares (nostrils) is filtered by the coarse hairs lining the nasal vestibule. A blanket of mucus (secreted by goblet cells and mucous glands in the upper respiratory tract) traps dust and fine particulate matter. The mucus and entrapped materials are swept toward the mouth by ciliary movements. The cough reflex provides a more forceful mechanism for the expulsion of secretions and particulate matter from the respiratory tract.

Alveolar macrophages ("dust cells") provide a major defense against bacterial invasion of the lungs. These unique phagocytic cells migrate freely over the alveolar surface, engulfing and lysing bacteria and other particulate matter.

Pulmonary Ventilation

Pulmonary ventilation operates on the principle that the pressure and volume of a closed cavity are inversely related. Therefore, if the volume of a closed cavity increases, the pressure within it will fall.

The lungs lie in separate airtight cavities within the thorax, surrounded by the pleura. The elastic recoil of the lungs tends to pull them away from the thoracic wall, creating a partial vacuum within the pleural cavity. The flow of air through the respiratory tract follows pressure gradients between the atmosphere and the lungs. Just before inspiration, the pressure inside the lungs (the *intrapulmonary pressure*) is equal to atmospheric pressure, whereas the pressure within the pleural cavity (the *intrapleural pressure*) is always below atmospheric.

Inspiration is an active process resulting from the expansion of the thorax. It is initiated by nervous activity leading to the contraction of respiratory muscles. During normal quiet inspiration the contraction and descent of the *diaphragm* increases the vertical dimensions of the thoracic cavity, while contraction of the *external intercostal muscles* widens the thorax by elevating the ribs and sternum. The lungs expand as they follow the movements of the thoracic wall because the surface tension generated by the serous fluid in the pleural cavity causes the visceral and parietal pleura to adhere closely, much as two moist plates of glass resist separation.

As the lungs expand and the pulmonary volume increases, the intrapulmonary pressure falls below atmospheric, creating a pressure gradient that causes air to flow from the atmosphere through the conducting passageways into the lungs. As the lungs expand, elastic components of the lung stretch and develop tension.

Quiet expiration occurs passively through relaxation of the inspiratory muscles. As the diaphragm ascends and the ribs and sternum return to their resting positions, the size of the thoracic cavity decreases. As the thorax assumes its original size, the potential energy stored in the elastic elements of the lung is converted into kinetic energy. These events cause the intrapulmonary pressure to temporarily exceed the atmospheric pressure, thus reversing the flow of air.

Accessory muscles of respiration include the scalene, and pectoralis minor, which contract during forceful inspiration

to further expand the thorax. During active, forceful expiration, coughing, and vomiting, the internal intercostal muscles contract to pull the ribs downward and inward, while the abdominal muscles contract to push the diaphragm upward.

Respiratory Compliance

Respiratory compliance, which may be defined as the lung volume change per unit of pressure, is a term often used to describe the ease with which the lungs may be inflated. Two major factors that affect respiratory compliance are *surface tension* and *resistance to airflow.*

Surface Tension

Surface tension is a phenomenon resulting from the forces of attraction between molecules on a fluid surface at a liquid–gas interface. The inner surface of the alveoli is coated with a thin film of fluid that exerts a surface tension tending to impair expansion of alveoli upon inspiration (and favor collapse on expiration).

The surface tension and tendency for collapse is particularly great in the smaller alveoli. Normally, the alveolar septal (type II) cells secrete a lipoprotein *surfactant* that reduces the surface tension and lowers the resistance of the alveoli to expansion on inspiration. Pulmonary surfactant therefore increases respiratory compliance and reduces the work required for breathing.

A deficiency of pulmonary surfactant characterizes *respiratory distress syndrome* (also known as *hyaline membrane disease*), a condition often afflicting premature infants.

Resistance to Airflow

Any obstruction or resistance to the flow of air would increase the force required to bring air into the alveoli. Airway resistance is encountered chiefly in the bronchi and bronchioles. It can be increased by the contraction of respiratory smooth muscle (*bronchoconstriction*) or by swelling of the respiratory mucosa (*mucosal edema*).

Reflex bronchoconstriction may follow mechanical or chemical stimulation of airway receptors. Parasympathetic stimulation, acetylcholine, and histamine cause bronchoconstriction. Sympathetic stimulation, epinephrine, and isoproterenol relax bronchiolar smooth muscle.

Bronchial asthma is a bronchospastic disease (frequently allergic in origin) characterized by great airway resistance. Major factors contributing to the heightened airway resistance are respiratory muscle spasm and mucosal edema leading to excessive accumulation of mucus.

The important mechanisms involved in bronchial constriction and relaxation are summarized in Figure 53-1.

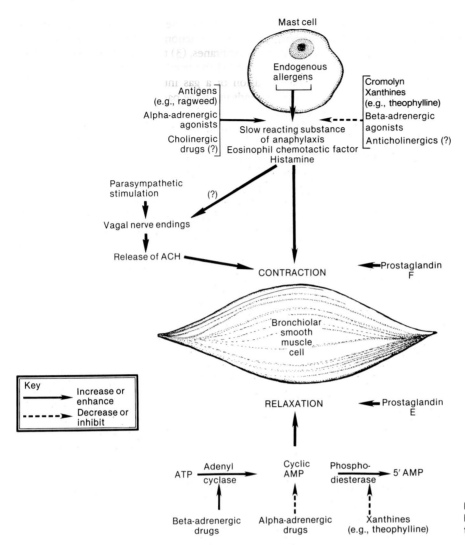

Figure 53-1 Factors regulating bronchiolar smooth muscle contraction and relaxation.

Volumes of Air Exchanged

The amount of air exchanged during normal, quiet respiration (*eupnea*) varies with the age, sex, and size of the person. In the average adult the *tidal volume* (volume of air inspired or expired) is approximately 500 ml. The product of *tidal volume* and *respiratory rate* equals the *minute respiratory volume,* which represents the volume of air entering the lungs in 1 minute.

The most critical factor in the total process of pulmonary ventilation is *alveolar ventilation.* Alveolar ventilation (the volume of air that enters the alveoli per minute) is a fraction of the total ventilation because with each breath some air remains in the conducting passages and is therefore unavailable to the alveoli for gaseous exchange. The total internal volume of these conducting passages is termed *anatomical dead space,* estimated to be 150 ml. The *physiologic dead space,* which in normally functioning lungs is essentially equal to the anatomical dead space, is more variable (and larger) in the presence of nonfunctioning alveoli.

Exchange and Transport of Respiratory Gases

In a mixture of gases (such as the atmosphere), the portion of the total pressure contributed by a particular gas in the mixture is termed the *partial pressure* or *tension.* The partial pressure exerted by each individual gas varies directly with its concentration in the mixture and with the total pressure of the mixture. For example, O_2, which makes up approximately 21% of atmospheric air, exerts a partial pressure (P_{O_2}) of 160 mm Hg under standard total atmospheric pressure of 760 mm Hg, that is, $0.21 \times 760 = 160$.

Atmospheric (inspired) air is composed primarily of nitrogen and O_2 with very small amounts of CO_2, water vapor, and inert gases. Alveolar air differs from atmospheric air in composition because the inspired air becomes saturated with water vapor and mixed with old anatomical dead space air during its passage through the conducting components of the respiratory tract. *Alveolar* P_{O_2} is 100 mm Hg in contrast with the *atmospheric* P_{O_2} of 160 mm Hg.

The exchange of gases within the body occurs through diffusion, with each gas diffusing according to its partial pressure gradient. As shown in Figure 53-2, pressure gradients cause O_2 to diffuse from the alveoli into the blood, and from the blood into the tissues. The pressure gradients are reversed for CO_2, causing it to diffuse from the tissues into the blood and subsequently into the alveoli.

Within the alveoli, large volumes of water-saturated air are exposed to a vast volume of blood to effect efficient exchange of gases. Pulmonary venous blood is not maximally oxygenated because alveolar ventilation and perfusion are not uniform throughout the lung. During normal ventilation (in an upright person at rest) the lower (basal) segments of the lungs receive a relatively greater blood flow than the upper (apical) portions due to gravitational forces. Most respiratory disorders are characterized by even greater ventilation–perfusion inequalities. Possible pathologic causes of uneven ventilation include obstruction of airways (as in asthma), altered elasticity of airways (as in advanced emphysema), and reduced pulmonary expansion (as in atelectasis). Uneven capillary perfusion may result from shunts, embolization, and compression of pulmonary blood vessels.

During pulmonary exchange of gases, O_2 and CO_2 must diffuse across a functional respiratory membrane composed of the following: (1) alveolar membrane, (2) interstitial fluid, (3) capillary endothelium and basement membrane, (4) plasma, and (5) erythrocyte (red blood cell) membrane.

The rate at which O_2 diffuses from the alveoli into the blood depends upon (1) the partial pressure gradient for oxygen, (2) the total functional surface area of the alveolar and capillary membranes, (3) the thickness of the respiratory membrane, and (4) the ventilation–perfusion ratio.

The diffusion of a gas into a liquid medium, such as plasma, depends upon the partial pressure gradient and the solubility of the gas in that fluid. Immediately upon entering the blood, the respiratory gases dissolve in the fluid portion of blood—the plasma (CO_2 is about 20 times more soluble in plasma than O_2).

Erythrocytes play an essential role in the transport of both O_2 and CO_2 because mere physical solution of these gases in blood plasma would not be adequate to meet even minimal body needs. The gas-carrying capacity of blood is greatly increased by rapidly reversible chemical reactions that remove O_2 and CO_2 from solution, thus steepening their gradients for diffusion.

Oxygen Transport

The amount of O_2 in the blood is essentially determined by three factors: (1) the amount of O_2 dissolved in the plasma, (2) the amount of *hemoglobin* (Hb) in the blood, and (3) the affinity of Hb for O_2.

Normally, the amount of O_2 physically dissolved in plasma is very small because of its low solubility in this fluid. Most

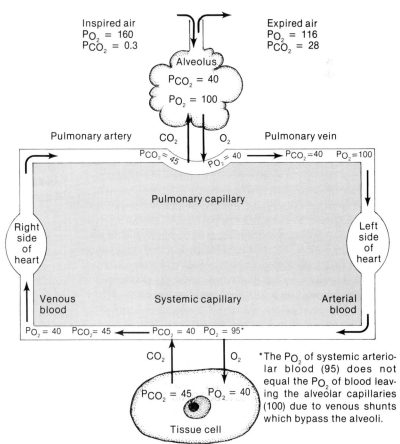

Figure 53-2 Gaseous exchange according to partial pressure gradients.

Inspired air
$P_{O_2} = 160$
$P_{CO_2} = 0.3$

Expired air
$P_{O_2} = 116$
$P_{CO_2} = 28$

Alveolus
$P_{CO_2} = 40$
$P_{O_2} = 100$

Pulmonary artery CO_2 O_2 Pulmonary vein

$P_{CO_2} = 45$ $P_{O_2} = 40$ $P_{CO_2} = 40$ $P_{O_2} = 100$

Pulmonary capillary

Right side of heart

Left side of heart

Venous blood   Systemic capillary   Arterial blood

$P_{O_2} = 40$ $P_{CO_2} = 45$ $P_{CO_2} = 40$ $P_{O_2} = 95*$

CO_2 O_2

*The P_{O_2} of systemic arteriolar blood (95) does not equal the P_{O_2} of blood leaving the alveolar capillaries (100) due to venous shunts which bypass the alveoli.

$P_{CO_2} = 45$ $P_{O_2} = 40$

Tissue cell

(approximately 98%) of the O_2 in the blood is transported in combination with Hb, a conjugated protein present in erythrocytes. Hb contains four iron atoms, each of which can reversibly bind one molecule of oxygen. While the oxygenation of Hb occurs in a stepwise fashion, the overall process is generally represented by the simple equation:

$$\underset{\text{hemoglobin}}{Hb} + \underset{\text{oxygen}}{O_2} \rightleftarrows \underset{\text{oxyhemoglobin}}{HbO_2}$$

When fully saturated with the gas, each gram of Hb can hold 1.34 ml of O_2. At an average Hb concentration of 15 g per 100 ml of blood, the O_2-carrying capacity of Hb is 20.1 volumes percent (15×1.34).

In arterial blood Hb is 97% saturated with O_2, whereas in venous blood the degree of saturation falls to 75%. The color of Hb reflects the degree of its saturation with O_2. HbO_2 is bright crimson, explaining the bright red color of arterial blood, whereas reduced Hb is dark purple, imparting a port wine color to venous blood.

The affinity of Hb for O_2 is greatly affected by the P_{O_2}. When the P_{O_2} is high, as it is in the lungs, Hb binds large amounts of O_2 and becomes nearly saturated with it. In the tissue capillaries, where P_{O_2} is substantially lower, the affinity of Hb for O_2 is reduced, and O_2 is released for diffusion into the tissues.

The amount of O_2 in combination with Hb also depends upon the P_{CO_2}, pH, and temperature of the blood. Under conditions of increased P_{CO_2}, low pH (acidity), or elevated temperature of the blood, the amount of O_2 that binds to hemoglobin at any given P_{O_2} is diminished.

The reduced affinity of Hb for O_2 that occurs when blood pH falls is termed the *Bohr effect*. The pH of the blood falls as its CO_2 content increases because CO_2 combines with water to form carbonic acid (H_2CO_3), which rapidly dissociates into hydrogen (H^+) and bicarbonate ions (HCO_3^-), as shown below:

$$CO_2 + H_2O \rightleftarrows H_2CO_3 \rightleftarrows H^+ + HCO_3^-$$

Another metabolic factor that favors the dissociation of O_2 from Hb is 2,3 diphosphoglycerate (2,3 DPG), an organic phosphate present in erythrocytes that binds to Hb and decreases its affinity for O_2. Erythrocyte 2,3 DPG concentration increases during prolonged exercise, anemia, and in various diseases marked by chronic hypoxia.

As the O_2 dissociates from Hb, it becomes available for diffusion into tissue cells. Metabolically active tissues tend to accumulate CO_2 and acidic metabolites and undergo temperature elevation—conditions that favor O_2 dissociation from Hb and increase availability of O_2 to the tissue cells.

Carbon Dioxide Transport

CO_2, a principal end product of cellular metabolism, diffuses from the tissues into the blood for transport to the lungs (for elimination). It is transported by the blood in three forms as follows:

1 *Dissolved* in the plasma
2 As *carbamino compounds*
3 As *bicarbonate ions*

CO_2 is highly soluble in plasma and nearly 10% of the total CO_2 in the blood is carried in physical solution within the plasma.

Approximately 20% of blood CO_2 combines with *amino* groups of various blood proteins (principally Hb) to form *carbamino compounds*. Some of the CO_2 that diffuses from the plasma into the erythrocytes combines with Hb to form the compound *carbaminohemoglobin*. However, most of the CO_2 in the erythrocytes is readily hydrated in the presence of carbonic anhydrase enzyme, forming H_2CO_3. H_2CO_3 rapidly dissociates into H^+ and HCO_3^- ions. The H^+ ions are buffered, principally by Hb, while the HCO_3^- ions diffuse into the plasma. Electrochemical neutrality is maintained by the rapid diffusion of chloride (Cl^-) ions into the erythrocytes (the so-called *chloride shift*). Approximately 70% of the CO_2 in the blood is transported in the form of HCO_3^- ions.

Regulation of Respiration

Neural Control of Respiration

The rhythmic pattern of normal respiration is maintained by the cyclic discharge of neurons located in the brain stem. Three bilateral interconnected respiratory "centers" (located in the medulla and pons) are generally recognized: the *medullary* center, the *apneustic* center, and the *pneumotaxic* center.

Medullary Respiratory Center

The medullary respiratory center consists of two anatomically intermingled but functionally distinct and reciprocally active aggregates of neurons: *inspiratory* neurons and *expiratory* neurons. The inspiratory neurons exhibit spontaneous bursts of activity during which the expiratory neurons are inhibited due to the operation of oscillating negative feedback circuits.

Simultaneously, impulses originating in the inspiratory neurons travel along the phrenic and intercostal nerves to the diaphragm and external intercostal muscles, respectively, causing their contraction and the subsequent enlargement of the thorax, leading to inspiration. The medullary respiratory center receives afferent (sensory) input from central chemoreceptors, various peripherally located receptors, and from higher brain centers (including the apneustic and pneumotaxic centers of the pons). The afferent input can modify the basic rhythmic discharge of the medullary respiratory neurons. For example, impulses originating in the cerebral cortex allow voluntary interruption of the normal breathing cycle for activities such as speaking, laughing, and breath-holding.

Apneustic Center

The apneustic center, located in the reticular formation of the lower pons, provides tonic stimulation to the medullary inspiratory neurons, thereby facilitating and prolonging inspiration. The apneustic center is not necessary for the maintenance of a basic respiratory rhythm, and its level of activity can be modified (inhibited) by afferent input from the pneumotaxic center and from pulmonary stretch receptors.

Pneumotaxic Center

The pneumotaxic center (located in the superior pons) periodically inhibits inspiration and facilitates expiration by inhibiting the apneustic center and possibly by inhibiting the medullary inspiratory neurons directly. The pneumotaxic center does not possess an inherent rhythmicity, but is activated by a feedback mechanism during discharge of medullary inspiratory neurons. Inhibition of the inspiratory neurons deprives the pneumotaxic center of its stimulation, causing it to become inactive.

Chemical Control of Respiration

The CO_2, O_2, and H^+ ion levels of the blood (and other body fluids) are of major importance in the control of respiration. CO_2 is the most potent physiologic stimulant of respiration, exerting its effects chiefly through central chemoreceptors. It must be noted, however, that very high concentrations of CO_2 (in excess of 30% in inspired air) produce central nervous system (and respiratory) depression and may be lethal.

Central Chemoreceptors

The ventral surface of the medulla contains chemosensitive cells that respond to elevations of CO_2 and H^+ ions in arterial blood and cerebrospinal fluid by stimulating the medullary respiratory center.

CO_2 readily diffuses from the blood plasma into the cerebrospinal fluid, where it combines with water to form H_2CO_3, which then dissociates into H^+ and HCO_3^- ions.

Because cerebrospinal fluid is not as well buffered as the blood, the H^+ ion concentration rises quickly, effectively stimulating the central chemoreceptors and thereby increasing pulmonary ventilation.

Peripheral Chemoreceptors

Located peripherally in the *carotid* and *aortic bodies* are chemoreceptors neurally connected to the medullary respiratory center by afferent glossopharyngeal and vagal nerve fibers.

These peripheral chemoreceptors are primarily sensitive to arterial O_2 levels, responding to lowered arterial Po_2 (hypoxemia) by stimulating respiration. They serve as an important emergency mechanism of respiratory stimulation in states of low O_2 intake.

Carotid and aortic chemoreceptors also respond to elevations in arterial Pco_2 and H^+ ion concentrations, mechanisms of importance in acidosis.

Reflex Regulation of Respiration

In addition to chemoreceptors, there are a number of peripheral receptors whose stimulation initiates reflex changes in respiration.

Sensory modalities such as pain, temperature, and touch affect respiration, with pain exerting a strong excitatory effect upon the medullary respiratory center.

Movements of joints, whether active or passive, stimulate respiration by way of afferent pathways originating in the proprioceptors of muscles, tendons, and joints. These pathways, which converge upon the respiratory center, augment pulmonary ventilation during exercise.

Sneezing and coughing are reflex, modified respiratory responses to irritants of the respiratory mucosa.

Inflation of the lungs stimulates pulmonary stretch receptors that lead to vagally mediated inhibition of inspiration. This "inflation reflex" (also termed the *vagal* or *Hering-Breuer reflex*) does not appear to be of great importance during normal respiration in humans.

54 Antitussives and Expectorants

Coughing is a protective mechanism initiated by chemical or mechanical stimulation of the tracheobronchial tree by which the body attempts to remove foreign particles or accumulated secretions from the respiratory tract. The cough reflex may be initiated by a number of factors, such as local inflammation of the bronchioles (*e.g.,* smoking), mechanical or physical obstruction (*e.g.,* foreign bodies, emboli), local or systemic disease states (*e.g.,* pulmonary edema, bronchogenic carcinoma, or congestive heart failure), and emotional stress. To the extent that the cough is annoying or debilitating, proper drug therapy should be undertaken to eliminate the condition. Not all coughing is undesirable, however, and the productive type of cough that aids in removing excessive bronchiolar mucus in the form of sputum generally should not be suppressed. Of course, if the cough is secondary to some other disease, every effort should be made to identify and eliminate the underlying pathologic condition, such as pneumonia, bronchitis, or tuberculosis.

The most frequently employed drugs for the control of coughing may be divided into the antitussives and the expectorants. Antitussives are cough suppressants that may act centrally at the level of the "cough center" in the brain stem or peripherally at various sites along the tracheobronchial tree. Antitussives are primarily indicated in the treatment of annoying, dry, unproductive coughing, especially where it interferes with other functions (*e.g.,* talking, sleeping) or leads to excessive weakness or progressive irritation.

Expectorants, on the other hand, increase and liquefy bronchial secretions, making it easier for the person to expel them. These drugs act either on the secretory glands of the respiratory tract or by irritation of the gastric mucosa, which reflexly increases respiratory secretions. They find their major clinical application in the treatment of obstructive pulmonary diseases associated with accumulation of excessive tenacious mucus, where they may reduce the viscosity of bronchial secretions, thus facilitating elimination. There is doubt, however, as to the efficacy of the usual amounts of expectorants found in over-the-counter cough formulations in reducing bronchial irritation or lessening the severity of nonproductive coughing. Exposure to humidified air and especially adequate fluid intake have proven as effective as most expectorants in relieving nonproductive coughing, liquefying thick, tenacious mucus, and facilitating removal of respiratory secretions.

Antitussives

The antitussive drugs are used to reduce the frequency of dry, unproductive coughing, and most act to depress the cough reflex by a direct inhibition of the cough center in the medulla. Drugs possessing antitussive activity can be divided into two groups, the narcotic and the non-narcotic cough suppressants. The effectiveness of narcotics as cough inhibitors generally parallels their analgesic efficacy; thus the most potent narcotic analgesics might be expected to provide the greatest degree of cough control. However, toxicity and potential for abuse likewise are functions of narcotic potency, and for this reason only the weaker narcotic analgesics are suitable for use as cough suppressants. Of the many narcotic drugs available (see Chap. 18), only codeine is routinely used for the relief of coughing, usually as a component of a combination product.

The non-narcotic antitussives are a structurally diverse group of pharmacologic agents that possess a variety of both central and peripheral mechanisms of action. In most cases, they are nearly as effective as codeine, with perhaps a somewhat lower incidence of disturbing side-effects. Because they have various mechanisms of action as well as different patterns of side-effects, they are discussed individually.

Narcotic Antitussives

The most commonly used narcotic antitussive is codeine, and although it is available in tablet form, it is most frequently administered as a component of liquid cough preparations, in which it may be combined with antihistamines, decongestants, expectorants, or analgesics.

▶ codeine

Mechanism
Suppresses cough reflex by a direct depressant effect on the cough center in the medulla

Use
1 Symptomatic relief of nonproductive coughing

Dosage
Adults: 10 mg to 20 mg every 4 hours to 6 hours; maximum 120 mg/day
Children: (6 yr–12 yr) 5 mg to 10 mg every 4 hours to 6 hours; maximum 60 mg/day
Children: (2 yr–6 yr) 2.5 mg to 5 mg every 4 hours to 6 hours; maximum 30 mg/day

Fate
Well absorbed when taken orally; onset of action is 10 minutes to 20 minutes; duration varies from 3 hours to 6 hours; metabolized in the liver and excreted largely in the urine

Common Side-Effects
(Frequent at excessive doses) Lightheadedness, dizziness, sedation, sweating, and nausea

Significant Adverse Reactions
GI—dry mouth, anorexia, constipation, biliary spasm
CNS—euphoria, weakness, insomnia, headache, anxiety, fear, mood changes, disorientation, agitation, tremors, impaired physical performance, psychological dependence, delirium, hallucinations, coma, visual disturbances, respiratory and cardiovascular depression (especially with large doses)

Other—allergic reactions (rash, urticaria, pruritus, edema), urinary retention, decreased libido or potency, flushing, tachycardia, palpitation, faintness, syncope, ureteral spasm

Contraindications
Patients with known or suspected narcotic addiction

Interactions
1 Profound sedation, hypotension, and respiratory depression may occur with combinations of codeine and other narcotics, sedatives, hypnotics, alcohol, phenothiazines, tricyclic antidepressants, general anesthetics, and other CNS depressants (see also Narcotic Analgesics, Chap. 18).

▶ NURSING ALERTS
See Chapter 18 for general nursing alerts concerning use of all narcotics. In addition:
▷ 1 Caution patients not to exceed recommended dosage, because antitussive effect is not significantly enhanced but untoward reactions and danger of habituation are increased.
▷ 2 Use with caution in patients with asthma or other pulmonary diseases, cardiac disease (including arrhythmias), convulsive disorders, renal or hepatic impairment, prostatic hypertrophy, severe CNS depression, toxic psychoses, head injuries, intracranial lesions, hypothyroidism, Addison's disease, and in alcoholics and pregnancy.

▶ NURSING CONSIDERATIONS
▷ 1 Inform patients that products may cause drowsiness but that some persons may experience restlessness, anxiety, or nervousness, especially with large doses.
▷ 2 Suggest that patients drink large amounts of fluids, for example, 2 liters/day, which may help to decrease the tenacity of bronchial secretions, and to use a humidifier or vaporizer during the night.
▷ 3 Advise patients to use hard candy, gum, or throat lozenges to soothe pharyngeal mucosa irritated by constant coughing.
▷ 4 Note that codeine alone in tablet form is a Schedule II drug, but it is most commonly used combined with other agents in cough syrups. Depending upon the amount of codeine contained in the mixture, these combination antitussives may be Schedule III or V. Observe proper handling and dispensing procedures for all controlled substances (see Appendix).
▷ 5 When used in syrup form, administer medications undiluted and do *not* immediately follow with water.

Non-narcotic Antitussives

▶ benzonatate
Tessalon Perles

Mechanism

Exerts a local anesthetic action on the stretch receptors in the respiratory passages, lungs, and pleural cavity, thus dampening the cough reflex

Uses

1 Symptomatic relief of nonproductive coughing, especially in chronic respiratory conditions
2 Adjunctive treatment in bronchoscopy and other procedures where coughing must be avoided

Dosage

100 mg orally three times a day; maximum 600 mg/day

Fate

Onset of action is 15 minutes to 20 minutes; effects last 4 hours to 8 hours

Significant Adverse Reactions

Drowsiness, dizziness, headache, nasal congestion, burning in the eyes, numbness in the chest, vague "chilly" sensation, skin eruptions, pruritus, nausea, constipation, and GI upset

Interactions

1 Benzonatate may intensify the effects of other CNS depressants.

▶ NURSING ALERT

▷ 1 Use cautiously in pregnant or nursing women.

▶ NURSING CONSIDERATIONS

▷ 1 Instruct patients to swallow the capsule (perle) whole, because release of drug in the mouth can produce temporary anesthesia in the oral mucosa.
▷ 2 Be aware that use of the drug in a patient who is vomiting can lead to aspiration and possible pneumonitis.
▷ 3 Suggest adjunctive measures (*e.g.,* adequate hydration, hard candy or gum, cessation of smoking) to assist in control of nonproductive coughing.
▷ 4 Note that benzonatate is reportedly as effective as codeine in controlling nonproductive coughing and does not have the danger of habituation.

▶ chlophedianol

Ulo

Mechanism

Not established; exhibits both local anesthetic and anticholinergic activity

Use

1 Symptomatic treatment of nonproductive cough

Dosage

Adults: 25 mg three to four times a day
Children: (6 yr–12 yr) 12.5 mg to 25 mg three to four times a day
Children: (2 yr–6 yr) 12.5 mg three to four times a day

Fate

Onset is 30 minutes to 60 minutes; duration may range from 4 hours to 8 hours

Significant Adverse Reactions

Excitation, irritability, hallucinations, nightmares, hypersensitivity reactions; large doses may elicit anticholinergic effects (dryness of the mouth, visual disturbances, drowsiness, constipation, vertigo)

Contraindications

Children under 2 years of age

Interactions

1 Chlophedianol may enhance the effects of both CNS depressants and CNS stimulants.

▶ NURSING ALERTS

▷ 1 Be alert for development of CNS excitation, occasionally accompanied by hallucinations. Discontinue drug immediately; symptoms should subside within a few hours.
▷ 2 Use cautiously in pregnant or nursing women and in elderly or debilitated patients who are more likely to experience untoward reactions.
▷ 3 Urge patient to use caution in driving or operating machinery, because drug may cause drowsiness.

▶ NURSING CONSIDERATIONS

▷ 1 Suggest use of gum or candy to assist in relieving coughing or throat irritation as well as to prevent dryness of the mouth due to use of the drug.
▷ 2 Note that potency is comparable to that of most narcotic antitussives with less danger of habituation. Effects are slower in developing, but persist longer than with narcotics.

▶ dextromethorphan

Benylin DM, Congespirin, Delsym, Pertussin, Romilar CF, and various other manufacturers

A widely used non-narcotic antitussive, dextromethorphan has minimal CNS depressant action and no analgesic effect, and its administration is unlikely to produce constipation or result in tolerance. It is commonly found in over-the-counter cough formulations, frequently combined with antihistamines, decongestants, and expectorants. A 30-mg dose is approximately equivalent to 15 mg of codeine.

Mechanism

Not conclusively established; appears to depress the cough center in the medulla

Use

1 Temporary relief of nonproductive coughing

Dosage

Lozenges/Syrup
Adults: 10 mg to 30 mg every 4 hours to 8 hours; maximum 120 mg/24 hours

Children: (6 yr–12 yr) 2.5 mg to 5 mg every 4 hours or 7.5 mg to 15 mg every 6 hours to 8 hours; maximum 60 mg/24 hours

Children: (2 yr–6 yr) 1.25 mg to 2.5 mg every 4 hours or 3.75 mg to 7.5 mg every 6 hours to 8 hours; maximum 30 mg/24 hours

Controlled-Release Liquid (Delsym Pennkinetic)

Adults: 60 mg twice a day
Children: (6 yr–12 yr) 30 mg twice a day
Children: (2 yr–6 yr) 15 mg twice a day

Fate

Onset of action is 15 minutes to 30 minutes and antitussive effects persist 3 hours to 6 hours depending on the dose (up to 12 hr with controlled release liquid)

Significant Adverse Reactions

Dizziness, GI distress, and drowsiness

Contraindications

Patients taking MAO inhibitors (see Chap. 24)

Interactions

1 Combinations of dextromethorphan and MAO inhibitors can result in hyperpyrexia, muscular rigidity, and laryngospasm.

▶ NURSING ALERT

▷ 1 Use cautiously in patients with chronic obstructive pulmonary disease, high fever, persistent headache, or vomiting, and where cough is accompanied by excessive secretions.

▶ NURSING CONSIDERATIONS

▷ 1 Administer syrup undiluted to enhance its local effect.
▷ 2 Be aware that drug is available over-the-counter. Do not administer to children under 2 years of age except under medical supervision.
▷ 3 Note that increasing the dose increases the duration of action.
▷ 4 Advise patients to consult physician if coughing persists longer than 7 days with dextromethorphan or any other antitussive therapy.
▷ 5 Note that the antitussive activity of dextromethorphan is comparable to that of codeine, and that the drug does not induce tolerance, hypnosis, respiratory depression, or analgesia in therapeutic doses. Constipation is much less frequent than with codeine.
▷ 6 Note that dextromethorphan is available in throat lozenge form alone and also combined with benzocaine (*e.g.,* Formula 44 Cough Control Discs, Spec-T Sore Throat Cough Suppressant, Vick's Cough Silencers) for control of spasmodic coughing. Lozenges are not as effective as the syrup.

▶ noscapine

Tusscapine

Mechanism

Not established; appears to block cough reflex at the brain stem level without affecting higher centers; structurally related to papaverine and claimed to be as effective as codeine in suppressing cough

Use

1 Relief of nonproductive cough

Dosage

Adults: 15 mg to 30 mg three or four times a day; maximum 120 mg/day
Children: (6 yr–12 yr) 15 mg three to four times a day; maximum 60 mg/day
Children: (2 yr–6 yr) 7.5 mg to 15 mg three to four times a day

Fate

Onset is approximately 15 minutes to 30 minutes and effects persist up to 4 hours

Significant Adverse Reactions

Nausea, drowsiness, dizziness, headache, and skin rash

▶ NURSING ALERTS

▷ 1 Advise patients to use caution in driving or operating other machinery, because drug may cause drowsiness or dizziness.
▷ 2 Do not administer to children under 2 years of age.

▶ NURSING CONSIDERATION

▷ 1 Note that the antitussive action of noscapine is reputed to be equivalent to that of codeine without the undesirable side-effects. The drug is available over-the-counter.

Expectorants

Expectorants are claimed to facilitate removal of viscous mucus from the respiratory tree, and provide a soothing, demulcent action on the respiratory mucosa by stimulating secretion of a lubricating fluid. While large doses of certain prescription-only expectorants (such as potassium iodide) may decrease the tenacity of mucus associated with chronic obstructive pulmonary diseases, the efficacy of most other nonprescription expectorants is subject to considerable debate. They are probably no more effective in providing relief of bronchial irritation or facilitating mucus liquefaction than high fluid intake, that is, 6 to 10 glasses/day, and humidification of the environment. There is little support for the claim that expectorants relieve dry, irritative coughing by increasing production of a soothing fluid any more than would be produced by use of a cough drop or throat lozenge. Therefore, their inclusion in cough/cold formulations containing antitussives, antihistamines, and decongestants among other medications is probably an example of therapeutic overkill.

On the other hand, adverse reactions are rare at usual therapeutic doses, the most frequent complaint being GI distress. Thus, the drugs are quite safe when taken as directed, and if patients believe the compounds are effective, it may be difficult to convince them otherwise.

▶ ammonium chloride

Ammonium chloride is primarily used as a systemic and urinary acidifier to treat metabolic alkalosis, to correct chloride depletion and to assist in the urinary excretion of certain basic drugs. These indications are considered in Chapter 77. The drug has also been used as an expectorant, and is found in a number of over-the-counter cough preparations, although its efficacy is subject to considerable doubt and its use in this manner should be discouraged.

Mechanism
May increase flow of respiratory fluid by reflex irritation of the gastric mucosa

Uses
1 Facilitation of productive cough (efficacy not conclusively established)
2 Acidification of the urine as an aid in excretion of certain basic drugs
3 Treatment of metabolic alkalosis and hypochloremic states (see Chap. 77)

Dosage
Expectorant: adults—200 mg to 400 mg every 4 hours; children—50 mg/kg to 75 mg/kg/day in divided doses
Urinary acidification: 3 g to 12 g a day in divided doses at 4-hour to 6-hour intervals

Fate
Absorption is slow but complete; metabolized to urea and hydrochloric acid, which are excreted primarily in the urine

Common Side-Effects
GI irritation, nausea (especially with large doses)

Significant Adverse Reactions
Metabolic acidosis (vomiting, thirst, weakness, hyperventilation, lethargy, drowsiness, confusion), skin rash, headache, hyper-reflexia, hypokalemia, hypocalcemia, and hyperglycemia
Too rapid IV administration can result in arrhythmias, tonic convulsions, and coma.

Contraindications
Severe renal, hepatic, or pulmonary disease

Interactions
1 Excretion of basic drugs (*e.g.*, amphetamines, antidepressants, antihistamines, anti-anxiety agents, catecholamines, narcotic analgesics, quinidine, theophylline) may be enhanced by ammonium chloride.

2 Acidic drugs (*e.g.*, barbiturates, clofibrate, mercurial diuretics, pyrazolones, salicylates, oral antidiabetics, thyroid hormones) may be potentiated by ammonium chloride, because their renal excretion may be retarded.

▶ NURSING ALERTS
▷ 1 Note rate and depth of respiration during drug therapy. Hyperventilation, weakness, and shortness of breath are possible early signs of acidosis. Advise physician.
▷ 2 Use cautiously in patients with chronic heart disease, and in small children.

▶ NURSING CONSIDERATIONS
▷ 1 Administer drug in a liquid or tablet form with a full glass of water (commonly used as a 10% solution), because fluids help to stimulate flow of respiratory secretions.
▷ 2 Do not use enteric-coated tablets as expectorants, because gastric irritation, the desired action, is eliminated.
▷ 3 Avoid administration of milk or other alkaline solutions with ammonium chloride.

▶ guaifenesin
Breonesin, Robitussin, and various other manufacturers—formerly known as glyceryl guaiacolate

Mechanism
May increase output of respiratory tract fluid by reducing its adhesiveness and surface tension, thus facilitating removal of mucus; increased fluid flow is also claimed to soothe dry, irritated membranes, thereby relieving dry, hacking cough

Use
1 Symptomatic relief of dry, unproductive coughing associated with common respiratory disorders, such as colds, bronchitis, bronchial asthma (efficacy not conclusively established)

Dosage
Adults: 100 mg to 400 mg every 4 hours to 6 hours; maximum 2.4 g/day
Children: (6 yr–12 yr) 50 mg to 100 mg every 4 hours to 6 hours; maximum 600 mg/day
Children: (2 yr–6 yr) 50 mg every 4 hours; maximum 300 mg/day

Significant Adverse Reactions
(Usually with large doses) Nausea, vomiting, GI distress, and drowsiness

Interactions
1 Guaifenesin may decrease platelet aggregation, thus increasing the risk of bleeding with anticoagulants.

▶ NURSING CONSIDERATIONS
▷ 1 Do not use for longer than 1 week if cough is persistent, and do not administer to patients with high fever, rash, or prolonged headache.

▷ 2 Note that guaifenesin may cause color interference with laboratory determinations of 5-hydroxyindole-acetic acid (a serotonin metabolite) and vanillylman-delic acid (a catecholamine metabolite). Discontinue drug for several days prior to performing these laboratory tests.

▷ 3 Recognize that although guaifenesin is widely used alone or in combination with other cough suppressants, antihistamines, analgesics, and other drugs, there is a lack of convincing evidence that it is a clinically effective expectorant.

▷ 4 Urge the use of adjunctive measures (*e.g.,* high fluid intake, humidification) to facilitate liquefaction of mucus and relief of dry, nonproductive coughing.

▶ iodinated glycerol

Organidin

Mechanism

A complex of iodine and glycerol that increases flow of respiratory tract fluid and helps liquefy thick, tenacious mucus; less effective than inorganic iodides, but less irritating to the GI tract

Use

1 Adjunctive treatment of respiratory conditions associated with increased mucus, such as bronchitis, asthma, emphysema, and cystic fibrosis, and following surgery to help prevent atelectasis (efficacy not conclusively established)

Dosage

Adults: 60 mg four times a day with liquid
Children: up to one half adult dosage based on weight

Significant Adverse Reactions

(Rare) Iodism (GI distress, rash, metallic taste, salivation, sore throat, parotid gland swelling); see Potassium Iodide

Contraindications

Hypersensitivity to inorganic iodides

▶ NURSING ALERT

▷ 1 Be alert for development of skin rash, itching, or other signs of hypersensitivity, and discontinue drug.

▶ NURSING CONSIDERATIONS

▷ 1 Administer all preparations (*e.g.,* tablets, elixir, solution) with additional liquids.

▷ 2 Be aware that use of large doses may interfere with laboratory determinations of protein-bound iodine (PBI).

▷ 3 Note that drug is commonly used in liquid form as Theo Organidin (with theophylline), Tussi Organidin (with codeine), or Tussi Organidin DM (with dextromethorphan).

▶ potassium iodide

Pima and various other manufacturers

Mechanism

Iodides enhance secretion of respiratory fluids, thus decreasing viscosity and tenacity of mucus.

Use

1 Symptomatic treatment of chronic pulmonary diseases complicated by tenacious mucus, such as bronchial asthma, chronic bronchitis, or emphysema

Dosage

Adults: 300 mg to 650 mg every 4 hours to 6 hours
Children: 150 mg to 300 mg every 4 hours to 6 hours

Common Side-Effects

GI distress

Significant Adverse Reactions

(Rare at recommended doses) Iodism (skin rash, fever, sore throat, metallic taste, nausea, vomiting, epigastric pain, parotid gland swelling, mucous membrane ulceration, salivation, coryza, and lacrimation)

Also, angioedema, mucosal hemorrhage, serum sickness, thyroid adenoma, goiter, and myxedema are possible.

Contraindications

Hyperthyroidism, hyperkalemia, goiter, sensitivity to iodides, tuberculosis, and acute bronchitis

Interactions

1 The hypothyroid and goitrogenic effects of potassium iodide may be potentiated by lithium or other antithyroid drugs.

2 Hyperkalemia can be intensified by potassium supplements or potassium-sparing diuretics.

▶ NURSING ALERTS

▷ 1 Discontinue use if skin rash, fever, sore throat, vomiting, epigastric pain, or other signs of iodism appear (see Significant Adverse Reactions).

▷ 2 Use cautiously in patients with high fever or persistent cough, and in pregnant or nursing women.

▷ 3 Administer enteric-coated tablets with caution, because small bowel lesions have occurred, resulting in obstruction, hemorrhage, and perforation. Discontinue immediately if abdominal pain, distention, vomiting, or GI bleeding occurs.

▷ 4 Note that potassium iodide may elevate levels of protein-bound iodine and interfere with 17-hydroxycorticosteroid determinations.

▶ NURSING CONSIDERATIONS

▷ 1 Administer liquid drug well diluted in water, juice, or other vehicle. Tablets are taken with food or milk to minimize GI distress.

▷ 2 Encourage increased fluid intake, cessation of smoking, and use of humidifier to increase expectorant action of iodides.

▷ 3 Note that hydrogen iodide syrup (hydriodic acid) is also used as an expectorant. Adult dose is 70 mg (5 ml) well diluted in water three to four times a day. Children receive 1 to 10 drops in water one to three times a day. This is an over-the-counter preparation whereas other iodide expectorants are by prescription only.

▷ 4   Be aware that prolonged use of iodides can lead to hypothyroidism and iodide-induced goiter. Do not exceed recommended doses and do not administer for prolonged periods of time.

▷ 5   See Chapter 40 for additional indications for iodide products.

▶ potassium iodide–niacinamide hydroiodide
Iodo-Niacin

A combination of two iodide salts, Iodo-Niacin is used in tablet form (135 mg KI and 25 mg niacinamide hydroiodide) to facilitate cough and to aid in bronchial drainage. Adult dosage is 2 tablets three times/day after meals, with water. Children over 8 receive 1 tablet three times/day. Efficacy is questionable and prolonged use should be avoided. The drug combination is also indicated for prophylaxis of goiter and management of mild hyperthyroidism, usually with an antithyroid drug.

Combination Cough Mixtures

Although this chapter has dealt with individual antitussive and expectorant drugs, the most frequent use of these products, as indicated, is in combination cough mixtures. Such formulations may contain several other types of drugs, in addition to an antitussive and an expectorant. The most commonly used of these other agents are listed below, along with the rationale for their inclusion.

1   *Analgesics*
    For example, aspirin, acetaminophen, sodium salicylate; used to provide relief of headache, fever, and muscle aches often accompanying an upper respiratory condition (see Chap. 19)

2   *Anticholinergics*
    For example, atropine, belladonna alkaloids, methscopolamine; employed for their drying action on mu-

cous membranes; thus are only beneficial in conditions characterized by excessive secretions (*e.g.,* rhinorrhea); should be avoided in chronic obstructive pulmonary diseases (see Chap. 10)

3   *Antihistamines*
    For example, chlorpheniramine, pyrilamine; provide symptomatic relief of running nose, sneezing, itching, watery eyes; may be effective in relieving chronic cough resulting from postnasal drip (*e.g.,* allergic rhinitis, chronic sinusitis); exhibit an anticholinergic (drying) action, therefore should not be used in respiratory conditions characterized by excessive congestion; most have a sedative effect (see Chap. 14)

4   *Bronchodilators*
    For example, ephedrine, theophylline; relax bronchiolar smooth muscle, thus are of greatest benefit in conditions characterized by excessive bronchiolar muscle tone (*e.g.,* asthma) rather than mucus accumulation (see Chap. 55)

5   *Decongestants*
    For example, phenylephrine, phenylpropanolamine, pseudoephedrine; used to reduce mucosal congestion by activating alpha-adrenergic receptor sites, thus eliciting vasoconstriction; probably not significantly effective and can lead to systemic side-effects (*e.g.,* hypertension) (see Chap. 11)

The principal disadvantage of combination products is that the fixed dosage ratio of the ingredients precludes individualization of the dosage of each drug according to the needs of the patient. Moreover, the "shotgun" approach to drug therapy—inclusion of several different kinds of drugs in one preparation—is usually unnecessary from a therapeutic standpoint and most often simply increases the likelihood of untoward reactions without significantly improving the *desired* therapeutic effect. Finally, the cost of combination formulas is frequently in excess of the cost of the necessary individual ingredients used separately. Nevertheless, antitussive and expectorant combinations remain the most widely used over-the-counter preparations for the relief of cough, and it is essential that users of such medications be advised of the potential hazards inherent in the indiscriminate consumption of these readily available cough mixtures.

Summary. Antitussives and Expectorants

Drug	Preparations	Usual Dosage Range
Narcotic Antitussives		
Codeine	Tablets—15 mg, 30 mg, 60 mg	Adults—10 mg to 20 mg every 4 hours to 6 hours
		Children (6 yr–12 yr)—5 mg to 10 mg every 4 hours to 6 hours
		Children (2 yr–6 yr)—2.5 mg to 5 mg every 4 hours to 6 hours
Non-narcotic Antitussives		
Benzonatate (Tessalon Perles)	Capsules (perles)—100 mg	100 mg 3 times a day (maximum 600 mg/day)

Summary. Antitussives and Expectorants (continued)

Drug	Preparations	Usual Dosage Range
Chlorphedianol (Ulo)	Syrup—25 mg/5 ml	Adults—25 mg 3 to 4 times a day Children (6 yr–12 yr)—12.5 mg to 25 mg 3 to 4 times a day Children (2 yr–6 yr)—12.5 mg 3 to 4 times a day
Dextromethorphan (Benylin DM, Delsym, Romilar CF, and various other manufacturers)	Syrup—2.5 mg, 5 mg, 10 mg 15 mg/5 ml Controlled-release liquid—30 mg/5 ml Chewable tablets—15 mg Lozenges—7.5 mg Lozenges (with benzocaine)—2.5 mg, 5 mg, 10 mg Lozenges (with phenol)	Adults—10 mg to 30 mg every 4 hours to 8 hours or 60-mg controlled-release liquid twice a day Children (6 yr–12 yr)—2.5 mg to 5 mg every 4 hours or 30-mg controlled-release liquid twice a day Children (2 yr–6 yr)—1.25 mg to 2.5 mg every 4 hours or 15-mg controlled-release liquid twice a day
Noscapine (Tusscapine)	Chewable tablets—15 mg	Adults—15 mg to 30 mg 3 to 4 times a day (maximum 120 mg/day) Children (6 yr–12 yr)—15 mg 3 to 4 times a day Children (2 yr–6 yr)—7.5 mg to 15 mg 3 to 4 times a day
Expectorants		
Ammonium chloride	Powder/Crystals Tablets—325 mg, 500 mg Enteric-coated tablets—0.5 g, 1 g	Expectorant: Adults—200 mg to 400 mg every 4 hours Children—50 to 75 mg/kg/day in divided doses Urinary acidifer: 3 g to 12 g/day in divided doses
Guaifenesin (Robitussin, Breonesin, and various other manufacturers)	Tablets—100 mg, 200 mg Capsules—200 mg Syrup—100 mg/5 ml	Adults—100 mg to 400 mg every 4 hours to 6 hours Children (6 yr–12 yr)—50 mg to 100 mg every 4 hours to 6 hours Children (2 yr–6 yr)—50 mg every 4 hours
Hydrogen iodide (Hydriodic acid)	Syrup—70 mg/5 ml	Adults—5 ml in water 3 to 4 times a day Children—1 to 10 drops in water 1 to 3 times a day
Iodinated glycerol (Organidin)	Tablets—30 mg Elixir—60 mg/5 ml Solution (sugar-free)—50 mg/ml	Adults—60 mg 4 times a day Children—Up to ½ adult dose based on weight
Potassium iodide (Pima and various other manufacturers)	Enteric-coated tablets—300 mg Liquid—500 mg/15 ml Saturated solution (SSKI)—1 g/ml Syrup—325 mg/5 ml	Adults—300 mg to 650 mg every 4 hours to 6 hours Children—150 mg to 300 mg every 4 hours to 6 hours
Potassium iodide—Niacinamide hydroiodide (Iodo-Niacin)	Tablets—135 mg potassium iodide and 25 mg niacinamide hydroiodide	Adults—2 tablets 3 times/day Children—1 tablet 3 times/day

55 Bronchodilators

Drugs capable of relaxing bronchiolar smooth muscle have their principal clinical application in three common respiratory disorders: bronchial asthma, chronic bronchitis, and emphysema. Although these three diseases differ in etiology and overall pathology, they share one important common characteristic, namely a reduced respiratory flow due to obstructed airways. The extent to which these chronic obstructive pulmonary diseases (COPDs) respond to bronchodilator therapy, however, is dependent in large measure on whether the increased resistance to airflow is primarily due to excessive bronchiolar smooth muscle tone or to the presence of mucus or other obstructive lesions within the bronchiolar network. The various mechanisms operative in the regulation of bronchiolar muscle tone are outlined in Chapter 53, Figure 53-1.

Bronchospasm associated with asthma is frequently due to increased responsiveness of bronchiolar smooth muscle to various external stimuli, such as dust and pollen, which trigger, *via* an antigen–antibody reaction, release of endogenous allergenic mediators (*e.g.,* histamine, eosinophil chemotactic factor) from mast cells. These substances then interact with the smooth muscle cells to cause contraction. A second important mechanism contributing to bronchospasm is activation of parasympathetic reflex pathways, which appear to become hypersensitive in many asthmatics. This reflex parasympathetic response results in release of acetylcholine (ACh) from vagal nerve endings, and may be elicited by the allergens extruded from the mast cells. ACh constricts bronchiolar smooth muscle cells, resulting in narrowing of the airways. Because the increased airway resistance is muscular in origin, it frequently responds well to systemic or local bronchodilators, and these drugs, in fact, represent the mainstay in the treatment of bronchial asthma.

Other chronic obstructive diseases of the respiratory tract may be the result of excessive mucus accumulation within the tracheobronchial tree, as in chronic bronchitis or in loss of elasticity of terminal bronchiolar walls with an increase in dead air space, as occurs in emphysema. These latter conditions respond much less favorably to bronchodilator drugs, although the drugs are of some benefit as part of an overall regimen which may also include mucolytics and expectorants.

Distinction must be made between the therapeutic aims in treating acute *versus* chronic bronchospastic conditions. Sudden bronchial constriction, as seen during acute attacks of asthma, requires immediate and vigorous therapy, and is usually treated with aminophylline IV, epinephrine SC or IM, or, in less acute situations, one of the inhaled adrenergic bronchodilators. Maintenance therapy of the COPDs, on the other hand, is directed toward decreasing the overall tone and responsiveness of bronchiolar smooth muscle and keeping the respiratory passages free of obstructions, thus reducing the incidence and severity of acute bronchospastic attacks. To accomplish these aims, a variety of pharmacologic agents are often employed, including oral or inhaled bronchodilators (*e.g.,* aminophylline, beta-adrenergic agonists), expectorants, mucolytics, corticosteroids, and cromolyn, an agent that has a prophylactic effect in certain asthmatic patients. In addition, persons with bronchospastic disorders should employ adjunctive measures such as adequate hydration, cessation of smoking, and avoidance of precipitating factors such as irritants, cold, and allergens to minimize the disturbing symptoms associated with these diseases and to avoid potentially dangerous complications.

Many of the drugs used in the management of COPDs have been reviewed in other chapters and are not considered here. Thus, adrenergic bronchodilators are discussed in Chapter 11; corticosteroids, in Chapter 43; expectorants, in Chapter 54, and mucolytics, in Chapter 56. Xanthine derivatives, of which the most widely used is theophylline, are discussed in detail in this chapter, including a listing (see Table 55-2) of individual drugs. Cromolyn, an agent used to prevent asthmatic attacks, is also reviewed in this chapter.

Xanthine Derivatives

The methylated xanthine derivatives (methylxanthines) include theophylline, its soluble salts (*e.g.,* aminophylline, oxtriphylline), and a chemically related derivative, dyphylline. These products are available in a number of different dosage forms. Theophylline itself has been used as an effective bronchodilator for over a quarter of a century, and many of the problems associated with its early use—GI upset, poor or erratic absorption—have been largely overcome by the synthesis of various theophylline salts as well as by the incorporation of theophylline into different dosage vehicles. Currently, theophylline and its derivatives are available in tablets, capsules, coated tablets, sustained-release tablets and capsules, aqueous solutions and suspensions, hydro-alcoholic elixirs, suppositories, rectal solutions, and IV and IM injections. This multiplicity of available preparations has frequently created confusion among clinicians concerning the appropriate dose and dosage form of theophylline to be employed for a particular clinical situation. Proper prescribing of methylxanthines, therefore, requires recognition of the many factors that may contribute to the often marked therapeutic variation observed in different patients using these products.

Clinical efficacy is a direct function of theophylline blood levels, the desired therapeutic range being 10 mcg to 20 mcg per milliliter of serum. Principal causes of difficulty in determining the appropriate dose of theophylline are (1) variations in anhydrous theophylline content among different preparations; (2) varying rates of absorption, metabolism, and elimination; (3) altered availability of theophylline from different dosage forms; and (4) age and health status of the patient. A closer look at some of these factors may aid in selecting the proper dose of theophylline for each patient.

Because of differences in anhydrous theophylline base content, the various available salt preparations are not therapeutically equal on a weight basis, and equivalent doses of the different theophylline products can vary by as much as 100%. Table 55-1 lists the percent of theophylline base and approximate equivalent doses for each clinically available preparation. These differences become important if patients are transferred from one theophylline product to an-

Table 55-1. Theophylline Content of Xanthine Derivatives

Preparation	Percent Theophylline Base	Equivalent Dosage
Theophylline, anhydrous	100%	100 mg
Aminophylline, anhydrous	86%	115 mg
Aminophylline dihydrate	79%	127 mg
Dyphylline*	70%	143 mg
Oxtriphylline	64%	156 mg
Theophylline sodium glycinate	49%	204 mg
Theophylline calcium salicylate	48%	208 mg

* A derivative of theophylline that is *not* metabolized to theophylline *in vivo*; contains 70% theophylline by molecular weight ratio, but therapeutic equivalence is not established.

other, because the plasma concentration, and thus clinical efficacy, varies directly with the intake of *theophylline base.*

Oral absorption of theophylline appears to be related primarily to the dosage form. Although it was formerly believed to be poorly or erratically absorbed from the GI tract, most data indicate that theophylline is inherently well absorbed, tablet disintegration being the major rate-limiting step. Thus, oral liquids are the most rapidly absorbed form of theophylline, followed very closely by uncoated tablets, especially if they are chewed. Enteric-coated or sustained-release forms of the drug, on the other hand, may be erratically or incompletely absorbed, and can yield variable plasma levels. However, newer continuous-release formulations have provided quite consistent serum drug levels for up to 24 hours, and represent a major advance in the chronic treatment of asthma. Food has little effect on theophylline availability, although oral absorption may be somewhat slower when food is present than from an empty stomach. Rectal absorption in adults is generally considered to be slow and unreliable with suppositories but nearly equivalent to oral absorption when concentrated rectal solutions are used. IM administration yields effective serum levels about equal to that of oral dosing, although not quite as rapid as with use of oral liquids.

Rates of metabolism and excretion of theophylline also vary widely. Hepatic metabolism is extensive (80%–90%), and the major metabolite is 3-methylxanthine, which exhibits approximately one third to one half the bronchodilator activity of theophylline itself. The plasma elimination half-life can range from 3 hours to 12 hours in adults and 1½ hours to 9 hours in children (see Fate). Decreased clearance is noted in patients with heart failure, liver dysfunction, and pulmonary edema, whereas smoking enhances plasma clearance. Children over 9 years of age generally respond to theophylline in a manner similar to adults, and should be given comparable doses. Younger children, however, require higher infusion rates and larger oral doses of theophylline than adults to maintain effective plasma concentrations. However, some children are unusually sensitive to the CNS-stimulating effects of theophylline, and caution is recommended when administering this drug to pediatric patients.

Dosage must, of course, be individualized and carefully titrated, and serum levels maintained in the range of 10 mcg to 20 mcg/ml for optimal therapeutic effect. To achieve a rapid effect, an initial loading dose can be given, although many clinicians prefer to start at lower doses and gradually increase the dosage based upon the response. Dosage adjustments are usually made on the basis of clinical signs and careful monitoring of toxicity. Once the plasma levels have stabilized, they tend to remain constant as long as the dose and dosage form are kept consistent. Dosage intervals with immediate-release products are usually maintained at 6 hours to 8 hours to provide stable blood levels, whereas sustained-release formulations may be given to nonsmokers every 12 hours to 24 hours depending on the preparation and the response. Smokers, however, may require sustained-release dosage forms every 8 hours due to the increased rate of theophylline clearance. IV administration of aminophylline is usually accomplished by giving an initial loading dose over a 20-minute to 30-minute period, followed by a continuous maintenance infusion (see Dosage, below).

Owing to the difficulties in individualizing theophylline dosage, the use of fixed combination bronchodilator products (*e.g.,* theophylline, ephedrine, sedatives, or expectorants) should be strongly discouraged. Although frequently employed, such combination formulations do not allow the dosage flexibility necessary in bronchodilator therapy, and may increase the overall incidence of untoward reactions. Moreover, inclusion of barbiturates in these preparations may enhance the hepatic metabolism of theophylline, necessitating use of larger doses to maintain steady-state blood levels. Ephedrine, another frequent inclusion in such formulations, may potentiate the CNS-excitatory action of the methylxanthines.

Xanthines

Aminophylline	Oxtriphylline
Dyphylline	Theophylline

Mechanism

Inhibit the enzyme phosphodiesterase, thus preventing breakdown of cyclic AMP; increased levels of cyclic AMP relax bronchiolar smooth muscle and may inhibit release of endogenous allergens such as histamine and slow-reacting substance of anaphylaxis (SRS-A) from sensitized mast cells; other actions include myocardial stimulation, mild diuresis, CNS excitation, increased respiration and gastric acid secretion, glycogenolysis, lipolysis, and epinephrine release from the adrenal medulla.

Uses

1 Symptomatic relief or prevention of bronchial asthma
2 Treatment of bronchospasm associated with chronic bronchitis, emphysema, and other obstructive pulmonary diseases.
3 Treatment of bradycardia and apnea in premature infants (investigational use only)

Dosage

Highly individualized, and adjusted based on theophylline serum levels (optimal range 10 mcg–20 mcg/ml); dosage should be calculated on the basis of *lean* body weight, because theophylline does not distribute into fatty tissue. (Following doses are for *anhydrous theophylline*—refer to Table 55-1 for conversion factors.)

Acute therapy (patients *not* receiving theophylline)
Adults: 6 mg/kg as a loading dose, then 3 mg/kg every 6 hours for 2 doses, then 3 mg/kg every 8 hours
Children (9 yr–16 yr) and adult smokers: 6 mg/kg as a loading dose, then 3 mg/kg every 4 hours for three doses, then 3 mg/kg every 6 hours
Children (under 9 yr): 6 mg/kg as a loading dose, then 4 mg/kg every 4 hours for three doses, then 4 mg/kg every 6 hours

Acute therapy (patients currently receiving theophylline)
Initially 2.5 mg/kg; subsequent doses based on serum theophylline levels; each 0.5 mg/kg will raise the serum theophylline concentration approximately 1.0 mcg/ml

Chronic therapy
Initially 16 mg/kg/day or 400 mg/day (whichever is less) in divided doses every 6 hours to 8 hours; increase in approximately 25% increments at 2-day to 3-day intervals, if tolerated, until optimal response or maximum dose is attained; maximum doses are the following:
Adults: 13 mg/kg/day, or 900 mg
Children (12 yr–16 yr): 18 mg/kg/day
Children (9 yr–12 yr): 20 mg/kg/day
Children (under 9 yr): 24 mg/kg/day
See Table 55-2 for recommended dosage schedules for individual preparations.

Fate

Well absorbed orally, except for enteric-coated and some sustained-release dosage forms; rectal absorption from suppositories is slow and unreliable while concentrated rectal solutions yield good absorption; peak effects differ among preparations and dosage forms, ranging from 1 hour with most liquids to 10 hours with sustained-release tablets and capsules; plasma elimination half-life of theophylline averages 7 hours to 9 hours in adult nonsmokers, 4 hours to 5 hours in adult smokers, and 3 hours to 5 hours in children; decreased plasma clearance occurs in patients with congestive heart failure, liver dysfunction, pulmonary edema, cor pulmonale, respiratory infections, and in alcoholism; metabolized in the liver to 3-methylxanthine, a weakly active metabolite, which is excreted largely in the urine; less than 15% of the drug is eliminated unchanged

Common Side-Effects

GI upset, nausea, nervousness, and urinary frequency

Significant Adverse Reactions

GI—vomiting, hematemesis, diarrhea, intestinal bleeding, activation of ulcer pain

CNS—restlessness, dizziness, insomnia, muscle twitching, headache, reflex hyperexcitability, muscle twitching, depression, speech difficulties, tonic or clonic convulsions

Cardiovascular—palpitations, tachycardia, flushing, hypotension, extrasystoles, circulatory failure

Renal—diuresis, dehydration, proteinuria

Other—tachypnea, respiratory arrest, fever, hyperglycemia, rectal irritation and strictures with use of suppositories

Rapid IV injection can result in flushing, palpitations, dizziness, hyperventilation, hypotension, and anginal-like pain.

Contraindications

Severe renal or liver impairment, peptic ulcer, active gastritis, and in patients in whom myocardial stimulation might prove dangerous

Interactions

1 Xanthines may increase the CNS stimulation seen with amphetamines, ephedrine, and other sympathomimetic drugs.
2 Increased theophylline plasma levels (decreased clearance) may occur with use of cimetidine, allopurinol, influenza virus vaccine, erythromycin, clindamycin, lincomycin, and troleandomycin.
3 The effects of theophylline may be decreased by nicotine, marijuana, and phenobarbital.
4 Xanthines can increase the excretion of lithium and phenytoin, and decrease their effectiveness.
5 Xanthines and beta-adrenergic blocking agents (*e.g.,* propranolol, metoprolol, nadolol) may be mutually antagonistic.
6 Xanthines can enhance the diuretic action of other types of diuretics.
7 The toxicity of digitalis glycosides may be increased by xanthines.
8 Tachycardia can result when xanthines are given together with reserpine.
9 Large doses of xanthines can increase plasma prothrombin and clotting factor 5, thus reducing effectiveness of oral anticoagulants.

▶ NURSING ALERTS

▷ 1 Use cautiously in patients with acute cardiac disease, severe hypoxemia, hypertension, myocardial damage, glaucoma, hyperthyroidism, peptic ulcer, diabetes, prostatic hypertrophy; during pregnancy or lactation, and in children and alcoholics.

▷ 2 Be alert for development of cardiac arrhythmias or convulsions, particularly if dosage is excessive. Theophylline products may worsen preexisting arrhythmias.

▷ 3 Warn patients, especially the elderly, that dizziness can occur, and use adequate precautions where possible (*e.g.,* bed rails, ambulatory aids).

▷ 4 Avoid use of liquid theophylline formulations containing alcohol, because it is *not* necessary for absorption and may be potentially harmful, especially in younger patients.

▷ 5 When switching from one xanthine preparation to another, make appropriate dosage adjustments based upon content of theophylline base (see Table 55-1).

▶ NURSING CONSIDERATIONS

▷ 1 Be alert for early signs of possible overdose (*e.g.,* vomiting, dizziness, restlessness, irritability) and advise physician.

▷ 2 Administer oral preparations with a full glass of water, and with food, if necessary, to minimize GI upset.

▷ 3 Caution patients not to chew or crush enteric-coated or other sustained-release formulations, because release of excessive amounts of free drug may result.

▷ 4 Make dosage adjustments carefully, based upon clinical responses (*e.g.,* respiratory function, pulse rate, urine output) and plasma levels if possible. When blood is difficult to obtain, saliva levels (approximately 60% of simultaneous plasma levels) may be used.

▷ 5 Be alert for appearance of CNS-stimulatory effects, especially in children.

▷ 6 Avoid IM injections because they are usually quite painful. With IV infusion, monitor vital signs and observe closely for development of untoward reactions such as hypotension, arrhythmias, or convulsions, which may be the *initial* signs of toxicity.

▷ 7 If rectal administration is employed, insert suppository before meals and keep patient recumbent for 15 minutes to 20 minutes or until defecation reflex subsides.

▷ 8 Note that children absorb drug rectally much faster than do adults. Be very cautious with use of suppositories in children.

▷ 9 Caution patients against indiscriminate use of over-the-counter preparations containing medications that can alter respiratory functions (*e.g.,* sympathomimetics, expectorants, antitussives).

▷ 10 Be aware that cigarette smoking may decrease the duration of action of theophylline, requiring dosage adjustment (see Dosage).

▷ 11 To improve respiratory function, suggest use of adjunctive measures such as adequate fluid intake, humidification, breathing exercises, postural drainage to remove secretions, and avoidance of smoking, irritants, or cold weather.

▷ 12 Note that theophylline is incompatible with many other drugs in solution (see remarks for aminophylline in Table 55-2).

▷ *Dietary precautions*

▷ 1 Charcoal-broiled foods may increase theophylline elimination.

▷ 2 Consumption of large amounts of caffeine-containing beverages (*e.g.,* coffee, tea, cocoa, cola drinks) may increase the side-effects of theophylline.

▶ cromolyn sodium

Intal

Table 55-2. Xanthine Bronchodilators

Drug	Preparations	Usual Dosage Range	Remarks
Aminophylline (Aminodur, Amoline, Lixaminol, Phyllocontin, Somophyllin, Truphylline)	Tablets—100 mg, 200 mg Timed-release tablets—225 mg, 300 mg Elixir—250 mg/15 ml Liquid (alcohol-free)—315 mg/15 ml Suppositories—250 mg, 500 mg Rectal solution—300 mg/5 ml Injection (IV)—250 mg/10 ml, 500 mg/20 ml Injection (IM)—500 mg/2 ml	Oral: Adults—500 mg initially, then 200 mg to 300 mg every 6 hours to 8 hours Children—7.5 mg/kg initially, then 5 mg/kg to 6 mg/kg every 6 hours to 8 hours Timed-release tablets—1 to 2 tablets every 8 hours to 12 hours before meals and at bedtime Rectal solutions: Adults—300 mg 1 to 3 times a day or 450 mg twice a day Children—5 mg/kg every 6 hours to 8 hours Suppositories: Adults—500 mg 1 to 2 times a day Children—7 mg/kg IM: Adults—500 mg IV: Initially 6 mg/kg loading dose at a rate not exceeding 25 mg/minute For continuous infusion, the rates (mg/kg/hr) are as follows: |	0–12 hr	>12 hr
---	---	---
Nonsmoking adults	0.7	0.5
Smoking adults and children 9 yr–16 yr	1.0	0.8
Children 1 yr–9 yr	1.2	1.0
Infants		0.2–0.8
Patients with congestive heart failure	0.5	0.1–0.2		Ethylenediamine salt of theophylline with similar pharmacologic properties; only xanthine derivative used IV for acute attacks of bronchial asthma; sensitivity reactions and dermatitis have occurred, especially with parenteral use; suppositories may produce rectal irritation; IM injections are very painful and should be avoided if possible; use only diluted solutions (25 mg/ml) for IV injection and warm to room temperature; inject very slowly (maximum 25 mg/min) to avoid cardiovascular disturbances, and closely monitor vital signs during infusion. Timed-release tablets are not recommended in children under 12; drug is incompatible in IV fluids with ascorbic acid, chlorpromazine, corticotropin, dimenhydrinate, hydralazine, hydroxyzine, insulin, meperidine, methadone, morphine, oxytetracycline, penicillin G potassium, phenobarbital, phenytoin, prochlorperazine, promethazine, tetracycline, and vancomycin
Dyphylline (Asminyl, Dilin, Dilor, Dyflex, Lufyllin, Neothylline, Oxystat)	Tablets—200 mg, 400 mg Sustained-action tablets—400 mg Liquid (alcohol-free)—100 mg/5 ml Elixir—100 mg/15 ml, 160 mg/15 ml Injection (IM)—250 mg/ml	Oral: Adults—up to 15 mg/kg every 6 hours depending on response Children—4.4 mg to 6.6 mg/kg/day in divided doses IM: Adults only—250 mg to 500 mg	A chemically related derivative of theophylline that is *not* metabolized to theophylline *in vivo;* equivalent to approximately 70% theophylline by molecular weight ratio; claimed to produce less GI upset and fewer overall side-effects, but blood levels and activity are somewhat lower than theophylline; peak plasma levels occur in 1 hour; short half-life (2 hr) requires frequent dosing to maintain effective blood levels; inject drug slowly IM and aspirate to avoid inadvertent IV injection; excreted essentially unchanged in the urine
Oxtriphylline (Choledyl)	Tablets (partially enteric coated)—100 mg, 200 mg Sustained-release tablets—400 mg, 600 mg Elixir—100 mg/5 ml Syrup—50 mg/5 ml (pediatric)	Adults—200 mg 4 times a day or 400 mg to 600 mg sustained action tablets every 12 hours Children—3.6 mg/kg 4 times a day (100 mg/60 lb)	Choline salt of theophylline containing 64% theophylline; claimed to be more uniformly absorbed and more stable than theophylline, and to produce less GI distress and

Table 55-2. Xanthine Bronchodilators *(continued)*

Drug	Preparations	Usual Dosage Range	Remarks
			tolerance; regular tablets are partially enteric coated, which delays onset but not completeness of absorption
Theophylline (Aerolate, Bronkodyl, Elixophyllin, Slo-Phyllin, Somophyllin, Theo-Dur, Theolair, Theo-24, and various other manufacturers)	Tablet—100 mg, 125 mg, 200 mg, 225 mg, 250 mg, 300 mg Timed-release tablets—100 mg, 130 mg, 200 mg, 250 mg, 260 mg, 300 mg, 500 mg Chewable tablets—100 mg Capsules—100 mg, 200 mg, 250 mg Timed-release capsules—50 mg, 60 mg, 65 mg, 100 mg, 125 mg, 130 mg, 200 mg, 250 mg, 260 mg, 300 mg Encapsulated powder (Theo-Dur Sprinkle)—50 mg, 75 mg, 125 mg, 200 mg Elixir—80 mg/15 ml, 112.5 mg/15 ml, 150 mg/15 ml Liquid (alcohol-free)—80 mg/15 ml, 150 mg/15 ml Syrup (alcohol-free)—80 mg/15 ml Suspension—100 mg/5 ml	Oral: Adults—100 mg to 250 mg every 6 hours or 1 to 2 timed-release preparations every 8 hours to 24 hours Children—4 mg to 6 mg/kg every 6 hours (see Dosage under general discussion of xanthines)	Standard xanthine derivative widely used as a bronchodilator; available in various dosage forms, allowing flexibility in dosing; sustained-release preparations provide for gradual release of active drug so that they may be given every 8 hours to 24 hours depending on formulation; liquid formulations may be hydro-alcoholic elixirs or alcohol-free syrups or suspensions; aqueous solutions provide similar serum levels as alcoholic elixirs, but lack CNS-depressant effects and are better tasting; some timed-release products may exhibit unpredictable absorption; found in many combination products with ephedrine, sedatives, or expectorants; fixed combination preparations do not allow individual dosage adjustments that are often necessary to obtain optimal action
Theophylline sodium glycinate (Synophylate)	Elixir—330 mg/15 ml	Adults—330 mg to 660 mg every 6 hours to 8 hours Children (6 yr–12 yr)—220 mg to 330 mg every 6 hours to 8 hours Children (under 6 yr)—55 mg to 165 mg every 6 hours to 8 hours	Mixture of sodium theophylline and glycine containing 47% theophylline; claimed to elicit fewer adverse GI effects; infrequently used preparation.

An adjunctive agent for the management of severe bronchial asthma, cromolyn may decrease the severity of the clinical symptoms of asthma, or reduce the requirements for concomitant drug therapy, or both. It is strictly a prophylactic drug and possesses no intrinsic bronchodilator, antihistaminic, or anti-inflammatory activity. It is of no value in the treatment of acute asthmatic attacks. The drug is available for oral inhalation as powder-containing capsules and a solution for nebulization, and *no* significant difference in effectiveness between these two dosage forms has been demonstrated. Cromolyn is also marketed as a nasal spray (Nasalcrom) for treatment of chronic allergic rhinitis. This latter indication is discussed later in the chapter.

Mechanism

Inhibits release of intrinsic allergens (*e.g.,* histamine, slow-reacting substance of anaphylaxis) from sensitized and nonsensitized mast cells in response to exposure to specific antigens

Uses

1 *Prophylactic* agent for the management of severe, perennial bronchial asthma (reduces severity of symptoms or bronchodilator drug dosage requirements)
2 Symptomatic treatment of food allergies (experimental use only)
3 Treatment of chronic allergic rhinitis—see discussion that follows

Dosage

20 mg inhaled four times a day; capsules are placed into inhaler (Spinhaler) and powder is administered according to package directions; nebulizer solution is administered using a power-assisted nebulizer equipped with a suitable face mask.

Fate
Approximately 8% to 10% of dose is absorbed by the lungs following inhalation, then rapidly excreted unchanged in the bile and urine; remainder of dose is either exhaled or swallowed and then excreted in the feces (GI absorption is poor); elimination half-life is 80 minutes to 90 minutes

Common Side-Effects
Cough, nasal congestion, pharyngeal irritation, wheezing

Significant Adverse Reactions
Lacrimation, parotid gland swelling, rash, urticaria, angioedema, dysuria, urinary frequency, joint swelling, dizziness; rarely, hoarseness, myalgia, vertigo, photosensitivity, peripheral neuritis, nephrosis, anemia, exfoliative dermatitis, vasculitis, pericarditis, eosinophilia, and anaphylactic reactions

Contraindications
Children under 5 years; acute asthmatic attack

▶ NURSING ALERTS
▷ 1 Initiate cromolyn therapy only after an acute attack has abated, the airway has cleared, and the patient is able to inhale adequately. An inhaled bronchodilator may be administered before each dose of cromolyn to aid penetration into lungs.

▷ 2 Once a patient is stabilized on cromolyn, attempts should be made to reduce dosage to lowest effective level. Be alert for worsening of symptoms as dose is lowered, and provide symptomatic therapy as necessary.

▷ 3 If improvement in steroid-dependent asthmatics is noted with cromolyn, gradually reduce corticosteroid dosage while closely observing patient for deterioration of condition or symptoms of adrenal insufficiency (see Beclomethasone, Chap. 43). Be prepared to reinstitute steroid therapy during periods of stress or loss of respiratory control.

▷ 4 Do not discontinue cromolyn therapy abruptly except under a physician's care, because exacerbation of asthmatic condition can occur.

▷ 5 Use cautiously in patients with impaired renal or hepatic function, and in pregnant women.

▶ NURSING CONSIDERATIONS
▷ 1 Ensure that patient understands the correct procedure for administering the powdered capsular form of the drug. Follow package instructions carefully. Caution patient not to swallow capsules.

▷ 2 Instruct patient to clear airway of as much mucus as possible before inhalation.

▷ 3 Caution patient against exhaling moisture into the capsule inhaler, because drug is in a powder form, and moisture may cause particle clumping and interfere with proper administration.

▷ 4 Do not administer inhalant solution with a hand-operated nebulizer. A power-operated nebulizer with an adequate flow rate and suitable face mask is necessary to ensure sufficient penetration.

▷ 5 Instruct patient to avoid inhaling drug during acute asthmatic attacks, because it may be irritating to respiratory passages, thus worsening symptoms.

▷ 6 Re-evaluate patient's drug regimen if no improvement is noted after 4 weeks of cromolyn therapy.

▶ cromolyn sodium intranasal
Nasalcrom

Cromolyn is also available as a nasal spray for the management of symptoms of allergic rhinitis. Repeated inhalation of the drug is believed to decrease the occurrence and severity of attacks of allergic rhinitis. One spray is administered into each nostril every 4 hours to 6 hours using the inhaler supplied with the drug cartridge. Side-effects are rare and the drug is well tolerated.

Summary. Bronchodilators

Drug	Preparations	Usual Dosage Range
Xanthine derivatives	See Table 55-2.	
Cromolyn sodium (Intal)	Capsules—20 mg (for inhalation)	20 mg inhaled 4 times a day
	Solution (for nebulizer)—20 mg/2 ml	
Cromolyn sodium, intranasal (Nasalcrom)	Nasal spray—40 mg/ml	1 spray each nostril 3 to 4 times/day

Mucolytic agents have the ability to liquefy mucus and thus facilitate its removal from the respiratory passages by normal physiologic processes such as ciliary action, bronchiolar peristalsis, coughing, or through suction. Although various proteolytic enzymes and detergents have been tried previously as mucolytic agents, most exhibited undesirable side-effects, and were unsuitable for clinical use. The only currently available mucolytic drug is acetylcysteine, an amino-acid derivative that disrupts the molecular structure of mucus. It is a relatively nontoxic compound when used by inhalation for adjunctive therapy of a number of broncho-obstructive conditions resulting from excessive or highly viscous mucus.

Acetylcysteine may be administered by nebulization, using a face mask or mouthpiece, or if large volumes are required, by use of a tent or croupette. The drug may also be instilled directly into the bronchial tree *via* a tracheostomy tube or intratracheal cannula. However, when administered by an ordinary aerosol nebulizer, its effectiveness is compromised by its inability to penetrate deeply enough into the obstructed bronchiolar passages. Acetylcysteine is also available in combination with the bronchodilator isoproterenol, for use in those patients with increased airway obstruction that impairs penetration of the mucolytic drug. However, acetylcysteine is *not* indicated for routine use in bronchial asthmatic patients with mucus accumulation, inasmuch as it is frequently irritating and may elicit reflex bronchospasm, further impairing the patients' respiratory function.

Prompt removal of the liquefied secretions is necessary following use of a mucolytic agent. When coughing is unsuccessful in eliminating the liquefied mucus, or in the case of elderly or debilitated patients who are unable to encourage productive coughing, the airway must be kept clear by mechanical suction.

Acetylcysteine has also been employed investigationally to prevent or to minimize hepatotoxicity associated with acetaminophen overdosage by blocking the formation of toxic metabolites. The drug is given orally for this indication, and the dosage is outlined below.

Mucolytics

56

▶ **acetylcysteine**

Mucomyst

Mechanism

Breaks disulfide linkages in the mucoprotein structure of mucus, thus lowering its viscosity; mucolytic activity increases with increasing *p*H, and is optimal between *p*H 7 and 9. In acetaminophen overdosage, retards formation of a hepatotoxic metabolite.

Uses

1 Adjunctive therapy for the relief of abnormal, viscous mucus accumulation associated with a variety of chronic respiratory conditions, such as emphysema, asthmatic bronchitis, bronchiectasis, tuberculosis, or amyloidosis of the lung

2 Minimization of bronchiolar obstructive complications associated with tracheostomy, cystic fibrosis, atelectasis, surgery, anesthesia, or trauma

3 Facilitation of diagnostic bronchial studies
4 Prevention of hepatotoxicity due to acetaminophen overdosage (experimental use only, see Dosage)

Dosage

Nebulization (face mask, mouthpiece, tracheostomy): 1 ml to 10 ml (20% solution) or 2 ml to 20 ml (10% solution) every 2 hours to 6 hours; usual dose is 6 ml to 10 ml of 10% solution three to four times a day

Nebulization (tent, croupette): volume of 10% to 20% solution sufficient to maintain a *heavy* mist in the area for the desired time period

Direct instillation: 1 ml to 2 ml of 10% to 20% solution every 1 hour to 4 hours *via* a tracheostomy tube or tracheal cannula

Diagnosis: 1 ml to 2 ml (20% solution) or 2 ml to 4 ml (10% solution) by nebulization or direct instillation before diagnostic procedure

Antidote to acetaminophen overdosage (experimental use only): *oral use only*—initially 140 mg/kg as a 5% solution mixed with soda, water, or juice, followed by 17 maintenance doses of 70 mg/kg every 4 hours; begin treatment within 12 hours after acetaminophen ingestion

Fate

Liquefaction of mucus following inhalation begins within 1 minute to 2 minutes and is maximal at 5 minutes to 10 minutes; with direct intratracheal application, onset is immediate.

Significant Adverse Reactions

Nausea, vomiting, rhinorrhea, stomatitis, fever, tracheal and bronchial irritation, chest tightness, bronchospasm, and dermal eruptions

Interactions

1 Acetylcysteine is incompatible in solution with many antibiotics (*e.g.,* tetracyclines, amphotericin B, sodium ampicillin, erythromycin), and should not be mixed in the same solution.

▶ NURSING ALERTS

▷ 1 Closely observe asthmatic patients receiving acetylcysteine, and discontinue drug at first sign of bronchospasm. If necessary, give a bronchodilator by inhalation.

▷ 2 Ensure that patients remove liquefied secretions by expectoration. If coughing is inadequate to expel mucus, consider use of mechanical aspiration.

▷ 3 Use cautiously in patients with bronchial asthma, and in elderly or debilitated patients with respiratory insufficiency.

▶ NURSING CONSIDERATIONS

▷ 1 Use only nebulizers with a compressed air source. Ordinary hand-held bulb nebulizers should not be used because output is too small and particle size of drug is too large.

▷ 2 With prolonged nebulization, dilute nebulizing solution with Sterile Water for Injection to prevent extreme concentration of solution, which might impair proper drug delivery.

▷ 3 Instruct patients to clear airway by productive coughing before inhaling drug.

▷ 4 Inform patient that a disagreeable rotten egg-like odor may be noticeable initially, but will soon become less apparent. Be prepared to assist patient if odor causes nausea or vomiting.

▷ 5 Following use, wash face, mask, and container with water, because drug leaves a sticky coating.

▷ 6 Note that the 20% solution may be diluted with sterile normal saline or Sterile Water for Injection, whereas the 10% solution is usually used undiluted.

▷ 7 Avoid contact of acetylcysteine solution with rubber, iron, or copper, because discoloration of solution can occur, with possible reduction in potency.

▷ 8 Store unused portion of solution in a refrigerator and use within 96 hours to minimize contamination. A light purple color may appear but does not impair drug's effectiveness.

▷ 9 Note that acetylcysteine (10%) is available in solution with isoproterenol (0.05%) as Mucomyst w/Isoproterenol. This solution should only be administered by nebulization or inhalation using a face mask or mouthpiece.

▷ 10 When used to prevent acetaminophen-induced hepatotoxicity, administer as soon as possible after ingestion of acetaminophen. Effectiveness of acetylcysteine is greatly reduced if given later than 18 hours after poisoning with acetaminophen.

Summary. Mucolytic Agents

Drug	Preparations	Usual Dosage Range
Acetylcysteine (Mucomyst)	Solution— 10%, 20%	Nebulization—1 ml to 10 ml (20%) or 2 ml to 20 ml (10%) every 2 hours to 6 hours
		Direct instillation—1 ml to 2 ml (10%–20%) every 1 hour to 4 hours
		Diagnostic procedures—1 ml to 2 ml (20%) or 2 ml to 4 ml (10%) before procedure
		Acetaminophen overdose— initially, 140 mg/kg *orally*, as a 5% solution; then, 10 mg/ kg every 4 hours for 17 doses

Drugs having the ability to enhance depressed respiratory function are termed respiratory stimulants or analeptics. Such agents act both at the level of the respiratory center in the brain stem as well as on the peripheral carotid chemoreceptors to increase the depth and, frequently, also the rate of respiration. They are primarily indicated to overcome respiratory depression due to drug overdosage with the various classes of CNS depressants (*e.g.,* hypnotics, narcotics) or overdosage resulting from general anesthesia. However, their clinical effectiveness in many cases of drug-induced respiratory depression has been questioned, and their potential for eliciting untoward reactions is rather high. Thus, they are much less frequently used today than in previous years.

Foremost among their disadvantages is that doses needed to elicit sufficient respiratory stimulation in cases of marked respiratory depression often stimulate other CNS areas as well (*e.g.,* vasomotor center, vomiting center, brain stem reticular formation), resulting in a variety of undesirable effects ranging from mild cardiovascular stimulation to marked central activation leading to vomiting, hyper-reflexia, and convulsions. Since respiratory stimulants have a rather narrow safety margin, they must be administered cautiously by trained personnel and only in conjunction with appropriate resuscitative measures (*e.g.,* oxygen, suction, anticonvulsants, muscle relaxants) as necessary.

Analeptics are merely *physiologic* antagonists of respiratory depressants, and do not specifically block the effects of narcotics, barbiturates, muscle relaxants, or other drugs. In fact, analeptics alone are often insufficient in arousing a severely depressed individual and should be used only in conjunction with adequate adjunctive measures, such as mechanical assistance, narcotic antagonists, or cholinergic drugs, depending upon the particular drug involved. Obviously, maintenance of an open airway is essential with use of respiratory stimulants.

Although these drugs are not routinely employed to overcome postanesthetic respiratory depression and to shorten recovery time, some clinicians advocate a single IV injection or a slow IV infusion of doxapram, the preferred analeptic, together with oxygen following surgery to encourage "deep breathing" and prevent development of postoperative atelectasis, especially in patients with compromised respiratory function. A danger in such a procedure is that the analeptic can mask the residual effects of a muscle relaxant if one was administered during surgery.

An additional application for doxapram is as an aid to prevent elevated arterial carbon dioxide when oxygen is being administered during an episode of acute respiratory insufficiency in patients with chronic obstructive pulmonary disease. The increased depth of respiration produced by infusion of this analeptic may improve alveolar ventilation and help arouse patients from their lethargic condition. Mechanical ventilation is not used during the period of analeptic administration, which should not exceed 2 hours.

The two available analeptic drugs are considered individually, owing to the differences in safety and efficacy between them. Caffeine and sodium benzoate injection has also been employed as a respiratory stimulant, and this combination is considered in Chapter 27 with other CNS stimulants.

Respiratory
Stimulants

57

▶ **doxapram**

Dopram

Mechanism

Enhances depth and rate of respiration by direct stimulation of medullary respiratory center and by increasing activation of peripheral carotid chemoreceptors; large doses stimulate vasomotor center (increase blood pressure and cardiac output); little direct action on cortex and exhibits a slightly greater margin of safety (increased respiratory stimulant/convulsive ratio) than similar drugs

Uses

1 Reversal of postanesthetic respiratory depression or apnea (except due to muscle relaxants) and facilitation of emergence from anesthesia
2 Adjunctive treatment of drug-induced CNS and respiratory depression, to hasten arousal and facilitate return of laryngopharyngeal reflexes (*Note:* Respiratory depression due to CNS-depressant overdosage is *best* managed by mechanical ventilation.)
3 Prevention of elevated arterial carbon dioxide tension during oxygen administration in patients with chronic obstructive pulmonary disease with acute respiratory insufficiency

Dosage

Postanesthesia: 0.5 mg to 1 mg/kg IV injection (maximum 2 mg/kg) or 1 mg to 5 mg/minute by IV infusion depending on response and vital signs

Drug-induced respiratory depression: 2 mg/kg IV injection; repeat in 5 minutes, then at 1-hour to 2-hour intervals until arousal is sustained (total maximum dose is 3 g); alternately 1 mg to 3 mg/minute by IV infusion following initial priming dose given above (total maximum dose is 3 g)

Chronic obstructive pulmonary disease: 1 mg to 3 mg/minute by IV infusion (2 mg/ml solution) for a maximum of 2 hours

Fate

Onset of action is 20 seconds to 40 seconds and peak effect occurs within 1 minute to 2 minutes; duration ranges from 5 minutes to 12 minutes

Common Side-Effects

Mild hypertension, variations in heart rate

Significant Adverse Reactions

CNS/autonomic—flushing, sweating, pruritus, paresthesias, headache, dizziness, disorientation, mydriasis, tremors, involuntary movements, muscle spasticity, convulsions, increased deep tendon reflexes

Respiratory—cough, dyspnea, bronchospasm, laryngospasm, hiccups, rebound hypoventilation

Cardiovascular—chest pain and tightness, phlebitis, depressed T waves, arrhythmias

GI—nausea, vomiting, diarrhea

Other—urinary retention, incontinence

Contraindications

Epilepsy or other convulsive states, airway obstruction, incompetence of the ventilatory mechanism, pneumothorax, extreme dyspnea, acute bronchial asthma, suspected or confirmed pulmonary embolism, respiratory failure due to neuromuscular disorders, pulmonary fibrosis, severe hypertension, head injury, coronary artery disease, and uncompensated heart failure

Interactions

1 Additive pressor effects may occur if doxapram is combined with sympathomimetics or MAO inhibitors.
2 Doxapram releases epinephrine, and thus may increase the incidence of arrhythmias with those general anesthetics that sensitize the myocardium (*e.g.,* halothane, enflurane, cyclopropane).
3 Doxapram may enhance the CNS effects of amantadine (see Chap. 26).

▶ **NURSING ALERTS**

▷ 1 Ensure patency of airway and adequacy of oxygenation before administering doxapram.
▷ 2 Have proper measures and drugs available (*e.g.,* oxygen, resuscitative equipment, anticonvulsants, antiarrhythmics) in case of doxapram overdosage.
▷ 3 Be alert for early signs of toxicity (tachycardia, hyperactive reflexes, tremors, hypertension), and reduce infusion rate or discontinue drug if necessary.
▷ 4 Delay administration of doxapram for 10 minutes to 15 minutes following discontinuation of anesthetics (*e.g.,* halothane, enflurane) known to sensitize the myocardium to catecholamines, because release of epinephrine by doxapram may elicit arrhythmias.
▷ 4 Discontinue drug if sudden dyspnea or hypotension occurs.
▷ 5 Use with caution and under close supervision in patients with cerebral edema, severe tachycardia, arrhythmias, cardiac disease, pheochromocytoma, history of bronchial asthma, hyperthyroidism, peptic ulcer, acute agitation; in pregnant women and in children under 12 years.
▷ 6 Use care to avoid extravasation of solution, because thrombophlebitis can result.

▶ **NURSING CONSIDERATIONS**

▷ 1 Monitor blood pressure, pulse, and deep tendon reflexes during administration to prevent overdosage.
▷ 2 Maintain close observation of patient for at least 1 hour after injection or until patient is fully alert and pharyngeal and laryngeal reflexes are restored.
▷ 3 Adjust flow rate of infusion to sustain the desired level of respiratory stimulation with minimal side-effects.
▷ 4 In patients with obstructive pulmonary disease, determine arterial blood gases before administration of doxapram, then at least every ½ hour during infusion. Do not infuse for more than 2 hours. Provide supplemental oxygen as needed.
▷ 5 Re-administer subsequent doses of doxapram only to those persons who have responded to the initial dose.
▷ 6 Do not mix doxapram injection with alkaline solutions, because precipitation will result. Injection is compatible with normal saline or Dextrose in Water.

▶ nikethamide
Coramine

Mechanism
Direct stimulation of medullary respiratory center and secondary stimulation of peripheral carotid chemoreceptors; no direct effect on the heart or blood vessels, but less effective and has a lower margin of safety than doxapram

Uses
1   Treatment of CNS, respiratory, and circulatory depression due to effects of depressant drugs (*Note:* Respiratory depression resulting from overdosage with CNS depressants is best managed by mechanical ventilation.)
2   Aid to restoration of respiration following electroshock therapy

Dosage
Anesthetic overdosage: 2 ml to 5 ml IV to increase amplitude of respiration; 5 ml to 15 ml to overcome respiratory depression. May repeat as needed.

   If cardiac arrest is present—0.5 ml to 1 ml intracardially
CNS-depressant poisoning: 5 ml to 10 ml IV initially, then 5 ml every 5 minutes for 1 hour, then once every hour thereafter as needed
Shock: 10 ml to 15 ml IV or IM, repeated as necessary
Acute alcoholism: 5 ml to 20 ml IV, repeated as necessary
Electroshock: 5 ml diluted with 5 ml of sterile water and injected rapidly IV prior to stimulus (oral maintenance dosage—3 ml to 5 ml every 4 hours to 6 hours)

Fate
Well absorbed following oral or IM administration, with a maximum effect in 20 minutes to 30 minutes; onset is rapid with IV injection and effects persist for 5 minutes to 10 minutes; converted to nicotinamide *in vivo* and excreted in the urine as the *N*-methyl metabolite

Common Side-Effects
(Usually with large doses) Burning and itching at the back of the nose, flushing, and feeling of warmth

Significant Adverse Reactions
Sweating, coughing, sneezing, nausea, vomiting, restlessness, tachycardia, increased blood pressure, muscle twitching, and convulsions

Contraindications
See Doxapram.

Interactions
See Doxapram.

▶ NURSING ALERTS
See Doxapram. In addition,
▷ 1   Do not inject intra-arterially, because arterial spasm and thrombosis may result.
▷ 2   Be aware that safety margin is low, and observe for development of any side-effects. Be prepared to administer a short-acting barbiturate to control convulsions and use other adjunctive measures as necessary.

▶ NURSING CONSIDERATIONS
See Doxapram. In addition,
▷ 1   Do not confuse 25% injection solution with 25% oral solution.
▷ 2   Note that drug is most effective (and most hazardous) when given by the IV route.

Summary. Respiratory Stimulants

Drug	Preparations	Usual Dosage Range
Doxapram (Dopram)	Injection—20 mg/ml	Postanesthesia—0.5 mg to 1 mg/kg IV injection or 1.5 mg/min IV infusion
		Drug-induced respiratory depression—2 mg/kg IV injection at 1-hour to 2-hour intervals or 1 mg to 3 mg/minute IV infusion after priming dose given above (maximum 3 g)
		Chronic obstructive pulmonary disease—1 mg to 3 mg/minute IV infusion for a maximum of 2 hours
Nikethamide (Coramine)	Injection—250 mg/ml Oral solution—250 mg/ml	Anesthetic and drug-induced CNS depression—2 ml to 15 ml IV (usually 5 ml–10 ml); repeat every 5 minutes for 1 hour, then once every hour as needed
		Electroshock—5 ml diluted with 5 ml sterile water and injected rapidly IV prior to stimulus; oral maintenance dose—3 ml to 5 ml every 4 hours to 6 hours

Anti-Infective and Chemotherapeutic Agents

VIII

Drugs used for the treatment of infectious diseases may be termed *antibiotics, anti-infectives, antimicrobials,* or *chemotherapeutic agents.* While these terms are often used interchangeably, the first three, that is, antibiotics, anti-infectives, and antimicrobials, are properly used to describe those drugs commonly employed for the treatment of infections. The designation *chemotherapeutic agent* has come to be more closely associated with those drugs used in the treatment of cancer.

Antibiotics are strictly defined as *natural* substances produced by various microorganisms and capable of inhibiting the growth of other microorganisms. Little distinction is made, however, between those substances having a natural origin and those with a synthetic origin. In fact, the term *semisynthetic* is often applied to the product of a chemical alteration of a naturally derived anti-infective compound.

Although the use of substances extracted from soil, plants, or living organisms to kill other organisms has been described for centuries, the modern age of chemotherapy had its origin in the late 1930s and early 1940s with the introduction of sulfonamides and penicillins, respectively. Since that time, a variety of antimicrobial agents have become available, and the overall morbidity and mortality due to infectious diseases has steadily diminished. Nevertheless, the search for newer anti-infective drugs continues unabated, because some infectious diseases still have not been completely eradicated, while other newer diseases are just beginning to appear. In addition, the treatment of some previously susceptible microorganisms by currently available antimicrobial drugs is becoming more difficult due to the emergence of increasing numbers of resistant strains. While many different antibiotics are now available to the clinician, enabling treatment of a wide range of bacterial infections, no single agent yet represents the "ideal" antimicrobial drug in terms of spectrum of action, efficacy, safety, and cost.

Anti-Infective Therapy— General Considerations

58

Classification

There are several different characteristics that may be used to classify the currently available antimicrobial drugs. However, no single classification is sufficient to completely categorize a particular drug; rather, complete description of any agent requires reference to a number of these characteristics. The most commonly used classifying characteristics are outlined below:

Spectrum of Activity

A broad classification of antibiotics divides them according to the range of their antimicrobial activity into *broad spectrum* and *narrow spectrum.* Broad-spectrum antibiotics exert their effects against a number of different types of bacteria and other microorganisms. Tetracyclines are, for example, active against a wide range of both gram-positive and gram-negative bacteria, as well as several other categories of microorganisms, such as *Rickettsia, Chlamydia,* and *Mycoplasma* species. Generally, if an agent is effective against both gram-positive and gram-negative organisms, it is referred to as *broad spectrum,* although some broad-spectrum antibiotics are active against a much wider range of organisms than others.

Antibacterial drugs that primarily affect only one group of microorganisms are termed *narrow-spectrum* antibiotics. For example, penicillin G affects only gram-positive bacteria and *Neisseria* at normal therapeutic doses and therefore is considered narrow spectrum. It is worth noting here, however, that *spectrum of activity* does not necessarily correlate with *antimicrobial effectiveness.* In fact, because of excessive use and subsequent emergence of resistant strains, many broad-spectrum antibiotics are much less active against many microorganisms than the more selective narrow-spectrum drugs.

Antimicrobial Activity

Antimicrobial agents may also be categorized on the basis of their antibacterial activity as either *bacteriostatic* or *bactericidal.* Bacteriostatic drugs (*e.g.,* tetracyclines, sulfonamides) suppress the growth of microorganisms without actually killing existing microbes. The invading microorganisms are removed by the host defense mechanisms. Bactericidal drugs (such as penicillins), on the other hand, are capable of directly destroying organisms, especially those in an active state of replication. Theoretically, bactericidal drugs are more desirable from a therapeutic standpoint, but it is important to recognize that their lethal action on microorganisms is dependent on their being present in sufficient concentrations. In subtherapeutic doses, bactericidal drugs are merely bacteriostatic, and conversely, at very high doses some bacteriostatic drugs may exert a bactericidal action. Nevertheless, even the most potent bactericidal drug is usually incapable of totally eliminating an infection without intervention of the patient's own natural defense mechanisms, such as antibody production, phagocytosis, and leukocyte proliferation. Impaired defense mechanisms can result from disease states (neoplasms, diabetes, hematologic disorders) or drugs (*e.g.,* antineoplastics, corticosteroids) and can severely compromise the action of antimicrobial drugs.

Mechanism of Action

Antimicrobial agents exhibit several different mechanisms of action and may also be categorized on this basis. Most antibiotics exert their effects on microorganisms in one of five ways:

1 Inhibition of Bacterial Cell Wall Synthesis

(*e.g.,* penicillins, cephalosporins, bacitracin) Unlike animal cells, bacteria possess a *rigid* cell wall composed of macromolecules cross-linked by peptide chains. This arrangement serves to maintain the shape of the cell and to prevent cell rupture, because most bacteria have a high internal osmotic pressure. Thus, the viability of these bacterial cells depends on the integrity of the cell wall. Drugs acting by inhibiting cell wall synthesis do so by interfering with various steps in the assembly of the peptide chains that impart rigidity to the wall. The weakened cell wall can then no longer support the internal pressure and the cells undergo lysis and disintegrate. Drugs acting in this manner are bactericidal.

2 Alteration in Cell Membrane Function

(*e.g.,* amphotericin, nystatin, polymyxins) The semipermeable bacterial cell membrane (located between the cell wall and cytoplasm) helps control the internal environment of the cell by functioning as a selective barrier to penetration of cell constituents and nutrients. Disruption of this membrane by antibiotics alters its permeability, allowing escape of proteins, nucleotides, sugars, amino acids, and so on, resulting in damage to the cell and ultimately cellular death. Drugs acting in this manner may be either bacteriostatic or bactericidal depending on the drug, dose, and organism.

3 Inhibition of Protein Synthesis

(*e.g.,* aminoglycosides, erythromycin, tetracyclines) Certain antibiotics can interfere with ribosomal-mediated protein synthesis in bacterial cells without affecting normal mammalian cells. It is believed that this occurs because the composition of the ribosomes in bacterial cells is different. Antibiotics may disrupt bacterial protein synthesis at several stages; for example, by binding to the ribosomes, blocking attachment of transfer RNA, causing a misreading of the genetic code, interfering with attachment of amino acids to the developing peptide chain, or tying up essential cofactors such as calcium, magnesium, or iron. Drugs inhibiting protein synthesis may be either bactericidal or bacteriostatic.

4 Inhibition of Nucleic Acid Metabolism

(*e.g.,* nalidixic acid, rifampin, trimethoprim) Although most agents interfering with nucleic acid metabolism are used as antineoplastic drugs, a few antibacterial compounds act in this manner as well. Nalidixic acid inhibits DNA synthesis, rifampin interferes with DNA-dependent RNA synthesis, and trimethoprim can inhibit dihydrofolate reductase, an enzyme essential for production of tetrahydrofolic acid, an intermediate in the formation of DNA. These drugs are bacteriostatic.

5   Interference with Intermediate Cell Metabolism

(*e.g.,* sulfonamides) All bacteria require dihydrofolic acid for production of nucleic acids; however, certain bacteria cannot assimilate preformed dihydrofolic acid but must synthesize it themselves from precursors within the cell. An essential precursor is para-aminobenzoic acid (PABA) and because sulfonamides are close structural analogs of PABA, they compete with it for active sites within bacterial cells, impairing synthesis of dihydrofolic acid and thus cell replication. Sulfonamides are bacteriostatic at normal dose levels.

Selection of Appropriate Drug

Several important considerations go into the choice of a suitable antimicrobial drug for use in a particular patient. The most important of these factors are examined below:

1   Necessity of Therapy

Even before a decision is made as to which antibiotic should be prescribed, the necessity for antibiotic therapy at all must be determined. Many infectious conditions do not require systemic antimicrobial therapy, and the clinician should make a careful assessment of the patient's status and the location and severity of the infection before undertaking antibiotic therapy. Unfortunately, overprescribing of antibiotics, especially in children with "colds" or "flu," occurs to a significant extent and is responsible for an undue number of untoward reactions as well as increased development of resistant strains of microorganisms. Likewise, indiscriminate medication of children by parents with "refillable" antibiotics has contributed to the reduced effectiveness of these drugs in many infectious conditions. While occupying a deservedly important place in pharmacotherapy, antibiotics are indeed frequently misused, usually to the detriment of the patient.

2   Diagnosis of the Pathogen

Accurate determination of the infecting organism or organisms is the cornerstone of safe and effective antimicrobial therapy. Appropriate anti-infective therapy is best accomplished by bacteriologic culture of the infected material (sputum, pus, urine), subsequent isolation and identification

of the pathogen, and selection of an antibiotic known to be effective against the offending organism. While it is always desirable to have the results of bacterial culturing before initiating antimicrobial treatment, this is not always practical or feasible. For example, in acute, life-threatening infections (such as septicemia, peritonitis, pneumonia), a delay in initiating treatment of 24 hours to 48 hours while awaiting results of culture testing can prove fatal and cannot be justified. In these situations, as well as others requiring immediate antibiotic therapy, the initial choice of an antibiotic should be made on the basis of a patient history, physical examination, clinical symptoms, and, most especially, an awareness on the part of the clinician as to what microorganisms are *likely* to be present based upon the site of infection and the circumstances under which it developed. In some cases, the probable organism can be determined by the attending physician by performing a simple Gram stain on smears of exudate from the infected area. However, proper bacteriologic culturing is essential for *accurate* diagnosis of the infecting pathogen, and should be ordered as soon as possible. Once the microbiological information has been obtained, definitive antimicrobial therapy can be initiated. The physician will either continue with the antibiotic prescribed initially if appropriate or switch to one that is more active or more selective against the bacterial species shown to be present.

3   Sensitivity Testing

Because many common microorganisms exhibit varying degrees of antibacterial resistance, once a pathogen has been identified by bacteriologic culturing, the *sensitivity* of the infecting organism to different antimicrobial drugs is often determined. Sensitivity testing, however, is not always necessary, because some microorganisms are uniformly susceptible to certain antibiotics. For example, *Pneumococcus,* group A beta-hemolytic *Streptococcus, Clostridia,* and *Treponema pallidum* respond predictably to penicillin G. Conversely, *Staphylococcus aureus, Streptococcus viridans,* and several gram-negative bacilli (such as *Escherichia coli, Pseudomonas aeruginosa, Klebsiella pneumoniae, Salmonella, Shigella, Hemophilus influenzae*) exhibit varying degrees of resistance to different antibiotics and should be tested for susceptibility *in vitro.*

The most widely used procedure for sensitivity testing is the disk method, in which paper disks containing known amounts of various antibiotics are placed on an agar surface that has been swabbed with bacteria isolated from the patient. After incubation, the size of the clear zone of inhibition around each disk is a measure of the activity of each antibiotic to inhibit the growth of the particular microorganism. While useful as an index of microbial susceptibility to various antibiotics, the disk method of sensitivity testing measures only growth inhibition, and thus is an indication of *bacteriostatic* activity only. Where a bactericidal action is essential (as for bacterial endocarditis), demonstration of sensitivity by the disk method is meaningless. In these situations, tube dilution sensitivity testing may be employed to determine both the minimum inhibitory concentration (MIC) and the minimum bactericidal concentration (MBC) of an antibiotic against a particular organism.

There is frequently a discrepancy between *in vitro* results and clinical response, due to a number of factors such as pH, temperature, and the ability of the drug to reach the site of infection. Demonstration of *in vitro* bacterial susceptibility does not guarantee clinical success but merely provides another parameter upon which to base selection of an antimicrobial agent.

4   Location of the Infection

Generally, once the offending pathogen has been identified and its susceptibility ascertained, a fairly selective choice of an antimicrobial agent can be made. However, consideration must also be given to the location of the infection when choosing an appropriate antibiotic. The distribution of an antibacterial drug in the body is an important determinant of its ultimate efficacy. Although the concentration of an antimicrobial agent in the body is usually defined in terms of blood or plasma levels, the critical concentration is that which is achieved in the infected tissues themselves. Plasma levels often do *not* accurately reflect tissue levels, and in spite of high plasma concentrations, some drugs may never attain sufficient tissue concentrations at the desired site of action. It is difficult to generalize about the distribution of antibiotics, because the attainment of adequate infected tissue levels is dependent on a multitude of factors such as dose and route of administration, protein binding, lipid solubility, presence of tissue fluid or abscesses, pH, site of infection, causative organism, and others. For example, drugs used in meningitis must be able to readily penetrate the CNS (meninges) while drugs excreted largely unchanged in the urine are quite effective in urinary tract infections (provided they are active at a pH of 5 to 6) in spite of the fact that they may exhibit very low plasma levels.

There are, of course, other factors that can influence the choice of an antibiotic; these include severity of the infection, a previous hypersensitivity or serious adverse reaction to a particular drug, patient acceptance of parenteral administration, and cost of the drug. While proper selection of antimicrobial agents can result in quick eradication of most infections with minimal adverse effects or complications, injudicious use of antibiotics may ultimately prove harmful to the patient. The decision to initiate antibacterial therapy must be based on careful assessment of the patient and the choice of drugs determined by accurate bacteriologic and sensitivity testing whenever possible. Antibiotic therapy in the absence of proper culturing should be undertaken only with those drugs most likely to be effective against the *suspected* pathogen, and modified if necessary as soon as the culture and sensitivity test results are known. Further, adequate dosage and duration of therapy are essential to ensure complete drug efficacy. These factors are considered next.

Dosage and Duration of Therapy

Anti-infective drug dosage should always be high enough and duration of treatment long enough to provide effective drug concentrations in infected tissues for a suitable period of time. As indicated earlier, blood levels of the antibiotic do not always reflect tissue concentrations at the infection site; nonetheless, they are frequently used as a guide to determine if proper dosage is being administered. Despite the importance of maintaining treatment long enough to completely eradicate the microorganism, antibiotics are sometimes discontinued too early. The result of this may be either reinfection with the same organism or emergence of mutant strains resistant to the drug being used.

Although different infections require variable treatment durations, oral antimicrobial therapy of most common respiratory and urinary infections should be continued for a minimum of 7 to 10 days. Patients may decide to discontinue antimicrobial drugs as soon as the overt symptoms (*e.g.,* fever, sore throat, painful urination) of their disease subside. For this reason, they should be carefully instructed to continue the drugs for at least 48 hours to 72 hours after symptoms disappear to ensure that the pathogen is completely eliminated. Follow-up cultures are also desirable to confirm the effectiveness of therapy.

More severe infections, such as endocarditis and staphylococcal pneumonia, generally require parenteral administration of higher doses of antibiotics and for longer periods than the more common infections, which can be treated orally. Large doses of antimicrobial drugs may also be necessary in debilitated patients or in patients with disease- or drug-impaired defense mechanisms.

In infections characterized by the presence of purulent exudates or large abscesses, drainage of these areas is often necessary; antibiotics frequently are unable to penetrate these infected lesions sufficiently to eradicate the large quantity of pathogens at these sites. Similarly, patients with urinary infections associated with the presence of renal stones will continue to suffer recurrent infections despite the use of antibiotics unless the stones are removed. It is important to recognize that no antibiotic alone can be expected to completely control every infection, and appropriate adjunctive measures are frequently necessary to treat certain types of infections.

Prophylactic Use of Antibiotics

The use of antimicrobial drugs to prevent rather than treat infections is a very controversial area of chemotherapy. While doubtless effective in certain situations, anti-infective prophylaxis is without proven value in many conditions and may, in fact, be detrimental in certain instances. There is general agreement that successful chemoprophylaxis is most often attained when a *single* drug known to be effective against a specific pathogen is used to prevent invasion of that pathogen before it has a chance to become established. Some generally accepted indications for antimicrobial prophylaxis are as follows:

1 *Penicillin G*—for prophylaxis of rheumatic fever, recurrent cellulitis in lymphedema, and subacute bacterial endocarditis
2 *Penicillin V*—prevention of infection in bite wounds
3 *Rifampin*—prophylaxis of meningococcal meningitis
4 *Isoniazid*—prophylaxis of tuberculosis
5 *Doxycycline*—prevention of "traveler's diarrhea"

In addition, there is some evidence that prophylactic use of antibiotics such as cephalosporins *during* certain abdominal, cardiac, and gynecologic surgical procedures can prevent development of secondary infections and reduce morbidity. However, there is no rationale for continuing the treatment beyond 4 hours to 6 hours after the end of the surgical procedure in the absence of a demonstrated susceptible organism. Prophylactic antimicrobial usage has also been advocated for preventing recurrent urinary tract infections and for reducing postoperative infections following surgery for head or neck cancer.

On the other hand, conclusive evidence is lacking on the effectiveness of antibiotics used prophylactically in patients with chronic obstructive pulmonary disease, in patients undergoing urologic, dental, or neurologic surgical procedures, and in patients with acute pancreatitis. Finally, chemoprophylaxis is considered to be ineffective in preventing (1) secondary bacterial infection in "common colds," influenza, or other viral diseases; (2) urinary infections in the presence of stones, obstruction, or indwelling urinary catheters; (3) recurring herpes simplex ulcers of the mouth; (4) secondary infections in burn patients; and (5) infections associated with prolonged use of corticosteroids, immunosuppressants, or antineoplastic drugs.

A major danger of chemoprophylaxis is the development of superinfections with drug-resistant strains, the incidence of which is closely related to the duration of exposure to the antibiotic. Therefore, short-term prophylaxis is preferred wherever possible, and antimicrobial drugs used for surgical prophylaxis generally should be given no more than 48 hours preoperatively and 4 hours to 6 hours postoperatively. Prolonged use of prophylactic antibiotics, as in rheumatic fever, endocarditis, or chronic bronchitis must be continually monitored and patients closely observed for signs of a developing superinfection (diarrhea, glossitis, perianal or vaginal itching).

Other disadvantages to antimicrobial chemoprophylaxis include an increased incidence of allergic reactions and diarrhea, and frequently a substantially higher cost to the patient.

Combined Antimicrobial Therapy

Although most infections can be adequately treated with a single anti-infective agent, simultaneous administration of two or more antimicrobial agents is justifiable under certain circumstances. When combination antimicrobial therapy is indicated, it should be accomplished by administration of two or more *individual* drugs whose doses can be titrated independently to provide an optimal effect. The once widespread use of "fixed-dose" antibiotic combinations has essentially been eliminated by the removal of most of these combinations from the market, on the grounds that many contained subtherapeutic amounts of antibiotic drugs, were often ineffective, and favored emergence of resistant bacterial populations.

The primary indications for combination anti-infective therapy are the following:

1 Treatment of Mixed Bacterial Infections

Some infections (*e.g.,* peritonitis, urinary infections, otitis media) may be complicated by the presence of two, or possibly more, microorganisms possessing different antimicrobial susceptibility. Although broad-spectrum antibiotics are occasionally successful when used alone in such infections, combination therapy is frequently necessary to ensure complete eradication of all pathogens present in mixed infections. Sensitivity testing is essential in such cases.

2 Initial Treatment of Severe Infections Where the Causative Agent Is Unknown

Before the results of bacteriologic culturing in an unknown infection are obtained, combination therapy is often undertaken to ensure that the widest range of possible organisms is covered. Such treatment, of course, should be modified if necessary as soon as culture and sensitivity data are available.

3 Postponement of the Emergence of Resistant Strains

Development of resistance to antibiotic agents is often delayed (but not necessarily prevented) when a sensitive pathogen is exposed to two drugs simultaneously. This is particularly apparent with the combined use of two or more antitubercular drugs (*e.g.,* isoniazid, rifampin) or combinations of carbenicillin and gentamicin or tobramycin for severe pseudomonal infections.

4 Enhancement of Antibacterial Activity

Increased antibacterial activity is frequently observed with simultaneous use of two antibiotics, compared to that observed with each drug alone. This synergistic effect is noted, for example, with isoniazid and ethambutol in treating tuberculosis, with tetracycline and streptomycin in treating brucellosis or glanders, and with amphotericin B and flucytosine in treating certain systemic fungal infections.

5 Reduction of Toxicity

Combined antimicrobial therapy is also used to reduce the untoward effects of one or more antibacterial agents. For example, several sulfonamides may be administered together to reduce the incidence of crystalluria.

On the other hand, combination anti-infective drug therapy can result in undesirable effects, reduced clinical effectiveness, and superinfections. For example, combined use of two or more aminoglycosides can increase the incidence of ototoxicity and nephrotoxicity above that observed with each drug alone. Therefore, other than those circumstances outlined above where combination antimicrobial therapy has proven beneficial, use of more than one carefully selected anti-infective drug to treat a particular infectious condition should be avoided.

Adverse Effects of Antimicrobial Drugs

A wide range of adverse reactions have been reported with the various classes of drugs used in the treatment of infections, and these are reviewed in detail in the individual chapters dealing with each group of drugs. The most frequently encountered untoward reactions with antibiotics are considered briefly at this time.

1 Hypersensitivity Reactions

Both acute and delayed allergic responses have occurred with a number of antimicrobial drugs, most frequently with the penicillins and sulfonamides. These may range from mild dermatologic manifestations such as skin rash, itching, and urticaria, to severe anaphylactic reactions, which have proved fatal in a number of instances. The importance of obtaining a careful patient history before administration of an antimicrobial agent known to be associated with hypersensitivity reactions cannot be overemphasized.

2 Organ Toxicity

Various classes of antibiotics are known to exert selective toxic effects upon certain structures or organs of the body. For example, aminoglycosides and vancomycin cause both renal and eighth cranial nerve damage. Amphotericin B and polymyxins, among others, impair kidney function while lincomycin and clindamycin often induce severe diarrhea and colitis. Tetracyclines may damage teeth, nails, or bones, and rifampin and the estolate salt of erythromycin can be hepatotoxic.

3 Superinfection

Development of secondary infections is a potentially serious problem connected with antibiotic usage. It occurs most often as a result of prolonged anti-infective therapy, insufficient drug dosage, impaired host defense mechanisms, concurrent therapy with immunosuppressive drugs, or a combination of these factors. Pathogens frequently responsible for secondary infections include *Pseudomonas, Proteus, Candida,* and drug-resistant staphylococci and fungi. These organisms may be especially difficult to eradicate because they often represent strains resistant to conventional antimicrobial agents. Although superinfection can theoretically occur anywhere in the body, it is usually found most commonly in the GI tract, and may be manifested by diarrhea, glossitis, stomatitis, "furry" tongue, and perineal irritation. Prompt recognition of a secondary infection is critical to its effective management. Therapy is best accomplished by discontinuing the initial antibiotic, culturing the infected area, and administering an antimicrobial drug shown by sensitivity testing to be effective against the new organism.

4 Resistance

Bacteria are susceptible to elimination by some anti-infective drugs but not others. The phenomenon whereby certain organisms are unaffected by a particular antimicrobial agent is called *resistance.* Bacterial resistance may be broadly categorized into either *natural* or *acquired* resistance. *Natural* resistance is genetically determined, and may be characteristic of either an entire species or only certain strains within a species. It is not a significant therapeutic problem, inasmuch as the resistance is usually to a particular mechanism of antimicrobial action, and there are other antibiotics with different mechanisms of action to which the organism is usually susceptible. *Acquired* resistance, on the other hand, can develop in previously susceptible pathogens for a number of reasons and is a major clinical problem with many anti-infective drugs. Development of bacterial resistance has severely limited the usefulness of many antibiotics in certain infections.

Unfortunately, the more an antimicrobial agent is employed in clinical practice, the greater the likelihood that resistant strains of once susceptible bacteria will develop. This further underscores the importance of sensitivity testing whenever there is doubt as to the susceptibility of an infecting microorganism to a chosen antibiotic. Complicating the picture is the problem of *cross-resistance,* that is, not only the resistance of a certain bacteria to all members of a particular antibiotic group (*e.g.,* penicillins, tetracyclines, sulfonamides) but resistance to other chemically related drugs (*e.g.,* penicillins and cephalosporins) or in some cases chemically unrelated drugs (*e.g.,* erythromycin and lincomycin). Microbial resistance has presented a serious dilemma in many hospitals where a variety of anti-infective agents must be used to control the many types of infections frequently encountered in this setting. As a result, secondary infections occur to a significant extent, and these are often caused, as indicated above, by strains or mutants of pathogens resistant to conventional therapy. Control of many of these hospital-acquired infections is therefore often difficult.

Microorganisms can develop resistance to antiinfective drugs in a number of ways, the most important of which are listed below:

1 Elaboration of enzymes (*e.g.,* penicillinases, cephalosporinases) that destroy the drug
2 Decreased permeability of the microbial cell membrane to certain antibiotics (*e.g.,* tetracyclines, aminoglycosides, chloramphenicol) that depend upon penetration into the bacteria for their effectiveness
3 Development of altered binding sites (*e.g.,* loss of specific ribosomal proteins) within the bacterial cell for certain antibiotic drugs (*e.g.,* aminoglycosides, erythromycins) that normally interrupt ribosomal function by chemically binding to ribosomal proteins
4 Development of altered enzymatic or metabolic pathways that either entirely bypass the reaction inhibited by the antimicrobial drug or that become less susceptible to interruption by antibiotic drugs such as sulfonamides
5 Production by bacteria of a direct antibiotic drug antagonist (*e.g.,* PABA *versus* sulfonamides)

In many cases, the emergence of resistant bacterial strains has necessitated the use of less effective and more toxic antimicrobial agents to treat an infection formerly controlled by a more desirable drug. Moreover, the increasing numbers of anti-infective drugs proving ineffective against certain infectious organisms (*e.g.,* staphylococci, gram-negative bacilli) has raised the specter of some diseases to eventually becoming largely uncontrollable by the currently available antibiotic drugs. To minimize this possibility, it is essential that antimicrobial drugs be used sensibly and that only those drugs necessary to eliminate the organisms known to be present should be prescribed.

Antibiotics in Renal Failure

Kidney function is a major determinant of the response to many antimicrobial drugs. Drugs eliminated principally by the kidney are potentially more hazardous when employed at normal doses in the patient with renal impairment, because serum levels are more elevated for longer periods of time due to the slowed elimination. Therefore, clinicians should

be aware of the mode of excretion of any anti-infective agent that they administer. Further, renal function should be determined not only before administration of an anti-infective agent that is cleared by the kidney, but throughout the course of therapy as well, particularly if the course of treatment is prolonged. Antibiotics eliminated largely by the kidneys include the penicillins, cephalosporins, aminoglycosides, polymyxins, vancomycin, trimethoprim–sulfamethoxazole, and most tetracyclines. The penicillins and cephalosporins are relatively nontoxic even at high plasma levels and therefore can be used safely in the presence of limited renal dysfunction. The tetracyclines are cleared by the kidney at varying rates, and those derivatives with extended half-lives (except doxycycline) should not be used when renal function is impaired. The aminoglycosides, polymyxins, and vancomycin will accumulate rapidly when kidney function is reduced; thus, the dosage or frequency of administration of these drugs must be reduced in the patient with renal impairment. Moreover, these latter drugs are themselves nephrotoxic, and thus can elicit or aggravate renal failure, further reducing their own excretion. It is unfortunate that patients with renal failure are often subject to precisely those infections (*e.g.,* gram-negative bacilli) that are usually most responsive to nephrotoxic drugs such as aminoglycosides, thus setting up a potentially vicious cycle. Nevertheless, there are a number of effective antimicrobial agents that may be employed with reasonable safety in patients with kidney impairment, provided that the appropriate dosage adjustments are undertaken. The excretion patterns and related cautions to be observed with the use of each class of antibiotic drugs are noted in the individual drug monographs in succeeding chapters.

Drugs of Choice for

Various Infections

The selection of an individual antimicrobial agent as a drug of choice for a particular infection is sometimes subject to debate, and opinions often change as new drugs become available or resistant strains of previously susceptible organisms emerge. Nevertheless, some agreement does exist on the first-line drugs for a number of common infections, providing sensitivity tests have confirmed pathogen susceptibility. While by no means definitive, Table 58-1 outlines recommended drugs of choice as well as alternative drugs for the treatment of infections resulting from a number of microorganisms, and also lists the type of organism and the most common illnesses associated with it. The recommendations made in Table 58-1 represent a distillate of several sources and are presented only as a guide to aid the clinician in choosing an appropriate antibiotic. They are not intended as a substitute for careful sensitivity testing, and the drug ultimately used to treat a specific infectious state should be chosen on the basis of as much laboratory and clinical data as can be obtained.

Table 58-1. Antimicrobial Drugs of Choice for Common Infections

Organism	Classification	Representative Clinical Illnesses	Drugs of First Choice	Alternate Drugs
Acinetobacter (*Mima, Herellea*) species	Gram (−) bacilli	Bacteremia, endocarditis, meningitis, urethritis	Gentamicin, tobramycin	Amikacin, kanamycin, netilmicin, doxycycline, minocycline, carbenicillin, ticarcillin, mezlocillin, piperacillin, azlocillin, ceftizoxime, chloramphenicol
Actinomyces israelli	Actinomycetes	Actinomycosis	Penicillin G	Tetracycline, erythromycin, clindamycin
Alcaligenes faecalis	Gram (−) bacilli	Urinary infections, wound infections	Chloramphenicol, tetracycline	Colistimethate, polymyxin B, gentamicin, kanamycin
Aspergillus	Fungi	Systemic fungal infections, (*e.g.,* skin, lung, bone)	Amphotericin B	Flucytosine
Bacillus anthracis	Gram (+) bacilli	Anthrax, pneumonia, meningitis	Penicillin G	Erythromycin, tetracycline, cephalosporins, chloramphenicol
Bacteroides (various strains)	Gram (−) bacilli	Bacteremia, brain and lung abscesses, genital infections, pulmonary infections, endocarditis	Penicillin G (oropharyngeal strains) or clindamycin (gastrointestinal strains)	Tetracycline, piperacillin, mezlocillin, azlocillin, chloramphenicol, cefoxitin, third generation cephalosporins, erythromycin, metronidazole
Blastomyces dermatitidis	Fungi	Blastomycosis	Amphotericin B	Hydroxystilbamidine, ketoconazole
Bordetella pertussis	Gram (−) bacilli	Whooping cough	Erythromycin	Ampicillin, tetracycline, trimethoprim–sulfamethoxazole
Borrelia recurrentis	Spirochetes	Relapsing fever	Tetracycline	Penicillin G
Brucella	Gram (−) bacilli	Brucellosis	Tetracycline with or without streptomycin	Chloramphenicol with or without streptomycin, trimethoprim–sulfamethoxazole
Calymmatobacterium granulomatis	Gram (−) bacilli	Granuloma inguinale	Tetracycline	Streptomycin, ampicillin
Candida (various species)	Fungi	Local and systemic fungal infections	Systemic—amphotericin B with or without flucytosine	Systemic—flucytosine alone
			Gastrointestinal—oral nystatin	
			Local—miconazole, clotrimazole, nystatin	
Chlamydia psittaci	Chlamydiae	Psittacosis, ornithosis	Tetracycline	Chloramphenicol
Chlamydia trachomatis	Chlamydiae	Inclusion conjunctivitis	Erythromycin	Tetracycline, sulfonamide
		Pneumonia	Erythromycin	Sulfonamide
		Trachoma	Tetracycline	Sulfonamide
		Urethritis	Tetracycline	Erythromycin
Clostridium perfringens	Gram (+) bacilli	Gas gangrene	Penicillin G	Chloramphenicol, clindamycin, tetracycline, metronidazole
Clostridium tetani	Gram (+) bacilli	Tetanus	Penicillin G	Tetracycline, cephalosporins, erythromycin
Clostridium difficile	Gram (+) bacilli	Pseudomembranous colitis (antibiotic associated)	Vancomycin	
Coccidioides immitis	Fungi	Systemic fungal infections	Amphotericin B	Miconazole, ketoconazole
Corynebacterium diphtheriae	Gram (+) bacilli	Laryngitis, pharyngitis, pneumonia, tracheitis	Erythromycin	Penicillin G

Table 58-1. Antimicrobial Drugs of Choice for Common Infections (continued)

Organism	Classification	Representative Clinical Illnesses	Drugs of First Choice	Alternate Drugs
Cryptococcus neoformans	Fungi	Systemic fungal infections	Amphotericin B, with or without flucytosine	Ketoconazole, miconazole
Dermatophytes (*tinea*)	Fungi	Infections of the skin, hair, and nails	Clotrimazole, miconazole	Oral—griseofulvin Topical—tolnaftate Topical—haloprogin
Enterobacter (*Aerobacter aerogenes*)	Gram (−) bacilli	Urinary infections, bacteremia, wound infections	Gentamicin, tobramycin, mezlocillin, piperacillin, azlocillin	Amikacin, netilmicin, carbenicillin, ticarcillin, tetracycline, cefonicid, third generation cephalosporins
Escherichia coli	Gram (−) bacilli	Urinary infections, bacteremia, meningitis, gastroenteritis	Gentamicin, tobramycin, mezlocillin, piperacillin, azlocillin	Ampicillin, carbenicillin, ticarcillin, netilmicin, amikacin, kanamycin, cephalosporin, trimethoprim–sulfamethoxazole
Francisella tularensis	Gram (−) bacilli	Tularemia	Streptomycin	Tetracycline, chloramphenicol
Hemophilus ducreyi	Gram (−) bacilli	Chancroid	Trimethoprim–sulfamethoxazole	Tetracycline, erythromycin, streptomycin, cephalothin
Hemophilus influenzae	Gram (−) bacilli	Pharyngitis, pneumonia, meningitis, otitis media, tracheobronchitis, epiglottiditis	Life-threatening—chloramphenicol plus ampicillin Other infections—ampicillin, amoxicillin	Moxalactam, trimethoprim–sulfamethoxazole Tetracycline, sulfonamide, cefonicid, cefaclor, third generation cephalosporins, trimethoprim–sulfamethoxazole
Hemophilus vaginalis	Gram (−) bacilli	Vaginal infections	Metronidazole	
Herpes simplex	Virus	Keratitis	Topical—acyclovir, trifluridine	Topical—idoxuridine, vidarabine
		Encephalitis	Vidarabine	Acyclovir (experimental)
Histoplasma capsulatum	Fungi	Pneumonia, meningitis, skin, lung, and bone lesions	Amphotericin B	Ketoconazole
Influenza A	Virus	Influenza	Amantadine (prophylaxis)	
Klebsiella pneumoniae	Gram (−) bacilli	Pneumonia, urinary and biliary infections, osteomyelitis	Gentamicin, tobramycin, mezlocillin, piperacillin, azlocillin	Cephalosporin, kanamycin, amikacin, netilmicin, tetracycline, trimethoprim–sulfamethoxazole, chloramphenicol
Legionella pneumophila	Gram (−) bacilli	Legionnaires' disease	Erythromycin with or without rifampin	Tetracycline
Leptospira	Spirochetes	Meningitis, Weil's disease	Penicillin G	Tetracycline
Leptotrichia buccalis	Gram (−) bacilli	Vincent's infection	Penicillin G	Tetracycline, erythromycin
Listeria monocytogenes	Gram (+) bacilli	Bacteremia, meningitis, endocarditis, recurrent abortion	Ampicillin or penicillin G with or without gentamicin or streptomycin	Tetracycline, chloramphenicol
Lymphogranuloma venereum (*Chlamydia trachomatis*)	Chlamydiae	Lymphogranuloma venereum	Tetracycline	Erythromycin, sulfonamide
Mucor	Fungi	Systemic fungal infections	Amphotericin B	
Mycobacterium (atypical)	Acid-fast bacilli	Lymphadenitis, pulmonary lesions	Isoniazid with rifampin with or without ethambutol	Erythromycin, cycloserine, ethionamide
Mycobacterium leprae	Acid-fast bacilli	Leprosy	Dapsone with rifampin	Ethionamide

(continued)

Table 58-1. Antimicrobial Drugs of Choice for Common Infections *(continued)*

Organism	Classification	Representative Clinical Illnesses	Drugs of First Choice	Alternate Drugs
Mycobacterium tuberculosis	Acid-fast bacilli	Pulmonary, renal, meningeal, or other tuberculosis infections	Isoniazid with rifampin	Streptomycin, pyrazinamide, ethambutol, cycloserine, ethionamide, kanamycin
Mycoplasma hominis	Mycoplasmas	Nonspecific urethritis, septicemia	Clindamycin, tetracycline	Erythromycin, chloramphenicol, gentamicin
Mycoplasma pneumoniae	Mycoplasmas	Atypical viral pneumonia	Erythromycin, tetracycline	
Neisseria gonorrhoeae	Gram (−) cocci	Gonorrhea, meningitis, urethritis, vaginitis, endocarditis, arthritis	Penicillin G, amoxicillin, tetracycline	Ampicillin, spectinomycin, cefoxitin, third generation cephalosporins
Neisseria meningitidis	Gram (−) cocci	Meningitis, bacteremia	Penicillin G	Chloramphenicol, sulfonamide, moxalactam
Nocardia	Actinomycetes	Pulmonary lesions, brain abscess	Trisulfapyrimidines with or without minocycline or ampicillin	Trimethoprim–sulfamethoxazole, cycloserine, ampicillin plus erythomycin
Pasteurella multocida	Gram (−) bacilli	Bacteremia, meningitis	Penicillin G	Tetracycline, cephalosporin
Proteus mirabilis	Gram (−) bacilli	Urinary and other infections	Ampicillin, gentamicin, tobramycin	Carbenicillin, ticarcillin, amikacin, mezlocillin, azlocillin, piperacillin, cephalosporin
Proteus (other species)	Gram (−) bacilli	Urinary and other infections	Gentamicin, tobramycin, amikacin	Carbenicillin, ticarcillin, mezlocillin, azlocillin, piperacillin, tetracycline, chloramphenicol, cefonicid, cefoxitin, third generation cephalosporins
Providencia (*Proteus inconstans*)	Gram (−) bacilli	Urinary and other infections	Amikacin	Gentamicin, tobramycin, carbenicillin, ticarcillin, mezlocillin, azlocillin, chloramphenicol, cefonicid, third generation cephalosporins
Pseudomonas aeruginosa	Gram (−) bacilli	Urinary and other infections (*e.g.,* respiratory, skin)	Antipseudomonal penicillins (*e.g.,* mezlocillin, azlocillin, piperacillin) with an aminoglycoside (such as gentamicin, amikacin, or tobramycin)	Aminoglycoside (*e.g.,* amikacin, gentamicin, tobramycin, netilmicin) with a third generation cephalosporin (*e.g.,* cefoperazone, cefotaxime, ceftizoxime, moxalactam)
Pseudomonas mallei	Gram (−) bacilli	Glanders	Streptomycin with tetracycline	Streptomycin with chloramphenicol
Pseudomonas pseudomallei	Gram (−) bacilli	Melioidosis	Trimethoprim–sulfamethoxazole	Sulfonamide, tetracycline with or without chloramphenicol, kanamycin
Rickettsia (various species)	Rickettsiae	Rocky Mountain spotted fever, typhus, Q fever, tick-bit fever	Tetracycline	Chloramphenicol
Salmonella typhosa	Gram (−) bacilli	Typhoid fever	Chloramphenicol	Ampicillin, amoxicillin, trimethoprim–sulfamethoxazole
Salmonella (other species)	Gram (−) bacilli	Paratyphoid fever, gastroenteritis, bacteremia	Ampicillin, amoxicillin	Chloramphenicol, trimethoprim–sulfamethoxazole

Table 58-1. Antimicrobial Drugs of Choice for Common Infections (continued)

Organism	Classification	Representative Clinical Illnesses	Drugs of First Choice	Alternate Drugs
Serratia	Gram (−) bacilli	Various systemic infections (usually secondary to immunosuppressive therapy)	Gentamicin, amikacin, netilmicin	Third generation cephalosporins, trimethoprim–sulfamethoxazole, carbenicillin, ticarcillin, mezlocillin, azlocillin, piperacillin
Shigella	Gram (−) bacilli	Acute gastroenteritis	Trimethoprim–sulfamethoxazole, ampicillin	Chloramphenicol, tetracycline
Spirillum minus	Gram (−) bacilli	Rat-bite fever	Penicillin G	Tetracycline, streptomycin
Sporothrix schenckii	Fungi	Sporotrichosis	Amphotericin B	Potassium iodide (for cutaneous form *only*)
Staphylococcus aureus	Gram (+) cocci	Pneumonia, meningitis, endocarditis, bacteremia, abscesses, osteomyelitis	Nonpenicillinase-producing—penicillin G or V Penicillinase-producing—penicillinase-resistant penicillin	Cephalosporin, clindamycin, vancomycin
Streptobacillus moniliformis	Gram (−) bacilli	Rat-bite fever, Haverhill fever, bacteremia	Penicillin G	Tetracycline, streptomycin
Streptococcus (anaerobic species)	Gram (+) cocci	Bacteremia, endocarditis, peritonitis, brain abscess	Penicillin G	Clindamycin, tetracycline, erythromycin, chloramphenicol, cephalosporins
Streptococcus bovis	Gram (+) cocci	Urinary infections, endocarditis, bacteremia, meningitis	Penicillin G	Cephalosporin, vancomycin
Streptococcus faecalis (enterococcus group)	Gram (+) cocci	Endocarditis, septicemia, meningitis, severe systemic infection	Ampicillin or Penicillin G with gentamicin or tobramycin	Vancomycin with gentamicin or streptomycin
		Urinary infections	Ampicillin, amoxicillin	Nitrofurantoin, tetracycline
Streptococcus (*Diplococcus*) *pneumoniae*	Gram (+) cocci	Pneumonia, meningitis, endocarditis, arthritis	Penicillin G or V	Erythromycin, cephalosporins, vancomycin chloramphenicol
Streptococcus pyogenes (groups A, C, G)	Gram (+) cocci	Various infections	Penicillin G or V	Erythromycin, cephalosporin
Streptococcus pyogenes (group B)	Gram (+) cocci	Various infections	Penicillin G, ampicillin	Chloramphenicol, erythromycin, cephalosporin, clindamycin
Streptococcus (viridans group)	Gram (+) cocci	Urinary infections, dental infections, endocarditis, meningitis	Penicillin G with or without streptomycin	Cephalosporin, vancomycin, clindamycin
Treponema pallidum	Spirochetes	Syphilis	Penicillin G	Tetracycline, erythromycin
Treponema pertenue	Spirochetes	Yaws	Penicillin G	Tetracycline
Vibrio cholerae	Gram (−) bacilli	Cholera	Tetracycline	Trimethoprim–sulfamethoxazole, chloramphenicol, erythromycin
Yersinia (*Pasturella*) *pestis*	Gram (−) bacilli	Plague	Streptomycin with or without tetracycline	Tetracycline, chloramphenicol

59 Sulfonamides

Sulfonamides were the first group of systemic antimicrobial agents to be effective when used clinically and were the mainstay of anti-infective therapy before the introduction of the penicillins in the 1940s. Sulfonamides are bacteriostatic against a broad spectrum of both gram-positive and gram-negative organisms, but their use has declined dramatically with the introduction of more potent and, in some cases, more specific antibacterial drugs. Nonetheless, they remain valuable therapeutic agents in certain infectious conditions, most notably acute urinary tract infections, because the high solubility in urine of certain derivatives allows them to reach effective concentrations without danger of kidney damage.

Significant differences exist among the various sulfonamide drugs in their rates of absorption, metabolism, and excretion, and these differences are important with regard to the indications, efficacy, and toxicity of the various compounds. Based upon such differences, the sulfonamides may be categorized into several groups; such a classification is presented in Table 59-1. Among the systemic agents, the short-acting compounds are rapidly absorbed and quickly eliminated by the kidney. Sulfamethoxazole, an intermediate-acting sulfonamide, is somewhat more slowly absorbed and excreted than the short-acting drugs, and thus may be used twice a day rather than four to five times a day, possibly improving dosing compliance.

While most systemic sulfonamide use is by oral ingestion, sulfisoxazole is available for injection. Parenteral use of sulfonamides should be undertaken only where oral administration is impractical (as in a comatose patient) and is best accomplished by slow IV injection. The solutions are highly alkaline and irritating, and the drug may precipitate out of solution.

Locally acting sulfonamides may be employed in several ways. Sulfasalazine is administered orally for the treatment of ulcerative colitis. The compound is split by the action of intestinal microflora into sulfapyridine and 5-aminosalicylate, the latter agent accumulating in significant amounts in the colon, where it may exert an anti-inflammatory action. Other indications for use of locally acting sulfonamides are eye and vaginal infections (sulfacetamide, sulfathiazole, sulfisoxazole) and prevention and treatment of sepsis in second- and third-degree burns (mafenide, silver sulfadiazine). Topical application of sulfonamides occasionally elicits allergic hypersensitivity reactions and local ocular irritation.

A major deterrent to the continuing use of sulfonamides has been the emergence of resistant strains of microorganisms that were once sensitive to the action of these drugs (*e.g.,* gonococci, beta-hemolytic streptococci, meningococci, coliform organisms). Development of sulfonamide resistance in these organisms has been greatly abetted by the previous widespread prophylactic use of the drugs in subtherapeutic doses for the attempted control of gonorrhea, upper respiratory infections, and urinary infections. Among the major causes of increased sulfonamide resistance among microorganisms are production of excessive amounts of para-aminobenzoic acid (PABA) by the bacteria (PABA is an essential component of folic acid synthesis necessary for cell growth and is competitively antagonized by sulfonamides); enhanced destruction of the sulfonamide molecule by the microorganism; or development of alternate metabolic pathways for handling essential amino acids (see Chap. 58). Acquired bacterial resistance plays a major role of therapeutic failures with sulfonamides, and the clinical usefulness of these agents, in spite of their relatively low cost, is rather limited. Cross-resistance between sulfonamides is very common as well. The principal indications for sulfonamides are listed under Uses in the discussion that follows, and their usefulness in certain infections is also documented in Chapter 58, Table 58-1.

Sulfonamides

Mafenide	Sulfamethoxazole
Sulfacetamide	Sulfapyridine
Sulfacytine	Sulfasalazine
Sulfadiazine	Sulfisoxazole
Sulfamethizole	Multiple sulfonamides

The sulfonamides, with the exception of those drugs used in the treatment of severe burns, are reviewed as a group, and then are listed in Table 59-2. Mafenide and silver sulfadiazine are then discussed individually as is trimethoprim–sulfamethoxazole, a synergistic combination of two antibacterial agents, one a sulfonamide, used in both acute and chronic urinary tract infections as well as for several other indications. Resistance has been shown to develop more slowly to this combination than to either drug alone. The sulfonamide discussion focuses principally on the sys-

temic effects of the drugs, with mention being made of specific points pertaining to their local application wherever necessary.

Mechanism

Bacteriostatic at normal doses; interfere with bacterial cell synthesis of folic acid, an essential precursor of nucleic acids, by competitively antagonizing PABA; by preventing PABA utilization, bacterial cell replication is halted

Table 59-1. Sulfonamides

I. Systemic

A. Short Acting

Sulfacytine
Sulfadiazine
Sulfamerazine
Sulfamethazine
Sulfamethizole
Sulfisoxazole

B. Intermediate Acting

Sulfamethoxazole
Sulfapyridine

II. Local

A. Intestinal

Sulfasalazine

B. Ophthalmic

Sulfacetamide
Sulfisoxazole

C. Vaginal

Sulfabenzamide
Sulfacetamide
Sulfathiazole
Sulfisoxazole

D. Topical

Mafenide
Silver sulfadiazine

Table 59-2. Sulfonamides

Drug	Preparations	Usual Dosage Range	Remarks
Sulfacetamide (Ak-Sulf, Bleph-10, Cetamide, Isopto Cetamide, Opthacet, Sebizon Lotion, Sodium Sulamyd, Sulf-10, Sulfacel-15, Sulten-10)	Ophthalmic drops—10%, 15%, 30% Ophthalmic ointment—10% Lotion—10%	Drops—1 to 2 drops every 1 hour to 4 hours as condition dictates Ointment—small amount in conjunctival sac 2 to 4 times a day Lotion—apply 2 to 4 times a day for bacterial infections or at bedtime for seborrheic dermatitis	Ophthalmic drops or ointment are indicated for treatment of conjunctivitis, corneal ulcers, superficial ocular infections and as adjunctive therapy with systemic sulfonamides for trachoma; lotion is used for seborrheic dermatitis and cutaneous bacterial infections with susceptible organisms; solutions are incompatible with silver preparations; nonsusceptible organisms may proliferate with use of sulfacetamide; drug may be inactivated by PABA produced by purulent exudates; ophthalmic ointment may impair corneal healing; 30% drops may be irritating upon application; do not use if ophthalmic solution is dark brown; discontinue drug if signs of hypersensitivity develop; apply topical lotion cautiously to abraded or denuded skin areas; available with phenylephrine as ophthalmic solution (Vasosulf) and combined with sulfathiazole and sulfabenzamide as vaginal creme and vaginal tablets (Sultrin, Triple Sulfa)

(continued)

Table 59-2. Sulfonamides (continued)

Drug	Preparations	Usual Dosage Range	Remarks
Sulfacytine (Renoquid)	Tablets—250 mg	Adults—500 mg initially, then 250 mg 4 times a day for 10 days	Short-acting sulfonamide not recommended in children under 14 years of age; only used for treatment of urinary tract infections
Sulfadiazine (Microsulfon)	Tablets—500 mg	Adults—2 g to 4 g initially, then 2 g to 4 g/day in 3 to 6 divided doses Children—75 mg/kg initially, followed by 150 mg/kg/day in 4 to 6 divided doses (maximum 6 g/day) Rheumatic fever prophylaxis—0.5 g to 1 g once daily	Short-acting sulfonamide used for prophylaxis of rheumatic fever; drug is poorly soluble in acid urine and danger of nephrotoxicity exists; high urine volume must be maintained; component of triple sulfa formulations with sulfamerazine and sulfamethazine; combination claimed to reduce chance of crystalluria
Sulfamethizole (Microsul, Proklar, Thiosulfil, Urifon)	Tablets—250 mg, 500 mg, 1000 mg	Adults—0.5 g to 1 g 3 to 4 times a day Children—30 mg to 45 mg/kg/day in 4 divided doses	Short-acting sulfonamide principally used for acute and chronic urinary infections; highly bound to plasma proteins; use with caution with other protein-bound drugs; rapidly excreted in urine, mostly in active form; drug may impart an orange–yellow color to urine or skin; available in combination with phenazopyridine (Thiosulfil-A, Microsul-A, Uremide) and tetracyclines (Urobiotic)
Sulfamethoxazole (Gantanol, Urobak)	Tablets—500 mg, 1000 mg Suspension—500 mg/5 ml	Adults—2 g initially, followed by 1 g 2 to 3 times a day Children—50 mg to 60 mg/kg initially, then 25 mg to 30 mg/kg morning and night (maximum 75 mg/kg/day)	Intermediate-acting sulfonamide similar to sulfisoxazole but with somewhat slower oral absorption and urinary excretion; used twice a day in most cases to prevent accumulation; available in combination with trimethoprim (Bactrim, Septra; see separate discussion) and phenazopyridine (Azo Gantanol), the latter drug serving as a urinary analgesic for relief of dysuria associated with urinary tract infection
Sulfapyridine	Tablets—500 mg	Adults—500 mg 4 times a day until improvement is noted, then reduce by 500 mg/day at 3-day intervals to effective maintenance level	Intermediate-acting agent used in the treatment of dermatitis herpetiformis (recurrent, inflammatory skin disease, herpetic in nature, characterized by erythema, vesicles, and pustules); slowly absorbed from GI tract (peak levels in 6 hr–8 hr); excreted both as intact drug and conjugated metabolites, largely within 3 days to 4 days; administer with sufficient fluids to prevent crystalluria
Sulfasalazine (Azulfidine, S.A.S.-500, Sulfadyne)	Tablets—500 mg Enteric-coated tablets (EN-Tabs)—500 mg Suspension—250 mg/5 ml	Adults—3 g to 4 g/day in divided doses initially (maximum 8 g/day); then reduce to maintenance levels of 1.5 g to 2 g/day in divided doses Children—40 mg to 60 mg/kg/day in 3 to 6 divided doses initially, followed by 30 mg/kg/day in 4 divided doses	Locally-acting sulfonamide used orally in the treatment of mild-to-moderate ulcerative colitis; hydrolyzed in intestinal tract to sulfapyridine (antibacterial) and 5-aminosalicylic acid (anti-inflammatory); systemic absorption of parent drug and hydrolysis products are variable (increased in the presence of severe ulceration); frequently

Table 59-2. Sulfonamides (continued)

Drug	Preparations	Usual Dosage Range	Remarks
			produces GI intolerance; if noted early in therapy, space daily dosage more evenly or use enteric-coated tablets; enteric-coated tablets have passed through GI tract without disintegrating, if this is noted, discontinue therapy; if GI distress is observed after several days of therapy, reduce dosage or stop drug for 5 days to 7 days, then resume at a lower dose; drug is often continued at reduced levels even when clinical symptoms, including diarrhea, are controlled; dosage and duration of therapy are primarily governed by endoscopic evaluation; if diarrhea recurs, increase dosage to previously effective level; infertility has been reported in men; withdrawal of drug reverses this effect; advise patient that drug may impart an orange–yellow color to skin and to alkaline urine; sulfasalazine may impair absorption of folic acid
Sulfisoxazole (Gantrisin, Koro-Sulf, Lipo Gantrisin, SK-Soxazole, Sulfizin)	Tablets—500 mg Syrup—500 mg/5 ml Pediatric suspension—500 mg/5 ml Emulsion (Lipo Gantrisin)—1 g/5 ml in homogenized vegetable oil (long acting) Ophthalmic drops—4% Ophthalmic ointment—4% Vaginal cream—10% Injection—400 mg/ml (diolamine salt)	Oral (except emulsion, see remarks): Adults—2 g to 4 g initially, then 4 g to 8 g/day in 3 to 6 divided doses Children—150 mg/kg/day in 4 to 6 divided doses (initial dose is ½ the 24-hr dose) Parenteral: 50 mg/kg initially, then 100 mg/kg/day as follows: IV—4 divided doses by slow IV injection or IV drip SC—3 divided doses IM—2 to 3 divided doses Ophthalmic: 1 to 3 drops every 1 hour to 4 hours as condition warrants or small amount of ointment 3 to 4 times a day Vaginal: ½ to 1 applicator twice a day for up to 2 weeks; repeat course if necessary	Short-acting sulfonamide used orally, parenterally, and locally (eye, vagina) for a number of bacterial infections; injections should be given only when oral administration is impractical and preferably by IV route. Peak blood levels occur within 3 hours to 4 hours following oral, IM, or SC administration and in 15 minutes to 30 minutes with IV injection; highly protein bound but rapidly excreted in the urine (95% within 24 hr); emulsion (Lipo Gantrisin) is long acting and is administered every 12 hours (adults 4 g to 5 g; children 60 mg to 75 mg/kg); see Sulfacetamide for remarks concerning ophthalmic and vaginal application; available in combination with phenazopyridine (*e.g.,* Azo Gantrisin), which provides an analgesic effect for relief of dysuria associated with urinary infections, or erythromycin (Pediazole), used for acute otitis media in children caused by *Hemophilus influenzae*
Multiple sulfonamides (Neotrizine, Terfonyl, and various other manufacturers)	Tablets—162 mg or 167 mg each of sulfadiazine, sulfamerazine, and sulfamethazine	Adults—2 g to 4 g initially, then 2 g to 4 g/day in 4 to 6 divided doses Children—75 mg/kg initially, then 150 mg/kg/day in 4 to 6 divided doses	A combination of three short-acting sulfonamides that provides the therapeutic effect of the total sulfonamide content, but reduces the risk of precipitation in the kidneys, because the solubility of each sulfonamide is independent of the others; infrequently used preparation, because other equally effective and more soluble sulfonamides are available, *e.g.,* sulfisoxazole

Uses

(Short- or intermediate-acting systemic drugs, *i.e.,* sulfadiazine, sulfisoxazole, sulfamethoxazole, multiple sulfonamides, unless otherwise indicated)

1 Acute, recurrent, or chronic urinary tract infections in the absence of obstruction
2 Chancroid
3 Trachoma
4 Nocardiosis
5 Toxoplasmosis (with pyrimethamine)
6 Acute otitis media due to *Hemophilus influenzae* (with penicillin or erythromycin)
7 Adjunctive therapy of malaria (chloroquine-resistant strains of *Plasmodium falciparum*)
8 Prophylaxis and treatment of sulfonamide sensitive group A strains of meningococcal menigitis
9 Prophylaxis of recurrent rheumatic fever (sulfadiazine only)
10 Conjunctivitis and superficial eye infections (sulfacetamide, sulfisoxazole)
11 *Hemophilus vaginalis* vaginitis (sulfabenzamide, sulfacetamide, sulfathiazole, sulfisoxazole)
12 Ulcerative colitis (sulfasalazine)
13 Dermatitis herpetiformis (sulfapyridine only)

Dosage

See Table 59-2.

Fate

Systemic sulfonamides are readily absorbed from the GI tract except for locally acting intestinal drugs (see Table 59-1); absorption from other sites (topical, vaginal) is variable; bound to plasma proteins in varying degrees and widely distributed in body fluids, including cerebrospinal fluid, eye, and in placenta and fetus; duration of action primarily depends upon rates of metabolism and excretion; half-life ranges from 4 hours to 12 hours; metabolized largely in the liver (except locally acting drugs) and eliminated by the kidney, both as intact drug and metabolites; urinary solubility of metabolites and unchanged drug is *p*H-dependent; alkaline urine favors excretion (increases solubility and ionization of molecule) and prevents crystallization in the urine.

Common Side-Effects

GI distress (nausea, abdominal discomfort)

Significant Adverse Reactions

(Incidence varies depending on drug)

GI—vomiting, diarrhea, anorexia, stomatitis, pancreatitis, jaundice, hepatitis, impaired folic acid absorption

CNS—headache, drowsiness, dizziness, insomnia, vertigo, tinnitus, ataxia, depression, convulsions, hallucinations, peripheral neuritis, hearing loss, psychosis

Renal—proteinuria, albuminuria, hematuria, oliguria, anuria, crystalluria, nephrotic syndrome

Hematologic—petechiae, hemolytic or macrocytic anemia, blood dyscrasias, hypoprothrombinemia, methemoglobinemia, purpura

Allergic-hypersensitivity—pruritus, urticaria, photosensitivity, arthralgia, periorbital edema, erythema multiforme, exfoliative dermatitis, serum sickness, anaphylactic reactions, myocarditis

Other—fever, chills, malaise, alopecia, cyanosis, goiter, diuresis, hypoglycemia, reduction in sperm count, periarteritis nodosum, lupus-like syndrome

Contraindications

Advanced kidney disease, near term of pregnancy or during the nursing period, porphyria, infants less than 2 months of age (except for treating congenital toxoplasmosis), group A beta-hemolytic streptococcal infections, hypersensitivity to sulfonylurea antidiabetics or thiazide diuretics

In addition, sulfasalazine is contraindicated in intestinal or urinary obstruction, in children under 2 years, and in patients with salicylate allergy.

Interactions

1 Due to competition for protein-binding sites, sulfonamides may potentiate or be potentiated by other protein-bound drugs, e.g., oral anticoagulants, oral antidiabetics, methotrexate, phenytoin, salicylates, anti-inflammatory agents, sulfinpyrazone, probenecid, and barbiturates.
2 Effects of sulfonamides may be impaired by local anesthetics that are derivatives of PABA, for example, benzocaine, procaine, and tetracaine.
3 Sulfonamides can displace bilirubin, possibly resulting in kernicterus (abnormal pigmentation of gray matter of CNS, leading to neuronal degeneration and, frequently, death) in premature and newborn infants.
4 Incidence of crystalluria with sulfonamides can be increased by paraldehyde, methenamine, or urinary acidifiers (*e.g.,* ammonium chloride).
5 Antacids and possibly mineral oil may decrease the effects of sulfonamides by impairing absorption.
6 Sulfonamides can enhance the toxic effects of alcohol by inhibiting oxidation of acetaldehyde.
7 Sulfasalazine can reduce the bioavailability of digoxin and can retard the absorption of folic acid.

▶ NURSING ALERTS

▷ 1 Caution patients to be aware of early signs of possible developing hematologic toxicity (sore throat, fever, mucosal ulceration, malaise, pallor, jaundice), and discontinue the drug, and consult physician should these signs occur.

▷ 2 Perform blood counts and urinalysis as well as liver and kidney function tests during extended therapy. Renal complications occur much less frequently with the more soluble sulfonamides (sulfisoxazole, sulfamethiazole).

▷ 3 Closely observe patients for appearance of severe headache, rhinitis, urticaria, conjunctivitis, stomatitis, or rash, because these may signal early development of Stevens–Johnson syndrome (*severe* erythema multiforme), which is occasionally fatal. Discontinue drug immediately.

▷ 4 Caution patients against prolonged exposure to sunlight or ultraviolet light, because photosensitization can occur.

▷ 5 Do not use sulfonamides in treating group A beta-hemolytic streptococcal infections, because they will not eradicate the organism nor prevent sequelae (*e.g.,* rheumatic fever, glomerulonephritis).

▷ 6 Use with caution in patients with kidney and liver disease, blood dyscrasias, severe allergy, bronchial asthma, or glucose 6-phosphate dehydrogenase deficiency (danger of hemolysis).

▷ 7 Monitor intake–output ratio and observe for symptoms of possible renal impairment (renal colic, oliguria, hematuria).

▷ 8 Advise patients applying sulfonamides topically to discontinue drug at first sign of local irritation or other allergic reaction.

▷ 9 Recognize that prolonged use of sulfonamides can result in hypoprothrombinemia and bleeding tendencies (due to decreased synthesis of vitamin K by intestinal microflora). Physician should be notified of any unusual bleeding.

▶ NURSING CONSIDERATIONS

(See Table 59-2 for specific information on each drug.)

▷ 1 Ensure that drugs, especially longer acting derivatives, are taken on an empty stomach with liberal amount of fluids to prevent crystalluria (urinary output should be at least 1500 ml/day).

▷ 2 Note that diabetic patients may require dosage adjustment of insulin or oral hypoglycemic drugs when taking sulfonamides. Monitor serum glucose levels. Note that sulfonamides can produce false-positive urinary glucose tests using Benedict's method.

▷ 3 Test urine for excessive acidity before administration of long-acting sulfonamides, and administer sodium bicarbonate if necessary to raise urine *p*H sufficiently to ensure drug solubility.

▷ 4 Be aware that topically applied sulfonamides may be inactivated by the presence of pus, blood, or cell breakdown products.

▷ 5 Caution patients against indiscriminate use of over-the-counter preparations during sulfonamide therapy, because some vitamin combinations and analgesic mixtures contain PABA, which can reduce sulfonamide effectiveness.

▷ 6 Be aware that *in vitro* sulfonamide sensitivity tests are not always reliable and data should be correlated with bacteriologic studies as well as with clinical response.

▷ 7 Note that increased systemic absorption of the "insoluble" sulfonamide sulfasalazine can occur following oral administration in patients with extensive ulceration of the colon.

▷ 8 Counsel patients to complete the *full course* of prescribed therapy even if symptoms have disappeared.

▷ 9 Stress the importance of good personal hygiene to the prevention of recurrent urinary tract infections.

▶ mafenide
Sulfamylon

A topical sulfonamide used to retard invasion of avascular burn sites by a variety of gram-positive and gram-negative organisms, mafenide is effective against proliferation of *Pseudomonas aeruginosa* and certain strains of anaerobes, even in the presence of pus and serum, and its activity is not altered by changes in *p*H. It facilitates spontaneous healing of deep, partial-thickness burns.

Mechanism
See general discussion of sulfonamides.

Use
1 Adjunctive therapy to prevent sepsis in second- and third-degree burns

Dosage
Applied aseptically twice a day over burned surface to a depth of 1 mm to 2 mm; should be reapplied whenever necessary to maintain continuous covering of area; continue application until healing is well along or skin is ready for grafting

Fate
Diffuses through devascularized areas and is quickly absorbed from burn surface, with peak plasma concentrations in 2 hours to 4 hours; rapidly metabolized and eliminated by the kidney

Common Side-Effects
Pain, burning, or stinging at application site

Significant Adverse Reactions
(Often difficult to distinguish between adverse drug reactions and secondary effects of burn) Bleeding of skin, allergic reactions (rash, itching, surface edema, urticaria, erythema, eosinophilia); rarely, hyperventilation, acidosis, excoriation of new skin, and superinfections

▶ NURSING ALERTS

▷ 1 Monitor acid–base balance in patients receiving mafenide, especially those with extensive burns or those who exhibit pulmonary or renal dysfunction. Drug and its metabolite inhibit carbonic anhydrase and may cause metabolic acidosis.

▷ 2 Observe for early signs of developing acidosis (*e.g.,* nausea, vomiting, abdominal pain, weakness, diarrhea, disorientation) and advise physician.

▷ 3 Use with caution in patients with acute renal failure, pulmonary infection, or impaired respiratory function, history of sulfonamide allergy (cross-sensitivity has *not* been demonstrated), and in pregnant women.

▷ 4 Be prepared to administer an appropriate analgesic should drug application result in significantly increased pain.

▶ **NURSING CONSIDERATIONS**

▷ 1 Cleanse and debride wound area before application of mafenide.

▷ 2 Although not required, if patient needs a dressing, use only a thin layer.

▷ 3 When feasible, bathe patient daily, preferably by whirlpool, to aid debridement of burn.

▷ 4 Do not discontinue mafenide therapy while the possibility of infection exists unless untoward reactions make it necessary. Therapy is usually continued until healing is advanced or site is ready for grafting.

▷ 5 Be alert for appearance of allergic reaction to drug application (rash, itching, urticaria). Temporary discontinuation of drug may be necessary.

▷ 6 Note that drug is bacteriostatic only, thus will not eradicate existing infection if present.

▶ **silver sulfadiazine**
Silvadene

A condensation product of silver nitrate with sulfadiazine, silver sulfadiazine possesses broad antimicrobial activity. Bactericidal against a number of both gram-positive and gram-negative bacteria as well as yeasts. Used topically to prevent invasion as well as to *eradicate* sensitive microorganisms from burns. Does not affect electrolyte or acid–base balance, and application is less painful than mafenide.

Mechanism

Not completely established; appears to exert its bactericidal effect on bacterial cell membranes and cell wall; sulfadiazine is released in body tissues, and may produce a bacteriostatic action by usual means, that is, antagonism of PABA.

Uses

1 Prevention and treatment of sepsis in second- and third-degree burns

Dosage

Apply aseptically one or two times a day to a thickness of 1 mm to 2 mm; re-apply as necessary to maintain continuous covering.

Fate

Hydrolyzed to a silver salt, which is poorly absorbed systemically, and sulfadiazine, which may attain significant plasma levels

Common Side-Effects

Burning at application site

Significant Adverse Reactions

Rash, itching, pain, interstitial nephritis (rare); also, because sulfadiazine may be absorbed in significant amounts, see general discussion of sulfonamides for possible systemic adverse effects.

Contraindications

Pregnancy at term, premature infants, and infants under 2 months of age

Interaction

1 Silver may inactivate topically applied proteolytic enzymes.

▶ **NURSING ALERTS**

▷ 1 Use cautiously in patients with a history of sulfonamide hypersensitivity, impaired renal or hepatic function, or glucose 6-phosphate dehydrogenase deficiency (danger of hemolysis), and during pregnancy.

▷ 2 Monitor serum and urine sulfonamide levels and perform kidney function tests during chronic treatment of burns involving large areas, because systemic sulfonamide concentration may approach the toxic level, due to continuous absorption.

▷ 3 Do not discontinue drug as long as infection remains a distinct possibility, unless a severe adverse reaction occurs.

▶ **NURSING CONSIDERATIONS**

See Mafenide. In addition,

▷ 1 Note that silver sulfadiazine, unlike mafenide, is bactericidal as well as bacteriostatic, and does not appear to significantly alter acid–base balance.

▷ 2 Do not use cream if its white color has darkened.

▶ **trimethoprim–sulfamethoxazole [co-trimoxazole]**
Bactrim, Bethaprim, Cotrim, Septra, TMP-SMZ, Sulfatrim

A synergistic combination of antimicrobial drugs that interfere with two sequential steps in an essential enzymatic reaction necessary for bacterial multiplication. Consequently, clinical efficacy is enhanced and development of resistance is significantly reduced when compared to the use of either agent alone. Its antibacterial spectrum includes common urinary pathogens (except *Pseudomonas aeruginosa*) and middle ear pathogens (*e.g., Hemophilus*) as well as several organisms associated with respiratory conditions such as acute bronchitis and pneumonitis.

Mechanism

Sulfamethoxazole inhibits synthesis of dihydrofolic acid by competitive antagonism of PABA; trimethoprim inhibits the dihydrofolate reductase enzyme, thus blocking production of tetrahydrofolic acid. Thus, two consecutive steps in the synthesis of essential proteins and nucleic acids in many bacteria are impaired.

Uses

1 Recurrent or chronic urinary tract infections due to susceptible organisms (*i.e., Escherichia coli, Klebsiella-Enterobacter, Proteus mirabilis, Proteus vulgaris, Proteus morgani*)

Initial episodes of uncomplicated acute urinary tract infections should be treated with a *single* agent (*e.g.,* a sulfonamide or cephalosporin) rather than this combination

2 Acute otitis media in children over 2 years of age due to susceptible strains of *Hemophilus influenzae* (including ampicillin- and amoxicillin-resistant strains) or *Streptococcus pneumoniae*

3 Acute exacerbations of chronic bronchitis in adults due to susceptible strains of *H. influenzae* or *S. pneumoniae*

4 Enteritis due to susceptible strains of *Shigella*

5 *Pneumocystis carinii* pneumonitis in children and adults immunosuppressed by cancer chemotherapy or other immunosuppressive therapy (drug of choice)

6 Treatment of *Nocardia asteroides* infections (usually for 6 mo to 12 mo)

7 Investigational uses include treatment of cholera, salmonella type infections, melioidosis, brucellosis, and prophylaxis of traveler's diarrhea

Dosage

(Dosage ratios given refer to the amount of trimethoprim/sulfamethoxazole in the preparation)

Urinary infections, bronchitis, shigellosis, otitis media
Adults: 160 mg/800 mg every 8 hours to 12 hours for 10 days to 14 days (5 days in shigellosis)
Children: 8 mg/kg//40 mg/kg per day in two or three divided doses for 10 days (5 days in shigellosis)

Severe urinary infections or shigellosis
8 mg to 10 mg/kg/day (trimethoprim equivalent) by IV infusion in three to four divided doses

Prevention of recurrent urinary infections in females
40 mg/200 mg daily at bedtime

Pneumocystis carinii pneumonitis
Adults: 20 mg/kg//100 mg/kg per day orally or IV infusion in equally divided doses every 6 hours for 14 days
Children: 160 mg/800 mg every 6 hours for 14 days

Fate

Rapidly absorbed when taken orally; peak serum levels occur in 1 hour with trimethoprim and 4 hours with sulfamethoxazole; half-lives for both drugs are 10 hours with oral administration and 11 hours to 13 hours with IV infusion; ratio for trimethoprim to sulfamethoxazole in the blood is 1:20; approximately 45% of trimethoprim and 70% of sulfamethoxazole are protein-bound; excreted primarily by kidneys; urine concentrations are significantly higher than serum concentrations.

Common Side-Effects

Nausea, diarrhea

Significant Adverse Reactions

GI—vomiting, abdominal pain, hepatitis, pancreatitis
CNS—Headache, tinnitus, vertigo, fatigue, insomnia, muscle weakness, ataxia, convulsions, peripheral neuritis, depression, hallucinations
Allergic—pruritus, urticaria, periorbital edema, generalized skin eruptions, photosensitivity, arthralgia, myocarditis, anaphylactic reactions, serum sickness, erythema multiforme, Stevens–Johnson syndrome, epidermal necrolysis
Hematologic—blood dyscrasias, purpura, hemolytic anemia, hypoprothrombinemia, methemoglobinemia
Other—chills, fever, oliguria, anuria, lupus-like syndrome, goiter, diuresis, hypoglycemia, periarteritis nodosa

Contraindications

Pregnancy, nursing mothers, infants less than 2 months of age, streptococcal pharyngitis

Interactions

See general sulfonamide discussion.

▶ NURSING ALERTS

See general sulfonamide discussion in this chapter and Trimethoprim (Chap. 66).

▶ NURSING CONSIDERATIONS

See general sulfonamide discussion in this chapter and Trimethoprim (Chap. 66).

Summary. Sulfonamides

Drug	Preparations	Usual Dosage Range
Systemic, Ophthalmic, and Vaginal Drugs		See Table 59-2
Mafenide (Sulfamylon)	Cream—85 mg/g	Apply twice a day to burn area to a thickness of 1 mm to 2 mm; re-apply as necessary as patient's activity dictates to ensure continuous covering
Silver sulfadiazine (Silvadene)	Cream—10 mg/g	Apply 1 to 2 times a day to burn to a thickness of 1 mm to 2 mm; re-apply as needed to maintain continuous covering

(continued)

Summary. Sulfonamides (continued)

Drug	Preparations	Usual Dosage Range
Trimethoprim–Sulfamethoxazole (Bactrim, Bethaprim, Cotrim, Septra, TMP–SMZ, Sulfatrim)	Tablets—80 mg/400 mg, 160 mg/800 mg Suspension—40 mg/200 mg per 5 ml Pediatric suspension (flavored)—40 mg/200 mg per 5 ml Infusion solution—80 mg/400 mg per 5 ml	Urinary infections, bronchitis otitis media: Adults—160 mg/800 mg every 8 to 12 hours for 10 days to 14 days Children—8 mg/kg//40 mg/kg per 24 hours in 2 or 3 divided doses for 10 days *Pneumocystis carinii* pneumonitis: Adults—20 mg/kg//100 mg/kg per day orally or IV in equally divided doses every 6 hours for 14 days Children—160 mg/800 mg every 6 hours for 14 days

The penicillin group of antibiotics includes natural extracts from several strains of the *Penicillium* mold and a number of semisynthetic derivatives. Of the many natural fermentation products first developed, penicillin G (benzylpenicillin) proved to be the most active and is still frequently used. Penicillin G, however, possesses several undesirable characteristics, such as instability in gastric acid, susceptibility to inactivation by penicillinase enzyme, rapid renal excretion, and a relatively narrow antimicrobial spectrum of action. Some of these problems have been at least partially eliminated in many of the newer semisynthetic penicillin derivatives. These semisynthetic penicillins have been prepared by incorporating specific precursors into the mold cultures (*e.g.,* penicillin V) or, more commonly, by chemically replacing a side chain on the 6-aminopenicillanic nucleus, as in ampicillin. Although these chemically modified derivatives of penicillin G each possess distinct advantages in certain aspects, it must be recognized that none of these agents represents the "ideal" penicillin in terms of activity and toxicity. In fact, penicillin G, by virtue of its good antibacterial activity, minimal toxicity, and low cost is still the preferred drug for a number of infections due to susceptible organisms, especially the more common gram-positive cocci such as streptococci, gonococci, and meningococci.

Many different penicillin derivatives are currently available, differing principally in stability in gastric acid, resistance to inactivation by penicillinase (a beta-lactamase enzyme produced by many bacteria), degree of protein binding, and spectrum of antimicrobial activity. The important characteristics of the various penicillins are outlined in Table 60-1. The usefulness of these derivatives in treating specific bacterial infections may be ascertained by reference to Chapter 58, Table 58-1, which presents a listing of the preferred antimicrobial drugs for treating a number of microorganisms.

Penicillins exert their antibacterial effects by blocking biosynthesis of cell wall mucopeptide, rendering the bacteria osmotically unstable and thus unable to survive. Penicillins, in adequate concentrations, are bactericidal, and are most effective when active bacterial cell multiplication is occurring. Moreover, the penicillins are virtually nontoxic toward human cells, inasmuch as these cells do not have rigid walls like those of bacteria but merely a limiting cytoplasmic membrane. The greater activity of most penicillins toward gram-positive organisms than toward gram-negative organisms is due to the higher proportion of mucopeptide in the cell walls of gram-positive bacteria and their higher internal osmotic pressure. Unlike some other antibiotics, such as sulfonamides, the activity of the penicillins is not inhibited by blood, pus, or other tissue breakdown products.

The major untoward reaction associated with use of the penicillins is hypersensitivity. This can range from mild skin rash and contact dermatitis to severe allergic reactions, including exfoliative dermatitis, serum sickness, and anaphylaxis. The incidence of allergic reactions to penicillin is higher in patients with previously demonstrated hypersensitivity to multiple allergens or a history of hay fever or asthma, and the drugs should be used with extreme caution in such persons. No one penicillin derivative is safer in this respect than any other. Penicillin-sensitive patients can also

Penicillins

60

Table 60-1. Penicillins—General Characteristics

Drug	Routes of Adminis- tration	Oral Absorption	Protein Binding	Acid Stable	Penicillinase Resistant	Remarks
Amoxicillin	Oral	Excellent	20%–25%	Yes	No	Similar to ampicillin but better absorbed, thus giving more rapid and higher serum levels
Ampicillin	Oral, IV, IM	Good	20%–25%	Yes	No	Broad spectrum; effective against many gram (−) organisms, but no real advantage over penicillin G for most gram (+) infections
Azlocillin	IV		20%–40%		No	Broad spectrum; good effectiveness against *Pseudomonas* and most other gram (−) bacilli
Bacampicillin	Oral	Excellent	20%–25%	Yes	No	Rapidly hydrolyzed to ampicillin during GI absorption; peak ampicillin blood levels 3 times those obtained with ampicillin itself
Carbenicillin	Oral, IV, IM	Good	50%	Yes	No	Broad spectrum with high activity against most strains of *Pseudomonas;* less active than ampicillin against gram (+) bacteria
Cloxacillin	Oral	Good	95%	Yes	Yes	Effective against penicillinase-producing staphylococci as well as most other gram (+) organisms
Cyclacillin	Oral	Excellent	20%	Yes	No	Broad spectrum but somewhat less active than ampicillin in spite of higher peak blood levels
Dicloxacillin	Oral	Good	95%–98%	Yes	Yes	Similar to but slightly more active than cloxacillin or oxacillin
Hetacillin	Oral	Good	20%–25%	Yes	No	Inactive drug hydrolyzed *in vivo* to ampicillin
Methicillin	IV, IM		40%–50%		Yes	Parenteral antibiotic active against penicillinase-producing staphylococci but less effective than penicillin G against most other gram (+) infections
Mezlocillin	IV, IM		20%–40%		No	Broad spectrum; highly active against *Enterobacter;* good activity *versus* most other gram (−) organisms
Nafcillin	Oral, IV, IM	Fair	90%	Yes	Yes	Highly resistant to penicillinase but erratically absorbed orally; good activity against gram (+) organisms
Oxacillin	Oral, IV, IM	Good	90%–95%	Yes	Yes	Similar to cloxacillin; most effective when given parenterally
Penicillin G	Oral, IV, IM	Poor	50%–60%	No	No	Highly active against gram (+) bacteria; much less active against gram (−) organisms
Penicillin V	Oral	Good	80%–90%	Yes	No	Similar to penicillin G; much more reliably absorbed but less potent
Piperacillin	IV, IM		20%–40%		No	Broad spectrum; very effective against *Pseudomonas* and *Enterobacter;* uniformly active against gram (−) bacilli
Ticarcillin	IV, IM		45%–50%		No	Broad spectrum, including *Pseudomonas, Serratia, Citrobacter;* only effective parenterally

exhibit *cross*-sensitivity to certain other antibacterial agents, notably cephalosporins, and caution must be exercised in using cephalosporins in penicillin-sensitive patients and *vice versa.*

Bacterial resistance to the penicillins is variable. In spite of extensive clinical use of penicillin for over 25 years, some species of bacteria have remained uniformly susceptible (*e.g., Diplococcus pneumoniae, Neisseria meningitidis*) whereas other species have developed progressively increasing resistance. This variability in development of resistance may be explained in part by the fact that there are several mechanisms responsible for resistance to penicillins. Most commonly, resistance occurs because some bacteria (such as staphylococci) can synthesize beta-lactamase en-

zymes, most notably penicillinase, which convert the drugs to inactive products. Such bacteria would display resistance to penicillins susceptible to enzyme activity, but not to penicillinase-resistant derivatives. On the other hand, certain bacteria may develop resistance to all penicillins, possibly because their cell surfaces have become impermeable to the drugs or because they have developed alternate metabolic pathways that avoid steps sensitive to the action of the drugs.

Discussion of the penicillins focuses on these agents as a group, inasmuch as the basic pharmacology and toxicology of all derivatives are identical. Drugs are listed in Table 60-2, where appropriate dosages and individual characteristics are given. A brief summary of the major types of penicillins follows the table, beginning on p. 564.

Table 60-2. Penicillins

Drug	Preparations	Usual Dosage Range	Remarks
Amoxicillin (Amoxil, Larotid, Polymox, Sumox, Trimox, Utimox, Wymox)	Capsules—250 mg, 500 mg Chewable tablets—125 mg, 250 mg Powder for oral suspension—125 mg/5 ml, 250 mg/5 ml Drops—50 mg/ml	Adults and children over 20 kg—250 mg to 500 mg every 8 hours Children under 20 kg—20 mg to 40 mg/kg/day in divided doses every 8 hours Uncomplicated gonorrhea (adults): 3 g with 1 g oral probenecid as a single dose Disseminated gonococcal infection: As above, followed by 500 mg oral amoxicillin 4 times/day for 7 to 10 days Pelvic inflammatory disease: As above, followed by 100 mg oral doxycycline twice daily for 14 days	Broad spectrum acid-stable penicillin rapidly and completely absorbed from the GI tract; absorption is not significantly affected by food; activity similar to ampicillin but less effective against *Shigella;* widely used in acute otitis media due to *Hemophilus,* although resistant strains are emerging; less likely to disturb GI flora than ampicillin; often used as initial therapy before culture and sensitivity tests because of broad spectrum of action; no more effective than penicillin G or V against susceptible gram (+) organisms; see ampicillin below
Ampicillin (Amcill, Omnipen, Polycillin, Principen, SK-Ampicillin, Totacillin, and various other manufacturers	Capsules—250 mg, 500 mg Capsules with probenecid—389 mg/111 mg Powder for oral suspension—125 mg/5 ml, 250 mg/5 ml, 500 mg/5 ml Drops—100 mg/ml Oral suspension with probenecid—3.5 g/1 g Powder for injection—125-mg, 250-mg, 500-mg, 1-g, 2-g, 10-g vials	Respiratory and soft tissue infections: Adults Oral—250 mg every 6 hours IM, IV—250 mg to 500 mg every 6 hours Children under 40 kg Oral—50 mg/kg/day in divided doses IM, IV—25 mg to 50 mg/kg/day in divided doses GI and urinary infections: Adults Oral, IM, IV—500 mg every 6 hours Children under 40 kg Oral—100 mg/kg/day in divided doses IM, IV—50 mg/kg/day in divided doses Bacterial meningitis and septicemia: Adults and children—150 mg to 200 mg/kg/day in divided doses every 3 hours to 4 hours; begin with IV administration, then continue with IM Gonorrheal urethritis: 3.5 g with 1 g probenecid orally or 500 mg IM every 8 hours to 12 hours Gonorrhea: 3.5 g with 1 g probenecid orally as single dose Disseminated gonococcal infection: As above, followed by 500 mg oral ampicillin 4 times/day for 7 days Pelvic inflammatory disease: As above, followed by 100 mg oral doxycycline twice a day for 14 days	Broad-spectrum penicillin widely used in respiratory, GI, urinary, and soft tissue infections including otitis media, septicemia, and bacterial meningitis; skin rash can occur, especially in patients with mononucleosis or hyperuricemia; parenteral form should be used only for severe infections or in patients unable to take oral medications; treatment should be continued 48 hours to 72 hours after symptoms have disappeared; administer on an empty stomach to enhance GI absorption; during extended therapy (*e.g.,* chronic urinary infections), frequent bacteriologic tests should be performed and sufficient doses must be given; clinical and bacteriologic follow up should be maintained for several months after cessation of therapy; use only freshly prepared solutions for parenteral administration, dilute according to package directions with suitable diluent, and use within 1 hour after preparation

(continued)

Table 60-2. Penicillins (continued)

Drug	Preparations	Usual Dosage Range	Remarks
Azlocillin (Azlin)	Powder for injection—2-g, 3-g, 4-g vials	Urinary infections: IV only—100 mg to 200 mg/kg/day (2 g–3 g every 6 hr) Serious systemic infections: 200 mg to 300 mg/kg/day in 4 to 6 divided doses (3 g every 4 hr) Life-threatening infections: Up to 350 mg/kg/day (4 g every 4 hr)	Extended spectrum antipseudomonal penicillin used either by slow IV injection (over 5 min–10 min) or by IV infusion (30 min); very effective *in vitro* against *Pseudomonas, Proteus, Salmonella,* and *Acinetobacter; rapid* IV administration has elicited transient chest discomfort; Contains 2.17 mEq/g of sodium, less than one half the amount in carbenicillin or ticarcillin; dosage should be reduced in patients with significant renal impairment; synergistic with aminoglycosides against pseudomonal infections but must be administered in a separate syringe; solutions are stable at room temperature for 24 hours
Bacampicillin (Spectrobid)	Tablets—400 mg Powder for oral suspension—125 mg/5 ml	Upper respiratory, urinary and skin infections: Adults—400 mg to 800 mg every 12 hours Children—25 mg to 50 mg/kg/day in 2 equally divided doses Lower respiratory infections: 800 mg every 12 hours Gonorrhea: 1.6 g with 1 g probenecid as a single dose	Rapidly hydrolyzed to ampicillin during GI absorption; each tablet equivalent to 280 mg ampicillin; more completely absorbed than ampicillin, yielding effective serum levels for up to 12 hours; much more costly than ampicillin; see Ampicillin for additional remarks; do not administer with disulfiram
Carbenicillin disodium (Geopen, Pyopen)	Powder for injection—1-g, 2-g, 5-g, 10-g, 20-g, 30-g vials	Urinary infections: Adults—200 mg/kg/day IV drip or 1 g to 2 g IM or IV every 6 hours Children—50 mg to 200 mg/kg/day IM or IV in divided doses Soft tissue or respiratory infections, septicemia: Adults—15 g to 40 g daily IV in divided doses or by continuous drip Children—250 mg to 500 mg/kg/day IM or IV in divided doses (maximum dose 40 g/day) Gonorrhea: 1 g probenecid orally followed in 1 hour by 4 g carbenicillin IM Presence of renal insufficiency: (creatinine clearance less than 5 ml/min)—2 g IV every 8 hours	Extended-spectrum penicillin especially effective against many gram (–) organisms, such as *Pseudomonas, Proteus, Acinetobacter, Escherichia, Salmonella,* and *Enterobacter;* attains very high levels in urine when given IM or IV; synergistic with aminoglycosides against *Pseudomonas;* may elicit increased bleeding tendencies associated with abnormal coagulation tests; be alert for signs of hemorrhage (bruising, petechiae); fairly high in sodium content; monitor serum electrolytes during extended administration; use very cautiously in patients with impaired renal function; IV therapy is recommended for serious urinary or systemic infections; IM injections should not exceed 2 g/dose; reconstitute solutions according to package directions and discard unused solutions after 24 hours at room temperature (72 hr in refrigerator); do not mix carbenicillin and gentamicin together in the same IV fluid; administer separately
Carbenicillin indanyl sodium (Geocillin)	Tablets—382 mg	382 mg to 764 mg 4 times a day	Indanyl ester of carbenicillin, suitable for oral use; primarily indicated for acute and chronic upper and

Table 60-2. Penicillins (continued)

Drug	Preparations	Usual Dosage Range	Remarks
			lower urinary tract infections and prostatitis, due to *Escherichia coli, Proteus, Pseudomonas, Enterobacter,* and Enterococcus; readily absorbed orally and hydrolyzed to carbenicillin, which is rapidly excreted in the urine, attaining high levels
Cloxacillin (Cloxapen, Tegopen)	Capsules—250 mg, 500 mg Powder for oral solution—125 mg/5 ml	Adults—250 mg to 500 mg every 6 hours Children—50 mg to 100 mg/kg/day in divided doses every 6 hours	Penicillinase-resistant penicillin primarily used to treat infections caused by penicillinase-producing staphylococci; may also be used to initiate therapy in patients in whom a staphylococcal infection is suspected; somewhat less effective than penicillin G against most other gram (+) cocci; best absorbed from an empty stomach; highly protein-bound
Cyclacillin (Cyclapen-W)	Tablets—250 mg, 500 mg Powder for oral suspension—125 mg/5 ml, 250 mg/5 ml	Adults—250 mg to 500 mg 4 times a day in equally spaced doses Children—125 mg to 250 mg 3 to 4 times a day in equally spaced doses	Broad spectrum agent, rapidly and completely absorbed when taken orally; peak serum levels within 30 minutes; rapidly excreted in the urine; dosage frequency must be reduced in renal impairment; indicated for treatment of bronchitis, pneumonia, upper respiratory infections, urinary infections, and otitis media due to susceptible organisms; not used in children under 2 months; somewhat lower incidence of skin rash and diarrhea than with ampicillin or amoxicillin; should not be used for infections caused by *Escherichia coli* or *Proteus mirabilis* other than urinary tract
Dicloxacillin (Dycill, Dynapen, Pathocil, Veracillin)	Capsules—125 mg, 250 mg, 500 mg Powder for oral suspension—62.5 mg/5 ml	Adults—125 mg to 250 mg every 6 hours Children under 40 kg—12.5 mg to 25 mg/kg/day in divided doses every 6 hours	Penicillinase-resistant penicillin similar to cloxacillin and oxacillin, but producing slightly higher plasma levels than equivalent doses of other related penicillins; do not use in neonates; see Cloxacillin
Hetacillin (Versapen)	Capsules—equivalent to 225 mg of ampicillin Powder for oral suspension—equivalent to 112.5 mg of ampicillin/5 ml	Adults—225 mg to 450 mg 4 times a day Children under 40 kg—22.5 mg to 45 mg/kg/day in divided doses	Broad-spectrum penicillin that is rapidly converted to ampicillin in the body; no significant advantage over ampicillin itself and more costly; see Ampicillin for additional remarks
Methicillin (Staphcillin)	Powder for injection—1-g, 4-g, 6-g, 10-g vials	Adults: IM—1 g every 4 hours to 6 hours IV—1 g every 6 hours in 50 ml Sodium Chloride Injection at a rate of 10 ml/min Children: IM—25 mg/kg every 6 hours	Penicillinase-resistant penicillin with same uses as cloxacillin but used by injection only; considerably less active than penicillin G against streptococci and pneumococci; well tolerated by deep IM injection, slow IV injection, or continuous IV infusion; observe injection sites for signs of irritation, inflammation, or hypersensitivity; be alert for development of drug-induced febrile reactions with IV administration; drug has produced interstitial nephritis within 2 weeks

(continued)

Table 60-2. Penicillins (continued)

Drug	Preparations	Usual Dosage Range	Remarks
			to 4 weeks of start of therapy; observe for early indications (*e.g.,* cloudy urine, oliguria, spiking fever) and discontinue drug; methicillin is incompatible in solution with a wide range of drugs; do not mix with other drugs, including antibiotics but administer separately; carefully follow instructions on container when diluting powder for injection; higher concentrations (10 mg–30 mg/ml) are stable for 8 hours at room temperature, but weaker dilutions (2 mg/ml) are only stable for 4 hours
Mezlocillin (Mezlin)	Powder for injection—1-g, 2-g, 3-g, 4-g vials or infusion bottles	Adults: IV—1.5 g to 4 g every 4 hours to 6 hours depending on the severity of infection (life-threatening infections—4 g every 4 hr) IM—1.5 g to 2 g every 6 hours Acute gonococcal urethritis: 1 g to 2 g, as a single IV or IM injection, together with 1 g probenecid orally Children: IV, IM—75 mg/kg every 6 hours to 12 hours	Extended-spectrum penicillin similar in activity to piperacillin, but somewhat less effective against *Pseudomonas;* may be used with an aminoglycoside or cephalosporin in severe infections in cases in which the causative agent is unknown; do not inject more than 2 g IM, and give slowly (15 sec) well into the body of a large muscle mass; inject IV over a period of 3 minutes to 5 minutes (concentration of drug in solution should not exceed 10% to minimize venous irritation); IV infusion should be given over 30 minutes; follow package directions for mixing and diluting, for dosage reductions in patients with impaired renal function (based on creatinine clearance), and for compatibility and stability data; low sodium content (1.85 mEq/g)
Nafcillin (Nafcil, Nallpen, Unipen)	Capsules—250 mg Tablets—500 mg Powder for oral solution—250 mg/5 ml Powder for injection—500-mg, 1-g, 2-g, 4-g, 10-g vials	Adults: Oral—250 mg to 1000 mg every 4 hours to 6 hours depending on severity of infection IM—500 mg every 4 hours to 6 hours IV—500 mg to 1000 mg every 4 hours Children: Oral—50 mg/kg/day in 4 divided doses Scarlet Fever/pneumonia: 25 mg/kg/day in 4 divided doses IM—25 mg/kg twice a day Neonates: IM—10 mg/kg twice a day	Penicillinase-resistant penicillin with same indications as cloxacillin; oral absorption is inferior to that of other similar penicillins; major route of elimination is by way of the bile; parenteral therapy is indicated initially in severe infections; change to oral therapy should be made as condition warrants; not as active as penicillin G against nonpenicillinase-producing organisms; for IV use, dilute powder in 15 ml to 30 ml Sterile Water for Injection or Sodium Chloride Injection and inject over 5 minutes to 10 minutes; avoid extravasation because tissue necrosis can occur; reconstitute solution for IM injection with Sterile or Bacteriostatic Water for Injection; administer immediately by deep intragluteal injection; solution may be kept refrigerated for up to 48 hours
Oxacillin (Bactocill, Prostaphlin)	Capsules—250 mg, 500 mg Powder for oral solution—250 mg/5 ml	Adults: Oral—500 mg to 1000 mg every 4 hours to 6 hours for	Penicillinase-resistant drug, similar in most respects to cloxacillin and dicloxacillin, but slightly less

Table 60-2. Penicillins (continued)

Drug	Preparations	Usual Dosage Range	Remarks
	Powder for injection—250-mg, 500-mg, 1-g, 2-g, 4-g, 10-g vials	a minimum of 7 days depending on severity of infection IM, IV—250 mg to 1000 mg every 4 hours to 6 hours depending on severity of infection Children under 40 kg: Oral—50 mg to 100 mg/kg/day in divided doses IM, IV—50 mg to 100 mg/kg/day in divided doses	potent orally; in serious infections, parenteral therapy is indicated, because oral absorption may be unreliable; following initial control of infection, oral therapy may then be substituted; drug should be taken on an empty stomach; solutions for IM or IV use should be prepared by diluting powder with Sterile Water for Injection or Sodium Chloride Injection; discard unused IM injection after 3 days at room temperature or 7 days with refrigeration; consult package for suitable diluents for IV infusion solutions; at concentrations of 0.5 mg to 40 mg/ml, dilutions are stable for approximately 6 hours to 8 hours at room temperature; adjust rate of infusion to deliver intended drug dose within this time; transient elevations in serum enzymes (SGOT, SGPT, LDH) may occur with oxacillin
Penicillin G, potassium or sodium (Pentids, Pfizerpen G, and various other manufacturers)	Tablets—200,000 U, 250,000 U, 400,000 U, 500,000 U, 800,000 U Powder for oral solution—200,000 U/5 ml, 250,000 U/5 ml, 400,000 U/5 ml Powder for injection—200,000 U/vial, 500,000 U/vial; 1-, 5-, 10-, 20-million U/vial (400,000 units = 250 mg)	Adults: Oral—200,000 U to 500,000 U every 6 hours to 8 hours for at least 10 days IM, IV—300,000 U to 8 million U daily (some severe infections, *e.g.,* meningococcal meningitis, gram-negative bacteremia, clostridial infections may require up to 20 to 30 million U/day) Children under 12: Oral—25,000 U to 90,000 U/kg/day in 3 to 6 divided doses IM, IV—300,000 U to 1.2 million U/day in divided doses (up to 10 million U/day may be required)	Natural penicillin preparation derived from the *Penicillium* mold; considered drug of choice for treating infections due to susceptible organisms (see Chap. 58); rapid-acting, inexpensive, and very effective against many organisms, but destroyed by gastric acid and penicillinase; administer orally on an empty stomach; refrigerate reconstituted oral solution and discard within 14 days; do not use oral penicillin G as prophylaxis for genitourinary instrumentation or surgery, lower intestinal surgery, sigmoidoscopy, or childbirth; IM is the preferred parenteral route; keep injection volume small and inject deeply into a large muscle mass; maximal plasma concentrations are attained within 30 minutes to 60 minutes; doses exceeding 10 million U/day must be given by IV infusion only; administer large doses slowly, because electrolyte overload may occur depending on which salt is used; use extreme caution in renal insufficiency; half-life (normally 30 min) increases to 10 hours in patients with anuria; perform periodic serum electrolyte determinations during high-dose therapy and be alert for symptoms of hyperkalemia (hyperreflexia, convulsions, arrhythmias) when using potassium salts
Penicillin G, benzathine (Bicillin, Permapen)	Tablets—200,000 U Injection—300,000 U/ml, 600,000 U/ml	Adults: Oral—400,000 U to 600,000 U every 4 hours to 6 hours	Benzathine salt of penicillin G providing a slowly absorbed and hence long-acting dosage form;

(continued)

Table 60-2. Penicillins (*continued*)

Drug	Preparations	Usual Dosage Range	Remarks
		IM—1,200,000 U as a single injection Children under 12: Oral—25,000 U to 90,000 U/kg/day in 3 to 6 divided doses IM—600,000 U to 1,200,000 U depending on weight Syphilis (early): 2.4 million units IM as a single dose Syphilis (of more than 1 year's duration: 2.4 million U IM/week for 3 successive weeks Prophylaxis of rheumatic fever: 200,000 U orally twice a day, 1.2 million U once a month, or 600,000 U every 2 weeks	oral preparations are less effective than IM forms due to unpredictable GI absorption; use a large-gauge needle for administration, inject deeply into a large muscle, and do not massage injection site; not for IV or SC use; when high sustained serum levels of penicillin are desired, use aqueous penicillin G, because benzathine salt provides fairly low serum concentrations; in small children, divide dose between two injection sites if necessary
Penicillin G, procaine (Crysticillin A.S., Duracillin A.S., Pfizerpen-AS, Wycillin)	Injection—300,000 U/ml, 500,000 U/ml Injection—300,000 U; 600,000 U; 1.2-, 2.4-million U per unit dose	600,000 U to 1.2 million U every 1 day to 3 days Gonorrheal infections: 1 g probenecid followed in 30 minutes by 4.8 million U divided into two doses and injected at different sites	Long-acting form of penicillin G, similar to benzathine penicillin G in most respects; indicated in moderately severe infections due to organisms sensitive to persistent, low serum levels of penicillin G; only given IM; contains procaine, which provides for slow release and absorption of penicillin; may be allergenic; procaine may impart a local anesthetic effect, making injections less painful than benzathine preparation; single-dose therapy for gonorrhea has elicited anxiety, confusion, depression, hallucinations, seizures, and extreme weakness
Penicillin G, benzathine and procaine (Bicillin C-R)	Injection—150,000 U–150,000 U; 300,000 U–300,000 U, and 900,000 U–300,000 U per ml each, respectively, benzathine and procaine penicillin G	Streptococcal infections: Adults—2.4 million U IM Children 30 to 60 lb—900,000 to 1.2 million U IM Children under 30 lb—600,000 U IM Pneumococcal infections: 600,000 U in children or 1.2 million U in adults every 2 to 3 days until patient is afebrile for 48 hours	Combination of long-acting forms of penicillin G, used to treat infections due to organisms susceptible to the lower serum levels common to this drug; only administered IM; not effective against streptococcal group D; do not use in venereal diseases; see benzathine penicillin G and procaine penicillin G
Penicillin V; penicillin V, potassium (Pen-Vee K, V-Cillin K, and various other manufacturers)	Tablets—125 mg, 250 mg, 500 mg Powder for oral suspension—125 mg/5 ml, 250 mg/5 ml Powder for oral solution (potassium salt)—125 mg/5 ml, 250 mg/5 ml	Adults—125 mg to 500 mg every 6 hours to 8 hours depending on severity of infection Children—15 mg to 50 mg/kg/day in 3 to 6 divided doses	Phenoxymethyl derivative of penicillin G, with identical range of activity but more resistant to inactivation by gastric acid, hence better absorbed, yielding 2 to 5 times higher blood levels; potassium salt is preferred due to better overall GI absorption; only used orally for mild infections of the throat, respiratory tract or soft tissues, and not indicated as initial therapy when parenteral penicillins are necessary (*e.g.*, in severe infections); highly bound to plasma proteins; rapidly excreted

Table 60-2. Penicillins *(continued)*

Drug	Preparations	Usual Dosage Range	Remarks
			in the urine; effective when given with food, but blood levels are higher if administered on an empty stomach
Piperacillin (Pipracil)	Powder for injection—2-g, 3-g, 4-g vials or infusion bottles	Adults: IV—6 g to 18 g a day in divided doses, depending on severity of infection IM—6 g to 8 g a day in 2 to 4 divided doses Uncomplicated gonorrheal infection: 2 g IM in a single dose	Extended-spectrum penicillin, used IM or IV for treatment of a variety of gram (+) and gram (−) infections; similar to mezlocillin in spectrum of activity and efficacy; synergistic with aminoglycosides against *Pseudomonas aeruginosa*, but do not mix in the same bottle; sodium content (1.88 mEq/g) is lower than that of carbenicillin or ticarcillin; reduce dose in patients with renal impairment according to creatinine clearance values; not recommended for use in children under 12; maximum adult daily dosage is 24 g; do not inject more than 2 g at any one IM injection site; refer to package insert for mixing, diluting, and storage instructions; solutions are stable for 24 hours at room temperature, and up to 1 week refrigerated
Ticarcillin (Ticar)	Powder for injection—1-g, 3-g, 6-g, 20-g vials	Adults: IV infusion—150 mg to 300 mg/kg/day in divided doses every 3 hours to 6 hours IV, IM injection—1 g every 6 hours Children: IV infusion—150 mg to 300 mg/kg/day in divided doses every 4 hours to 6 hours IV, IM injection—50 mg to 100 mg/kg/day in divided doses every 6 hours to 8 hours Neonates: Initially 100 mg/kg, followed by 75 mg/kg in 4 hours to 8 hours	Extended spectrum penicillin, not absorbed when taken orally; similar in activity to carbenicillin, but more active against most strains of *Pseudomonas*; synergistic with gentamicin and tobramycin against *Pseudomonas* organisms; high in sodium content, therefore monitor serum electrolytes during prolonged therapy and use with caution in sodium-restricted patients; IM injections should not exceed 2 g/dose; children weighing more than 40 kg should receive the adult dose; administer IM deeply into large muscle mass; discard IM solutions after 24 hours at room temperature or 72 hours if refrigerated; inject slowly IV to avoid vein irritation; reduce dosage according to package instructions in patients with renal insufficiency based on creatinine clearance; do not mix ticarcillin and gentamicin or tobramycin in same solution, because latter drugs may be inactivated

Natural Products

1 Penicillin G

First penicillin in extensive clinical use; still considered a first-line drug against most gram-positive bacteria (except penicillinase-producing staphylococci) when given by IM injection. Virtually nontoxic to human cells, thus can be given safely in large amounts. Widely distributed in the body, especially following IM injections and rapidly bactericidal. Very low cost. Major disadvantages are irregular oral absorption, destruction by gastric acid, inactivation by penicillinase enzyme, and rather narrow antimicrobial spectrum of action. Effects may be prolonged by parenteral (IM) use of benzathine or procaine salts of penicillin G, repository forms of the drug producing lower serum blood levels but longer duration of action.

Semisynthetic Derivatives

1 Penicillin V

Semisynthetic analog of penicillin G with similar spectrum of activity. More completely absorbed orally than penicillin G and not destroyed by gastric acid, thus yielding three to five times higher blood levels. Preferred over penicillin G for oral therapy of mild infections of the throat, upper respiratory tract, or soft tissues caused by non-penicillinase-producing staphylococci and other gram-positive cocci, but ineffective for gonorrhea. Only used orally, therefore not indicated during *acute* stages of serious infections with susceptible organisms, because these usually require parenteral penicillin G. Potassium salt is the preferred form, because it is better absorbed than plain penicillin V.

2 Penicillinase-Resistant Penicillins

(Cloxacillin, Dicloxacillin, Methicillin,

Nafcillin, Oxacillin)

Resistant to inactivation by penicillinase, and used in the treatment of infections due to penicillinase-producing *Staphylococcus aureus.* Cloxacillin or dicloxacillin is indicated for oral use, because they are acid stable and well absorbed, although their GI absorption is reduced by food. Parenteral methicillin, nafcillin, or oxacillin should be employed in serious infections. Less effective than penicillin G against *non*-penicillinase-producing staphylococci and other gram-positive organisms. Inactive against gram-negative organisms.

3 Broad-Spectrum Penicillins

(Amoxicillin, Ampicillin, Bacampicillin,

Cyclacillin, Hetacillin)

Effective against a range of both gram-positive and gram-negative organisms. No real advantage over the less costly penicillin G or V in treating most gram-positive infections, but significantly more active against many gram-negative organisms, especially *Hemophilus influenzae, Escherichia coli, Proteus mirabilis, Salmonella,* and *Shigella.* Thus, frequently employed as initial drugs where the identity of the microorganism has not been determined, for example, urinary infections, respiratory infections such as sinusitis or bronchitis, and otitis media. Drugs are not resistant to penicillinase enzyme.

4 Extended-Spectrum Penicillins

(Antipseudomonal Penicillins)

(Azlocillin, Carbenicillin, Mezlocillin,

Piperacillin, Ticarcillin)

Wide antimicrobial spectrum, including *Pseudomonas* and many other gram-negative bacilli resistant to the broad spectrum penicillins. In addition to the organisms listed under Broad-Spectrum Penicillins, above, carbenicillin and ticarcillin are *also* effective against *Pseudomonas,* several *Proteus* species, *Acinetobacter, Enterobacter,* and *Serratia.* Azlocillin, mezlocillin, and piperacillin have the broadest *in vitro* spectrum of all penicillins, including *Klebsiella* and *Citrobacter,* and contain less than one half the sodium content of carbenicillin and ticarcillin. Their activity is nearly comparable to that of the aminoglycosides, but they are considerably less toxic. Extended-spectrum penicillins are not penicillinase-resistant.

Penicillins

Amoxicillin	Methicillin
Ampicillin	Mezlocillin
Azlocillin	Nafcillin
Bacampicillin	Oxacillin
Carbenicillin	Penicillin G
Cloxacillin	Penicillin V
Cyclacillin	Piperacillin
Dicloxacillin	Ticarcillin
Hetacillin	

Mechanism
Interfere with the synthesis of bacterial cell wall mucopeptide, thus rendering the cells osmotically unstable; the high internal osmotic pressure then causes the bacterial cells to swell and burst; in adequate concentrations, penicillins are bactericidal and most effective during active cellular multiplication; lower concentrations may produce only bacteriostatic activity

Uses
(See Chap. 58, Table 58-1, for specific indications for different penicillins in various infections; see also Table 60-2.)
1 Treatment of infections due to organisms sensitive to normal serum levels of the drugs

Dosage

See Table 60-2.

Fate

Oral absorption ranges from excellent (amoxicillin, cyclacillin) to fair-to-poor (nafcillin, penicillin G); most other orally effective derivatives are reasonably well absorbed. Following IM injection, most drugs yield rapid and high serum levels, except for the procaine and benzathine salts of penicillin G, which provide lower blood levels but more prolonged effects. Drugs diffuse readily into most body tissues, and tissue levels equal serum levels at most sites except the CNS and the eye where significant penetration occurs only when the meninges are inflamed. All derivatives are protein-bound to varying degrees (20% with cyclacillin to 98% with dicloxacillin). Penicillin V and oxacillin are the only derivatives metabolized to any extent; others are rapidly excreted largely unchanged in the urine. Elimination half-life is less than 1 hour for most drugs, slightly longer for ampicillin and amoxicillin. Also secreted into the bile, which is only a minor route of elimination for all drugs except nafcillin and oxacillin, which are excreted in significant amounts in the bile.

Common Side-Effects

Allergic reactions (*e.g.,* skin rash, urticaria, itching), especially in patients with a past history of allergies

Significant Adverse Reactions

(Most adverse reactions are rare and are usually only seen with large doses. Hypersensitivity reactions, however, can occur with small doses of any penicillin derivative.)

Hypersensitivity—severe reactions (wheezing, laryngeal edema, macropapular rash, serum sickness, exfoliative dermatitis, erythema multiforme, arthralgia, prostration, anaphylaxis)

GI—nausea, vomiting, epigastric distress, glossitis, stomatitis, dry mouth, abnormal taste, "hairy" tongue, diarrhea, flatulence, enterocolitis (due to secondary microbial overgrowth), abdominal pain, GI bleeding

Electrolyte—hypokalemia (extended-spectrum penicillins), hypernatremia (especially carbenicillin, ticarcillin)

Renal–hepatic—interstitial nephritis (most frequently with methicillin), glomerulonephritis, cholestatic hepatitis

CNS—neurotoxicity (irritability, lethargy, hallucinations, seizures), anxiety, confusion, agitation, depression

Hematologic—blood dyscrasias, bone marrow depression, hemolytic anemia, hemorrhagic manifestations associated with abnormalities of coagulation tests

Other—pain and irritation at injection site, phlebitis, oral and rectal candidiasis, overgrowth of nonsusceptible organisms, vaginitis, neuropathy, sciatic neuritis

Contraindications

History of previous hypersensitivity to any penicillin or cephalosporin

Interactions

1 Concurrent use of *bacteriostatic* antibiotics (*e.g.,* tetracyclines, erythromycin) may diminish the effectiveness of penicillins by slowing the rate of bacterial growth, because penicillins are most effective during rapid multiplication.
2 Probenecid prolongs blood levels of penicillins by blocking their elimination by renal tubular secretion.
3 Highly protein-bound penicillins, for example, cloxacillin, dicloxacillin, nafcillin, and oxacillin, can be potentiated by other highly protein-bound drugs (*e.g.,* salicylates, oral anticoagulants, anti-inflammatory agents).
4 Antacids and other alkalinizing agents can inhibit the action of oral penicillins by impairing absorption.
5 Oral neomycin can reduce the oral absorption of penicillin V.
6 Increased incidence of skin rash can occur with combined use of ampicillin and allopurinol.
7 The effectiveness of oral contraceptives may be reduced by ampicillin or penicillin V.
8 Penicillins mixed in solution with an aminoglycoside may inactivate the aminoglycoside.

▶ NURSING ALERTS

▷ 1 Obtain a careful medical history before using any penicillin and do not administer to anyone with a previous history of hypersensitivity to any penicillin or cephalosporin without skin testing for hypersensitivity. The incidence of cross-sensitivity between penicillins and cephalosporins is approximately 10%.

▷ 2 Use with caution in patients with asthma, hay fever, history of any allergy, or renal impairment, and in neonates (reduced elimination). Always skin test for allergenicity if doubt exists.

▷ 3 Observe patients for development of allergic reactions, which may be immediate or delayed several days or weeks, and discontinue drug.

▷ 4 In severe infections, administer drug parenterally because oral administration cannot always be relied upon to provide sufficiently high serum levels.

▷ 5 Be aware that large doses of nafcillin or the extended-spectrum penicillins may induce coagulation test abnormalities associated with bleeding tendencies. Upon drug withdrawal, bleeding should cease and test results should revert to normal.

▷ 6 Do not use an *oral* penicillin to treat severe pneumonia, empyema, bacteremia, pericarditis, meningitis, or purulent or septic arthritis during the acute stage.

▷ 7 During prolonged therapy, periodically monitor renal, hepatic, and hematopoietic function, especially in small children or if large doses are used.

▷ 8 Be alert for overgrowth of bacteria and yeasts in the GI tract (*e.g.,* loose, foul-smelling stools, cramping), and advise physician if these symptoms occur.

▷ 9 During injection, watch for appearance of a wheal or flaring, indications of hypersensitivity. Discontinue administration.

▷ 10 Ensure that drugs are taken in adequate dosage for a

sufficient period of time (minimum 7 days–10 days) to eliminate completely the infecting organism and to prevent emergence of resistant strains. Stress the importance of taking *all* of the prescribed dosage, even if symptoms disappear. In treating group A beta-hemolytic streptococcal infections, administer drugs for *at least* 10 days to prevent development of acute glomerulonephritis or rheumatic fever.

▷ 11 If desired clinical response does not occur within 24 hours to 48 hours with oral administration, consider adding or substituting a parenteral penicillin.

▷ 12 In suspected staphylococcal infections, because there are a number of resistant strains, perform appropriate culture and sensitivity tests to ensure use of proper antibiotic.

▷ 13 Be aware that serious anaphylactic reactions are not controllable with antihistamines and may require epinephrine, aminophylline, oxygen, corticosteroids, and mechanical respiratory assistance.

▷ 14 Aspirate syringe prior to injecting a penicillin IM, because intravascular administration has resulted in severe neurovascular damage, including gangrene and paralysis. Injection into or near a nerve has resulted in permanent neurologic damage.

▶ **NURSING CONSIDERATIONS**

(See Table 60-2 for specific information on each drug.)

▷ 1 Administer oral preparation 1 hour to 2 hours before meals or 2 hours to 3 hours after meals to improve GI absorption (penicillin V, bacampicillin, and amoxicillin are apparently not significantly affected by presence of food, and may be given with meals to reduce GI distress).

▷ 2 Stress the importance of maintaining a rigid dosing schedule (around the clock if necessary) to maintain sufficient plasma levels.

▷ 3 Do not use *oral* penicillin preparations in patients who are vomiting, or who have intestinal hypermotility, gastric dilatation, or cardiac spasm.

▷ 4 Suggest that patients allergic to penicillin always carry this information either in their wallet or on a tag or bracelet.

▷ 5 Note that penicillinase-resistant penicillins are commonly used as *initial* therapy for any suspected staphylococcal infection until culture and sensitivity results are known. Recognize, however, that strains of staphylococci resistant to penicillinase-resistant penicillins have been reported, and are capable of producing serious disease and death. Accurate early sensitivity studies are essential.

▷ 6 Always check expiration date on container before administering a penicillin.

▷ 7 Inject drugs deeply IM into body of a large muscle (*e.g.,* gluteus) and aspirate before delivery. Do *not* massage site after injection. Rotate injection sites with prolonged drug administration.

▷ 8 Note that high-dose IV therapy with the sodium or potassium salts of various penicillins can result in electrolyte overload. Serum electrolyte monitoring is necessary during prolonged infusion or repeated administration with these salts.

▷ 9 Recognize that IV administration of penicillins can be irritating. Dilute drug according to manufacturer's directions, and closely observe patient for signs of thrombophlebitis.

▷ 10 Advise patients to keep reconstituted oral suspensions in a cool place (*e.g.,* refrigerator), and to discard contents after period of time indicated on the bottle (usually 10 days–14 days).

▷ 11 Be aware that results of the following laboratory tests can be altered by the indicated penicillins: urine glucose using Clinitest (false positive with ampicillin); serum uric acid (decreased with azlocillin); serum proteins (false positive with azlocillin or mezlocillin); plasma estrogens (decreased with ampicillin); Coombs' tests (positive with IV carbenicillin or piperacillin).

The cephalosporins are a rapidly proliferating group of semisynthetic, broad-spectrum antibiotics mostly derived from cephalosporin C, a natural product of the fungus *Cephalosporium acremonium.* In addition to the various cephalosporin C derivatives, cefoxitin (a semisynthetic derivative of cephamycin C) and moxalactam (a beta-lactam) are also viewed as cephalosporins due to their structural and pharmacologic similarities to the other derivatives.

Cephalosporins are divided into first-, second- and third-generation drugs. As outlined in Table 61-1, differences among the three groups are primarily noted in their antibacterial spectrum of action. Activity against gram-negative bacilli *increases* from first- to third-generation drugs, as does efficacy against resistant organisms as well as drug cost. Conversely, efficacy against gram-positive organisms is greatest with the first-generation drugs and progressively *decreases* through the second- and third-generation compounds. The organisms susceptible to each of the three groups of cephalosporins are also indicated in Table 61-1. Within each group of drugs, the individual agents differ primarily in their pharmacokinetic properties, such as oral *versus* parenteral efficacy, half-lives, protein binding, and principal routes of excretion. Some of these differences are also presented in Table 61-1.

Cephalosporin antibiotics are usually bactericidal against most gram-positive cocci (except enterococci, which are unaffected by all drugs except possibly cefoperazone) and many gram-negative bacilli. In general, the older, first-generation drugs are the most effective against staphylococci and streptococci, whereas the newer, second- and third-generation drugs display increased activity against the gram-negative enterobacteria. However, although widely prescribed, cephalosporins are seldom drugs of choice for any specific infection, due to the availability of more specific, more effective, or less costly alternatives.

Cephalosporins are indicated for surgical prophylaxis when extended gram-negative activity is desired, and for treatment of gram-positive infections (except enterococci) in patients allergic to penicillin. However, cross-allergenicity exists between the penicillins and the cephalosporins (estimated incidence is 5%–15%), so caution is indicated when cephalosporins are given to patients with a history of penicillin allergy.

Second- and third-generation drugs should *not* be used for gram-positive infections, because they are less effective than first-generation agents and significantly more expensive as well. More specific, more active, and less costly alternatives (*e.g.,* penicillins, erythromycins) are readily available.

Because many gram-negative bacilli are susceptible to the second- and third-generation cephalosporins (see Table 61-1), these drugs are frequently used in respiratory, genitourinary, skin, and soft-tissue infections due to a variety of gram-negative microorganisms. In addition, the third-generation drugs display varying degrees of activity against *Pseudomonas, Serratia,* and possibly *Salmonella* and *Acinetobacter* and are often employed as alternatives to the more toxic (however more effective) aminoglycosides. Cefoxitin, as well as the four third-generation drugs are also active against *Bacteroides fragilis,* but this activity is not as great or as predictable as with other non-cephalosporin drugs. Moreover, many gram-negative bacilli develop resis-

Cephalosporins

61

Table 61-1. Characteristics of Cephalosporins

Drug	Routes of Administration	Protein Binding	Plasma Half-life (min)	Urinary Excretion (%)	Sodium Content (mEq/g)	Susceptible Microorganisms*
First Generation						
Cefadroxil	Oral	20	70–80	90–95		Staphylococci
Cephalexin	Oral	10–15	30–50	80–100		Streptococci (including beta-hemolytic)
Cephradine	Oral/IM/IV	10–15	45–60	80–90	6	*Escherichia coli*
Cephapirin	IM/IV	40–50	20–40	50–75	2.4	*Hemophilus influenzae*
Cephalothin	IM/IV	65–75	30–60	50–75	2.8	*Klebsiella*
Cefazolin	IM/IV	75–85	90–120	75–100	2	*Neisseria gonorrhoeae*
						Neisseria meningitidis
						Proteus mirabilis
						Salmonella
						Shigella
						Clostridium
						Peptococcus
						Peptostreptococcus
Second Generation						**All the above, plus:**
Cefaclor†	Oral	25	40–50	60–80		*Proteus morganii*
Cefamandole	IM, IV	65–75	30–60	60–80	3.3	*Proteus vulgaris*
Cefonicid	IM, IV	90–95	240–300	99	3.7	
Cefoxitin	IM, IV	65–75	30–60	90–100	2.3	*Providencia*
Cefuroxime	IM, IV	40–50	60–120	70–95	2.4	*Enterobacter*
Ceforanide	IM, IV	80	150–180	80–95	0	*Citrobacter* (cefuroxime *only*)
						Bacteroides fragilis (cefoxitin only)
						Fusobacterium
Third Generation						**All the above, plus:**
Cefotaxime	IM, IV	30–50	60–70	50–60	2.2	*Pseudomonas aeruginosa*
Ceftizoxime	IM, IV	30	100–120	75–80	2.6	*Serratia*
Cefoperazone	IM, IV	80–90	100–150	20–25	1.5	*Acinetobacter* (ceftizoxime and
Moxalactam	IM, IV	45–55	120–210	70–90	3.8	cefoperazone *only*)
						Eubacterium
						Clostridium difficile (cefoperazone *only*)

* Susceptibility may vary with individual members of the group, and in some cases has only been demonstrated *in vitro*.
† Cefaclor is *only* active against microorganisms listed under first-generation drugs.

tance to the cephalosporins, greatly restricting their usefulness in many infections.

Most first- and second-generation drugs are susceptible to inactivation by beta-lactamase (*i.e.,* cephalosporinase) enzymes. Newer agents, such as cefoxitin (second generation) and the third-generation cephalosporins, display greater resistance to enzymatic inactivation, including the cephalosporinases produced by many gram-negative pathogens, such as *Pseudomonas, Hemophilus, Acinetobacter, Neisseria,* and some strains of *Bacteroides.*

Compared to many other antibacterial drugs, cephalosporins are relatively nontoxic. The most commonly occurring adverse reactions are allergic in nature, and include rash, urticaria, fever, angioedema, and occasionally serum sickness, eosinophilia, and anaphylaxis (for additional untoward reactions, refer to the general discussion of cephalosporins which follows).

A major factor in the selection of cephalosporins is their cost, which has been mentioned before in this discussion. Parenterally administered cephalosporins are among the most expensive antibiotics in use today, and their cost increases substantially with broadened spectrum. Thus, second-generation drugs are approximately twice as expensive as first-generation drugs, while third-generation drugs can exceed the cost of first-generation drugs by a factor of four or

five. It becomes cost imperative, then, to use the least expensive cephalosporin that is effective against the microorganisms shown to be present. Empiric therapy with third-generation cephalosporins is a frightfully expensive undertaking, and considerable justification should be established for this procedure, such as the presence of severe ototoxicity or nephrotoxicity that would contradict the use of aminoglycosides.

The cephalosporins are considered here as a group. Individual drugs are then listed in Table 61-2, together with specific information pertaining to each drug. In addition, reference should be made to Table 58-1, Chapter 58, for the recommended indications for the cephalosporins.

Cephalosporins

Cefaclor	Cefoxitin
Cefadroxil	Ceftizoxime
Cefamandole	Cefuroxime
Cefazolin	Cephalexin
Cefonicid	Cephalothin
Cefoperazone	Cephapirin
Ceforanide	Cephradine
Cefotaxime	Moxalactam

Table 61-2. Cephalosporins

Drug	Preparations	Usual Dosage Range	Remarks
Cefaclor (Ceclor)	Capsules—250 mg, 500 mg Oral suspension—125 mg/5 ml, 250 mg/5 ml	Adults—250 mg to 500 mg every 8 hours (maximum 4 g/day) Children—20 mg to 40 mg/kg/day in divided doses every 8 hours (maximum 1 g/day)	Orally effective, short-acting cephalosporin used in respiratory, urinary, skin, and soft-tissue infections and otitis media; classified as second-generation, but spectrum of activity is essentially identical to first-generation drugs; a single 2-g dose has been used in acute, uncomplicated urinary tract infections
Cefadroxil (Duricef, Ultracef)	Capsules—500 mg Tablets—1 g Oral suspension—125 mg/5 ml, 250 mg/5 ml, 500 mg/5 ml	Adults—1 g to 2 g/day in a single or divided doses Children—30 mg/kg/day in divided doses every 12 hours	Orally effective drug used principally to treat urinary tract infections due to *Escherichia coli, Proteus mirabilis,* or *Klebsiella;* also used in staphylococcal and streptococcal infections of skin, pharynx, and tonsils; not metabolized to any extent and excreted essentially intact in the urine; oral absorption is not significantly affected by food; adjust dosage according to package instructions in patients with renal impairment
Cefamandole (Mandol)	Injection—500 mg, 1 g, 2 g, 10 g	Adults—500 mg to 1000 mg IM or IV every 4 hours to 8 hours (up to 2 g/4 hr in severe infections) Children—50 mg to 100 mg/kg/day in divided doses every 4 hours to 8 hours Perioperative prophylaxis: Adults—1 g to 2 g one hour prior to incision, then 1 g to 2 g every 6 hours for 24 hours to 48 hours Children—50 mg to 100 mg/kg/day in equally divided doses according to above schedule	Second-generation parenteral cephalosporin indicated for infections of the respiratory or urinary tracts and skin, for surgical prophylaxis, and for septicemia and peritonitis caused by susceptible organisms; effective against anaerobic organisms (*Clostridium, Peptococcus*), indole-positive *Proteus* and some strains of *Bacteroides fragilis;* also used in combination with an aminoglycoside for gram-positive or gram-negative sepsis (danger of nephrotoxicity, see Drug Interactions); reduce dose as indicated in package insert in patients with renal impairment; do not mix with aminoglycoside in same container; dilute drug solution as instructed with appropriate diluent; reconstituted cefamandole is stable for 24 hours at room temperature and 96 hours under refrigeration; IV dosage can be up to 12 g/day depending on severity of infection (*e.g.,* bacterial septicemia)
Cefazolin (Ancef, Kefzol)	Injection—250 mg/10 ml, 500 mg/10 ml, 1 g/10 ml; 5 g/100 ml, 10 g/100 ml	Adults—250 mg to 1.5 g IV or IM every 6 hours to 12 hours depending on severity of infection (maximum 12 g/day) Children—25 mg to 100 mg/kg/day divided into 3 or 4 doses depending on severity of infection Perioperative prophylaxis: 1 g one hour before surgery, 0.5 g to 1 g during surgery of 2 hours or longer, then 0.5 g to 1 g every 6 hours to 8 hours for up to 5 days	Parenteral cephalosporin similar to cephalothin but claimed to be less irritating and less nephrotoxic; used in treatment of respiratory, urinary, and biliary tract infections, skin and soft-tissue infections, septicemia, bone and joint infections, and endocarditis; also indicated as alternative therapy for gonorrhea in pregnant patients allergic to penicillin and perioperatively to reduce risk of infection following certain surgical procedures; highly protein bound; do not use in children under 1 month; follow manufacturer's recommendations for dosing in renal impairment; pain on injection is infrequent; diluted solutions are stable for 24 hours at room temperature and 96 hours under refrigeration

(continued)

Table 61-2. Cephalosporins (continued)

Drug	Preparations	Usual Dosage Range	Remarks
Cefonicid (Monocid)	Injection—500 mg, 1 g, 10 g (bulk–vial)	Adults—0.5 g to 1 g IM or slow IV injection once every 24 hours (maximum dose is 2 g once daily) Perioperative prophylaxis: Adults—1 g given 1 hour prior to incision	Long-acting second-generation cephalosporin given once daily for respiratory, urinary, skin, bone, and joint infections, and septicemia; not active against *Pseudomonas, Serratia, Enterococcus, Acinetobacter,* and most strains of *B. fragilis;* may cause pain on injection; doses larger than 1 g should be divided and given at two different IM sites; reduce dosage in patients with impaired renal function according to package directions; dilutions are stable for 24 hours at room temperature and 72 hours if refrigerated
Cefoperazone (Cefobid)	Powder for injection—1-g, 2-g vials	Adults—2 g to 4 g/day IM or IV in equally divided doses every 12 hours; up to 16 g/day has been given by constant infusion in severe infections	Third-generation cephalosporin with an extensive spectrum of action; used in respiratory, intra-abdominal, and urogenital infections, bacterial septicemia, and infections of the skin and associated structures; highly protein-bound; extensively excreted in the bile, do not exceed 4 g/day in patients with hepatic disease or biliary obstruction; no dosage adjustment is required in the presence of renal failure; long half-life requires only twice a day dosing, although more frequent administration can be used in severe infections; highly resistant to beta-lactamase enzymes produced by most gram (−) pathogens; pseudomembranous colitis has occurred, be alert for development of diarrhea; symptoms of hepatitis have been reported
Cefotaxime (Claforan)	Injection—500 mg, 1 g, 2 g	Adults—1 g every 6 hours to 8 hours IV or IM (maximum dose 12 g/day) Children—50 mg to 180 mg/kg/day in 4 to 6 divided doses Perioperative prophylaxis: 1 g IV or IM 30 minutes to 90 minutes before surgery, then 1 g 60 minutes to 120 minutes later, then 1 g within 2 hours following surgery Gonorrhea: 1 g IM as a single injection Disseminated gonorrhea: 500 mg IV 4 times/day for at least 7 days	Third-generation, parenteral cephalosporin used in the treatment of serious infections of the abdomen, lower respiratory tract, urinary tract, skin, and genital tract; also indicated as a surgical prophylactic agent and for penicillinase-producing *Neisseria gonorrhoeae* infections resistant to spectinomycin; Many strains of *Pseudomonas* and enterococci are resistant; most common adverse reactions are pain, tenderness, and inflammation at injection site; reduce dose according to package instructions in patients with renal impairment; does not appear to be nephrotoxic; may be used concurrently with an aminoglycoside, but do not mix in same syringe
Cefoxitin (Mefoxin)	Injection—1 g, 2 g	Adults—1 g to 2 g every 6 hours to 8 hours IV or IM (maximum is 12 g/day) Gonorrhea (see remarks): 2 g IM with 1 g probenecid Disseminated gonorrhea: 1 g IV 4 times/day for at least 7 days Acute pelvic inflammatory disease: 2 g IV 4 times/day with 100 mg doxycycline IV twice a day	Second-generation cephalosporin effective against a variety of organisms susceptible to first-generation cephalosporins as well as anaerobic organisms, indole-positive *Proteus, Bacteroides fragilis,* and some gram-negative bacteria resistant to other cephalosporins and broad-spectrum penicillins; may reduce incidence of postoperative infections in patients undergoing surgical procedures that are classified as potentially contaminated (*e.g.,* GI

Table 61-2. Cephalosporins (continued)

Drug	Preparations	Usual Dosage Range	Remarks
		for at least 4 days; continue 100 mg doxycycline, orally, twice a day for an additional 10 to 14 days Perioperative prophylaxis: 2 g IV or IM ½ hour to 1 hour before surgery and every 6 hours thereafter for up to 24 hours Children—160 mg/kg/day in 4 to 6 divided doses maximum 1 g/day	surgery, vaginal hysterectomy); also indicated for penicillinase-producing *Neisseria gonorrheae* resistant to spectinomycin and for acute pelvic inflammatory disease; highly resistant to beta-lactamase; reconstituted solutions maintain potency for 24 hours at room temperature, 1 week under refrigeration, and up to 26 weeks frozen; dry material may darken with time but potency is not affected; frequently painful upon IM injection; follow package directions for dosing patients with renal impairment
Ceftizoxime (Cefizox)	Powder for injection—1-g, 2-g vials	Adults—1 g to 2 g IM or IV every 8 hours to 12 hours (maximum dose is 12 g/day) Uncomplicated gonorrhea: 1 g IM as a single dose	Third-generation drug used in a variety of infections due to both gram (+) and gram (−) organisms; long half-life allows twice daily dosing in less severe infections, but serious infections require administration every 8 hours; stable *against* beta-lactamase enzymes and only slightly (30%) protein-bound; newer derivative that may be active against some microorganisms that have developed resistance to other cephalosporins; dosage must be reduced in patients with impaired renal function; may be injected directly IV (3 min–5 min) or given by intermittent or continuous infusion; reconstitute powder in Sterile Water for Injection; stable for 8 hours at room temperature and 48 hours if refrigerated
Cefuroxime (Zinacef)	Powder for injection—750 mg, 1.5-g vials	Adults—2.25 g to 6 g/day IM or IV in divided doses every 6 hours to 8 hours (maximum dose is 9 g/day in bacterial meningitis) Uncomplicated gonorrhea: 1.5 g IM as a single dose with 1 g oral probenecid Perioperative prophylaxis: 1.5 g IV just prior to surgery, then 750 mg IV or IM every 8 hours for 24 hours Children (over 3 mo)—50 mg to 100 mg/kg/day in divided doses every 6 hours to 8 hours Bacterial meningitis: 200 mg to 240 mg/kg/day IV in divided doses every 6 hours to 8 hours, reduce to 100 mg/kg/day IV upon improvement	Second-generation cephalosporin which, unlike other first- and second-generation drugs, attains significant concentrations in the cerebrospinal fluid, especially if the meninges are inflamed; effective against many gram (−) bacilli, including *Enterobacter* and *Citrobacter* (some strains, however, are resistant); administer single 1.5-g IM dose for gonorrhea at two different sites; dosage is reduced, according to package instructions, in patients with renal dysfunction; inject slowly (3 min–5 min) IV or infuse either intermittently or continuously; do not mix with aminoglycosides; powder and solutions may darken with time, but potency of solution is unaffected for 24 hours at room temperature and 48 hours refrigerated
Cephalexin (Keflex)	Capsules—250 mg, 500 mg Tablets—1 g Oral suspension—125 mg/5 ml, 250 mg/5 ml Pediatric drops—100 mg/ml	Adults—250 mg to 500 mg every 6 hours (maximum dose is 4 g/day) Children—25 mg to 100 mg/kg/day in 4 divided doses depending on severity of infection	Orally effective first-generation cephalosporin indicated for respiratory, urinary, skin, bone, and soft-tissue infections, and otitis media in penicillin-sensitive patients; some staphylococci are resistant; stable in gastric acid, well absorbed, and only slightly protein-bound; if doses

(continued)

Table 61-2. Cephalosporins (continued)

Drug	Preparations	Usual Dosage Range	Remarks
			greater than 4 g/day are necessary, parenteral cephalosporins should be used; refrigerate oral suspension and discard unused portion in 14 days
Cephalothin (Keflin, Seffin)	Powder for injection—1 g, 2 g, 4 g, 20 g/vial Injection—1 g/50 ml, 2 g/50 ml, 10 g/10 ml	Adults—500 mg to 1000 mg IM or IV injection every 4 hours to 6 hours (up to 2 g every 4 hours IV in life-threatening infections) Children—80 mg to 160 mg/kg/day IM in divided doses Perioperative prophylaxis: Adults—1 g to 2 g IM or IV ½ hour to 1 hour before surgery, during surgery as needed, and every 6 hours following surgery for 24 hours Children—20 mg/kg to 30 mg/kg following the above schedule	Prototype first-generation parenteral cephalosporin used to treat respiratory, GI, urinary, skin, bone, joint, and soft-tissue infections as well as septicemia and meningitis; not effective against *Pseudomonas, Serratia,* indole-positive *Proteus* or *Enterococcus;* may be employed perioperatively to reduce incidence of certain infections in high-risk situations (*e.g.,* vaginal hysterectomy, intestinal or colorectal surgery, open heart surgery, cholecystectomy, prosthetic arthroplasty); IM injection often elicits pain, induration, and sloughing; IV administration may lead to phlebitis or other inflammatory reactions; may be added to peritoneal dialysis fluid in concentrations up to 6 mg/100 ml and instilled throughout the dialysis procedure; due to short half-life (30 min–45 min), initial perioperative dose should be given just before start of surgery and re-administered at appropriate intervals throughout procedure to maintain sufficient blood levels; prophylactic use should be discontinued within 24 hours following surgery; maintenance dose must be reduced in patients with impaired renal function based upon creatinine clearance; solutions are stable for 12 hours to 24 hours at room temperature and 96 hours under refrigeration; slight darkening does not affect potency
Cephapirin (Cefadyl)	Powder for injection—500 mg, 1 g, 2 g, 4 g, 20 g	Adults—500 mg to 1000 mg IM or IV every 4 hours to 6 hours (up to 12 g/day IV in serious infections) Children—40 mg to 80 mg/kg/day IM in divided doses Perioperative prophylaxis: 1 g to 2 g IM or IV ½ hour to 1 hour before surgery, during surgery if needed, and every 6 hours after surgery for 24 hours	Parenteral cephalosporin similar to cephalothin in action but causing less tissue irritation; clinical evidence of renal damage has not been reported; do not use in children under 3 months of age; dilutions are stable for 24 hours at room temperature and up to 10 days with refrigeration; check package instructions for compatibility with various infusion solutions
Cephradine (Anspor, Velosef)	Capsules—250 mg, 500 mg Tablets—1 g Oral suspension—125 mg/5 ml, 250 mg/5 ml Powder for injection—250 mg, 500 mg; 1 g, 2 g, 4 g	Oral: Adults—250 mg to 500 mg every 6 hours or 1 g every 12 hours Children (over 9 mo)—25 mg to 100 mg/kg/day in divided doses every 6 hours to 12 hours (maximum 4 g/day) IV, IM: Adults—500 mg to 1000 mg 4 times a day (maximum 8 g/day) Children (over 12 mo)—50 mg to 100 mg/kg/day in 4 divided doses	Only cephalosporin available in both oral and parenteral dosage forms; oral preparations are primarily used as follow-up therapy to parenteral treatment; may be given without regard to meals, because drug is acid-stable; excreted largely unchanged in urine, mostly within 6 hours, thus is effective in urinary infections due to susceptible organisms; very slightly protein-bound; following reconstitution, IM, or direct IV solutions should be used within 2 hours at room temperature; continuous IV solutions retain potency for 10 hours at room

Table 61-2. Cephalosporins (continued)

Drug	Preparations	Usual Dosage Range	Remarks
		Perioperative prophylaxis: 1 g IV or IM 30 min to 40 min before surgery, then 1 g every 4 hours to 6 hours thereafter up to 24 hours Cesarean section: 1 g IV when cord is clamped, then again at 6 hours and 12 hours	temperature, infusion solution should be replaced at that time; do not combine cephradine solutions with those of other antibiotics; doses smaller than those indicated should not be used; persistent infections may require several weeks therapy
Moxalactam (Moxam)	Powder for injection—1 g, 2 g	Adults—250 mg to 2 g IV or IM every 8 hours to 12 hours for most mild to moderate infections; serious or life-threatening infections—up to 4 g every 8 hours Children—50 mg/kg every 6 hours to 8 hours Infants—50 mg/kg every 6 hours Neonates—50 mg/kg every 8 hours to 12 hours	Long-acting, third-generation cephalosporin, highly resistant to inactivation of beta-lactamases; indicated in lower respiratory, urinary, intra-abdominal, CNS (penetrates blood–brain barrier), skin, bone, and joint infections due to susceptible organisms; effective against many strains of *Pseudomonas* but high doses are necessary and other therapy (*e.g.,* aminoglycosides) should be instituted if a clinical response does not occur promptly; may be given concomitantly with an aminoglycoside; probenecid does *not* alter the elimination of moxalactam; hypoprothrombinemia and increased bleeding tendency has been reported; monitor bleeding time (especially if dose exceeds 4 g/day) and observe for signs of bleeding; discontinue drug or provide supplemental vitamin K (10 mg/week); IV administration of moxalactam is preferred for more serious infections, *i.e.,* slow injection (3 min–5 min) or infusion; reconstituted solution is stable for 90 hours if stored under refrigeration

Mechanism

Inhibit mucopeptide synthesis in the bacterial cell wall, resulting in a defective, osmotically unstable wall; may be bactericidal or bacteriostatic depending on dose, tissue concentrations of drug, organism susceptibility, and rate of bacterial replication; most effective against rapidly growing organisms

Uses

1 Alternates to penicillins for treatment of infections of the respiratory tract, skin and soft tissues, genitourinary tract, middle ear, and bloodstream caused by susceptible organisms (see Chap. 58, Table 58-1, and Table 61-1 for susceptible microorganisms)
2 Surgical prophylaxis when expanded gram-negative activity is desired
3 Adjunctive treatment (with an aminoglycoside) of bacteremia of unknown origin in debilitated or immunosuppressed patients
4 Adjunctive therapy in septicemia, acute endocarditis, meningitis, and bone and joint infections

Dosage

See Table 61-2.

Fate

Oral drugs are well absorbed from GI tract, but absorption may be delayed by food. Absorption from IM sites is good. Peak blood levels are attained rapidly (usually 30 min–60 min). Half-lives are given in Table 61-1. Cephalosporins are distributed extensively, but only cefuroxime and the third-generation drugs diffuse into the cerebrospinal fluid, especially when the meninges are inflamed. Penetration into bone is variable (highest levels seen with cephradine, cefamandole, cefuroxime, ceftizoxime, and cefoperazone). Drugs readily cross placental barrier, and are secreted into milk of nursing mothers. Most derivatives (except cefotaxime, cephalothin, and cephapirin) are not appreciably metabolized and are excreted largely unchanged in the urine. Cefoperazone, however, is eliminated predominantly in the bile.

Common Side-Effects

Nausea and diarrhea with oral administration, hypersensitivity reactions in persons with a history of allergy

Significant Adverse Reactions

(Most reactions occur more commonly with large doses or during prolonged therapy.)

GI—anorexia, abdominal pain, dyspepsia, heartburn, vomiting, severe diarrhea, oral candidiasis, glossitis, GI bleeding, enterocolitis

Allergic—urticaria, pruritus, skin rash, fever, chills, serum sickness, eosinophilia, angioedema, exfoliative dermatitis, anaphylactic reactions

Hematologic—neutropenia, leukopenia, thrombocytopenia, agranulocytosis, hemolytic anemia, bleeding due to hypoprothrombinemia, positive direct Coombs' test

Genitourinary—dysuria, elevated BUN, proteinuria, hematuria, vaginal discharge, candidal vaginitis, genitoanal pruritus, genital candidiasis

Hepatic—elevated SGOT, SGPT, bilirubin, alkaline phosphatase and LDH levels; hepatitis (rare)

Other—headache, weakness, dizziness, dyspnea, paresthesia, candidal overgrowth, hepatomegaly; IM administration may cause pain, induration, tenderness, fever, and tissue sloughing

Interactions

1 Use of bacteriostatic antibiotics (*e.g.,* tetracyclines, erythromycins) may reduce cephalosporin effectiveness, especially in acute infections where the organisms are proliferating rapidly.

2 The nephrotoxic effects of cephalosporins may be augmented by aminoglycosides, colistin, vancomycin, polymyxin B, ethacrynic acid, furosemide, probenecid, and sulfinpyrazone.

3 Cephalosporins are incompatible in parenteral mixtures with tetracyclines, erythromycins, calcium chloride, and magnesium salts.

4 Probenecid may increase and prolong cephalosporin plasma levels (except moxalactam) by inhibiting renal tubular secretion of the drugs.

5 Alcohol may elicit a disulfiram-like reaction (see Chap. 80) with cefamandole, cefoperazone, or moxalactam.

▶ NURSING ALERTS

▷ 1 Obtain a detailed patient history before initiating cephalosporin therapy, especially relating to previous allergic reactions to penicillins or other related drugs.

▷ 2 Use with caution in patients with a history of allergies, asthma, hay fever, penicillin sensitivity (see introductory comments), or impaired renal function, and in small children, during pregnancy, and in nursing mothers.

▷ 3 Be aware that cephalosporins (especially moxalactam, cefamandole, and cefoperazone) can interfere with hemostasis by decreasing availability of vitamin K and interfering with normal platelet function. Use smallest effective doses to minimize effect on platelet function, and administer supplemental vitamin K (10 mg/week) if necessary, based on prothrombin times.

▷ 4 During prolonged therapy, perform periodic (*i.e.,* 3 mo–6 mo) hematologic, renal, and hepatic function tests.

▷ 5 Be alert for development of hypersensitivity reactions (*e.g.,* pruritus, fever, rash), and advise physician.

▷ 6 In beta-hemolytic streptococcal infections, continue therapy for at least 10 days to prevent development of rheumatic fever or glomerulonephritis.

▷ 7 Advise patients who develop severe or prolonged diarrhea with cephalosporin use to consult a physician. Pseudomembranous colitis can occur due to alteration in the normal intestinal flora, allowing proliferation of *Clostridium difficile,* which elaborates a toxin.

▷ 8 Observe for signs of diminished renal function (*e.g.,* decreased urine output, proteinuria, elevated BUN or serum creatinine) because nephrotoxicity has occurred with cephalosporin usage.

▶ NURSING CONSIDERATIONS

(See Table 61-2 for specific information on each drug.)

▷ 1 Continue treatment of all infections at least 48 hours after symptoms disappear or evidence of bacterial presence is lacking. Treatment course should extend at least 7 days.

▷ 2 During prolonged or repeated therapy, observe for development of superinfection by nonsusceptible organisms (especially in the GI or genitourinary tracts). Obtain cultures and treat with appropriate antibiotic.

▷ 3 Note that oral absorption may be delayed by food but drug may have to be taken with meals if GI upset occurs.

▷ 4 Inject IM deeply into a large muscle and rotate injection sites during re-administration to minimize pain and inflammation.

▷ 5 Use small IV needles, inject into large veins, and alternate infusion sites to minimize danger of phlebitis during IV infusion.

▷ 6 Note that IV administration is preferable to IM injection in patients with bacteremia, septicemia or other severe infections.

▷ 7 Monitor electrolyte levels during prolonged infusion, because sodium overload can occur with those drugs that contain significant amounts of sodium (see Table 61-1).

▷ 8 Be aware that cephalosporins may give false reading with the following laboratory measurements: urinary glucose using Benedict's or Fehling's solution or Clinitest tablets; urinary protein with acid and denaturization–precipitation tests; urinary 17-ketosteroids; positive direct Coombs' test.

▷ 9 In patients with impaired renal function, reduce dose of cephalosporin as indicated in the package instructions. Note that cefoperazone is not excreted significantly in the urine, and a dosage adjustment is not required.

▷ 10 Do not add solutions of cephalosporins to aminoglycoside solutions, but administer separately when indicated.

The tetracycline group of antibiotics is composed of a number of naturally derived and semisynthetic compounds possessing similar pharmacologic properties. These bacteriostatic anti-infective agents exhibit a broad spectrum of activity, but because of their extensive and often indiscriminate use in past years, their current clinical usefulness has been restricted by the emergence of a number of resistant bacterial strains. Many previously sensitive staphylococcal, streptococcal, pneumococcal, and other gram-positive organisms are now largely resistant to the tetracyclines, and *in vitro* laboratory susceptibility tests are necessary to determine the usefulness of a given tetracycline in a particular patient.

While essentially alike in their antimicrobial activity, the various tetracyclines differ in some of their pharmacokinetic properties, and these differences are indicated in Table 62-1. Oral absorption is generally good, but except for doxycycline and minocycline, may be reduced by many factors, including elevated gastric *p*H and the presence of food or polyvalent cations such as iron, calcium, magnesium, and aluminum. Plasma protein binding varies throughout a wide range. Tetracyclines diffuse readily into most body tissues, attaining highest concentrations in the lungs, liver, kidney, spleen, bone marrow, and lymph. Penetration of the drugs into the CNS is largely determined by their lipid solubility, minocycline and doxycycline being the most lipophilic derivatives and thus best able to enter the CNS. In addition, minocycline attains high levels in saliva, making it useful in eliminating meningococci from the nasopharynx of carriers.

The drugs cross the placental barrier and concentrations in the fetal circulation may reach as high as 70% of the maternal circulation. Due to the high affinity of tetracyclines for calcium, any fetal tissue undergoing active calcification (*e.g.,* bone, teeth) may have its development impaired by the presence of tetracyclines. Likewise, prolonged use of tetracyclines during the entire period of tooth development (fourth fetal month through the eighth year of life) may cause inadequate calcium deposition and discoloration of both deciduous and permanent teeth. Therefore, these drugs should be avoided if possible during pregnancy and lactation (because they are secreted in breast milk), and in young children.

With the exception of minocycline, the other tetracyclines are not metabolized to an appreciable extent, and except for doxycycline, are excreted largely in the urine. Doxycycline is secreted into the intestinal lumen and is eliminated in the feces, as is minocycline and its metabolites. Renal clearance of tetracyclines is by glomerular filtration, and varies widely among the different derivatives (see Table 62-1). Drugs having a high renal clearance (*e.g.,* oxytetracycline, tetracycline) are more effective in treating urinary tract infections than drugs with low renal clearances, but they may be more dangerous in the presence of renal impairment because of accumulation of drug in the body.

The systemic tetracyclines can be divided arbitrarily into two broad groups based upon their serum half-lives. Tetracycline and oxytetracycline are considered short-acting drugs, having half-lives of 6 hours to 10 hours. The remaining derivatives possess half-lives of approximately 10 hours to 20 hours and thus exhibit a longer duration of action. There

Tetracyclines

62

Table 62-1. Characteristics of Tetracyclines

Drug	Routes of Administration	Approximate Percent Oral Absorption	Protein Binding	Plasma Half-life	Major Route of Elimination	Renal Clearance
Chlortetracycline	Ophthalmic Topical					
Demeclocycline	Oral	60%–70%	50%–90%	10 hr–16 hr	Kidney	30 ml–35 ml/min
Doxycycline	Oral, IV	90%–95%*	70%–90%	12 hr–24 hr	Feces	16 ml–25 ml/min
Meclocycline	Topical					
Methacycline	Oral	30%–60%	75%–90%	12 hr–16 hr	Kidney	30 ml–32 ml/min
Minocycline	Oral, IV	95%–100%*	60%–75%	12 hr–20 hr	Kidney/feces (metabolites)	9 ml–10 ml/min
Oxytetracycline	Oral, IV, IM	50%–60%	20%–30%	6 hr–10 hr	Kidney	85 ml–90 ml/min
Tetracycline	Oral, IV, IM Ophthalmic Topical	70%–80%	20%–60%	6 hr–10 hr	Kidney	60 ml–65 ml/min

* Absorption is not significantly decreased by the presence of food, dairy products, or antacids.

is no convincing evidence, however, that one derivative is significantly more effective than any other for most susceptible infections. The more completely absorbed, longer acting drugs (*i.e.,* doxycycline, minocycline) require less frequent administration (twice a day *versus* three or four times a day) than the other derivatives, and thus may improve patient compliance; however, they are considerably more expensive, and minocycline is associated with a high incidence of vestibular disturbances (*e.g.,* dizziness, ataxia, lightheadedness). Because doxycycline and minocycline are not appreciably excreted by the kidney, they are the preferred tetracyclines for use in patients with renal impairment.

As noted previously, the emergence of resistant strains has severely limited the clinical application of the tetracyclines. Currently they are considered first-choice drugs for only the following infections: cholera, brucellosis, granuloma inguinale, melioidosis, chlamydial infections (ornithosis, psittacosis, trachoma, urethritis, cervicitis, lymphogranuloma venereum), *Mycoplasma pneumoniae* infections, rickettsial infections (Rocky Mountain spotted fever, endemic typhus, tick-bite fever, typhus, Q fever), relapsing fever, and gonorrhea and syphilis in penicillin-sensitive patients. Tetracyclines are also indicated as alternate drugs for a number of gram-positive and gram-negative infections (see Chap. 58, Table 58-1), although sensitivity tests are necessary to confirm susceptibility. Although active *in vitro* against many gram-positive cocci, tetracyclines should not be used to treat staphylococcal, group A beta-hemolytic streptococcal or *Streptococcus pneumoniae* infections because of the occurrence of many resistant strains. Oral tetracyclines have been used as adjunctive therapy for severe acne, because they reduce the amount of free fatty acids in acne lesions as well as decrease the population of *Corynebacterium acnes* in sebaceous glands. Topical application of tetracycline solution or meclocycline cream is also effective in the treatment of acne vulgaris lesions, although the mechanism is not well established. Both oral and topical tetracyclines may be employed for treatment of inclusion conjunctivitis. Finally, doxycycline appears to be useful in preventing "travelers' diarrhea" caused by *Escherichia coli,* and minocycline can

be used to treat asymptomatic carriers of *Neisseria meningitidis.*

Tetracyclines

Chlortetracycline	Methacycline
Demeclocycline	Minocycline
Doxycycline	Oxytetracycline
Meclocycline	Tetracycline

The following discussion considers the tetracyclines as a group. Individual members of the class are then listed in Table 62-2.

Mechanism
Bacteriostatic at recommended doses; inhibit protein synthesis in microbial cells by blocking binding of transfer RNA to the messenger RNA–ribosome complex; may also inhibit replication of DNA on the cell membrane at high doses

Uses
1 Treatment of infections due to susceptible organisms (see above introduction and also Chap. 58, Table 58-1)
2 Adjunctive therapy for severe acne or inclusion conjunctivitis
3 Adjunctive therapy (with amebicides) in the treatment of acute intestinal amebiasis
4 Treatment of uncomplicated urethral, endocervical, or rectal infections in adults caused by *Chlamydia trachomatis*
5 Alternate therapy for gonorrhea or syphilis in penicillin-sensitive patients
6 Elimination of meningococci from the nasopharynx of asymptomatic carriers of *Neisseria meningitidis* (oral minocycline only)
7 Prevention of travelers' diarrhea due to enterotoxic *Escherichia coli* (doxycycline only)
8 Management of chronic inappropriate antidiuretic

Table 62-2. Tetracyclines

Drug	Preparations	Usual Dosage Range	Remarks
Chlortetracycline (Aureomycin)	Ophthalmic ointment—1% Topical ointment—3%	Ophthalmic—place small amount of ointment into lower conjunctival sac every 3 hours as needed Topical—apply small amount every 3 hours to 6 hours as needed	Tetracycline derivative not given systemically and infrequently used topically due to risk of sensitization; be alert for appearance of allergic reactions and discontinue drug; ophthalmic ointment may retard corneal healing; topical use should be supplemented by appropriate systemic antibiotics
Demeclocycline (Declomycin)	Tablets—150 mg, 300 mg Capsules—150 mg	Adults—150 mg 4 times a day or 300 mg twice a day Children—3 mg to 6 mg/lb (6.6 mg–13.2 mg/kg) divided into 2 to 4 doses Gonorrhea in penicillin-sensitive patients—600 mg initially, followed by 300 mg every 12 hours for 5 days Uncomplicated chlamydial infections—300 mg 4 times/ day for at least 7 days	Orally effective tetracycline that is slowly excreted in part because of enterohepatic circulation; among tetracyclines, produces highest incidence of photosensitivity reactions; may result in diabetes insipidus-like syndrome (polyuria, polydipsia, weakness) on prolonged therapy; syndrome is caused by interference with action of vasopressin (ADH) on the kidneys, is dose-dependent, and is reversible upon discontinuation of drug; intake–output ratio should be monitored routinely
Doxycycline (Doxy-Caps, Doxychel, Doxy-Tabs, Vibramycin, Vibra Tabs)	Tablets—100 mg Capsules—50 mg, 100 mg Oral suspension—25 mg/5 ml Syrup—50 mg/5 ml Injection—100 mg/vial, 200 mg/vial	Oral: Adults—200 mg in 2 divided doses initially followed by 100 mg/day in single or 2 divided doses; severe infections require 100 mg every 12 hours Children—2 mg/lb (4.4 mg/kg) in divided doses the first day; then 1 mg to 2 mg/lb (2.2 mg–4.4 mg/kg) as a single dose or 2 divided doses each day. IV infusion: Adults—200 mg the first day; then 100 mg to 200 mg/day in 1 to 2 infusions Children—2 mg/lb (4.4 mg/kg) first day in 1 to 2 infusions; then 1 mg to 2 mg/lb (2.2 mg to 4.4 mg/kg) in 1 to 2 infusions each day Gonococcal infections: 200 mg initially orally, then 100 mg at bedtime first day; thereafter, 100 mg twice a day for 7 days Syphilis: 300 mg/day orally or IV for at least 10 days Uncomplicated chlamydial infections: 100 mg twice a day for at least 7 days	Semisynthetic tetracycline that is well absorbed orally, exhibits a prolonged duration of action, and is slowly excreted, primarily in the feces; may be used safely in patients with renal impairment, IV infusion is not recommended in children under 8 years of age; oral absorption is not significantly affected by food or milk; low incidence of photosensitivity; duration of IV infusion varies with the dose, and ranges from 1 hour to 4 hours; minimum infusion time for 100 mg of a 0.5 mg/ml solution is 1 hour; therapy should be continued for at least 24 hours to 48 hours after symptoms have subsided; follow package instructions for preparation and storage of IV infusion solutions; do not inject solutions IM or SC and avoid extravasation, because solutions are irritating
Meclocycline (Meclan)	Cream—1%	Apply twice a day in generous amounts until skin is thoroughly wet	Locally acting tetracycline that is not absorbed to a significant extent; used in the treatment of mild to moderate acne vulgaris; avoid contact with eyes, nose, or mouth; may produce skin

(continued)

Table 62-2. Tetracyclines (continued)

Drug	Preparations	Usual Dosage Range	Remarks
			irritation; slight yellowing of the skin can occur but may be removed by washing; cosmetics may be applied in the usual manner during treatment
Methacycline (Rondomycin)	Capsules—150 mg, 300 mg	Adults—600 mg/day in 2 to 4 divided doses Children—3 mg to 6 mg/lb/day (6.6 mg–13.2 mg/kg/day) in 2 to 4 divided doses Gonorrhea—900 mg initially, then 300 mg 4 times/day to a total of 5.4 g Syphilis—18 g to 24 g in equally divided doses over 10 days to 15 days	Semisynthetic, orally effective tetracycline; incompletely absorbed orally; highly bound to plasma proteins; excreted largely in urine; use with caution in presence of renal impairment; similar to tetracycline in most other respects, and significantly more expensive
Minocycline (Minocin)	Capsules—50 mg, 100 mg Tablets—50 mg, 100 mg Syrup—50 mg/5 ml Powder for injection—100 mg/vial	Oral: Adults—200 mg initially, then 100 mg every 12 hours or 50 mg 4 times a day Children (over 8 yr)—4 mg/kg initially; then 2 mg/kg every 12 hours Gonorrhea—200 mg initially then 100 mg every 12 hours for a minimum of 5 days Syphilis—100 mg every 12 hours for 10 days to 15 days Meningococcal carrier state—100 mg every 12 hours for 5 days Chlamydial infections—100 mg twice a day for at least 7 days IV injection: Adults—200 mg initially then 100 mg every 12 hours (maximum 400 mg/day) Children—4 mg/kg initially, then 2 mg/kg every 12 hours	Semisynthetic tetracycline that is almost completely absorbed orally; very lipid soluble and possesses a long half-life (up to 24 hr); low renal clearance; oral absorption is not appreciably altered by food or dairy products; only tetracycline drug metabolized to any extent; photosensitivity occurs rarely; vestibular side-effects are very common (lightheadedness, dizziness, vertigo); therefore, urge caution in driving or operating machinery; indicated in treatment of asymptomatic carriers of *Neisseria meningitidis* to eliminate organism from nasopharynx; *not* recommended for treatment of meningococcal infection; also used in treatment of nocardiosis; IV solutions are stable at room temperature for 24 hours
Oxytetracycline (E.P. Mycin, Oxymycin, Terramycin, Uri-Tet)	Capsules—125 mg, 250 mg Tablets—250 mg Syrup—125 mg/5 ml IM injection—50 mg/ml, 125 mg/ml with 2% lidocaine Powder for IV injection—250 mg/vial, 500 mg/vial	Oral: Adults—1 g to 2 g/day in 2 to 4 equally divided doses Children—10 mg to 20 mg/lb/day (22 mg–44 mg/kg/day) in 2 to 4 equally divided doses IM: Adults—250 mg/day in a single dose or 300 mg/day in divided doses every 8 hours to 12 hours Children—15 mg to 25 mg/kg/day in divided doses every 8 to 12 hours (maximum 250 mg/day) IV: Adults—250 mg to 500 mg every 12 hours (maximum 2 g/day) Children—12 mg/kg/day in 2 divided doses (range 10 mg–20 mg/kg/day)	Naturally derived tetracycline with actions similar to tetracycline itself; oral absorption is incomplete, half-life is 6 hours to 10 hours, and protein binding is minimal; renal clearance is highest of all tetracyclines, thus drug may be more effective than other derivatives in urinary infections; use with caution in presence of renal impairment, because drug may accumulate rapidly; IM solution contains 2% lidocaine; do *not* inject IV; use only injection marked "IV" for IV administration; reconstituted solutions for injection are stable for 48 hours with refrigeration

Table 62-2. Tetracyclines (continued)

Drug	Preparations	Usual Dosage Range	Remarks
Tetracycline (Achromycin, Panmycin, Sumycin, Tetrex, and various other manufacturers)	Capsules—100 mg, 250 mg, 500 mg Tablets—250 mg, 500 mg Syrup—125 mg/5 ml Powder for IM injection—100 mg/vial, 250 mg/vial with 2% procaine Powder for IV injection—250 mg/vial, 500 mg/vial Ophthalmic drops—1% Ophthalmic ointment—1% Topical ointment—3% Topical solution—2.2 mg/ml	Oral: Adults—1 g to 2 g/day in 2 to 4 equal doses Children—25 mg to 50 mg/kg/day in 2 to 4 equal doses Gonorrhea—1.5 g initially; then 0.5 g every 6 hours for 5 to 7 days Syphilis—30 g to 40 g in equally divided doses over 10 days to 15 days Chlamydial infections—500 mg 4 times/day for at least 7 days Acne—500 mg to 2 g/day initially (maintenance 125 mg–500 mg/day) IM: Adults—250 mg/day in a single dose or 300 mg/day in divided doses every 8 hours to 12 hours (maximum 800 mg/day) Children—15 mg to 25 mg/kg/day in divided doses every 8 hours to 12 hours IV: Adults—250 mg to 500 mg every 12 hours (maximum 2 g/day) Children—10 mg to 20 mg/kg/day in 2 divided doses Ophthalmic: 1 to 2 drops or small amount of ointment in affected eye 2 to 4 times a day Topical: Apply 2 to 4 times a day	Semisynthetic tetracycline produced from chlortetracycline or obtained naturally; most widely used and least expensive of the tetracyclines; used orally, parenterally, or locally; drug is available as a phosphate complex (Tetrex), which is more rapidly and completely absorbed orally than the free base or hydrochloride salt, may yield slightly higher blood levels; also available in combination with amphotericin B (Mysteclin-F) and nystatin (Terrastatin, Tetrastatin); combinations are claimed to reduce the incidence of *Candida* superinfections; topical application may result in hypersensitivity reactions; discontinue drug at first sign of allergic response; ophthalmic use may retard corneal healing; IM injections contain procaine and are not suitable for IV administration; injection of IM solution into subcutaneous layer may cause pain and induration; do not dilute injectable solutions with calcium-containing diluents, because precipitate can form

hormone secretion (SIADH); investigational use for demeclocycline only

9 Alternative to sulfonamides in treatment of nocardiosis (investigational use for minocycline)

Dosage

See Table 62-2.

Fate

Oral absorption is generally good but, except for doxycycline and minocycline, can be impaired by food, milk and other dairy products, iron, antacids, or alkali. Widely distributed in the body, except for the CNS, where only highly lipophilic derivatives (*e.g.,* doxycycline, minocycline) attain appreciable levels. Minocycline is highly concentrated in saliva and tears. Plasma half-lives vary from 6 hours to 24 hours (see Table 62-1), and extent of protein binding differs considerably among the different drugs. Other than minocycline, the drugs are not metabolized to a significant extent. Doxycycline and minocycline are excreted largely in the feces whereas all other derivatives are eliminated primarily by the kidneys (see Table 62-1 for renal clearance rates).

Common Side-Effects

Diarrhea, nausea, anorexia, vestibular disturbances (minocycline only), and photosensitivity (especially with demeclocycline)

Significant Adverse Reactions

GI—stomatitis, glossitis, sore throat, dysphagia, vomiting, enterocolitis, steatorrhea, inflammation in the anogenital region, esophageal ulceration

Dermatological—macropapular and erythematous rash, exfoliative dermatitis

Hypersensitivity—fever, urticaria, angio-edema, headache, impaired vision, papilledema, pericarditis, anaphylaxis, exacerbation of systemic lupus erythematosus

Hematological—hemolytic anemia, eosinophilia, neutropenia, thrombocytopenia, leukopenia, leukocytosis

Other—increased BUN, permanent discoloration of teeth, enamel hypoplasia, impaired calcification of bony structures, increased intracranial pressure and bulging fontanels in young infants, nephrogenic diabetes insipidus (demeclocycline only), irritation at IM injection sites, thrombophlebitis with IV administration, overgrowth of nonsusceptible organisms (*e.g., Candida*)

Contraindications

Severe renal or liver impairment (except doxycycline), pregnancy, in nursing mothers, and children under 8 years of age (unless no other drugs are effective for a particular infection).

Interactions

1 Oral absorption of tetracyclines (except doxycycline and minocycline) may be impaired by the presence of food, dairy products, antacids, iron, or other polyvalent cations (*e.g.,* calcium, magnesium, aluminum), and alkali (*e.g.,* sodium bicarbonate).
2 Because they are bacteriostatic, tetracyclines can reduce the effectiveness of penicillins and other bactericidal antibiotics.
3 The action of doxycycline may be shortened by barbiturates, other sedative–hypnotics, phenytoin, and carbamazepine because of hepatic enzyme induction.
4 BUN elevation can occur with combined tetracycline–diuretic use.
5 Tetracycline may enhance the effects of oral anticoagulants by interfering with synthesis of vitamin K by intestinal microorganisms.
6 Plasma levels of digoxin and lithium can be increased by tetracyclines.
7 Tetracyclines may enhance methoxyflurane-induced nephrotoxicity.
8 The effects of oral contraceptives may be reduced by tetracyclines, possibly resulting in breakthrough bleeding or pregnancy.
9 Theophylline and tetracyclines can result in increased GI side-effects.

▶ NURSING ALERTS

▷ 1 Avoid use of tetracyclines in young children (under 8 yr) and in pregnant or nursing patients unless absolutely necessary to treat a specific infection not controlled by other antibiotics, because danger of permanent tooth discoloration and impaired calcification is considerable.

▷ 2 Do not use outdated or stale tetracycline products, because the incidence of nephrotoxicity is much higher than with fresh preparations. Tetracyclines readily decompose, frequently to toxic products, with age or exposure to excess light, heat, or humidity.

▷ 3 In patients with renal impairment, decrease dosage or increase dosage intervals to prevent excessive accumulation of drug (except with doxycycline and minocycline). Be alert for vomiting, azotemia, acidosis, weight loss, or dehydration, and discontinue drug should these symptoms occur.

▷ 4 Advise patients to avoid prolonged contact with direct sunlight or other ultraviolet light during therapy, especially with demeclocycline, to prevent photosensitization. Discontinue drug if skin discomfort or allergic reaction persists.

▷ 5 Administer IV very cautiously in the presence of renal dysfunction or pregnancy, and do not exceed 2 g/day. High-dose IV tetracycline therapy has been associated with liver failure and death. When the drug is used IV, frequent liver and kidney function tests are essential.

▷ 6 Be alert for signs of overgrowth of nonsusceptible organisms (*e.g.,* black or "furry" tongue; sore mouth; rectal, vaginal, or perineal itching; diarrhea), and institute appropriate clinical measures and anti-infective drugs. Be careful to distinguish between tetracycline-induced diarrhea (first few days of therapy) and that resulting from intestinal superinfection (later in therapy and frequently more intense).

▷ 7 Caution patients to avoid concurrent use of tetracycline and antacids, antidiarrheals, milk or other dairy products, and calcium-containing drugs or foods, because oral absorption of the antibiotic is significantly impaired.

▶ NURSING CONSIDERATIONS

▷ 1 Administer oral drugs at least 1 hour before or 2 hours after meals. If nausea, GI distress, or diarrhea occurs, drug may be given with small quantities of most foods (except those high in calcium) without significantly impairing efficacy. Absorption of doxycycline and minocycline is not appreciably altered by food.

▷ 2 Continue drug administration at least 48 hours to 72 hours after fever and other symptoms of infection have subsided.

▷ 3 During long-term therapy, monitor renal, hepatic, and hematopoietic function at regular intervals.

▷ 4 Urge patients to maintain good hygienic care of the mouth, skin, and perineal area to minimize the occurrence of candidal superinfections.

▷ 5 Inject IM deeply into the body of a large muscle. Avoid SC injection, which is very painful. Use care not to inject IV, because IM preparations contain lidocaine a local anesthetic that may be hazardous if injected IV.

▷ 6 Inquire about a possible allergy to lidocaine before administering drug solution IM.

▷ 7 Administer IV at a slow rate and observe site of injection for redness or swelling. Prolonged IV administration can result in thrombophlebitis.

▷ 8 Note that tetracyclines may increase serum levels of creatinine, urea nitrogen, bilirubin, alkaline phosphatase, SGPT, SGOT, and urinary levels of catecholamines and protein, and may decrease hemoglobin and platelet values. They may also yield a false negative with Clinistix or Tes-Tape and a false positive urinary glucose test with Clinitest.

The erythromycins are members of the macrolide group of antibiotics, so named because the chemical structure of the compounds consists of a large lactone ring to which one or more sugars are attached. Erythromycin itself as a base is an orally effective antibiotic originally isolated from a strain of *Streptomyces erythreus*. Although erythromycin base is a biologically active form, it is unstable in gastric acid and thus must be formulated in an enteric-coated preparation for oral administration. Absorption of enteric-coated products is occasionally less than adequate, however, and blood levels may not reach sufficient concentrations. Therefore, to avoid destruction of the drug by gastric juices, while maintaining good oral absorption, erythromycin has also been formulated in several salts (estolate, ethylsuccinate, stearate), all of which are largely acid-stable and yield biologically effective plasma levels of free erythromycin base. The strength of erythromycin products is expressed in terms of base equivalents. Thus, 400 mg of the ethylsuccinate salt provides serum levels of free erythromycin equivalent to those resulting from administration of 250 mg of erythromycin base or the stearate or estolate salts. Two other soluble salts of erythromycin (gluceptate, lactobionate) are available for IV use and are indicated mainly in severe infections where high serum levels of the drug are required immediately. The other clinically available macrolide antibiotic is troleandomycin, an agent resembling erythromycin in both structure and pharmacologic activity, but somewhat less effective and more toxic, and hence infrequently used today. It is discussed briefly at the end of the chapter.

Erythromycins inhibit protein synthesis and are bacteriostatic at normal therapeutic doses, although they may be bactericidal against certain organisms at high concentrations. Their antibacterial spectrum of action is similar to that of the penicillins, being most effective against certain gram-positive cocci, such as staphylococci, streptococci, enterococci, and pneumococci. Although used principally as *alternatives* to penicillin in treating susceptible organisms, the erythromycins may be considered the drugs of choice against the following organisms: *Bordetella pertussis* (whooping cough), *Corynebacterium diphtheriae, Legionella pneumophila* (Legionnaires' disease), *Mycoplasma pneumoniae* (atypical viral pneumonia), and strains of *Chlamydia trachomatis* causing pneumonia and inclusion conjunctivitis (refer to Chap. 58, Table 58-1, for a listing of the organisms for which erythromycin is considered an alternate drug).

Microbial resistance has become a problem with use of the erythromycins and is especially frequent in staphylococci. Prolonged use of erythromycin in staphylococcal infections is almost invariably associated with the emergence of resistance, and alternative drugs should be used in treating severe staphylococcal infections. Erythromycin-resistant streptococci and pneumococci are likewise developing with increasing frequency. Although cross-resistance is not a significant problem between erythromycin and most other antibiotics, it has been reported with lincomycin and clindamycin, and is virtually complete among all the members of the macrolides.

As noted earlier, erythromycin is used as the free base as well as several salts, and the various preparations are

Erythromycins

63

available for oral, IV, topical, and ophthalmic administration. Absorption of the base and the stearate preparations are impaired by the presence of food, and these drugs should be administered on an empty stomach, if possible. Conversely, absorption of the estolate and ethylsuccinate salts are either unaffected or enhanced by the presence of food. However, the estolate salt has been associated with cholestatic hepatitis, especially in adults, and its use in this group cannot be justified. Erythromycins in general, however, are among the safest antibiotics, and their administration is accompanied by relatively few and predominately minor adverse effects. For this reason, these agents are commonly prescribed in children, although as previously mentioned, they should not be considered first-line drugs except in those few infections listed above.

Following a general discussion of erythromycin, the various salts, their doses and dosage forms, and pertinent comments are presented in Table 63-1. The other macrolide antibiotic, troleandomycin, is then reviewed at the end of the chapter.

Table 63-1. Erythromycins

Drug	Preparations	Usual Dosage Range	Remarks
Erythromycin base (E-Mycin, Ery-Tab, Eryc, Ilotycin, Robimycin, RP-Mycin)	Enteric-coated tablets—250 mg, 333 mg, 500 mg Film-coated tablets—250 mg, 500 mg Capsules (enteric-coated pellets)—250 mg Ointment—1% Ophthalmic ointment—0.5%	Oral: Adults—250 mg to 500 mg every 6 hours to 12 hours up to 4 g/day for severe infections Children—30 mg/kg to 50 mg/kg/day in 3 to 4 divided doses, up to 100 mg/kg/day Syphilis—30 g to 40 g in divided doses over 10 days to 15 days Topical—apply to skin or eye 2 to 4 times/day as necessary	Free-base form of erythromycin, which is acid-labile and thus administered orally in enteric-coated form; absorption is variable depending upon product used; should be administered on an empty stomach if possible; do not break or crush enteric-coated tablets; ophthalmic ointment may retard corneal healing; be alert for hypersensitivity reactions with topical application
Erythromycin base, topical solution (A/T/S, Eryderm, Erymax, Staticin)	Topical solution—1.5%, 2%	Apply morning and evening to areas usually affected by acne	Alcohol solution of erythromycin base used in the treatment of acne vulgaris; avoid contact with eyes, nose, mouth, or other mucous membranes; use cautiously with other topical acne treatment, because severe irritation can occur; most common side-effect is excessive drying of treated area; erythema, pruritus, burning, and desquamation have also been reported; wash, rinse, and dry area to be treated before application
Erythromycin estolate (Ilosone)	Tablets—250 mg, 500 mg Chewable tablets—125 mg, 250 mg Capsules—125 mg, 250 mg Drops—100 mg/ml Suspension—125 mg/5 ml, 250 mg/5 ml Powder for suspension—125 mg/5 ml	Adults—250 mg every 6 hours (or 500 mg every 12 hr) up to 4 g/day Children—30 mg/kg to 50 mg/kg/day orally in divided doses, up to 100 mg/kg/day Syphilis—20 g over 10 days in divided doses	Ester salt of erythromycin that is acid-stable, well absorbed in the presence of food, and yields higher and more sustained blood levels than other derivatives; may produce hepatotoxicity; thus be alert for early signs of liver dysfunction (vomiting, malaise, cramping, right upper quadrant pain, fever, jaundice), and discontinue drug; symptoms usually occur with 1 week to 2 weeks of continuous therapy and are reversible upon discontinuation of medication; not indicated for prolonged administration (*e.g.,* acne, prophylaxis of rheumatic fever) or for treatment of syphilitic infections in pregnant women; do not confuse regular tablets (250 mg, 500 mg) with chewable tablets (125 mg, 250 mg); regular tablets should be swallowed whole; liquid should be kept refrigerated and unused portion discarded after 14 days

Table 63-1. Erythromycins (continued)

Drug	Preparations	Usual Dosage Range	Remarks
Erythromycin ethylsuccinate (E.E.S., E-Mycin E, EryPed, Pediamycin, Wyamycin-E)	Film-coated tablets—400 mg Chewable tablets—200 mg Drops—100 mg/2.5 ml Suspension—200 mg/5 ml, 400 mg/5 ml Powder for suspension—200 mg/5 ml, 400 mg/5 ml	Adults—400 mg every 6 hours, up to 4 g/day for severe infections Children—30 mg/kg to 50 mg/kg/day up to 100 mg/kg/day Syphilis—64 g over 10 days in divided doses	Acid-stable salt of erythromycin that is reliably absorbed from the GI tract; requires a higher dose (*i.e.*, 400 mg *vs* 250 mg) than other oral salts to yield comparable blood levels of erythromycin base, the active form; oral liquids are stable for 14 days with refrigeration; reconstituted powder is stable for 10 days
Erythromycin gluceptate (Ilotycin Gluceptate)	Powder for injection—250 mg/20 ml, 500 mg/30 ml, 1 g/50 ml	Adults and children—15 mg/kg to 20 mg/kg/day by continuous (preferred) or intermittent infusion; up to 4 g/day can be used in severe infections	Soluble salt of erythromycin indicated in severe infections requiring immediate, high serum levels, or when oral administration is not possible or feasible; may produce pain, irritation, and possibly phlebitis upon administration; solution is prepared initially by adding Sterile Water for Injection to the vial according to package directions and shaking until dissolved; no preservatives should be used; reconstituted solution should be stored in refrigerator and used within 7 days; intermittent infusion is performed by administering 250 mg to 500 mg in 100 ml to 250 ml of Sodium Chloride Injection or 5% Dextrose over 30 minutes to 60 minutes 4 times a day; initial solution may be added to Sodium Chloride Injection or 5% Dextrose in Water to give 1 g/liter for slow IV infusion; *p*H of diluted solution should be kept between 6 and 8; do *not* give by IV push, because irritation is common; high doses have resulted in alterations in liver function; periodic hepatic function tests are required during prolonged therapy
Erythromycin lactobionate (Erythrocin Lactobionate-IV)	Powder for injection—500 mg/vial, 1 g/vial Piggyback single dose vial—500 mg powder/vial when reconstituted	Adults and children—15 mg/kg to 20 mg/kg/day by continuous (preferred) or intermittent infusion; up to 4 g/day may be given in severe infections	Soluble salt of erythromycin used in a similar manner as the gluceptate salt; see Gluceptate for mixing and diluting instructions; IV infusion of 4 g/day or more has caused reversible hearing loss; *do not exceed this dose;* intermittent IV administration is accomplished by giving ¼ the daily dose over 30 minutes to 60 minutes every 6 hours by slow injection of 250 mg to 500 mg in 100 ml to 250 ml of Sodium Chloride or 5% Dextrose; IV therapy should be replaced by oral therapy as soon as is feasible
Erythromycin stearate (Bristamycin, Eramycin, Erypar, Erythrocin, Ethril, Pfizer-E, SK-Erythromycin, Wyamycin-S)	Film-coated tablets—250 mg, 500 mg	Adults—250 mg every 6 hours (or 500 mg every 12 hr) up to 4 g/day in divided doses Children—30 mg/kg to 50 mg/kg/day in divided doses 4 times a day, up to 100 mg/kg/day Syphilis—30 g to 40 g in divided doses over 10 days to 15 days	Acid-stable salt of erythromycin claimed to be the most completely and reliably absorbed of all the derivatives when taken on an empty stomach; may be associated with a slightly higher incidence of allergic reactions than other forms of erythromycin

Erythromycins

Erythromycin base	Erythromycin gluceptate
Erythromycin estolate	Erythromycin lactobionate
Erythromycin ethylsuccinate	Erythromycin stearate

Mechanism

Inhibit bacterial protein synthesis by attaching to 50 S ribosomal subunits of sensitive microorganisms, thereby blocking binding of t–RNA to donor site; do not affect nucleic acid synthesis nor act on the cell wall; bacteriostatic at normal therapeutic levels but may be bactericidal against some organisms at high concentrations

Uses

1 Treatment of respiratory infections caused by susceptible organisms, such as the following: *Mycoplasma pneumoniae* (drug of choice), *Legionella pneumophila* (drug of choice), *Streptococcus pneumoniae*, group A beta-hemolytic *Streptococcus* (in penicillin-sensitive patients), and *Bordetella pertussis*
2 Treatment of acute skin and soft-tissue infections due to *Staphylococcus aureus*
3 Prophylaxis of subacute bacterial endocarditis and recurrence of acute rheumatic fever in penicillin-sensitive patients
4 Treatment of *Neisseria gonorrhoeae* (gonorrhea) and *Treponema pallidum* (syphilis) in penicillin- and tetracycline-sensitive patients
5 Treatment of chlamydial infections (*e.g.,* urethritis, endocervicitis, conjuncivitis, pneumonia) in tetracycline-sensitive patients
6 Treatment of *Campylobacter jejuni* gastroenteritis
7 Adjunctive treatment of *Corynebacterium* infections (with antitoxin)
8 Topical control of mild to moderate acne vulgaris
9 Reduction of wound complications when given with neomycin prior to colorectal surgery

Dosage

See Table 63-1.

Fate

Oral absorption of base and salts is good, but base and stearate absorption may be impaired by food; base is destroyed by gastric acid, thus is formulated in enteric-coated tablets or capsules; drug diffuses readily into most body tissues, except CNS unless meninges are inflamed, and passes through the placental barrier, although fetal blood levels remain rather low; peak serum levels occur in 1 hour to 4 hours with oral use; drug is approximately 70% protein-bound; concentrated in the liver and excreted in active form primarily in the bile; less than 5% of an oral dose and 15% of an IV dose is excreted in the urine

Common Side-Effects

Abdominal discomfort and cramping (usually with elevated doses)

Significant Adverse Reactions

Vomiting, diarrhea, allergic reactions (rash, urticaria, fever, eosinophilia, anaphylaxis); superinfections by nonsusceptible organisms; cholestatic hepatitis (primarily from estolate salt); pain, irritation, or phlebitis with IV injection; impaired hearing with IV infusion of lactobionate or gluceptate salts (4 g/day or more)

Contraindications

Estolate salt in liver disease

Interactions

1 The activity of erythromycins may be enhanced by urinary alkalinizers (*e.g.,* sodium bicarbonate, acetazolamide) and decreased by urinary acidifiers (*e.g.,* ammonium chloride, citric acid beverages).
2 The effects of lincomycin and clindamycin may be antagonized by erythromycin, which competes for ribosomal binding sites.
3 Tetracyclines and cephalothin are incompatible with erythromycin in parenteral mixtures.
4 Erythromycin can elevate serum digoxin levels in a small percentage of patients who metabolize digoxin in the GI tract by slowing its metabolism in the gut.
5 Erythromycins can increase serum theophylline and carbamazepine levels by reducing their hepatic clearance.
6 Erythromycin, being primarily bacteriostatic, may impair the antimicrobial activity of penicillins or other bactericidal antibiotics.
7 The effects of oral anticoagulants may be increased by erythromycins.

▶ NURSING ALERTS

▷ 1 Administer cautiously to patients with impaired liver function and to pregnant or nursing women. Perform periodic hepatic function tests during prolonged (*i.e.,* several weeks) therapy.
▷ 2 Observe patients closely for early signs of hepatic dysfunction (malaise, nausea, vomiting, cramping, fever). Jaundice (dark urine, pale stools, pruritus, yellow skin or sclerae) may or may not occur. Discontinue drug immediately should these signs occur.
▷ 3 Use with caution during pregnant and in nursing mothers and patients with a history of liver dysfunction or allergic diseases.

▶ NURSING CONSIDERATIONS

▷ 1 Administer oral drugs with a full glass of water on an empty stomach unless gastric distress is present. Avoid fruit juice or other acidic beverages. Estolate and ethylsuccinate salts may be taken without regard for meals.
▷ 2 Instruct patients to swallow enteric-coated tablets whole.
▷ 3 Observe patients for indication of overgrowth of nonsusceptible organisms (fever, black or "furry" tongue, diarrhea, perianal irritation or itching, vaginal discharge), and advise physician immediately should these symptoms occur.

▷ 4 Be alert for signs of local hypersensitivity when drug is applied topically.

▷ 5 Continue therapy for at least 48 hours after clinical signs of infection have disappeared (minimum 7 days–10 days).

▷ 6 Note that erythromycins can elevate serum levels of SGPT, SGOT, and alkaline phosphatase, decrease serum levels of glucose and cholesterol, and give false elevations of urinary catecholamines and 17-ketosteroids.

▷ 7 Consider administration of one half of total daily dose on a twice-a-day basis rather than every 6 hours to improve patient compliance.

▷ 8 Note that 400 mg of erythromycin ethylsuccinate produces the same free erythromycin serum levels as 250 mg of the base, stearate or estolate.

▷ 9 Give IM deeply into a large muscle mass, because injections can cause considerable pain. Rotate injection sites, and do not administer more than 600 mg at a single site.

▷ 10 When administering IV, use only dilute solutions and closely observe patient for signs of phlebitis.

▷ 11 Cleanse affected area of skin before application of topical solution or ointment unless directed otherwise by physician. Keep solution or ointment away from eyes, nose, mouth, and other mucous membranes.

▶ troleandomycin

Tao

A semisynthetic derivative of oleandomycin, troleandomycin is a macrolide antibiotic obtained from *Streptomyces antibioticus*. It is similar to erythromycin in activity but somewhat less effective and more toxic, hence its clinical usefulness is limited. Troleandomycin is generally effective in eradicating streptococci from the nasopharynx.

Mechanism
Inhibits protein synthesis in susceptible bacteria

Uses
1 Treatment of upper respiratory infections due to susceptible strains of *Diplococcus pneumoniae* and *Streptococcus pyogenes* (alternative therapy *only*)

Dosage
Adults: 250 mg to 500 mg four times a day
Children: 125 mg to 250 mg every 6 hours

Fate
Well absorbed orally; widely distributed in the body, including the CNS; metabolized in the liver and excreted in the bile and urine

Common Side-Effects
Abdominal discomfort and cramping

Significant Adverse Reactions
Nausea, vomiting, diarrhea, allergic reactions (rash, fever, pruritis, urticaria, anaphylaxis), overgrowth of nonsusceptible organisms, and cholestatic hepatitis

Contraindications
Liver impairment

Interactions
1 Combined use of ergotamine and troleandomycin can induce ischemic reactions.
2 Troleandomycin may elevate serum levels of theophylline, carbamazepine, and corticosteroids if used concurrently.
3 Concomitant use of troleandomycin and oral contraceptives can result in cholestatic jaundice.

▶ NURSING ALERTS
See Erythromycin.

▶ NURSING CONSIDERATIONS
See Erythromycin.

Summary. Erythromycins–Troleandomycin

Drug	Preparations	Usual Dosage Range
Erythromycins	See Table 63-1	
Troleandomycin (Tao)	Capsules—250 mg Suspension—125 mg/5 ml	Adults—250 mg to 500 mg 4 times/day Children—125 mg to 250 mg every 6 hours

64 Aminoglycosides

The aminoglycosides are a group of broad-spectrum bactericidal antibiotics that exhibit similar pharmacologic, antimicrobial, and toxicologic properties. Despite their extended spectrum of action, however, their use is generally restricted to treatment of serious systemic gram-negative infections caused by *Pseudomonas, Proteus, Klebsiella, Enterobacter, Serratia,* and *Escherichia* species. Aminoglycoside treatment of infections due to other organisms, both gram-negative and gram-positive is generally reserved for those instances where less toxic agents have failed. The major limitation to the routine use of aminoglycoside antibiotics is their potential for eliciting serious untoward reactions, most notably ototoxicity (both auditory and vestibular) and nephrotoxicity. Toxicity with aminoglycosides can develop even with conventional therapeutic doses, although it is much more common at higher doses, especially in patients with impaired renal function. Adverse effects are considered in more detail below. Due to the narrow margin between efficacy and toxicity with aminoglycosides, serum concentrations should be monitored frequently in critically ill patients and in persons with renal impairment. Peak serum concentrations are determined 30 minutes after completion of IV infusion or one hour after IM injection. Minimum (*i.e.,* trough) levels are taken immediately prior to the next dose. Unlike most drugs, dosage adjustments are usually made according to the trough, rather than peak, levels.

Absorption of aminoglycosides from the GI tract is negligible, and the drugs must be administered parenterally for treatment of systemic infections. Several aminoglycosides may also be given orally for localized intra-intestinal infections or as adjunctive therapy in the treatment of hepatic coma. Some drugs are also applied topically to the eye, skin, or mucous membranes for treatment of superficial infections due to susceptible organisms. Thus, despite similar chemical and pharmacologic properties, the aminoglycosides do *not* share similar modes of administration or clinical indications. Table 64-1 lists the various routes of administration for each of the aminoglycosides, as well as their major antimicrobial spectrum of action. The aminoglycosides, while active against a variety of gram-positive organisms, are rarely used clinically against these organisms due to the availability of more effective and less toxic antibacterial agents. As indicated above, their principal application is in treating severe systemic infections caused by a number of gram-negative aerobic bacilli (see Table 64-1). Gentamicin and tobramycin are usually considered the drugs of first choice against the following susceptible organisms: *Acinetobacter, Enterobacter aerogenes, Escherichia coli, Klebsiella pneumoniae, Proteus* species, and *Pseudomonas aeruginosa.* Gentamicin or amikacin are drugs of choice for *Serratia* infections, and amikacin may be viewed as a first-line drug against *Providencia.* Netilmicin is similar to gentamicin in spectrum of activity, but has been reported to be considerably less active against *Pseudomonas aeruginosa.* However, netilmicin may be somewhat less ototoxic and nephrotoxic than the other aminoglycosides. Streptomycin is the agent of choice for treating infections due to *Francisella tularensis* (tularemia), *Pseudomonas mallei* (melioidosis), and *Yersinia pestis* (plague). The various aminoglycosides are also employed as alternative agents against a wide variety of organisms as outlined in Chapter 58, Table 58-1. The drugs are more active in an

Table 64-1. Administration and Antimicrobial Spectrum of Aminoglycosides

Drug	Routes of Administration	Plasma Half-life (hr)	Principal Antimicrobial Spectrum of Action*
Amikacin	IM, IV	1–3	1, 2, 3, 7, 8, 10, 11, 12, 15, 17
Gentamicin	IM, IV, intrathecal, ophthalmic, topical	1–4	1, 2, 3, 7, 10, 11, 12, 13, 14, 15, 17
Kanamycin	IM, IV, intraperitoneal, aerosol, oral	2–3	1, 3, 6, 7, 8, 9, 10, 13, 14, 15, 17
Neomycin	IM, ophthalmic, topical, oral	3	3, 7, 10, 12
Netilmicin	IM, IV	2–3	1, 2, 3, 7, 10, 11, 12, 13, 14, 15, 17
Paromomycin	Oral	3–4	Intestinal amebiasis (see Chap. 71)
Streptomycin	IM	2–3	3, 4, 5, 6, 7, 8, 9, 10, 16, 17
Tobramycin	IM, IV, ophthalmic	1–2	1, 2, 3, 7, 10, 11, 12, 15, 16, 17

Organisms

1. *Acinetobacter* species
2. *Citrobacter freundii*
3. *Escherichia coli*
4. *Francisella tularensis*
5. *Hemophilus ducreyi*
6. *Hemophilus influenzae*
7. *Klebsiella–Enterobacter–Serratia* species
8. *Mycobacterium tuberculosis*
9. *Neisseria gonorrhoeae*
10. *Proteus* species
11. *Providencia* species
12. *Pseudomonas aeruginosa*
13. *Salmonella* species
14. *Shigella* species
15. *Staphylococcus* species
16. *Streptococcus* (group D)
17. *Yersinia pestis*

* Does *not* necessarily indicate drug of choice; see Chapter 58, Table 58-1.

alkaline medium; thus alkalinization of the urine will enhance their activity in treating urinary infections.

Resistance to the aminoglycosides is becoming more prevalent as their use increases. This resistance can occur in a number of ways, the most common being decreased penetration of the drug into the bacterial cell, a deficiency of the ribosomal receptor (see Mechanism), or increased enzymatic destruction of the drug. The newer derivatives (tobramycin, amikacin, netilmicin) may still be effective, however, against certain organisms that have become resistant to the action of the older agents such as kanamycin and gentamicin. For example, amikacin is not degraded by most aminoglycoside-inactivating enzymes that affect other derivatives, and thus may be useful against enzyme-producing organisms resistant to the other systemic aminoglycosides. Nevertheless, culture and sensitivity tests should be performed to determine the susceptibility of an infecting organism to a particular aminoglycoside.

The possibility of serious adverse reactions is a major limitation to the routine use of the aminoglycosides and all derivatives exhibit essentially the same range of toxic effects, although some effects occur less frequently with some of the newer agents. Foremost among the untoward reactions seen with aminoglycoside use is ototoxicity, which can involve both the auditory and vestibular functions of the eighth cranial nerve. The risk is greatest in patients with renal impairment or preexisting hearing loss, and although the incidence of ototoxicity is generally related to the dose and duration of treatment, it has occasionally occurred with normal therapeutic doses. Patients should be observed closely for early signs of impending toxicity (tinnitus, vertigo, high-frequency deafness), and the dosage lowered or the drug discontinued to prevent irreversible deafness. Vestibular toxicity is more common with gentamicin and streptomycin, whereas auditory toxicity is more prevalent with kanamycin, neomycin, amikacin, and netilmicin. The relative ototoxicity

of aminoglycosides is neomycin > streptomycin, kanamycin > amikacin, gentamicin, tobramycin, netilmicin.

Because aminoglycosides are eliminated almost entirely by the kidneys, they may accumulate in patients with compromised renal function. Moreover, the drug's own toxic effects may further reduce the organ's ability to excrete nitrogenous wastes. The result is increased nitrogen retention (*i.e.,* elevated BUN or serum creatinine), frequently accompanied by oliguria, proteinuria, azotemia, and the presence of red and white cell casts in the urine. Because renal tubular damage is usually reversible if detected early enough, careful monitoring of renal function and serum creatinine levels is essential during prolonged aminoglycoside therapy, especially in the patient with pre-existing renal dysfunction. Decreased creatinine clearance necessitates a reduction in drug dosage or an increase in dosing intervals, or both; the presence of casts in the urine suggests that hydration of the patient should be increased; the appearance of symptomatic azotemia or a progressive decrease in urine output is usually an indication to discontinue the drug. It should be noted, however, that when patients are well hydrated and kidney function is normal, the risk of nephrotoxicity with aminoglycosides is comparatively *low* provided dosage limits are not exceeded. The relative nephrotoxicity of these agents is approximately neomycin > amikacin, gentamicin, kanamycin, netilmicin > tobramycin > streptomycin.

Interference with neuromuscular transmission, possibly leading to respiratory depression or paralysis, has occurred with the aminoglycosides, especially when given either simultaneously with or shortly after general anesthetics or muscle relaxants. Reversal of aminoglycoside-induced neuromuscular blockade, characterized by apnea and muscle paralysis, may be accomplished with either neostigmine or calcium salts.

Inasmuch as the different aminoglycosides share the same properties, they are considered as a group. Characteristics

Table 64-2. Aminoglycosides

Drug	Preparations	Usual Dosage Range	Remarks
Amikacin (Amikin)	Injection—100 mg/2 ml; 500 mg/2 ml; 1 g/4 ml	IM, IV: Adults and older children—15 mg/kg/day in 2 to 3 divided doses (maximum 1.5 g/day) Urinary tract infections: 250 mg IM twice a day Neonatal sepsis: Initially 10 mg/kg, followed by 7.5 mg/kg every 12 hours	Semisynthetic aminoglycoside derived from kanamycin, exhibiting a similar spectrum of action; *not* degraded by most aminoglycoside-inactivating enzymes, therefore may be effective against organisms resistant to other derivatives; amikacin resistance is emerging, however, as its use increases; duration of treatment should be 7 days to 10 days; longer therapy necessitates daily monitoring of renal and auditory function; if a clinical response does *not* occur within 5 days, stop drug and re-evaluate; may be used in uncomplicated urinary tract infections (dose: 250 mg IM twice a day) due to organisms not susceptible to other, less toxic agents; urine should be examined during treatment for the presence of protein, blood cells, or casts; maintain high degree of hydration to minimize renal irritation; solution for IV use is prepared by adding contents of 500-mg vial to 200 ml of appropriate diluent (see package instructions) and administered over a 30-minute to 60-minute period (1 hr–2 hr for neonates); do not premix with other drugs; stable for extended period of time at room temperature
Gentamicin (Apogen, Bristagen, Garamycin, Genoptic, Jenamicin)	Injection—10 mg/ml, 40 mg/ml Piggyback injection—60 mg/dose, 80 mg/dose, 100 mg/dose Intrathecal injection—2 mg/ml Ophthalmic drops—0.3% Ophthalmic ointment—0.3% Topical ointment—0.1%	IM, IV: Adults—3 mg/kg to 5 mg/kg/day in 3 to 4 divided doses Children—6 mg/kg to 7.5 mg/kg/day in 3 divided doses Infants and neonates—7.5 mg/kg/day in 3 divided doses Premature infants and neonates (less than 1 wk)—5 mg/kg/day in 2 equal doses Intrathecal: Adults—4 mg to 8 mg/day in a single dose Children and infants (over 3 mo)—1 mg to 2 mg once/day Ophthalmic: 1 to 2 drops or small amount of ophthalmic ointment 2 to 4 times/day Topical: Apply sparingly to affected area 3 to 4 times/day	Broad-spectrum aminoglycoside obtained from an *Actinomyces* organism; drug of choice against several gram-negative organisms (see Chap. 58, Table 58-1), synergistic with extended-spectrum penicillins against *Pseudomonas* infections; may be used in combination with a penicillin or cephalosporin in treating serious unknown infections before sensitivity testing; also used with antistaphylococcal penicillins for treatment of staphylococcal endocarditis; generally given IM, but may be used IV in patients with septicemia, shock, congestive heart failure, severe burns, or hematologic disorders; do not mix with other drugs before injection; intrathecal administration is used as an adjunct to systemic administration in serious CNS infections (*e.g.*, meningitis, ventriculitis) due to *Pseudomonas* species; topical application is used to treat superficial infections of the skin and mucous membranes due to susceptible organisms; photosensitivity reactions have

Table 64-2. Aminoglycosides (continued)

Drug	Preparations	Usual Dosage Range	Remarks
			occurred following topical use; systemic toxicity can result from application to large abraded areas of skin; use cautiously on burns or large wounds
Kanamycin (Kantrex, Klebcil, Lypho Med)	Injection—500 mg/2 ml; 1 g/3 ml Pediatric injection—75 mg/2 ml Capsules—500 mg	IM: Adults and children—7.5 mg/kg every 12 hours (maximum 1.5 g/day) IV: Up to 15 mg/kg/day in 2 to 3 divided doses infused over a 30-minute to 60-minute period Intraperitoneal: 500 mg/20 ml Sterile Distilled Water instilled into peritoneal cavity through a wound catheter Aerosol: 250 mg (1 ml) diluted with 3 ml saline 2 to 4 times/day, using a nebulizer Oral: Suppression of intestinal bacteria—1 g every hour for 4 hours, then 1 g every 6 hours for 36 hours to 72 hours Hepatic coma—8 g to 12 g/day in divided doses	Aminoglycoside derived from a species of *Streptomyces;* similar in activity to neomycin but not as toxic; effective against many common gram (−) organisms (except *Pseudomonas*) but not considered drug of choice for any infection; primarily used as alternate to gentamicin or tobramycin; occasionally used as adjunctive therapy of *Mycobacterium tuberculosis;* inject deeply IM and rotate sites; discontinue drug if a clinical response does not occur within 5 days; prepare IV solutions by adding 500 mg to 200 ml, or 1 g to 400 ml, of sterile diluent, and infuse over 30 minutes to 60 minutes 2 to 3 times a day; do not mix dilution with other drug solutions; solution in vials may darken on shelf with no loss of potency, intraperitoneal instillation should be postponed until patient has recovered from effects of anesthesia and muscle relaxants (danger of respiratory depression and muscle paralysis); may be used as an irrigating solution (0.25%) in abscess cavities, peritoneal, ventricular, or pleural spaces; when used orally, be alert for malabsorption syndrome (*e.g.,* increased fecal fat) or secondary bacterial or fungal infections (*e.g.,* diarrhea, stomatitis); used with caution orally in patients with GI ulceration, because enhanced systemic absorption can occur
Neomycin (Mycifradin, Myciguent, Neobiotic)	Powder for injection—500 mg Tablets—500 mg Oral solution—125 mg/5 ml Topical ointment—0.5% Topical cream—0.5%	IM: Adults—15 mg/kg/day in 4 divided doses Oral: Preoperative bowel preparation—88 mg/kg (40 mg/lb) in 6 equally divided doses every 4 hours before surgery Hepatic coma— Adults—4 g to 12 g/day in divided doses Children—50 mg to 100 mg/kg/day in divided doses Infectious diarrhea—50 mg/kg/day in divided doses for 2 days to 3 days Topical: Apply 2 to 4 times a day	Broad-spectrum antibiotic obtained from a species of *Streptomyces;* similar in action to kanamycin, but is the most potent neuromuscular blocker and reportedly the most toxic of all aminoglycosides; many organisms exhibit moderate to marked resistance against neomycin; seldom used IM due to toxicity; generally reserved for hospital cases in which no other antimicrobial agent is effective; daily IM dose should not exceed 1 g nor should drug be given longer than 10 days; principal indications for oral neomycin are severe diarrhea due to *Escherichia coli* and preoperative bowel sterilization in conjunction with a low-residue diet; a saline cathartic is administered before

(continued)

Table 64-2. Aminoglycosides *(continued)*

Drug	Preparations	Usual Dosage Range	Remarks
			first dose of neomycin; may interfere with absorption of other drugs, *e.g.,* digitalis glycosides, methotrexate, penicillins (see Interactions); nausea and diarrhea are fairly common with oral administration; widest application is topically, either alone or more commonly with bacitracin and polymyxin (*e.g.,* Neosporin, Mycitracin, Neo-Polycin) for superficial infections of eye, skin, and mucous membranes; hypersensitivity reactions are common with topical application; discontinue drug if irritation, redness, or itching occurs; do not use over large body surface areas, or if skin is broken or abraded, because increased systemic absorption and toxicity can occur
Netilmicin (Netromycin)	Injection—100 mg/ml Pediatric injection—25 mg/ml Neonatal injection—10 mg/ml	IM, IV: Adults—3 mg/kg to 6.5 mg/kg/day in divided doses every 8 hours to 12 hours Children—5.5 mg/kg to 8 mg/kg/day in divided doses every 8 hours to 12 hours Neonates—4 mg/kg to 6 mg/kg/day in divided doses every 12 hours	Semisynthetic derivative similar to gentamicin in activity but somewhat less effective against *Pseudomonas;* may be slightly less nephrotoxic and ototoxic than other aminoglycosides; used in serious staphylococcal infections where penicillins are contraindicated, and in suspected or confirmed gram (−) infections; usual duration of treatment is 7 to 14 days; for longer therapy, carefully monitor renal, auditory, and vestibular functions; follow package instructions for dosage adjustment in the presence of impaired renal function
Paromomycin (Humatin)	Capsules—250 mg	Intestinal amebiasis: Adults and children—25 mg/kg to 35 mg/kg/day in 3 divided doses, with meals for 5 days to 10 days Hepatic coma: Adults—4 g/day in divided doses for 5 days to 6 days	Antimicrobial agent obtained from a species of *Streptomyces,* with antibacterial activity similar to kanamycin and neomycin; only used orally (not absorbed) for treatment of acute and chronic intestinal amebiasis (not effective in *extra-intestinal* amebiasis); see Chapter 71; also reduces concentration of ammonia-forming organisms in the GI tract, thus is used adjunctively in hepatic coma to decrease blood ammonia levels; diarrhea and cramping frequently occur; be alert for overgrowth of nonsusceptible organisms
Streptomycin (Streptomycin)	Powder for injection—1 g/vial, 5 g/vial Injection—400 mg/vial, 500 mg/vial	IM use only: Tuberculosis—1 g/day, together with other antitubercular drugs (*e.g.,* isoniazid, ethambutol, rifampin); may reduce to 1 g 2 to 3 times a week as condition improves	Aminoglycoside isolated from a species of *Streptomyces;* fairly high toxicity and rapid development of resistance limits its usefulness to those infections not controlled by other less toxic drugs, except in tularemia, plague, and melioidosis, where it

Table 64-2. Aminoglycosides (continued)

Drug	Preparations	Usual Dosage Range	Remarks
		Tularemia—1 g to 2 g/day in divided doses for 7 days to 10 days Plague—2 g to 4 g/day in divided doses Bacterial endocarditis—0.5 g to 1 g twice a day Prophylaxis of bacterial endocarditis in patients undergoing intestinal or urinary tract surgery—1 g IM ½ hour to 1 hour before surgery in combination with 2 million U penicillin G or 1 g ampicillin IM or IV Other infections—1 g to 4 g/day in divided doses depending on severity of infection Children—20 mg to 40 mg/kg/day in divided doses every 6 hours to 12 hours	is the drug of choice, and tuberculosis, where it is commonly used in combination with several other tuberculostatic agents; (See Chap. 68); total treatment period for tuberculosis is a minimum of 1 year; also indicated for prophylaxis of bacterial endocarditis in high-risk patients undergoing respiratory, gastrointestinal, or genitourinary surgery or instrumentation, in combination with penicillin G or ampicillin; most frequent adverse effect is vestibular toxicity; observe for headache, vomiting, dizziness, difficulty in reading, or ataxia, and consult physician; incidence of nephrotoxicity is lowest of all aminoglycosides, but use with caution in renal impairment, and perform frequent determinations of serum drug concentration; adequate hydration is important, especially during prolonged therapy (e.g., tuberculosis therapy); commercially available IM solutions contain a preservative and should not be injected IV or SC; solution may darken during storage but potency is not affected
Tobramycin (Nebcin, Tobrex)	Injection—60 mg/1.5 ml; 80 mg/2 ml Pediatric injection—20 mg/2 ml Powder for injection—40 mg/ml when reconstituted Ophthalmic solution—0.3% Ophthalmic ointment—3 mg/g	IM, IV: Adults and children—3 mg/kg to 5 mg/kg/day in 3 to 4 equally divided doses depending on severity of infection Children—6 mg/kg to 7.5 mg/kg/day in 3 or 4 equally divided doses Neonates (1 wk or less)—up to 4 mg/kg/day in 2 equal doses every 12 hours Ophthalmic: 1 to 2 drops or ½-inch ribbon of ointment every 4 hours; in severe infections 2 drops every hour until improvement is noted	Aminoglycoside antibiotic with pharmacologic properties, indications, and overall toxicity similar to gentamicin; somewhat lower incidence of vestibular toxicity has been reported; do not exceed 5 mg/kg/day unless serum levels are monitored; prolonged serum concentrations above 12 mcg/ml should be avoided; urine should be observed for presence of protein, cells, and casts; follow package directions for dosage reduction in patients with renal impairment; reduced doses may be calculated based upon creatinine clearance or serum creatinine; IV dose should be diluted to 50 ml to 100 ml for adults (and proportionately less for children) with sodium chloride or 5% Dextrose Injection and infused over 20 minutes to 60 minutes do not premix with other drugs but administer separately; usual duration of treatment is 7 days to 10 days; in severe or complicated infections, a longer course of therapy may be necessary; auditory, vestibular, and renal function should be monitored frequently during prolonged therapy

of individual drugs are then presented in Table 64-2. The discussion focuses primarily on the parenteral use of the drugs, with references to their oral and topical application where appropriate.

Aminoglycosides

Amikacin	Netilmicin
Gentamicin	Paromomycin
Kanamycin	Streptomycin
Neomycin	Tobramycin

Mechanism

Inhibit protein synthesis in the bacterial cell; bind to the 30 S ribosomal subunit, causing a misreading of the genetic code and thus formation of improper peptide sequences in the protein chain

Uses

(See Tables 58-1 and 64-1 for susceptible organisms.)

1   Treatment of severe gram-negative infections of the GI, respiratory or urinary tracts, CNS, skin, bone, and soft tissues due to susceptible organisms (parenteral use only)
2   Suppression of intestinal bacteria (kanamycin or neomycin orally)
3   Treatment of acute or chronic intestinal amebiasis (paromomycin orally, see Chap. 71)
4   Adjunctive therapy of hepatic coma to reduce concentration of ammonia-forming bacteria in the GI tract (kanamycin, neomycin, or paromomycin orally)
5   Treatment of superficial infections of the eye, skin, or mucous membranes due to susceptible organisms (gentamicin or neomycin)
6   Treatment of severe diarrhea due to *Escherichia coli* (neomycin orally)

Dosage

See Table 64-2.

Fate

Not appreciably absorbed from the GI tract; absorption following IM injection is rapid; peak blood levels occur in 1 hour to 2 hours; plasma half-life is 1 hour to 4 hours with normal kidney function (see Table 64-1), but may be longer in infants (5 hr–8 hr), in elderly persons, or in patients with renal impairment (up to 96 hr); widely distributed in the body, except for the CNS (unless meninges are inflamed); drugs are not significantly protein-bound; serum levels in febrile patients are generally lower than those in afebrile patients given the same dosage, and half-lives are shorter; not metabolized to a significant extent, but eliminated largely unchanged by the kidneys following parenteral injection (up to 98% of a single IV dose is excreted within 24 hr); orally administered drugs are excreted almost completely in the feces

Common Side-Effects

Oral—nausea, diarrhea
Parenteral—headache, tinnitus, dizziness (especially at high doses)
Topical—hypersensitivity reactions (especially with neomycin)

Significant Adverse Reactions

Oral—"malabsorption syndrome" (*i.e.,* decreased absorption of vitamins, minerals, electrolytes, fats), steatorrhea, anorexia, stomatitis, salivation
Parenteral
CNS—ototoxicity (vertigo, ataxia, impaired hearing, irreversible deafness), confusion, disorientation, lethargy, depression, visual disturbances, amblyopia, nystagmus, optic neuritis, numbness and paresthesias, muscle twitching, tremor, convulsions
Renal—proteinuria, oliguria, azotemia, red and white cell casts in urine, increased BUN and serum creatinine.
Allergic—rash, pruritus, urticaria, alopecia, laryngeal edema, fever, exfoliative dermatitis, anaphylaxis
Hematologic—agranulocytosis, leukopenia, thrombocytopenia, eosinophilia, pancytopenia, anemia
Hepatic—increased serum transaminase and bilirubin, hepatomegaly, hepatic necrosis
Other—palpitations, myocarditis, splenomegaly, arthralgia, hypotension, pulmonary fibrosis, superinfections, muscle weakness, respiratory depression, pain and irritation with IM injection
Topical—burning, itching, urticaria, erythema, photosensitivity, macropapular dermatitis

Contraindications

Oral use in patients with bowel obstruction, long-term parenteral therapy in patients with renal impairment, and concurrent administration with other ototoxic or nephrotoxic drugs (see Interactions)

Interactions

1   Concurrent use of aminoglycosides and amphotericin, bacitracin, cephalothin, colistimethate, polymyxin, or vancomycin can increase the incidence of nephrotoxicity.
2   The ototoxic effects of the aminoglycosides can be enhanced by potent diuretics such as ethacrynic acid, bumetanide, furosemide, and mannitol.
3   Dimenhydrinate, meclizine, cyclizine, and other antivertigo drugs may mask the ototoxic effects of aminoglycosides.
4   Aminoglycosides can enhance the muscle-relaxing effects of neuromuscular blocking agents and general anesthetics, possibly leading to respiratory depression.
5   Aminoglycosides exert a synergistic effect with antipseudomonal penicillins (*e.g.,* carbenicillin, ticarcillin, piperacillin, mezlocillin, azlocillin) against *Pseudomonas* infections at normal concentrations; however, high concentrations of the penicillins may inhibit the antibacterial activity of aminoglycosides.

6 Orally administered neomycin and possibly other aminoglycosides may decrease the absorption of digoxin, penicillin V, and vitamin B$_{12}$.

▶ **NURSING ALERTS**

Warning: Aminoglycoside administration can result in serious ototoxicity, even with normal therapeutic doses, especially if renal function is impaired. Closely observe patients receiving aminoglycosides for evidence of ototoxicity (dizziness, tinnitus, vertigo, ataxia, nystagmus, hearing loss at high frequencies), and report immediately. Determine vestibular and auditory function before and at regular intervals during therapy, *especially* in patients with impaired kidney function or during prolonged treatment. Continue monitoring vestibular and auditory function for 3 weeks to 4 weeks after discontinuation of drug, because onset of hearing loss may be delayed.

▷ 1 Assess kidney function before initiating therapy, monitor intake–output ratio during therapy, and determine BUN and serum creatinine values as a guide to dosage adjustments. Decreased urinary output and urinary creatinine levels, increased BUN or serum creatinine levels are signs of possible nephrotoxicity and indicate the need for dosage reduction or discontinuation of therapy.

▷ 2 Use with caution in patients with impaired renal function (reduce dose or increase dosage interval or both), in young children, in elderly patients, and in pregnant or nursing women. Also administer cautiously to patients with neuromuscular disorders (*e.g.,* myasthenia, parkinsonism) or following use of general anesthetics or skeletal muscle relaxants, because respiratory paralysis can occur.

▷ 3 Monitor trough drug levels at regular intervals and adjust dosage as necessary to ensure that drug cumulation does not occur.

▷ 4 Avoid concurrent or sequential administration of other potentially ototoxic or nephrotoxic drugs (see Interactions).

▷ 5 Keep patients well hydrated to prevent irritation of the renal tubules. If signs of renal irritation are noted (red or white cells, albumin, or casts in urine), increase fluid intake (*i.e.,* 2000 cc–3000 cc per day) to prevent further damage.

▷ 6 Be alert for signs of bacterial or fungal overgrowth (superinfections) as indicated by diarrhea, "furry" tongue, stomatitis, glossitis, or perianal itching or irritation, and treat with appropriate anti-infective.

▷ 7 Administer oral drugs cautiously to patients with ulcerative lesions of the bowel, because systemic absorption may be enhanced, increasing renal toxicity.

▷ 8 Infuse slowly IV, to minimize the possibility of severe neuromuscular blockade and subsequent development of apnea.

▶ **NURSING CONSIDERATIONS**
(See Table 64-2 for additional information on each drug.)

▷ 1 In treating urinary infections, consider administering an alkalinizing agent (*e.g.,* sodium bicarbonate) to elevate urinary *p*H, because drugs are more active in an alkaline medium.

▷ 2 Inject deeply IM into large muscle mass, observe for signs of irritation, and rotate injection sites as necessary.

▷ 3 Be aware that normal duration of therapy for most infections is 7 days to 10 days. Severe or complicated infections may require prolonged aminoglycoside treatment. In such cases, frequently monitor renal, auditory, and vestibular function, because likelihood of toxicity increases with extended therapy.

▷ 4 Advise patients to report immediately any ringing in the ears, decreased hearing acuity, dizziness, or unsteady gait, because these may be signs of ototoxicity.

▷ 5 Advise patients using drugs topically to discontinue medication and inform physician if allergic symptoms develop (rash, pruritus, urticaria, angioedema).

▷ 6 Use topical neomycin-containing products with caution in treating extensive burns or ulcerated skin areas where significant systemic absorption is possible.

▷ 7 Do not apply topical neomycin or gentamicin ointment to the eyes or to the external ear canal if eardrum is perforated. Use only ophthalmic preparations (ophthalmic ointment or drops) in the eye.

▷ 8 Note that bacterial resistance to aminoglycosides develops slowly, with the exception of streptomycin, in which case resistance can occur very rapidly (see Chap. 68).

▷ 9 Consult package instructions for appropriate dosage modifications in patients with impaired renal function. Parameters used to determine proper dosage adjustments include trough serum levels of aminoglycoside and creatinine clearance.

▷ 10 Use reconstituted solutions as soon as possible after mixing because drugs are relatively unstable in solution. Check manufacturer's instructions for stability data.

65 Polypeptides

The polypeptide group of antibiotics comprises polymyxin B, colistin (polymyxin E), the methanesulfonate salt of colistin (colistimethate), and bacitracin. The first three of these drugs are commonly termed the *polymyxins,* and while certain similarities exist between these agents and bacitracin, significant differences are noted as well.

The polymyxins are a group of strongly basic polypeptides obtained from *Bacillus polymyxa* and variants, and are designated as polymyxins A, B, C, D, and E. Of these, only polymyxins B and E are employed clinically, because the remaining derivatives are too toxic for human use. Shortly after introduction of the polymyxins, another polypeptide was isolated from the colistinus strain of *Bacillus polymyxa* and was named colistin. Subsequent work revealed colistin to be identical to polymyxin E.

The polymyxins are bactericidal, primarily against gram-negative bacilli such as *Pseudomonas, Escherichia coli, Klebsiella, Enterobacter, Salmonella, Shigella,* and *Hemophilus.* However, most strains of *Proteus* and *Neisseria* and virtually all gram-positive organisms are unaffected by the polymyxins. They exert their antibacterial action by disrupting the bacterial cell membrane, thus allowing cell constituents to escape. The drugs are not absorbed orally, and following parenteral administration, they do not reach the CNS (unless given intrathecally), the joints, or the eye in appreciable amounts. Excretion is by the kidney (except oral colistin), thus cumulation toxicity can occur in the presence of renal impairment. The polymyxins are used systemically only for severe infections, especially of the urinary tract, caused by susceptible gram-negative organisms not sensitive to other less toxic antimicrobial drugs. The drugs find their widest application for topical treatment of skin and mucous membrane infections (including the eye and ear), especially if *Pseudomonas* is the offending pathogen. Principal adverse effects are of two major types, neurotoxicity and nephrotoxicity, and the incidence and severity of these untoward reactions severely limit the systemic usefulness of the polymyxins to all but very severe infections.

Polymyxin B is available as an injection, a powder for preparing ophthalmic drops, and in several combination products (*e.g.,* with neomycin, bacitracin, and corticosteroids) for ophthalmic or otic use. Colistin sulfate (polymyxin E) can be used either as an oral suspension for control of diarrhea and gastroenteritis or in combination with hydrocortisone and neomycin as ear drops (ColyMycin S Otic). Colistimethate, as a powder for injection, may be administered either IV or IM for serious systemic or urinary infections, particularly when caused by *Pseudomonas.* Because there are many differences among these three polymyxin preparations, they are considered individually in this chapter.

Bacitracin is a mixture of several polypeptides isolated from a strain of *Bacillus subtilis,* the major constituent being bacitracin A. This antibiotic appears to inhibit bacterial cell wall formation and is bactericidal against a variety of gram-positive bacteria as well as a few gram-negative organisms. The drug is available for IM injection, and as a topical and ophthalmic ointment. Because of its potential for serious toxicity, however, it is used parenterally *only* for treatment of staphylococcal pneumonia or empyema in infants. Bacitracin is most often used topically, alone or in combination with neomycin and polymyxin, for treatment of cutaneous or ocular infections, because it is highly effective against susceptible organisms and rarely causes hypersensitivity reactions. Kidney damage is a major danger with parenteral use of bacitracin and renal function must be closely monitored during therapy.

▶ bacitracin
Baciguent

Mechanism
Not completely established; probably acts by inhibiting bacterial cell wall synthesis and may alter cell membrane permeability as well; bactericidal at therapeutic doses; spectrum of action *in vitro* is similar to that of penicillin G

Uses
1 Treatment of staphylococcal pneumonia or empyema in infants (IM use)
2 Treatment of superficial infections of the skin, mucous membranes, and eye due to susceptible organisms (topical use only)

Dosage
IM: (infants under 2.5 kg) 900 U/kg/day in two or three divided doses; (infants over 2.5 kg) 1000 U/kg/day in two or three divided doses
Topical: apply two or three times a day to affected area
Ophthalmic: apply to lower conjuctival sac several times a day

Fate
Rapidly absorbed from IM injection site; distributed widely in the body, except in CNS; duration of action is 6 hours to 8 hours with single IM doses; excreted largely in the urine

Common Side-Effects
Pain and irritation at IM injection site

Significant Adverse Reactions

Warning: Bacitracin (IM) can result in renal failure, due to glomerular injury or tubular necrosis. Use only when indicated (see Uses), monitor renal function daily, and maintain adequate fluid intake.

Renal—proteinuria, azotemia, urinary frequency, oliguria, hematuria, increased BUN, uremia, renal failure
Other—neuromuscular weakness, hypersensitivity reactions (rash, urticaria, hypotension), nausea, vomiting, tinnitus, diarrhea, altered taste sensations, allergic contact dermatitis (with topical use)

Contraindications
Severe renal impairment

Interactions
1 Nephrotoxic effects of bacitracin may be additive to those of other antibiotics having similar toxicity, for example, aminoglycosides, polymyxins, vancomycin.
2 Bacitracin can enhance or prolong the muscle-relaxing effects of neuromuscular blocking agents and anesthetics, or other drugs with neuromuscular blocking actions, that is, aminoglycosides, procainamide, succinylcholine.

▶ NURSING ALERTS
▷ 1 Be aware that parenteral use of bacitracin may cause renal failure due to tubular or glomerular necrosis. Use only for infections specified (see Uses), and have patients under constant supervision during treatment.
▷ 2 Perform renal function tests before initiation of therapy and daily throughout the course of treatment. Closely monitor urinary output and maintain fluid intake at a sufficient level to avoid renal toxicity.
▷ 3 Observe for early indications of renal dysfunction (hematuria, proteinuria, oliguria, increased BUN, frequent urination), and discontinue drug immediately.

▶ NURSING CONSIDERATIONS
▷ 1 Dissolve drug in Sodium Chloride Injection containing 2% procaine hydrochloride, because IM injections are painful.
▷ 2 Note that bacitracin solutions are rapidly inactivated at room temperature but are stable up to 1 week if refrigerated.
▷ 3 Be alert for the development of hypersensitivity reactions with topical application (rash, pruritus, urticaria) and advise physician should these reactions develop.

▶ colistimethate
Coly-Mycin M

Mechanism
Disrupts the bacterial cell membrane, probably through a surface action, thus allowing escape of cell constituents

Uses
1 Treatment of acute or chronic infections due to sensitive strains of certain gram-negative organisms, especially *Pseudomonas aeruginosa, Escherichia coli, Klebsiella pneumoniae,* and *Enterobacter aerogenes* (not effective against *Proteus* or *Neisseria*)

Dosage
Adults and children: 2.5 mg/kg to 5 mg/kg/day, IM or IV, in two to four divided doses (maximum 5 mg/kg/day in patients with normal renal function)
IV administration may be by direct injection (one half daily dose over 3 min–5 min every 12 hr) or by infusion (one half dose over 3 min–5 min, then 5 mg–6 mg/hr starting 1 hr–2 hr after initial injection)

Fate

Absorption from IM sites is good; blood levels are maximum 1 hour to 2 hours after IM injection, 10 minutes to 15 minutes after IV administration; serum half-life is 2 hours to 3 hours; does not enter CNS, even if meninges are inflamed; excreted primarily in the urine, mostly within 18 hours to 24 hours.

Common Side-Effects

Pain at IM injection site

Significant Adverse Reactions

Renal—decreased urine output, increased BUN, proteinuria, azotemia, renal failure

Neurologic—paresthesias; numbness in the extremities; visual, auditory, or speech disturbances; dizziness; ataxia

Allergic—pruritus, urticaria, drug fever, dermatoses

Other—neuromuscular blockade (muscle weakness, respiratory depression or paralysis), GI upset, agranulocytosis, superinfections

Contraindications

Severe renal failure

Interactions

See Bacitracin.

▶ NURSING ALERTS

▷ 1 Perform baseline renal function tests before therapy and monitor renal function during drug treatment. Be alert for changes in urinary output or elevations in BUN, serum creatinine, or plasma drug levels, possible indications of renal toxicity.

▷ 2 Instruct patients to report immediately any changes in visual, auditory, or verbal function, drowsiness, dizziness or paresthesias, possible early signs of developing toxicity. Urge caution in driving or operating machinery.

▷ 3 Use cautiously in patients with myasthenia gravis, renal impairment, or in persons receiving muscle relaxants or potentially nephrotoxic drugs (*e.g.,* aminoglycosides, vancomycin).

▷ 4 Be aware that respiratory arrest has occurred following injection. Have appropriate resuscitative equipment and drugs available, and observe closely for dyspnea, chest pain, or restlessness, signs of respiratory distress.

▷ 5 Do not exceed 5 mg/kg/day, even in patients with normal renal function, because overdosage can result in severe muscle weakness, apnea, and renal insufficiency.

▶ NURSING CONSIDERATIONS

▷ 1 Administer deeply IM into a large muscle and rotate injection sites. Injections may be painful.

▷ 2 Prepare IV infusion solution with appropriate diluent according to package instructions and use within 24 hours.

▷ 3 Note that reconstituted IM drug solution is stable for 7 days, either at room temperature or refrigerated.

▷ 4 Be alert for signs of superinfection with drug-resistant strains (diarrhea, perianal irritation, fever), and initiate appropriate therapy.

▶ colistin sulfate

Coly-Mycin S

Mechanism

Disrupts bacterial cell membrane, causing loss of cellular constituents; bactericidal against most gram-negative enteric pathogens, except *Proteus*

Uses

1 Control of diarrhea in infants and children due to susceptible strains of enteropathogenic *Escherichia coli* (oral suspension)

2 Treatment of gastroenteritis due to *Shigella* organisms (oral suspension)

3 Treatment of superficial infections of the ear canal (combination with neomycin and hydrocortisone as Coly-Mycin S Otic)

Dosage

Oral—adults and children: 5 mg/kg to 15 mg/kg/day in three divided doses; higher doses may be required in severe infections

Otic—three or four drops into external ear canal three or four times a day

Fate

Not absorbed to a significant extent from the GI tract; effects are localized; excreted in the feces

Significant Adverse Reactions

None reported at recommended doses; superinfection can occur with prolonged use

Contraindications

(Topical use only) Fungal or viral infections of the ear, herpes simplex, vaccinia, varicella

Interactions

See Bacitracin for *potential* drug interactions; actual incidence is minimal, because drug is not absorbed systemically

▶ NURSING ALERT

▷ 1 Recognize that slight systemic absorption may occur in some instances and renal toxicity is possible, especially if large doses are employed or azotemia is present. Use cautiously in patients with pre-existing kidney damage.

▶ NURSING CONSIDERATIONS

▷ 1 Reconstitute powder for oral suspension with distilled water. Store in refrigerator and discard any unused portion after 2 weeks.

▷ 2 Clean and dry external ear canal before instillation of drops.

▷ 3 Note that otic solution contains neomycin and should therefore be used very cautiously where eardrum is perforated or chronic otitis media exists, because neomycin is ototoxic.

▶ polymyxin B sulfate
Aerosporin

Mechanism
Disrupts the lipoprotein cell membrane of susceptible bacteria, resulting in leakage of cellular constituents and cell death

Uses
1 Treatment of acute infections due to susceptible strains of *Pseudomonas aeruginosa* (IM, IV)
2 Alternate treatment of severe infections of the blood, meninges, or urinary tract due to *Escherichia coli, Klebsiella pneumoniae, Enterobacter aerogenes,* or *Hemophilus influenzae,* when less toxic drugs are ineffective (IM, IV)
3 Treatment of superficial infections of the eye, ear, mucous membranes, or skin due to susceptible organisms (topical combination products containing polymyxin B)

Dosage
IV infusion:
Adults and children—15,000 U/kg to 25,000 U/kg/day; infusions may be given every 12 hours
Infants—Up to 40,000 U/kg/day
IM:
Adults and children—25,000 U/kg to 30,00 U/kg/day, divided and given at 4-hour to 6-hour intervals
Infants—up to 40,000 U/kg/day
Intrathecal (*e.g.,* in pseudomonal meningitis):
Adults and children (over 2 yr)—50,000 U once daily for 3 days to 4 days; then 50,000 U every other day for at least 2 weeks after cultures of the cerebrospinal fluid are negative and glucose content has returned to normal.
Children (under 2 yr)—20,000 U once daily for 3 days to 4 days; then 25,000 U every other day
Ophthalmic:
One or two drops in affected eye several times a day, as necessary
Topical:
Apply several times a day to affected area

Fate
Not significantly absorbed from the GI tract or mucous membranes; peak plasma concentrations are reached within 2 hours after IM injection; plasma half-life is 4 hours to 6 hours; active blood levels are low, because drug loses up to one half its activity in the serum; activity levels are higher in infants and children than in adults; diffusion into many tissues is poor, and drug does not enter CNS unless given intrathecally; slowly excreted by the kidneys, largely in unchanged form

Common Side-Effects
Pain on IM injection

Significant Adverse Reactions

Warning: Nephrotoxicity and neurotoxicity can occur, especially with IM or intrathecal administration. Administer only to hospitalized patients and provide constant supervision.

Renal—proteinuria, hematuria, azotemia, cellular casts, increasing blood levels of drug without increases in dosage
Neurologic—flushing, paresthesias, drowsiness, dizziness, neuromuscular blockade (muscle weakness, respiratory depression, apnea)
Hypersensitivity—pruritis, dermatoses, urticaria, drug fever, local burning or irritation with topical application
Other—meningeal irritation (headache, stiff neck, fever) with intrathecal administration, thrombophlebitis with IV infusion, GI disturbances, overgrowth of nonsusceptible organisms

Contraindications
Severe renal impairment, concurrent use of other nephrotoxic or neurotoxic drugs (*e.g.,* bacitracin, aminoglycosides, colistimethate)

Interactions
See Bacitracin.

▶ NURSING ALERTS
▷ 1 Administer IM or intrathecally to hospitalized patients only, because constant supervision is necessary.
▷ 2 Be aware that IM injection may cause severe pain, especially in infants and children. Avoid IM administration if possible.
▷ 3 Perform baseline renal function tests and monitor kidney function closely during therapy. Renal toxicity usually occurs within several days after start of treatment. Note any reductions in urinary output or increases in BUN, serum creatinine, plasma drug levels, or urinary proteins and discontinue drug if these occur.
▷ 4 Advise patients to immediately report signs of neuromuscular blockade (shortness of breath, dyspnea, muscle weakness). Discontinue drug and treat symptoms as necessary. Resuscitative measures (*e.g.,* respiratory aids, oxygen, calcium chloride) should be readily available.
▷ 5 Inform patients that signs of neurotoxicity may develop (irritability, paresthesias, dizziness, numbness, blurring of vision) but generally can be eliminated by a dosage reduction. Urge prompt recognition and reporting.

▶ NURSING CONSIDERATIONS
▷ 1 Be alert for overgrowth of nonsusceptible organisms and administer appropriate anti-infective agents.

▷ 2 Administer polymyxin only by the intrathecal route in treating meningeal infections, because drug does not penetrate the blood–brain barrier.

▷ 3 Reconstitute drug with the following diluents:
IM—Sterile Water for Injection, Sterile Physiologic Saline, or 1% Procaine Hydrochloride Solution
IV—5% Dextrose in Water
Intrathecal—Sterile Physiologic Saline
Opthalmic drops—Sterile Physiologic Saline or Sterile Distilled Water

▷ 4 Store reconstituted parenteral solutions under refrigeration and discard unused portion after 72 hours.

▷ 5 Avoid *total* systemic and ophthalmic dosage of greater than 30,000 U/kg/day.

▷ 6 Urge maintenance of a daily fluid intake sufficient to produce an output of at least 1500 ml/day.

▷ 7 Note that polymyxin is available as either a solution or ointment for ophthalmic use with neomycin (Statrol), bacitracin (Polysporin), oxytetracycline (Terramycin), neomycin plus bacitracin (Neosporin Ophthalmic, Ak-Sporin), and neomycin plus a corticosteroid (Cortisporin Ophthalmic, Maxitrol).

▷ 8 Be aware that polymyxin is also available as an otic solution or suspension with hydrocortisone (Pyocidin-Otic Solution), and hydrocortisone plus neomycin (Cortisporin Otic, Otobione) for treatment of superficial ear infections.

▷ 9 Warm ear drops before instilling into auditory canal but avoid heating beyond body temperature, because loss of potency can occur.

▷ 10 Note that polymyxin is not available *alone* for topical application, but is found in combination with various other antibiotics in many different ointments, aerosols, and powders.

▷ 11 Be aware that polymyxin and neomycin are available as a genitourinary irrigant solution (Neosporin G. U. Irrigant) for use with catheter systems, permitting continuous irrigation of the urinary bladder. Solution contains 40 mg neomycin and 200,000 U polymyxin B sulfate per milliliter.

Summary. Polypeptides

Drug	Preparations	Usual Dosage Range
Bacitracin (Baciguent)	Injection—10,000 U/vial, 50,000 U/vial Ophthalmic ointment—500 U/g Topical ointment—500 U/g	IM: 900 U/kg to 1000 U/kg/day in 2 to 3 divided doses Topical: Apply 2 to 3 times a day Ophthalmic: Apply to lower conjunctival sac several times a day
Colistimethate (Coly-Mycin M)	Powder for injection—150 mg/vial	Adults and children—2.5 mg/kg to 5 mg/kg/day IM or IV in 2 to 4 divided doses
Colistin sulfate (Coly-Mycin S)	Oral suspension—25 mg/5 ml Otic suspension—3 mg/ml with neomycin and hydrocortisone	Oral: 5 mg/kg to 15 mg/kg/day in 3 divided doses Otic: 3 to 4 drops into ear canal 3 to 4 times a day
Polymyxin B sulfate (Aerosporin)	Injection—500,000 U/vial Powder for ophthalmic drops—500,000 U (50 mg)/vial Otic solution—10,000 U/ml	IV infusion: 15,000 U/kg to 25,000 U/kg/day; infants—up to 40,000 U/kg/day; infusions given every 12 hours IM: 25,000 U/kg to 30,000 U/kg/day divided and given every 4 hours to 6 hours; infants—up to 40,000 U/kg/day Intrathecal: Adults and children (over 2 yr)—50,000 U once daily for 3 days to 4 days, then 50,000 U every other day Children (under 2 yr)—20,000 U once daily for 3 days to 4 days, then 25,000 U every other day Ophthalmic: 1 to 2 drops several times/day Topical: Apply several times a day to affected area

Although the term *urinary anti-infective* refers theoretically to any drug capable of eradicating pathogens present in the urinary tract, it is generally applied only to those agents specific for urinary infections by virtue of their lack of significant *systemic* antibacterial action. Thus, while other antimicrobial drugs, such as broad-spectrum penicillins, cephalosporins, tetracyclines, sulfonamides, aminoglycosides, and polypeptides, have all been employed successfully in the treatment of urinary tract infections, they are not considered specific urinary anti-infectives because most attain significant plasma levels throughout the body and can therefore be used to treat a number of systemic infections as well. The drugs considered to be selective urinary anti-infectives are cinoxacin, methenamine, nalidixic acid, nitrofurantoin, and trimethoprim. Although specific for urinary infections by virtue of their rapid elimination in the urine and their lack of significant systemic antimicrobial activity, these agents are usually not considered drugs of choice for acute uncomplicated urinary tract infections, inasmuch as they are not as effective against many common urinary pathogens as sulfonamides, broad-spectrum penicillins, or cephalosporins. The urinary anti-infectives are most often reserved for those persons who are either intolerant of or unresponsive to one of the first-line drugs. Urinary anti-infectives are also of value for the control of *chronic* urinary infections due to organisms that have developed resistance to commonly used antibiotics. For example, low doses of nitrofurantoin, administered once a day at bedtime, have been used successfully for long-term prophylaxis in chronic urinary infections. Likewise, trimethoprim–sulfamethoxazole and methenamine have also been employed for chemoprophylaxis of chronic urinary infections.

The fact that urinary anti-infectives generally do not attain effective antibacterial blood levels does not mean that they are free of systemic toxic effects. On the contrary, with the exception of methenamine, the other agents in this group all have the potential to elicit serious untoward reactions, and their use should be accorded the same respect as any other antimicrobial drug.

Patients receiving a urinary anti-infective drug should be advised to continue taking the prescribed dose for the recommended period of time (usually 10 days–14 days) even though the symptoms of the infection, such as low back pain, burning on urination, or fever, have disappeared. *Complete* eradication of the infecting organism, not simply symptomatic relief, is the goal of urinary chemotherapy, because relapses and re-infection are major problems in the treatment of urinary infections. A relapse, the result of failure to eliminate completely the original pathogen from the urinary system with the initial course of therapy, is most often due to insufficient dose or duration of therapy, or both. Recurring infections are frequently noted some time after successful recovery from an initial attack, and are often caused by microorganisms different from those responsible for the initial infection. These may include resistant forms that have emerged during the first course of therapy.

Perhaps the most troublesome situation is the chronic urinary infection that often complicates an anatomic or physiologic abnormality such as urinary stones, urethral strictures, or prostate enlargement. Treatment of these con-

Urinary
Anti-Infectives

66

ditions requires prolonged therapy with a urinary anti-infective capable of interfering with bacterial growth without favoring emergence of resistant organisms. The most commonly employed drugs for chronic urinary conditions are trimethoprim–sulfamethoxazole (see Chap. 59), nitrofurantoin, and methenamine. Of course, surgical intervention is often necessary when a blockage or some other anatomic lesion is present.

In addition to the urinary anti-infectives mentioned above, several other drugs may be employed in urinary infections. Methylene blue, a dye, is a weak germicide and is occasionally used orally as a mild urinary antiseptic. Phenazopyridine, another dye, is excreted in the urine following oral ingestion and exerts a mild analgesic effect. It is used to relieve irritation and pain in conjunction with an appropriate anti-infective. Acetohydroxamic acid (AHA) inhibits the urease-mediated hydrolysis of urea and the subsequent production of ammonia in urine infected with urea-splitting organisms. It is indicated as adjunctive therapy in chronic urea-splitting urinary infections.

Inasmuch as significant differences exist among the various urinary anti-infective agents with respect to actions, indications, and toxicity, they are reviewed individually below.

▶ cinoxacin
Cinobac

Mechanism
Inhibits DNA replication in susceptible bacteria within the range of urinary *p*H; bactericidal at normal dose levels; active against most strains of *Escherichia coli, Klebsiella* species, *Enterobacter* species, and *Proteus* species; not effective against *Pseudomonas,* staphylococci, or enterococci.

Use
1 Treatment of initial and recurrent urinary tract infections in adults caused by susceptible organisms (see above)

Dosage
1 g/day, orally, in two to four divided doses for 7 days to 14 days; reduce dosage in patients with impaired renal function according to package directions

Fate
Rapidly absorbed from GI tract; peak serum concentrations occur within 1 hour to 2 hours, and detectable levels persist for 10 hours to 12 hours; excreted almost entirely in the urine, 60% as unaltered drug and the remainder as metabolites; peak urine levels are noted within 2 hours to 4 hours

Common Side-Effects
Nausea, cramping

Significant Adverse Reactions
GI—anorexia, vomiting, diarrhea
CNS—headache, tinnitus, photophobia, insomnia, dizziness, tingling sensation, nervousness, confusion
Hypersensitivity—rash, pruritus, urticaria, edema
Other—altered BUN, SGOT, SGPT, serum creatinine, and alkaline phosphatase

Contraindications
Pregnancy, prepubertal children, and anuria

Interactions
See Nalidixic Acid. Cinoxacin is chemically related to nalidixic acid and may exhibit the same potential drug interactions.

▶ NURSING ALERTS
▷ 1 Use cautiously in patients with impaired renal or hepatic function and in nursing mothers.
▷ 2 Reduce dosage in patients with decreased renal function. An initial dose of 500 mg is followed by maintenance doses determined on the basis of creatinine clearance (or serum creatinine) according to the package instructions.

▶ NURSING CONSIDERATIONS
▷ 1 Tell patient to take drug for the *entire* prescribed course of therapy even though clinical symptoms may disappear within a few days.
▷ 2 Administer drug with food if GI distress occurs.
▷ 3 Perform *in vitro* susceptibility tests before administration and during treatment if clinical response is unsatisfactory.

▶ methenamine

Methenamine is a urinary antibacterial agent whose action depends on its hydrolysis to ammonia and formaldehyde in an acidic urine. Formaldehyde is bactericidal against a variety of gram-positive and gram-negative organisms (see Mechanism below). Methenamine is most often used in the form of an acid salt (hippurate, mandelate), which helps maintain a low urinary *p*H. Characteristics of the different methenamine salts, as well as methenamine base (which is also clinically available), are presented in Table 66-1.

Mechanism
In an acid urine (*p*H 5.5 or lower), drug is hydrolyzed to form ammonia and formaldehyde, the latter being bactericidal; acid liberated from the salt (*i.e.,* mandelic or hippuric) may also exert a weak antibacterial action; susceptible organisms include *Escherichia coli,* staphylococci, and enterococci. *Enterobacter aerogenes* is resistant, as are *Pseudomonas* and *Proteus* species, the latter two being urea-splitting organisms that can raise urinary *p*H above the effective level.

Uses
1 Treatment of chronic bacteriuria associated with cystitis, pyelonephritis, or other chronic urinary conditions
2 Prophylaxis before urinary instrumentation or catheterization

Table 66-1. Methenamine Derivatives

Drug	Preparations	Usual Dosage Range	Remarks
Methenamine	Tablets—0.5 g	Adults—1 g 4 times a day Children (6 yr–12 yr)—500 mg 4 times a day Children (under 6 yr)—50 mg/kg/day in 3 divided doses	Over-the-counter preparation; infrequently used, because lack of acid salt reduces its clinical effectiveness
Methenamine hippurate (Hiprex, Urex)	Tablets—1 g	Adults—1 g twice a day Children (6 yr–12 yr)—0.5 g to 1 g twice a day	Effective in lower daily doses than mandelate salt; safe use in early pregnancy has not been established; may transiently elevate serum transaminase levels; periodic liver function tests are indicated
Methenamine mandelate (Mandelamine)	Tablets—0.5 g, 1 g Enteric-coated tablets—0.25 g, 0.5 g, 1 g Oral suspension—0.25 g/5 ml Suspension forte—0.5 g/5 ml Granules—0.5 g/packet, 1 g/packet	Adults—1 g 4 times a day Children (6 yr–12 yr)—0.5 g 4 times a day Children (under 6 yr)—0.25 g/30 lb 4 times a day	Most commonly used methenamine salt; enteric-coated tablets are claimed to lower incidence of GI upset; oral suspensions have a vegetable oil base; use cautiously in elderly or debilitated patients due to danger of aspiration (lipid) pneumonia; granules are orange flavored

3 Adjunctive treatment of patients with anatomic abnormalities of the urinary tract

Dosage

See Table 66-1.

Fate

Readily absorbed orally; excreted largely unchanged (75%–90%) in the urine within 24 hours; formation of formaldehyde is dependent on urinary pH, level of methenamine, and length of time urine is retained in the bladder; peak formaldehyde concentrations occur at a urine pH of 5.5 or less; a level of 25 mcg/ml or greater is necessary for antimicrobial activity

Common Side-Effects

GI upset with large doses

Significant Adverse Reactions

Cramping, vomiting, diarrhea, stomatitis, anorexia, urinary frequency or urgency, bladder irritation, dysuria, proteinuria, hematuria, hypersensitivity reactions (rash, pruritus), and abdominal pain

Contraindications

Renal insufficiency, severe hepatic disease (because ammonia is liberated), and severe dehydration

Interactions

1 Sulfonamides can form insoluble precipitates with formaldehyde in the urine.
2 Effectiveness of methenamine can be reduced by drugs that raise urinary pH, for example, sodium bicarbonate, acetazolamide, thiazide diuretics.
3 Methenamine salts may increase the urinary excretion of amphetamines, lowering their activity.

▶ **NURSING ALERTS**

▷ 1 Do not use alone for acute infections or infections with renal parenchymal involvement associated with systemic symptoms.
▷ 2 Use cautiously in pregnant or nursing mothers, and in patients with gout, because methenamine salts may cause precipitation of urate crystals in the urine.

▶ **NURSING CONSIDERATIONS**

▷ 1 Monitor intake–output ratio. Provide adequate fluids (8–10 glasses of water per day), but be aware that *excessive* hydration and the resultant increased urinary flow can reduce the amount of free formaldehyde in the urine.
▷ 2 Monitor urinary pH (*e.g.,* with Nitrazine paper; see Chap. 78). Provide supplementary acidification (*e.g.,* ascorbic acid, 4 g–12 g/day in divided doses) if urinary pH exceeds 5.5.
▷ 3 If dysuria occurs, reduce dosage and acidify urine. Large doses (8 g/day for several weeks) have caused bladder irritation, painful urination, and hematuria.
▷ 4 Recognize that methenamine is *not* suitable for prevention of urinary infections in patients with indwelling catheters, because the bladder does not retain the drug long enough to form sufficient levels of formaldehyde.
▷ 5 To minimize GI distress, administer drug with food around the clock at regular intervals, if possible. Complete entire prescribed course of therapy.
▷ 6 Inform physician if skin rash or painful urination occurs.
▷ 7 Note that bacteria and fungi do *not* develop resistance to formaldehyde, making methenamine suitable for long-term prophylaxis in chronic infections.
▷ 8 Be aware that methenamine can interfere with laboratory urine determination of catecholamines, 17-hy-

droxycorticosteroids, estriol, and 5-hydroxyindole-
acetic acid (5-HIAA), a serotonin metabolite.
▷ 9 Perform periodic liver function studies in patients with
liver dysfunction undergoing prolonged therapy.
▷ 10 Note that methenamine is also available in many combination products with anticholinergics, urinary acidifiers, methylene blue, and salicylates.

▷ *Dietary precaution*
▷ 1 Advise patients to avoid excessive intake of alkalinizing
foods such as milk or citrus fruits.

▶ methylene blue
Urolene Blue

Mechanism
Exerts a weak germicidal action; it is primarily bacteriostatic; high concentrations convert the ferrous iron of reduced
hemoglobin to the ferric state, resulting in formation of
methemoglobin; this latter action is the basis for its use as
an antidote in cyanide poisoning

Uses
1 Symptomatic treatment of cystitis and urethritis (infrequent use)
2 Treatment of idiopathic and drug-induced methemoglobinemia and as an antidote for cyanide poisoning
(oral or IV)

Dosage
Oral: 65 mg to 130 mg 3 times/day
IV: 1 mg/kg to 2 mg/kg injected over several minutes

Common Side-Effects
Discoloration of the urine

Significant Adverse Reactions
Nausea, vomiting, diarrhea, bladder irritation; large doses
can cause abdominal pain, fever, dizziness, headache,
sweating, and confusion

Contraindications
Renal insufficiency, intraspinal injection

▶ NURSING ALERTS
▷ 1 Use cautiously in patients with glucose-6-phosphate
dehydrogenase deficiency, anemia, and decreased hemoglobin levels.
▷ 2 Be aware that cyanosis and cardiovascular abnormalities have been noted, especially with IV administration.

▶ NURSING CONSIDERATIONS
▷ 1 Administer oral drug after meals with a full glass of
water.
▷ 2 Inform patients that drug may discolor urine and possibly the stool blue–green.
▷ 3 Give slowly IV (over several minutes) and do not
exceed recommended dosage.

▶ nalidixic acid
Neg Gram

Mechanism
Bactericidal over the entire urinary *p*H range against most
gram-negative bacteria causing urinary infections; probably
acts by inhibiting DNA polymerization, and may impair RNA
synthesis as well; exhibits good activity against *Proteus* species, *Escherichia coli*, *Enterobacter*, and *Klebsiella*; ineffective against *Pseudomonas*; resistance has developed in
some cases

Use
1 Treatment of urinary tract infections caused by susceptible organisms (see above); disk susceptibility
testing should be performed; see Chapter 58

Dosage
Adults: initially 1 g four times a day for 2 weeks; reduce
to 2 g/day in divided doses for prolonged therapy
Children (over 3 mo): initially 55 mg/kg/day in four
divided doses for at least 2 weeks; maintenance dose
is 33 mg/kg/day

Fate
Rapidly absorbed orally; peak serum levels occur in 1
hour to 2 hours, and peak urine levels in 3 hours to 4 hours;
highly (90%–95%) protein-bound in plasma; partially metabolized in the liver and rapidly excreted by the kidneys
both as unchanged drug and several metabolites; hydroxy-
nalidixic acid, an active metabolite, represents 85% of the
biologically active drug in the urine

Common Side-Effects
Nausea, diarrhea, and abdominal distress

Significant Adverse Reactions
CNS—drowsiness, dizziness, weakness, headache, vertigo, visual disturbances (*e.g.,* difficulty in focusing,
double vision, altered color perception), convulsions
(with large doses)
Infants and children may experience increased intracranial pressure, papilledema, severe headache, and
bulging anterior fontanel.
Allergic—rash, pruritus, urticaria, angio-edema, eosinophilia, arthralgia, photosensitivity reactions, anaphylactic reaction (rare)
Other—(rare) GI bleeding, cholestasis, paresthesias,
metabolic acidosis, blood dyscrasias, glucose 6-phos-
phate dehydrogenase deficiency, toxic psychosis

Contraindications
History of convulsive disorders, early pregnancy, and in
infants under 3 months

Interactions
1 Nalidixic acid may potentiate the action of other
strongly protein-bound drugs (*e.g.,* oral anticoagulants,
phenytoin, oral hypoglycemics, anti-inflammatory
agents).

2 Nitrofurantoin may inhibit the antibacterial activity of nalidixic acid.

3 Urinary acidifiers can potentiate the antibacterial activity of nalidixic acid by reducing its urinary excretion *rate*.

4 Antacids may impair GI absorption of nalidixic acid, reducing its activity.

5 Cross-resistance has occurred between nalidixic acid and cinoxacin.

▶ **NURSING ALERTS**

▷ 1 Use with caution in patients with liver disease, epilepsy, cerebral arteriosclerosis, severe renal failure, and in young children, because cartilage erosion can occur in weight-bearing joints.

▷ 2 Perform periodic blood counts and liver function tests during prolonged (greater than 2 wk) therapy.

▷ 3 Caution patients receiving the drug to avoid excessive exposure to sunlight. Discontinue drug if photosensitivity reactions occur.

▷ 4 Be alert for development of CNS reactions (irritability, headache, vomiting, excitement, drowsiness, vertigo, bulging of anterior fontanel in children) especially in infants, children, or elderly patients. Such reactions often occur rapidly and are usually reversible shortly after the discontinuation of drug.

▷ 5 Urge caution in driving or operating other machinery, because drowsiness and dizziness can occur.

▶ **NURSING CONSIDERATIONS**

▷ 1 Administer with food or milk if GI intolerance occurs.

▷ 2 Perform disk sensitivity tests before administration. If clinical response is unsatisfactory or relapse occurs, repeat culture and sensitivity tests, because resistance can develop within 48 hours, especially if dosage is inadequate.

▷ 3 Advise patients to report any visual disturbances immediately. These disturbances usually disappear quickly with a reduction in dosage.

▷ 4 Note that nalidixic acid can yield a false positive reaction in urinary glucose testing with Benedicts' or Fehling's solutions or Clinitest Reagent tablets. Tes-Tape or Clinistix can still be used reliably. Urinary 17-ketosteroids may also be falsely elevated by nalidixic acid.

▶ **nitrofurantoin**

Furadantin, Furalan, Furan, Furanite, Furatoin, Nitrex, Nitrofan

▶ **nitrofurantoin sodium injection**

Ivadantin

▶ **nitrofurantoin macrocrystals**

Macrodantin

A synthetic nitrofuran derivative, nitrofurantoin is a specific urinary antibacterial agent effective against a range of gram-positive and gram-negative organisms. It is available as a sodium salt for parenteral administration and in macro-crystalline form for oral administration, which causes less GI distress than the normal oral dosage forms.

Mechanism

Bacteriostatic in low concentrations and bactericidal in higher concentrations; probable mechanism is interference with carbohydrate metabolism by inhibition of acetyl coenzyme A; may also impair bacterial cell wall formation; most effective against *Escherichia coli, Klebsiella, Enterobacter,* and *Citrobacter* species, group B streptococci, enterococci, and staphylococci; some strains of *Enterobacter* and *Klebsiella* are resistant, as are most strains of *Proteus, Serratia,* and *Acinetobacter; Pseudomonas* is highly resistant; acquired resistance of susceptible organisms is minimal

Uses

1 Treatment of urinary tract infections due to susceptible organisms (see above)

2 Prophylaxis against recurrent bacteriuria (Macrodantin—small dose)

Dosage

Oral: Adults—50 mg to 100 mg four times a day for 10 days to 14 days; chronic therapy 25 mg to 50 mg four times a day

Children (over 3 mo)—5 mg/kg to 7 mg/kg/day in four divided doses

Prophylaxis of recurrent infections (Macrodantin)—50 mg daily at bedtime for at least 6 months.

IV infusion:

Over 120 lb—180 mg twice a day

Under 120 lb—3 mg/lb/day (6.6 mg/kg/day) in two equal doses

Infusion solution is prepared by adding 20 ml 5% Dextrose Injection to the vial containing 180 mg nitrofurantoin sodium; each ml of this solution is added to at least 25 ml of parenteral fluid; final solution is administered at a rate of 2 ml to 3 ml/min

Fate

Well absorbed orally (macrocrystalline form is absorbed more slowly than other oral forms but causes less GI distress); absorption is *enhanced* by ingestion of food; therapeutic serum and tissue levels are not attained, except in the urinary tract; plasma half-life is 15 minutes to 30 mintues; approximately one half of a dose is rapidly inactivated in tissues and excreted unchanged in the urine; activity is increased in an acid urine

Common Side-Effects

Nausea, anorexia, and vomiting

Significant Adverse Reactions

GI—diarrhea, abdominal pain, pancreatitis, parotitis

Pulmonary—chills, cough, chest pain, dyspnea, pulmonary infiltration with consolidation or pleural effusion, diffuse interstitial pneumonitis or fibrosis (with prolonged therapy)

Dermatologic—rash, pruritus, urticaria, angioedema, alopecia; rarely, exfoliative dermatitis, erythema multiforme

Hematologic—hemolytic anemia, megaloblastic anemia, leukopenia, granulocytopenia, eosinophilia, thrombocytopenia, agranulocytosis

Allergic—drug fever, asthmatic attack, cholestatic jaundice, arthralgia, anaphylaxis

Neurologic—dizziness, paresthesias, headache, drowsiness, nystagmus, peripheral neuropathy

Other—Hypotension, myalgia, superinfections, tooth staining from oral suspension

Contraindications

Anuria, oliguria, significant renal impairment (creatinine clearance less than 40 ml/min) and pregnancy at term; in infants under 3 months (possibility of hemolytic anemia due to immature enzyme systems)

Interactions

1 Nitrofurantoin can antagonize the action of nalidixic acid.
2 Acidifying agents (*e.g.,* ammonium chloride, ascorbic acid) may potentiate nitrofurantoin, whereas alkalinizing agents (*e.g.,* acetazolamide, sodium bicarbonate) can reduce its effectiveness.
3 Probenecid reduces the renal clearance of nitrofurantoin, and may increase its toxicity.
4 Antacids can reduce the effectiveness of nitrofurantoin by impairing its GI absorption.
5 Anticholinergics, other GI antispasmodic drugs, and food may increase GI absorption of nitrofurantoin by prolonging gastric emptying time.

▶ NURSING ALERTS

▷ 1 Observe carefully for development of acute pulmonary sensitivity reaction during early days (up to 3 wk) of therapy. Common symptoms are fever, chills, cough, dyspnea, chest pain, and eosinophilia. Discontinuation of drug usually results in rapid resolution of symptoms.
▷ 2 During prolonged therapy, be alert for insidious development of subacute or chronic pulmonary reactions (cough, malaise, dyspnea on exertion, x-ray findings of diffuse pneumonitis or pulmonary fibrosis). Early recognition is important to prevent serious pulmonary impairment.
▷ 3 Alert patients to note development of early neurologic symptoms (numbness, paresthesias, muscle weakness) because drug should be discontinued to prevent severe and possibly irreversible peripheral neuropathy.
▷ 4 Perform periodic hematologic evaluations and liver function tests during extended therapy, because hemolytic anemia or hepatitis has resulted from use of nitrofurantoin.
▷ 5 Monitor intake–output and observe patients for signs of renal impairment (oliguria, anuria, creatinine clearance below 40 ml/min). If present, terminate therapy to minimize risk of serious toxicity.
▷ 6 Use parenteral form of nitrofurantoin only in those patients with clinically significant urinary infections to whom oral dosage forms cannot be given.
▷ 7 Use with caution in patients with anemia, diabetes, vitamin B deficiency, electrolyte imbalances, or a debilitating disease, because these conditions may predispose to peripheral neuropathy. Cautious use is also indicated in pregnant or nursing mothers, and IV use should be undertaken with caution in children under 12 years of age.

▶ NURSING CONSIDERATIONS

▷ 1 Administer oral drug with meals or milk to reduce GI distress and possibly to improve absorption. Consider use of macrocrystalline dosage form to further minimize GI upset.
▷ 2 Ensure that drug is taken at evenly spaced intervals, around the clock if possible.
▷ 3 Inform patients that drug may impart a harmless brownish color to the urine.
▷ 4 Instruct patients to rinse mouth thoroughly after use of the oral suspension to prevent staining of teeth.
▷ 5 Be alert for signs of urinary tract superinfections (foul smelling urine, dysuria, fever), and treat with appropriate antibiotic, based upon disk susceptibility testing. *Pseudomonas* is the pathogen most commonly implicated in superinfections during nitrofurantoin therapy.
▷ 6 Protect drug from strong light (*i.e.,* dispense in amber bottles because darkening and possible loss of potency can occur).
▷ 7 Note that nitrofurantoin may cause false positive tests for serum glucose, bilirubin, alkaline phosphatase, and BUN levels.

▶ trimethoprim

Proloprim, Trimpex

A synthetic antibacterial agent, trimethoprim has demonstrated activity against common urinary tract pathogens, *except Pseudomonas aeruginosa.*

Mechanism

Blocks production of tetrahydrofolic acid by reversible inhibition of dihydrofolate reductase, thus interfering with synthesis of proteins and nucleic acids in susceptible bacteria.

Uses

1 Treatment of initial episodes of uncomplicated urinary tract infections due to susceptible strains of *Escherichia coli, Proteus mirabilis, Klebsiella pneumoniae, Enterobacter* species, and coagulase-negative *Staphylococcus* species

Dosage

Adults and children (over 12 yr): 100 mg every 12 hours for 10 days, or 200 mg once daily

Fate

Rapidly absorbed orally; peak serum levels occur in 1 hour to 4 hours; half-life is 8 hours to 10 hours; approximately one half is protein-bound in plasma; excreted in the urine; largely as unmetabolized drug, 50% to 60% of an oral dose within 24 hours

Common Side-Effects
Pruritic rash

Significant Adverse Reactions
GI—epigastric distress, nausea, vomiting, glossitis
Dermatologic—macropapular or morbilliform rash, exfoliative dermatitis
Hematologic—thrombocytopenia, leukopenia, neutropenia, megaloblastic anemia, methemoglobinemia
Other—fever; elevations in BUN, serum creatinine, serum transaminase, and bilirubin

Contraindications
Megaloblastic anemia due to folate deficiency, severe renal impairment (creatinine clearance below 15 ml/min)

Interactions
1 Trimethoprim may potentiate the action of oral anticoagulants.

▶ **NURSING ALERTS**
▷ 1 Caution patients to note appearance of signs of possible blood dyscrasias (sore throat, fever, bruising, mucosal ulceration, pallor), and advise physician immediately if these signs occur.
▷ 2 Perform complete blood counts during prolonged therapy. If signs of bone marrow depression are noted (thrombocytopenia, leukopenia, megaloblastic anemia), discontinue drug and administer 3 mg to 6 mg leucovorin IM daily for 3 days to restore normal hematopoiesis.
▷ 3 Use cautiously in patients with liver impairment, reduced renal function, folate deficiency, and in pregnant or nursing women.

▶ **NURSING CONSIDERATIONS**
▷ 1 Observe for development of skin rash, commonly appearing 7 days to 14 days after initiation of therapy. Symptoms usually disappear following discontinuation of drug.
▷ 2 Recognize that while culture and sensitivity tests should be performed to determine susceptibility of the pathogens to trimethoprim, therapy can be initiated before obtaining the results.
▷ 3 Note that trimethoprim is also available in combination with sulfamethoxazole (Bactrim, Septra) for treatment of both acute and chronic urinary infections, acute otitis media, acute exacerbations of chronic bronchitis, and enteritis (see Chap. 59).

Urinary Analgesic

▶ **phenazopyridine**
Pyridium and various other manufacturers

Phenazopyridine is an azo dye that is excreted in the urine, where it exerts a mild analgesic action. It is usually given in combination with a urinary anti-infective.

Mechanism
Not established; may exert a local anesthetic effect on mucosal membranes

Use
1 Symptomatic relief of pain, burning, irritation, and urinary urgency or frequency resulting from lower urinary tract infections

Dosage
200 mg three times a day

Fate
Adequately absorbed orally; partially metabolized, but mainly excreted unchanged in the urine

Significant Adverse Reactions
(Rare) GI distress, hemolytic anemia, methemoglobinemia, renal or hepatic damage

Contraindications
Renal insufficiency, uremia, and chronic glomerulonephritis

▶ **NURSING CONSIDERATIONS**
▷ 1 Advise patients that drugs may produce a reddish orange discoloration of the urine, which can stain fabrics.
▷ 2 Caution patients to observe for appearance of yellowish tinge to sclera or skin, possible indication of reduced renal excretion and accumulation toxicity. Advise physician immediately.
▷ 3 Be aware that drugs can interfere with laboratory test results based on urinary colorimetric procedures.
▷ 4 Recognize that relief of symptoms produced by the drugs can delay recognition, diagnosis, and proper treatment of underlying pathology.
▷ 5 Note that phenazopyridine is available in fixed combination with sulfamethizole (Uremide, Thiosulfil-A), sulfamethoxazole (Azo Gantanol) and sulfisoxazole (Azo Gantrisin and others).
▷ 6 Be aware that phenazopyridine may be discontinued as soon as the discomfort is relieved; *however,* the accompanying anti-infective must be continued for the duration of the prescribed therapy.

Urease Inhibitor

▶ **acetohydroxamic acid**
Lithostat

Acetohydroxamic acid is used to enhance the effectiveness of antimicrobial agents used to treat chronic urinary infections resulting from urea-splitting organisms.

Mechanism
Inhibits the bacterial enzyme urease, thus retarding hydrolysis of urea to ammonia in the presence of urea-splitting organisms; decreased ammonia levels and reduced pH enhance the action of antimicrobial agents and improve the

cure rate; the drug does not acidify the urine directly, nor does it possess an antibacterial action.

Use

1 *Adjunctive* treatment of urinary infections due to urea-splitting organisms

Dosage

Adults: 250 mg three to four times/day to a maximum of 1.5 g/day

Children: 10 mg/kg/day, initially, in divided doses; titrate to desired response

Fate

Oral absorption is good; approximately one half of a dose is excreted unchanged in the urine; therapeutic effects occur at a urinary concentration of 10 mcg/ml; higher levels provide more complete urease inhibition

Common Side-Effects

Headache (30%); anxiety, nervousness, mild tremor, depression, nausea, vomiting, anorexia, malaise (20%); reticulocytosis (5%)

Significant Adverse Reactions

Hemolytic anemia, superficial phlebitis, palpitations, nonpruritic skin rash, alopecia, teratogenicity

Contraindications

Decreased renal function (serum creatinine greater than 2.5 mg %), urinary infections due to *non*-urease-producing organisms, pregnancy, and females not using contraceptive methods

Interactions

1 Alcohol has produced a rash in the presence of acetohydroxamic acid.
2 Acetohydroxamic acid can reduce oral absorption of iron by forming a chelate with the metal.

▶ NURSING ALERTS

▷ 1 Recognize that acetohydroxamic acid should not be used in lieu of appropriate antimicrobial or surgical treatment, nor in the treatment of non-urease-splitting infections.

▷ 2 Perform a complete blood count two weeks after beginning therapy and every three months thereafter. If reticulocyte count is greater than 6%, reduce the dosage. Most patients develop a *mild* reticulocytosis, but hemolytic anemia has occurred in about 30% of patients, usually accompanied by nausea, vomiting, anorexia, and malaise

▷ 3 Advise women of childbearing potential receiving the drug to use appropriate contraceptive measures, because acetohydroxamic acid may cause fetal damage.

▷ 4 Closely monitor patients with renal impairment, because acetohydroxamic acid is eliminated primarily by the kidneys. A dosage reduction may be necessary in patients with reduced renal function.

▷ 5 Use with caution in patients with anemia, blood dyscrasias, bone marrow depression, thrombophlebitis, skin rash, depression, and in nursing mothers.

▶ NURSING CONSIDERATIONS

▷ 1 Inform patients that headache is very common during the first 48 hours to 72 hours of treatment, but will usually disappear spontaneously. Mild analgesics can be used, if necessary.

▷ 2 Caution patients that alcohol ingestion during acetohydroxamic acid therapy frequently results in development of a nonpruritic macular skin rash, which may range from mild and transient to severe.

▷ 3 Advise patients taking oral iron supplements that iron absorption is impaired by acetohydroxamic acid. If iron is necessary, parenteral iron is recommended.

▷ 4 Note that treatment may have to be continued for extended periods of time, as long as the urea-splitting organism is present.

Summary. Urinary Anti-infectives and Analgesics

Drug	Preparations	Usual Dosage Range
Anti-infectives		
Cinoxacin (Cinobac)	Capsules—250 mg, 500 mg	1 g/day in 2 to 4 divided doses for 7 days to 14 days
Methenamine	See Table 66-1	
Methylene Blue (Urolene Blue)	Tablets—65 mg	Oral—65 mg to 130 mg 3 times/day
	Injection—10 mg/ml	IV—1 mg/kg to 2 mg/kg over several minutes
Nalidixic acid (NegGram)	Tablets—250 mg, 500 mg, 1 g	Adults—1 g 4 times/day (maintenance 2 g/day)
	Suspension—250 mg/5 ml	Children (over 3 mo)—55 mg/kg/day in 4 divided doses (maintenance 33 mg/kg/day)

Summary. Urinary Anti-infectives and Analgesics *(continued)*

Drug	Preparations	Usual Dosage Range
Nitrofurantoin (Ivadantin, Furadantin, Furalan, Furan, Furanite, Furatoin, Nitrex, Nitrofan)	Tablets—50 mg, 100 mg Capsules—50 mg, 100 mg Oral suspension—25 mg/5 ml Powder for injection—180 mg/vial	Oral: Adults—50 mg to 100 mg 4 times a day Children—5 mg/kg to 7 mg/kg/day in 4 divided doses (Chronic—25 mg to 50 mg 4 times/day)
Nitrofurantoin macrocrystals (Macrodantin)	Capsules—25 mg, 50 mg, 100 mg	IV: Over 120 lb—180 mg twice a day Under 120 lb—3 mg/lb/day (6.6 mg/kg/day) in 2 equal doses
Trimethoprim (Proloprim, Trimpex)	Tablets—100 mg, 200 mg	100 mg every 12 hours for 10 days or 200 mg once daily
Analgesics		
Phenazopyridine (Pyridium and various other manufacturers)	Tablets—100 mg, 200 mg	200 mg 3 times/day
Urease Inhibitor		
Acetohydroxamic acid (Lithostat)	Tablets—250 mg	Adults—250 mg 3 to 4 times/day to a maximum of 1.5 g/day Children—initially, 10 mg/kg/day; titrate as necessary

67 Miscellaneous Antibiotics

A number of antimicrobial drugs in clinical use today cannot be precisely categorized based upon their chemical structure or biologic activity. These drugs are most conveniently grouped under a miscellaneous heading and are reviewed here individually.

▶ chloramphenicol

Antibiopto, Chloromycetin, Chloroptic, Econochlor, Mychel, Ophthochlor

Chloramphenicol is a synthetic, broad-spectrum, bacteriostatic antibiotic effective against a wide range of gram-positive and gram-negative bacteria, rickettsiae, and chlamydiae. Its potential for eliciting serious toxicity, however, largely restricts its systemic use to *severe* infections in which other, less toxic drugs are ineffective or contraindicated. The drug is also commonly employed locally in the eye for treating superficial ocular infections and in the ear for infections of the external auditory canal. Currently, it is considered to be the drug of choice for acute *Salmonella typhi* infections (typhoid fever), but should not be used for routine treatment of the typhoid "carrier state." Other organisms against which it is quite active are *Hemophilus influenzae, Bacteroides fragilis,* other *Salmonella* species, *Rickettsiae,* lymphogranuloma–psittacosis group and various gram-negative bacteria causing bacteremia or meningitis. The major danger associated with chloramphenicol is bone marrow depression, and fatal blood dyscrasias have occurred following both its short-term and long-term use. Frequent blood studies are therefore essential during its administration. Other untoward reactions noted with chloramphenicol are neurotoxicity and the "gray syndrome" in newborns (see Adverse Reactions). While it is a valuable anti-infective for certain severe infections, chloramphenicol should never be used for minor infections (*e.g.,* colds, flu, throat infections) or as a prophylactic agent.

Mechanism
Binds to the 50 S ribosomal subunits of bacteria and inhibits bacterial protein synthesis by cellular ribosomes; bacteriostatic at normal concentrations

Uses
1 Treatment of acute infections caused by *Salmonella typhi* (drug of choice)
2 Alternative treatment of severe infections due to susceptible organisms for which less toxic drugs are ineffective or contraindicated (see Chap. 58, Table 58-1). Principal indications include *Hemophilus influenzae* meningitis, pneumococcal or meningococcal meningitis in penicillin-sensitive patients, *Bacteroides fragilis* infections, and rickettsial infections in tetracycline-sensitive patients.
3 Adjunctive therapy in cystic fibrosis regimens
4 Superficial infections of the skin, eye, and external auditory canal due to susceptible microorganisms (topical application only)

Dosage
Oral, IV:
Adults and children—50 mg/kg/day in divided doses every 6 hours (maximum 100 mg/kg/day)

Newborns and infants with immature metabolic processes—25 mg/kg/day in two equally divided doses

Topical:

Apply several times a day to affected area

Ophthalmic:

One or two drops or small amount of ointment to infected eye two to four times a day

Otic:

Two to three drops three times a day

Fate

Rapidly absorbed orally; peak serum levels occur in 1 hour to 2 hours; distribution is variable; highest concentrations occur in the liver and kidney, while lowest amounts are found in the brain and cerebrospinal fluid (about one half the levels in the blood); approximately 50% to 60% protein-bound; elimination half-life is 2 hours to 3½ hours; metabolized by the liver and excreted in the urine, largely as glucuronic acid conjugate, with small amounts (8%–12%) of unchanged drug; minor quantities of active drug are found in the bile and feces; readily crosses placental barrier and appears in breast milk

Common Side-Effects

GI distress

Significant Adverse Reactions

Warning: Serious and potentially fatal blood dyscrasias (*e.g.,* aplastic anemia, thrombocytopenia, granulocytopenia) have occurred with both short-term and prolonged use of chloramphenicol. Thus, it should be employed only in severe infections unresponsive to other, less hazardous antibiotics, and careful blood studies should be performed at least every 2 days during therapy. A dose-related *reversible* type of bone marrow depression may occur during treatment. It is readily detectable by blood studies, and responds promptly to discontinuation of the drug. An *irreversible* type of bone marrow depression leading to aplastic anemia which may terminate in leukemia with a high mortality rate has also been reported (1:25,000–40,000), but does not appear to be dose-related. It may occur weeks or even months following therapy and is characterized by bone marrow aplasia or hypoplasia. Most importantly, it is not readily predictable by routine blood studies performed *during* treatment. Follow-up blood tests and close observation of the patient are necessary.

Hematologic—blood dyscrasias (leukopenia, reduction in erythrocytes, granulocytopenia, hypoplastic anemia, thrombocytopenia, aplastic anemia)

Neurologic—headache, confusion, depression, delirium, optic and peripheral neuritis

Hypersensitivity—fever, rash, urticaria, angio-edema, anaphylaxis; itching or burning with topical application.

GI—vomiting, glossitis, stomatitis, diarrhea, enterocolitis (rare)

Other—jaundice, superinfections, gray syndrome in premature infants and newborns (abdominal distention, emesis, pallid cyanosis, vasomotor collapse, irregular respiration, hypothermia; occurs in 3 days–4 days, usually after initiation of high-dose therapy within the first 48 hrs of life and can be fatal)

Contraindications

Treatment of trivial infections (colds, flu, sore throat), prophylactic use, infections other than those indicated as susceptible by testing, and concurrent therapy with other bone marrow depressive drugs

Interactions

1 Chloramphenicol can inhibit the metabolism of oral anticoagulants, oral antidiabetic drugs, cyclophosphamide, barbiturates, and phenytoin, thus potentiating their effects.

2 Chloramphenicol may inhibit the hematinic activity of vitamin B_{12}, folic acid, and iron.

3 The bactericidal action of other antibiotics (*e.g.,* penicillins) may be reduced by chloramphenicol.

4 Chloramphenicol can interfere with the immune response to diphtheria and tetanus toxoids.

5 Concomitant administration of acetaminophen may elevate serum levels of chloramphenicol.

6 A disulfiram-like reaction to alcohol may occur with use of chloramphenicol (see Chap. 80).

▶ **NURSING ALERTS**

(See Warning under Adverse Reactions)

▷ 1 Perform baseline blood studies (differential, leukocyte, and reticulocyte counts) before initiation of therapy, at 48-hour intervals during therapy, and periodically for *several months* after termination. Discontinue drug immediately if any abnormality is noted.

▷ 2 Advise patients to notify physician immediately if any signs of blood dyscrasias are noted (fever, sore throat, bruising or bleeding, fatigue), even after drug has been discontinued.

▷ 3 Use cautiously in patients with renal or hepatic impairment, glucose-6-phosphate dehydrogenase deficiency, acute intermittent porphyria; in infants and in pregnant or nursing women.

▷ 4 Avoid repeated courses of therapy and do not extend treatment longer than the time required to effect a cure with little risk of relapse (*e.g.,* a normal temperature for 48 hr).

▷ 5 Caution patients to report any visual disturbances; drug should be discontinued to minimize the danger of optic neuritis.

▶ **NURSING CONSIDERATIONS**

▷ 1 Administer on an empty stomach (unless GI distress occurs) at evenly spaced intervals, around the clock if possible.

▷ 2 Be alert for indications of superinfection (diarrhea, perianal irritation, vaginal discharge, fever, glossitis), and initiate proper antibiotic therapy.

▷ 3 Monitor blood glucose of diabetic patients receiving oral hypoglycemics and prothrombin time of patients receiving oral anticoagulants during chloramphenicol therapy, because loss of control may occur.

▷ 4 Observe for indications of hypersensitivity reactions during topical chloramphenicol treatment. Avoid prolonged topical (*i.e.,* skin, eye, ear) application.

▷ 5 Note that chloramphenicol *base* solution is used by IV infusion in adults only, whereas the *sodium succinate salt* may be given by slow (1 min–2 min) IV injection to both adults and children. Do not administer the salt IM, because it is largely ineffective. Substitute oral dosage as soon as possible.

▶ **clindamycin**
  Cleocin

▶ **lincomycin**
  Lincocin

Clindamycin and lincomycin are two chemically related, primarily bacteriostatic antibiotics frequently termed lincosamides. They exhibit antibacterial activity similar to but not identical to that of the erythromycins. Lincomycin and its chlorine-substituted derivative clindamycin are effective against most of the common gram-positive pathogens, particularly *Staphylococcus, Pneumococcus, Streptococcus, Corynebacterium,* and *Nocardia,* as well as many anaerobic organisms, such as *Bacteroides, Actinomyces, Peptococcus,* and most strains of *Clostridium* (except *Clostridium difficile*). Most gram-negative organisms, on the other hand, are resistant. Because of their toxic potential, however, lincomycin and clindamycin are usually recommended only for treatment of serious anaerobic infections for which penicillin or erythromycin is ineffective or inappropriate (*e.g.,* when penicillin hypersensitivity is present). The major dangers associated with use of clindamycin and lincomycin are related to the GI tract, and include persistent profuse diarrhea, severe abdominal cramping, and pseudomembranous colitis. These effects, although most frequent with systemic use, have occurred upon topical application of clindamycin as well. Clindamycin is generally regarded as the preferred drug of the two for systemic use, because it is better absorbed orally, has a somewhat broader spectrum of action, including *Bacteroides fragilis,* and is reported to elicit fewer GI side-effects. Although the two drugs are alike enough in their pharmacologic properties to be discussed together, some important differences do exist and these are noted whenever appropriate in the following discussion as well as in Table 67-1.

Mechanism
Interfere with protein synthesis in susceptible organisms by binding to the 50 S subunits of bacterial ribosomes; resistance develops slowly, possibly due to chromosomal alterations; possess neuromuscular blocking activity; both drugs are active against most common gram-positive pathogens; clindamycin demonstrates a slightly wider range of action against anaerobic gram-positive organisms (*e.g., Actinomyces, Peptococcus, Clostridia,* micro-aerophilic streptococci) and anaerobic gram-negative bacilli (*e.g., Bacteroides, Fusobacterium*).

Uses
1 Alternate therapy for serious streptococcal, pneumococcal, or staphylococcal infections in patients in whom penicillins and erythromycins are ineffective or inappropriate
2 Alternate treatment of serious infections due to anaerobic organisms, such as *Bacteroides, Fusobacterium, Peptococcus,* or *Actinomyces* species, in penicillin-sensitive patients (clindamycin is most effective)
3 Treatment of acne (topical application of clindamycin solution)

Dosage
See Table 67-1.

Fate
Oral absorption is rapid and virtually complete (90%) for clindamycin, whereas only about 20% to 30% of an oral dose of lincomycin is absorbed. Food markedly impairs absorption of lincomycin but not clindamycin. Peak plasma levels occur within 45 minutes with oral clindamycin and 2 hours to 4 hours with oral lincomycin. IM injection yields peak serum levels within 30 minutes with lincomycin and 1 hour to 3 hours with clindamycin. Plasma half-lives are 2 hours to 3 hours for clindamycin and 4 hours to 6 hours for lincomycin. Both drugs are widely distributed in the body and are approximately 70% protein-bound. Effective antibacterial blood levels are maintained for 6 hours to 8 hours after oral administration, and up to 12 hours following IM injection or IV infusion; excreted in the urine, bile, and feces, primarily (90%) as inactive metabolites

Common Side-Effects
Nausea, diarrhea, and skin rash

Significant Adverse Reactions

Warning: Severe persistent diarrhea and pseudomembranous colitis, occasionally fatal, have occurred with these drugs. The colitis is probably due to toxins secreted by resistant strains of *Clostridium difficile.* Do not use for minor infections, and discontinue drug if diarrhea, bloody stools, severe abdominal pain, or high fever occurs. Vancomycin, 2 g/day in divided doses, is effective for *Clostridium difficile*-induced colitis.

GI—vomiting, persistent or severe diarrhea, abdominal pain, glossitis, esophagitis, stomatitis, acute enterocolitis, or pseudomembranous colitis (occasionally fatal)
Hypersensitivity—urticaria, angioedema, serum sickness, erythema multiforme (rare), Stevens–Johnson syndrome (rare), exfoliative dermatitis (rare)
Hematologic—eosinophilia, infrequent blood dyscrasias (neutropenia, leukopenia, thrombocytopenia, agranulocytosis, aplastic anemia)
Cardiovascular—hypotension (parenteral injection), cardiopulmonary arrest following IV injection

Table 67-1. Clindamycin–Lincomycin

Drug	Preparations	Usual Dosage Range	Remarks
Clindamycin (Cleocin)	Capsules—75 mg, 150 mg Granules for suspension—75 mg/5 ml Injection—300 mg/2 ml, 600 mg/4 ml, 900 mg/6 ml Topical solution—10 mg/ml (Cleocin-T)	Oral: Adults—150 mg to 450 mg every 6 hours depending on severity of infection Children—8 mg/kg to 12 mg/kg/day in 3 to 4 divided doses (up to 25 mg/kg/day in severe infections) IM, IV: Adults—600 mg to 2700 mg/day in 2 to 4 equally divided doses depending on severity of infection Children—15 mg/kg to 40 mg/kg/day in 3 to 4 equal doses depending on severity of infection or 350 mg to 450 mg/M^2/day Topical: Apply thin film to affected area twice a day	Do not use in children under 1 month; minimum recommended oral dose in children weighing 10 kg or less is 37.5 mg 3 times a day; do *not* refrigerate reconstituted granules, because it may thicken and become difficult to pour; solution is stable for 2 weeks at room temperature; use parenteral therapy initially in children to treat anaerobic infections; follow with oral administration when appropriate; in severe infections children should receive no less than 300 mg a day parenterally, regardless of body weight; adults may be given up to 4.8 g a day IV in life-threatening infections; single IM injections of more than 600 mg are not recommended; do not give more than 1200 mg an hour by IV infusion; physically incompatible with ampicillin, phenytoin, aminophylline, barbiturates, calcium gluconate, and magnesium sulfate; applied topically to acne vulgaris lesions; alcohol base may be irritating to sensitive surfaces (eye, mucous membranes, wounds)
Lincomycin (Lincocin)	Capsules—250 mg, 500 mg Syrup—250 mg/5 ml Injection—300 mg/ml	Oral: Adults—500 mg 3 to 4 times a day Children—30 mg/kg to 60 mg/kg/day in 3 to 4 divided doses IM: Adults—600 mg every 12 hours to 24 hours Children—10 mg/kg every 12 hours to 24 hours IV infusion: Adults—600 mg to 1 g every 8 hours to 12 hours Children—10 mg/kg to 20 mg/kg/day in divided doses Subconjunctival injection: 0.25 ml (75 mg)	Do not use in children under 1 month; administer orally on an empty stomach; IM injections should be made deeply and slowly to minimize pain; severe cardiopulmonary reactions have occurred when drug has been given IV at higher than recommended doses or rates; in life-threatening situations, daily IV doses of up to 8 g have been used; dilute 1 g lincomycin in 100 ml of a compatible infusion solution (see package insert) and infuse over a period of not less than 1 hour; repeat as often as needed to a maximum of 8 g a day; subconjunctival injection results in effective ocular fluid levels of antibiotics for 5 hours; drug is incompatible with novobiocin and kanamycin, as well as phenytoin sodium and protein hydrolysates

Other—vaginitis, pruritus ani, jaundice, abnormal liver function tests, tinnitus, vertigo, pain or induration on IM injection; topical application of clindamycin can result in contact dermatitis, skin dryness, oily skin, facial swelling, stinging sensation, gram-negative folliculitis

Contraindications

Minor systemic bacterial or viral infections or meningitis, pregnancy, liver disease; in nursing mothers and in neonates

Interactions

1 The activity of clindamycin and lincomycin may be antagonized by concurrent use of erythromycin or chloramphenicol.
2 Clindamycin and lincomycin can enhance the action of neuromuscular blocking drugs.

3 Use of antiperistaltic drugs such as opiates, loperamide, and diphenoxylate may prolong or aggravate the diarrhea observed with clindamycin and lincomycin.
4 The oral absorption of clindamycin and lincomycin can be impaired by kaolin, pectin, other antidiarrheal medications, and cyclamates.

▶ NURSING ALERTS

▷ 1 Caution patients to note development of abdominal cramps or prolonged, excessive diarrhea or bloody stools, and contact physician immediately should these occur. This may occur after just a few days of therapy. Discontinue drug and perform endoscopic examination of the large bowel.
▷ 2 Use drugs cautiously in patients with mild liver impairment, history of GI disease, asthma or other allergic diseases, or renal dysfunction, and in elderly or debilitated persons.

▷ 3 Do not administer systemic antiperistaltic drugs such as opiates, diphenoxylate, or loperamide to patients experiencing drug-induced diarrhea, because condition may be worsened. Fluid and electrolyte supplementation is indicated. Corticosteroids may help relieve colitis.

▷ 4 Perform periodic blood studies and liver and kidney function tests during prolonged therapy.

▷ 5 Reduce dosage by 50% to 75% in the presence of impaired renal function.

▶ NURSING CONSIDERATIONS

▷ 1 Administer lincomycin orally 1 hour to 2 hours before meals or 2 hours to 3 hours after meals, because food retards absorption; clindamycin absorption is largely unaffected by food.

▷ 2 Obtain a careful history of previous drug sensitivity before administration. Use with caution in patients with a prior allergic reaction to any drug.

▷ 3 Be alert for signs of overgrowth of nonsusceptible organisms. Recognize, however, that diarrhea, normally an indication of GI superinfection with a resistant organism, is a common side-effect of clindamycin and lincomycin and may not indicate a secondary infection.

▷ 4 Be aware that drugs can increase serum levels of SGOT, SGPT, and alkaline phosphatase and can decrease platelet counts.

▶ dapsone
DDS

Sulfones, of which the sole clinically available representative is dapsone, are chemical analogs of the sulfonamides that are used in the treatment of all forms of leprosy (Hansen's disease). Although clinical benefit is often noted within a few months, the more severe skin lesions characteristic of the disease may require several years for complete resolution. Because of its high potential for toxicity, dapsone is usually used only for the treatment of leprosy, although it has been shown to be effective in the treatment of dermatitis herpetiformis and in the management of relapsing polychondritis.

Mechanism
Probably similar to the sulfonamides, that is, interference with essential components of bacterial nutrition; also possesses immunosuppressant action and may inhibit certain bacterial enzymes

Uses
1 Treatment of leprosy
2 Treatment of dermatitis herpetiformis
3 Management of relapsing polychondritis (investigational use only)
4 Prophylaxis of malaria (investigational use only)

Dosage
Leprosy
Adults: 6 mg to 10 mg/kg per week (50 mg to 100 mg per day); Children: ¼ to ½ adult dose

Dermatitis herpetiformis
Initially 50 mg/day; increase gradually until desired effect (usual dosage range 50 mg to 300 mg daily)

Fate
Slowly and completely absorbed orally; peak plasma concentrations occur in 4 hours to 8 hours; dapsone is 50% to 60% protein-bound; well distributed in the body; metabolized in the liver by acetylation and slowly excreted in the urine (70%–85%) as both unchanged drug and metabolites; plasma half-life averages 25 hours to 30 hours

Common Side-Effects
Anorexia, pallor, skin rash, hemolysis, and back or leg pain

Significant Adverse Reactions
Dermatologic—dermatitis, phototoxicity, drug-induced lupus erythematosus
Hematologic—hemolytic anemia, leukopenia, granulocytopenia, agranulocytosis
GI—nausea, vomiting
CNS—headache, paresthesias, tinnitus, insomnia, vertigo, psychotic reactions (rare)
Other—muscle weakness, drug fever, methemoglobinemia, blurred vision, hematuria, albuminuria, nephrotic syndrome, renal papillary necrosis, liver damage, motor neuropathy, infertility, infectious mononucleosis-like syndrome

Contraindications
Advanced renal amyloidosis

Interactions
1 Probenecid inhibits the renal tubular secretion of dapsone, thus elevating its plasma level.
2 Rifampin and barbiturates can reduce the effects of dapsone by increasing hepatic microsomal enzyme activity.
3 The leprostatic effects of dapsone can be antagonized by para-aminobenzoic acid (PABA).

▶ NURSING ALERTS

▷ 1 Observe patients for signs of developing hypersensitivity, advise physician, and temporarily discontinue drug. Resume at low dosage after reaction has subsided.

▷ 2 Be alert for indications of possible blood dyscrasias (fever, sore throat, bruising, malaise). Perform blood counts at frequent intervals, and discontinue drug if blood picture is abnormal or if signs of severe anemia are present.

▷ 3 Determine hepatic function at regular intervals and note early signs of developing hepatotoxicity (anorexia, vomiting, abdominal pain, light colored stools). Evidence of liver impairment necessitates immediate drug withdrawal.

▷ 4 Use with caution in patients with anemia, liver or kidney disease, glucose-6-phosphate dehydrogenase deficiency, or hypersensitivity to sulfonamides, and in pregnant or nursing women.

▶ **NURSING CONSIDERATIONS**
▷ 1 Administer tablets with food to minimize GI distress.
▷ 2 Note that because bacterial resistance can develop when sulfones are used alone, concurrent administration of rifampin or ethionamide is frequently carried out during the initial months of therapy.
▷ 3 Recognize that sulfone therapy may have to be continued for several years in most cases, and occasionally for a lifetime in severe, complicated forms of leprosy. Stress the importance of dosage compliance.
▷ 4 Provide emotional support as necessary, because many leprosy patients have to deal with severe surface disfigurement.

▶ **furazolidone**
Furoxone

Furazolidone is a synthetic nitrofuran with both antibacterial and antiprotozoal activity. It is effective against many common GI pathogens, such as *Escherichia coli, Salmonella, Shigella, Enterobacter aerogenes, Proteus, Vibrio cholerae,* staphylococci, as well as the protozoan *Giardia lamblia.* Furazolidone is poorly absorbed orally and its action is largely restricted to the GI tract.

Mechanism
Interferes with several bacterial enzyme systems; development of resistance is minimal; does not alter normal bowel flora nor lead to fungal overgrowth; possesses an MAO-inhibitory action if used for longer than 4 days to 5 days, which is probably due to accumulation of a metabolite, 2-hydroxyethylhydrazine

Use
1 Treatment of bacterial or protozoal diarrhea and enteritis due to susceptible organisms

Dosage
Adults: 100 mg four times a day
Children (over 5 yr): 25 mg to 50 mg four times a day
Children (1–4 yr): 17 mg to 25 mg four times a day
Children (under 1 yr): 8 mg to 17 mg four times a day (maximal daily dose 8.8 mg/kg/day)

Common Side-Effects
Nausea, anorexia

Significant Adverse Reactions
Vomiting, headache, malaise, hypersensitivity reactions (fever, skin rash, urticaria, arthralgia), hypotension, hypoglycemia, reversible intravascular hemolysis, disulfiram-like reaction to alcohol (see Chap. 80).

Contraindications
In infants under 1 month; concurrent use of alcohol, other drugs having an MAO-inhibitory action, sympathomimetic amines, or tyramine-containing foods (see MAO Inhibitors, Chap. 24)

Interactions
1 Alcohol may elicit a mild disulfiram-like reaction (flushing, hyperthermia, sweating, dyspnea, tachycardia, palpitations) in the presence of furazolidone.
2 Hypertension can result from concurrent use of furazolidone with other MAO inhibitors, sympathomimetic amines, methyldopa, antihistamines, or tyramine-containing foods (see below).
3 Furazolidone can potentiate the effects of antiparkinsonian drugs, CNS depressants, cocaine, insulin, narcotics, phenothiazines, thiazide diuretics.
4 A toxic psychosis can result from concurrent use of furazolidone and tricyclic antidepressants.

▶ **NURSING ALERTS**
▷ 1 Caution patients to avoid alcohol during treatment and for at least 4 days following therapy to prevent development of a disulfiram-like reaction.
▷ 2 During extended therapy (*i.e.,* greater than 5 days), advise patients to limit or avoid foods high in tyramine (*e.g.,* unpasteurized cheeses, beer, wine, broad beans, yeasts, and fermented products) to minimize the danger of a hypertensive reaction due to the MAO-inhibitory action of furazolidone.
▷ 3 Do not administer to infants under 1 month, because hemolytic anemia due to immature enzyme systems can occur.
▷ 4 Be alert for signs of dehydration or electrolyte depletion (hypotension, "sunken" eyes, irregular pulse, cramping) during episodes of diarrhea, and advise physician should these signs occur.
▷ 5 Counsel patients to adhere to recommended doses and to advise physician if diarrhea persists longer than 5 days or if it worsens. Discontinue drug after 7 days if a satisfactory clinical response has not been attained.

▶ **NURSING CONSIDERATIONS**
▷ 1 Warn patients to avoid over-the-counter drugs unless specifically directed by the physician. Preparations containing vasopressor substances can result in elevations in blood pressure with furazolidone.
▷ 2 Inform patients that drug may discolor urine brown but that this effect is not harmful.
▷ 3 Monitor blood sugar closely in the diabetic patient receiving furazolidone, because hypoglycemia has been reported. Adjust dose of antidiabetic medication, if necessary.
▷ 4 Be alert for indications of weakness, faintness, or dizziness, possible signs of hypotension or hypoglycemia. Dosage adjustment may be necessary.

▶ **hydroxystilbamidine**

An antifungal, antiprotozoal agent, hydroxystilbamidine is active against *Leishmania donovani* and *Blastomyces dermatitidis* and is useful in the treatment of visceral leishmaniasis (kala-azar), American mucocutaneous leishmaniasis, and North American blastomycosis, although the rate of relapse in North American blastomycosis is very high.

Mechanism

Combines with bacterial ribonucleic acid, perhaps disrupting normal bacterial cell replication

Uses

1 Treatment of visceral leishmaniasis (kala-azar) and American mucocutaneous leishmaniasis
2 Alternate treatment of North American blastomycosis

Dosage

Adults: 225 mg/day IV as a single dose infused over 2 hours to 3 hours
Children: 3 mg/kg to 4.5 mg/kg/day IV infused over 2 hours to 3 hours

Fate

Drug is stored in body tissues and slowly released; excretion is by way of the urine and bile

Common Side-Effects

Anorexia, nausea, malaise, diarrhea

Significant Adverse Reactions

Headache, dizziness, drowsiness, paresthesias, pruritus, chills, fever, rash, arthralgia, leukopenia, thrombophlebitis, hypotension, tachycardia, hepatitis, and renal insufficiency

▶ NURSING ALERTS

▷ 1 Perform liver and kidney function studies before and at regular intervals during therapy.
▷ 2 Infuse drug slowly, because hypotension, tachycardia, dyspnea, and anaphylaxis are more common with rapid administration.
▷ 3 Use cautiously in patients with liver or kidney dysfunction.

▶ NURSING CONSIDERATIONS

▷ 1 Prepare fresh solution for each injection, and protect from heat and light to avoid rapid decomposition.
▷ 2 Divide total course of therapy into two treatment periods, with an intervening rest period. Recognize that clinical effects persist for some time after drug is discontinued.
▷ 3 Note that while IV is the preferred route of administration, the drug may be given IM if necessary, but injection is painful.

▶ nitrofurazone

Furacin, Furazyme

A synthetic nitrofuran, nitrofurazone exhibits a broad antibacterial spectrum of action. It is used topically to prevent infection in burns or skin grafts, and rarely used systemically for the treatment of African trypanosomiasis (sleeping sickness).

Mechanism

Inhibits function of enzymes necessary for carbohydrate metabolism in bacteria; bactericidal against both aerobic and anaerobic organisms, although some strains of *Pseudomonas* and *Proteus* are resistant; virtually nontoxic to human cells

Uses

1 Adjunctive therapy to prevent bacterial contamination of second-degree or third-degree burns or skin grafts
2 Alternate therapy of African trypanosomiasis (systemic administration—experimental use only)

Dosage

Soluble dressing or cream: apply directly to lesion or place on sterile gauze; re-apply once daily or every few days as necessary

Significant Adverse Reactions

Contact dermatitis, irritation, and superinfections

▶ NURSING ALERTS

▷ 1 Use cautiously in patients with a glucose-6-phosphate dehydrogenase deficiency (danger of hemolytic anemia if significant systemic absorption occurs) and in pregnant women.

▶ NURSING CONSIDERATIONS

▷ 1 Do not use for treatment of minor burns, wounds, or skin infections, because effectiveness has not been demonstrated in these conditions.
▷ 2 Observe for signs of allergic hypersensitivity (itching, burning, swelling, rash), and discontinue drug if these signs occur.
▷ 3 Apply only to affected area. Protect surrounding skin with petrolatum or zinc oxide.
▷ 4 Be aware that solutions used to impregnate gauze may become discolored upon autoclaving or exposure to light but this does not affect the potency of the drug. Do not autoclave gauze more than once.
▷ 5 Use with caution topically in patients with marked renal impairment, because certain components (*e.g.,* polyethylene glycols) of the base can be absorbed through the denuded skin and may not be excreted by a poorly functioning kidney.

▶ novobiocin

Albamycin

A bacteriostatic antibiotic effective against certain gram-positive cocci, especially *Staphylococcus aureus* and some strains of *Proteus vulgaris,* novobiocin is infrequently used because resistance usually develops rapidly and there is a high incidence of hypersensitivity reactions (such as urticaria, dermatitis) associated with this drug. Blood dyscrasias and hepatic dysfunction have also occurred.

Mechanism

Not completely established; inhibits protein and nucleic acid synthesis and interrupts bacterial cell wall synthesis; may also alter stability of cell membrane by complexing with magnesium within the bacterial cell

Use

1 Treatment of serious infections due to susceptible strains of *Staphylococcus aureus* or *Proteus* species in patients unresponsive or sensitive to other, less toxic antibiotics, such as penicillins, cephalosporins, tetracyclines, or erythromycin

Dosage

Adults: 250 mg every 6 hours or 500 mg every 12 hours (maximum 1 g every 12 hr)

Children: 15 mg/kg to 45 mg/kg/day in divided doses every 6 hours to 12 hours depending on severity of infection

Fate

Well absorbed orally; peak plasma levels occur within 2 hours; highly (90%–95%) bound to plasma proteins; diffuses poorly into most body tissues; excreted primarily in the bile and feces

Common Side-Effects

Hypersensitivity reactions (urticarial, erythematous, maculopapular, or scarlatiniform rash)

Significant Adverse Reactions

Erythema multiforme (rare), liver dysfunction, jaundice, nausea, vomiting, diarrhea, intestinal hemorrhage, alopecia, and blood dyscrasias (leukopenia, eosinophilia, anemia, pancytopenia, agranulocytosis, thrombocytopenia)

Contraindications

Newborn or premature infants

Interactions

1 Tetracyclines may reduce the effectiveness of novobiocin.
2 Lincomycin is incompatible in solution with novobiocin.

▶ NURSING ALERTS

▷ 1 Be alert for the development of hypersensitivity reactions (rash, urticaria, fever) and discontinue drug if reactions cannot be managed by usual measures.

▷ 2 Caution patients to be aware of early signs of possible blood dyscrasias (fever, sore throat, bruising, or bleeding), and to discontinue therapy should these signs occur. Routine blood studies are indicated.

▷ 3 Perform periodic hepatic function studies during treatment and terminate therapy if signs of liver disease are noted (yellowish discoloration of skin or eyes, abdominal pain, elevated serum bilirubin).

▶ NURSING CONSIDERATIONS

▷ 1 Be aware that because of rapid emergence of resistance to novobiocin, the drug is rarely used alone but may be given with penicillin, because no cross-resistance has been demonstrated.

▷ 2 Do not use for minor infections or for infections caused by organisms other than those with demonstrated sensitivity to novobiocin.

▶ spectinomycin

Trobicin

An antibiotic related to the aminoglycosides, spectinomycin is used IM for alternate treatment of gonorrhea in patients hypersensitive to penicillins, or for eradication of organisms resistant to penicillins.

Mechanism

Inhibits protein synthesis in the bacterial cell at the 30 S ribosomal subunit; bacteriostatic at normal doses; active against most strains of *Neisseria gonorrhoeae;* not effective against *Treponema* (syphilis)

Uses

1 Treatment of acute gonorrheal urethritis, proctitis, and cervicitis due to susceptible strains of *Neisseria gonorrhoeae* (usually in patients sensitive to penicillins or tetracyclines or when organisms are resistant to these drugs)

Dosage

Adults and children over 100 lb: usually 2 g (5 ml) IM in a single dose; in areas where antibiotic resistance is known to be present, 4 g (10 ml) divided into two equal parts and injected at different sites

Children under 100 lb (safety has *not* been established): 40 mg/kg IM

Fate

Absorption from IM injection site is rapid; serum levels peak in 1 hour to 2 hours and effective levels are still present at 8 hours; not significantly protein-bound; excreted by the kidneys in a biologically active form

Common Side-Effects

Irritation and soreness at injection site

Significant Adverse Reactions

Urticaria, fever, dizziness, nausea, chills, insomnia, and reduced urine output

Multiple doses have elicited decreases in hemoglobin and hematocrit and creatinine clearance, and elevations in BUN, alkaline phosphatase, and SGPT.

▶ NURSING ALERTS

▷ 1 Be aware that drug may mask or delay the symptoms of incubating syphilis. Perform a serologic test for syphilis at the time of diagnosis and again after 3 months.

▷ 2 Use cautiously in persons with a history of allergies and in pregnant or nursing women.

▷ 3 Do not use to treat pharyngeal infections due to *Neisseria gonorrhoeae.*

▶ NURSING CONSIDERATIONS

▷ 1 Recognize that persons known to have had recent exposure to gonorrhea should be treated the same as those proven to have gonorrhea by culture.

▷ 2 Inject IM deeply into upper outer quadrant of the

buttocks. Use a 20-gauge needle and do not administer more than 5 ml at one injection site.

▷ 3 Reconstitute powder for injection with accompanying diluent and mix thoroughly. Use within 24 hours.

▶ vancomycin
Vancocin

Vancomycin is a bactericidal glycopeptide antibiotic active against many gram-positive organisms, such as streptococci, staphylococci (including penicillinase-producing), *Clostridium difficile, Corynebacterium,* and *Listeria.* The potential for serious toxicity, however, limits its systemic usefulness to treatment of life-threatening infections in patients allergic or unresponsive to less toxic antibacterial drugs. It may be administered orally for treatment of staphylococcal enterocolitis and antibiotic-induced pseudomembranous colitis (for which it is generally considered to be the drug of choice), because it is poorly absorbed from the GI tract.

Mechanism
Inhibits cell wall mucopeptide synthesis and may also damage the bacterial cell membrane

Uses
1 Treatment of serious staphylococcal infections (*e.g.,* endocarditis, septicemia, pneumonia, osteomyelitis) in patients who cannot tolerate or who do not respond to penicillins, cephalosporins, or other less toxic antibiotics
2 Treatment of staphylococcal enterocolitis (oral use only)
3 Treatment of antibiotic-induced (*e.g.,* clindamycin, lincomycin) pseudomembranous colitis caused by *Clostridium difficile* (drug of choice)

Dosage
Oral, IV:
Adults—500 mg every 6 hours or 1 g every 12 hours
Children—44 mg/kg/day in divided doses
Prevention of bacterial endocarditis in penicillin-allergic patients undergoing dental procedures or upper respiratory tract surgery:
Adults—1 g IV infused over 30 minutes to 60 minutes ½ hour to 1 hour before surgery; then oral erythromycin 500 mg every 6 hours for 8 doses
Children—20 mg/kg IV infused over 30 minutes to 60 minutes as above; then 10 mg/kg oral erythromycin every 6 hours for 8 doses
Prevention of bacterial endocarditis in penicillin-allergic patients undergoing GI or genitourinary surgery:
Adults—1 g IV infused over 30 minutes to 60 minutes *plus* 1 g streptomycin IM ½ hour to 1 hour prior to procedure
Children—20 mg/kg each of vancomycin and streptomycin, ½ hour to 1 hour prior to procedure
Pseudomembranous colitis:
Adults—500 mg to 2 g *orally* every 6 hours to 8 hours for 7 to 10 days

Fate
Poorly absorbed orally; IV administration yields rapid attainment of effective serum levels; half-life is 4 hours to 8 hours in adults and 2 hours to 3 hours in children; half-life increases in renal failure; widely distributed in the body, but does not readily cross the blood–brain barrier; penetrates into pleural, pericardial, ascitic, and synovial fluid in the presence of inflammation; approximately 80% of injected drug is excreted by the kidneys

Common Side-Effects
Nausea with oral administration

Significant Adverse Reactions
(Parenteral administration) "Red-neck" syndrome (fever, chills, erythema of the neck and back, paresthesias—usually seen with too-rapid injection); macular rash, urticaria, eosinophilia, ototoxicity, nephrotoxicity, anaphylactoid reactions, pain and thrombophlebitis with IV injection, and superinfections

Contraindications
Renal impairment, hearing disturbances, concurrent use with other ototoxic or nephrotoxic drugs (see Interactions)

Interactions
1 Increased ototoxicity and nephrotoxicity can result from concurrent use of vancomycin with aminoglycosides, polymyxin B, colistin, furosemide, and ethacrynic acid.
2 The action of vancomycin may be antagonized by concurrent use of bacteriostatic antibiotics, for example, tetracyclines, erythromycins.
3 Antivertigo and antinausea drugs (*e.g.,* meclizine, dimenhydrinate, promethazine) may mask the ototoxic effects of vancomycin.

▶ NURSING ALERTS
▷ 1 Caution patients receiving vancomycin to report tinnitus or other auditory disturbances *immediately,* because drug must be discontinued to prevent deafness, which may be progressive despite cessation of therapy.
▷ 2 Perform serial tests of auditory function and vancomycin serum levels in patients with borderline renal function and in elderly persons.
▷ 3 Perform periodic hematologic studies, urinalyses, and liver and kidney function tests in all patients receiving the drug.
▷ 4 Observe for signs of possible nephrotoxicity (oliguria, proteinuria, urinary casts) and advise physician immediately should these signs occur.

▶ NURSING CONSIDERATIONS
▷ 1 Do not administer orally for systemic infections, because drug is poorly absorbed from GI tract.
▷ 2 To prepare oral solution, dilute contents of one vial (500 mg) in 30 ml water and administer by mouth or by a nasogastric tube.
▷ 3 Administer IV by *intermittent* infusion where possible.

Dilute powder for injection with 10 ml Sterile Water for Injection, then add to 100 ml to 200 ml infusion solution. Infuse over 20 minutes to 30 minutes every 6 hours.

▷ 4 If *continuous* IV infusion is necessary, dilute 1 g to 2 g powder in sufficient vehicle, and administer by slow IV drip over 24 hours.

▷ 5 Avoid extravasation of infusion solution; severe irritation and necrosis can result.

▷ 6 When administering IV, instruct patient to report any pain in the extremity and closely observe patient for signs of thrombophlebitis. The risk of thrombophlebitis can be reduced by mixing with 200 ml or more of glucose or saline solution.

Summary. Miscellaneous Antibiotics

Drug	Preparations	Usual Dosage Range
Chloramphenicol (Antibiopto, Chloromycetin, Chloroptic, Econochlor, Mychel, Ophthochlor)	Capsules—100 mg, 250 mg Oral suspension—150 mg/5 ml Injection (base)—500 mg/2 ml Injection (sodium succinate)—100 mg/ml Ophthalmic drops—0.5% Powder for ophthalmic solution—25 mg/vial Ophthalmic ointment—10 mg/g Otic solution—0.5% Topical cream—1%	Oral, IV: Adults and children—50 mg/kg/day in divided doses (maximum 100 mg/kg/day) Newborns—25 mg/kg/day in 4 equally divided doses Topical: Apply several times a day Ophthalmic: 1 to 2 drops or a small amount of ointment in affected eye 2 to 4 times a day Otic: 2 to 3 drops 3 times a day
Clindamycin (Cleocin)	See Table 67-1	
Lincomycin (Lincocin)	See Table 67-1	
Dapsone	Tablets—25 mg, 100 mg	Leprosy: Adults—6 mg to 10 mg/kg per week (50 mg to 100 mg/day) Children—¼ to ½ adult dose Dermatitis herpetiformis: initially 50 mg/day; increase gradually until desired effect (usual range 50 mg to 300 mg daily)
Furazolidone (Furoxone)	Tablets—100 mg Liquid—50 mg/15 ml	Adults—100 mg 4 times a day Children (over 5 yr)—25 mg to 50 mg 4 times a day Children (1 yr–4 yr)—17 mg to 25 mg 4 times a day Children (under 1 yr)—8 mg to 17 mg 4 times a day
Hydroxystilbamidine (Hydroxystilbamidine)	Powder for injection—225 mg/20 ml	Adults—225 mg/day, infused over 2 hours to 3 hours Children—3 mg/kg to 4.5 mg/kg/day, infused over 2 horus to 3 hours
Nitrofurazone (Furacin, Furazyme)	Soluble dressing—0.2% Topical cream—0.2%	Dressing and cream: Apply directly to lesions or place on sterile gauze; re-apply daily or several times a week
Novobiocin (Albamycin)	Capsules—250 mg	Adults—250 mg every 6 hours or 500 mg every 12 hours (maximum 2 g/day) Children—15 mg/kg to 45 mg/kg/day dependent upon severity of infection

(continued)

Summary. Miscellaneous Antibiotics *(continued)*

Drug	Preparations	Usual Dosage Range
Spectinomycin (Trobicin)	Powder for injection—2 g with 3.2 ml diluent or 4 g with 6.2 ml diluent (400 mg/ml when reconstituted)	2 g (5 ml) IM in a single dose; when resistance is known to be present, 4 g (10 ml) IM in 2 equally divided doses at different sites
Vancomycin (Vancocin)	Powder for injection—500 mg/10-ml vial Powder for oral solution—10 g/container	Oral, IV: Adults—500 mg every 6 hours or 1 g every 12 hours Children—44 mg/kg/day in divided doses Prevention of bacterial endocarditis: See text Pseudomembranous colitis: 500 mg to 2 g orally every 6 hours to 8 hours for 7 days to 10 days

Tuberculosis, an infection caused by *Mycobacterium tuberculosis,* is most commonly confined to the lungs, and is characterized by severe inflammation, tissue necrosis, and frequently by the development of open cavities, all of which can impair pulmonary function. In some cases, the offending pathogen gains access to the blood or lymph, and the infection may spread to other body tissues as well. Transmission of the disease is usually by inhalation of droplets of cough from infected persons.

Current chemotherapy for tuberculosis is very effective, provided strict patient compliance can be ensured, but it may be complex, difficult, and prolonged. Infections tend to be chronic, and the microorganisms can exhibit extended periods of inactivity, making complete eradication difficult. The pathogen rapidly develops resistance to single-drug antitubercular therapy and, perhaps even more serious, increasing numbers of bacterial strains are proving resistant to some multiple-drug regimens. To minimize the emergence of resistant strains, therefore, antitubercular agents are almost always administered as combinations of two or three drugs. Moreover, combination therapy allows use of lower doses of each individual drug than would be required if each were used alone, thereby reducing the likelihood of adverse effects.

Antitubercular drugs vary markedly, both in efficacy and toxicity, and based on these differences, may be divided into first-line drugs and second-line drugs. The first-line drugs are almost always used to initiate treatment of a newly diagnosed infection, inasmuch as they are the most dependable and least toxic agents when employed in low to moderate dose combination therapy. Second-line drugs, on the other hand, are often less effective and usually more toxic than the first-line drugs, and thus are reserved for treatment of resistant infections. Classification of the available antitubercular drugs is as follows:

First-line drugs
    1 Ethambutol
    2 Isoniazid (INH)
    3 Rifampin
    4 Streptomycin
Second-line drugs
    1 Aminosalicylic acid and salts
    2 Capreomycin
    3 Cycloserine
    4 Ethionamide
    5 Pyrazinamide

Antitubercular Agents

68

Note: Some references group the antitubercular agents into three categories, that is, primary (isoniazid, rifampin), secondary (ethambutol, pyrazinamide, streptomycin), and tertiary (aminosalicylic acid, capreomycin, cycloserine, ethionamide)

Treatment of an active case of tuberculosis is almost always initiated with isoniazid (INH), the most active antitubercular drug, usually in combination with rifampin, both given in single daily doses. Clinical effectiveness (*i.e.,* cessation of *Mycobacterium tuberculosis* growth in culture of sputum) is usually demonstrated within one month with this regimen. However, approximately one fourth of these patients show laboratory evidence of impaired liver function, although only about 5% of these persons develop symptoms (nausea, anorexia, vomiting, jaundice). The drug regimen should be discontinued if the above symptoms persist.

Other treatment regimens used successfully are (1) INH–rifampin for 20 weeks followed by INH–ethambutol, (2) INH–streptomycin–ethambutol initially, followed by INH–ethambutol, and (3) INH–ethambutol–rifampin for 2 to 3 months, then INH–ethambutol for 18 to 24 months.

Although para-aminosalicylic acid (PAS) was formerly widely used with INH, it is poorly tolerated by many patients, and the GI distress resulting from the large doses that are required reduced patient compliance. PAS is still a valuable adjunctive drug, but as indicated above, it has been replaced in many INH drug regimens by ethambutol or rifampin. Streptomycin is likewise an effective antitubercular drug, but must be given only in combination with other drugs such as INH, PAS, ethambutol, and rifampin, because resistance develops rapidly. It is used primarily for extensive pulmonary or disseminated tuberculosis. The second-line drugs, because of their toxicity, are indicated only where treatment with the first-line drugs has failed. In addition, pyrazinamide is only effective for approximately two months, and should not be continued for longer periods of time.

Because there are numerous differences among the various clinically available antitubercular drugs, they are considered individually.

▶ para-aminosalicylate sodium

P.A.S. Sodium, Teebacin

The sodium salt of PAS contains 73% aminosalicylic acid equivalent and 10.9% sodium. It is used in combination with isoniazid, rifampin, and/or streptomycin to delay the emergence of bacterial resistance to these first-line antitubercular drugs. PAS should never be used as the sole therapeutic agent in treating tuberculosis.

Mechanism
Inhibits bacterial folic acid synthesis by competing with enzyme systems for incorporation of para-aminobenzoic acid (PABA)

Uses
1 Adjunctive treatment of tuberculosis in combination with isoniazid, rifampin, and/or streptomycin to delay development of resistance.

Dosage
Adults: 14 g to 16 g/day in two to three divided doses
Children: 275 mg/kg to 420 mg/kg/day in three to four divided doses

Fate
Well absorbed orally; widely distributed, concentrating in pleural tissue but attaining low cerebrospinal fluid levels; half-life is about 1 hour; rapidly excreted in the urine, 80%

to 90% within 8 hours to 10 hours, both as intact drug and metabolites

Common Side-Effects
GI distress, nausea, and anorexia

Significant Adverse Reactions
GI—diarrhea, vomiting, abdominal pain, epigastric burning, ulceration, gastric hemorrhage
Hypersensitivity—fever, skin rash, malaise, joint pain, mononucleosis-like syndrome, jaundice, hepatitis, pancreatitis
Hematologic—leukopenia, agranulocytosis, thrombocytopenia, hemolytic anemia
Other—goiter, hypokalemia, acidosis, vasculitis, Löffler's syndrome (fever, cough, dyspnea), encephalopathy, crystalluria

Contraindications
Salicylate hypersensitivity

Interactions
1 PAS plasma levels may be increased by probenecid, salicylates, or sulfinpyrazone.
2 PAS may decrease absorption of rifampin, folic acid, and vitamin B_{12}.
3 PAS may increase INH plasma levels by reducing its rate of metabolism.
4 Urinary acidifiers (*e.g.,* ammonium chloride, ascorbic acid) increase the possibility of PAS crystalluria.
5 PAS may potentiate the action of oral anticoagulants.

▶ NURSING ALERTS
▷ 1 Be alert for signs of hypersensitivity (*e.g.,* skin eruptions, fever, malaise, fatigue, pruritus, joint pain), and, if necessary, discontinue all drugs to prevent development of liver or kidney damage or pancreatitis. Resume therapy with low doses once symptoms have abated, and observe patient carefully.
▷ 2 Use with caution in persons with impaired renal or hepatic function, gastric ulcer, congestive heart failure and other situations requiring sodium restriction, goiter, or hematologic abnormalities.
▷ 3 Advise patients to notify physician if fever, sore throat, unusual bleeding or bruising, or skin eruptions occur, because these may indicate a developing blood dyscrasia.

▶ NURSING CONSIDERATIONS
▷ 1 Maintain high fluid intake and keep urine neutral or slightly alkaline, for example, with sodium bicarbonate or antacids, to prevent crystalluria.
▷ 2 Administer drug with food to minimize GI upset. Suggest use of gum or candy to eliminate sour or bitter taste in mouth that often results from oral administration of PAS.
▷ 3 Do not use tablets or solutions (made from powder) that are brown or purple in color, because discoloration indicates deterioration of the drug.
▷ 4 Protect drug from heat and moisture, because it is very unstable. Use solutions of drug within 24 hours.

▷ 5 Be aware that drug may interfere with certain laboratory tests, for example, urinary protein, urobilinogen, and VMA and urinary glucose determinations with copper sulfate reagents (Clinitest tablets).
▷ 6 Note that the sodium salt is freely soluble in water and may be administered by dissolving powder in water. Powder is available in preweighed packets and in bulk containers.

▷ *Dietary precaution*
▷ 1 Avoid excessive intake of cranberry or prune juice, because these tend to acidify urine, increasing the danger of crystalluria.

▶ capreomycin
Capastat

Capreomycin is a polypeptide antibiotic used in combination with other appropriate drugs as an alternate antitubercular agent when the first-line drugs are ineffective. Capreomycin is both ototoxic and nephrotoxic and must be administered cautiously.

Mechanism
Not established; bacteriostatic against human strains of *Mycobacterium tuberculosis;* exhibits a neuromuscular blocking action in large doses; no cross-resistance with other tuberculostatic drugs

Uses
1 Alternate therapy of pulmonary tuberculosis in patients intolerant of or resistant to first-line drug regimens (*i.e.,* INH, ethambutol, rifampin, streptomycin)

Dosage
IM only: 1 g/day for 60 days to 120 days, followed by 1 g two to three times a week (maximum 20 mg/kg/day)

Fate
Not appreciably absorbed when administered orally; peak serum levels in 1 hour to 2 hours following IM injection; excreted essentially unchanged in the urine, 50% within 12 hours

Common Side-Effects
Elevated BUN and nonprotein nitrogen (NPN), subclinical hearing loss (5–10 decibels), and eosinophilia

Significant Adverse Reactions
Hematuria, proteinuria, abnormal urinary sediment, renal tubular necrosis, tinnitus, vertigo, anorexia, clinically apparent hearing loss, leukocytosis, leukopenia, abnormal liver function tests, pain and induration of IM injection site, urticaria, maculopapular skin rash, hypokalemia

Contraindications
Concurrent administration with streptomycin or other ototoxic drugs (*e.g.,* aminoglycosides, polymyxin, colistin), and severe renal impairment

Interactions
1 Capreomycin may enhance the muscle-relaxing action of neuromuscular blocking agents, polypeptide antibiotics, aminoglycosides, and general anesthetics.
2 The potential for nephrotoxicity is increased by combined use of capreomycin with aminoglycosides, cephalothin, ethacrynic acid, furosemide, polymyxins, and vancomycin.
3 Ototoxic effects of capreomycin can be potentiated by aminoglycosides, ethacrynic acid, furosemide, and vancomycin.

▶ NURSING ALERTS
▷ 1 Urge patients to report immediately any signs of hearing impairment or vertigo. Discontinue drug immediately to prevent development of serious ototoxicity. Perform periodic audiometric and vestibular function tests during therapy.
▷ 2 Use with caution in patients with renal or hepatic dysfunction, auditory impairment, history of allergies, and in children and during pregnancy.
▷ 3 Monitor intake–output ratio and observe for signs of renal toxicity (*e.g.,* urinary casts or presence of red or white cells; elevation of BUN, *e.g.,* above 30 mg/100 ml; proteinuria; hematuria). Discontinue drug to prevent serious kidney damage. Perform regular renal function tests during therapy.

▶ NURSING CONSIDERATIONS
▷ 1 Make IM injections deeply into a large muscle and observe for inflammation and bleeding. Rotate injection sites.
▷ 2 Make frequent determinations of serum potassium levels, because hypokalemia has occurred during prolonged therapy. Observe for signs of potassium deficiency, for example, paresthesias, muscle cramping, palpitations.
▷ 3 Be aware that therapy for tuberculosis is usually continued for 18 months to 24 months. Consider a change to oral therapy as soon as is feasible, because patient compliance is frequently much better than with long-term parenteral therapy.
▷ 4 Prepare solution by dissolving powder for injection in 2 ml of Sodium Chloride Injection or Sterile Water for Injection. Complete dissolution may require 2 to 3 minutes of mixing. Solution may darken over time, without affecting potency. Store for 48 hours at room temperature or up to 14 days refrigerated.

▶ cycloserine
Seromycin

A broad-spectrum antibiotic, cycloserine is effective against a variety of gram-positive and gram-negative bacteria as well as *Mycobacterium tuberculosis*. A second-line drug in the treatment of tuberculosis, it can also be used for acute urinary tract infections unresponsive to commonly employed drugs. Major untoward reactions are CNS toxicity (*e.g.,* convulsions, psychosis, depression) and allergic reactions.

Mechanism

Inhibits cell wall synthesis in susceptible bacteria by antagonizing D-alanine, an essential factor in bacterial cell wall synthesis; bactericidal at usual therapeutic doses

Uses

1 Alternate treatment of active tuberculosis in conjunction with other tuberculostatic drugs when first-line therapy has failed
2 Alternate treatment of acute urinary tract infections, especially those due to *Enterobacter* and *Escherichia coli,* only where other antimicrobial agents are ineffective and the infecting organism has demonstrated sensitivity to cycloserine

Dosage

Oral: initially 250 mg twice a day for 2 weeks; maintenance dose is 500 mg to 1000 mg/day in divided doses as necessary; do not exceed 1 g/day

Fate

Well absorbed orally; peak plasma levels attained in 3 hours to 4 hours; widely distributed, including the CNS; half-life is 10 hours; excreted primarily in the urine, both as active drug and metabolites

Significant Adverse Reactions

Neurotoxicity (dose-related; symptoms include vertigo, paresthesias, irritability, headache, aggression, hyperreflexia, drowsiness, tremor, dysarthria, confusion, disorientation, loss of memory, convulsions, localized clonic seizures, psychoses, suicidal tendencies, coma)

Other adverse reactions are skin rash, allergic dermatitis, photosensitivity, elevated serum transaminase, vitamin B_{12} or folic acid deficiency, megaloblastic anemia.

Contraindications

Epilepsy, severe anxiety, psychoses, excessive alcohol consumption, depression, and severe renal insufficiency

Interactions

1 Cycloserine can potentiate the effects of MAO inhibitors and phenytoin
2 Ethionamide, isoniazid, and alcohol can enhance the neurotoxic effects of cycloserine.
3 Cycloserine can increase the excretion of the B-complex vitamins.

▶ NURSING ALERTS

▷ 1 Inform physician immediately if symptoms of allergic dermatitis or CNS toxicity occur (see Adverse Reactions). Reduce dosage or discontinue drug to avoid more serious untoward reactions. Anticonvulsants, pyridoxine, or sedatives may be effective in controlling CNS toxicity.
▷ 2 Be aware that CNS toxicity is related to serum drug levels. High dosage (greater than 500 mg/day) or inadequate renal clearance predisposes to neurotoxic effects.
▷ 3 Urge patients to exercise caution in driving or performing hazardous tasks, because drowsiness, dizziness, and confusion may occur.
▷ 4 Caution patients to avoid excessive alcohol consumption, because risk of convulsions is increased by ingestion of large amounts of alcohol.

▶ NURSING CONSIDERATIONS

▷ 1 Perform periodic hematologic, renal excretion, liver function, and blood level studies during therapy. Blood levels should be determined at least weekly in patients who receive large doses or who exhibit reduced renal function. Adjust dosage to keep blood level below 30 mcg/ml.
▷ 2 Reduce dosage in patients with renal impairment based upon creatinine clearance (see package instructions).
▷ 3 Be alert for signs of a developing anemia and institute appropriate therapy (*e.g.,* vitamin B_{12}, folic acid).
▷ 4 Be prepared to administer oxygen, artificial respiration, IV fluids, vasopressors, and anticonvulsants should convulsions or other manifestations of CNS toxicity occur.

▶ ethambutol
Myambutol

A synthetic orally administered tuberculostatic drug effective against actively divided mycobacteria, ethambutol is a first-line drug for treatment of pulmonary tuberculosis. It is most often used in combination with INH, with or without rifampin or streptomycin, depending on the severity of the condition because it is somewhat less active alone than other first-line drugs. Previously unexposed microorganisms are uniformly sensitive to ethambutol, but resistance does develop in a stepwise manner. Ethambutol may have adverse effects on visual acuity, thus monthly eye examinations are recommended during therapy.

Mechanism

Inhibits protein synthesis and impairs cellular metabolism, thus blocking multiplication of bacterial cells; does not exhibit cross-resistance with other agents

Use

1 Initial treatment of pulmonary tuberculosis, usually in combination with INH and possibly rifampin or streptomycin

Dosage

Initial treatment: 15 mg/kg as a single oral dose every 24 hours with INH
Retreatment: (patients having previous antituberculosis treatment) 25 mg/kg as a single oral dose every 24 hours with at least one other antitubercular drug to which the organism is susceptible; decrease to 15 mg/kg after 60 days

Fate

Readily absorbed from GI tract and unaffected by the presence of food; peak serum level occurs in 2 hours to 4 hours; no accumulation has been reported in patients with normal kidney function; approximately 50% excreted unchanged in the urine, 20% to 25% eliminated unchanged in the feces, and the remainder excreted as metabolites in the urine

Significant Adverse Reactions
CNS—decreased visual acuity due to optic neuritis (*e.g.*, altered color perception, blurred vision), fever, malaise, headache, dizziness, confusion, disorientation, paresthesias, hallucinations
GI—abdominal pain, GI upset, vomiting, anorexia
Allergic—pruritus, dermatitis, joint pain, anaphylactic reactions
Other—elevated serum uric acid, acute gout, transient impairment of liver function, epidermal necrolysis, thrombocytopenia

Contraindications
Optic neuritis; in children under 12 years of age

Interactions
1 Ethambutol may reduce the effectiveness of uricosuric drugs such as probenecid and sulfinpyrazone.
2 Aluminum-containing antacids may impair oral absorption of myambutol.

▶ NURSING ALERTS
▷ 1 Advise patients to report promptly any change in visual acuity or color perception. Discontinue drug and inform patient that recovery may take several weeks to several months. Effects are generally readily reversible, but in rare cases may be prolonged or permanent.
▷ 2 Test for visual function before beginning therapy and then periodically during treatment (monthly if drug is administered in high doses).
▷ 3 Use cautiously in patients with hepatic or renal dysfunction, hyperuricemia, or history of acute gout, and during pregnancy.

▶ NURSING CONSIDERATIONS
▷ 1 Administer with food to minimize GI upset. Absorption is not altered by the presence of food.
▷ 2 Reduce dosage in patients with impaired renal function, based upon desired serum levels of the drug (*i.e.*, 2 mcg–5 mcg/ml).
▷ 3 Note that the drug can increase levels of SGPT, SGOT, and serum uric acid.

▶ ethionamide
Trecator-SC

Mechanism
Not established; probably similar to that of isoniazid

Use
1 Alternate therapy of active tuberculosis in combination with other effective antitubercular drugs when treatment with first-line drugs (INH, ethambutol, rifampin, streptomycin) has failed

Dosage
Adults: 0.5 g to 1 g/day in divided doses with at least one other antitubercular drug
Children: optimum dosage is not established; 4 mg/kg to 5 mg/kg every 8 hours has been suggested.

Fate
Well absorbed orally and distributed widely in the body, including the CNS; peak serum levels attained in 3 hours to 4 hours; excreted largely in the urine, almost entirely as metabolites

Common Side-Effects
GI upset (nausea, vomiting, cramping), salivation, diarrhea, anorexia, drowsiness, asthenia.

Significant Adverse Reactions
Neurotoxicity—blurred vision, diplopia, optic neuritis, peripheral neuritis, olfactory disturbances, dizziness, headache, restlessness, tremors, convulsions, psychosis
GI—metallic taste, stomatitis, hepatitis, jaundice
Other—orthostatic hypotension, impotence, gynecomastia, acne, skin rash, alopecia, pellagra-like syndrome, thrombocytopenia

Contraindications
Severe hepatic dysfunction

Interactions
1 Ethionamide can enhance the neurotoxicity of cycloserine and may intensify the adverse effects of other tuberculostatic agents.
2 Ethionamide may increase the neurotoxic effects of alcohol.
3 Ethionamide may potentiate the hypotensive effects (especially orthostatic) of antihypertensive drugs.
4 Ethionamide may interfere with the management of diabetes by antidiabetic drugs.

▶ NURSING ALERTS
▷ 1 Use cautiously in patients with diabetes mellitus, liver or renal impairment, in children, and during pregnancy (fetal damage has been reported in experimental animals).
▷ 2 Caution patients to avoid excessive use of alcohol during drug therapy to minimize danger of neurotoxicity.

▶ NURSING CONSIDERATIONS
▷ 1 Administer with food to reduce GI upset.
▷ 2 Measure serum transaminase (SGOT, SGPT) before and at 2-week to 4-week intervals throughout therapy.
▷ 3 Be aware that ethionamide therapy may make management of diabetes mellitus more difficult. Adjust dosage of antidiabetic drugs as necessary based on blood glucose determinations.
▷ 4 Note that ethionamide may contribute to the vitamin B_6 (pyridoxine) deficiency produced by isoniazid when these drugs are used concurrently. Administer 50 mg/day of vitamin B_6 during therapy with ethionamide.

▶ **isoniazid**

INH, Laniazid, Nydrazid, Teebaconin

A first-line drug of choice for most cases of active tuberculosis, isoniazid is usually prescribed in combination with ethambutol or rifampin, or both, to delay the emergence of resistant strains. It is also indicated for prophylactic use in high-risk patients, such as household members of infected persons or persons with positive tuberculin skin test reactions. A major danger associated with INH is severe and sometimes fatal hepatitis. The risk of developing hepatitis increases with advancing age (see Significant Adverse Reactions).

Mechanism

Not completely established; drug is bactericidal; may interfere with biosynthesis of lipids, proteins, and nucleic acid in susceptible organisms; resistance frequently develops rapidly when INH is used alone; can antagonize the activity of vitamin B_6.

Uses

1 Treatment of all forms of active tuberculosis due to susceptible organisms, usually in combination with other tuberculostatic drugs
2 Prophylaxis in high-risk patients such as household members or close associates of actively infected individuals or persons evidencing positive tuberculin skin test reactions in the absence of positive bacteriologic findings; also used in persons under 35 (especially children under 7 yr) with positive skin test reactions, patients with hematologic diseases (*e.g.,* leukemia, Hodgkin's disease) or diabetes, persons undergoing immunosuppressive therapy or prolonged treatment with corticosteroids, and following a gastrectomy.

Dosage

Acute tuberculosis

Adults: 5 mg/kg/day in a single dose (maximum 300 mg/day)

Children: 10 mg/kg to 20 mg/kg/day in a single dose (maximum 500 m/day)

Prophylaxis

Adults: 300 mg/day in a single dose
Children: 10 mg/kg/day in a single dose

Fate

Adequately absorbed from the GI tract; absorption is reduced by food; peak blood levels in 1 hour to 2 hours, declining to 50% or less within 6 hours; widely distributed in the body including cerebrospinal, pleural, and ascitic tissues; less than one half is excreted unchanged in the urine; most of the remainder is acetylated or hydrolyzed by the liver and metabolites are removed by the kidney; rate of acetylation is genetically determined, and may be slow (in approximately 50% of Blacks and Caucasians) or rapid (rest of Blacks and Caucasians, Orientals, and Eskimos); rate of acetylation does *not* alter clinical efficacy of INH but may

influence toxicity (*i.e.,* slow acetylators are more prone to elevated blood levels and increased toxic reactions, including peripheral neuropathies, rapid acetylators are more likely to develop hepatitis); liver disease can prolong clearance of INH

Common Side-Effects

Paresthesias, peripheral neuropathy (especially in malnourished, diabetic, or alcoholic persons), and mild hepatic dysfunction (transient elevation of serum transminase)

Significant Adverse Reactions

CNS—optic neuritis, toxic encephalopathy, memory impairment, toxic psychosis, convulsions
GI—nausea, vomiting, epigastric distress
Hepatic—bilirubinemia, bilirubinuria, jaundice, severe (occasionally fatal) hepatitis
Hematologic—hemolytic or aplastic anemia, agranulocytosis, eosinophilia, thrombocytopenia
Allergic—fever, skin rashes (morbilliform, maculopapular, purpuric, exfoliative), vasculitis, lymphadenopathy
Other—vitamin B_6 deficiency, hyperglycemia, metabolic acidosis, gynecomastia, pellagra, rheumatoid or systemic lupus-like symptoms, irritation at IM injection site

Contraindications

Acute liver disease, previous adverse reaction with isoniazid

Interactions

1 INH can increase serum levels of phenytoin by reducing its metabolism.
2 The efficacy of INH may be reduced when given concurrently with corticosteroids.
3 Alcohol increases the risk of INH-induced hepatitis.
4 INH can potentiate the pharmacologic and toxicologic effects of carbamazepine and benzodiazepine antianxiety agents.
5 Antacids reduce GI absorption of INH if they are given together.
6 Disulfiram and INH can impair coordination and produce behavioral changes.
7 Concurrent use of INH and rifampin may increase the likelihood of hepatotoxicity, while combined use of INH and cycloserine can increase CNS toxicity.
8 INH may exhibit MAO inhibitory activity and can potentiate sympathomimetic amines, leading to increased blood pressure.
9 INH has been reported to potentiate anesthetics, anticoagulants, anticonvulsants, antidiabetics, antihypertensives, antiparkinsonian agents, anticholinergics, antidepressants, narcotics, and sedatives, although the clinical importance of these potential interactions has not been definitely established.

▶ **NURSING ALERTS**

▷ 1 Closely observe patients for indications of hepatic dysfunction (anorexia, malaise, nausea, vomiting, darkening of the urine, paresthesias, jaundice), and discontinue drug immediately. Monthly liver function tests should be performed during therapy.

▷ 2 Be alert for development of hypersensitivity reactions, and discontinue drug. If therapy is reinstituted, do so in very small doses and withdraw immediately if hypersensitivity recurs.

▷ 3 Closely monitor and use with caution in patients with chronic liver impairment, renal disease, alcoholism, history of convulsive disorders or psychoses, and in pregnant or nursing women.

▷ 4 Urge patients to reduce intake of alcohol during INH therapy to minimize the risk of hepatitis.

▶ NURSING CONSIDERATIONS

▷ 1 Perform periodic ophthalmic examinations during therapy and advise physician if visual disturbances occur during treatment.

▷ 2 Administer drug on an empty stomach if possible and avoid simultaneous administration of antacids. Food may be given to minimize GI irritation, but will slow GI absorption as well.

▷ 3 Use supplemental vitamin B_6 (10 mg–100 mg/day) to minimize the neurotoxic effects of INH, especially in malnourished or diabetic persons and "slow" acetylators of INH (see Fate). INH is available in fixed combinations with vitamin B_6 (100 mg INH/5 mg vitamin B_6; 100 mg/10 mg; 300 mg/30 mg) as Teebaconin and vitamin B_6 and P-I-N Forte

▷ 4 Recognize that adverse effects with INH, especially those affecting the liver and nervous system, are more prevalent at higher doses. Do not exceed recommended doses.

▷ 5 Stress the importance of adherence to dosage regimen. Caution against missing doses or discontinuing therapy without physician's knowledge, because relapse rates are high if treatment is terminated too early, and resistant strains emerge if the dose is insufficient.

▷ 6 Monitor diabetic patients closely and adjust dose of antidiabetic medication as needed to maintain control, because INH can elevate blood sugar or potentiate the action of hypoglycemic drugs.

▷ 7 Administer IM only when oral route is unavailable or impractical. Inform patient that IM injections may be irritating or painful.

▷ 8 Note that INH is also available in fixed combinations with rifampin as Rifamate or Rimactane/INH Dual Pack.

▶ pyrazinamide

Pyrazinamide is a second-line tuberculostatic agent, used only in combination with primary drugs (INH, ethambutol, rifampin, streptomycin) in resistant patients or for short-term therapy before pulmonary surgery in advanced cases to minimize further spread of infection. Principal adverse effects are hepatotoxicity (the incidence of which ranges from 2%–20% and is dependent on the dosage) and hyperuricemia.

Mechanism

Not established; primarily bacteriostatic, possibly due to interference with protein synthesis; active only at slightly acidic *p*H

Uses

1 Adjunctive therapy of tuberculosis in combination with other first-line drugs in patients in whom these primary agents are ineffective

Dosage

20 mg/kg to 35 mg/kg/day in three or four divided doses (maximum dose 3 g/day)

Fate

Readily absorbed orally; peak serum levels in 2 hours; half-life is 9 hours to 10 hours; widely distributed in the body, partially metabolized by the liver and excreted in the urine primarily (70%) as metabolites with some unchanged drug

Significant Adverse Reactions

Hepatic dysfunction (fever, anorexia, malaise, hepatomegaly, abdominal tenderness, splenomegaly, jaundice, yellow atrophy of the liver), GI distress, arthralgia, anemia, dysuria, urinary retention, hyperuricemia, acute gout, skin rash, urticaria, and photosensitivity

Contraindications

Severe liver damage; in children

Interactions

1 Pyrazinamide can interfere with the uricosuric action of probenecid and sulfinpyrazone.
2 Pyrazinamide may alter the dosage requirements for insulin or oral hypoglycemic drugs in diabetics.

▶ NURSING ALERTS

▷ 1 Be alert for signs of liver dysfunction (see Significant Adverse Reactions) and discontinue drug immediately should they appear. Perform liver function tests before beginning drug and then every 2 weeks to 4 weeks during therapy. Hepatotoxicity can range from an asymptomatic abnormality of liver cell function to severe jaundice and fulminating acute yellow atrophy.

▷ 2 Monitor serum uric acid before and during treatment, and advise patients to report development of pain in toes, ankle, heel, or other joints.

▷ 3 Use cautiously in patients with a history of gout or hyperuricemia, diabetes mellitus, impaired renal function, peptic ulcer, and acute intermittent porphyria.

▶ NURSING CONSIDERATIONS

▷ 1 Use only when close observation of patients is possible and laboratory facilities are available to monitor liver function and serum uric acid.

▷ 2 Adjust dose of antidiabetic medication as necessary to maintain stable blood glucose levels, because pyrazinamide can affect control of the diabetic condition.

▶ streptomycin

An aminoglycoside antibiotic effective against *Mycobacterium tuberculosis,* streptomycin is considered a primary drug. It is most often used in combination with INH, rifampin, or ethambutol for control of more severe infections. Resistance develops rapidly; hence combination therapy is necessary to maintain effectiveness. It is administered IM only, thus patient compliance during prolonged therapy may be poor. The principal danger associated with use of streptomycin is ototoxicity, both vestibular and auditory, and patients receiving the drug must be observed carefully. Streptomycin has been discussed in detail in Chapter 62, and only the dosage regimen for use in tuberculosis will be given here.

Dosage
Usual regimen is 1 g streptomycin IM with an appropriate
   dose of additional antitubercular drugs, such as INH,
   ethambutol, or rifampin; reduce streptomycin dose to
   1 g two or three times a week as symptoms improve.
Use smaller doses in the elderly or in patients with impaired renal function.

▶ rifampin
Rifadin, Rimactane

A derivative of the antibiotic rifamycin B, rifampin is a first-line bacteriostatic antitubercular drug. It is most often used in combination with INH and ethambutol, because resistance develops rapidly if it is given alone. The drug should be taken on an uninterrupted schedule, because intermittent therapy has resulted in a higher incidence of adverse reactions, especially involving the liver and kidneys.

Mechanism
Inhibits DNA-dependent RNA polymerase activity in bacterial cells, thus interfering with nucleic acid synthesis; active against a number of gram-positive and gram-negative organisms

Uses
1 Treatment of pulmonary tuberculosis in conjunction with at least one other tuberculostatic drug (*e.g.,* INH, ethambutol, streptomycin)
2 Treatment of asymptomatic carriers of *Neisseria meningitidis* to eliminate meningococci from the nasopharynx (*not* indicated for meningococcal infections)
3 Investigational uses include treatment of staphylococcal infections, Legionnaire's disease not responsive to erythromycin, gram-negative bacteremia in infancy, leprosy (with dapsone), and prophylaxis of *Hemophilus* meningitis.

Dosage
Pulmonary tuberculosis
Adults: 600 mg/day in a single oral dose
Children (over 5 yr): 10 mg/kg to 20 mg/kg/day in a single dose

Meningococcal carriers
Adults: 600 mg/day for 4 consecutive days
Children (over 5 yr): 10 mg/kg to 20 mg/kg/day for 4 consecutive days

Fate
Oral absorption is adequate; peak blood levels vary widely and occur between 2 hours to 4 hours; half-life is approximately 3 hours; 70% to 80% protein-bound; metabolized in the liver and excreted both in the feces (via bile) and to a lesser extent in the urine as both free drug and deacetylated metabolites

Common Side-Effects
Elevation of liver enzymes, "flu-like" syndrome at high doses

Significant Adverse Reactions
GI—anorexia, vomiting, diarrhea, cramping, flatulence, sore mouth, pancreatitis, pseudomembranous colitis
CNS—headache, drowsiness, fatigue, dizziness, ataxia, confusion, visual disturbances, muscle weakness, generalized numbness, hearing disturbances
Allergic—pruritus, urticaria, rash, acneiform lesions, fever
Hepatic/renal—abnormal liver function tests (elevated BUN, serum bilirubin, serum transaminase, alkaline phosphatase), hepatitis, hemoglobinuria, hematuria, proteinuria, renal insufficiency, acute renal failure
Hematologic—transient leukopenia, thrombocytopenia, decreased hemoglobin, hemolytic anemia, eosinophilia
Other—conjunctivitis, elevated serum uric acid, menstrual irregularities, osteomalacia, myopathy

Interactions
1 Rifampin induces microsomal enzymes and thus may decrease the effects of other drugs metabolized by these liver enzymes, for example, oral anticoagulants, estrogens, progestins, metoprolol, propranolol, quinidine, clofibrate, corticosteroids, oral antidiabetics, and methadone.
2 PAS administered concurrently can impair GI absorption of rifampin and can reduce rifampin serum levels.
3 The action of rifampin can be potentiated by probenecid, which competes for hepatic uptake.
4 Concomitant use of rifampin and alcohol may increase the incidence of hepatotoxicity.

▶ NURSING ALERTS
▷ 1 Observe closely for development of flu-like symptoms (fever, chills, headache, muscle aches), especially if drug has been used intermittently, because these may signal impending hepatorenal dysfunction.
▷ 2 Advise patients to note occurrence of sore throat, unusual bleeding or bruising, or excessive weakness, indications of possible blood dyscrasias, and to inform physician immediately should they occur. Hematologic studies should be performed.
▷ 3 Caution patients to report appearance of jaundice-like symptoms immediately (yellowing of skin or sclerae, pruritus, darkened urine, light colored stools). Liver function must be evaluated periodically during therapy.

▷ 4 Administer carefully to persons with hepatic or renal disease or a history of alcoholism, and to pregnant women and children under 5 years of age.

▷ 5 Discuss the use of alternate contraceptive methods with women using oral contraceptive drugs during rifampin therapy, because the effectiveness of oral contraceptives may be reduced by rifampin.

▶ **NURSING CONSIDERATIONS**

▷ 1 Inform patients that the drug may impart a harmless red orange color to urine, feces, saliva, sputum, sweat, and tears.

▷ 2 Stress the importance of taking the drug on a continual basis, because interruptions in therapy may increase the likelihood of adverse reactions.

▷ 3 Administer on an empty stomach if possible, because food may delay absorption and reduce peak serum drug concentration.

▷ 4 Alert female patients to the fact that menstrual irregularities can occur during rifampin therapy.

▷ 5 Be aware that rifampin can interfere with standard assays for serum folate and vitamin B_{12}. Alternative methods must be used to perform these determinations.

Summary. Antitubercular Drugs

Drug	Preparations	Usual Dosage Range
Para-aminosalicylate sodium (P.A.S. Sodium, Teebacin)	Tablets—0.5 g, 1 g Powder	Adults—14 g to 16 g/day in 2 to 3 divided doses
		Children—275 mg/kg–420 mg/kg/day in 3 to 4 divided doses
Capreomycin (Capastat)	Powder for injection—1 g/5-ml	1 g/day IM for 60 days to 120 days, then 1 g 2 to 3 times a week
Cycloserine (Seromycin)	Capsules—250 mg	250 mg twice a day for 2 weeks, then 500 mg to 1000 mg/day in divided doses
Ethambutol (Myambutol)	Tablets—100 mg, 400 mg	Initially 15 mg/kg/day as a single dose
		Retreatment: 25 mg/kg/day as a single oral dose
Ethionamide (Trecator-SC)	Tablets—250 mg	Adults—0.5 g to 1 g/day in divided doses
Isoniazid (INH, Laniazid, Nydrazid, Teebaconin)	Tablets—50 mg, 100 mg, 300 mg Injection—100 mg/ml Powder	Treatment: Adults—5 mg/kg/day in a single dose (maximum 300 mg a day)
		Children—10 mg to 20 mg/kg/day in a single dose (maximum 500 mg a day)
		Prophylaxis: Adults—300 mg/day in a single dose
		Children—10 mg/kg/day in a single dose
Pyrazinamide (Pyrazinamide)	Tablets—500 mg	20 mg to 35 mg/kg/day in 3 to 4 divided doses (maximum 3 g/day)
Streptomycin (Streptomycin)	Injection—1 g, 5 g	1 g IM with an appropriate dose of INH, rifampin, or ethambutol
Rifampin (Rifadin, Rimactane)	Capsules—150 mg, 300 mg	Tuberculosis: Adults—600 mg/day in a single dose
		Children—10 mg/kg to 20 mg/kg/day in a single dose
		Meningococcal carrier state: Adults—600 mg/day for 4 consecutive days
		Children—10 mg to 20 mg/kg/day for 4 consecutive days

69 Antimalarial Agents

Malaria is a parasitic disease that is still prevalent in many areas of the world, especially Southeast Asia, Africa, and Central and South America. Four species of the protozoan *Plasmodium* can cause malaria in man and these are described briefly below.

1 *Plasmodium falciparum*—cause of malignant tertian (MT) malaria; a severe, often fulminating infection that may progress to a fatal outcome if not treated quickly and vigorously; prompt therapy is usually highly successful, however, and relapses generally do not occur

2 *Plasmodium vivax*—cause of benign tertian (BT) malaria; a less severe disease than that produced by the *Plasmodium falciparum* strain, having a low mortality rate but characterized by periodic relapses that may continue for years if untreated

3 *Plasmodium malariae*—cause of quartan malaria; so named because the attacks of chills and high fever recur every 4 days rather than every 3 days as in the tertian form of the disease; outbreaks tend to appear in localized regions of the tropics; clinical signs may remain dormant for many years, and relapses do occur, but less frequently than with the *Plasmodium vivax* organism

4 *Plasmodium ovale*—cause of ovale tertian malaria, a rare form of relapsing malaria similar to but milder and more readily cured than the vivax infection

Malaria is usually transmitted to man by the bite of the female Anopheles mosquito, which deposits the infective sporozoites, formed in the blood of the mosquito by the union of male and female gametocytes, into the human. The sporozoites localize in the liver, where they form primary tissue schizonts. These then grow and multiply into merozoites. This is the pre-erythrocytic or symptom-free stage of the infection. When mature, the merozoites are released from the liver and invade the erythrocytes (red blood cells) to begin the blood-cycle phase of the infection. Young parasites in the red blood cell are termed trophozoites, and they grow and divide into mature schizonts, also known as blood merozoites. Periodically, the blood merozoites burst from the ruptured cells and invade a new group of erythrocytes, beginning the process anew. This periodic (every 3 days–4 days) rupturing of infected erythrocytes is responsible for the characteristic fever and chills that accompany acute attacks of malaria.

In all but falciparum malaria, another important phase of the plasmodial life cycle is the exoerythrocytic cycle; this is responsible for the relapses frequently seen in many patients. A portion of the released merozoites make their way back to the liver as well as other tissue sites, rather than invade more erythrocytes. There they may persist for long periods, multiply, and periodically send forth new erythrocyte invaders. Thus, acute malarial attacks can occur for several years unless these exoerythrocytic forms are eradicated during the primary treatment phase.

Finally, some of the merozoites that invade erythrocytes do not undergo the above described process of *asexual* reproduction, but instead differentiate into male and female gametocytes. Upon ingestion into a female mosquito (*via* a bite of an infected human), *sexual* fertilization of the female gametocyte by the male gametocyte occurs in the gut of the mosquito, giving rise to new infective sporozoites.

Drug therapy of malaria may be directed either toward prevention of infection, suppression of clinical symptoms, treatment of acute attacks, or prevention of relapses. These methods are reviewed below:

1 *Prevention of infection*—drugs that kill the malarial organisms during their pre-erythrocytic stages are termed *causal prophylactics;* however, no drug is currently available that can *selectively* destroy sporozoites at therapeutic levels that are considered safe. Prophylaxis of malaria is best accomplished by mosquito control.

2 *Suppression of clinical symptoms*—inhibition of the erythrocytic stage of the cycle can prevent development of clinical symptoms in an infected individual. Several antimalarial drugs (*i.e.,* chloroquine, hydroxychloroquine, pyrimethamine) act in this manner, but acute attacks can occur when therapy is discontinued if exoerythrocytic forms of the organism are still present.

3 *Treatment of acute attacks*—interruption of erythrocytic parasite multiplication can terminate the symptoms of an acute malarial attack, and drugs acting in this way are termed *schizonticides.* The 4-aminoquinolines are generally considered drugs of choice in this case, but they do not completely eliminate the parasite from the body; hence the possibility of relapse exists, especially with the vivax strains.

4 *Prevention of relapse*—drugs that eradicate the exoerythrocytic parasites (secondary tissue forms) can prevent relapse infections, and such treatment is sometimes referred to as a *radical cure.* The only currently available drug producing a radical cure in vivax malaria is primaquine and it is usually given in combination with a drug (*e.g.,* chloroquine) that suppresses the erythrocyte cycle as well.

Combination suppressive therapy and radical cure (*e.g.,* with chloroquine and primaquine) is widely employed in travelers to areas in which malaria is endemic. Therapy is begun before arrival and repeated at weekly intervals during and for at least 2 months after returning from the malarial region to ensure that in the event infection occurs, clinical symptoms are suppressed and any secondary tissue forms are eradicated.

Prophylaxis may also be accomplished by use of the combination product sulfadoxine and pyrimethamine (Fansidar) beginning 1 day to 2 days before exposure to an endemic area, continuing during the stay, and then for 4 weeks to 6 weeks following departure.

Owing to the many differences among them, the available antimalarial drugs are considered individually here.

▶ 4-aminoquinolines

Chloroquine
Hydroxychloroquine

The 4-aminoquinolines are synthetic drugs that are particularly active against the erythrocytic forms of *Plasmodium* *vivax* and *Plasmodium malariae* and against most forms of *Plasmodium falciparum.* Because they are ineffective against the exoerythrocytic forms, they do not prevent initial infection nor do they prevent relapses in infected persons. Their principal indications are as suppressive agents in vivax or malariae malaria and for terminating acute attacks of all types of malaria. The two drugs are reviewed together, then listed individually in Table 69-1.

Mechanism

Not entirely known; appear to complex with DNA molecules of the parasite, thereby inhibiting RNA replication and subsequent nucleic acid synthesis; may also exert an amebicidal action and may exhibit anti-inflammatory and antihistaminic activity as well

Uses

1 Suppression and treatment of acute attacks of malaria due to *Plasmodium vivax, Plasmodium malariae, Plasmodium ovale,* and susceptible strains of *Plasmodium falciparum*

2 Treatment of extra-intestinal amebiasis (chloroquine, see Chap. 71)

3 Treatment of systemic lupus erythematosus and rheumatoid arthritis (hydroxychloroquine—see Table 69-1)

Dosage

See Table 69-1.

Fate

Rapidly and completely absorbed orally; widely distributed in the body, attaining high concentrations in many tissues; partially metabolized in the liver and slowly excreted by the kidneys; urinary elimination is enhanced by acidification of the urine; tissue levels are detectable for months and occasionally years, especially after termination of prolonged therapy

Common Side-Effects

Mild and transient headaches, GI distress

Significant Adverse Reactions

(Usually seen with prolonged high-dose therapy)

CNS—visual disturbances (blurring, difficulty in focusing), corneal edema or opacity, retinal changes, scotomata, optic atrophy, vertigo, tinnitus, impaired hearing, fatigue, psychic stimulation, convulsions, psychotic episodes

Cardiovascular—hypotension, ECG changes (T wave inversion, widening of the QRS complex)

Dermatologic—skin eruptions, pruritus, alopecia, dermatoses, skin and mucosal pigmentary changes

Hematologic—blood dyscrasias

Other—vomiting, diarrhea, stomach pain, anorexia, neuromyopathy, muscle weakness

Contraindications

Retinal damage, visual field changes, pregnancy, prolonged therapy in children, in patients receiving bone marrow depressants or hemolytic drugs

Table 69-1. 4-Aminoquinolines

Drug	Preparations	Usual Dosage Range	Remarks
Chloroquine (Aralen)	Tablets (phosphate)—250 mg, 500 mg (equivalent to 150 mg, 300 mg of base) Injection (hydrochloride)—50 mg/ml (equivalent to 40 mg/ml base)	Treatment of acute attack: Adults Oral—600 mg (base) initially followed by 300 mg (base) 6 hours, 24 hours, and 48 hours later IM—160 mg to 200 mg (base) initially; repeat in 6 hours; (maximum 800 mg base/24 hr) Children Oral—10 mg/kg (base) initially, followed by 5 mg/kg (base) 6 hours, 24 hours and 48 hours later IM—5 mg/kg (base) initially; repeat in 6 hours (maximum 10 mg/kg base in a 24-hr period) Suppression (oral only): Adults and children 5 mg/kg (base) once weekly, beginning 2 weeks before exposure (maximum 300 mg weekly); continue for 8 weeks after leaving endemic area Treatment of Amebiasis: Oral—600 mg (base) daily for 2 days, then 300 mg (base) daily for 2 weeks to 3 weeks IM—160 mg to 200 mg (base) injected daily for 10 days to 12 days	Indicated for treatment of acute attacks and suppressive therapy of all forms of malaria; also used with an amebicide for treatment of extra-intestinal amebiasis (see Chap. 71); for radical cure of vivax malaria, should be combined with primaquine; parenteral therapy should be terminated and oral therapy initiated as soon as possible; children and infants are very susceptible to adverse attacks from parenteral chloroquine; do not exceed 5 mg/ kg base for any single injection in young children; may be used for treating symptoms of rheumatoid arthritis (150 mg of base in a single daily dose) but hydroxychloroquine is preferred
Hydroxychloroquine sulfate (Plaquenil)	Tablets—200 mg (equivalent to 155 mg base)	Treatment of acute attack: Adults 620 mg (base) initially, followed by 310 mg (base) 6 hours, 24 hours, and 48 hours later Children 10 mg/kg (base) initially, followed by 5 mg/kg (base) 6 hours, 24 hours, and 48 hours later Suppression: Adults and children 5 mg/kg (base) once weekly beginning 2 weeks before exposure (maximum 310 mg base per week); continue for 8 weeks after leaving endemic area Rheumatoid arthritis: Initially 400 mg to 600 mg/day in a single dose; reduce to 200 mg to 400 mg/day when optimum response is observed Lupus erythematosus: Initially 400 mg once or twice a day; continue for weeks or months, but reduce to 200 mg to 400 mg/day when possible	Used for suppression and treatment of all forms of susceptible malaria and for treatment of rheumatoid arthritis and systemic lupus erythematosus; children's dose should never exceed adult dose; radical cure of vivax and malariae malaria requires concomitant therapy with primaquine; several weeks may be required to demonstrate an effect in rheumatoid arthritis; safe use in juvenile arthritis has not been established.

Interactions

1 Liver toxicity may be increased by combined use of other known hepatotoxic drugs.

2 Gold compounds, anti-inflammatory drugs, and other agents known to cause drug sensitization and dermatitis may increase the dermatologic side-effects of the 4-aminoquinolines.

3 Excretion of the 4-aminoquinolines may be enhanced

by urinary acidifiers (*e.g.,* ammonium chloride) and reduced by urinary alkalinizers (*e.g.,* sodium bicarbonate).

4 The action of antipsoriatic drugs may be antagonized by the 4-aminoquinolines, and a severe psoriatic attack can be precipitated.

5 MAO inhibitors can increase the toxicity of 4-aminoquinolines by impairing their hepatic inactivation.

▶ **NURSING ALERTS**

▷ 1 Perform baseline and periodic ophthalmologic examinations during and following prolonged therapy. Advise patients to report at once any visual disturbances, because retinal damage is frequently irreversible and may progress even after cessation of therapy.

▷ 2 Obtain blood counts regularly during therapy and discontinue drug if any severe abnormality is detected.

▷ 3 Use with caution in patients with neurologic or hepatic disease, glucose 6-phosphate dehydrogenase deficiency, blood disorders, psoriasis, porphyria, severe GI disorders, or alcoholism, in infants or small children, and in pregnant or nursing women.

▷ 4 Be alert for development of muscular weakness or impaired reflexes especially during prolonged therapy, and discontinue treatment should this develop.

▷ 5 Do not exceed 5 mg/kg IM of chloroquine as a single dose in children, because they are very susceptible to adverse reactions.

▶ **NURSING CONSIDERATIONS**

▷ 1 Recognize that certain strains of *Plasmodium falciparum* are resistant to 4-aminoquinolines and may require treatment with quinine or other appropriate antimalarial drugs.

▷ 2 Observe for appearance of dermatologic reactions (rash, pruritus, pigmentary changes) and advise physician; dosage should be lowered or alternate drug employed.

▷ 3 Inform patients that drug may discolor urine yellow brown.

▷ 4 Begin weekly suppressive treatment at least 2 weeks before anticipated exposure and continue for at least 8 weeks after leaving endemic area. Give drug on the same day each week.

▷ 5 Administer oral drugs with meals to minimize GI irritative effects.

▶ **primaquine phosphate**

Primaquine

Primaquine phosphate is a synthetic 8-aminoquinoline derivative that eliminates the tissue or exoerythrocytic forms of the organism, thereby preventing relapse of vivax malaria. Primaquine is not effective alone during an acute attack, but is administered in combination with chloroquine or hydroxychloroquine, which destroy the blood or erythrocytic forms.

Mechanism

Not completely established; appears to produce mitochondrial swelling in parasitic cells, thereby disrupting energy metabolism and impairing protein synthesis; prevents development of blood (erythrocytic) forms of vivax malaria; also active against gametocytes of *Plasmodium falciparum*

Use

1 Prevention of relapse (radical cure) of vivax malaria

Dosage

Adults: 26.3 mg (equivalent to 15 mg base) daily for 14 days, *or* 79 mg (45 mg base) once a week for 8 weeks

Children: 0.3 mg (base)/kg/day for 14 days *or* 0.9 mg (base)/kg/week for 8 weeks

Fate

Well absorbed orally; plasma levels are maximum within 2 hours to 3 hours, but fall rapidly thereafter; relatively low levels are found in the lung, liver, heart, skeletal muscles, or brain; rapidly and completely metabolized and excreted largely in the urine; metabolism is impaired by quinacrine (see Interactions)

Common Side-Effects

Epigastric distress

Significant Adverse Reactions

Nausea, vomiting, abdominal cramping, headache, impaired visual accommodation, pruritus, granulocytopenia, leukopenia, hemolytic anemia, and methemoglobinemia

Contraindications

In patients receiving quinacrine (see Interaction), acutely ill patients; rheumatoid arthritis, lupus erythematosus, granulocytopenia, concurrent therapy with potentially hemolytic drugs or bone-marrow depressants

Interactions

1 Quinacrine can potentiate the toxicity of primaquine, presumably by impairing its metabolism

▶ **NURSING ALERTS**

▷ 1 Observe for signs of developing hemolytic anemia (darkened urine, fall in hemoglobin or erythrocyte count, chills, fever, precordial pain) and discontinue drug.

▷ 2 Perform regular routine blood cell counts and hemoglobin determinations during therapy, and do not exceed recommended doses.

▷ 3 Be aware that dark-skinned persons are particularly prone to develop hemolytic anemia due to a congenital deficiency of erythrocytic glucose 6-phosphate dehydrogenase.

▶ **NURSING CONSIDERATIONS**

▷ 1 Administer drug with meals to minimize gastric irritation.

▷ 2 Do not use alone to treat acute attacks of vivax malaria or in patients with parasitized red blood cells; chloroquine should be given concurrently with primaquine in these patients to destroy the erythrocytic parasites.

▷ 3 Note that primaquine (45 mg base) is available in fixed combination with chloroquine (300 mg base) as Aralen Phosphate with Primaquine Phosphate for prophylaxis of malaria in areas where the disease is endemic. Adult dosage is one tablet weekly during exposure and for 8 weeks after leaving endemic area.

▶ **pyrimethamine**
Daraprim

A folic acid antagonist that interferes with development of fertilized gametes in the mosquito, pyrimethamine is used for prophylaxis of malaria due to susceptible strains. Its slow onset of action reduces its usefulness in treating acute attacks. Commonly given with a fast-acting schizonticide such as chloroquine to provide both transmission control and suppressive (*not* radical) cure.

Mechanism
Selectively inhibits the enzyme dihydrofolate reductase, in protozoal cells, thereby blocking conversion of dihydrofolic acid to tetrahydrofolic acid, an essential step in protozoal cell metabolism; reduces sporogony (*i.e.,* reproduction of spores) in the mosquito, but does not destroy gametocytes; plasmodial resistance can develop rapidly when pyrimethamine is used alone

Uses
1 Prophylaxis of malaria due to susceptible strains of *Plasmodia* (usually in combination with a 4-aminoquinoline during acute attacks)
2 Treatment of toxoplasmosis, in combination with a sulfonamide

Dosage
Prophylaxis
Adults and children: (over 10 yr): 25 mg once a week
Children (4 yr–10 yr): 12.5 mg once a week
Children (under 4 yr): 6.25 mg (or 0.5 mg/kg) once a week for at least 10 weeks after leaving exposure area

Treatment of acute attacks
With a rapid-acting schizonticide, for example chloroquine—25 mg/day for 2 days, then 12.5 mg to 25 mg/week

Toxoplasmosis
Adults: 50 mg to 75 mg/day with 1 g to 4 g/day of a sulfapyrimidine for 1 week to 3 weeks; reduce dose by one half and continue for another 4 weeks to 5 weeks
Children: 1 mg/kg/day in two divided doses with appropriate dose of a sulfonamide for 2 days to 4 days; reduce by one half and continue for 30 days

Fate
Well absorbed orally; plasma half-life is about 4 days, but effective levels are maintained for up to 2 weeks; excreted mainly in the urine, slowly over a period of several weeks

Significant Adverse Reactions
Usually with larger doses, as used for toxoplasmosis) Anorexia, vomiting, skin rash, atrophic glossitis, megaloblastic anemia, leukopenia, thrombocytopenia, pancytopenia, hemolytic anemia in patients with a glucose 6-phosphase dehydrogenase deficiency, convulsions with overdosage

Interactions
1 The action of pyrimethamine can be impaired by folic acid or para-aminobenzoic acid (PABA)
2 Pyrimethamine can increase quinine blood levels by competing for protein-binding sites.

▶ **NURSING ALERTS**
▷ 1 Note that the dose of pyrimethamine used in toxoplasmosis is 10 to 20 times the dosage used for malaria, and approaches the toxic level. Monitor patients very closely.
▷ 2 Perform weekly blood counts (including platelet counts) during high-dose therapy and discontinue drug if hematologic abnormalities appear. Folinic acid (leucovorin) may be given (3 mg–9 mg IM daily for 3 days) to return depressed platelet or white blood cell count to normal.
▷ 3 Caution patients to report signs of possible developing blood dyscrasia immediately (fever, sore throat, mucosal ulceration, bruising or bleeding).
▷ 4 Use cautiously in patients with convulsive disorders and during pregnancy.

▶ **NURSING CONSIDERATIONS**
▷ 1 Administer with food to minimize stomach upset.
▷ 2 Do not exceed recommended doses for malaria suppression, because incidence of untoward reactions is significantly higher at elevated dose levels.

▶ **sulfadoxine and pyrimethamine**
Fansidar

A fixed combination of sulfadoxine (500 mg) and pyrimethamine (25 mg) is available for prophylaxis of malaria and for treatment of susceptible strains of *Plasmodia* resistant to chloroquine.

Mechanism
The two drugs block sequential enzymatic steps involved in the biosynthesis of folinic acid, a necessary intermediate in the parasitic cellular synthesis of purines, pyrimidines, and certain amino acids. Thus, protein and nucleic acid production is impaired in the plasmodial organisms.

Uses
1 Treatment of malaria due to susceptible strains of plasmodia resistant to chloroquine
2 Prophylaxis of malaria in persons in endemic areas

Dosage
Acute attacks
Adults: 2 to 3 tablets (500 mg/25 mg) as a single dose, either alone or in sequence with quinine or prima-

quine, followed by primaquine for 2 weeks to prevent relapse

Children: ½ to 2 tablets, according to age, given as outlined above

Prophylaxis

Once a week or once every two weeks, according to the schedule below; give first dose 1 day to 2 days before entering endemic area, continue during the stay, and then for 4 weeks to 6 weeks following return.

	Weekly	Biweekly
Adults	1 tablet	2 tablets
Children (9 yr–14 yr)	¾ tablet	1½ tablet
Children (4 yr–8 yr)	½ tablet	1 tablet
Children (under 4 yr)	¼ tablet	½ tablet

Fate

Both drugs are well absorbed orally; peak serum concentrations are attained in 2 hours to 8 hours; elimination half-life is prolonged, averaging 7 days for sulfadoxine and 4.5 days for pyrimethamine

Significant Adverse Reactions

See sulfonamides (Chap. 59) and pyrimethamine (this chap.).

Note: While all adverse reactions reported for the sulfonamides and pyrimethamine are *theoretically* possible with Fansidar, not all have been documented thus far for this combination drug.

Contraindications

Megaloblastic anemia due to folate deficiency, pregnancy at term, nursing mothers, infants less than 2 months of age, and sulfonamide hypersensitivity

Interactions

See sulfonamides (Chap. 59) and pyrimethamine (this chapter).

▶ NURSING ALERTS

(See also discussion of individual drugs.)

▷ 1 Discontinue prophylactic use if a significant reduction is noted in the count of any formed blood element or if patient develops an active bacterial or fungal infection. Leukopenia has occurred with prophylactic treatment of 2 months or longer.

▷ 2 Use with caution in patients with renal or hepatic impairment, folate deficiency, severe allergy, or bronchial asthma.

▷ 3 Urge patients to notify physician at first sign of fever, sore throat, abnormal bruising, pallor, jaundice, or glossitis, all possible indications of developing toxicity.

▷ 4 Advise women of childbearing potential receiving the drug to use contraceptive measures during therapy.

▶ NURSING CONSIDERATIONS

(See also discussion of individual drugs.)

▷ 1 Maintain adequate fluid intake to prevent crystalluria or stone formation.

▷ 2 If folate deficiency develops during therapy, discontinue drug and administer folinic acid (Leucovorin), 3 mg to 9 mg/day IM for 3 days or longer to restore depressed platelet or white cell count.

▶ quinacrine

Atabrine

Although quinacrine is an effective antimalarial, its use in malaria has been supplanted largely by more active and less toxic drugs. It has been used for both treatment and suppression of malaria, inasmuch as it destroys both erythrocytic forms of vivax, falciparum, and quartan malaria as well as gametocytes of vivax and quartan malaria. Quinacrine is ineffective, however, against falciparum gametocytes and all sporozoites. The drug finds its principal application today in the treatment of tapeworm infestations and giardiasis and is discussed more fully in Chapter 70.

Mechanism

Not completely established; may interfere with nucleic acid synthesis by blocking DNA replication and interfering with transcription of RNA

Uses

1 Treatment and suppression of susceptible strains of *Plasmodia*

2 Treatment of giardiasis and cestodiasis (tapeworm infestations; see Chap. 70)

Dosage

Treatment of malaria

Adults: 200 mg (with 1 g sodium bicarbonate) every 6 hours for five doses, then 100 mg three times a day for 6 days

Children: 100 mg to 200 mg three times a day the first day, then 100 mg one or two times a day for 6 days

Suppression of malaria

Adults: 100 mg/day for 1 month to 3 months
Children: 50 mg/day for 1 month to 3 months

Fate

Readily absorbed from GI tract; maximum plasma levels occur in 1 hour to 3 hours; highly protein-bound; widely distributed in the body and binds to many tissues; slowly excreted by the kidney, and cumulation of drug in the body is gradual

Common Side-Effects

Nausea, abdominal cramping, diarrhea, headache, dizziness, and yellowing of the urine, skin, and nails

Significant Adverse Reactions

GI—vomiting

Dermatologic—skin eruptions, contact dermatitis, exfoliative dermatitis

CNS—nervousness, vertigo, irritability, insomnia, emotional changes, nightmares, transient psychosis, convulsions (rare)

Hematologic—(rare) aplastic anemia, agranulocytosis, bone marrow depression

Other—hepatitis, corneal edema or deposits

Contraindications

Psoriasis, porphyria, and combined use with primaquine (see Interactions)

Interactions

1 Quinacrine increases the toxicity of primaquine and may potentiate the effects of other hepatotoxic drugs.
2 Quinacrine may produce a disulfiram-like reaction with alcohol (see Chap. 80)
3 The anticoagulant effects of heparin, an acidic drug, may be antagonized by quinacrine, a basic drug.
4 The adverse effects of quinacrine can be potentiated by MAO inhibitors, which reduce its hepatic metabolism.
5 Urinary alkalinizers can increase the effects of quinacrine by delaying its urinary excretion.

▶ NURSING ALERTS

▷ 1 Use with caution in patients with hepatic or renal disease, alcoholism, history of psychosis, glucose 6-phosphate dehydrogenase deficiency, during pregnancy, and in small children and patients over 60.
▷ 2 Be alert for signs of CNS toxicity (emotional instability, insomnia, irritability, vertigo) and advise physician. Dosage should be reduced or drug discontinued.
▷ 3 Perform periodic blood counts during prolonged therapy and discontinue drug if any significant abnormality is detected.

▶ NURSING CONSIDERATIONS

▷ 1 Caution patients to report promptly the onset of any visual changes. Perform ophthalmologic examinations at regular intervals during prolonged treatment.
▷ 2 Administer drug daily for at least 1 month to 2 months to effect suppression of malaria.

▶ quinine sulfate

Coco-Quinine, QM-260, Quinamm, Quine, Quiphile

A natural alkaloid from the bark of the cinchona tree, quinine is an effective antimalarial drug that has been replaced largely by more active and less toxic drugs. However, it is used in conjunction with pyrimethamine and sulfadiazine or tetracycline for treatment of *Plasmodia* resistant to other antimalarials, especially chloroquine-resistant falciparum strains. Due to its skeletal muscle relaxant effects, it is also occasionally used for relief of nocturnal leg cramps.

Mechanism

Not completely established; may inhibit protein synthesis in malarial organisms by complexing with parasite DNA, and interfere with cellular metabolism; suppresses oxygen uptake and carbohydrate metabolism of *Plasmodia;* actively schizonticidal for all forms of malaria and gametocidal for *Plasmodium vivax* and *Plasmodium malariae* strains; also possesses an analgesic, antipyretic, skeletal muscle relaxant, oxytocic, and hypoprothrombinemic action; its muscle-relaxing action is due to increased refractory period of muscle cells, decreased excitability of the motor end plate, and altered distribution of calcium within the muscle fiber

Uses

1 Adjunctive treatment of chloroquine-resistant falciparum malaria, along with pyrimethamine and sulfadiazine or tetracycline and in combination with other antimalarials for radical cure of relapsing vivax malaria
2 Relief of nocturnal leg cramps

Dosage

Malaria

Adults: 650 mg every 8 hours for 10 days to 14 days
Children: 25 mg/kg/day in divided doses every 8 hours for 10 days to 14 days

Leg Cramps

200 mg to 300 mg at bedtime

Fate

Rapidly absorbed orally; peak plasma levels occur in 2 hours to 3 hours; highly (70%–80%) protein-bound; widely distributed in the body, except to the CNS; metabolized by the liver and excreted in the urine, largely as metabolites with some (10%) unchanged drug

Common Side-Effects

Cinchonism (tinnitus, headache, dizziness, GI upset, visual disturbances)—frequently seen at full therapeutic doses

Significant Adverse Reactions

CNS—temporary deafness, fever, apprehension, restlessness, excitement, confusion, delirium, syncope, hypothermia, convulsions
Ophthalmic—photophobia, amblyopia, scotomata, diplopia, mydriasis, altered color perception, optic atrophy
GI—vomiting, stomach cramps, diarrhea
Allergic—rash, pruritus, flushing, urticaria, facial edema, asthmatic-like reaction.
Hematologic—hypoprothrombinemia, hemolytic anemia, thrombocytopenia, agranulocytosis
Other—(usually observed with very large doses) hypotension, respiratory depression, muscle paralysis

Contraindications

Pregnancy, myasthenia gravis, glucose 6-phosphate dehydrogenase deficiency, tinnitus, and optic neuritis

Interactions

(Because quinidine is an isomer of quinine, the interactions listed for quinidine in Chap. 30 are theoretically possible with quinine as well.)

1 Pyrimethamine may increase quinine blood levels, possibly leading to toxic effects.
2 Quinine can enhance the effects of skeletal muscle relaxants and increase their respiratory depressant action.
3 Quinine may potentiate the effects of oral anticoagulants due to its hypoprothrombinemic action.
4 The urinary excretion of quinine can be reduced by urinary alkalinizers (*e.g.,* sodium bicarbonate, acetazolamide).
5 Aluminum-containing antacids can delay or reduce the oral absorption of quinine.

▶ **NURSING ALERTS**
▷ 1 Use carefully in patients with cardiac arrhythmias (quinine has cardiovascular actions similar to quinidine), angina, or renal impairment, and in nursing mothers.

▶ **NURSING CONSIDERATIONS**
▷ 1 Observe for symptoms of cinchonism (tinnitus, dizziness, visual disturbances, headache, GI distress), and reduce dose or discontinue drug. Effects usually disappear quickly when drug is stopped.
▷ 2 Administer with food, and caution patient not to break capsule, because drug powder has a very bitter taste.
▷ 3 Urge caution in driving or operating other machinery, because blurred vision or dizziness can occur.
▷ 4 Note that a chocolate flavored suspension is available (Coco-Quinine) for use especially in children.
▷ 5 Be aware that quinine may interfere with determination of 17-hydroxycorticosteroids, and may produce elevated 17-ketogenic steroid values.

Summary. Antimalarial Agents

Drug	Preparations	Usual Dosage Range
4-Aminoquinolines	See Table 69-1	
Primaquine (Primaquine)	Tablets—26.3 mg (equivalent to 15 mg base)	Adults—26.3 mg daily for 14 days or 79 mg once a week for 8 weeks
		Children—0.3 mg (base)/kg/day for 14 days *or* 0.9 mg (base)/kg/week for 8 weeks
Pyrimethamine (Daraprim)	Tablets—25 mg	Prophylaxis: Adults—25 mg/wk
		Children—6.25 mg to 12.5 mg/week
		Acute attacks: 25 mg/day for 2 days with a rapid-acting schizonticide, then 12.5 mg to 25 mg/week
		Toxoplasmosis: Adults—50 mg to 75 mg/day for 1 week to 3 weeks then one half dose for another 4 weeks to 5 weeks
		Children—1 mg/kg/day for 2 days to 4 days; then one half dose for another 30 days (given with an appropriate sulfonamide)
Sulfadoxine and pyrimethamine (Fansidar)	Tablets—500 mg sulfadoxine/ 25 mg pyrimethamine	Acute attacks: Adults—2 to 3 tablets as a single dose followed by primaquine for 2 weeks
		Children—½ to 2 tablets, as outlined above
		Prophylaxis: Adults—1 tablet/week or 2 tablets every other week during and for 4 weeks to 6 weeks following exposure
		Children—¼ to ¾ tablet/week or ½ to 1½ tablets every other week during and for 4 weeks to 6 weeks following exposure

(continued)

Summary. Antimalarial Agents (continued)

Drug	Preparations	Usual Dosage Range
Quinacrine (Atabrine)	Tablets—100 mg	Treatment: Adults—200 mg with 1 g sodium bicarbonate every 6 hours for 5 doses, then 100 mg 3 times a day for 6 days
		Children—100 mg to 200 mg 3 times a day first day, then 100 mg 1 to 2 times a day for 6 days
		Suppression: Adults—100 mg/day
		Children—50 mg/day
Quinine (Coco-Quinine, QM-260, Quinamm, Quine, Quiphile)	Capsules—130 mg, 195 mg, 200 mg, 260 mg, 300 mg, 325 mg	Malaria: Adults—650 mg every 8 hours for 10 days to 14 days
	Tablets—260 mg, 325 mg	Children—25 mg/kg/day in divided doses every 8 hours for 10 days to 14 days
	Suspension—110 mg/5 ml	Leg cramps: 200 mg to 300 mg at bedtime

Anthelmintics are drugs used to facilitate the expulsion from the body of parasitic worms or helminths. Helminthiasis or worm infection is the most common disease in the world today. While endemic in many tropical countries, helminthiasis is by no means limited to these areas, but is found in increasing numbers in many temperate climates as well. Poor living conditions, inadequate sanitation, lack of careful hygiene, and malnutrition are major contributory factors to the high incidence of helminthiasis in underdeveloped countries.

Helminthic infections are caused by two principal types of worms, roundworms (nematodes) and flatworms (cestodes, trematodes). Table 70-1 lists the major species of each type of worm and the drugs that are most effective against each helminth. Most nematodal infections are confined to the intestinal tract and include parasites such as roundworms, pinworms, whipworms, hookworms, and threadworms. However, tissue-invading nematodes such as filarial worms and pork roundworms (trichinella) can enter body organs, including the heart, liver, lungs, skeletal muscle, and CNS, in which case eradication is often quite difficult.

Cestodal infestations can occur with several types of tapeworms, the most common being the beef tapeworm (*Taenia saginata*). These infections are usually localized in the GI tract, although larvae of the pork tapeworm (*Taenia solium*) can occasionally gain access to the systemic circulation, resulting in other organ involvement.

Tissue-invading trematodes or blood flukes are responsible for a chronic infection termed schistosomiasis, or bilharziasis, which is widespread throughout Africa and parts of South America. Complications may range from minor conditions such as rash, itching, or headache to severe damage to vital organs. Other trematodes include the lung, liver, and intestinal flukes.

Accurate diagnosis of the invading helminth is essential for the successful treatment of the infestation, because many anthelmintic drugs are highly specific for a particular infection. Diagnosis is usually accomplished by obtaining a stool specimen. Once the type of worm involved has been determined, selection of an appropriate anthelmintic drug can be made. Although a large number of different kinds of chemicals have been used in the past for treating the various types of worm infestations, they have been replaced today by a few newer, more effective, and less toxic agents. Most of these newer anthelmintic drugs are not appreciably absorbed following oral administration, and thus attain high levels in the GI tract while largely avoiding systemic toxicity. Another advantage of certain of the newer drugs (mebendazole, thiabendazole, praziquantel) is that they have a broad spectrum of action and thus are effective against several types of helminths. These drugs are particularly valuable in mixed infections or when the diagnosis is uncertain.

An important aspect of successful anthelmintic therapy is proper patient education with regard to personal hygiene. Because many worms are primarily transmitted by transfer of eggs (ova) *via* hands, food, or contaminated articles such as toilet paper, towels, clothes, or sheets, it is imperative that patients be instructed in the necessary procedures for minimizing spread of the infection. Important measures that should be stressed are careful washing of hands following

Table 70-1. Helminthiasis Classification and Treatment

Class of Helminth	Disorder	Suggested Drugs of Choice	
		Primary	*Secondary*
Nematodes			
Roundworm (*Ascaris lumbricoides*)	Ascariasis	Mebendazole, pyrantel pamoate	Piperazine, thiabendazole
Hookworm (*Necator americanus*) (*Ancylostoma duodenale*)	Uncinariasis	Mebendazole	Pyrantel pamoate, thiabendazole
Whipworm (*Trichuris trichiura*)	Trichuriasis	Mebendazole	Thiabendazole
Threadworm (*Strongyloides stercoralis*)	Strongyloidiasis	Thiabendazole	Pyrvinium pamoate
Pinworm (*Enterobius vermicularis*)	Enterobiasis	Mebendazole, pyrantel pamoate	Thiabendazole, piperazine, pyrvinium pamoate
Pork roundworm (*Trichinella spiralis*)	Trichiniasis, trichinosis	Corticosteroids	Thiabendazole
Filarial worms			
(*Wuchereria bancrofti*)	Filariasis	Diethylcarbamazine	
(*Brugia malayi*)	Filariasis	Diethylcarbamazine	
(*Loa loa*)	Loiasis	Diethylcarbamazine	
(*Onchocerca volvulus*)	Onchocerciasis	Diethylcarbamazine and suramin*	
Guinea worm (*Dracunculus medinensis*)		Niridazole*	Mebendazole, thiabendazole
Cestodes			
Tapeworms			
Beef			
(*Taenia saginata*)	Taeniasis	Niclosamide	Paromomycin, praziquantel
Pork			
(*Taenia solium*)	Taeniasis	Niclosamide	Paromomycin, praziquantel
Fish			
(*Diphyllobothrium latum*)	Diphyllobothriasis	Niclosamide	Dichlorophen, praziquantel
Dwarf			
(*Hymenolepis nana*)	Hymenolepiasis	Niclosamide, praziquantel	Mebendazole
Trematodes			
Blood flukes			
(*Schistosoma haematobium*)	Schistosomiasis (Bilharziasis)	Praziquantel, metrifonate*	Niridazole,* stibocaptate*
(*Schistosoma mansoni*)	Schistosomiasis	Praziquantel, oxamniquine	Niridazole,* stibocaptate*
(*Schistosoma japonicum*)	Schistosomiasis	Praziquantel, niridazole*	Stibocaptate*
Lung flukes			
(*Paragonimus westermani*)	Paragonimiasis	Bithionol*	Chloroquine
(*Paragonimus kellicotti*)	Paragonimiasis	Praziquantel	
Liver fluke (*Fasciola hepatica*)	Fascioliasis	Bithionol*	Emetine plus sulfonamides, praziquantel
Intestinal fluke (*Fasciolopsis buski*)	Fasciolopsiasis	Niclosamide, praziquantel	Tetrachloroethylene, hexylresorcinol

* Available only by request from the Parasitic Disease Drug Service, Centers for Disease Control, Atlanta, Georgia 30333.

each bowel movement, daily or more frequent changes of underwear, towels, and bedding, and avoidance of scratching of the perianal area. Nail biting should also be strongly discouraged. Diagnosis of pinworm infection in one family member makes it imperative that all other family members be tested as well, because this infection commonly affects an entire family.

Most drugs used to treat the principal nematodal and cestodal infections (see Table 70-1) are readily available and are discussed in detail in this chapter. Certain other anthelmintic drugs, such as niridazole, bithional, stibocaptate, and suramin, are used primarily for certain filarial or trematodal infections, and are currently available only upon request from the Parasitic Disease Drug Service of the Centers for Disease Control. These agents are reviewed briefly at the end of the chapter in Table 70-2. Still other drugs that are occasionally used in certain helminthic infections (*e.g.,* emetine, chloroquine, paromomycin) have additional therapeutic actions as well and are reviewed elsewhere in the book.

▶ antimony compounds

Antimony compounds were the major antischistosomal drugs for many years, but are seldom used today because of their toxicity and the availability of other more effective drugs. Antimony potassium tartrate (tartar emetic) is a highly effective drug for the treatment of *Schistosoma japonicum,* but because of its high toxicity (*e.g.,* dizziness, vomiting, tachycardia, arrhythmias, renal damage, blood dyscrasias), instability in solution, and the necessity for IV administration, it is seldom employed today. Antimony sodium dimercaptosuccinate (stibocaptate) is an alternate drug in the treatment of schistosomal infections (see Table 70-1) and is available as Astiban from the Centers for Disease Control in Atlanta. Stibocaptate is stable in solution, can be administered IM, and is considerably less toxic than antimony potassium tartrate. The dose of stibocaptate is 40 mg/kg for *Schistosoma haematobium* and *Schistosoma mansoni* infections and 50 mg/kg for *Schistosoma japonicum* infections. The total dosage is divided into 5 equal parts, and given once a week for 5 weeks. The course of therapy can be repeated in 2 months if necessary.

▶ diethylcarbamazine
Hetrazan

Mechanism
Sensitizes the small worms (microfilaria), increasing their susceptibility to phagocytosis by fixed tissue macrophages; does not appear to alter phagocytosis in the bloodstream; considered the drug of choice for filarial infections

Uses
1 Treatment of filarial worm infections (Bancroft's filariasis, loiasis, onchocerciasis)
2 Treatment of roundworm infections (ascariasis)
3 Treatment of tropical eosinophilia

Dosage
Filarial Worm Infections
2 mg/kg orally three times a day for 3 weeks to 4 weeks

Roundworm infections
Adults: 13 mg/kg/day in a single dose for 7 days
Children: 6 mg/kg to 10 mg/kg 3 times a day for 7 days to 10 days)

Tropical Eosinophilia
13 mg/kg/day for 4 days to 7 days.

Fate
Well absorbed orally; peak blood levels occur in 3 hours to 4 hours; widely distributed in the body; excreted primarily in the urine, both as metabolites and unchanged drug

Common Side-Effects
Headache, weakness, lassitude, malaise, nausea, joint pain, and leukocytosis

In patients with onchocerciasis, facial edema and pruritus of the eyes are common.

Significant Adverse Reactions
Vomiting, skin rash, lymphadenopathy, tachycardia, visual disturbances, GI upset, abdominal pain, anorexia, fever, and severe allergic reactions due to release of helminthic proteins

▶ NURSING ALERT
▷ 1 Be alert for development of allergic reactions, especially in treating onchocerciasis. Have antihistamines, epinephrine, and corticosteroids available in case of severe allergic response. Oral antihistamines may be given during the first several days of therapy to reduce the incidence of allergic reactions.

▶ NURSING CONSIDERATIONS
▷ 1 Stress the need for good personal hygiene to minimize the danger of re-infection.
▷ 2 Consider use of corticosteroid eye drops if ocular inflammation occurs.
▷ 3 Note that when diethylcarbamazine is used to treat onchocerciasis, it is usually combined with suramin to kill the adult worms as well as the microfilaria.

▶ hexylresorcinol

Hexylresorcinol is a broad-spectrum, relatively nontoxic, orally effective anthelmintic active against a variety of nematodes as well as the beef tapeworm. It may be used as an alternative drug in treating roundworm or hookworm infections where patients cannot tolerate more toxic agents or it can be employed in treating mixed helminthic infections. Although essentially devoid of serious systemic toxicity, GI irritation is common, and buccal and mucosal ulceration can occur if the gelatin-coated capsules are chewed or broken rather than swallowed whole. Hexylresorcinol should not be used in patients with peptic ulcers, ulcerative colitis, or intestinal obstruction. Usual adult oral dose is 1 g, followed in 2 hours to 4 hours by a saline cathartic. The drug is administered following an overnight fast. Children's doses range from 400 mg to 800 mg. Hexylresorcinol can also be given by way of a retention enema (1:100 in water) for trichuriasis, although perineal irritation is quite common following this method of administration. Hexylresorcinol is no longer distributed in the United States, but is available in several other countries.

▶ mebendazole
Vermox

Mechanism
Blocks uptake and utilization of glucose by worms, thereby depleting endogenous glycogen, reducing energy supply below that necessary for survival

Uses

1 Treatment of single or mixed whipworm, pinworm, roundworm, and hookworm infestations

Dosage

(Adults and children)

Whipworm, hookworm, roundworm

Adults and children: 100 mg twice a day for 3 consecutive days; if necessary repeat in 2 weeks

Pinworm

Adults and children: 100 mg as single dose

Fate

Only 5% to 10% of an oral dose is generally absorbed; approximately 2% of an administered dose is excreted in the urine, both as unchanged drug and a metabolite; the remainder is excreted in the feces.

Significant Adverse Reactions

(Usually with massive infections) Abdominal pain, nausea, vomiting, and diarrhea due to expulsion of worms; fever

Contraindications

Pregnancy

▶ **NURSING ALERT**

▷ 1 Use cautiously in children under 2 years of age.

▶ **NURSING CONSIDERATIONS**

▷ 1 Inform patients that tablets may be chewed, swallowed whole, or crushed and mixed with food.

▷ 2 Note that fasting or post-treatment purging is not required with mebendazole.

▷ 3 Initiate a second course of treatment if patient is not cured 3 weeks after initial treatment.

▶ **niclosamide**

Niclocide

Mechanism

Inhibits oxidative phosphorylation in the mitochondria of cestodal parasites, and may also stimulate ATPase; the head (scolex) and proximal segments of the worm are killed on contact, and the parasite is released from its attachment on the intestinal wall; the partially digested worms are then expelled in the feces; drug does not appear to produce any hematologic, renal, or hepatic abnormalities

Uses

1 Treatment of cestodal (tapeworm) infections—see Table 70-1 (drug of choice)

Dosage

(Tablets are thoroughly chewed and swallowed with a little water.)

Taenia/Diphyllobothrium infections

Adults: 2 g in a single dose

Children: 1.0 g to 1.5 g in a single dose depending on weight

Hymenolepis nana infections

Adults: 2 g as a single dose daily for 7 days

Children (over 75 lb): 1.5 g the first day, then 1 g daily for 6 days

Children (under 75 lb): 1.0 g the first day, then 0.5 g daily for 6 days

Fate

Not absorbed from the GI tract; excreted in the feces

Common Side-Effects

Nausea, vomiting, and anorexia

Significant Adverse Reactions

GI—diarrhea, constipation, rectal bleeding
CNS—headache, drowsiness, dizziness
Dermatologic—skin rash
Other—fever, oral irritation, bad taste in mouth, sweating, palpitations, weakness, backache, irritability, alopecia

Contraindications

Children under 2 years of age

▶ **NURSING ALERTS**

▷ 1 If *Taenia* or *Diphyllobothrium* segments or ova are still present in the stool 7 days after treatment, repeat the treatment. A cure is considered to be a negative stool for at least 3 months.

▷ 2 Use with caution in pregnant and nursing mothers and only where the benefits *clearly* outweigh the risks.

▶ **NURSING CONSIDERATIONS**

▷ 1 Administer tablets following a light meal (*e.g.,* breakfast). In young children, tablets may be crushed and mixed with a little water to form a paste.

▷ 2 Use a mild laxative, if needed, to relieve constipation.

▷ 3 Continue treatment of *Hymenolepis* infections for the entire 7 days as recommended, to ensure complete destruction of both mature and larval stages of the worm.

▶ **oxamniquine**

Vansil

Mechanism

Not completely established; may cause a shift in worms from the mesentery to the liver, where they die; appears to be more toxic to male schistosomes than to females, but surviving female worms no longer lay eggs

Uses

1 Treatment of all stages (acute, subacute, chronic) of *Schistosoma mansoni* infections

Dosage

Adults: 12 mg/kg to 15 mg/kg as a single oral dose

Children (under 30 kg): 20 mg/kg in two divided doses with a 2-hour–8-hour interval between doses.

Fate

Readily absorbed orally; peak serum concentration in 2 hours to 3 hours; plasma half-life is approximately 1½ hours to 3 hours; extensively metabolized and excreted in the urine, largely as inactive metabolites

Common Side-Effects

Drowsiness, dizziness

Significant Adverse Reactions

Headache, anorexia, abdominal pain, nausea, vomiting, urticaria, convulsions, and liver enzyme elevations

▶ **NURSING ALERTS**

▷ 1 Use with caution in patients with a history of convulsive episodes and in pregnant or lactating women.

▷ 2 Advise caution in performing hazardous tasks, because drug causes drowsiness and dizziness in approximately one third of patients.

▶ **NURSING CONSIDERATIONS**

▷ 1 Administer with food to improve patient tolerance.

▷ 2 Advise patients that drug may color urine a harmless orange red.

▶ **piperazine**

Antepar, Vermizine

Mechanism

Produces muscle paralysis in worms, possibly by blocking acetylcholine, resulting in expulsion of the helminths by normal peristaltic movement

Uses

1 Alternative treatment of roundworm and pinworm infestations

Dosage

Roundworm

Adults: 3.5 g once daily for 2 days

Children: 75 mg/kg/day as a single dose for 2 days; may repeat in 1 week in severe infections; if repeat therapy is impractical or for mass therapy as a public health measure, 150 mg/kg may be given in a single dose

Pinworm

Adults and children: 65 mg/kg/day for 7 consecutive days (maximum daily dose 2.5 g)

Fate

Oral absorption is variable; a portion of the absorbed drug is metabolized and excreted in the urine; remainder is eliminated in the feces or urine as unchanged drug

Significant Adverse Reactions

(Usually with high doses)

GI—nausea, vomiting, diarrhea, abdominal cramping

CNS—headache, vertigo, muscular weakness, hyporeflexia, blurred vision, paresthesias, tremors, choreiform movements, convulsions, impaired memory, EEG abnormalities, worsening of epileptic seizures

Allergic—fever, urticaria, arthralgia, purpura, lacrimation, eczematous skin eruptions, rhinorrhea, bronchospasm, erythema multiforme

Contraindications

Renal or hepatic impairment, convulsive disorders

Interaction

1 Piperazine may increase the severity of extrapyramidal reactions due to phenothiazine administration.

▶ **NURSING ALERTS**

▷ 1 Do not exceed recommended dose and duration of therapy, because potential for neurotoxicity is increased, especially in children.

▷ 2 Use cautiously in patients with anemia, severe malnutrition, or neurologic disorders, and in pregnant women.

▶ **NURSING CONSIDERATIONS**

▷ 1 Advise physician if CNS, GI, or hypersensitivity reactions occur.

▷ 2 Recognize that dietary restrictions, enemas, or laxatives are not required with piperazine.

▷ 3 Educate patients in the proper methods for preventing spread of the infection (*e.g.,* careful hand washing; daily changes of underwear, towels, and bedding; proper disposal of fecal matter) because pinworm infections are easily transmitted from person to person.

▷ 4 Note that piperazine is available as the citrate salt, but is converted to the hexahydrate in solution. The dosage is therefore given in hexahydrate equivalents.

▶ **praziquantel**

Biltricide

Praziquantel is a relatively new anthelmintic that exhibits a rather broad spectrum of activity and a low overall incidence of serious adverse effects. It is considered a first-line drug in schistosomal infections, and is also active against other trematodes as well as cestodes (see Table 70-1). In addition, praziquantel also shows promise as being useful in the treatment of cysticercosis, a serious complication of cestodal infections where the larvae of *Taenia* invade other organs of the body, leading to fatigue, muscle pain, weakness, nervousness, and possibly convulsions or general paralysis.

Mechanism

Produces vacuolization and subsequent disintegration of the surface tegumentum of the parasite, leading to death of the schistosomal organism

Uses

1 Treatment of schistosomal infections (*i.e., S. haematobium, S. mansoni, S. japonicum*)—drug of choice
2 Alternative treatment of lung, liver, and intestinal flukes and cestodal (tapeworm) infections (see Table 70-1)

Dosage

Schistosomiasis
20 mg/kg 3 times a day for 1 day, at intervals of 4 hours to 6 hours

Cestodal infections
10 mg/kg to 25 mg/kg as a single dose

Fate

Rapidly and almost completely (80%) absorbed orally; peak serum levels occur within 1 hour to 3 hours; metabolized in the liver and excreted largely in the kidney

Common Side-Effects

Headache, dizziness, and anorexia

Significant Adverse Reactions

Abdominal discomfort, fever, urticaria, pruritus, diarrhea, arthralgia, myalgia (more frequent in heavily infected patients and those receiving high doses)

Contraindications

Ocular cysticercosis (parasite destruction may cause irreparable lesions)

▶ NURSING ALERTS

▷ 1 Urge caution in driving or operating other machinery, because drowsiness and dizziness can occur.
▷ 2 Use cautiously in pregnant or nursing women and in children under 4 years of age.
▷ 3 Note that in cases where schistosomiasis or other trematodal infections are associated with cysticercosis, the patient should be hospitalized.

▶ NURSING CONSIDERATION

▷ 1 Instruct patients to swallow the tablet whole with a little liquid, preferably during a meal. Tablets are bitter and can produce gagging or vomiting if chewed or kept in the mouth too long.

▶ pyrantel pamoate
Antiminth

Mechanism

Paralyzes worms, probably by a depolarizing neuromuscular blocking action, facilitating their expulsion by peristalsis

Uses

1 Treatment of roundworm and pinworm infections

Dosage

Adults and children: 11 mg (base)/kg in a single dose (1 ml suspension/10 lb of body weight) (maximum dose 1 g)

Fate

Poorly absorbed orally; plasma levels are maximum in 1 hour to 3 hours, but are quite low; metabolized in the liver; greater than 50% of an oral dose is excreted unchanged in the feces, and less than 7% in the urine as both unchanged drug and metabolites

Significant Adverse Reactions

GI—nausea, vomiting, anorexia, abdominal cramps, diarrhea, tenesmus, elevated SGOT (transient)
CNS—headache, dizziness, drowsiness, insomnia
Allergic—rash, fever

▶ NURSING ALERTS

▷ 1 Use with caution in patients with liver dysfunction, in pregnant women, and in children under 2 years of age.

▶ NURSING CONSIDERATIONS

▷ 1 Note that the drug may be given without regard to presence of food or time of day and that use of a laxative is not necessary.
▷ 2 Stress the importance of meticulous hygiene for complete eradication of the parasites, because pinworm infections are readily transmitted from person to person.

▶ pyrvinium pamoate
Povan

Mechanism

Not completely established; may interfere with carbohydrate utilization by worms; death of worms occurs when endogenous carbohydrate stores are depleted

Use

1 Alternate treatment of pinworm infections

Dosage

Adults and children: 5 mg/kg as a single dose; repeat in 2 weeks to 3 weeks if necessary

Fate

Not significantly absorbed from GI tract; excreted largely as unchanged drug in feces, with small amounts appearing in the urine

Significant Adverse Reactions

Nausea, vomiting, diarrhea, abdominal cramps, dizziness, photosensitivity, allergic skin reactions, and erythema multiforme (rare)

Contraindications
Use of tablets in patients with aspirin and salicylate hypersensitivity (possible cross-sensitivity with tartrazine dye in tablet coating)

▶ NURSING ALERTS
▷ 1 Use cautiously in patients with intestinal inflammation or ulceration, and in pregnant women and infants.
▷ 2 Be aware that pyrvinium has been found to contain a substance that can be converted to a mutagenic metabolite. Use only as an alternate drug where other drugs have failed to eradicate the infection.

▶ NURSING CONSIDERATIONS
▷ 1 Inform patients that drug will stain anything it contacts a bright red. This includes feces, vomitus, and teeth as well as clothing. Reassure patients that the discoloration of the stools is not harmful.
▷ 2 Caution patients to swallow tablets whole to avoid staining of teeth.
▷ 3 Be aware that vomiting occurs more frequently with the oral suspension than with oral tablets, and GI distress is noted more commonly at the higher doses needed in older children and adults.
▷ 4 Note that a table giving convenient doses for both tablets and oral suspension based on body weight is included with each package.
▷ 5 Ensure that all family members of an infected individual be examined for pinworm infestation and treated accordingly.
▷ 6 Stress the importance of proper adjunctive measures (*e.g.,* hygiene, bathing, daily laundering of sheets, towels, clothing) for the complete eradication of the infection and prevention of re-infection.

▶ quinacrine
Atabrine

Quinacrine may occasionally be employed as an alternate drug in the management of tapeworm infections, but has largely been replaced by other more effective, less toxic agents such as niclosamide, praziquantel, paromomycin, or mebendazole. It apparently acts by causing the head of the worm to detach from the intestinal wall; the worm is then expelled by use of a purgative. Because rather high doses of quinacrine are required to treat tapeworm infections, side-effects are common. Nausea and vomiting are frequently produced by the drug, as well as dizziness, headache, abdominal cramping, and signs of CNS stimulation (*e.g.,* anxiety, restlessness, confusion, aggression, and psychotic behavior). Treatment with quinacrine is best carried out in the hospital. Dosage depends on the type of parasite present, and is usually administered in divided amounts, followed by a saline purge to remove the worm from the intestinal tract. Quinacrine has also been employed in the treatment of malaria, and this application is discussed in Chapter 69.

▶ thiabendazole
Mintezol

Mechanism
Not established; broad-spectrum anthelmintic that also possesses anti-inflammatory and analgesic activities; appears to enhance T-cell function; may interfere with enzyme systems in helminths; suppresses egg and larval production by *Trichinella spiralis* (pork roundworm) and reduces fever and eosinophilia; it is a first-line drug against threadworm infections and cutaneous larva migrans, but in spite of its broad spectrum of activity, is not recommended as first choice in other nematodal infections.

Uses
1 Treatment of threadworm (*Strongyloides*) infections (drug of choice)
2 Treatment of cutaneous larva migrans (creeping eruption) (drug of choice)
3 Alternate treatment of pinworm, whipworm, hookworm, roundworm, and guinea worm infections
4 Symptomatic treatment of invasive trichinosis

Dosage
Threadworm
25 mg/kg, up to 1.5 g, orally twice a day for 2 days depending on patient's weight; if infection is systemic, continue for 5 days to 7 days.

Trichinosis/Cutaneous Larva Migrans
25 mg/kg twice daily for 2 days to 5 days

Fate
Well absorbed orally; peak plasma levels occur in 1 hour to 2 hours; metabolized in the liver and excreted largely (90%) within 24 hours in the urine

Common Side-Effects
Anorexia, nausea, vomiting, and dizziness

Significant Adverse Reactions
GI—diarrhea, epigastric distress, cramping, perianal rash
CNS—lethargy, drowsiness, giddiness, headache, tinnitus, irritability, blurred vision, numbness
Allergic—pruritus, fever, flushing, chills, angioedema, erythema multiforme, lymphadenopathy, anaphylaxis
Renal/hepatic—enuresis, malodor of the urine, crystalluria, hematuria, cholestasis, jaundice, parenchymal liver damage, elevated SGOT
Other—hypotension, bradycardia, hyperglycemia, leukopenia

▶ NURSING ALERTS
▷ 1 Be alert for development of hypersensitivity reactions (fever, chills, skin rash) and discontinue drug. Fatalities have occurred from severe erythema multiforme (Stevens–Johnson syndrome)
▷ 2 Caution patients against performing hazardous tasks

during therapy, because dizziness, drowsiness, and other CNS side-effects may occur.

▷ 3 Use carefully in patients with impaired kidney or liver function, anemia, or malnutrition, and in pregnant or nursing women.

▶ **NURSING CONSIDERATIONS**

▷ 1 Note that dietary restrictions and laxatives or enemas are not necessary with thiabendazole.

▷ 2 Instruct patients to chew tablets well. Drug is best given after meals.

Table 70-2. Anthelmintic Drugs Available by Request to Centers for Disease Control*

Drug	Principal Indications	Preparation	Usual Dosage Range	Remarks
Bithionol (Actamer, Bitin, Lorothidol)	Lung fluke (*Paragonimus*) and liver fluke (*Fasciola*) infections	Powder	30 mg/kg to 50 mg/kg orally in 2 or 3 divided doses on alternate days for 10 to 15 days	Drug of choice for treating lung fluke infections; GI side-effects are common; use with caution in children under 8 years of age
Metrifonate (Bilarcil)	Schistosomiasis	Tablet—100 mg	7.5 mg/kg to 10 mg/kg as a single dose; repeat twice at 2-week intervals	One of the drugs of choice for *Schistosoma haematobium* infections; *not* effective against *S. mansoni* or *S. japonicum*; well tolerated; minimal side-effects
Niridazole (Ambilhar)	Schistosomiasis, guinea worm infections	Tablets—100 mg, 500 mg	25 mg/kg/day orally for 7 days	Primary drug for *Schistosoma japonicum* infections and alternate drug for other schistosomal infections; high incidence of side-effects (70%) especially GI and allergic; CNS toxicity can occur, especially at high doses; patients must be hospitalized; generally contraindicated in cardiac, liver, or renal disease, hypertension, epilepsy, psychiatric disorders, GI ulceration, or hemorrhage
Stibocaptate (Astiban)	Schistosomiasis	Powder for injection— 0.5 g/vial (5 ml saline added to prepare a 10% solution)	40 mg/kg to 50 mg/kg total dose divided into 5 injections given at weekly intervals	Highly effective in treating schistosomal infections; antimony-containing compound with high incidence of side-effects, but less toxic than antimony potassium tartrate; do not use in the presence of bacterial or viral infections hepatic, renal, or cardiac insufficiency, or anemia
Suramin (Bayer 205, Belganyl, Germanin, Moranyl, Naphuride)	Onchocerciasis (filarial worm infection), African trypansomiasis (sleeping sickness)	Powder for injection— 0.5 g/vial, 1 g/vial	1 g by *slow* IV injection weekly for 4 weeks to 7 weeks	Used to eradicate adult filariae of *Onchocerca volvulus* following treatment with diethylcarbamazine to eliminate microfilariae; proteinuria can occur; avoid extravasation, because severe pain can result

* Parasitic Disease Drug Service, Bureau of Epidemiology, Centers for Disease Control, Atlanta, Georgia 30333.

Summary. Anthelmintic Drugs

Drug	Preparations	Usual Dosage Range
Diethylcarbamazine (Hetrazan)	Tablets—50 mg	Filariasis: 2 mg/kg 3 times a day for 3 weeks to 4 weeks

Summary. Anthelmintic Drugs *(continued)*

Drug	Preparations	Usual Dosage Range
		Ascariasis: 13 mg/kg/day for 7 days or 6 mg/kg to 10 mg/kg 3 times a day for 7 days Tropical eosinophilia: 13 mg/kg/day for 4 days to 7 days
Hexylresorcinol*	Coated tablets—100 mg	1 g orally, followed in 2 hours to 4 hours by a saline cathartic Children—400 mg to 800 mg
Mebendazole (Vermox)	Chewable tablets—100 mg	Pinworm: 100 mg as a single dose Whipworm, hookworm, roundworm: 100 mg twice a day for 3 days; repeat in 3 weeks if necessary
Niclosamide (Niclocide)	Chewable tablets—500 mg	Taenia/Diphyllobothrium: Adults—2 g (single dose) Children—1.0 g to 1.5 g (single dose) depending on weight Hymenolepsis: Adults—2 g/day for 7 days Children—1.0 g to 1.5 g the first day, then 0.5 g to 1.0 g daily for 6 days
Oxamniquine (Vansil)	Capsules—250 mg	Adults—12 mg to 15 mg/kg as a single dose Children (under 30 kg)—20 mg/kg in 2 divided doses 2 hours to 8 hours apart
Piperazine (Antepar, Vermizine)	Tablets—250 mg, 500 mg hexahydrate equivalent Syrup—500 mg/5 ml hexahydrate equivalent	Roundworm: Adults—3.5 g/day for 2 days Children—75 mg/kg/day for 2 days; may repeat in 1 week in severe infections; alternately, 150 mg/kg as a single dose (less effective) Pinworm: Adults and children—65 mg/kg/day for 7 days
Praziquantel (Biltricide)	Tablets—600 mg	Schistosomiasis: 20 mg/kg 3 times a day for 1 day, at 4-hour to 6-hour intervals Cestodal infections: 10 to 25 mg/kg as a single dose
Pyrantel pamoate (Antiminth)	Suspension—50 mg (base)/ml	11 mg (base)/kg as a single dose (maximum 1 g)
Pyrvinium pamoate (Povan)	Coated tablets—50 mg	5 mg/kg as a single dose; repeat in 2 weeks to 3 weeks if necessary
Quinacrine (Atabrine)	Tablets—100 mg	800 mg as a single dose by a duodenal tube or 200 mg orally every 10 minutes for 4 doses with 600 mg sodium bicarbonate; follow in 1 hour to 2 hours with a saline purgative
Thiabendazole (Mintezol)	Chewable tablets—500 mg Suspension—500 mg/5 ml	22 mg/kg up to 1.5 g twice a day for 2 days to 4 days depending on infection and patient's weight

* No longer distributed in the United States.

71 Amebicides

Amebiasis refers to infection with the organism *Entamoeba histolytica,* a protozoan that usually invades the lower intestinal tract but may be found in the liver, lungs, brain, and other organs as well. Amebiasis affects approximately 10% of the world's population, is endemic in many tropical regions, and is present in as many as 5% of the people in the United States, especially those exposed to poor sanitary conditions.

The disease can be manifested in one of several ways as follows:

1 *Asymptomatic intestinal amebiasis*—presence of the organism in the intestinal tract without evidence of clinical symptoms; treatment is indicated because these patients are at risk for developing GI pathology and can serve as carriers, spreading the infection to other less resistant persons.

2 *Symptomatic intestinal amebiasis*—presence of overt clinical symptoms ranging from mild manifestations (such as diarrhea, cramping, and flatulence) to severe dysentery with accompanying bloody diarrhea, vomiting, fever, and dehydration. Intestinal mucosal scarring and ulceration can promote systemic absorption of the protozoa, leading to the third stage of the disease, extra-intestinal amebiasis.

3 *Extra-intestinal amebiasis*—presence of organisms in other body organs, most commonly the liver and lungs; may result in liver necrosis, amebic hepatitis, lung abscesses, and empyema; organisms can also invade the heart, causing pericarditis, and the CNS, leading to brain abscesses.

The drugs used in the treatment of amebiasis can be characterized on the basis of their predominant site of action. That is, some agents are only active against organisms present in the lumen of the intestine, others are effective against parasites found in the bowel wall and other tissues, whereas still other drugs are claimed to affect both intestinal and extra-intestinal protozoa. In order to better understand the rationale for the use of a particular drug in the various stages of amebiasis, it is helpful to briefly review the two-stage life cycle of *Entamoeba histolytica.*

The organism is transmitted from person to person via ingestion of amebic cysts, a form in which the protozoa are extremely resistant to destruction outside the body. The cysts are likewise unaffected by gastric juice, and pass intact to the small intestine where some develop into motile trophozoites that can invade the intestinal mucosa, be absorbed systemically, and find their way to other organs in the body. The remaining cysts are excreted intact, and they can thus continue the re-infective cycle in another person.

Interruption of this cycle can be accomplished in several ways. Most drugs for treating amebiasis are amebicidal, either directly killing or inhibiting the growth and maturation of the trophozoites, whereas some drugs exhibit a cystocidal action. Because most of the currently effective amebicides have the potential to elicit serious untoward reactions, their use should be undertaken only upon a definitive diagnosis of *Entamoeba histolytica* as the causative agent, and patients must be closely observed during therapy for development of adverse reactions.

There is lack of general agreement as to the preferred

drug regimens for treating the various forms of amebiasis. Treatment of symptomatic amebiasis, whether intestinal or extra-intestinal, generally requires either concomitant or sequential use of two or more drugs, especially if the infection is severe and the parasites are present in extra-intestinal sites.

Metronidazole is effective against both intestinal and extra-intestinal parasites, and therefore is considered by some as the drug of choice for moderate to severe intestinal infections, usually in combination with diloxanide or diiodohydroxyquin. However, metronidazole has been demonstrated to be carcinogenic in mice and rats, and many clinicians feel that it should be used only in *severe acute* intestinal amebiasis with hepatic abscesses. Emetine is also active against both intestinal and extra-intestinal organisms, but is also a potentially dangerous drug and must be administered parenterally in a hospital setting under close supervision. The remaining currently marketed amebicides may be divided into those recommended for either intestinal infections (carbarsone, diiodohydroxyquin, paromomycin) or extra-intestinal (*i.e.,* hepatic) infections (chloroquine). Two other drugs, dehydroemetine and diloxanide, are not available for general use in the United States, but may be obtained by request from the Parasitic Disease Drug Service of the Centers for Disease Control. They are briefly discussed in Table 71-1. Interestingly, diloxanide alone is viewed by some as the drug of choice for eradication of microorganisms from asymptomatic carriers of the disease, and is also considered as a primary drug for treatment of milder intestinal infections, sometimes combined with diiodohydroxyquin.

The amebicides are discussed individually in this chapter. Several drugs used in amebiasis (*e.g.,* paromomycin, chloroquine) are also effective in other disease states and have been reviewed elsewhere. Only those aspects of their pharmacology related to the treatment of amebic infections are considered here.

▶ carbarsone
Carbarsone

An organic arsenical with amebicidal action against the trophozoite form of *Entamoeba histolytica*, carbarsone is infrequently used, only as an alternative drug for acute intestinal amebiasis. It is not effective in extra-intestinal forms.

Mechanism
Not established; may interfere with enzymes necessary for growth of trophozoites

Uses
1 Alternative treatment of acute intestinal amebiasis without hepatic involvement, usually in combination with other amebicides

Dosage
Adults: 250 mg two to three times a day for 10 days; may repeat in 2 weeks
Children: 75 mg/kg total dose over a 10-day period divided into three daily doses

Fate
Readily absorbed when taken orally; accumulates in body tissues and is very slowly eliminated in the urine and bile

Common Side-Effects
Nausea, epigastric distress

Significant Adverse Reactions
Diarrhea, abdominal cramping, weight loss, sore throat, skin rash, pruritus, icterus, mucosal ulceration, hepatitis, neuritis, visual disturbances, polyuria, edema, splenomegaly, liver necrosis, exfoliative dermatitis, and kidney damage

Contraindications
Liver or kidney impairment, amebic hepatitis, and contracted visual or color fields

▶ NURSING ALERTS
▷ 1 Do not exceed recommended dose or duration of therapy (*i.e.,* 10 days). If further treatment is necessary, a rest period of 10 days to 14 days must be allowed to prevent cumulation toxicity, because drug is excreted very slowly.
▷ 2 Discontinue drug immediately at first evidence of intolerance or toxicity (see Significant Adverse Reactions). Advise patient to report any unusual symptoms during and for several weeks following discontinuation of therapy.

▶ NURSING CONSIDERATIONS
▷ 1 Advise patients to notify physician if GI upset, sore throat, visual disturbances, or skin lesions are noted.

▶ chloroquine
Aralen

Primarily employed as an antimalarial drug, chloroquine is also effective in the treatment of amebic liver abscesses (often with emetine), because chloroquine localizes in the liver in a concentration several hundred times greater than in the plasma. The drug is largely ineffective against intestinal organisms, because it is rapidly absorbed, therefore it is always given either in combination with or following other drugs active against intestinal amebiasis. When used in hepatic amebiasis, chloroquine may also be combined with metronidazole or diloxanide or both to ensure that all protozoa are eradicated. Chloroquine is discussed fully in Chapter 69 and only information pertinent to its use in amebiasis is presented here.

Uses
1 Treatment of extra-intestinal amebiasis, in combination with other amebicides active against intestinal forms

Dosage
Oral: (phosphate salt) 1 g/day for 2 days, then 500 mg/day for at least 2 weeks to 3 weeks

IM: (hydrochloride salt) 200 mg to 250 mg/day for 10 days to 12 days; oral therapy should be substituted as soon as possible

Children: maximum single dose is 5 mg (base)/kg

▶ **diiodohydroxyquin**

Iodoquinol, Moebiquin, Yodoxin

An iodinated hydroxyquinoline, diiodohydroxyquin is effective in intestinal amebiasis, especially in asymptomatic carriers. It is relatively nontoxic and inexpensive and has been used for mass treatment.

Mechanisms

Not established; exerts a direct amebicidal action against both motile and cystic forms of trophozoites; action is restricted to the intestinal tract

Uses

1 Treatment of asymptomatic or mild to moderate acute or chronic intestinal amebiasis
2 Treatment of giardiasis

Dosage

Adults: 650 mg orally three times a day for 20 days

Children: 40 mg/kg/day in three divided doses for 20 days (maximum 2 g/day)

Fate

Largely unabsorbed from the GI tract; distribution and fate in man is unknown

Common Side-Effects

Gastric distress (diarrhea, nausea, abdominal discomfort)

Significant Adverse Reactions

(Rare at usual doses) Vomiting, abdominal cramping, pruritus ani, urticaria, skin eruptions, headache, vertigo, fever, chills, thyroid enlargement, optic neuritis, optic atrophy, and peripheral neuropathy

Contraindications

Hypersensitivity to iodides, hepatic damage

▶ **NURSING ALERTS**

▷ 1 Be alert for the development of ocular or neurologic disturbances, especially during prolonged high-dose therapy, and advise physician. Drug should be discontinued. Avoid long-term therapy.

▷ 2 Perform periodic ophthalmologic examinations during therapy, especially in young children.

▷ 3 Use cautiously in patients with thyroid disorders and in pregnant or lactating women.

▶ **NURSING CONSIDERATIONS**

▷ 1 Observe for the development of hypersensitivity reactions (pruritus, urticaria, chills, fever), and advise physician if they occur.

▷ 2 Note that the drug can interfere with certain thyroid function tests by increasing protein-bound serum iodine levels.

▷ 3 Recognize that diiodohydroxyquin is *not* indicated for prophylaxis or treatment of nonspecific or "travelers" diarrhea, although it has been used in these conditions.

▷ 4 Determine if patient has an iodide hypersensitivity before administering the initial dose.

▶ **emetine**

Emetine

Emetine is a potent amebicide effective against both intestinal and extra-intestinal tissue parasites. Its use is restricted to severe cases of amebic dysentery and amebic hepatitis or liver abscesses, inasmuch as the drug can cause serious untoward reactions due to cumulative toxicity as well as a wide range of milder adverse effects.

Mechanism

Exerts a direct lethal action on trophozoites, probably blocking protein synthesis by interfering with attachment of t-RNA to the ribosomes; much more effective against motile forms than against cysts

Uses

1 Symptomatic treatment of acute amebic dysentery or acute episodes of chronic amebic dysentery, in combination with other amebicides

2 Treatment of amebic hepatitis and amebic abscesses in other tissues, in combination with an amebicide effective against intestinal parasites

3 Alternative treatment of balantidiasis, fascioliasis, and paragonimiasis.

Dosage

(Deep SC injection is preferred; may be given IM)

Acute amebic dysentery

65 mg/day SC or IM 3 days to 5 days, in a single or two divided doses

Amebic hepatitis or abscesses

65 mg/day SC or IM for 10 days

Children (under 8 yr): maximum 10 mg/day

Children (over 8 yr): maximum 20 mg/day

Fate

Well absorbed from SC or IM injection sites; widely distributed in the body (*e.g.*, kidney, spleen, lungs), highest concentrations being found in the liver; excreted very slowly by the kidney, some drug still present in the body 60 days after administration; danger of cumulative toxicity is appreciable

Common Side-Effects

Pain, tenderness, stiffness, and local muscle weakness at injection sites, nausea, diarrhea, abdominal pain, dizziness, and fainting

Significant Adverse Reactions

GI—vomiting

Cardiovascular—hypotension, tachycardia, precordial pain, cardiac dilatation, ECG abnormalities (T wave

inversion, Q–T prolongation), gallop rhythm, dyspnea, congestive heart failure, and arrhythmias
Neuromuscular—muscle stiffness and weakness, tremors
Dermatologic—urticarial, eczematous, or purpuric skin lesions

Contraindications

Organic heart or kidney disease, pregnancy; in children (except those with *severe* dysentery not controlled by other amebicides) and persons receiving a course of emetine therapy within the previous 2 months; IV injection of the drug

▶ NURSING ALERTS

▷ 1 Confine patients to bed during therapy and for several days thereafter. Observe patients very carefully, record pulse and blood pressure several times a day, and perform an ECG before initiating therapy, after the fifth dose, upon completion of treatment, and again 1 week later.

▷ 2 Discontinue drug if tachycardia, neuromuscular symptoms, marked drop in blood pressure, muscle weakness, or severe GI symptoms occur.

▷ 3 Advise physician if fatigability, listlessness, muscle stiffness, pain, or tenderness occurs, especially in the neck or upper extremities, because these often are early signs of more serious neuromuscular toxicity. Drug should be discontinued.

▷ 4 Monitor intake–output, and note any change in renal function. Report immediately.

▷ 5 Do not extend therapy beyond 10 days or exceed a total dose of 650 mg in adults, because cumulative toxicity can occur. Do not repeat a course of therapy within 6 weeks to 8 weeks.

▷ 6 Use cautiously in elderly or debilitated patients and in patients with liver disease.

▶ NURSING CONSIDERATIONS

▷ 1 Caution patients against strenuous activity for several weeks after termination of therapy.

▷ 2 Always administer emetine in combination with other amebicides effective in the treatment of intestinal parasites, because emetine alone produces a cure in only 10% to 15% of the cases of intestinal amebiasis.

▷ 3 Administer by deep IM or SC injection and avoid inadvertent IV injection, because severe toxic effects can result.

▷ 4 Observe for any ECG changes, which are common with emetine therapy. Although these are not an absolute indication for discontinuing therapy, patients must be carefully observed for additional complications (*e.g.,* dyspnea, arrhythmias).

▷ 5 Avoid contact of solution with eyes and mucous membranes, because drug is very irritating. Handle carefully.

▷ 6 Note number, consistency, and any unusual characteristics of the stools. Perform repeated fecal examinations up to 3 months following therapy to ensure elimination of parasites.

▶ metronidazole

Flagyl, Metro I.V., Metryl, Protostat, Satric

Metronidazole exerts a direct amebicidal and trichomonacidal action against *Entamoeba histolytica* and *Trichomonas vaginalis,* respectively. It is considered the drug of choice for oral treatment of trichomoniasis in both females and males. In addition, it is employed in treating acute intestinal amebiasis, both symptomatic and asymptomatic as well as amebic liver abscess. In spite of its broad-spectrum amebicidal action, reports of its carcinogenicity in mice and rats have somewhat dampened enthusiasm for the drug. Nevertheless, metronidazole remains a valuable drug for the therapy of both amebiasis and trichomoniasis.

In addition to its use as both an amebicide and trichomonicide, metronidazole is also available both orally and IV for the treatment of serious infections caused by susceptible anaerobic bacteria. Parenteral metronidazole has demonstrated clinical activity against the following organisms: *anaerobic gram-negative bacilli,* including *Bacteroides* and *Fusobacterium* species; *anaerobic gram-positive bacilli,* including *Clostridium* species; and *anaerobic gram-positive cocci,* including *Peptococcus* and *Peptostreptococcus* species. Necessary surgical procedures should always be performed in conjunction with drug treatment, and in mixed aerobic–anaerobic infections, appropriate antibiotics should be included in the drug regimen. The principal hazard connected with parenteral metronidazole therapy is the possibility of convulsive seizures and development of peripheral neuropathy. The benefit–risk ratio must be critically evaluated in patients who show evidence of abnormal neurologic signs.

Mechanism

Not entirely established; appears to disrupt the structure of DNA in susceptible organisms, causing strand breakage and loss of helical structure; destroys most organisms within 24 hours to 48 hours

Uses

1 Treatment of acute intestinal amebiasis (amebic dysentery) and amebic liver abscess
2 Treatment of symptomatic and asymptomatic trichomoniasis in both sexes (oral only)
3 Treatment of serious infections caused by susceptible anaerobic bacteria, especially *Bacteroides, Clostridium, Eubacterium, Peptococcus,* and *Peptostreptococcus* species (IV)
4 Investigational uses include (1) hepatic encephalopathy, (2) prophylaxis of infection in gynecologic, abdominal, or colonic surgery, (3) treatment of giardiasis or *Gardnerella vaginalis.*

Dosage

Amebiasis
Adults: 500 mg to 750 mg three times a day orally for 5 days to 10 days
Children: 35 mg/kg to 50 mg/kg/day orally in three divided doses for 10 days

Trichomoniasis
250 mg three times a day orally for 7 days for males and females; alternately 2 g in a single dose or two divided doses

Anaerobic infections

Initially 15 mg/kg infused over 1 hour; maintenance doses, 7.5 mg/kg infused over 1 hour every 6 hours for 7 days to 10 days; maximum dose, 4 g/24-hour period; may change to oral therapy (7.5 mg/kg every 6 hr) as condition warrants

Fate

Well absorbed from GI tract; peak serum levels occur in 1 hour to 2 hours; widely distributed in the body and diffuses well into all tissues; slightly (20%) bound to plasma proteins; plasma half-life is approximately 8 hours; excreted largely in the urine, both as unchanged drug (20%) and 2-hydroxy methyl metabolite; both parent compound and metabolite have antibacterial activity

Common Side-Effects

(Especially orally) Nausea, metallic taste, anorexia, and epigastric distress

Significant Adverse Reactions

Oral

GI—vomiting, diarrhea, abdominal cramping, furry tongue, glossitis, stomatitis, candidal overgrowth

CNS—dizziness, vertigo, incoordination, ataxia, paresthesia, numbness, confusion, depression, irritability, insomnia

Allergic—pruritus, flushing, urticaria, fever

Urinary—dysuria, cystitis, polyuria, incontinence, darkened urine

Other—leukopenia, nasal congestion, xerostomia, dyspareunia, decreased libido, proctitis, pyuria, flattened T wave, joint pain

IV

See Oral; in addition, convulsions, peripheral neuropathy, thrombophlebitis with IV infusion.

Contraindications

Blood dyscrasias, organic CNS disease, first trimester of pregnancy (unless absolutely necessary, *e.g., severe,* life-threatening infections)

Interactions

1 Alcohol ingestion may elicit a disulfiram-like reaction (abdominal cramps, vomiting, severe headache, hypotension); see Chap. 80

2 Metronidazole may potentiate the effects of oral anticoagulants

3 The effectiveness of metronidazole may be reduced if given concurrently with phenobarbital or phenytoin, drugs that may increase its rate of metabolism.

▶ NURSING ALERTS

▷ 1 Observe for symptoms of CNS toxicity (incoordination, ataxia, tremors, paresthesias), and discontinue drug if these symptoms occur.

▷ 2 Recognize that demonstration of the carcinogenic potential of metronidazole in mice and rats at rather low doses demands a cautious approach to the use of the drug in humans. Use only where necessary and stress the importance of adherence to the prescribed dosage.

▷ 3 Observe patients carefully for signs of abnormal neurologic function, especially with IV administration. Persistent peripheral neuropathy has occurred in some patients on prolonged therapy. Benefit–risk ratio of continued therapy must be critically evaluated.

▷ 4 Inform patients that ingestion of alcohol in any form (*e.g.,* cough preparations, mouthwashes) can result in a disulfiram-like reaction (vomiting, diarrhea, flushing, hypotension, abdominal pain).

▷ 5 Use cautiously in young children, pregnant women during the second and third trimester of pregnancy, nursing mothers, and in patients with persistent fungal infections or CNS diseases. Reduce IV dose in patients with hepatic dysfunction.

▶ NURSING CONSIDERATIONS

▷ 1 Perform total and differential leukocyte counts before and periodically during therapy, because drug can elicit leukopenia.

▷ 2 Be aware that use of the drug can result in secondary fungal (candidal) overgrowth. Observe for signs of glossitis, stomatitis, vaginitis, vaginal discharge, proctitis, or furry tongue, and institute appropriate antifungal medication.

▷ 3 In treating trichomoniasis, recognize that concurrent treatment of the male sexual partner is usually necessary to prevent reinfection.

▷ 4 Advise patients that drug may darken the urine but this phenomenon is of no clinical significance.

▷ 5 Closely follow package instructions for preparing IV infusion solution. Order of mixing is important. Do not refrigerate neutralized solution because precipitation may occur. Use within 24 hours.

▷ 6 Administer oral drug with food to minimize GI upset. Complete the full course of prescribed therapy.

▷ 7 Inform patients that drug may cause an unpleasant metallic taste.

▶ paromomycin

Humatin

An aminoglycoside-like drug, paromomycin exhibits an antibacterial action resembling that of neomycin. In addition, it exerts an amebicidal action in the intestinal tract, but is not appreciably absorbed orally; therefore it is ineffective in extra-intestinal amebiasis. Paromomycin is reviewed in Chapter 64 and only its antiamebic properties will be discussed in this chapter.

Mechanism

Direct amebicidal action *in vivo* and *in vitro;* may also reduce the population of intestinal microbes essential for proliferation of protozoa

Uses

1 Treatment of acute and chronic intestinal amebiasis, usually as an alternative drug to other more potent and specific amebicides

2 Adjunctive therapy in management of hepatic coma (see Chap. 64)

Table 71-1. Amebicides Available by Request from the Centers for Disease Control*

Drug	Preparations	Usual Dosage Range	Remarks
Dehydroemetine (Mebadin)	Injection—30 mg/ml	Adults and children—1 mg/kg to 1.5 mg/kg/day IM or SC for up to 5 days (maximum 100 mg/day)	Clinical indications are the same as for emetine, but the incidence and severity of cardiovascular complications may be somewhat less; usually given in combination with diloxanide, and a tetracycline, followed by chloroquine if hepatic amebiasis is present; daily dosage may be divided into 2 parts; use very cautiously in patients with cardiac disease or neuromuscular disorders
Diloxanide furoate (Furamide)	Tablets—500 mg	Adults—500 mg 3 times a day for 10 days Children—20 mg/kg/day in 3 divided doses for 10 days; repeat in several weeks if necessary	A relatively nontoxic intestinal amebicide regarded by many as the drug of choice for asymptomatic and mild symptomatic intestinal amebiasis; ineffective alone against extra-intestinal parasites; may be combined with metronidazole in moderate to severe intestinal disease; mild GI distress and flatulence have been reported; GI absorption is appreciable, and much of an oral dose is excreted in the urine within 48 hours, largely as metabolites

* Parasitic Disease Drug Service, Centers for Disease Control, Atlanta, Georgia 30333.

Dosage

Amebiasis

25 mg/kg to 35 mg/kg/day in three divided doses for 5 days to 10 days

Hepatic coma

4 g/day in divided doses for 5 days to 6 days

Fate

Not significantly absorbed orally; excreted largely in the feces; systemically absorbed drug is excreted very slowly *via* the kidney

Common Side-Effects

Nausea, anorexia, GI upset, and diarrhea

Significant Adverse Reactions

Abdominal cramps, pruritus ani, headache, vertigo, skin rash, malabsorption state, and overgrowth of nonsusceptible organisms

Contraindications

Intestinal obstruction, ulcerative bowel lesions

▶ NURSING CONSIDERATIONS

▷ 1 Be alert for indications of fungal overgrowth (glossitis, vaginitis, furry tongue, diarrhea) and advise physician. Appropriate antifungal therapy should be instituted.

▷ 2 Administer drug with meals to minimize GI upset.

▷ 3 Examine stools weekly during and for at least 6 weeks following termination of therapy.

▷ 4 Because paromomycin is an aminoglycoside derivative, recognize that it has the potential to elicit serious untoward reactions (nephrotoxicity, ototoxicity) as well as interact with a number of other drugs. (See Chap. 64 for complete discussion of aminoglycosides.) Note, however, that the incidence of these reactions with paromomycin is quite low, because the drug is generally absorbed poorly.

Summary. Amebicides

Drug	Preparations	Usual Dosage Range
Carbarsone (Carbarsone)	Capsules—250 mg	Adults—250 mg 2 to 3 times a day for 10 days; may repeat in 2 weeks Children—75 mg/kg over 10 days in 3 daily divided doses
Chloroquine (Aralen)	Tablets (phosphate)—250 mg, 500 mg Injection (hydrochloride)—50 mg/ml	Oral—1 g/day for 2 days, then 500 mg/day for at least 2 weeks to 3 weeks IM—200 mg to 250 mg/day for 10 days to 12 days
Diiodohydroxyquin (Iodoquinol, Moebiquin, Yodoxin)	Tablets—210 mg, 650 mg	Adults—630 mg to 650 mg 3 times a day for 20 days Children—30 mg to 40 mg/kg/day in 3 divided doses for 20 days (maximum 2 g/day)

(continued)

Summary. Amebicides *(continued)*

Drug	Preparations	Usual Dosage Range
Emetine (Emetine)	Injection—65 mg/ml	65 mg/day, in a single dose, or divided doses, SC or IM, for 3 days to 5 days in amebic dysentery or for 10 days in amebic hepatitis
Metronidazole (Flagyl, Metro I.V., Metryl, Protostat, Satric)	Tablets—250 mg, 500 mg Powder for injection—500 mg/vial Injection—500 mg/100-ml single-dose containers	Amebiasis: Adults—500 mg to 750 mg 3 times a day orally for 5 days to 10 days Children—35 mg to 50 mg/kg/day orally in 3 divided doses for 10 days Trichomoniasis: 250 mg 3 times a day orally for 7 days or 2 g in a single dose or 2 divided doses Anaerobic infections: Initially 15 mg/kg infused over 1 hour Maintenance 7.5 mg/kg infused over 1 hour every 6 hours for 7 days to 10 days (maximum 4 g in 24 hr)
Paromomycin (Humatin)	Capsules—250 mg	25 mg to 35 mg/kg/day in 3 divided doses for 5 days to 10 days Hepatic coma: 4 g/day in divided doses for 5 days to 6 days

Fungal, or mycotic, infections are responsible for a number of pathologic conditions in man that, with few exceptions, remain a difficult-to-treat group of diseases. Fungal diseases are conventionally categorized as either topical (cutaneous, superficial) or deep (systemic) infections. Although this classification is convenient, it should be recognized that organisms responsible for local infections of the skin, nails, vagina, or GI tract (such as *Candida*) can also invade deeper body organs, resulting in systemic involvement and serious complications. Because there are only a few effective systemic antifungal drugs, most of which are relatively toxic in the doses needed to eliminate deep mycotic infections, successful treatment of systemic fungal diseases is one of the most difficult tasks in chemotherapy. The need for specific, safe, and effective systemic antifungal agents is acute; until such drugs become available, it is imperative that the currently available drugs be prescribed properly and monitored closely.

Reflecting the classification of fungal diseases into topical or deep infections, antifungal drugs can be categorized in much the same way, although it should be noted that some drugs are utilized in treating *both* superficial as well as systemic infections. A useful classification of antifungal agents is as follows:

Drugs for treating systemic infections only
  Flucytosine
Drugs for treating both systemic and topical infections
  Amphotericin B
  Ketoconazole
  Miconazole
  Nystatin
Drugs for treating topical infections only
  1 *Oral only*
     Griseofulvin
  2 *Cutaneous only*
     Acrisorcin
     Ciclopirox
     Econazole
     Haloprogin
     Iodochlorhydroxyquin
     Tolnaftate
     Triacetin
     Undecylenic acid
  3 *Vaginal only*
     Candicidin
  4 *Cutaneous and vaginal*
     Clotrimazole
Drugs for treating ophthalmic infections only
  Natamycin

The various organisms responsible for the common fungal infections, together with the preferred drugs for treating each disease, are listed in Table 58-1, Chapter 58. Most systemic fungal infections respond best to amphotericin B. Flucytosine is indicated for serious candidal or cryptococcal infections and is synergistic with amphotericin B against these organisms. Miconazole and ketaconazole are viewed as rather broad-spectrum antifungal agents, but some questions exist as to their clinical efficacy in many fungal diseases. In addition, relapses have frequently occurred with use of these agents. Oral nystatin is indicated solely for intestinal

Antifungal Agents

72

candidasis. Topical or vaginal monilial infections due to *Candida* species can be effectively controlled by several antifungal drugs, such as candicidin, clotrimazole, miconazole, and nystatin. Cutaneous dermatophytal infections (*e.g.,* tinea) of the skin, hair, or nails (including ringworm, athlete's foot, jock itch) can be controlled either by oral griseofulvin (severe ringworm) or one of the topically effective antifungal drugs such as ciclopirox, econazole, haloprogin, tolnaftate, triacetin, or undecylenic acid. Natamycin is an antifungal agent used locally in the eye for treatment of fungal conjunctivitis, blepharitis, and keratitis.

The systemic antifungal agents are reviewed individually in detail in this chapter. The topically effective drugs are then listed in Table 72-1, along with their indications, dosage ranges, and specific information relating to each drug.

Systemic Antifungal Agents

▶ amphotericin B
Fungizone

An antibiotic produced by a strain of *Streptomyces,* amphotericin is a first-line drug for many severe progressive and potentially fatal systemic fungal infections, but because of its serious toxicity, it should never be used to treat trivial or clinically insignificant fungal diseases. It is also used topically to treat cutaneous or mucosal candidal (monilial) infections.

Mechanism
Fungistatic or fungicidal depending on organism and concentration of drug; binds to sterols (*e.g.,* ergosterol) in fungal cell membrane, thus increasing cell permeability and allowing leakage of cellular constituents; no effect on bacteria, viruses, or rickettsiae; potentiates the effects of flucytosine and other antibiotics by allowing penetration of these drugs into the fungal cell.

Uses
1 Treatment of serious and potentially fatal systemic fungal infections, such as aspergillosis, blastomycosis, coccidioidomycosis, cryptococcosis, disseminated candidiasis (moniliasis), histoplasmosis, mucormycosis, and sporotrichosis (see Table 58-1)
2 Alternative treatment of American mucocutaneous leishmaniasis (IV only)
3 Treatment of cutaneous and mucocutaneous candidal (monilial) infections (topically only)

Dosage
IV infusion: initially 0.25 mg/kg/day infused over 6 hours; may increase gradually to 1 mg/kg/day or 1.5 mg/kg every other day as tolerance permits; total treatment time is usually several months, although some serious infections can require 9 months to 12 months of ther-

apy; maximum daily dose is 1.5 mg/kg; total dosage can range from 1.5 g for blastomycosis up to 4 g for life-threatening infections such as rhinocerebral phycomycosis
Intrathecal/intraventricular: 0.1 mg initially, increased gradually up to 0.5 mg every 48 hours to 72 hours (investigational use only)
Topical: apply liberally to lesions 2 to 4 times a day for 1 week to 4 weeks depending on response

Fate
Poorly absorbed from GI tract and not given orally; following IV infusion, drug is highly (90%–95%) bound to plasma proteins, and has a plasma half-life of 24 hours; diffuses well into inflamed pleural and peritoneal cavities and joints, but poorly into most other body tissues; slowly excreted by the kidneys (elimination half-life is 15 days), a small fraction in a biologically active form; drug can be detected in the urine for at least 7 weeks after termination of therapy.

Common Side-Effects
IV—fever, chills, nausea, vomiting, diarrhea, headache, dyspepsia, impaired renal function (hypokalemia, azotemia, renal tubular acidosis, nephrocalcinosis), anorexia, weight loss, malaise, muscle and joint pain, abdominal cramping, pain at injection site, phlebitis, normochromic–normocytic anemia

Significant Adverse Reactions
IV—maculopapular rash, pruritus, tinnitus, hearing loss, blurred vision, vertigo, flushing, peripheral neuropathy, blood pressure alterations, arrhythmias, cardiac arrest, blood dyscrasias, coagulation defects, anuria, oliguria, hemorrhagic gastroenteritis, convulsions, anaphylactic reaction, acute liver failure
Topical—drying of the skin, irritation, pruritus, erythema, burning, contact dermatitis, skin discoloration

Contraindications
No absolute contraindications if the situation being treated is potentially life-threatening

Interactions
1 Hypokalemia produced by amphotericin B may be increased by diuretics or corticosteroids, and poses a danger in patients receiving digitalis drugs.
2 Amphotericin B can enhance the effect of peripherally acting muscle relaxants, for example, curare, gallamine, succinylcholine.
3 Concomitant use of corticosteroids, antibiotics, or antineoplastics with amphotericin B can increase the incidence of superinfections and blood dyscrasias.
4 Aminoglycosides and other nephrotoxic or ototoxic drugs can have additive toxic effects with amphotericin B.
5 Flucytosine, minocycline, and rifampin can potentiate the antifungal activity of amphotericin B.

▶ **NURSING ALERTS**

▷ 1 Recognize that amphotericin B is potentially a very toxic drug and should never be used to treat trivial fungal infections.

▷ 2 Administer IV under close supervision, only to hospitalized patients following a confirmed diagnosis of progressive, potentially fatal fungal disease.

▷ 3 Determine BUN and serum creatinine levels at least weekly during therapy. Perform hemograms, serum potassium determinations, and liver function tests at weekly intervals as well. Discontinue drug if liver function is abnormal, if BUN exceeds 40 mg/100 ml, or if serum creatinine exceeds 3 mg/100 ml.

▷ 4 Monitor intake–output and observe for oliguria, hematuria, or cloudy urine. Advise physician of any change in renal function, because nephrotoxicity develops after a few months in most patients. The azotemia that develops during therapy is usually reversible, but if total dose exceeds 4 g, *persistent* renal damage often ensues.

▷ 5 Advise patients to report immediately any changes in auditory or vestibular function, because drug is potentially ototoxic.

▷ 6 Observe for signs of hypokalemia (muscle weakness or cramping, drowsiness, paresthesias), and provide necessary potassium supplementation.

▷ 7 Use with extreme caution in pregnant women and in patients with renal impairment, blood dyscrasias, neurologic disorders, or peptic ulcer.

▶ **NURSING CONSIDERATIONS**

▷ 1 Infuse IV at a slow rate and observe injection site for signs of inflammation. Avoid extravasation, because thromboses and thrombophlebitis can occur.

▷ 2 Use aseptic technique in reconstituting powder, because no preservative or bacteriostatic agent is present. Add 10 ml Sterile Water for Injection to powder, shake, then dilute further (1:50) with 5% Dextrose Injection of pH above 4.2. Do not reconstitute with saline solution, because precipitation may result.

▷ 3 If an in-line membrane filter is used during IV infusion, ensure that the mean pore diameter is greater than 1μ to allow passage of the colloidal dispersion of the drug.

▷ 4 Store vials in refrigerator, protect against exposure to light, and use IV infusion solutions immediately upon preparation.

▷ 5 Whenever therapy is interrupted for longer than 7 days, resume at lowest dosage level (0.25 mg/kg/day) and increase gradually.

▷ 6 Consider administration of aspirin, antihistamines, antiemetics, or small doses of corticosteroids as needed to lessen the severity of adverse reactions (*e.g.,* fever, headache, vomiting) to amphotericin B. Simultaneous infusion of heparin may decrease the incidence of thrombophlebitis.

▷ 7 Be aware that use of amphotericin can interfere with a number of laboratory test results (*e.g.,* SGOT, SGPT, BUN, serum creatinine, hematocrit, hemoglobin, platelet count).

▷ 8 Note that amphotericin B is available in combination with tetracycline (Mysteclin-F) to prevent fungal overgrowth that can occur with use of oral tetracyclines.

▷ 9 Watch for the development of hypersensitivity reactions to topical amphotericin (rash, pruritus, erythema) and notify physician.

▷ 10 Inform patients that some skin drying and discoloration may occur with use of cream preparation, but generally not with the lotion or ointment. Lotion may stain nail lesions, however.

▷ 11 Advise patients that topical preparations can stain clothes or other fabrics, but that the stain can be removed easily by washing with soap and water or by using a standard cleaning fluid.

▷ 12 Apply topical preparations liberally and rub gently but well into lesions.

▶ **flucytosine**
Ancobon

A synthetic pyrimidine, structurally related to the antineoplastic drug fluorouracil, flucytosine is an orally effective systemic antifungal drug that is considered a secondary agent in treating deep-seated mycotic infections due to *Candida* and *Cryptococcus* species. It is much less toxic than amphotericin B, but is less effective as well, and resistance frequently develops rapidly. Thus it is used mainly in combination with amphotericin B for treating cryptococcal infections such as meningitis.

Mechanism
Probably converted to 5-fluorouracil in fungal cells (but not normal mammalian cells); acts as a competitive inhibitor of nucleic acid synthesis; host cells apparently lack the enzyme that converts drug to active metabolite and are thus unaffected.

Uses
1 Treatment of serious systemic candidal infections (endocarditis, septicemia, urinary) or cryptococcal infections (meningitis, septicemia, pulmonary or urinary)—frequently given in combination with amphotericin B

Dosage
50 mg/kg to 150 mg/kg/day orally in divided doses every 6 hours

Fate
Well absorbed orally; peak plasma concentrations occur within 1 hour to 2 hours; minimally bound to plasma proteins; widely distributed in the body; drug levels in cerebrospinal fluid reach 50% to 100% of those in the serum; not significantly metabolized, but excreted largely unchanged (90%) in the urine; serum half-life is 3 hours to 6 hours.

Common Side-Effects
Nausea, diarrhea

Significant Adverse Reactions

Rash, anemia, leukopenia, thrombocytopenia, pancytopenia, vomiting, hepatomegaly, enterocolitis, elevation of SGOT, SGPT, BUN, and serum creatinine; less frequently, headache, vertigo, drowsiness, confusion, and hallucinations

Interactions

1 Flucytosine can potentiate the antifungal effects of amphotericin B.
2 Concurrent use with other bone marrow-depressing drugs (*e.g.,* antineoplastics, pyrazolones) may increase the toxic effects of both drugs.

▶ NURSING ALERTS

▷ 1 Use with extreme caution in patients with impaired renal function, bone marrow depression, hematologic disorders; during pregnancy or lactation; and in persons receiving radiation therapy or cancer chemotherapy.

▷ 2 Determine the renal, hepatic, and hematologic status of the patient before initiating therapy, and monitor these parameters at frequent intervals during therapy. Liver enzyme levels should be assessed frequently during therapy.

▷ 3 Monitor urinary function (intake–output) closely during therapy and perform frequent assays of blood level of drug to ensure normal excretion.

▶ NURSING CONSIDERATIONS

▷ 1 Administer capsules a few at a time over a 15-minute period to minimize the incidence of nausea and vomiting.

▷ 2 Periodically perform culture and sensitivity tests during therapy, because drug resistance has been reported with prolonged therapy.

▶ griseofulvin

Fulvicin, Grifulvin, Grisactin, Gris-PEG

An orally administered fungistatic antibiotic that is only effective against dermatophyte infections of the skin, hair, and nails, griseofulvin is available as either a microsize or ultramicrosize particle formulation. Ultramicrosize griseofulvin exhibits approximately 1.5 times the biological activity of microsize griseofulvin largely because of improved GI absorption; thus a 330-mg dose of ultramicrosize yields antifungal activity comparable to a 500-mg dose of the microsize formulation. However, there is no evidence that the ultramicrosize formulation is clinically superior with regard to efficacy or safety.

Mechanism

Localizes in keratin precursor cells in skin, nails, and hair and disrupts the mitotic spindle, thus arresting cell division; new keratin that is subsequently formed strongly binds griseofulvin, and becomes resistant to fungal invasion; no effect on bacteria, yeasts, or fungi other than dermatophytal organisms

Uses

1 Treatment of fungal infections of the skin, hair, or nails caused by the following dermatophytes: *Epidermophyton, Microsporum,* or *Trichophyton*

Dosage

Adults: 500 mg to 1 g microsize or 330 mg to 660 mg ultramicrosize daily in a single dose or divided doses
Children: 10 mg/kg microsize daily, in a single dose or divided doses

Fate

Oral absorption is somewhat variable, the ultramicrosize preparation being absorbed more efficiently than the microsize formulation. Peak plasma levels occur in about 4 hours, and drug is detectable in the skin within 4 hours to 8 hours. Griseofulvin exhibits a greater affinity for diseased skin than normal skin. Its plasma half-life is approximately 24 hours and it is metabolized in the liver and slowly excreted in the urine, mainly as metabolites.

Common Side-Effects

Skin rash, urticaria

Significant Adverse Reactions

GI—nausea, vomiting, diarrhea, epigastric distress, flatulence, stomatitis
Neurologic—paresthesias, fatigue, headache, dizziness, insomnia, confusion, peripheral neuritis, blurred vision, impaired motor skills, syncope
Hematologic—leukopenia, neutropenia, granulocytopenia
Allergic—angioedema, serum sickness, photosensitivity, erythema multiforme, lupus-like syndrome
Other—proteinuria, estrogen-like effects in children

Contraindications

Porphyria, severe liver disease, systemic lupus erythematosus, prophylaxis of *non*established fungal infections

Interactions

1 Griseofulvin can reduce the activity of oral anticoagulants.
2 Activity of griseofulvin may be diminished by barbiturates, glutethimide, diphenhydramine, orphenadrine, and phenylbutazone through enzyme induction.
3 The effects of alcohol may be potentiated by griseofulvin, producing tachycardia and flushing.

▶ NURSING ALERTS

▷ 1 Perform hematologic studies at least weekly during therapy, and monitor renal and hepatic function periodically during prolonged treatment.

▷ 2 Be aware that griseofulvin has produced hepatocellular necrosis and liver tumors in mice, impaired spermatogenesis in rats, and embryotoxicity and teratogenic effects in rats and dogs. Although these effects have not been demonstrated in humans, caution is required when using the drug for extended periods of time.

▷ 3 Do not use griseofulvin for minor or trivial fungal infections, nor for infections due to organisms other than susceptible dermatophytes.

▷ 4 Use cautiously in penicillin-sensitive patients (danger of cross-sensitivity) and during pregnancy.

▷ 5 Counsel patients to report the development of fever, sore throat, mucosal ulceration, or extreme malaise, because these might indicate a developing blood dyscrasia.

▶ **NURSING CONSIDERATIONS**

▷ 1 Warn patients to avoid exposure to intense sunlight, because photosensitivity can occur.

▷ 2 Be alert for indications of nonsusceptible fungal overgrowth (diarrhea, perianal itching, stomatitis, "black tongue") and advise physician.

▷ 3 Stress the necessity of continuing treatment until the infecting organism is completely eradicated, as indicated by clinical and laboratory examinations. Beneficial effects may not be noticeable for several weeks to months. Average durations of treatment are 4 weeks to 6 weeks for scalp ringworm, and at least 4 months to 6 months for fingernail and toenail fungal infections.

▷ 4 Note that a high-fat diet increases absorption of the drug, and administering drug with meals reduces GI irritation.

▷ 5 Urge good hygiene to control sources of re-infection and keep infected areas dry, because moisture enhances fungal growth.

▷ 6 Inform patients taking the drug that flushing and tachycardia can occur with ingestion of alcohol.

▷ 7 Note that cross-sensitivity to penicillins can occur.

▶ **ketoconazole**

Nizoral

Ketoconazole is an orally effective antifungal agent used for treating a variety of oral and systemic fungal infections. It is less toxic than amphotericin B, but somewhat less effective as well. Gastrointestinal complaints are common, and serious hepatotoxicity has been reported.

Mechanism

Not completely established; impairs the synthesis of ergosterol, which is a vital component of fungal cell membranes, resulting in increased permeability and subsequent leakage of cellular components.

Uses

1 Treatment of the following fungal infections: candidiasis, oral thrush, chronic mucocutaneous candidiasis, candiduria, histoplasmosis, blastomycosis, coccidioidomycosis, paracoccidioidomycosis, and chromomycosis.

2 Investigational uses include treatment of dermatophytosis, onychomycosis, pityriasis versicolor, and vaginal candidiasis.

Dosage

Adults: 200 mg to 400 mg (1 to 2 tablets) once a day, depending on severity of infection

Children (over 40 kg): 200 mg once a day

Children (20 kg–40 kg): 100 mg once a day

Children (under 20 kg): 50 mg once a day

Treatment is continued for at least 6 months in systemic mycotic infections.

Fate

Well absorbed orally; peak serum levels occur in 1 hour to 2 hours; tablet dissolution requires an acidic environment; highly (95%–99%) protein-bound; cerebrospinal fluid penetration is negligible; undergoes extensive hepatic metabolism; excreted largely (80%–90%) in the bile and feces (*via* enterohepatic circulation) with about 10% to 15% of drug excreted in the urine

Common Side-Effects

Nausea, vomiting, GI upset, pruritus, and gynecomastia

Significant Adverse Reactions

Abdominal pain, diarrhea, dizziness, lethargy, headache, fever, chills, photophobia, impotence, thrombocytopenia, hepatic dysfunction, and oligospermia

Interactions

1 GI absorption may be impaired by antacids, cimetidine, anticholinergics, and other drugs that reduce stomach acidity.

▶ **NURSING ALERTS**

▷ 1 Do not use ketoconazole for fungal meningitis, because the drug passes poorly into the cerebrospinal fluid.

▷ 2 Perform liver function tests before initiating therapy and at several week intervals thereafter during treatment. *Transient* elevations in liver enzymes frequently occur, and do not require discontinuation of therapy. Persistent elevations or presence of clinical signs of hepatic injury, however, require immediate termination of treatment, because the rare occurrence of liver disorders can be potentially fatal.

▶ **NURSING CONSIDERATIONS**

▷ 1 Continue treatment until *all* clinical and laboratory tests indicate that the active fungal infection has abated. In general, candidiasis requires a minimum of 2 weeks of therapy, whereas systemic mycotic infections may require 6 months or more of therapy.

▷ 2 Do not administer other drugs or substances that may reduce gastric acidity within 2 hours of ketoconazole, because GI absorption is impaired (see Interactions).

▷ 3 Use cautiously in pregnant or nursing women, and in children under 2 years of age.

▷ 4 Note that ketoconazole can decrease synthesis of cortisol and testosterone, especially with higher doses. The clinical significance of these effects remains to be determined.

▶ miconazole
Monistat I.V.

A broad-spectrum antifungal agent, miconazole is used intravenously for treatment of severe systemic fungal infections as well as topically and vaginally for control of cutaneous and mucocutaneous candidal and dermatophytal infections. The discussion that follows focuses on the systemic use of miconazole; its topical application is considered in Table 72-1.

Mechanism
Alters the permeability of the fungal cell membrane, resulting in loss of cell constituents and ultimately cellular death

Uses
1   Treatment of coccidioidomycosis, paracoccidioidomycosis, cryptococcosis, petriellidiosis, and chronic mucocutaneous candidiasis
2   Topical treatment of cutaneous and mucocutaneous candidal and dermatophytal infections (see Table 72-1)

Dosage
Intravenous
Adults: 200 mg to 3600 mg/day depending on disease and severity, divided over three infusions of 30 minutes to 60 minutes each; dilute standard injection (10 mg/ml) in 200 ml fluid before infusing
Coccidioidomycosis—1800 mg to 3600 mg/day
Cryptococcosis—1200 mg to 2400 mg/day
Petriellidiosis—600 mg to 3000 mg/day
Candidiasis—600 mg to 1800 mg/day
Paracoccidioidomycosis—200 mg to 1200 mg/day
Children: 20 mg to 40 mg/kg/day in divided infusions
Maximum is 15 mg/kg/infusion

Intrathecal
20 mg undiluted solution every 3 days to 7 days as adjunct to IV infusion in fungal meningitis

Bladder Instillation
200 mg diluted solution (10 mg/200 ml)

Fate
Highly bound to plasma protein; penetration into cerebrospinal fluid is poor; rapidly metabolized in the liver and excreted both in the urine and feces, mainly as inactive metabolites

Common Side-Effects
(IV use only) Phlebitis, pruritus, nausea, febrile reactions, rash, and vomiting

Significant Adverse Reactions
(IV use only) Diarrhea, drowsiness, flushing, anorexia, hyponatremia, decreased hematocrit, thrombocytopenia,

hyperlipemia (due to the castor oil vehicle), and arrhythmias (with too-rapid IV administration)

Interactions
1   Effects of oral anticoagulants may be enhanced by IV miconazole.
2   Miconazole and amphotericin B are mutually antagonistic and the antifungal activity of the combination is less than that of either drug used alone.

▶ NURSING ALERTS
▷ 1   Administer by slow IV infusion to minimize the danger of tachycardia and arrhythmias.
▷ 2   Begin treatment in a hospital setting, and closely monitor the patient during therapy. Given an initial dose of 200 mg to assess the patient's reaction.
▷ 3   Use cautiously in pregnant women and in young children.
▷ 4   Perform hemoglobin, hematocrit, electrolyte, and lipid determinations at the beginning of therapy and regularly thereafter.
▷ 5   Continue treatment until clinical and laboratory tests no longer indicate the presence of an active fungal infection (usually a minimum of 3 weeks–4 weeks), because inadequate treatment can result in recurrence of the infection.

▶ NURSING CONSIDERATIONS
▷ 1   Dilute injection in 200 ml sodium chloride or 5% dextrose solution and infuse over a 30-minute to 60-minute period.
▷ 2   Rotate intrathecal injections between lumbar, cervical, and cisternal sites every 3 days to 7 days.
▷ 3   Note that nausea and vomiting can be minimized by slowing the infusion rate, reducing the dose, avoiding mealtime drug administration, or by using prophylactic antiemetic medication.
▷ 4   Observe patient for signs of phlebitis.

▶ nystatin, oral
Mycostatin, Nilstat

Nystatin is a fungicidal antibiotic obtained from a species of *Streptomyces* that is used primarily in the treatment of candidal infections of the skin, mucous membranes, and intestinal tract. Following oral administration, it is poorly absorbed and thus is only effective against candidal infections of the oral cavity and intestinal tract. The drug is available as an oral tablet (which is swallowed whole) for the treatment of intestinal candidiasis and also as an oral suspension (which is retained in the mouth as long as possible before swallowing) for the treatment of candidiasis of the oral cavity. Those indications are discussed here, while the topical use of nystatin is considered in Table 72-1.

Mechanism
Binds to sterols in the membrane of fungal cells, altering its permeability; the resultant leakage of intracellular components leads to cellular death.

Uses
1 Treatment of intestinal candidiasis (oral tablet)
2 Treatment of candidiasis of the oral cavity (oral suspension)
3 Treatment of cutaneous and mucocutaneous candidal infections (for topical and vaginal application, see Table 72-1)

Dosage
Intestinal Candidiasis
500,000 U to 1 million U (1 or 2 tablets) three times a day; continue for at least 48 hours after clinical cure

Oral Candidiasis
Adults and children: 400,000 U to 600,000 U (4 ml–6 ml oral suspension) four times a day (one half dose in each side of mouth—retain for as long as possible before swallowing); continue for at least 48 hours after symptoms have disappeared
Infants: 200,000 U four times a day, as above

Fate
No detectable systemic blood levels following oral administration; excreted largely unchanged in the stool

Significant Adverse Reactions
Nausea, vomiting, GI distress, and diarrhea with large oral doses

▶ **NURSING CONSIDERATIONS**
▷ 1 Urge patients to complete the entire prescribed course of therapy to minimize the danger of reinfection or relapse.
▷ 2 Instruct patients using the oral suspension to place one half of the dose in each side of the mouth, retain there as long as possible (at least several minutes), then swallow.
▷ 3 Note that oral nystatin is also available in combination with tetracycline (Tetrastatin), and oxytetracycline (Terrastatin) to prevent fungal overgrowth that can occur with tetracyclines.

Topical/Vaginal Antifungal Agents

Acrisorcin
Amphotericin B
Candicidin
Ciclopirox
Clotrimazole
Econazole
Haloprogin
Iodochlorhydroxyquin
Miconazole
Nystatin
Tolnaftate
Triacetin
Undecylenic acid

A number of drugs possessing antifungal activity are employed topically or intravaginally for the treatment of cutaneous infections, for example, ringworm, athlete's foot, "jock itch," or mucocutaneous infections, such as vulvovaginal moniliasis. They are listed alphabetically in Table 72-1 along with dosage and other relevant information. Griseofulvin, an orally administered drug discussed earlier in the chapter, is also employed for treating ringworm (*Tinea*) infections of the skin, hair, or nails.

Ophthalmic Antifungal Agent

▶ **natamycin**
Natacyn

An antibiotic obtained from a species of *Streptomyces*, natamycin is fungicidal against a variety of organisms. It is not absorbed orally, and is only used in the eye for treatment of localized fungal infections.

Mechanism
Binds to sterols in fungal cell membrane, altering the cell permeability, thus allowing escape of essential cell constituents; not effective against bacteria

Uses
1 Treatment of fungal blepharitis, conjunctivitis, and keratitis due to susceptible organisms (drug of choice for *Fusarium solani* keratitis)

Dosage
One drop in affected eye every 1 hour to 2 hours for 3 days to 4 days, then reduce to one drop six to eight times a day for 14 days to 21 days depending on the severity of the infection

Fate
No appreciable systemic absorption following topical administration

Significant Adverse Reactions
Conjunctival hyperemia or chemosis, blurred vision, and photosensitivity

▶ **NURSING CONSIDERATIONS**
▷ 1 If clinical improvement is not observed within 7 days to 10 days, re-evaluate patient's status and perform additional laboratory tests to determine if other organisms are present.
▷ 2 Explain the proper dosage procedure and the importance of completing the entire course of therapy to prevent recurrence.
▷ 3 Inform patients that bottle must be shaken well before use and dropper should not be contaminated by touching eye, fingers, or other surfaces.
▷ 4 Advise physician if irritation occurs or condition appears to deteriorate.
▷ 5 Wait at least 5 minutes before using any other drops in the eyes.

Table 72-1. Topical/Vaginal Antifungal Agents

Drug	Preparations	Usual Dosage Range	Remarks
Acrisorcin (Akrinol)	Cream—2 mg/g	Apply small quantity twice a day, for at least 6 weeks	Indicated for the treatment of tinea versicolor, a superficial fungal infection caused by *Malassezia furfur;* may cause blisters, skin eruptions, hives, and a burning sensation following application; do not use near the eyes; evening application follows a warm, soapy bath and use of a stiff brush on the lesions; photosensitivity may occur
Amphotericin B, topical (Fungizone)	Cream—3% Ointment—3% Lotion—3%	Apply liberally 2 to 4 times a day; duration of therapy ranges from 1 week to 2 weeks for simple infections (*e.g.,* candidiasis) to several months for onychomycoses	Used for treating cutaneous and mucocutaneous candidal infections; similar to nystatin in activity; cream may have a drying effect and discolor the skin; lotion and ointment may, stain nail lesions; redness, itching, and burning have occurred with all preparations; discoloration of clothing or fabrics is removable by washing in soap and water or cleaning fluid; also used parenterally; see separate discussion
Candicidin (Vanobid)	Vaginal tablets—3 mg Vaginal ointment—0.6 mg/g	1 tablet or 1 vaginal applicatorful of ointment into vagina twice a day for 14 days	Antifungal activity is similar to nystatin; used in treatment of vaginitis due to *Candida* organisms; insert high into vagina; during pregnancy, tablets should be used rather than ointment, and inserted manually, not with applicator; continue use even during menstruation; irritation and sensitization are rare
Ciclopirox (Loprox)	Cream—1%	Apply twice a day	Broad-spectrum antifungal used for tinea pedis, tinea cruris, tinea corporis, candidiasis and tinea versicolor due to *Malassezia furfur;* penetrates hair, hair follicles, sebaceous glands, and dermis; do *not* use occlusive dressings; if no clinical improvement occurs within 4 weeks, re-evaluate therapy; very low incidence of irritation, sensitization, or phototoxicity; safety and efficacy in children less than 10 years of age have not been established
Clotrimazole (Gyne-Lotrimin, Lotrimin, Mycelex)	Cream—1% Solution—1% Vaginal tablets—100 mg Vaginal cream—1%	Topical—massage into infected area twice a day Vaginal—1 tablet inserted at bedtime for 7 days or 1 applicatorful of vaginal cream inserted at bedtime for 7 days to 14 days	Broad-spectrum antifungal used topically for dermatophytal infections, candidiasis, and tinea versicolor and vaginally for vulvovaginal candidiasis; topical application may cause burning, stinging, peeling, itching, urticaria, and edema; clinical improvement usually occurs within 7 days; discontinue if severe irritation or hypersensitivity reactions occur; vaginal application has resulted in mild burning, rash, urinary frequency, and lower abdominal cramping; use of a sanitary pad will prevent staining of clothing; in case of treatment failure,

Table 72-1. Topical/Vaginal Antifungal Agents *(continued)*

Drug	Preparations	Usual Dosage Range	Remarks
			presence of other pathogens (*e.g., Trichomonas, Hemophilus vaginalis*) should be suspected; stress importance of taking full course of therapy
Econazole (Spectazole)	Cream—1%	Apply once or twice a day	Broad spectrum antifungal with good activity against dermatophytes, yeasts, and some gram (+) bacteria; following topical application, inhibitory concentrations of drug were found as deep as the middle region of the dermis; low incidence of burning, itching, and erythema; apply after cleansing affected area; treat candidal infections, tinea cruris and tinea corporis for 2 weeks, and tinea pedis for 4 weeks
Haloprogin (Halotex)	Cream—1% Solution—1%	Apply liberally 2 times a day for 2 weeks to 4 weeks	Indicated for superficial fungal infections of the skin and for tinea versicolor; side-effects include irritation, burning, vesicle formation, and pruritus, may worsen pre-existing lesions; avoid contact with eyes; if no improvement is noted within 4 weeks, patient's condition should be re-evaluated
Iodochlorhydroxyquin (Clioquinol, Torofor, Vioform)	Cream—3% Ointment—3%	Apply 2 to 3 times a day for a maximum of one week	Antibacterial and antifungal agent used in treatment of cutaneous fungal infections and inflammatory skin conditions, *e.g.,* eczema; do not use in the presence of superficial viral conditions, tuberculosis, vaccinia, or varicella; infrequently elicits skin irritation, but can stain skin, hair, or fabrics; may be absorbed systemically if used on widespread areas, and can interfere with thyroid function tests, because drug contains iodine; available in combination with hydrocortisone (Vioform-HC) as prescription only, but can be sold over the counter when used alone
Miconazole (Micatin, Monistat-Derm, Monistat 7)	Cream—2% Lotion—2% Powder—2% Vaginal cream—2%	Topical—apply twice a day for 2 weeks to 4 weeks Vaginal—1 applicatorful vaginally at bedtime for 7 days	Indicated for cutaneous dermatophytal and candidal infections, tinea versicolor, and vulvovaginal candidiasis; rarely causes burning or irritation topically; avoid eyes; use lotion rather than cream between the toes or fingers to avoid maceration effects; clinical improvement should occur in 1 week to 2 weeks; diagnosis should be re-evaluated after 4 weeks if good response is not evident; pathogens other than *Candida* should be ruled out before using drug for vaginitis, because it is only effective against candidal vulvovaginitis; advise patient to insert high into vagina, *(continued)*

Table 72-1. Topical/Vaginal Antifungal Agents *(continued)*

Drug	Preparations	Usual Dosage Range	Remarks
			to use sanitary napkin to prevent staining, to complete full course of therapy, and to avoid sexual intercourse during treatment to prevent re-infection; burning, itching, and irritation can occur; advise physician; use cautiously during pregnancy, especially the first trimester; perform urine and blood glucose studies in patients who do not respond to treatment, because persistent candidal vulvovaginitis may result from unrecognized diabetes mellitus; also used IV for severe systemic fungal infections; see separate discussion
Nystatin (Korostatin, Mycostatin, Nilstat, O-V Statin)	Cream—100,000 U/g Ointment—100,000 U/g Powder—100,000 U/g Vaginal tablets—100,000 U	Topical—apply 2 to 3 times a day for at least 1 week after clinical cure Vaginal—1 tablet inserted vaginally daily for 14 days	Used in treating cutaneous and vaginal infections due to *Candida* species; no detectable blood levels are noted following topical application; irritation is rare and drug does not stain skin or mucous membranes; avoid contact with eyes; powder may be dusted into shoes and socks as well as onto feet; symptomatic relief of cutaneous infections usually occurs within 72 hours; vaginal application should be continued for entire 14 days, even though clinical symptoms disappear within a few days; lack of response suggests presence of other pathogens besides *Candida;* no adverse effects or complications have been reported when drug is used during pregnancy; also available in oral tablets and oral suspension for treatment of intestinal and oral candidiasis, respectively; see separate discussion
Tolnaftate (Aftate, Tinactin)	Cream—1% Gel—1% Solution—1% Liquid aerosol—1% Powder—1% Powder aerosol—1%	Apply small amount 2 to 3 times a day for 2 weeks to 6 weeks as necessary	Effective in treating cutaneous dermatophytal infections, *e.g.,* athlete's foot, jock itch, or ringworm; inactive systemically, virtually nontoxic, nonirritating, and nonsensitizing; serious or chronic fungal infections may require concomitant use of griseofulvin; powder is preferred in moist areas (*e.g.,* between toes), whereas liquids or solutions are preferred in hairy areas; not effective against *Candida,* therefore if patient does not improve within several weeks, additional antifungal therapy is indicated; discontinue treatment if irritation occurs or condition worsens; available over the counter
Triacetin (Enzactin, Fungacetin, Fungoid)	Cream—25% Ointment—25% Liquid (Fungoid)—with cetylpyridinium and chloroxylenol	Apply twice a day for at least 1 week after symptoms have subsided	Indicated for milder superficial fungal infections, *e.g.,* athlete's foot; cleanse affected area with alcohol or soap and water before application; cover treated areas;

Table 72-1. Topical/Vaginal Antifungal Agents (continued)

Drug	Preparations	Usual Dosage Range	Remarks
			avoid eyes; use cautiously in patients with impaired circulation; may stain certain fabrics; available over the counter, except Fungoid, which contains additional antiseptics
Undecylenic Acid and Salts (Caldesene, Cruex, Desenex, NP-27, Quinsana, Ting, and various other manufacturers)	Ointment—5% undecylenic acid and 20% zinc undecylenate Cream—20% zinc undecylenate Solution—10% undecylenic acid and 47% isopropyl alcohol Liquid—10% undecylenic acid Powder and aerosol powder—10% calcium undecylenate, 20% zinc undecylenate, or 2% undecylenic acid plus 20% zinc undecylenate Soap—2% undecylenic acid Foam—10% undecylenic acid and 35% isopropyl alcohol	Apply as needed several times a day	Fungistatic and weak antibacterial activity; mainly used for athlete's foot, jock itch, or ringworm, *exclusive* of nails and hairy areas; also employed for relief or prevention of diaper rash, prickly heat, groin irritation, and other minor skin irritations; do not use if skin is broken or severely abraded; area should be cleansed well before application; use with caution in patients with impaired circulation; powder is recommended on moist areas, while liquids or solutions are preferred on hairy areas

Summary. Antifungal Agents

Drug	Preparations	Usual Dosage Range
Systemic		
Amphotericin B (Fungizone)	Injection—50 mg/vial Cream—3% Ointment—3% Lotion—3%	IV infusion—initially 0.25 mg/kg/day infused over 6 hours; increase gradually to 1 mg/kg/day or 1.5 mg/kg every other day (maximum daily dose 1.5 mg/kg) Intrathecal/intraventricular—0.1 mg initially, increased gradually up to 0.5 mg every 48 hours to 72 hours Topical—apply liberally 2 to 4 times a day for 1 week to 4 weeks
Flucytosine (Ancobon)	Capsules—250 mg, 500 mg	50 mg to 150 mg/kg/day in divided doses at 6-hour intervals
Griseofulvin (Fulvicin, Grifulvin, Grisactin, Gris-PEG)	*Microsize* Tablets—125 mg, 250 mg, 500 mg Capsules—125 mg, 250 mg Suspension—125 mg/5 ml *Ultramicrosize* Tablets—125 mg, 165 mg, 250 mg, 330 mg (ultramicrosize tablets have 1.5 times the activity of microsize tablets)	Adults—500 mg to 1 g microsize or equivalent daily in a single dose or divided doses Children—10 mg/kg/day microsize or equivalent, daily in a single dose or divided doses
Ketoconazole (Nizoral)	Tablets—200 mg	Adults—200 mg to 400 mg once a day Children (over 40 kg)—200 mg once a day

(continued)

Summary. Antifungal Agents *(continued*

Drug	Preparations	Usual Dosage Range
		Children (20 kg–40 kg)—100 mg once a day
		Children (under 20 kg)—50 mg once a day
Miconazole IV (Monistat IV)	Injection—10 mg/ml	Adults—200 mg to 3600 mg/day (depending on disease) by 3 equally divided IV infusions
		Children—20 mg/kg to 40 mg/ kg/day in divided IV infusions (maximum 15 mg/kg/infusion)
		Intrathecal—20 mg undiluted injection every 3 days to 7 days
		Bladder instillation—200 mg diluted solution (10 mg/200 ml)
Nystatin, Oral (Mycostatin, Nilstat)	Tablets—100,000 U; 500,000 U Oral suspension—100,000 U/ml	Intestinal candidiasis—500,000 U to 1 million U (1–2 tablets) 3 times a day
		Oral candidiasis—400,000 U to 600,000 U (4 ml–6 ml suspension) 4 times a day; one half dose in each side of the mouth
		Infants—200,000 U 4 times a day
Topical/Vaginal	See Table 72-1	
Ophthalmic		
Natamycin (Natacyn)	Ophthalmic suspension—5%	1 drop every 1 hour to 2 hours for 3 days to 4 days, then 1 drop 6 to 8 times a day for 14 days to 21 days

Although viruses are responsible for a large number of diseases, few clinically effective antiviral drugs are currently available, and they have a rather limited therapeutic application. The principal obstacle to effective antiviral treatment is the fact that virus particles replicate within host (*i.e.,* human) cells by utilizing the enzyme systems of the invaded cell. Thus, drugs interfering with intracellular viral replication are likely to damage the host cell as well, and are therefore usually quite toxic if given systemically. In addition, most viral diseases are of short duration and are often clinically asymptomatic until the infectious process within the host cells is well advanced, by which time the body's own defense mechanisms have already come into play. Thus, in order to be maximally effective, drugs that block viral replication should be administered *before* the onset of the disease. Such is the case with use of amantadine as a prophylactic agent against influenza A virus. On the other hand, some viral infections, such as herpesvirus, continue to manifest viral replication even after symptoms have appeared. In these diseases, inhibition of *further* viral replication may speed healing and thus serves as the basis for use of drugs such as acyclovir, idoxuridine, and vidarabine in herpetic infections.

Viral diseases are best managed prophylactically, either by active (attenuated or killed virus vaccines) or in some cases passive (viral antibodies) immunization. Once the disease has appeared, however, immunization is of no value and most common viral infections (such as colds, or "flu") are usually best treated symptomatically. Specific antiviral drugs have a limited therapeutic application, largely for the reasons outlined above. Only a handful of viral infections have been shown to be responsive to the few available antiviral agents.

Antiviral Agents

73

▶ **acyclovir**
Zovirax

Acyclovir is a nucleoside of guanine with *in vitro* antiviral activity against herpes simplex types 1 and 2, varicella–zoster, Epstein–Barr, and cytomegalovirus. Normal cellular thymidine kinase enzyme does not utilize acyclovir; hence, the drug *selectively* inhibits viral cell replication with minimal toxicity for normal uninfected cells. Thus, the drug is well tolerated by most patients. It is currently available as an ointment and as a powder for preparing an IV infusion.

Mechanism
Converted by herpes simplex virus-coded thymidine kinase into acyclovir monophosphate, which is further transformed into the diphosphate and triphosphate, the latter representing the active form of the drug; acyclovir triphosphate interferes with herpes simplex virus DNA polymerase, thus blocking viral replication, and can also be incorporated into growing chains of DNA by viral DNA polymerase, thereby terminating further growth of the DNA chain.

Uses
Ointment
1 Management of initial episodes of herpes genitalis and limited, non-life-threatening mucocutaneous

herpes simplex infections in immunocompromised patients

Intravenous infusion
1   Treatment of initial and recurrent mucosal and cutaneous herpes simplex (HSV-1 and HSV-2) infections in immunocompromised patients
2   Treatment of *severe* initial episodes of herpes genitalis in patients who are *not* immunocompromised

Dosage
Ointment
Apply sufficient quantity to cover all lesions every 3 hours six times a day for 7 days

Intravenous infusion
Adults: 5 mg/kg infused at a constant rate over 1 hour every 8 hours for 5 days to 7 days
Children (under 12 yr): 250 mg/M² infused at a constant rate over 1 hour every 8 hours for 5 days to 7 days

Fate
IV infusion—widely distributed into most body tissues; concentrations in cerebrospinal fluid are approximately one half those in plasma; protein binding is low (10%–30%); plasma half-life is 2 hours to 3 hours in patients with normal kidney function; excreted primarily unchanged by the kidney (60%–90%), with approximately 15% of dose excreted as a metabolite
Systemic absorption after topical application is minimal.

Common Side-Effects
IV—inflammation at injection site following extravasation, elevated serum creatinine
Topical—burning or stinging at application site, pruritus

Significant Adverse Reactions
IV—rash, urticaria, sweating, hypotension, headache, nausea, hematuria, thrombocytosis, nervousness, and renal damage; *rarely,* lethargy, confusion, tremors, agitation, seizures, hallucinations, and coma
Topical—rash, vulvitis

Interactions
1   Probenecid increases the half-life of acyclovir and reduces the rate of urinary elimination.

▶ NURSING ALERTS
▷ 1   Administer only by *slow* IV infusion, because bolus injection can result in precipitation of acyclovir crystals in the renal tubules. Ensure adequate hydration during infusion and establish sufficient urine flow to minimize danger of precipitation.
▷ 2   Be alert for development of encephalopathic changes (see Significant Adverse Reactions). Use with caution in patients with underlying neurologic abnormalities.
▷ 3   Administer with caution to patients with renal, hepatic or electrolyte abnormalities, hypoxia, dehydration, and to pregnant or nursing women.

▷ 4   Observe infusion sites closely for signs of phlebitis or inflammation.

▶ NURSING CONSIDERATIONS
▷ 1   Initiate therapy as soon as possible following onset of symptoms.
▷ 2   Dissolve powder in 10 ml Sterile Water for Injection, yielding a final concentration of 50 mg/ml, and shake well. Remove the desired dose and add it to appropriate infusion solution. Infusion concentrations of 7 mg/ml or less are recommended, because higher concentrations are more likely to cause inflammation and phlebitis upon extravasation.
▷ 3   Use prepared solution (50 mg/ml) within 12 hours. Once diluted, each dose should be used within 24 hours.
▷ 4   Refer to enclosed package information for dosage modifications based on creatinine clearance in patients with renal impairment.
▷ 5   Recognize that the ointment is for cutaneous use only; do not use in the eye.
▷ 6   Do not exceed the recommended dose, frequency of application, or length of treatment; acyclovir ointment has not been demonstrated to prevent transmission of infection or prevent recurrent infections.
▷ 7   Use a finger cot or rubber glove when applying ointment.

▶ amantadine
Symmetrel

An orally effective drug that exhibits antiviral activity against influenza A viruses as well as an antiparkinsonian action, amantadine is used for the *prevention* of Asian (A) type viral infections in high-risk patients and as adjunctive therapy in Parkinson's disease and in drug-induced extrapyramidal reactions. There is some evidence that the drug might also be effective in *relieving* viral symptoms (fever, chills) if taken early in the course of infection. The antiviral activity of amantadine appears to be specific for A virus strains, and there is no evidence that the drug is effective for either prophylaxis or treatment of other viral diseases. The antiparkinsonian actions of the drug are discussed in detail in Chapter 26, and only its antiviral activity is considered here.

Mechanism
Inhibits viral replication at an early stage, probably by preventing the uncoating of viral nucleic acid and blocking the release of nucleic acids into host cells; increases release of dopamine from nerve endings in the CNS (see Chap. 26)

Uses
1   Prevention and symptomatic management of Asian (A) influenza infections, especially in high-risk patients or in cases in which contact with the virus is likely, for example, in hospital wards, infected households
2   Symptomatic treatment of parkinsonism or drug-in-

duced extrapyramidal reactions, usually in combination with levodopa (see Chap. 26)

Dosage

Influenza
Adults: 200 mg/day, in a single dose or two divided doses
Children (1 yr–9 yr): 4.4 mg/kg to 8.8 mg/kg/day (maximum 150 mg/day) in two or three equally divided doses
Children (9 yr–12 yr): 100 mg twice a day

Parkinson's Disease
100 mg twice a day; may increase to 400 mg/day if necessary

Fate

Readily absorbed orally; peak serum levels occur in 2 hours to 4 hours but 48 hours is required for drug to reach maximal tissue concentrations; excreted largely unchanged in the urine, 50% of a dose within 20 hours to 24 hours

Common Side-Effects

Dizziness, lightheadedness, anxiety, irritability, confusion, mild depression, orthostatic hypotension, urinary hesitancy, and constipation

Significant Adverse Reactions

Cardiovascular—congestive heart failure
Neurologic—fatigue, weakness, headache, nervousness, insomnia, tremors, convulsions, slurred speech, psychotic disturbances, blurred vision, oculogyric crisis, hallucinations
GI—nausea, vomiting, anorexia, dry mouth
Others—leukopenia, neutropenia, livedo reticularis (skin mottling), skin rash, eczematoid dermatitis, peripheral edema

Contraindications

Pregnant or nursing women

Interactions

1 Amantadine may exhibit additive atropine-like effects with anticholinergic drugs, tricyclic antidepressants, or antihistamines.
2 Excessive CNS stimulation may occur with combined use of amantadine and other CNS stimulants (*e.g.*, amphetamines, methylphenidate).

▶ NURSING ALERTS

(see also Chap. 26)
▷ 1 Use with caution in patients with epilepsy or a history of convulsive disorders, congestive heart failure, peripheral edema, renal impairment, orthostatic hypotension, liver disease, history of skin rash or other allergic dermatoses, or psychoses, and in elderly or debilitated patients.
▷ 2 Caution patients against engaging in hazardous activities, because dizziness, confusion, and blurred vision can occur, especially in the early stages of therapy.

▶ NURSING CONSIDERATIONS

(see also Chap. 26)
▷ 1 Be aware that amantadine does *not* suppress antibody response, and can therefore be used in conjunction with influenza A virus vaccine until antibody response develops. Administer for 2 weeks to 3 weeks after vaccine has been given. When given alone for prophylaxis, drug should be continued for the duration of the epidemic, usually 6 weeks to 8 weeks.
▷ 2 Advise patients to make positional changes slowly to minimize the danger of orthostatic hypotension.
▷ 3 Avoid administering drug too close to bedtime, because insomnia may occur.
▷ 4 Inform patients that should livedo reticularis (mottling of skin, usually of lower extremities) occur, it will subside upon discontinuation of the drug or lowering of the dose.

▶ idoxuridine

Herplex, Stoxil

Idoxuridine (IDU) is a structural analog of thymidine, an essential intermediate in DNA synthesis. Because it is rapidly inactivated by enzymes, IDU is used only locally in the eye for the treatment of herpes simplex keratitis, a viral disease that affects the cornea.

Mechanism

Incorporated into viral DNA, producing a faulty molecule incapable of reproduction, thus blocking herpes viral cell replication

Uses

1 Treatment of herpes simplex (herpetic) keratitis

Dosage

Ophthalmic solution: one drop in infected eye every hour during the day and every 2 hours at night; reduce to every 2 hours during the day and every 4 hours at night when improvement is noted; continue for 5 days to 7 days after healing is complete
Ophthalmic ointment: instill into lower conjunctival sac five times a day, every 4 hours; continue for 5 days to 7 days after healing is complete

Fate

Short acting and quickly inactivated by nucleotidases

Common Side-Effects

Periorbital burning, irritation, or lacrimation

Significant Adverse Reactions

Pain, inflammation, pruritus, and edema of eyes and eyelids; photophobia; local allergic reactions; corneal clouding, vascularization or stippling; prolonged use can result in follicular conjunctivitis, blepharitis, conjunctival hyperemia, and corneal epithelial staining.

Interaction

1 Concurrent use of boric acid with IDU may increase local irritation.

▶ **NURSING ALERTS**

▷ 1 Be aware that IDU has been demonstrated to be both mutagenic and carcinogenic in laboratory animals. The implication of this activity to humans remains to be established. Squamous cell carcinoma has been reported at the site of topical application.

▷ 2 Use cautiously in pregnant or lactating women.

▶ **NURSING CONSIDERATIONS**

▷ 1 Stress the importance of continuing therapy for at least 5 days to 7 days after healing is complete to prevent recurrence of infection, which is common with short courses of therapy.

▷ 2 Avoid contaminating dropper tip during instillation of drug. Apply light pressure on lacrimal sac for 1 minute after instillation.

▷ 3 Notify physician if improvement is not noted within 7 days to 8 days, in epithelial infections, or if pain, itching, or swelling occurs, because drug should be discontinued.

▷ 4 Store ophthalmic solution in refrigerator, except for Herplex Liquifilm, which requires no refrigeration.

▷ 5 Note that improvement of keratitic lesions may be enhanced by concomitant use of topical corticosteroids. Withdraw steroid several days before discontinuing idoxuridine. Do *not* use corticosteroids without IDU.

▶ **trifluridine**

Viroptic

A halogenated pyrimidine, trifluridine exhibits *in vivo* antiviral activity against herpes simplex virus types 1 and 2 and vaccinia virus. The drug is also active *in vitro* against some strains of adenovirus. Its clinical application is presently restricted to ophthalmic infections due to sensitive organisms, and the drug is often effective in patients unresponsive to IDU and vidarabine.

Mechanism

Not established; interferes with DNA synthesis in cultured mammalian cells

Uses

1 Treatment of primary keratoconjunctivitis and recurrent epithelial keratitis due to herpes simplex viruses 1 and 2

2 Treatment of epithelial keratitis in patients intolerant of or unresponsive to IDU or vidarabine

3 Treatment of ophthalmic infections due to vaccinia virus or adenovirus (clinical efficacy not definitely established)

4 Prophylaxis of herpes simplex virus keratoconjunctivitis and epithelial keratitis (efficacy not definitely established)

Dosage

One drop onto cornea every 2 hours *while awake* (maximum 9 drops/day) until corneal ulcer has completely re-epithelialized, then one drop every 4 hours (maximum 5 drops/day) for an additional 7 days

Fate

Intra-ocular penetration following topical application is good; systemic absorption is negligible; half-life is approximately 15 minutes.

Common Side-Effects

Mild, transient burning or stinging

Significant Adverse Reactions

Palpebral edema, superficial punctate keratopathy, epithelial keratopathy, stromal edema, irritation, hypersensitivity reactions, hyperemia, and increased intra-ocular pressure

▶ **NURSING ALERTS**

▷ 1 Do not use unless a clinical diagnosis of herpetic keratitis has been established; drug is not effective against bacterial, fungal, or chlamydial infections. Do not exceed recommended dosage and frequency of administration.

▷ 2 Use cautiously in patients with glaucoma and in pregnant or nursing women.

▶ **NURSING CONSIDERATIONS**

▷ 1 Consider alternative forms of therapy if clinical improvement has not occurred within 7 days or if *complete* re-epithelialization is not evident within 14 days. To avoid ocular toxicity, do not use for longer than 21 days under any circumstances.

▷ 2 Instruct patients in the proper method of administration and compression of lacrimal sac for 1 minute after instillation.

▷ 3 Avoid contaminating the dropper tip.

▷ 4 Store under refrigeration, because elevated temperatures accelerate degradation of the drug.

▷ 5 Inform patients that a stinging sensation may occur upon instillation, but that this is a transient effect.

▶ **vidarabine**

Vira-A

Vidarabine is a pyrimidine derivative that possesses antiviral activity against herpes simplex virus types 1 and 2. It may be used systemically in the treatment of herpes simplex virus encephalitis, or ophthalmically for keratoconjunctivitis and epithelial keratitis. Prompt diagnosis of herpes encephalitis, a frequent complication of cancer immunosuppressive therapy, and treatment by vidarabine can reduce mortality from 70% to approximately 25%. However, patients already in a comatose state at the time therapy is initiated do not appear to benefit from the drug. When applied locally in the eye, vidarabine is often effective in patients resistant to or intolerant of idoxuridine.

Mechanism

Converted into nucleotides, which can inhibit viral DNA synthesis, presumably by interfering with viral DNA polymerase; mammalian cell DNA synthesis is also inhibited, but to a lesser extent; metabolized to hypoxanthine arabinoside, which may act synergistically with the parent compound against DNA viruses

Uses

1 Treatment of herpes simplex virus encephalitis (IV only)
2 Treatment of superficial and recurrent epithelial keratitis and acute keratoconjunctivitis due to herpes simplex virus types 1 and 2 (ophthalmic only)

Dosage

IV: 15 mg/kg/day for 10 days, infused slowly over a 12-hour to 24-hour period

Ophthalmic: one half inch of ophthalmic ointment into lower conjunctival sac five times a day at 3-hour intervals until re-epithelialization has occured, then twice a day for an additional 7 days

Fate

IV infusion—rapidly deaminated to hypoxanthine arabinoside, the principal metabolite, which is quickly distributed in the body but possesses only one-tenth the *in vitro* antiviral activity of vidarabine; half-life of vidarabine is 1 hour, and hypoxanthine arabinoside is 3.5 hours; excreted primarily by the kidneys; if cornea is normal, only trace amounts of drug or metabolite are detectable in the aqueous humor. Systemic absorption following ocular administration is negligible.

Common Side-Effects

Temporary visual haze with ophthalmic application

Significant Adverse Reactions

IV—anorexia, nausea, vomiting, diarrhea, tremor, dizziness, ataxia, confusion, hallucinations, psychosis, decreased hemoglobin and hematocrit values, reduced white blood cell count and platelet count, weight loss, malaise, rash, pruritus, pain at injection site, and elevated total bilirubin and SGOT

Ophthalmic—irritation, ocular pain, photophobia, lacrimation, burning, superficial punctate keratitis, punctal occlusion, foreign body sensation, hypersensitivity reactions

▶ NURSING ALERTS

▷ 1 Do not use to treat trivial infections and do not exceed recommended dose and duration of therapy, because vidarabine has exhibited a mutagenic and carcinogenic potential in laboratory animals, although the significance of these findings in humans remains to be assessed.

▷ 2 Notify physician if improvement is not observed within 7 days or if condition worsens during therapy.

▷ 3 Use IV infusion very cautiously during pregnancy and lactation, and in patients with impaired renal or liver function or in CNS infections other than herpes encephalitis.

▷ 4 Avoid rapid or bolus IV injections, and do not administer SC or IM, because drug is poorly soluble and erratically absorbed.

▷ 5 Confirm diagnosis of herpes simplex virus before initiating therapy, because drug is ineffective against infections due to other viral species, for example, varicella–zoster, vaccinia, adenovirus, cytomegalovirus, as well as bacterial and fungal infections.

▶ NURSING CONSIDERATIONS

▷ 1 Perform periodic hematologic tests during systemic therapy, because vidarabine can alter blood picture (*e.g.,* hemoglobin, hematocrit, white blood cells, platelets). Report any changes immediately.

▷ 2 Before infusing, dilute drug in an appropriate IV solution. Solubility in IV infusion fluids is limited (1 mg/2.22 ml IV fluid), therefore 1 liter will solubilize about 450 mg vidarabine.

▷ 3 Transfer desired dose of drug (available as suspended injection, 200 mg/ml) into appropriate prewarmed (35°C–40°C) IV infusion fluid, and thoroughly agitate until completely clear. Dilution should be performed just prior to administration. Perform final filtration with an in-line membrane filter if necessary (0.45μ or smaller). Do not refrigerate final dilution and use within 48 hours.

▷ 4 Note that any IV solution is suitable for dilution *except* biological or colloidal fluids, such as protein solutions or blood products.

▷ 5 Advise patients that ophthalmic application may produce photophobia or a temporary clouding of vision. Urge caution in operating machinery or performing other hazardous tasks.

▷ 6 Explain technique to be followed in applying ophthalmic ointment (*i.e.,* small ribbon into lower conjunctival sac) and avoid contaminating dropper tip.

▷ 7 Stress importance of adhering to prescribed ophthalmic dosage and frequency of administration. If complete re-epithelialization has not occurred within 21 days, consider alternative treatment.

Summary. Antiviral Agents

Drug	Preparations	Usual Dosage Range
Acyclovir (Zovirax)	Powder for injection—500 mg/vial Topical ointment—5%	IV infusion: Adults—5 mg/kg infused over 1 hour every 8 hours for 5 to 7 days

(continued)

Summary. Antiviral Agents *(continued)*

Drug	Preparations	Usual Dosage Range
		Children (under 12 yr)—250 mg/M^2 infused over 1 hour every 8 hours for 5 to 7 days
		Ointment:
		Apply sufficient quantity to cover all lesions every 3 hours 6 times a day for 7 days
Amantadine (Symmetrel)	Capsules—100 mg Syrup—50 mg/5 ml	Adults—200 mg/day, either as a single dose or 2 equally divided doses
		Children (1 yr–9 yr)—4.4 mg/kg to 8.8 mg/kg/day in 2 to 3 divided doses (maximum 150 mg/day)
		Children (9 yr–12 yr)—100 mg twice a day
Idoxuridine (Herplex, Stoxil)	Ophthalmic solution—0.1% Ophthalmic ointment—0.05%	Solution:
		1 drop every hour during the day and every 2 hours at night; reduce to every 2 hours during the day and every 4 hours at night when improvement is noted
		Ointment:
		Instill into lower conjunctival sac 5 times a day, every 4 hours
Trifluridine (Viroptic)	Ophthalmic solution—1%	1 drop every 2 hours while awake until corneal ulcer has healed, then 1 drop every 4 hours for an additional 7 days
Vidarabine (Vira-A)	Injection—200 mg/ml Ophthalmic ointment—3%	IV:
		15 mg/kg/day for 10 days, infused over 12 hours to 24 hours
		Ophthalmic:
		½ inch of ointment into lower conjunctival sac 5 times a day at 3-hour intervals until re-epithelialization occurs, then twice a day for an additional 7 days

Cancer is a disease occurring in all human and animal populations that affects tissues composed of dividing cells. The exact etiology of most cancers is still unknown; however, infections as well as environmental (chemicals, fiber particles, radiation) and genetic factors are all capable of inducing a normal cell to become neoplastic.

Cancer may be characterized by the following:

1 Excessive cell growth due to permanent impairment of normal growth-controlling mechanisms.
2 Cells and tissues are undifferentiated.
3 Cells exhibit invasiveness and have the ability to metastasize (*i.e.,* establish themselves at sites distant from their original location).
4 Cells have acquired heredity (*i.e.,* properties of the original cancerous cells).
5 Cells demonstrate increased synthesis of macromolecules from nucleosides and amino acids.

Treatment of cancer may involve surgery, radiation, immunotherapy, or chemotherapy. Until recently, chemotherapy with antineoplastic drugs was used primarily as an adjunct to surgery or radiation therapy largely in an attempt to eradicate any remaining metastatic tumor cell foci. At present, however, chemotherapy is an accepted and vital part of most cancer regimens. Some neoplastic diseases are, in fact, treated primarily with chemotherapy, and many patients undergoing cancer chemotherapy have achieved a significantly prolonged survival time and, in some cases, complete remission (see Table 74-1).

The antineoplastic agents may be classified in a variety of ways. The broadest classification and the one used for this discussion is based on mechanism of action and source of the drug. Thus, the antineoplastic drugs include the following:

I. Alkylating agents
II. Antimetabolites
III. Natural products
IV. Hormones
V. Miscellaneous agents

Antineoplastic agents may also be classified on the basis of their differential effects on normal and malignant cell metabolism. To understand this classification it is important to review the phases of cell division:

G_1—*post*mitotic phase; various enzymes synthesized during this phase
S—period of DNA synthesis for chromosomes
G_2—*pre*mitotic phase; specialized protein and RNA synthesis and formation of mitotic spindle
M—mitosis
G_0—temporarily nondividing cells, cell differentiation, or cell death

Some antineoplastic agents inhibit cells during a specific phase of the above cycle and are referred to as cell-cycle specific (CCS). The therapeutic response to cell-cycle specific agents is usually schedule dependent; that is, therapeutic blood levels must be maintained for a sufficient period of time to allow large numbers of cells to enter the S phase, thus producing a larger cell kill. Other antineoplastic agents are cytotoxic during any phase of the cell cycle and are referred to as cell-cycle nonspecific (CCNS). Cell-cycle nonspecific agents are dose-dependent and are usually more

Antineoplastic Agents

74

Table 74-1. Neoplastic Diseases Showing a Good Response to Chemotherapy

Disease	Antineoplastic Agents*
Acute lymphocytic leukemia (pediatric)	Induction—vincristine + prednisone ± asparaginase or doxorubicin
	Maintenance—methotrexate + 6-mercaptopurine
Acute myelogenous leukemia (adult)	Doxorubicin or daunorubicin + cytarabine
	or cytarabine + thioguanine
	or cytarabine + vincristine + prednisone
Breast cancer	Estrogens and tamoxifen
	Cyclophosphamide + methotrexate + fluorouracil ± prednisone
	or cyclophosphamide + doxorubicin ± fluorouracil
Burkitt's lymphoma	Cyclophosphamide
	or cyclophosphamide + methotrexate + vincristine
Choriocarcinoma	Methotrexate ± dactinomycin
Diffuse histiocytic lymphoma	CHOP (cyclophosphamide, doxorubicin, vincristine, prednisone)
	or BACOP (bleomycin, doxorubicin, cyclophosphamide, vincristine, prednisone)
	or COMA (cyclophosphamide, vincristine, methotrexate, cytarabine)
	or COPP (cyclophosphamide, vincristine, procarbazine, prednisone)
Ewing's sarcoma	Cyclophosphamide + doxorubicin + vincristine
Hodgkin's disease	MOPP (mechlorethamine, vincristine, procarbazine, prednisone)
	or ABVD (doxorubicin, bleomycin, vinblastine, dacarbazine)
Nodular lymphomas	CVP (cyclophosphamide, vincristine, prednisone)
Retinoblastoma	Cyclophosphamide
Rhabdomyosarcoma	VAC (vincristine, dactinomycin, cyclophosphamide) ± doxorubicin
Testicular cancer	Vinblastine + bleomycin + cisplatin
Wilms' tumor	Dactinomycin + vincristine

* (±) indicates a possibly beneficial addition.

effective if given in large intermittent doses. The various cell-cycle specific and cell-cycle nonspecific agents are listed in Tablet 74-2.

In order to more fully understand the complex pharmacology of the antineoplastic agents, it is necessary to review the general principles of cancer chemotherapy.

1 The goal of cancer therapy is to destroy or remove all neoplastic cells with minimal effect upon normal host cells.

2 The maximum chance for cure exists when the tumor cell burden is at a minimum and tumors have a high growth fraction (*i.e.,* a high proportion of tumor cells are actively dividing).

3 A given dose of antineoplastic agent kills a constant *percentage* of cells, not a constant *number*.

4 Cell-cycle specific agents are more effective than cell-

cycle nonspecific agents in tumors with a large bulky mass.

5 Before a change to another agent, treatment with an antineoplastic agent should continue until either the desired response is obtained or toxicity occurs.

6 Toxicity is often the limiting factor in the usefulness of an antineoplastic agent and the risk of toxicity is increased if the patient has received prior chemotherapy or radiation treatment. However, the highly fatal nature of the disease makes the risk of serious toxicity relatively acceptable in most instances.

7 Malignant cells may exhibit resistance to some antineoplastic agents, thus limiting their usefulness. Resistance may be natural or acquired, that is, either the tumor is resistant from the start of therapy (natural), or resistance occurs after therapy has begun and results from drug-induced adaptation or mutation of malignant cells (acquired).

8 Drug scheduling is very important. High-dose intermittent therapy is usually more effective, less toxic, and less immunosuppressive than low-dose, continuous therapy. Toxicity may be reduced and cell resistance delayed by administering combinations of drugs in cycles or sequence (see discussion of combination chemotherapy at the end of the chapter).

9 Patient factors such as age, sex, physical condition, prior treatment, and altered renal or hepatic function can influence the outcome of chemotherapy.

10 When dosage of antineoplastic agents is based on weight, children tolerate relatively larger doses of drugs than do older patients. Dosage may be more accurately calculated in adults and children using body surface area; mg/kg doses may be conveniently converted to mg/m² doses by multiplying by 40.

Table 74-2. Cell-Cycle Specific and Cell-Cycle Nonspecific Agents

Cell-Cycle Specific	Cell-Cycle Non-specific
1. *Antimetabolites*	1. *Alkylating agents*
Cytarabine	Busulfan
Mercaptopurine	Carmustine
Methotrexate	Chlorambucil
Thioguanine	Cisplatin
	Cyclophosphamide
	Dacarbazine
	Lomustine
	Mechlorethamine
	Melphalan
	Pipobroman
	Streptozocin
	Triethylenethiophosphoramide
2. *Natural products*	2. *Natural products*
Bleomycin	Dactinomycin
Etoposide	Daunorubicin
Vinblastine	Doxorubicin
Vincristine	
3. *Miscellaneous*	3. *Antimetabolites*
Hydroxyurea	Floxuridine
	Fluorouracil
	4. *Miscellaneous*
	Procarbazine

Although a variety of drugs are employed in cancer chemotherapy, there are a number of nursing alerts and nursing considerations common to all antineoplastic drugs, and these are outlined below. Specific alerts and considerations pertaining to individual drugs are given with the respective discussions of each group.

▶ **NURSING ALERTS—ANTINEOPLASTIC DRUGS**

▷ 1 Be alert for signs of developing myelosuppression (unusual bleeding or bruising, fever, sore throat, mucosal ulceration, weakness), and inform physician immediately.

▷ 2 Advise patients to report possible signs of pulmonary fibrosis (fever, cough, shortness of breath).

▷ 3 Observe patient for swelling of feet or lower legs, joint pain, or stomach pain, because these may be indicative of hyperuricemia, which can lead to uric acid nephropathy.

▷ 4 Note symptoms of developing hepatic dysfunction (jaundice, yellowing of eyes, hepatomegaly, anorexia, tenderness in the right hypochondrium, clay-colored stools, dark urine), and advise physician.

▷ 5 Use cautiously in the presence of renal or hepatic dysfunction and in pregnant or lactating women.

▷ 6 Be alert for signs of CNS toxicity (dizziness, headache, convulsions, confusion, tiredness, slurred speech, paresthesias).

▷ 7 Advise patients to report loss of taste or tingling in face, fingers, or toes, symptoms of possible peripheral neuropathy; notify physician immediately.

▷ 8 Immediately stop IV administration of any medication at the first sign of swelling, redness, pain, or burning of the injection site, indications of extravasation or hypersensitivity.

▷ 9 Observe patient carefully during daily skin care for any signs of rash or dermatitis, which may signal hypersensitivity to a particular drug.

▶ **NURSING CONSIDERATIONS— ANTINEOPLASTIC DRUGS**

▷ 1 Perform baseline and periodic blood, liver, and renal studies in order to assess the effectiveness and toxicity of therapy. The frequency at which the studies are done varies with the agent or agents used and the clinical state of the patient.

▷ 2 Inform both male and female patients of the possibility of birth defects or sterility; these can occur both while taking the drug as well as following discontinuation of the medication.

▷ 3 Be aware that the concurrent use of other chemotherapeutic agents or radiation therapy may potentiate myelosuppression.

▷ 4 Take patient's temperature frequently, especially when granulocyte count is very low. Patients are very susceptible to infection. Avoid rectal temperatures because thermometer may be irritating to rectal mucosa.

▷ 5 Place patients with bone marrow suppression in reverse isolation and observe carefully for signs of infection.

▷ 6 Notify physician immediately if a patient vomits after receiving an oral antineoplastic agent. The medication may not have been absorbed and dosage adjustment may be necessary. Use of an antiemetic agent 30 minutes to 60 minutes before administration of an antineoplastic agent may minimize the nausea and vomiting caused by some agents.

▷ 7 Note that bland food or antacids given before an oral agent is taken may decrease the nausea and vomiting resulting from local irritation. Recognize, however, that the absorption of some agents may be impaired by the presence of food in the stomach.

▷ 8 Monitor fluid intake and output, and force fluids up to 2 liters to 3 liters/day to ensure adequate urine output for drug excretion, and to prevent dehydration caused by excessive vomiting.

▷ 9 Maintain adequate hydration to minimize effects of hyperuricemia and uric acid nephropathy.

▷ 10 Calculate dosages of medications based on the patient's *lean* body weight, particularly in obese patients and those with edema or ascites.

▷ 11 Avoid giving IM injections when platelet count is low.

▷ 12 Be prepared to treat hypersensitivity reactions with antihistamines, steroids, and epinephrine, and oxygen as necessary.

▷ 13 Recognize that good mouth care is essential to minimize or treat stomatitis.
   a. Use a soft-bristled toothbrush.
   b. To reduce discomfort, rinse mouth frequently with any of the following:
      (1) Hydrogen peroxide and water (1:1)
      (2) Benadryl Elixir and Kaopectate (1:1)
      (3) Benadryl 0.5% and Dyclone 0.5% aqueous solution
      (4) Lidocaine viscous and water (1:1)
      (5) Xero-Lube solution
   c. Avoid tart, acid, spicy, hot, and rough-textured foods. Bland and soft foods are usually better tolerated.
   d. Clotrimazole troches, nystatin suspension, nystatin vaginal tablets dissolved as a lozenge, or nystatin "pops" can be used to treat fungal overgrowth of the mouth.

▷ 14 Inform patients that if alopecia occurs, it is usually transient; encourage the use of wigs, scarves, and hats until normal regrowth occurs, commonly 4 weeks to 8 weeks after therapy ends. Transient regrowth may occur during therapy but hair is often of a different texture and color and will be lost as therapy continues. Hair loss may be minimized by the following:
   a. Applying a scalp tourniquet before drug administration and retaining for at least 5 minutes after termination of therapy
   b. Applying an ice compress to the scalp 15 minutes before and for 30 minutes after administration of the agent
   Note: The above procedures are useful only when the medication is given by IV push and widely metastatic tumors (*i.e.,* leukemia) are *not* being treated.

▷ 15 Take care to avoid extravasation during the administration of any antineoplastic agent. Certain agents such as carmustine, dacarbazine, dactinomycin, daunorubicin, doxorubicin, etoposide, mechlorethamine, mithramycin, mitomycin, streptozocin, vinblastine, and vincristine cause thrombophlebitis and tissue necrosis.

Guidelines to Reduce the Risk of Extravasation

a. Choose a vein that travels a straight course long enough to accept the length of the needle. Veins of the dorsum of the hand, ventral surface of the forearm, or anticubital fossa are preferred.

b. Avoid bruised, sclerosed, inflamed veins and veins traveling through hematomas or ecchymotic areas.

c. Avoid using an arm where axillary node dissection has been performed or an arm affected by the superior vena cava syndrome.

d. Alternate sites of drug administration.

e. Prepare the skin with alcohol or povidone solution and dry completely with a sterile sponge.

f. A 21-, 23-, or 25-gauge butterfly needle is preferred because it may be secured easily, and causes minimal irritation. The small needle is easy to position and the tubing allows one to note the presence of blood return.

g. When securing the butterfly catheter, or tubing, allow for visualization of the injection site, the proximal portion of the butterfly tubing, and the surrounding area, including most of the arm. Observe for local infiltration and distant vein irritation.

h. Always check the position and flow of the needle by administering 5 ml to 10 ml normal saline before injecting an antineoplastic agent.

i. Administer the drug by slow steady IV push or by IV infusion through the injection port of the tubing.

j. Flush the tubing and vein with 5 ml to 10 ml normal saline after administration of the agent.

k. Instruct the patient to immediately report any discomfort or other unusual sensation.

l. If there is any doubt about the patency of the vein, stop the injection and administer the drug via another site.

Guidelines for the Treatment of Extravasation

a. Stop the infusion and leave needle in place.

b. Aspirate as much of the drug as possible.

c. Administer specific antidote if available.

d. Through the *same* needle, administer 100 mg to 200 mg hydrocortisone or 4 mg dexamethasone.

e. Inject 1% to 2% lidocaine into the area to decrease pain (optional).

f. Apply ice packs for 24 hours to 36 hours.

g. Apply warm, moist compresses after the first 24 hours to 36 hours and check site frequently.

h. Elevate the injection site above the level of the heart.

i. Tissue necrosis may be treated by surgical excision of the ulcer and covering with a xenograft (usually pigskin) for 48 hours to 72 hours. The xenograft is then removed and replaced by a split-thickness skin graft and the extremity immobilized for 5 days to 7 days.

▷ 16 Advise patient that drug effects may take several weeks to become manifest. Stress adherence to the prescribed regimen and urge avoidance of all other nonprescribed drugs (including over-the-counter medications).

▷ 17 Provide necessary emotional supportive care during drug therapy. Encourage physical and mental activities on a regular basis. Observe carefully for the development of side-effects and advise physician, because dosage adjustment can often reduce the incidence and severity of untoward reactions.

▷ 18 Tailor dose to patient needs wherever possible, based on clinical response and development of adverse reactions, for example, myelosuppression.

▷ 19 Inform the patient to notify the physician if a dose of medication is missed. Do not double the next dose; instead resume the regular dosing schedule.

I Alkylating Agents

Busulfan	Mechlorethamine
Carmustine	Melphalan
Chlorambucil	Pipobroman
Cisplatin	Streptozocin
Cyclophosphamide	Thiethylenethiophosphoramide
Dacarbazine	Uracil mustard
Lomustine	

The alkylating agents were developed during the 1940s as a result of research on chemical warfare agents, notably the mustard gases. Of these compounds, the nitrogen mustards were found to have a marked cytotoxic action on lymphoid tissue, and clinical research was then initiated that led to development of chemically related derivatives.

The alkylating agents used in chemotherapy may be divided into six different chemical groups as follows:

1 *Nitrogen mustards*—chlorambucil, cyclophosphamide, mechlorethamine, melphalan, uracil mustard

2 *Ethylenimines*—thiotepa

3 *Alkyl sulfonates*—busulfan

4 *Triazenes*—dacarbazine

5 *Nitrosoureas*—carmustine, lomustine, streptozocin

6 *Miscellaneous alkylator-like agents*—cisplatin, pipobroman

The alkylating agents are discussed as a group, then individual drugs are listed in Table 74-3.

Mechanism

Alkylating agents are polyfunctional compounds that produce highly reactive carbonium ions that form covalent linkages with nucleophilic centers such as amino, carboxyl, hydroxyl, imidazole, phosphate, and sulfhydryl groups. The most important site of alkylation is the number 7 nitrogen in the purine base guanine. This may cause cross-linking of DNA strands and miscoding of the genetic message, resulting in abnormal base pairing. Destruction of the guanine ring

(Text continues on p. 679.)

Table 74-3. Alkylating Agents

Drug	Preparations	Usual Dosage Range	Uses	Remarks
Busulfan (Myleran)	Tablets—2 mg	Initially—4 mg to 12 mg/day Maintenance—2 mg once or twice a week to 1 mg to 4 mg/day Children—induction: 0.06 mg/kg to 0.12 mg/kg/day or 1.8 mg to 4.6 mg/m²/day	Chronic myelogenous leukemia (DOC) Polycythemia vera	May increase uric acid levels in blood and urine; pulmonary fibrosis usually occurs with long-term therapy; onset after 8 months to 10 years (average 4 yr) Treatment is usually unsatisfactory and death usually occurs within 6 months of diagnosis
Carmustine (BiCNU, BCNU)	Injection—100 mg/vial	75 mg to 100 mg/m² by IV infusion over 1 hour to 2 hours for 2 consecutive days or 200 mg/m² in a single dose no more frequently than every 6 weeks to 8 weeks A suggested guide for subsequent dosage adjustment is the following: *Nadir After Prior Dose* Leukocytes / Platelets / *% of Prior Dose to Be Given* Above 4000 / Above 100,000 / 100% 3000–3999 / 75,000–99,999 / 100% 2000–2999 / 25,000–74,999 / 70% Below 2000 / Below 25,000 / 50%	Brain tumors (DOC) Multiple myeloma (in combination with prednisone) Hodgkin's disease (in combination with other approved drugs in patients who relapse while on primary therapy or fail to respond to the primary therapy) Non-Hodgkin's lymphomas (in combination with other drugs; see above) May also be useful in Burkitt's tumor, Ewing's sarcoma, malignant melanoma, mycosis fungoides	Unopened vials of dry powder must be stored under refrigeration; oily film on bottom of the vial is sign of decomposition, and vial should be discarded. Preparation of solution: dissolve contents of vial with 3 ml absolute alcohol diluent and then add 27 ml of Sterile Water for Injection. The resulting solution contains 3.3 mg/ml. Further dilution in 500 ml of Dextrose 5% or Sodium Chloride 0.9% results in a solution stable for 48 hours when refrigerated and protected from light. Contact with skin may cause transient hyperpigmentation; may increase bilirubin, alkaline phosphatase, SGOT and BUN levels; a 0.1% to 0.4% solution in 95% alcohol applied topically 1 to 2 times/day for 2 weeks has been used to treat mycosis fungoides
Chlorambucil (Leukeran)	Tablets—2 mg	Initially—0.1 mg/kg to 0.2 mg/kg/day for 3 weeks to 6 weeks (4 mg–12 mg/day for the average patient) Maintenance—2 mg to 6 mg/day, not to exceed 0.1 mg/kg/day; may be as low as 0.03 mg/kg/day Children—0.1 mg/kg to 0.2 mg/kg/day or 4.5 mg/m²/day	Chronic lymphocytic leukemia (DOC) Malignant lymphomas Hodgkin's disease Choriocarcinoma Ovarian carcinoma Breast carcinoma	Give dose 1 hour before breakfast or 2 hours after evening meal; may increase serum and urine uric acid levels
Cisplatin (Platinol)	Injection—10 mg/vial, 50 mg/vial	As a single agent: 100 mg/m² IV once every 4 weeks Testicular tumors—20 mg/m² IV for 5 days every 3 weeks for 3 courses in combination with Bleomycin—30 U IV on day 2 of each week for 12 doses + Vinblastine—0.15 mg/kg to 0.2 mg/kg IV on days 1 and 2 of each week every 3 weeks for 4 courses Maintenance for patients who respond—vinblastine 0.2 mg/kg IV every 4 weeks for 2 years Ovarian tumors—50 mg/m² IV once every 3 weeks on day 1 in combination with	Metastatic testicular tumors (DOC) Metastatic ovarian tumors (DOC) Lymphoma Squamous cell carcinoma of head and neck Advanced bladder carcinoma (DOC)	Unopened vials of dry powder must be stored under refrigeration. Preparation of solution: dissolve contents of vial in 10 ml Sterile Water for Injection. Solution is stable for 20 hours at room temperature. Do *not* refrigerate. Hydrate patient with 1 liter to 2 liters fluid infused over 8 hours to 12 hours before treatment. Dilute drug in 1 liter to 2 liters 5% Dextrose in 0.3% or 0.45% saline containing 37.5 g mannitol, and infuse over 6 hours to 8 hours. Maintain urinary output of 100 ml/hour for 24 hours after therapy to reduce danger of

(continued)

Table 74-3. Alkylating Agents (continued)

Drug	Preparations	Usual Dosage Range	Uses	Remarks
		Doxorubicin—50 mg/m² IV once every 3 weeks on day 1 A repeat dose should not be given until serum creatinine is below 1.5 mg/100 ml or BUN is below 25 mg/100 ml, platelets are over 100,000/mm³, and WBCs are over 4000/mm³ Advanced bladder carcinoma—50 mg to 70 mg/m² IV once every 3 weeks to 4 weeks; patients receiving prior radiation or chemotherapy should start at 50 mg/m² IV once every 4 weeks		nephrotoxicity. Do not use needles, IV sets, or equipment containing aluminum to administer cisplatin: a black precipitate of platinum will form. May increase BUN, serum creatinine, SGOT, and serum uric acid levels. May decrease creatinine clearance and serum calcium, magnesium, and potassium levels. High frequency hearing loss may occur in one or both ears; more common in children
Cyclophosphamide (Cytoxan, Neosar)	Tablets—25 mg, 50 mg Injection—100 mg/vial, 200 mg/vial, 500 mg/vial, 1 g/vial, 2 g/vial	**Oral:** Adult—1 mg/kg to 5 mg/kg/day Children—induction:2 mg/kg to 8 mg/kg or 60 mg to 250 mg/m² for 6 or more days Maintenance—2 mg/kg to 5 mg/kg or 50 mg to 150 mg/m² twice a week **IV:** Adult—induction: 40 mg/kg to 50 mg/kg in divided doses over 2 days to 5 days Maintenance—10 mg/kg to 15 mg/kg every 7 days to 10 days or 3 mg/kg to 5 mg/kg twice a week or 1.5 mg/kg to 3 mg/kg daily Children—induction: 2 mg/kg to 8 mg/kg or 60 mg to 250 mg/m² in divided doses for 6 or more days Maintenance—10 mg/kg to 15 mg/kg every 7 days to 10 days or 30 mg/kg every 3 weeks to 4 weeks Reduce induction dose by ⅓ to ½ in patients with bone marrow depression Hepatic impairment—bilirubin 3.1 mg% to 5.0 mg% or SGOT > 180, reduce dose by 25%; bilirubin > 5.0 mg%, omit dose Renal impairment—GFR < 10 ml/minute, decrease dose by 50%	Hodgkin's disease Non-Hodgkin's lymphomas (DOC) Follicular lymphomas Lymphocytic lymphosarcoma Reticulum cell sarcoma Lymphoblastic lymphosarcoma Burkitt's lymphoma (DOC) Multiple myeloma (DOC) Leukemias: Chronic lymphocytic leukemia Chronic granulocytic leukemia Acute myelogenous and monocytic leukemia Acute lymphoblastic leukemia Mycosis fungoides Neuroblastoma Adenocarcinoma of ovary Retinoblastoma (DOC) Carcinoma of breast or lung (DOC)	Preparation of solution: Reconstitute with Sterile Water for Injection or Bacteriostatic Water for Injection (paraben preserved only). Use 5 ml for the 100-mg vial, 10 ml for the 200-mg vial, 25 ml for the 500-mg vial, 50 ml for the 1-g vial, and 100 ml for the 2-g vial. Solution is stable for 24 hours at room temperature or 6 days refrigerated. Solution may be given IM, IV push, intraperitoneally, intrapleurally, or by IV infusion in 5% Dextrose, 5% Dextrose in 0.9% saline, or 0.9% saline. May suppress positive reactions to skin tests. May increase uric acid levels of urine and serum. May produce false-positive PAP test. Secondary malignancies have been observed, most frequently of the urinary bladder. May cause syndrome of inappropriate antidiuretic hormone secretion (SIADH); manifested as tiredness, weakness, confusion, agitation. An oral solution may be prepared by dissolving the Powder for Injection in Aromatic Elixir to a concentration of 1 mg to 5 mg/ml; refrigerate and use within 14 days; tablets contain tartrazine
Dacarbazine (DTIC-Dome)	Injection—100-mg vial, 200-mg vial	IV—2 mg/kg to 4.5 mg/kg/day for 10 days, repeated every 28 days or 250 mg/m²/day for 5 days, repeated every 21 days	Metastatic malignant melanoma (DOC) Investigational uses include: Hodgkin's disease Soft-tissue sarcomas Neuroblastoma	Preparation of solution: add 9.9 ml Sterile Water for Injection to 100 mg vial or 19.7 ml Sterile Water for Injection to 200-mg vial giving a concentration of 10 mg/ml; solution, colorless or clear yellow in color, is stable 8 hours at room temperature or 72 hours refrigerated, protected from light; a change in color to pink indicates decomposition; may be given by IV push over 1 minute or by IV infusion over 30 minutes, diluted in 250 ml 5% Dextrose in Water or 0.9% Sodium Chloride; severe pain along injected vein can occur;

Table 74-3. Alkylating Agents *(continued)*

Drug	Preparations	Usual Dosage Range	Uses	Remarks
				dilute drug, infuse slowly, and avoid extravasation; may increase alkaline phosphatase, BUN, SGOT, SGPT

Lomustine (CCNU, CeeNU)	Capsules—10 mg, 40 mg, 100 mg	Oral: Adults and children—100 mg to 130 mg/m² as a single dose, repeated every 6 weeks. A suggested guide for subsequent dosage adjustment is the following:
		
		Nadir After Prior Dose / % of Prior Dose to Be Given
		Leukocytes — Platelets — Given
		Above 4000 — Above 100,000 — 100%
		3000–3999 — 75,000–99,999 — 75%–100%
		2000–2999 — 25,000–74,999 — 50%–75%
		Below 2000 — Below 25,000 — 0%–50%
			Brain tumors (DOC)
			Hodgkin's disease
			Investigational uses include:
			  Lung and breast carcinoma
			  Malignant melanoma
			  Multiple myeloma
			  Gastrointestinal carcinoma
			  Renal cell carcinoma
				May cause transient elevation of liver function tests; available as a Dose Pack containing two 10-mg capsules, two 40-mg capsules, and two 100-mg capsules.

Mechlorethamine (Mustargen, Nitrogen Mustard)	Injection—10 mg/vial	IV—0.4 mg/kg as a single dose or in divided doses of 0.1 mg/kg to 0.2 mg/kg/day; repeat every 3 weeks to 6 weeks Intracavitary—0.4 mg/kg diluted in 50 ml to 100 ml 0.9% saline; 0.2 mg/kg may be used intrapericardially	Hodgkin's disease (DOC) Lymphosarcoma Chronic myelocytic and lymphocytic leukemia Bronchogenic carcinoma Polycythemia vera Mycosis fungoides Intracavitary injection to control malignant effusions	Do not use drug if vial contains water droplets before reconstitution Preparation of solution: reconstitute with 10 ml Sterile Water for Injection or 0.9% Sodium Chloride injection; use immediately; discard unused portion after neutralizing with aqueous solution containing equal parts of 5% sodium bicarbonate and 5% sodium thiosulfate; any equipment used for administration (gloves, tubing, glassware) should be neutralized for 45 minutes in this solution; avoid inhalation of powder or vapors. Avoid contact with skin or mucous membranes. If contact occurs, wash 15 minutes with water, followed by 2% sodium thiosulfate solution; administer IV dose by injection into tubing of running IV; change position of patient every 5 minutes to 10 minutes for 1 hour after intracavitary injection A topical solution may be prepared by dissolving 10 mg in 20 ml to 60 ml of water or sodium chloride and applied daily initially, then 2 to 3 times a week to treat mycosis fungoides or psoriasis; an ointment may be prepared (0.01%–0.04%) by dissolving drug in absolute alcohol and mixing into an anhydrous ointment base May increase uric acid levels in blood and urine
Melphalan (Alkeran, PAM, L-PAM, Phenylalanine Mustard)	Tablets—2 mg	0.15 mg/kg/day for 7 days followed by a rest period of 2 weeks to 6 weeks then 0.05 mg/kg/day maintenance *or* 0.1 mg/kg to 0.15 mg/kg/day for 2 weeks to 3 weeks or 0.25 mg/	Multiple myeloma (DOC) Malignant melanoma Breast, lung, and ovarian carcinoma Testicular seminoma	May increase uric acid levels in blood and urine; acute, nonlymphatic leukemia has developed in some patients with multiple myeloma treated with melphalan; benefit/risk

(continued)

Table 74-3. Alkylating Agents (continued)

Drug	Preparations	Usual Dosage Range	Uses	Remarks
		kg/day for 4 days followed by a rest period of 2 weeks to 4 weeks, then 2 mg to 4 mg a day maintenance *or* 0.2 mg/kg/day for 5 days followed by a rest period of 4 weeks to 5 weeks (for ovarian carcinoma) *or* 7 mg/m²/day for 5 days every 5 wk to 6 wk	Reticulum cell and osteogenic sarcoma	ratio must be determined on an individual basis
Pipobroman (Vercyte)	Tablets—10 mg, 25 mg	Polycythemia vera—1 mg/kg/day for 30 days, then increase to 1.5 mg/kg to 3 mg/kg/day if no response. Maintenance—0.1 mg/kg to 0.2 mg/kg/day when hematocrit has been reduced to 50% to 55% Chronic myelocytic leukemia—1.5 mg/kg to 2.5 mg/kg/day until leukocyte count approaches 10,000, then maintenance dose of 7 mg to 175 mg a day as required.	Polycythemia vera Chronic myelocytic leukemia	May increase uric acid levels in blood and urine; may increase serum potassium. Not recommended for children under 15 years
Streptozocin (Zanosar)	Injection—1 g/vial	IV—500 mg/m² daily for 5 consecutive days every 4 weeks to 6 weeks or 1 g/m² once a week for 2 weeks; thereafter, dosage may be increased to a maximum of 1.5 g/m² weekly for 2 weeks to 4 weeks; may be given by rapid IV injection, short infusion (10 min–15 min) or long infusion (6 hr)	Metastatic islet cell carcinoma of the pancreas (DOC) Investigational use: malignant carcinoid tumors	Dry powder must be stored under refrigeration and protected from light. Preparation of solution: reconstitute with 9.5 ml of 5% Dextrose in Water or 0.9% sodium chloride; solution is stable for 12 hours at room temperature; solution is preservative-free and should not be used for more than one dose; a change in color from pale gold to brown indicates decomposition; adequate patient hydration may reduce renal toxicity; hypophosphatemia may be first sign of renal toxicity
Triethylenethiophosphoramide (Thiotepa)	Injection—15 mg/vial	IV—0.3 mg/kg to 0.4 mg/kg at 1-week to 4-week intervals, or 0.5 mg/kg every 1 week to 4 weeks, or 0.2 mg/kg/day for 5 days repeated every 2 weeks to 4 weeks; may be given by IV push Local, intratumor—0.6 mg/kg to 0.8 mg/kg; maintenance dose 0.07 mg/kg to 0.8 mg/kg every 1 week to 4 weeks Intracavitary—0.6 mg/kg to 0.8 mg/kg diluted in 10 ml to 20 ml 0.9% saline Bladder instillation—60 mg diluted in 30 ml to 60 ml Sterile Water for Injection; patient should retain for 2 hours with frequent repositioning; repeat once weekly for 4 weeks; volume may be reduced to 30 ml if discomfort occurs	Superficial papillary carcinoma of the urinary bladder (DOC) Adenocarcinoma of the breast and ovary Intracavitary injection to control malignant effusions	Dry powder must be stored under refrigeration Preparation of solution: reconstitute with 1.5 ml Sterile Water for Injection; solution should be clear to slightly opaque; if *grossly* opaque, discard; solution is stable 5 days under refrigeration; compatible with procaine 2% and epinephrine HCl 1:1000 for local injection; dehydrate patients 8 hours to 12 hours before bladder instillation; may increase uric acid levels in blood and urine; has been used IM, although not approved by the FDA
Uracil mustard	Capsules—1 mg	1. Initially 1 mg to 2 mg/day until improvement or bone marrow depression occurs; then 1 mg/day for 3 weeks out of 4 week maintenance	Chronic lymphocytic leukemia Non-Hodgkin's lymphomas Chronic myelocytic leukemia Polycythemia vera (early stage)	May increase uric acid levels in blood and urine Total dosage of 1 mg/kg greatly increases the risk of

Table 74-3. Alkylating Agents (continued)

Drug	Preparations	Usual Dosage Range	Uses	Remarks
		2. Initially 3 mg to 5 mg/day for 7 days not to exceed 0.5 mg/kg during this period, then 1 mg/day for 3 weeks out of 4-weeks maintenance	Mycosis fungoides	irreversible bone marrow depression Capsules contain tartrazine

DOC = Drug of choice.

and DNA chain breakage ensues, inhibiting DNA replication, transcription of RNA, and normal nucleic acid function. Cross-linking of DNA strands thus appears to be the major cytotoxic effect of the alkylating agents.

Uses
See Table 74-3.

Dosage
See Table 74-3.

Fate
The oral agents busulfan, chlorambucil, cyclophosphamide, lomustine, melphalan, pipobroman, and uracil mustard generally exhibit rapid absorption, but melphalan and uracil mustard may be incompletely absorbed. All alkylating agents are widely distributed throughout the body and exhibit some protein binding. Carmustine and lomustine are rapidly transported across the blood–brain barrier. Most agents are metabolized in the liver to inactivate metabolites; however, cyclophosphamide must be metabolized in order to become active. All alkylating agents are eliminated by way of the kidney as both inactive metabolites and unchanged drug.

Common Side-Effects
Myelosuppression (leukopenia, thrombocytopenia, anemia), nausea, vomiting, and anorexia
Cisplatin—nephrotoxicity and hyperuricemia
Cyclophosphamide—gonadal suppression
Streptozocin—nephrotoxicity

Significant Adverse Reactions
(Not all reactions observed with all drugs)
GI—diarrhea, abdominal cramping, stomatitis, glossitis, colitis
Renal—hyperuricemia, uric acid nephropathy, hemorrhagic cystitis
Hypersensitivity—dermatitis, maculopapular skin eruption, urticaria, fever, alopecia, pruritus, facial edema, anaphylactic-like reaction, erythema multiforme
Neurologic—headache, confusion, tinnitus, weakness, ataxia, peripheral neuropathies, dizziness, paralysis, depression, hyperactivity, convulsions
Respiratory—pulmonary fibrosis, dyspnea, wheezing
Cardiovascular—tachycardia, hypotension, flushing, sweating
Other—hepatic dysfunction, jaundice, hepatitis, gynecomastia, impotence, myxedema, myalgia, metallic taste, melanoderma, hyperpigmentation, pain at IV injection site or along vein
Note: All alkylating agents have been shown to be teratogenic, carcinogenic (due to a direct cellular action or immunosuppression), and to cause testicular and ovarian suppression.

Contraindications
Leukopenia, thrombocytopenia or anemia caused by previous chemotherapy or radiation therapy, hepatoxicity, renal toxicity, and known hypersensitivity

Interactions
1 The toxicity of *chlorambucil* and *cyclophosphamide* may be increased when used concurrently with barbiturates, chloral hydrate, or phenytoin due to induction of liver microsomal enzymes.
2 *Cisplatin* used concurrently with aminoglycosides may increase nephrotoxicity and ototoxicity.
3 Allopurinol and chloramphenicol may increase the toxicity of *cyclophosphamide.*
4 Corticosteroids may decrease the activity of *cyclophosphamide* due to inhibition of microsomal enzymes.
5 *Cyclophosphamide* and *thiotepa* may decrease serum pseudocholinesterase and therefore enhance the effect of succinylcholine.
6 *Cyclophosphamide* used concurrently with daunorubicin or doxorubicin may increase cardiotoxicity.
7 *Dacarbazine* may potentiate the activity of allopurinol by inhibiting xanthine oxidase.
8 The metabolism of *dacarbazine* may be enhanced by phenobarbital and phenytoin due to induction of liver microsomal enzymes.
9 Most *alkylating agents* may antagonize the effects of antigout medications by increasing serum uric acid levels; dosage adjustment of the antigout medications may be necessary.
10 *Alkylating agents* cause immunosuppression, which may result in a generalized vaccinia following immunization with smallpox vaccine.
11 Corticosteroids used concurrently with *streptozocin* may increase the hyperglycemic effect of *streptozocin.*
12 *Streptozocin* should not be used concurrently with nephrotoxic medications such as aminoglycoside antibiotics, cephalothin, cisplatin, or polymyxins.

13 Phenytoin may protect pancreatic beta cells from the cytotoxic effects of *streptozocin*, thus reducing its therapeutic effect in patients with islet cell tumors.

▶ **NURSING ALERTS**

See general discussion of nursing alerts for all antineoplastic drugs. In addition

▷ 1 Observe patient for tachycardia, hypotension, or shortness of breath when administering cisplatin or mechlorethamine; anaphylactoid reactions can occur, and require supportive measures.

▷ 2 Monitor patients on cyclophosphamide for hematuria or dysuria; discontinue medication at first sign of hemorrhagic cystitis and notify physician.

▷ 3 Caution patients receiving cisplatin or mechlorethamine to report development of tinnitus or impaired hearing. Periodic audiometric testing is recommended to detect ototoxicity.

▷ 4 Closely monitor patients receiving the first dose of streptozocin for signs of hypoglycemia due to a sudden release of insulin; have IV dextrose available.

▶ **NURSING CONSIDERATIONS**

See general discussion of nursing considerations for all antineoplastic drugs. In addition

▷ 1 Maintain adequate hydration in patients receiving cyclophosphamide to reduce the possibility of hemorrhagic cystitis. Give medication early in the morning to prevent accumulation of the drug in the bladder during the night.

II Antimetabolites

Cytarabine	Mercaptopurine
Floxuridine	Methotrexate
Fluorouracil	Thioguanine

The antimetabolites are structural analogs of normally occurring metabolites that interfere with the synthesis of nucleic acids by competing with purines or pyrimidines in metabolic pathways. The antimetabolites themselves may also be incorporated into nucleic acids, resulting in a cell product that fails to function. Antimetabolites act during the S phase of the cell cycle (see introduction). They can be divided into three groups: folic acid antagonists (methotrexate); purine antagonists (mercaptopurine, thioguanine); and pyrimidine antagonists (floxuridine, fluorouracil, cytarabine). They are considered here as a group, then listed individually in Table 74-4.

Mechanism

Folic acid antagonists bind to the enzyme dihydrofolate reductase, thereby preventing reduction of folic acid to tetrahydrofolic acid. This limits the availability of one-carbon fragments necessary for purine and thymidine synthesis, thus blocking DNA synthesis and cell replication.

Purine antagonists—analogs of the natural purines hypoxanthine, guanine, and adenine, these agents must be metabolized to active nucleotides, which then can interfere with the synthesis of natural purines, thus preventing normal nucleic acid synthesis.

Pyrimidine antagonists—floxuridine and fluorouracil compete for the enzyme thymylate synthetase, preventing synthesis of thymidine, an essential substrate of DNA, thus blocking DNA synthesis.

Cytarabine is metabolized by deoxycytidine kinase to the nucleotide triphosphate (ARA–CTP), which is an inhibitor of DNA polymerase, an enzyme necessary for the conversion of RNA into DNA.

Uses

See Table 74-4.

Dosage

See Table 74-4.

Fate

The oral agents mercaptopurine and methotrexate are well absorbed from the GI tract while thioguanine is poorly absorbed. Cytarabine and methotrexate are widely distributed and cross the blood–brain barrier. Mercaptopurine and methotrexate are moderately protein-bound. All agents are largely metabolized in the liver (except methotrexate) and are excreted by the kidney as inactive metabolites and unchanged drug. Floxuridine and fluorouracil are also partially eliminated by the lungs as carbon dioxide.

Common Side-Effects

Myelosuppression (leukopenia, thrombocytopenia, anemia), nausea; vomiting; diarrhea; stomatitis; glossitis; hepatotoxicity (thioguanine and methotrexate); gastritis (fluorouracil and methotrexate); hyperuricemia, renal toxicity; interstitial pneumonitis; and CNS disturbances (methotrexate)

Significant Adverse Reactions

(Not all reactions observed with all drugs)
Dermatologic—skin rash, freckling, dermatitis, hyperpigmentation, alopecia
CNS—ataxia, vertigo, anorexia
Ocular—blurred vision, photophobia, lacrimation
Renal/hepatic—hyperuricemia, uric acid nephropathy, hepatic dysfunction, cholestasis
Cardiovascular—myocardial ischemia, angina
Allergic—fever, anaphylaxis, arthralgia
Other—GI ulceration, osteoporosis, pneumonia, thrombophlebitis, cellulitis, Guillain–Barré syndrome
Note: Antimetabolite agents have been shown to be carcinogenic in animal studies, and thus may present an oncogenic risk in humans. The antimetabolites are potential mutagens and teratogens and also cause ovarian and testicular suppression.

Contraindications

Leukopenia, thrombocytopenia or anemia caused by previous chemotherapy or radiation therapy; hepatoxicity; and renal toxicity

Table 74-4. Antimetabolites

Drug	Preparations	Usual Dosage Range	Uses	Remarks
Cytarabine (Cytosine Arabinoside, ARA-C, Cytosar-U)	Injection—100-mg vial, 500-mg vial	Induction—IV infusion: 100 mg to 200 mg/m²/day or 3 mg/kg/day as a continuous IV infusion over 24 hours (or in divided doses by rapid IV injection) for 5 to 10 days and repeated approximately every 2 weeks

Maintenance—IM, SC: 1 mg/kg to 1.5 mg/kg once or twice a week at 1-week to 4-week intervals or 70 mg to 100 mg/m²/day by rapid IV injection in divided doses or continuous IV infusion for 2 days to 5 days repeated every 30 days

Investigational use for refractory acute myelogenous leukemia—3 gm/m² IV infusion over 1 hour–2 hours every 12 hours for 4 to 12 doses

Combination therapy: Cytarabine and Thioguanine

Cytarabine 3 mg/kg every 12 hours by injection + thioguanine 2.5 mg/kg every 12 hours; give both drugs until bone marrow depression occurs; repeat cycle after 10 days to 20 days rest

Cytarabine, cyclophosphamide, vincristine, and prednisone

Cytarabine, 100 mg/m²/day in 3 divided doses for 5 days

Cyclophosphamide 100 mg/m²/day rapid IV injection in 3 divided doses for 5 days

Vincristine 2 mg IV day 1 only

Prednisone 25 mg 4 times a day orally for 5 days; repeat every 2 weeks

Stop therapy if leukocyte count falls below 1000 or platelet count below 50,000; resume usually after 5 to 7 drug-free days, when above levels are reached

Intrathecal injection (investigational)—5 mg to 75 mg/m² or 30 mg to 100 mg every 3 days to 7 days | Acute myelogenous leukemia (DOC)

Also useful for: Acute lymphocytic leukemia

Chronic myelogenous leukemia | Store freeze-dried powder under refrigeration; reconstitute vials with Bacteriostatic Water for Injection (0.9% benzyl alcohol) 5 ml/100-mg vial; 10 ml/500-mg vial. Use 5 ml to 10 ml Elliott's B Solution, Lactated Ringer's Solution or patient's own cerebrospinal fluid to reconstitue for intrathecal injection; solution may be stored at room temperature for 48 hours; discard any hazy or cloudy solution; infusion solutions may be prepared in 0.9% Sodium Chloride or Dextrose 5%; solutions are stable at room temperature for 7 days; reconstitute with smaller volumes (1 ml–2 ml) for SC injection; may increase SGOT levels, and uric acid levels in blood and urine; usual pediatric dose is equivalent to the adult dose; less nausea, vomiting, diarrhea if given IV infusion rather than IV injection, but danger of hematologic toxicity is increased |
| Floxuridine (FUDR) | Injection—500 mg/vial | Intra-arterial infusion only: 0.1 mg/kg to 0.6 mg/kg/day by continuous infusion; 0.4 mg/kg to 0.6 mg/kg/day for hepatic artery infusion; continue therapy until toxicity occurs, usually 14 days to 21 days, with 2 weeks rest between each course | Palliative management of GI adeno-carcinoma metastatic to liver, pancreas, or biliary tract

Head and neck tumors | Reconstitute with 5 ml Sterile Water for Injection; solution stable for 14 days under refrigeration; further dilution in 0.9% Sodium Chloride or Dextrose 5% is necessary for infusion; dilution is stable for 24 hours; may increase serum alkaline phosphatase, LDH, SGOT, SGPT, and bilirubin levels |
| Fluorouracil (5-Fluorouracil, 5-FU, Adrucil) | Injection—500 mg/10 ml | Initially, 12 mg/kg IV injection over 1 minute to 2 minutes once daily for 4 days; maximum daily | Palliative management of carcinoma of | Solution may discolor slightly during storage, but may still be used safely; crystal |

(continued)

Table 74-4. Antimetabolites (continued)

Drug	Preparations	Usual Dosage Range	Uses	Remarks
		dose 800 mg; if no toxicity, give 6 mg/kg on days 6, 8, 10, and 12 (For poor-risk patients, reduce dose 50%) Maintenance—repeat above schedule every 30 days after last day of previous treatment or 10 mg/kg to 15 mg/kg IV once a week, not to exceed 1 g/week; dosage based on actual body weight unless patient is obese or has fluid retention Oral—15 mg/kg to 20 mg/kg/day for 5 days to 8 days; dilute in water or bicarbonate buffer solution rather than juice	colon, rectum, stomach, and pancreas (DOC) Treatment of breast, ovarian, cervical, and liver carcinomas	precipitate may be redissolved by heating to 60°C; allow to cool to body temperature before using; infusions may be prepared using 0.9% Sodium Chloride or Dextrose 5%; solutions are stable for 24 hours; incompatible with cytarabine and methotrexate; may increase 5-hydroxyindole acetic acid (5-HIAA) in urine; may decrease plasma albumin; FDA has *not* approved the drug for oral use
Mercaptopurine (6-Mercaptopurine, 6-MP, Purinethol)	Tablets—50 mg	Adult—initially 2.5 mg/kg or 80 mg to 100 mg/m² daily in single or divided doses; if no response and no toxicity after 4 weeks increase to 5 mg/kg/day Maintenance—1.5 mg to 2.5 mg/kg or 50 mg to 100 mg/m² daily Children—2.5 mg/kg or 50 mg/m² daily (Calculate all doses to nearest 25 mg)	Acute lymphocytic (DOC) and myelogenous leukemia Chronic myelogenous leukemia	Decrease dose of mercaptopurine to ⅓ to ¼ usual dose if given concurrently with allopurinol; may increase uric acid levels in blood and urine; rarely used as a single agent for maintenance of remissions in acute leukemia; may falsely increase serum glucose and uric acid levels when the SMA (sequential multiple analyzer) is used
Methotrexate (Amethopterin, Folex, MTX, Mexate)	Tablets—2.5 mg Injection—2.5 mg/ml, 25 mg/ml Powder for injection—20 mg/vial, 50 mg/vial, 100 mg/vial, 250 mg/vial	Choriocarcinoma—15 mg to 30 mg/day orally or IM for 5 days; repeat for 3 to 5 courses with 1 week to 2 weeks rest between each course Leukemia—induction: 3.3 mg/m² IM, IV or orally daily for 4 weeks to 6 weeks combined with prednisone 60 mg/m² daily Maintenance—30 mg/m² orally or IM twice a week or 2.5 mg/kg IV every 14 days Children—20 mg to 30 mg/m² orally or IM once a week Meningeal leukemia—10 mg to 15 mg/m² intrathecally every 2 days to 5 days; maximum 15 mg; maximum pediatric dose, 12 mg Burkitt's lymphoma—Stage I–II: 10 mg to 25 mg orally daily for 4 days to 8 days then rest 1 week Stage III: Up to 1 g/m²/day combined with cyclophosphamide and vincristine Mycosis fungoides: Oral—2.5 mg to 5 mg/day for weeks or months as needed IM—50 mg once a week or 25 mg twice a week	Trophoblastic tumors such as gestational choriocarcinoma, chorioadenoma destruens, or hydatidiform mole (DOC) Acute lymphocytic leukemia (DOC), prophylaxis of meningeal leukemia (DOC), breast, lung, and epidermoid cancers of head and neck, Burkitt's lymphoma (DOC), lymphosarcoma, mycosis fungoides, severe psoriasis, rheumatoid arthritis (investigational use)	Monitor urinary chorionic gonadotropin to determine effectiveness of therapy in choriocarcinoma; level should return to less than 50 IU/24 hours after 3 to 4 courses of therapy; use preservative-free solution in treating meningeal leukemia; reconstitute with Elliott's B Solution, 0.9% Sodium Chloride, Lactated Ringer's Solution, or patient's own cerebrospinal fluid; powders may be reconstituted with Sterile Water for Injection, 0.9% Sodium Chloride Injection, or Dextrose 5% in Water; solution is stable for 7 days at room temperature but should be used within 24 hours because it is not preserved; for high-dose methotrexate therapy use preservative-free solution and dilute in 0.9% Sodium Chloride or Dextrose 5% in Water; patient should be well hydrated and urine alkalinized with sodium bicarbonate (3 g every 3 hr for 12 hr before therapy) to prevent renal toxicity; may

Table 74-4. Antimetabolites (continued)

Drug	Preparations	Usual Dosage Range	Uses	Remarks
		Psoriasis: Oral—Three schedules may be used: 1. 10 mg to 25 mg once a week to a maximum of 50 mg/wk 2. 2.5 mg every 12 hours for 3 doses or every 8 hours for 4 doses once a week, to a maximum of 30 mg/wk 3. 2.5 mg/day for 5 days, skip 2 days, and repeat; maximum 6.25 mg/day (this schedule may cause increased liver toxicity) IM, IV—10 mg to 25 mg once a week to a maximum of 50 mg/wk High-dose methotrexate: IV infusion—100 mg/m² to 10 g/m² over 6 hours to 24 hours every 1 week to 3 weeks; follow with calcium leucovorin rescue. Oral, IV, IM—10 mg to 15 mg/m² every 6 hours starting 1 hour to 24 hours after methotrexate and continue for 24 hours to 72 hours; (dosage and schedule varies according to protocol and methotrexate dose)		increase uric acid levels in blood and urine; Calcium leucovorin is used as "rescue" because it is metabolized to tetrahydrofolic acid, which blocks the effect of methotrexate; CNS toxicity is commonly associated with intrathecal injection; methotrexate is excreted in breast milk
Thioguanine (TG, 6-Thioguanine)	Tablets—40 mg	Adults and children—2 mg/kg/day as a single dose; if no response in 3 weeks to 4 weeks and no toxicity, increase dose to 3 mg/kg/day (calculate dose to nearest 20 mg)	Acute lymphocytic and myelogenous leukemia (DOC) Chronic myelogenous leukemia	May increase uric acid levels of blood and urine

DOC = Drug of choice

In addition, do not use mercaptopurine or thioguanine in a patient who has demonstrated prior resistance to either of the two agents because there is usually complete cross-resistance.

Interactions

1 *Cytarabine* and *methotrexate* used concurrently can have either a synergistic or antagonistic effect.
2 *Fluorouracil* is incompatible with cytarabine, diazepam, doxorubicin, and methotrexate. Complete flushing of IV line between injections is recommended.
3 The absorption of *fluororuracil* when given orally is decreased by the presence of food.
4 Concomitant administration of *mercaptopurine* and allopurinol increases both the antineoplastic and toxic effects of mercaptopurine. Reduce the dose of mercaptopurine to one third to one fourth the usual dose.
5 Alcohol may enhance the possibility of *methotrexate*-induced hepatotoxicity.
6 Chloramphenicol, phenylbutazone, phenytoin, para-aminobenzoic acid, salicylates, sulfonamides, and tet-racyclines can displace *methotrexate* from binding sites and cause increased toxicity.
7 Probenecid and salicylates can block the tubular secretion of *methotrexate* and thus increase its toxicity.
8 Pyrimethamine used concurrently with *methotrexate* can cause increased toxicity because of similar folic acid antagonist actions.
9 *Methotrexate* may enhance the hypoprothrombinemic effect of oral anticoagulants such as warfarin.
10 Concurrent use of *methotrexate* and asparaginase may block the antineoplastic action of methotrexate by inhibiting cell synthesis. Administer asparaginase 9 days to 10 days before or within 24 hours after administering methotrexate; the toxic effect of methotrexate may also be reduced.
11 Vitamin preparations containing folic acid may decrease the effect of *methotrexate.*
12 Most *antimetabolite agents* may antagonize the effects of antigout medications by increasing serum uric acid levels; dosage adjustments of the antigout medications may be necessary.

13 *Antimetabolite agents* cause immunosuppression, which may result in a generalized vaccinia following immunization with smallpox vaccine.

14 Concurrent use of *fluorouracil* and allopurinol may reduce the hematologic toxicity of fluorouracil.

15 *Mercaptopurine* may increase or decrease the anticoagulant effect of warfarin.

▶ **NURSING ALERT**

See general discussion of nursing alerts for all antineoplastic drugs. In addition

▷ 1 Observe for tachycardia, hypotension, and shortness of breath when administering cytarabine or methotrexate; anaphylactoid reactions can occur and require supportive measures.

▶ **NURSING CONSIDERATIONS**

See general discussion of nursing considerations for all antineoplastic drugs. In addition

▷ 1 Fluorouracil, mercaptopurine, and thioguanine may be ordered as 5-FU, 6-MP, and 6-thioguanine, respectively. Be aware that the numbers *5* and *6* are part of the drug name and should *not* be confused with the number of vials or tablets to be administered.

▷ 2 Use an IV infusion pump for the intra-arterial administration of floxuridine.

▷ 3 Calcium leucovorin is the antidote for overdosage with methotrexate. For large methotrexate doses, give up to 75 mg calcium leucovorin by IV infusion within 12 hours of methotrexate dose, then follow with 12 mg IM every 6 hours for four doses. For smaller doses of methotrexate, use 6 mg to 12 mg IM every 6 hours for four doses. In general, for best results, the dose of calcium leucovorin should be equal to or higher than the dose of methotrexate and be administered within the first hour.

III Natural Products

Asparaginase	Etoposide
Bleomycin	Mithramycin (Plicamycin)
Dactinomycin	Mitomycin
Daunorubicin	Vinblastine
Doxorubicin	Vincristine

The natural products commercially available for use as chemotherapeutic agents include an enzyme, antibiotics, and plant derivatives. Asparaginase is an enzyme isolated from *Escherichia coli* and is used to treat acute lymphocytic leukemia. Bleomycin, dactinomycin, daunorubicin, doxorubicin, mithramycin, and mitomycin are antineoplastic antibiotics produced from fermentation processes of several different strains of the *Streptomyces* fungus and are used to treat a wide range of malignant diseases. Vinblastine and vincristine are plant alkaloids isolated from periwinkle (*Vinca rosea*); both agents have a broad spectrum of anti-

tumor activity. Etoposide is a semisynthetic podophyllotoxin derived from the root of the May apple or mandrake plant (*Podophyllum*) and is used to treat testicular and lung carcinomas.

Mechanism

Asparaginase—due to a lack of the enzyme asparagine synthetase, some tumor cells are unable to synthesize asparagine, an amino acid necessary for the synthesis of DNA and essential cellular proteins. Such cells must rely on an exogenous source of asparagine from the blood stream. The administration of asparaginase hydrolyzes serum asparagine to aspartic acid, which the tumor cells can not use. Normal cells are able to synthesize asparagine and are therefore much less affected by the agent.

Antibiotics—the antibiotics work by inhibiting DNA or RNA synthesis. Bleomycin causes rupture of DNA strands, thereby inhibiting DNA synthesis. Dactinomycin and mithramycin anchor to DNA and inhibit DNA-dependent RNA synthesis. Daunorubicin and doxorubicin bind to adjoining nucleotide pairs of DNA and inhibit DNA and DNA-dependent RNA synthesis. Mitomycin acts like an alkylating agent causing cross-linking between DNA strands, thus inhibiting duplication.

Plant derivatives—vinblastine and vincristine inhibit mitosis during the metaphase by binding to or crystallizing microtubular proteins, thus preventing their proper polymerization. At high concentrations, these agents also inhibit DNA-dependent synthesis. Etoposide inhibits mitosis at high concentrations (>10 mcg/ml) by causing lysis of cells entering mitosis, and at low concentrations (0.3 mg–10 mcg/ml) by inhibiting cells from entering prophase; the net effect is inhibition of DNA synthesis.

Uses
See Table 74-5.

Dosage
See Table 74-5.

Fate
All of the natural products are administered parenterally and for the most part are widely distributed to most body tissues and organs, primarily the liver, kidney, heart, and lungs. Asparaginase is not extensively distributed and its metabolic fate is not well known. Mithramycin is the only natural product that crosses the blood–brain barrier. The agents are metabolized in the liver to some degree and are excreted in the urine or feces (*via* the bile) as inactive metabolites or unchanged drug.

Common Side-Effects
Myelosuppression (leukopenia, thrombocytopenia, anemia; less commonly, agranulocytosis and pancytopenia), nausea, vomiting, alopecia, and anorexia

Daunorubicin and doxorubicin—congestive heart failure

Asparaginase—hypersensitivity reactions, pancreatitis, hepatotoxicity, and hypofibrinogenemia

Bleomycin—pneumonitis, hyperpigmentation, erythema, cutaneous edema and tenderness, and hyperthermia

(*Text continues on p. 689.*)

Table 74-5. Natural Products

Drug	Preparations	Usual Dosage Range	Uses	Remarks
Asparaginase (Elspar, L-Asparaginase)	Injection: 10,000 IU/vial	**Children** *Regimen I* Asparaginase—1000 IU/kg/day IV for 10 days starting day 22 Vincristine—2 mg/m² IV once a week on days 1, 8, 15; maximum single dose is 2 mg Prednisone—40 mg/m²/day in 3 divided doses for 15 days, then 20 mg/m² for 2 days, 10 mg/m² for 2 days, 5 mg/m² for 2 days, and 2.5/m² for 2 days *Regimen II* Asparaginase—6000 IU/m² IM every 3 days for 9 doses starting day 4 Vincristine—1.5 mg/m² IV for 4 doses on days 1, 8, 15, 22 Prednisone—40 mg/m²/day in 3 divided doses for 28 days, then taper over 14 days Sole induction agent—200 IU/kg IV daily for 28 days Adult induction—10,000 IU/m² every 1 week to 2 weeks Intra-arterial—20,000 IU/day for 7 days to 10 days	Acute lymphocytic leukemia	Adult usage is primarily investigational; may be administered *via* the hepatic artery for insulin-secreting pancreatic islet cell tumors; store intact vial under refrigeration; for IV use, reconstitute with 5 ml 0.9% Sodium Chloride and inject over at least 30 minutes into running IV of 0.9% Sodium Chloride or Dextrose 5%; for IM use reconstitute with 2 ml 0.9% Sodium Chloride; do not inject more than 2 ml into one site; avoid vigorous shaking during reconstitution; solution is stable for 8 hours at room temperature; discard solution if cloudy; *not* recommended as the sole induction agent unless combined chemotherapy is inappropriate due to toxicity or other factors; intradermal skin test is recommended prior to initiation of therapy and when more than 7 days have elapsed between doses (up to 35% of patients exhibit hypersensitivity reactions); give 0.1 ml (2 IU) of test solution and observe for at least 1 hour for erythema or wheal; to prepare skin test solution reconstitute vial with 5 ml 0.9% sodium chloride; withdraw 0.1 ml (200 IU) and inject into 9.9 ml 0.9% Sodium Chloride Injection giving test solution of 20 IU/ml; densensitiza-tion should be used on any positive reactors; inject 1 IU IV and double the dose every 10 minutes, provided there is no reaction, until total accumulated dose is equal to the dose for that day; may increase SGOT, SGPT, alkaline phosphatase, bilirubin values; may increase blood ammonia, glucose, and uric acid levels; may increase urine uric acid levels and decrease serum albumin and calcium; gelatinous fiber-like particles may develop in IV infusion on standing; solution may be administered through a 5-micron filter to remove particles without loss of

(continued)

Table 74-5. Natural Products (continued)

Drug	Preparations	Usual Dosage Range	Uses	Remarks
				potency; do not administer thru a 0.2-micron filter, loss of potency may result
Bleomycin (Blenoxane)	15 U/ampule	Squamous cell carcinoma, lymphosarcoma, reticulum cell sarcoma, testicular carcinoma—0.25 U to 0.5 U/kg (10 U–20 U/m²) IV, IM, or SC weekly or twice a week to a total of 300 U to 400 U Hodgkin's disease—as above until 50% response occurs, then 1 U daily or 5 U weekly IV or IM Intra-arterial infusion for squamous cell carcinoma of head, neck, and cervix—30 U to 60 U/day over 1 hour to 24 hours Reduce dose in patients with impaired renal function *Serum Creatinine* *Dose* 1.5–2.5 ½ normal dose 2.5–4.0 ¼ normal dose 4.0–6.0 ⅕ normal dose 6.0–10.0 1/10 to 1/20 normal dose	Squamous cell carcinoma of head and neck (DOC), mouth, tongue, nasopharynx, oropharynx, sinus, palate, lip, buccal mucosa, gingiva, epiglottis, skin, larynx, penis, cervix, vulva Lymphomas: Hodgkin's disease Reticulum cell sarcoma Lymphosarcoma Testicular carcinomas: Embryonal cell carcinoma Choriocarcinoma Teratocarcinoma (DOC)	For IM or SC use, reconstitute with 1 ml to 5 ml of Sterile Water for Injection, 0.9% Sodium Chloride, 5% Dextrose or Bacteriostatic Water for Injection; for IV use, reconstitute with 5 ml 0.9% Sodium Chloride or 5% Dextrose and administer slowly over 10 minutes; solution is stable 14 days at room temperature and 28 days refrigerated; give test dose of 2 U for first 2 doses in lymphoma patients because of possibility of anaphylactoid reaction; pneumonitis occurs in 10% to 40% of patients; be alert for symptoms such as dry cough, dyspnea, and fine rales; fatal in 10% of patients; cutaneous allergic reactions are also common; hypothermia occurs in 25% of patients 3 hours to 6 hours after administration and lasts 4 hours to 12 hours; becomes less frequent with continued use
Dactinomycin (Actinomycin D, Cosmegen)	Injection—0.5 mg/vial	Adults—0.01 mg/kg to 0.015 mg/kg/day IV for 5 days every 4 weeks to 6 weeks, or 0.5 mg/m² (maximum 2 mg) IV once a week for 3 weeks Children—0.01 mg/kg to 0.015 mg/kg/day IV for 5 days or a total dose of 2.5 mg/m² IV in divided doses over 7 days; may repeat every 4 weeks to 6 weeks Isolation perfusion: Upper extremity—0.035 mg/kg Lower extremity—0.05 mg/kg	Wilms' tumor (DOC) Rhabdomyosarcoma Carcinoma of testis and uterus Ewing's sarcoma	Reconstitute with 1.1 ml Sterile Water for Injection (preservative-free); administer directly into tubing of running IV of 0.9% Sodium Chloride or 5% Dextrose; may dilute and infuse over 10 minutes to 15 minutes; AVOID EXTRAVASATION; NEVER administer IM or SC; solution is *theoretically* stable at room temperature for long periods but should be discarded within 24 hours to prevent bacterial contamination; may increase uric acid levels of blood and urine; hyperpigmentation occurs if skin has been previously irradiated; nausea and vomiting are common during first few hours and may persist for up to 24 hours
Daunorubicin (Cerubidine)	Injection—20 mg/vial	Single agent: 30 mg to 60 mg/m²/day IV on days 1, 2, and 3 every 3 weeks to 4 weeks or 0.8 mg/kg to 1 mg/kg/day IV for 3 days to 6 days repeated every 3 weeks to 4 weeks	Acute myelogenous leukemia (DOC)	Reconstitue with 4 ml Sterile Water for Injection; solution is stable for 24 hours at room temperature and 48 hours under refrigeration; protect from exposure to sunlight; administer into the

Table 74-5. Natural Products (continued)

Drug	Preparations	Usual Dosage Range	Uses	Remarks
		Combination: Daunorubicin—45 mg/m²/day IV on days 1, 2, 3 of first course and days 1 and 2 of subsequent courses Cytarabine—100 mg/m²/day IV infusion daily for 7 days for the first course and daily for 5 days for subsequent courses Total cumulative dose of daunorubicin should not exceed 550 mg/m² Reduce dose in patients with impaired hepatic or renal function.		tubing of a rapidly flowing IV of 0.9% Sodium Chloride or 5% Dextrose; AVOID EXTRAVASATION; NEVER administer IM or SC; may increase uric acid levels of blood and urine
		Serum Bilirubin / Serum Creatinine / Dose 1.2 mg to 3 mg/dl — ¾ normal dose above 3 mg/dl / above 3 mg/dl / ½ normal dose		
Doxorubicin (Adriamycin)	Injection—10 mg/vial, 50 mg/vial	Adult—60 mg to 75 mg/m²/day IV repeated every 21 days or 25 mg to 30 mg/m²/day IV for 3 days repeated every 4 weeks Children—30 mg/m²/day IV for 3 days repeated every 4 weeks Total cumulative dose should not exceed 550 mg/m² Reduce dose in patients with impaired hepatic function. Serum Bilirubin / BSP Retention / Dose 1.2 mg–3 mg/dl / 9%–15% / ½ normal dose above 3 mg/dl / above 15% / ¼ normal dose	Acute lymphocytic and myelogenous leukemia Wilms' tumor Neuroblastoma (DOC) Soft-tissue and bone sarcomas (DOC) Thyroid carcinoma Hodgkin's disease Non-Hodgkin's lymphomas (DOC) Breast and ovarian carcinoma Bronchogenic carcinoma (DOC)	Reconstitute with 0.9% Sodium Chloride Injection (5 ml/10-mg vial and 25 ml/50-mg vial); solution is stable for 24 hours at room temperature and 48 hours under refrigeration; protect from exposure to sunlight; administer into the tubing of a rapidly flowing IV of 0.9% Sodium Chloride or 5% Dextrose; local erythematous streaking along the vein or facial flushing may indicate too rapid administration; AVOID EXTRAVASATION; NEVER administer IM or SC; may increase uric acid levels of blood and urine; cardiotoxic effects can occur at cumulative doses above 550 mg/m² in most patients, but may be seen at lower doses in patients who have received previous irradiation or cyclophosphamide therapy
Etoposide (VePesid, VP-16-213)	Injection—100 mg/5 ml	IV—50 mg to 100 mg/m²/day for 5 days repeated every 3 weeks to 4 weeks In combination with other agents: 100 mg/m²/day on days 1, 3, and 5 repeated every 3 weeks to 4 weeks	Refractory testicular tumors Investigational uses: Acute lymphocytic leukemia, small cell lung carcinoma, Hodgkin's disease	Do not give by rapid IV push: severe hypotension may result. IV infusion prepared in 5% Dextrose or 0.9% Sodium Chloride Injection may be given over 30 minutes to 60 minutes; infusion concentrations of 0.2 mg/ml are stable for 96 hours at room temperature, and concentrations of 0.4 mg/ml are stable for 48 hours in both glass and plastic containers

(continued)

Table 74-5. Natural Products *(continued)*

Drug	Preparations	Usual Dosage Range	Uses	Remarks
Mithramycin (Mithracin) (Note: generic name is also known as Plicamycin)	Injection—2.5 mg/vial	Testicular carcinoma—0.025 mg/kg to 0.03 mg/kg/day IV infusion for 8 days to 10 days or 0.025 mg/kg to 0.05 mg/kg/day IV on alternate days for 3 to 8 doses; repeat every 4 weeks Hypercalcemia and hypercalciuria—0.025 mg/kg/day for 3 days to 4 days; may repeat at 1-week intervals (see Chap. 41); reduce dose (by 25%–50%) in patients with impaired hepatic and renal function	Testicular carcinoma Hypercalcemia and hypercalciuria (not responsive to conventional treatment) associated with advanced neoplasms (see Chap. 41)	Store intact vial under refrigeration; alternate-day dosing may reduce toxicity; reconstitute with 4.9 ml Sterile Water for Injection; stable 24 hours at room temperature and 48 hours refrigerated; dilute in 5% Dextrose or 0.9% Sodium Chloride, and infuse over 4 hours to 6 hours; AVOID EXTRAVASATION; may increase SGOT, SGPT, LDH, BUN, serum creatinine levels; may decrease serum calcium, phosphorous, and potassium levels; be alert for epistaxis or hematemesis, early signs of possible hemorrhagic diathesis; advise physician immediately
Mitomycin (Mutamycin)	Injection—5 mg/vial, 20 mg/vial	IV—20 mg/m^2 as a single dose repeated every 6 weeks to 8 weeks *or* 2 mg/m^2/day IV for 5 days, skip 2 days, and repeat 2 mg/m^2/day for 5 days; cycle may be repeated every 6 weeks to 8 weeks A suggested guide for subsequent dosage adjustment is the following: Nadir after Prior Dose Leukocytes / Platelets / % of Prior Dose to be Given Above 4000 / Above 100,000 / 100% 3000–3999 / 75,000–99,999 / 100% 2000–2999 / 25,000–74,999 / 70% Below 2000 / Below 25,000 / 50% Doses greater than 20 mg/m^2 are no more effective than lower doses, but increase toxicity	Adenocarcinoma of stomach, pancreas, colon, rectum, and breast. Squamous cell carcinoma of head, neck, lungs, and cervix Malignant melanoma Chronic myelogenous leukemia	Reconstitute with Sterile Water for Injection: 10 ml/5-mg vial, 40 ml/20-mg vial; solution is stable 7 days at room temperature and 14 days if refrigerated; protect from light; may be diluted for IV infusion (5% Dextrose, stable for 3 hours at room temperature; 0.9% Sodium Chloride, stable 12 hours; Sodium Lactate, stable 24 hours; AVOID EXTRAVASATION; NEVER administer IM or SC; may increase BUN and serum creatinine levels; vomiting is usually transient (3 hr–4 hr), but nausea may persist up to 72 hours; if disease shows no response after 2 courses of therapy, discontinue because likelihood of response is minimal; bladder instillation of 20 mg 3 times a week for 20 doses has been used to treat bladder papillomas
Vinblastine (Velban)	Injection—10 mg vial	Adult—initially, 0.1 mg/kg or 3.7 mg/m^2 once every 7 days; increase in increments of 0.05 mg/kg or 1.8 mg to 1.9 mg/m^2 until tumor size decreases, leukocyte count falls to 3000, or a maximum dose of 0.5 mg/kg or 18.5 mg/m^2 is reached (usual range is 0.15 mg to 0.2 mg/kg or 5.5 mg to 7.4 mg/m^2); maintenance dose is 1 increment smaller than final initial dose repeated every 7 days to 14 days or 10 mg once or twice a month	Frequently responsive: Hodgkin's disease Lymphosarcoma Reticulum cell sarcoma Neuroblastoma Advanced mycosis fungoides Histiocytosis X (Letterer–Siwe disease) Testicular carcinoma (DOC)	Store unopened vial under refrigeration; reconstitute with 10 ml 0.9% Sodium Chloride; Solution is stable 30 days under refrigeration; administer by IV push or through tubing of a running IV (0.9% Sodium Chloride or 5% Dextrose) over 1 minute; AVOID EXTRAVASATION; rinse syringe and needle with venous blood before withdrawing. If extravasation occurs, damage may be minimized

Table 74-5. Natural Products (continued)

Drug	Preparations	Usual Dosage Range	Uses	Remarks
		Children—initially, 2.5 mg/m² once every 7 days; increase in increments of 1.25 mg/m² until leukocyte count falls to 3000, tumor size decreases, or maximum dose of 7.5 mg/m² is reached; maintenance dose is 1 increment smaller than final initial dose repeated every 7 days to 14 days; subsequent maintenance doses should not be given to adults or children until leukocyte count exceeds 4000.	Less responsive: Choriocarcinoma Breast carcinoma	by local injection of hyaluronidase and by following guidelines for treatment of extravasation outlined in general nursing considerations at the beginning of the chapter; may increase uric acid levels of blood and urine; Raynaud's phenomenon is seen with combined use of vinblastine and bleomycin for testicular carcinoma; response may not be seen in some patients until 4 weeks to 12 weeks of therapy has been completed
Vincristine (Oncovin)	Injection—1 mg/ml, 2 mg/ 2 ml, 5 mg/5 ml	Adult—0.01 mg/kg to 0.03 mg/kg or 1.4 mg/m² IV every 7 days as a single dose Children—1.5 mg to 2 mg/m² IV every 7 days as a single dose	Acute lymphocytic leukemia (DOC) Hodgkin's disease (DOC) Lymphosarcoma Rhabdomyosar-coma (DOC) Neuroblastoma (DOC) Wilms' tumor (DOC) Carcinoma of lung and breast	Store unopened vial under refrigeration; protect from light; administer by IV push or through tubing of running IV (0.9% Sodium Chloride or 5% Dextrose) over 1 minute; AVOID EXTRAVASATION (see Vinblastine); neurotoxicity (numbness, weakness, myalgia, jaw pain, loss of deep tendon reflexes, motor difficulties, visual disturbances) can occur as soon as 2 months after start of therapy and is usually progressive as long as treatment is continued; paralytic ileus can occur, more commonly in young children; intrathecal injection of vincristine can be fatal; syndrome of inappropriate antidiuretic hormone secretion has been noted, resulting in hyponatremia

DOC = Drug of choice

Dactinomycin—GI ulceration
Dactinomycin and doxorubicin—stomatitis and esophagitis
Mithramycin—hemorrhagic diathesis
Vincristine—neurotoxicity, hyperuricemia, paralytic ileus, and constipation

Significant Adverse Reactions
(Not all reactions observed with all drugs)
GI—diarrhea, cheilitis, pharyngitis, esophagitis, hemorrhagic colitis, rectal bleeding
Allergic—skin rash, fever, chills, urticaria, angioedema, pruritus, anaphylactic reaction
CNS—agitation, drowsiness, headache, hypothermia, lethargy, malaise, irritability, confusion, syncope, paresthesias, peripheral neuritis, convulsions, motor incoordination
Ocular—blurred vision, conjunctivitis, lacrimation
Dermatologic—acne, hyperpigmentation, hyperkeratosis, thickening of nail beds, photosensitivity
Renal/hepatic—cystitis, polyuria, dysuria, uric acid nephropathy, electrolyte abnormalities, hepatotoxicity
Other—hyperglycemia, ototoxicity, Raynaud's phenomenon, pain at tumor or injection site, phlebitis, tissue necrosis upon extravasation, pulmonary fibrosis
Note: Natural products have been shown to be carcinogenic in animal studies and may present oncogenic risk. These agents are also potential mutagens and teratogens and can cause ovarian and testicular suppression.

Contraindications

Leukopenia, thrombocytopenia, or anemia caused by previous chemotherapy or radiation therapy; hepatotoxicity; renal toxicity; and known hypersensitivity

The use of daunorubicin and doxorubicin in patients with pre-existing cardiac disease may increase the risk of cardiotoxicity (toxicity may occur at cumulative doses higher than 550 mg/m²). Daunorubicin and doxorubicin are contraindicated in patients who have received previous treatment with complete cumulative doses of one of the agents. Asparaginase should not be used in patients with a history of pancreatitis.

Interactions

1 Most *natural products* may antagonize the effects of antigout medications by increasing serum uric acid levels; dosage adjustment of the antigout medications may be necessary.

2 Concurrent use of *asparaginase* and methotrexate may block the antineoplastic action of methotrexate by inhibiting cell synthesis. Administer asparaginase 9 days to 10 days before or within 24 hours after administering methotrexate; the toxic effect of methotrexate may also be reduced.

3 The concurrent administration of *asparaginase*, *vincristine*, and prednisone may enhance the hyperglycemic effect, neurotoxicity, and myelosuppression of asparaginase. Toxicity does not appear to be enhanced when asparaginase is administered *after* vincristine and prednisone.

4 Because *asparaginase* causes hyperglycemia, dosage adjustment of hypoglycemic medications may be necessary during asparaginase therapy.

5 Raynaud's phenomenon has occurred in patients with testicular carcinoma being treated with a combination of *bleomycin* and *vinblastine*. It is unknown whether the cause is the disease, the chemotherapeutic agents, or a combination of these factors.

6 *Dactinomycin* may decrease the effect of vitamin K, requiring an increase in the dose of vitamin K and close observation of the patient.

7 *Daunorubicin* is incompatible with heparin sodium and dexamethasone phosphate when mixed together.

8 Concurrent use of cyclophosphamide, *dactinomycin*, or *mitomycin* with *doxorubicin* may result in increased cardiotoxicity. The total dose of doxorubicin should not exceed 400 mg/m².

9 *Doxorubicin* is incompatible in solution with aminophylline, cephalothin, dexamethasone, fluorouracil, hydrocortisone, and sodium heparin.

10 Concurrent use of cyclophosphamide with *daunorubicin* may increase cardiac toxicity. The total dose of daunorubicin should not exceed 450 mg/m².

11 Administration of *doxorubicin* to a patient who has received *daunorubicin*, or *vice versa*, increases the risk of cardiotoxicity. Neither agent should be used in a patient who has previously received complete cumulative doses of the other agent.

12 Concurrent use of *vincristine* with *doxorubicin* and prednisone can increase myelosuppression; avoid this combination.

▶ NURSING ALERTS

See general discussion of nursing alerts for all antineoplastic drugs. In addition

▷ 1 Asparaginase may frequently cause hypersensitivity or acute anaphylactic reactions. Observe patient for laryngeal constriction, hypotension, diaphoresis, facial edema, respiratory distress, fever, aches, chills, loss of consciousness. Be prepared to treat with epinephrine, diphenhydramine, steroids, and oxygen.

▷ 2 Be alert for severe stomach pain with nausea and vomiting, possible indications of pancreatitis due to asparaginase. Perform frequent determinations of serum amylase.

▷ 3 Observe patients receiving asparaginase for polyuria and polydipsia, potential signs of hyperglycemia.

▷ 4 Observe patients receiving bleomycin or mitomycin for cough or shortness of breath, indications of possible pulmonary toxicity.

▷ 5 Idiosyncratic anaphylactoid reactions occur in 1% of patients receiving bleomycin. Observe for wheezing, hypotension, and mental confusion during first 12 hours to 24 hours after first two doses.

▷ 6 Local burning or stinging at the injection site during the administration of dactinomycin, daunorubicin, doxorubicin, mitomycin, vinblastine, or vincristine may indicate extravasation. Stop immediately and use another vein. See guidelines for preventing and managing extravasation under general discussion of nursing considerations.

▷ 7 Observe patients receiving daunorubicin and doxorubicin for dyspnea, tachycardia, hepatomegaly, and swelling of feet and lower legs, indications of possible cardiotoxicity.

▷ 8 Note development of facial flushing and erythematous streaking along the vein, indications of too-rapid injection of daunorubicin and doxorubicin.

▷ 9 Monitor patients receiving mithramycin for episodes of epistaxis or hematemesis, signs of impending hemorrhagic syndrome.

▷ 10 Note development of tetany or muscle cramps during therapy with mithramycin, possible indications of hypocalcemia.

▷ 11 Observe patients receiving vincristine (and also vinblastine) for signs and symptoms of neurotoxicity (peripheral neuropathy, loss of deep tendon reflexes, numbness, weakness, myalgias, motor difficulties, and visual disturbances).

▷ 12 Monitor bowel habits of patients receiving vincristine and be alert for complaints of constipation or stomach cramps. Consider use of bulk-forming laxatives and/or stool softeners.

▷ 13 Anaphylactic-like reactions have occurred in 1% to 2% of patients receiving etoposide. Observe for chills, fever, tachycardia, bronchospasm, dyspnea, and hypotension.

▶ NURSING CONSIDERATIONS

See general discussion of nursing considerations for all antineoplastic drugs. In addition

▷ 1 Do not inject more than 2 ml asparaginase IM at one site.

▷ 2 Be aware that the incidence of hypersensitivity reactions with asparaginase increases with repeated doses. Repeat the intradermal skin test if more than 1 week has passed between doses.

▷ 3 Obtain frequent serum amylase determinations to monitor pancreatic function. Notify physician of any increase in serum amylase, possible evidence of pancreatitis.

▷ 4 Monitor blood sugar and urine glucose for hyperglycemia or glucosuria in patients receiving asparaginase.

▷ 5 Perform pulmonary function studies before bleomycin therapy. Repeat chest x-rays every 2 weeks. Monitor carbon dioxide diffusion capacity monthly and discontinue therapy when capacity falls below 30% to 35% of pretreatment value.

▷ 6 Note that administration of diphenhydramine before bleomycin therapy may reduce the risk of an anaphylactoid reaction.

▷ 7 Perform chest x-ray, electrocardiogram (ECG) and echocardiogram before initiating therapy and every month during therapy with daunorubicin and doxorubicin.

▷ 8 Warn patients receiving daunorubicin and doxorubicin that urine will be red for 24 hours to 48 hours after administration.

▷ 9 Obtain platelet count, bleeding time, and prothrombin time before and frequently during therapy with mithramycin.

▷ 10 Obtain serum calcium, phosphorus, and potassium levels before and at regular intervals during therapy with mithramycin.

▷ 11 Inform patients receiving mitomycin that purple colored bands in the nail beds can occur with repeated doses of the medication.

▷ 12 Provide a routine prophylactic regimen against constipation for all patients receiving vincristine.

IV Hormonal and Antihormonal Agents

Hormonal agents have been used to successfully treat a variety of different types of neoplasms. Tumors that are sensitive to hormones may respond to the administration of natural or synthetic hormonal agents that delay tumor growth. Hormonal agents are not curative, however, because most lack a cytoxic action. Still, they may provide the patient with prolonged palliation without major toxicities.

The principal hormones used as antineoplastic drugs are the sex hormones (androgens, estrogens, progestins) and the corticosteroids. Androgens, derivatives of testosterone, are used for the palliative treatment of advanced or disseminated breast cancer in *post*menopausal women when hormonal therapy is indicated. The androgens discussed in this section include the 17-alkylated compounds (dromostanolone, fluoxymesterone, testolactone) and testosterone propionate.

Estrogens are used for the palliative treatment of *post*menopausal breast cancer, advanced prostatic cancer, and male breast cancer in selected patients. The estrogens reviewed in this section include the estradiol compounds whose steroidal structures closely resemble the natural hormone, estramustine, a phosphorylated combination of estradiol and mechlorethamine, and several nonsteroidal agents possessing estrogenic activity, such as chlorotrianisene and diethylstilbestrol (DES).

Progestins are steroidal compounds related to the natural hormone progesterone. Progestins have been used in the palliative treatment of carcinoma of the breast, endometrium, and renal cells. The progestational agents discussed in this section include hydroxyprogesterone caproate, medroxyprogesterone acetate, and megestrol acetate.

Corticosteroids are synthetic steroidal agents derived from the natural adrenal hormone cortisol (hydrocortisone). Corticosteroids, primarily prednisone, are used frequently in combination chemotherapy regimens for the treatment of acute and chronic lymphocytic leukemia, Hodgkin's and non-Hodgkin's lymphomas, multiple myeloma, and some breast cancers.

In addition to the hormonal drugs, two antihormonal agents are considered in this section as well. Mitotane, a derivative of the insecticide DDT, is used in the palliative treatment of inoperable adrenal cortical carcinoma. Tamoxifen, a nonsteroidal anti-estrogen, is used for the palliative treatment of advanced breast cancer in *post*menopausal women with estrogen receptor (ER)-positive tumors.

The general discussion of these agents presented below is followed by a listing of individual agents in Table 74-6, where specific characteristics of each drug are given.

Mechanism
Hormonal agents
Androgens—the exact mechanism of the antitumor effect of androgens is unknown. In most cases, hormone receptors must be present in the tumor cell cytosol. Androgens bind to the receptor site, are transported into the cell nucleus, and block normal cell growth by inhibiting the transport of the natural growth hormone into the cell. In addition, androgens may inhibit estrogen synthesis, thus causing androgen-induced estrogen depletion.

Estrogens—the mechanism is thought to be essentially the same as proposed for androgens; the estrogens bind to the cell cytosol receptor and this complex then translocates to the cell nucleus and blocks normal growth of the cell. Estrogens can also cause regression of some tumors by suppressing normal pituitary function. In males with prostatic cancer, estrogens decrease the amount of luteinizing hormone (*i.e.,* interstitial cell-stimulating hormone) secreted by the pituitary, which in turn decreases the amount of androgen secreted by the testes. The antitumor effect of estramustine may be due to (1) estradiol, (2) the alkylating activity of mechlorethamine, (3) a direct effect of estramustine, or to a combination of these effects.

Progestins—they may have a direct local effect on hormonally sensitive endometrial cells, and may also decrease the amount of luteinizing hormone secreted by the pituitary gland. The antineoplastic effect of progestins on carcinoma of the breast is unclear.

Corticosteroids—corticosteroids produce their antitumor effects by binding to corticosteroid receptors present in high numbers on lymphoid tumors. This binding appears to inhibit both cellular glucose transport and phosphorylation, which decreases the amount of energy available for mitosis and protein synthesis, ultimately resulting in cell lysis.

Antihormonal agents

Mitotane—an adrenal cytoxic agent that causes adrenal inhibition, apparently without cellular destruction, its primary action is upon the mitochondria of the adrenal cortex, although the exact biochemical mechanism of action is unknown. Mitotane modifies the peripheral metabolism of steroids and directly suppresses the adrenal cortex. Mitotane also alters the extra-adrenal metabolism of cortisol, even though plasma levels of corticosteroids do not fall. The drug apparently causes increased formation of 6-beta-hydroxycortisol.

Tamoxifen—tamoxifen is a nonsteroidal estrogen antagonist that binds to estrogen receptor sites in the cytosol of the cell. This complex is translocated to the nucleus of the cell where it acts as a false messenger and ultimately inhibits DNA synthesis. Tamoxifen is unlikely to cause a response in patients who have had a negative estrogen receptor (ER) assay.

Uses

See Table 74-6.

Dosage

See Table 74-6.

Fate

The fate of the androgen, estrogen, progestin, and corticosteroid agents are reviewed in Chapters 43, 44, and 46. The antihormonal agent mitotane is approximately 40% absorbed from the GI tract and is excreted by the kidney (10%–25%) as a water-soluble metabolite, in the bile (a very small amount), and largely unchanged in the feces (60%). Mitotane is stored primarily in fatty tissues throughout the body and blood levels are detectable up to 10 weeks after the medication has been discontinued. Tamoxifen is well absorbed orally, metabolized in the liver, and excreted primarily in the feces.

Common Side-Effects

See Chapters 43, 44, and 46 for common side-effects of corticosteroids, estrogens and progestins, and androgens, respectively.

Mitotane—anorexia, nausea, vomiting, diarrhea, skin rash, skin darkening, and CNS toxicity (drowsiness, dizziness, depression)

Tamoxifen—nausea, vomiting, "hot flashes"

Significant Adverse Reactions

See Chapters 43, 44, and 46 for significant adverse reactions of corticosteroids, estrogens and progestins, and androgens, respectively.

Mitotane—visual disturbances, hypersensitivity reactions (dyspnea, wheezing), generalized aching, hyperpyrexia, muscle twitching, hematuria, proteinuria, hemorrhagic cystitis

Tamoxifen—leukopenia, thrombocytopenia, hypercalcemia, increased bone pain, vaginal bleeding, menstrual irregularities, lactation, alopecia, photosensitivity, dizziness, headache, depression, anorexia, retinopathy, corneal changes, decreased visual acuity

Contraindications

(Especially as they apply to the use of these agents as antineoplastic drugs)

1 *Androgens* are contraindicated in carcinoma of the male breast, known or suspected prostatic cancer, and premenopausal women.
2 *Estrogens* are contraindicated in men or women with known or suspected cancer of the breast, except in appropriately selected patients being treated for metastatic disease.
3 *Estrogen* usage is contraindicated in known or suspected estrogen-dependent neoplasia.
4 *Estrogen* and *progestin* usage is contraindicated in active thrombophlebitis or thromboembolic disorders and in markedly impaired liver function.
5 The progestins *hydroxyprogesterone* and *medroxyprogesterone* are contraindicated in known or suspected breast carcinoma, known or suspected genital malignancy, and undiagnosed vaginal bleeding.

(See Chaps. 43, 44, and 46 for additional information on contraindications of hormonal agents.)

Interactions

1 The androgens, particularly *fluoxymesterone* and *methyltestosterone,* may increase sensitivity to anticoagulants. The dosage of the anticoagulant may have to be decreased.
2 *Androgens* may enhance the hypoglycemic effect of antidiabetic agents.
3 *Estrogens* may reduce the effect of oral anticoagulants by increasing certain clotting factors in the blood.
4 The anticonvulsants carbamazepine, phenobarbital, phenytoin and primidone may reduce the effect of *estrogens* due to increased estrogen metabolism caused by the induction of liver enzymes.
5 Concurrent use of rifampin and *estrogens* may result in decreased estrogenic activity due to enzyme induction.
6 Large doses of *estrogens* may enhance the side-effects of tricyclic antidepressants and decrease their antidepressant effect.
7 *Corticosteroids,* when used concurrently with amphotericin B, may cause increased potassium depletion leading to hypokalemia.
8 *Corticosteroids* may increase or decrease the response to oral anticoagulants.
9 *Corticosteroids* cause hyperglycemia and thus may increase requirements for insulin or oral hypoglycemic agents.
10 Ephedrine, phenobarbital, phenytoin, and rifampin enhance the metabolism of *corticosteroids* through enzyme induction, thus decreasing corticosteroid activity.
11 Patients taking potassium-depleting diuretics and *corticosteroids* concomitantly may develop hypokalemia.

Table 74-6. Hormonal and Antihormonal Agents

Drug	Preparations	Usual Dosage Range	Uses	Remarks
Androgens				
Dromostanolone Proprionate (Drolban)	Injection—50 mg/ml	IM—100 mg 3 times a week	Advanced breast carcinoma	Indicated for women with inoperable cancer who are 1-year to 5-year *post*menopausal; continue treatment 8 weeks to 12 weeks to determine efficacy; if disease progresses during first 6 weeks to 8 weeks of therapy, consider alternate therapy; fewer androgenic side-effects than testosterone; do not refrigerate; precipitation may occur
Fluoxymesterone (Halotestin, Ora-Testryl)	Tablets—2 mg, 5 mg, 10 mg	10 mg to 30 mg/day in divided doses (0.05 mg/kg–1 mg/kg/day)	Advanced breast carcinoma	See Dromostanolone; higher incidence of biliary stasis and jaundice than other androgens
Testolactone (Teslac)	Tablets—50 mg, 250 mg Injection—100 mg/ml	Oral—250 mg 4 times a day IM—100 mg 3 times a week	Advanced breast carcinoma in women only	See Dromostanolone; administer by deep IM injection into upper outer quadrant of gluteal area; may be used in premenopausal women whose ovarian function has been terminated; shake injection well before use and inject immediately; devoid of androgenic activity in normal doses
Methyltestosterone (Oreton Methyl, Metandren)	Tablets—10 mg, 25 mg Buccal tablets—5 mg, 10 mg	Oral—200 mg/day Buccal—100 mg/day	Advanced breast carcinoma	See Dromostanolone; androgenic side-effects are more common; painful, erythematous local reactions can occur at injection site; hypercalcemia may result if patient is immobilized or if bony metastases are present
Testosterone cypionate (Depo-Testosterone)	Injection—50 mg/ml, 100 mg/ml, 200 mg/ml	IM—4 mg/kg to 7 mg/kg/wk		
Testosterone enanthate (Delatestryl)	Injection—100 mg/ml, 200 mg/ml	IM—600 mg to 1,200 mg/wk		
Testosterone propionate	Injection—25 mg/ml, 50 mg/ml, 100 mg/ml	IM—50 mg to 100 mg 3 times a week		
Estrogens				
Chlorotrianisene (Tace)	Capsules—12 mg, 25 mg, 72 mg	Oral—12 mg to 25 mg/day	Advanced prostatic carcinoma (DOC)	Also used for symptomatic treatment of menopausal symptoms and relief of postpartum breast engorgement (72-mg capsules); (see Chap. 44)
Diethylstilbestrol (DES)	Tablets—0.1 mg, 0.25 mg, 0.5 mg, 1 mg, 5 mg	Breast cancer: Oral—1 mg to 5 mg 3 times a day Prostatic cancer: Oral—1 mg to 3 mg/day initially, then decrease to 1 mg/day	Advanced breast and prostatic carcinoma (DOC)	Dosage may be increased in advanced prostatic carcinoma, but incidence of thromboembolic complications increases with doses above 1 mg
Diethylstilbestrol diphosphate (Stilphostrol)	Tablets—50 mg Injection—250 mg/5 ml	Oral—50 mg to 200 mg 3 times a day IV—500 mg on day 1, 1000 mg on days 2 to 5, then 250 mg to 500 mg 1 to 2 times a week	Advanced prostatic carcinoma (DOC)	Mix drug in 300 ml 5% Dextrose or normal saline solution; administer slowly for 10 minutes to 15 minutes at 20 to 30 drops/minute; then increase rate

(continued)

Table 74-6. Hormonal and Antihormonal Agents (continued)

Drug	Preparations	Usual Dosage Range	Uses	Remarks
		Maintenance—250 mg to 500 mg IV once or twice a week		to run entire infusion in over 1 hour
Estradiol	Tablets—1 mg, 2 mg	Breast cancer: 10 mg 3 times a day Prostatic cancer: 1 mg to 2 mg 3 times a day	Advanced breast and prostatic carcinoma	Continue breast cancer treatment for a minimum of 3 months to determine efficacy
Estradiol cypionate (Depo-Estradiol)	Injection—1 mg/ml, 5 mg/ml	IM—initially, 1 mg to 5 mg/wk Maintenance—2 mg to 5 mg every 3 weeks to 4 weeks	Advanced prostatic carcinoma (DOC)	
Estradiol valerate (Delestrogen)	Injection—10 mg/ml, 20 mg/ml, 40 mg/ml	IM—30 mg or more every 1 week to 2 weeks	Advanced prostatic carcinoma (DOC)	
Estramustine phosphate sodium (EMCYT)	Capsules—140 mg	14 mg/kg/day in 3 or 4 divided doses; maintenance therapy 10 mg/kg to 16 mg/kg/day in divided doses	Advanced prostatic carcinoma	Store in refrigerator and protect from light; continue treatment 1 month to 3 months to determine efficacy; may increase serum bilirubin, LDH, and SGOT concentrations
Estrogens, conjugated (Premarin)	Tablets—0.3 mg, 0.625 mg, 1.25 mg, 2.5 mg	Breast cancer: 10 mg 3 times a day Prostatic cancer: 1.25 mg to 2.5 mg 3 times a day	Advanced breast and prostatic carcinoma (DOC)	Continue breast cancer treatment 8 weeks to 12 weeks to determine efficacy; determine effectiveness in prostatic cancer by monitoring serum phosphate levels, which should decrease
Estrone	Injection—2 mg/ml, 5 mg/ml	IM—2 mg to 4 mg 2 to 3 times a week	Advanced prostatic carcinoma (DOC)	Continue treatment for 3 months to determine efficacy
Ethinyl estradiol (Estinyl, Feminone)	Tablets—0.02 mg, 0.05 mg, 0.5 mg	Breast cancer: 1 mg 3 times a day Prostatic cancer: 0.15 mg to 2 mg/day	Advanced breast and prostatic carcinoma (DOC)	
Polyestradiol phosphate (Estradurin)	Injection—40 mg	IM—40 mg every 2 weeks to 4 weeks; may increase to 80 mg	Advanced prostatic carcinoma (DOC)	Continue treatment for 3 months to determine efficacy, reconstitute with sterile diluent provided; do *not* agitate violently; store at room temperature away from light for 10 days and discard at first sign of cloudiness or precipitate
Progestins				
Hydroxyprogesterone caproate (Delalutin)	Injection—125 mg/ml, 250 mg/ml	IM—1 g to 7 g/wk	Advanced endometrial carcinoma (stage III or IV) (DOC)	Stop therapy when relapse occurs or after 12 weeks with no objective response.
Medroxyprogesterone acetate (Provera, Depo-Provera)	Tablets—2.5 mg, 10 mg Injection—100 mg/ml, 400 mg/ml	Oral, IM—400 mg to 1000 mg/wk Maintenance—400 mg/mo or adjusted to patient's needs	Endometrial and renal carcinoma (DOC)	Recommended only as adjunctive and palliative therapy in advanced inoperable cases; usually well tolerated even in large doses; gluteal abscesses have occurred

Table 74-6. Hormonal and Antihormonal Agents *(continued)*

Drug	Preparations	Usual Dosage Range	Uses	Remarks
Megestrol acetate (Megace, Pallace)	Tablets—20 mg, 40 mg	Breast cancer: 40 mg 4 times a day Endometrial cancer: 40 mg to 320 mg/day in 4 divided doses	Breast and endometrial carcinoma (DOC)	Continue treatment at least 2 months to determine efficacy
Corticosteroids				
Prednisone (Deltasone, Orasone)	Tablets—1 mg, 2.5 mg, 5 mg, 10 mg, 20 mg, 50 mg	Acute and chronic lymphocytic leukemia: 40 mg to 60 mg/m²/day Hodgkin's disease and non-Hodgkin's lymphomas: 40 mg to 100 mg/m²/day Multiple myeloma: 75 mg/m²/day Breast cancer: 40 mg/m²/day	Acute and chronic lymphocytic leukemia (DOC) Hodgkin's disease (DOC) Non-Hodgkin's lymphomas (DOC) Multiple myeloma (DOC) Some breast cancers	Never used alone but always as a part of combination chemotherapy regimens; side-effects are minimized by alternate-day or intermittent therapy
Antihormonal Agents				
Mitotane (Lysodren)	Tablets—500 mg	Adult—initially, 8 g to 10 g/day in 3 to 4 divided doses; adjust dosage to maximum tolerated dose (usually 2 g to 16 g/day); maximum dose 18 g to 19 g/day Children—0.1 mg/kg to 0.5 mg/kg/day in divided doses or 1 g to 2 g/day in divided doses; may be gradually increased to 5 g to 7 g/day	Functional and nonfunctional adrenal cortical carcinoma (DOC)	Continue therapy 3 months to determine efficacy; may decrease protein-bound iodine and urinary 17-hydroxycorticosteroid levels; adrenocortical insufficiency can occur; replacement therapy may be necessary
Tamoxifen (Nolvadex)	Tablets—10 mg	10 mg to 20 mg twice a day	Advanced breast carcinoma (DOC)	May increase serum calcium levels; transient "flaring" of disease may occur during initial therapy, usually subsides rapidly; ocular toxicity is associated with long-term, high-dose therapy

DOC = Drug of choice

12 *Corticosteroids* may decrease blood salicylate levels by increasing glomerular filtration rate and by decreasing tubular reabsorption of water.

13 *Mitotane* alters *corticosteroid* metabolism and higher doses of corticosteroids may be needed to treat adrenal insufficiency.

14 *Mitotane* and CNS depressants used concurrently may cause additive CNS depression.

▶ **NURSING ALERTS**

See individual Nursing Alerts for androgens, estrogens, progestins, and corticosteroids. In addition

▷ 1 Be alert for signs and symptoms of hypercalcemia (polyuria, polydipsia, weakness, constipation, mental sluggishness or disorientation) in patients with met-astatic breast cancer being treated with androgens, estrogens, or progestins. Perform periodic serum calcium determinations.

▷ 2 Notify physician if a patient receiving testolactone complains of numbness or tingling of fingers, toes, or face, as these are possible symptoms of peripheral neuropathy.

▷ 3 Observe patients receiving androgens and oral anticoagulants concomitantly for signs of increased anticoagulant activity such as bruising, nose bleeds, or hematuria, and notify physician immediately.

▷ 4 Recognize that diabetic patients receiving androgens may have an enhanced response to the hypoglycemic agents. Symptoms of hypoglycemia include anxiety, chills, cold sweats, cool pale skin, drowsiness, excessive hunger, headache, nausea, nervousness, rapid pulse, shakiness, and weakness. Be prepared to give the patient some type of sugar or administer 50% Dextrose Solution.

▷ 5 Diabetic patients receiving estrogens, progestins, or corticosteroids may have a decreased glucose tolerance. Monitor urine sugar closely and notify physician immediately of any abnormalities.

▷ 6 Be aware that androgens, estrogens, and progestins may cause acute intermittent porphyria manifested by moderate to severe abdominal pain; notify physician immediately.

▷ 7 Be prepared to discontinue mitotane and administer exogenous steroids following shock or severe trauma to patients; adrenal suppression caused by mitotane may prevent the normal response.

▶ **NURSING CONSIDERATIONS**

See individual Nursing Considerations for androgens, estrogens, progestins, and corticosteroids. In addition

▷ 1 Inform female patients receiving androgens that signs and symptoms of virilization (hoarseness, deepening of the voice, hirsutism, enlarged clitoris, increased libido, oily skin, acne, menstrual irregularities) can occur.

▷ 2 Monitor serum calcium levels of breast cancer patients receiving androgens, estrogens, progestins, or tamoxifen. Notify physician immediately of any increase.

▷ 3 Monitor serum bilirubin of patients receiving androgens; fluoxymesterone and methyltestosterone can cause liver dysfunction.

▷ 4 Estrogens, progestins, and corticosteroids may elicit sodium and fluid retention. Monitor fluid intake and output, and be aware that patients with asthma, epilepsy, mental depression, migraine headaches, or cardiac or renal disease require careful observation.

▷ 5 Monitor serum cholesterol levels of patients receiving androgens and notify physician of any increase.

▷ 6 Oral androgen tablets may cause GI upset; administer with meals or a snack. Patients receiving *buccal* androgen tablets should not swallow the tablets but should allow them to dissolve between the gum and cheek (preferred) or under the tongue; they should avoid eating, drinking, or smoking while the tablet is in place.

▷ 7 Inform males receiving estrogens that gynecomastia can occur; low-dose breast irradiation before treatment may prevent development of gynecomastia.

▷ 8 Recommend contraceptive measures for patients receiving estrogens, progestins, tamoxifen, and mitotane.

▷ 9 Be aware that tamoxifen may cause a *transient* flare of the disease with increased tumor and bone pain. Advise the patient that this is not uncommon, and provide additional analgesics if needed.

▷ 10 Recognize that immobilized patients are most susceptible to hypercalcemia; encourage ambulation and adequate fluid intake to aid calcium excretion.

▷ 11 Ensure that patient package inserts are available to patients to read before initiation of therapy with any estrogen or progestin agent.

V Miscellaneous Agents

Hydroxyurea   Procarbazine

The two agents discussed in this section, hydroxyurea and procarbazine, are classified as miscellaneous agents because their mechanism of action does not correspond with the other classes of antineoplastic drugs.

Mechanism

Hydroxyurea—the exact mechanism of action is not completely established. Hydroxyurea causes an immediate inhibition of DNA synthesis without interfering with the synthesis of RNA or protein. It is a cell-cycle specific agent for the S phase of cell division.

Procarbazine—the exact mechanism of action is not completely established. Procarbazine may inhibit DNA, RNA, and protein synthesis; however, no cross-resistance with other alkylating agents has been demonstrated. It is cell-cycle specific for the S phase of cell division.

Uses

See Table 74-7.

Dosage

See Table 74-7.

Fate

Hydroxyurea is readily absorbed from the GI tract and readily crosses the blood–brain barrier. It is metabolized in the liver and excreted by the kidney as urea and hydroxyurea and by the lungs as carbon dioxide.

Procarbazine is rapidly and completely absorbed from the GI tract and readily crosses the blood–brain barrier. It is metabolized by the liver to active metabolites and excreted by the kidneys and lungs.

Common Side-Effects

Hydroxyurea—myelosuppression (leukopenia), drowsiness

Procarbazine—myelosuppression (leukopenia, thrombocytopenia, anemia), nausea, vomiting, diarrhea, fever, chills, sweating, myalgia, arthralgia

Significant Adverse Reactions

Hydroxyurea—GI disturbances, stomatitis, neurotoxicity (headache, dizziness, disorientation, hallucinations, convulsion), hyperuricemia, dysuria, uric acid nephropathy, maculopapular rash, facial edema, alopecia

Procarbazine—neurotoxicity (paresthesias, decreased tendon reflexes, peripheral neuropathies, depression, insomnia, nightmares, tremors, ataxia, convulsions), dermatological toxicity (pruritus, dermatitis, alopecia, photosensitivity, hyperpigmentation), ophthalmic toxicity (diplopia, nystagmus, photophobia, papilledema, retinal hemorrhage), pneumonitis, hepatotoxicity, dysuria, orthostatic hypotension, tachycardia, hypertensive crisis, impaired hearing

Table 74-7. Miscellaneous Antineoplastic Agents

Drug	Preparations	Usual Dosage Range	Uses	Remarks
Hydroxyurea (Hydrea)	Capsules—500 mg	Solid tumors: Intermittent therapy—80 mg/kg as a single dose every third day Continuous therapy—20 mg/kg to 30 mg/kg daily as a single dose Carcinoma of head and neck: 80 mg/kg as a single dose every third day; used concomitantly with radiation Myelocytic leukemia: 20 mg/kg to 30 mg/kg daily as a single dose.	Acute and chronic myelocytic leukemia Malignant melanoma Ovarian carcinoma Squamous cell carcinoma of head and neck (excluding the lip)	Discontinue therapy if leukocytes are less than 2500 and platelets are less than 100,000; drowsiness occurs with large doses; hydroxyurea should be started at least 7 days before radiation therapy and continued during and after radiation therapy; contents of capsules may be emptied into a glass of water and taken immediately if patient is unable to swallow capsules (some inert material may not dissolve and may float on the surface); may increase serum uric acid, BUN, and creatinine levels; dysuria may occur, but is usually temporary; intermittent therapy causes less toxicity; continue therapy 6 weeks to determine efficacy
Procarbazine (Matulane)	Capsules—50 mg	Adults—initially 2 mg/kg to 4 mg/kg/day (to the nearest 50 mg) in single or divided doses the first week; then 4 mg/kg to 6 mg/kg/day until leukocytes fall below 4000, platelets below 100,000, or a maximum clinical response is obtained Following recovery from hematologic toxicity, 1 mg to 2 mg/kg/day; maintenance—1 mg/kg to 2 mg/kg/day Children—initially, 50 mg/day for 1 week; then 100 mg/m² daily (to the nearest 50 mg) until hematological toxicity occurs or maximum response occurs, then 50 mg/day after recovery; maintenance—50 mg/day	Hodgkin's disease (DOC) Non-Hodgkin's lymphomas (DOC) Lung carcinoma Malignant melanoma Brain tumors Multiple myeloma	Tolerance to GI side-effects usually develops within several days; fever, chills, and sweating are most common during early stages of therapy; use in children is limited; undue toxicity such as tremors, coma, and convulsions have occurred; dosage must be individualized

DOC = Drug of choice

Contraindications

Hydroxyurea and procarbazine therapy should not be initiated in any patient with marked bone marrow depression.

Interactions

1 *Hydroxyurea* may antagonize the effects of antigout medications by increasing serum uric acid; dosage adjustment of the antigout medications may be necessary.
2 *Procarbazine* and ethanol ingestion may cause a disulfiram-like reaction and have an additive CNS depressant effect.
3 Concurrent use of *procarbazine* with tricyclic antidepressants, monoamine oxidase (MAO) inhibitors, or phenothiazines, may cause a severe hypertensive crisis.
4 Thiazide diuretics administered concurrently with *procarbazine* may cause enhanced hypotension.
5 CNS depressants such as narcotic analgesics and barbiturates used concurrently with *procarbazine* may cause enhanced CNS depression and hypotension in some patients but may cause excitation, rigidity, sweating, hyperpyrexia, and hypertension in others.

6 *Procarbazine* may enhance the effects of insulin and oral hypoglycemic medications; dosage adjustment of hypoglycemic agents may be necessary.

7 Guanethidine, levodopa, methyldopa, or reserpine used concurrently with *procarbazine* may result in hypertension and excitation.

8 Sympathomimetics such as amphetamines, epinephrine, ephedrine, isoproterenol, methylphenidate, and phenylpropanolamine used concurrently with *procarbazine* may cause hyperpyrexia and a severe hypertensive crisis.

9 Ingestion of foods with a high tyramine content (see Nursing Alerts) may cause a severe hypertensive crisis in a patient on *procarbazine* therapy.

▶ NURSING ALERTS

See general discussion of nursing alerts for all antineoplastic agents. In addition

▷ 1 Be aware that hydroxyurea may cause temporary impairment of renal function; carefully monitor patient's input and output, as well as BUN and serum creatinine levels. Patients with renal impairment who receive hydroxyurea may develop auditory and visual hallucinations or increased hematologic toxicity.

▷ 2 Notify physician immediately if a patient complains of chest pain, severe headache, or stiff neck, indications of a possible hypertensive reaction.

▷ 3 Be aware that the following foods and beverages are high in tyramine content: alcohol (chianti, sherry, hearty red wines, beer), aged and natural cheeses, sour cream, pickled herring, broad beans, yeast extract, chicken liver, raisins, canned figs, chocolate, excessive amounts of caffeine (coffee, cola beverages), soy sauce, yogurt, avocados, ripe bananas, pineapple, and meats prepared with tenderizers. Advise patients receiving procarbazine to avoid these foods.

▷ 4 When initiating procarbazine therapy, be sure that patients have not taken any MAO inhibitors within the last 14 days or tricyclic antidepressants within the last 7 days.

▷ 5 Be aware that many prescription and nonprescription cough and cold, asthma, hay fever, and allergy medications, appetite depressants, and antiemetics contain sympathomimetic agents, which must be avoided while taking procarbazine; check the ingredients of all medications before administration.

▶ NURSING CONSIDERATIONS

See general discussion of nursing considerations for all antineoplastic agents. In addition

▷ 1 Inform patients receiving hydroxyurea and who have previously received radiation therapy that they may have an exacerbation of postirradiation erythema.

▷ 2 Monitor diabetic patients receiving procarbazine for signs of hypoglycemia.

▷ 3 Urge patients to continue to avoid previously listed foods, drugs, or drinks for at least 14 days after discontinuing procarbazine.

▷ 4 Inform patients on procarbazine therapy to avoid over-the-counter cough syrups and mouthwashes that contain alcohol.

▷ 5 Inform patients on procarbazine to exercise caution while driving or performing other tasks requiring mental alertness, due to development of possible drowsiness, dizziness, or blurred vision.

▷ 6 Note that flu-like symptoms that may occur during initiation of procarbazine therapy will generally abate after 7 days to 10 days.

VI Combination Chemotherapy

Combination chemotherapy is widely used today in many neoplastic diseases to produce higher response rates and longer periods of remission than that obtained with single-agent therapy. Combinations of agents are also used to delay the emergence of resistance in the tumor cells and to obtain a synergistic therapeutic effect with minimal toxicity.

The general principles used for the selection of agents to be used for a combination chemotherapeutic regimen are as follows:

1 Each agent used in the regimen must be *clinically active* in the specific disease.

2 To obtain synergism, each agent must have a *different mechanism* of action. Agents are used to block different sites in biochemical pathways or to inhibit critical cell functions. Three different types of blockade have been described:
   a Sequential blockade—the inhibition of two different steps of the same biochemical pathway
   b Concurrent blockade—the blockade of parallel metabolic pathways leading to a common end product
   c Complementary inhibition—inhibition at different sites in the synthesis of large polymeric molecules

3 Agents are used that have *different toxicities* or different timing of a similar toxicity. This reduces cumulative toxicity to a single organ system and allows for individual agents to be used in full clinical doses.

4 Agents are *scheduled* with respect to tumor cell kinetics to potentiate the effect of each agent in the regimen. Both cell-cycle specific and cell-cycle nonspecific agents are used in regimens to simultaneously kill both dividing and nondividing cell fractions in the tumor. Careful intermittent scheduling has also proved to be less immunosuppressive and less toxic than continuous daily therapy.

Table 74-8 lists a number of currently used combination chemotherapeutic regimens, according to their commonly known acronym. Individual drug components of the combination are given along with the recommended dosage and indications.

Table 74-8. Combination Chemotherapeutic Regimens

Acronym	Drug	Dosage	Indication
ABVD	A—Doxorubicin B—Bleomycin V—Vinblastine D—Dacarbazine	25 mg/m^2 IV days 1 and 14 10 mg/m^2 IV days 1 and 14 6 mg/m^2 IV days 1 and 14 375 mg/m^2 IV days 1 and 14 Repeat every 28 days for 6 to 8 cycles	Hodgkin's disease
AC–BCG	A—Doxorubicin C—Cyclophosphamide BCG—Bacillus Calmette- Guérin	40 mg/m^2 IV day 1 200 mg/m^2 IV days 3 to 6 1 vial by scarification on days 8 and 15 Repeat every 3 weeks to 4 weeks	Ovarian carcinoma
A Ce	A—Doxorubicin Ce—Cyclophosphamide	40 mg/m^2 IV day 1 200 mg/m^2 PO days 3 to 6 Repeat every 21 days to 28 days	Breast carcinoma
A-COPP	A—Doxorubicin C—Cyclophosphamide O—Vincristine P—Procarbazine P—Prednisone	60 mg/m^2 IV day 1 300 mg/m^2 IV days 14 and 20 1.5 mg/m^2 IV days 14 and 20 (maximum 2 mg) 100 mg/m^2 PO days 14 to 28 40 mg/m^2 PO days 1 to 27 (1st and 4th cycles) days 14 to 27 (2nd, 3rd, 5th, and 6th cycles) Repeat every 42 days for 6 cycles	Hodgkin's disease
Ad–OAP	Ad—Doxorubicin O—Vincristine A—Cytarabine P—Prednisone	40 mg/m^2 IV day 1 2 mg IV day 1 70 mg/m^2 continuous infusion days 1 to 7 100 mg/day days 1 to 5 Repeat after 2 weeks	Acute myelocytic leukemia
Adria + BCNU	Adria—Doxorubicin BCNU—Carmustine	30 mg/m^2 IV day 1 30 mg/m^2 IV day 1 Repeat every 21 days to 28 days	Multiple myeloma
Ara-C + ADR	Ara-C—Cytarabine ADR—Doxorubicin	100 mg/m^2 continuous IV infusion for 7 days to 10 days 30 mg/m^2 IV days 1 to 3	Acute myelocytic leukemia
Ara-C + DNR + PRED + MP	Ara-C—Cytarabine DNR—Daunorubicin PRED—Prednisolone MP—Mercaptopurine	80 mg/m^2 IV days 1 to 3 25 mg/m^2 IV day 1 40 mg/m^2 PO daily 100 mg/m^2 PO daily Repeat weekly until remission, then monthly for maintenance	Acute myelocytic leukemia (in children)
Ara-C + 6-TG	Ara-C—Cytarabine 6-TG—Thioguanine	100 mg/m^2 IV every 12 hours for 10 days 100 mg/m^2 PO every 12 hours for 10 days Repeat every 30 days until remission, then repeat monthly for 5 days for maintenance	Acute myelocytic leukemia
AV	A—Doxorubicin V—Vincristine	60 mg/m^2 day 1 1.4 mg/m^2 day 1 Repeat every 3 weeks	Breast carcinoma
BACON	B—Bleomycin A—Doxorubicin C—Lomustine O—Vincristine N—Mechlorethamine	30 U IV (6 hr after vincristine) 40 mg/m^2 IV day 1; Repeat every 4 weeks 65 mg/m^2 PO day 1 Repeat every 4 weeks to 8 weeks 0.75 mg to 1 mg IV day 2 Repeat every week for 6 weeks 8 mg/m^2 IV day 1 (30 min after lomustine) Repeat every 4 weeks	Squamous cell carcinoma of lung
BACOP	B—Bleomycin A—Doxorubicin C—Cyclophosphamide O—Vincristine P—Prednisone	5 mg/m^2 IV days 15 and 22 25 mg/m^2 IV days 1 and 8 650 mg/m^2 IV days 1 and 8 1.4 mg/m^2 IV days 1 and 8 60 mg/m^2 PO days 15 to 28 Repeat every 28 days for 6 cycles	Non-Hodgkin's lymphomas

(continued)

Table 74-8. Combination Chemotherapeutic Regimens (continued)

Acronym	Drug	Dosage	Indication
BCAP	B—Carmustine C—Cyclophosphamide A—Doxorubicin P—Prednisone	50 mg/m² IV day 1 200 mg/m² IV day 1 20 mg/m² IV day 2 60 mg/m² PO days 1 to 5 Repeat every 4 weeks	Multiple myeloma
B–CAVe	B—Bleomycin C—Lomustine A—Doxorubicin Ve—Vinblastine	5 mg/m² IV days 1, 28, 35 100 mg/m² PO day 1 60 mg/m² IV day 1 5 mg/m² IV day 1 Repeat every 6 weeks for 9 cycles	Hodgkin's disease
BCMF	B—Bleomycin C—Cyclophosphamide M—Methotrexate F—Fluorouracil	7.5 mg/m² continuous infusion days 1 to 3 300 mg/m² IV day 5 30 mg/m² IV day 5 300 mg/m² IV day 5 Repeat every 3 weeks	Squamous cell carcinoma of head and neck
BCNU + 5-FU	BCNU—Carmustine 5–FU—Fluorouracil	40 mg/m² IV days 1 to 5 10 mg/kg IV days 1 to 5 Repeat every 6 weeks	Gastric carcinoma
BCOP	B—Carmustine C—Cyclophosphamide O—Vincristine P—Prednisone	100 mg/m² IV day 1 600 mg/m² IV day 1 1 mg/m² IV days 1 and 14 40 mg/m² PO days 1 to 7 Repeat every 28 days	Non-Hodgkin's lymphomas
BCVPP	B—Carmustine C—Cyclophosphamide V—Vinblastine P—Procarbazine P—Prednisone	100 mg/m² IV day 1 600 mg/m² IV day 1 5 mg/m² IV day 1 100 mg/m² PO days 1 to 10 60 mg/m² PO days 1 to 10 Repeat every 28 days for 6 cycles	Hodgkin's disease
B–DOPA	B—Bleomycin D—Dacarbazine O—Vincristine P—Prednisone A—Doxorubicin	4 U mg/m² IV days 2 and 5 150 mg/m² IV days 1 to 5 1.5 mg/m² IV days 1 and 5 40 mg/m² PO days 1 to 6 60 mg/m² IV day 1 Repeat every 21 days	Hodgkin's disease
BHD	B—Carmustine H—Hydroxyurea D—Dacarbazine	100 mg or 150 mg/m²/day IV day 1 Repeat every 6 weeks 1480 mg/m²/day PO days 1 to 5 Repeat every 3 weeks 100 mg or 150 mg/m²/day IV days 1 to 5 Repeat every 3 weeks	Malignant melanoma
BM	B—Bleomycin M—Mitomycin	5 mg/day IV days 1 to 7 10 mg IV day 8 Repeat every 2 weeks	Carcinoma of cervix
BOPP	B—Carmustine O—Vincristine P—Procarbazine P—Prednisone	80 mg/m² IV day 1 1.4 mg/m² IV days 1 and 8 50 mg PO day 1; 100 mg PO day 2; 100 mg/m²/day PO days 3 to 14 40 mg/m²/day PO days 1 to 14 Repeat every 28 days for 6 cycles	Hodgkin's disease
BVD	B—Carmustine V—Vincristine D—Dacarbazine	65 mg/m² IV days 1, 2, 3 1 mg to 1.5 mg IV weekly 250 mg/m² IV days 1, 2, 3 Repeat every 6 weeks	Malignant melanoma
CAF	C—Cyclophosphamide A—Doxorubicin F—Fluorouracil	100 mg/m² PO days 1 to 14 30 mg/m² IV days 1 and 8 500 mg/m² IV days 1 and 8 Repeat every 4 weeks until total dose of 450 mg/m² doxorubicin is administered; then discontinue doxorubicin and replace with methotrexate 40 mg/m² IV and increase fluorouracil to 600 mg/m² IV	Breast carcinoma
CAMP	C—Cyclophosphamide A—Doxorubicin M—Methotrexate	300 mg/m² IV days 1 and 8 20 mg/m² IV days 1 and 8 15 mg/m² IV days 1 and 8	Lung carcinoma (non-oat cell)

Table 74-8. Combination Chemotherapeutic Regimens *(continued)*

Acronym	Drug	Dosage	Indication
	P—Procarbazine	100 mg/m^2 PO days 1 to 10 Repeat every 28 days	
CAP	C—Cyclophosphamide A—Doxorubicin P—Cisplatin	400 mg/m^2 IV day 1 40 mg/m^2 IV day 1 40 mg/m^2 IV day 1 Repeat every 4 weeks for 10 cycles	Adenocarcinoma of lung
CAVe	C—Lomustine A—Doxorubicin V—Vinblastine	100 mg/m^2 PO day 1 60 mg/m^2 IV day 1 5 mg/m^2 IV day 1 Repeat every 6 weeks for 9 cycles	Hodgkin's disease
CCV	C—Cyclophosphamide C—Lomustine V—Vincristine	700 mg/m^2 IV days 1 and 22 70 mg/m^2 PO day 1 2 mg IV days 1 and 22 Repeat every 6 weeks	Oat-cell carcinoma of lung
CCV–AV	C—Lomustine C—Cyclophosphamide V—Vincristine AV—Doxorubicin	100 mg/m^2 PO day 1 1 g/m^2 IV days 1 and 22 2 mg IV days 1, 22, 42, 63 75 mg/m^2 IV days 42 and 63 Repeat every 12 weeks	Oat-cell carcinoma of lung

CHL + PRED	CHL—Chlorambucil
	
	PRED—Prednisone
		0.4 mg/kg PO 1 day every other week,
		    increase by 0.1 mg/kg every 2 weeks
		    until toxicity or control
		100 mg/PO days 1 and 2 every other week
			Chronic lymphocytic leukemia

CHOP	C—Cyclophosphamide
	H—Doxorubicin
	O—Vincristine
	
	P—Prednisone
		750 mg/m^2 IV day 1
		50 mg/m^2 IV day 1
		1.4 mg/m^2 IV day 1
		    (maximum 2 mg)
		60 mg/day PO days 1 to 5
		Repeat every 21 days to 28 days for 6
		    cycles
			Non-Hodgkin's lymphoma

CHOP–BCG	CHOP (as above) *plus* BCG—Bacillus Calmette– Guérin	 1 vial by scarification days 7 and 14	Non-Hodgkin's lymphoma
CHOP–Bleo	C—Cyclophosphamide H—Doxorubicin O—Vincristine P—Prednisone Bleo—Bleomycin	750 mg/m^2 IV day 1 50 mg/m^2 IV day 1 1.4 mg/m^2 IV day 1 (maximum 2 mg) 100 mg/m^2/day days 1 to 5 4 U IV days 1 and 8 Repeat every 21 days to 28 days	Non-Hodgkin's lymphoma
CHOR	C—Cyclophosphamide H—Doxorubicin O—Vincristine R—Radiation	750 mg/m^2 IV days 1 and 22 50 mg/m^2 IV days 1 and 22 1 mg IV days 1, 8, 15, 22 3000 rad total dose in daily fractions over 2 weeks starting day 36	Lung carcinoma

CISCA	CIS—Cisplatin
	
	C—Cyclophosphamide
	
	A—Doxorubicin
		100 mg/m^2 IV infusion over 2 hours
		    day 2
		650 mg/m^2 IV day 1
		Increase to 1000 mg/m^2 when doxorubicin
		    discontinued
		50 mg/m^2 IV day 1; discontinue at 450 mg/
		    m^2 total dose; repeat every 21 days.
			Urinary carcinoma

CMC—High dose	C—Cyclophosphamide M—Methotrexate C—Lomustine	1000 mg/m^2 IV days 1 and 29 15 mg/m^2 IV twice a week for 6 weeks 100 mg/m^2 PO day 1	Lung carcinoma

CMC–V	C—Cyclophosphamide
	M—Methotrexate
	C—Lomustine
	
	V—Vincristine
		700 mg/m^2 IV day 1
		20 mg/m^2 PO days 18 and 21
		70 mg/m^2 PO day 1; repeat every 28 days
		2 mg IV days 1, 8, 15, 22 then 1.3 mg/m^2
		    IV every 4 weeks
			Small-cell carcinoma of the
			    lung

CMF	C—Cyclophosphamide M—Methotrexate F—Fluorouracil	100 mg/m^2 PO days 1 to 14 40 mg to 60 mg/m^2 IV days 1 and 8 600 mg/m^2 IV days 1 and 8 Repeat every 28 days	Breast carcinoma

(continued)

Table 74-8. Combination Chemotherapeutic Regimens (continued)

Acronym	Drug	Dosage	Indication
CMFP	C—Cyclophosphamide M—Methotrexate F—Fluorouracil P—Prednisone	100 mg/m^2 PO days 1 to 14 60 mg/m^2 IV days 1 and 8 700 mg/m^2 IV days 1 and 8 40 mg/m^2 PO days 1 to 14	Breast carcinoma

CMFVP
  (Cooper's regimen)
	C—Cyclophosphamide
	M—Methotrexate
	F—Fluorouracil
	V—Vincristine
	
	P—Prednisone
		2 mg/kg PO daily
		0.75 mg/kg IV weekly
		12 mg/kg IV weekly
		0.025 mg/kg IV weekly
		  (maximum 2 mg)
		0.75 mg/kg PO days 1 to 21 then taper
			Breast carcinoma

COMA	C—Cyclophosphamide
	O—Vincristine
	M—Methotrexate
	
	A—Cytarabine
		1.5 g/m^2 IV
		1.4 mg/m^2 IV days 1, 8, 15
		120 mg/m^2 PO
		Give leucovorin 25 mg PO every 6 hours
		  for 4 doses starting 6 hours after
		  methotrexate
		300 mg/m^2 IV bolus 16 hours after
		  methotrexate
		Repeat every 7 days to 14 days for 8
		  cycles through days 22 to 71
			Non-Hodgkin's lymphoma

COAP	C—Cyclophosphamide O—Vincristine A—Cytarabine P—Prednisone	100 mg/m^2 IV days 1 to 5 1 mg IV days 1, 8, 15, 22 200 mg/m^2 IV days 1 to 5 or 100 mg/m^2 IV days 1 to 10 100 mg/day PO days 1 to 5 Repeat after 2-week interval	Acute myelocytic leukemia
COP	C—Cyclophosphamide O—Vincristine P—Prednisone	1,000 mg/m^2 IV day 1 1.4 mg/m^2 IV day 1 (maximum 2 mg) 60 mg/m^2 PO days 1 to 5 Repeat every 21 days for 6 cycles	Non-Hodgkin's lymphoma
COP–BLAM	C—Cyclophosphamide O—Vincristine P—Prednisone B—Bleomycin A—Doxorubicin M—Procarbazine	400 mg/m^2 IV day 1 1 mg/m^2 IV day 1 40 mg/m^2 PO days 1 to 10 15 U IV day 14 40 mg/m^2 IV day 1 100 mg/m^2 PO days 1 to 10 Repeat every 21 days	Histiocytic lymphoma
COPP or C–MOPP	C—Cyclophosphamide O—Vincristine P—Procarbazine P—Prednisone	650 mg/m^2 IV days 1 and 8 1.4 mg/m^2 IV days 1 and 8 (maximum 2 mg) 100 mg/m^2 PO days 1 to 14 40 mg/m^2 PO days 1 to 14 Repeat every 28 days for 6 cycles	Non-Hodgkin's lymphoma
CVB	C—Cisplatin V—Vinblastine B—Bleomycin	20 mg/m^2 IV days 1 to 5 Repeat every 3 weeks for 3 cycles 0.2 mg/kg IV days 1 and 2 Repeat every 3 weeks for 12 weeks; then 0.3 mg/kg IV every 4 weeks for 2 years 30 U IV weekly for 12 weeks	Testicular carcinoma
CVB	C—Lomustine V—Vinblastine B—Bleomycin	100 mg/m^2 PO day 1 6 mg/m^2 IV days 1 and 8 15 U/m^2 IV days 1 and 8 Repeat every 28 days	Hodgkin's disease
CVP	C—Cyclophosphamide V—Vincristine P—Prednisone	400 mg/m^2 PO days 2 to 6 1.4 mg/m^2 IV day 1 (maximum 2 mg) 40 mg/m^2 PO days 1 to 14 Repeat every 28 days for 6 cycles	Non-Hodgkin's lymphoma
CVPP	C—Cyclophosphamide V—Vinblastine P—Procarbazine P—Prednisone	300 mg/m^2 IV days 1 and 8 10 mg/m^2 IV days 1, 8, and 15 100 mg/m^2 PO days 1 to 15 40 mg/m^2 PO days 1 to 15 (cycles 1 and 4 only) Repeat every 28 days	Hodgkin's disease

Table 74-8. Combination Chemotherapeutic Regimens (continued)

Acronym	Drug	Dosage	Indication
CVPP/CCNU	C—Cyclophosphamide V—Vinblastine P—Procarbazine P—Prednisone CCNU—Lomustine	600 mg/m² IV day 1 6 mg/m² IV day 1 100 mg/m² PO days 1 to 14 40 mg/m² PO days 1 to 14 75 mg/m² day 1 (alternate cycles) Repeat every 28 days	Hodgkin's disease
CY–VA–DIC	CY—Cyclophosphamide V—Vincristine A—Doxorubicin DIC—Dacarbazine	500 mg/m² IV day 1 1.4 mg/m² IV days 1 and 5 (maximum 2 mg) 50 mg/m² IV day 1 250 mg/m² IV days 1 to 5 Repeat every 21 days	Soft-tissue sarcomas
DA	D—Daunorubicin A—Cytarabine	45 mg/m² IV days 1 to 3 100 mg/m² IV days 1 to 10 Repeat as needed	Acute myelocytic leukemia
DOAP	D—Daunorubicin O—Vincristine A—Cytarabine P—Prednisone	60 mg/m² IV day 1 1 mg IV days 1, 8, 15, 22 200 mg/m² IV days 1 to 5 or 100 mg/m² IV days 1 to 10 100 mg/day PO days 1 to 5 Repeat after 2-week interval	Acute myelocytic leukemia
FAC	F—Fluorouracil A—Doxorubicin C—Cyclophosphamide	500 mg/m² IV days 1 and 8 50 mg/m² IV day 1 500 mg/m² IV day 1 Repeat every 3 weeks	Breast carcinoma
FAM	F—Fluorouracil A—Doxorubicin M—Mitomycin or F—Fluorouracil A—Doxorubicin M—Mitomycin	600 mg/m² IV days 1, 2, 28, 36 30 mg/m² IV days 1 and 28 10 mg/m² IV day 1 Repeat every 8 weeks 600 mg/m² IV week 1, 2, 5, 6, 9 30 mg/m² IV week 1, 5, 9 10 mg/m² IV week 1 and 9	Lung or gastric carcinoma Pancreatic carcinoma
FAP	F—Fluorouracil A—Doxorubicin P—Cisplatin	500 mg/m² IV day 1 50 mg/m² IV day 1 100 mg/m² IV day 1 Reduce to 50 mg to 75 mg/m² after 3 doses Repeat every 4 weeks	Bladder carcinoma
FIVB	F—Fluorouracil I—Dacarbazine V—Vincristine B—Carmustine	10 mg/kg IV days 1 to 5 3 mg/kg IV days 1 and 2 0.025 mg/kg IV day 1 1.5 mg/kg IV day 1 Repeat every 6 weeks	Colorectal carcinoma
FOMi	F—Fluorouracil O—Vincristine Mi—Mitomycin	300 mg/m² IV days 1 to 4 2 mg IV day 1 10 mg/m² IV day 1 Repeat every 3 weeks for 3 cycles then every 6 weeks	Lung carcinoma (non-small cell)
HOP	H—Doxorubicin O—Vincristine P—Prednisone	80 mg/m² IV day 1 1.4 mg/m² IV day 1 (maximum 2 mg) 100 mg/m² PO days 1 to 5 Repeat every 3 weeks	Non-Hodgkin's lymphoma
M–2 Protocol	Vincristine Carmustine Cyclophosphamide Melphalan Prednisone	0.03 mg/kg IV day 1 (maximum 2 mg) 0.5 mg/kg IV day 1 10 mg/kg IV day 1 0.25 mg/kg PO days 1 to 14 1 mg/kg PO days 1 to 7, then taper to day 21 Repeat every 35 days	Multiple myeloma
MA	M—Mitomycin A—Doxorubicin	10 mg/m² IV day 1 50 mg/m² IV days 1 and 22 Repeat every 6 weeks	Breast carcinoma Adenocarcinoma of lung

(continued)

Table 74-8. Combination Chemotherapeutic Regimens (continued)

Acronym	Drug	Dosage	Indication
MAC	M—Methotrexate A—Dactinomycin C—Chlorambucil	15 mg IM days 1 to 5 8 mcg to 10 mcg/kg IV days 1 to 5 8 mg to 10 mg PO days 1 to 5 Repeat every 10 days to 14 days	Choriocarcinoma
MACC	M—Methotrexate A—Doxorubicin C—Cyclophosphamide C—Lomustine	40 mg/m² IV day 1 40 mg/m² IV day 1 400 mg/m² IV day 1 30 mg/m² PO day 1 Repeat every 21 days	Lung carcinoma (non-oat cell)
MACM	M—Mitomycin A—Doxorubicin C—Lomustine M—Methotrexate	8 mg/m² IV day 1 60 mg/m² IV day 1 60 mg/m² PO day 1 40 mg/m² IV day 1 Repeat every 4 weeks	Squamous cell carcinoma of lung
MAP	M—Melphalan A—Doxorubicin P—Prednisone	6 mg/m² PO days 1 to 4 25 mg/m² IV day 1 60 mg/m² PO days 1 to 4 Repeat every 4 weeks	Multiple myeloma
MCBP	M—Melphalan C—Cyclophosphamide B—Carmustine P—Prednisone	4 mg/m² PO days 1 to 4 300 mg/m² IV day 1 30 mg/m² IV day 1 60 mg/m² PO days 1 to 4 Repeat every 4 weeks	Multiple myeloma
MCP	M—Melphalan C—Cyclophosphamide P—Prednisone	6 mg/m² PO days 1 to 4 500 mg/m² PO day 1 60 mg/m² PO days 1 to 4 Repeat every 4 weeks	Multiple myeloma
MF	M—Mitomycin F—Fluorouracil	15 mg to 20 mg/m² IV day 1 Repeat every 8 weeks Reduce dose 50% after second dose 1 g/m² continuous IV infusion over 24 hours days 1 to 4 Repeat every 4 weeks	Colorectal carcinoma
MOB	M—Mitomycin O—Vincristine B—Bleomycin	20 mg/m² IV day 1 0.5 mg/m² IV twice a week for 12 weeks 6 U/m² IM or IV 6 hours after vincristine twice a week for 12 weeks Repeat every 6 weeks	Squamous cell carcinoma of cervix
MOPP	M—Mechlorethamine O—Vincristine P—Procarbazine P—Prednisone	6 mg/m² IV days 1 and 8 1.4 mg/m² IV days 1 and 8 (maximum 2 mg) 100 mg/m² PO days 1 to 14 40 mg/m² PO days 1 to 14 Repeat every 28 days for 6 to 8 cycles	Hodgkin's disease
MOPP–LO BLEO	M—Mechlorethamine O—Vincristine P—Procarbazine P—Prednisone BLEO—Bleomycin	6 mg/m² IV days 1 and 8 1.5 mg/m² IV days 1 and 8 (maximum 2 mg) 100 mg/m² PO days 2 to 7, 9 to 12 40 mg/m² PO days 2 to 7, 9 to 12 2 mg/m² IV days 1 and 8 Repeat every 28 days for 6 cycles	Hodgkin's disease
MP	M—Melphalan P—Prednisone	0.25 mg/kg days 1 to 4 2 mg/kg days 1 to 4 Repeat every 6 weeks	Multiple myeloma
MPL + PRED (MP)	MPL—Melphalan PRED—Prednisone	8 mg/m² PO days 1 to 14 75 mg/m² PO days 1 to 7	Multiple myeloma
MTX + MP	MTX—Methotrexate MP—Mercaptopurine	20 mg/m² IV weekly 50 mg/m²/day PO Continue until relapse or remission for 3 years	Acute lymphocytic leukemia
MTX + MP + CTX	MTX—Methotrexate MP—Mercaptopurine CTX—Cyclophosphamide	20 mg/m² IV weekly 50 mg/m²/day PO 200 mg/m² IV weekly Continue until relapse or remission for 3 years	Acute lymphocytic leukemia

Table 74-8. Combination Chemotherapeutic Regimens *(continued)*

Acronym	Drug	Dosage	Indication
MVPP	M—Mechlorethamine V—Vinblastine P—Procarbazine P—Prednisone	6 mg/m² IV days 1 to 8 6 mg/m² IV days 1 and 8 100 mg/m² PO days 1 to 14 40 mg/day PO days 1 to 14 Rest 28 days and repeat for 6 or more cycles	Hodgkin's disease
MVVPP	M—Mechlorethamine V—Vincristine V—Vinblastine P—Procarbazine P—Prednisone	0.4 mg/kg IV day 1 1.4 mg/m² IV days 1, 8, 15 6 mg/m² IV days 22, 29, 36 100 mg/m² PO days 22 to 43 40 mg/m² PO days 1 to 22, (taper over 14 days) Repeat every 57 days	Hodgkin's disease
OAP	O—Vincristine A—Cytarabine P—Prednisone	1 mg IV days 1, 8, 15, 22 200 mg/m² IV days 1 to 5 or 100 mg/m² IV days 1 to 10 100 mg PO days 1 to 5 Repeat after 2-week interval	Acute myelocytic leukemia
PA	P—Cisplatin A—Doxorubicin	50 mg to 60 mg/m² IV 50 mg to 60 mg/m² IV Repeat every 3 weeks to 4 weeks	Adenocarcinoma of prostate

PAC–5	P—Cisplatin
	
	A—Doxorubicin
	
	C—Cyclophosphamide
		20 mg/m² IV days 1 to 5
		  (total dose 300 mg/m²)
		50 mg/m² IV day 1
		  (total dose 450 mg/m²)
		750 mg/m² IV day 1
		  (increase dose 20% after stopping cisplatin and doxorubicin)
		Repeat every 3 weeks
			Ovarian carcinoma

PCV	P—Procarbazine C—Lomustine V—Vincristine	60 mg/m² PO days 8 to 21 110 mg/m² PO day 1 1.4 mg/m² IV days 8 and 29 Repeat every 6 weeks to 8 weeks	Primary malignant brain tumors
POCC	P—Procarbazine O—Vincristine C—Cyclophosphamide C—Lomustine	100 mg/m² PO days 1 to 14 2 mg IV days 1 and 8 600 mg/m² IV days 1 and 8 60 mg/m² PO day 1 Repeat every 28 days	Lung carcinoma
SCAB	S—Streptozocin C—Lomustine A—Doxorubicin B—Bleomycin	500 mg/m² IV days 1 and 15 100 mg/m² PO day 1 45 mg/m² IV day 1 15 U/m² IV days 1 and 8 Repeat every 28 days	Hodgkin's disease
SMF	S—Streptozocin M—Mitomycin F—Fluorouracil	600 mg/m² IV days 1, 8, 29, 36 10 mg/m² IV day 1 1000 mg/m² IV day 1 Repeat every 8 weeks	Pancreatic carcinoma

T–2 Protocol	*Cycle No. 1*
	Month 1
	  Dactinomycin
	  Doxorubicin
	  Radiation
	
	Month 2
	  Doxorubicin
	  Vincristine
	
	  Cyclophosphamide
	  Radiation
	
	Month 3
	  Vincristine
	
	  Cyclophosphamide
		
		0.45 mg/m² IV days 1 to 5
		20 mg/m² IV days 20 to 22
		Days 1 to 21, then rest 2 weeks
		
		20 mg/m² IV days 8 to 10
		1.5 mg to 2 mg/m² IV day 24
		  (maximum 2 mg)
		1200 mg/m² IV day 24
		Days 8 to 28
		
		1.5 mg to 2 mg/m² IV days 3, 9, 15
		  (maximum 2 mg)
		1200 mg/m² IV day 1
			Ewing's sarcoma

(continued)

Table 74-8. Combination Chemotherapeutic Regimens (continued)

Acronym	Drug	Dosage	Indication
	Cycle No. 2 Repeat cycle No. 1 without radiation		
	Cycle No. 3 *Month 1*		
	Dactinomycin	0.45 mg/m^2 IV days 1 to 5	
	Doxorubicin	20 mg/m^2 IV days 20 to 22	
	Month 2		
	Vincristine	1.5 mg to 2 mg/m^2 IV days 8, 15, 22, 28 (maximum 2 mg)	
	Cyclophosphamide	1200 mg/m^2 IV days 8 and 22	
	Month 3 No drugs given for 28 days		
	Cycle No. 4 Repeat Cycle No. 3		
TODD	T—Thioguanine	2 mg/kg PO days 1 to 5	Acute lymphocytic leukemia
	O—Vincristine	2 mg/m^2 IV day 1	
	D—Pyrimethamine	1.5 mg/kg PO days 1 to 5	
	D—Dexamethasone	2 mg/m^2 PO 3 times a day days 1 to 5 Repeat every 11 days with 6 days rest period	
TRAMPCO(L)	T—Thioguanine	100 mg/m^2 PO days 1 to 3 Increase to 4 days to 5 days after first course	Acute leukemias
	R—Daunorubicin	40 mg/m^2 IV day 1	
	A—Cytarabine	100 mg/m^2 IV days 1 to 3 Increase to 4 days to 5 days after first course	
	M—Methotrexate	7.5 mg/m^2 IV or IM days 1 to 3 Increase to 4 days to 5 days after first course	
	P—Prednisolone	200 mg PO days 1 to 3 Increase to 4 days to 5 days after first course	
	C—Cyclophosphamide	100 mg/m^2 IV days 1 to 3 Increase to 4 days to 5 days after first course	
	O—Vincristine	2 mg IV day 1	
	L—L-Asparaginase	8,000 U/m^2 IV days 1 to 28 in first two courses Repeat every 2 weeks, 3 weeks, or 4 weeks with wider spacing in patients with good response	
VAC Pulse	V—Vincristine	2 mg/m^2 IV weekly for weeks 1 to 12 (maximum 2 mg)	Sarcoma
	A—Dactinomycin	0.015 mg/kg IV days 1 to 5 of weeks 1 and 13, then every 3 months for 5 to 6 courses (maximum 0.5 mg a day)	
	C—Cyclophosphamide	10 mg/kg IV or PO for 7 days Repeat every 6 weeks for 2 years	
VAC Standard	V—Vincristine	2 mg/m^2 IV weekly for weeks 1 to 12 (maximum 2 mg)	Sarcoma
	A—Dactinomycin	0.015 mg/kg IV days 1 to 5 Repeat every 3 months for 5 to 6 courses (maximum 0.5 mg a day)	
	C—Cyclophosphamide	2.5 mg/kg PO daily for 2 years	
VBAP	V—Vincristine	1 mg IV day 1	Multiple myeloma
	B—Carmustine	30 mg/m^2 IV day 2	
	A—Doxorubicin	30 mg/m^2 IV day 2	
	P—Prednisone	60 mg/m^2 PO days 2 to 5 Repeat every 3 weeks	

Table 74-8. Combination Chemotherapeutic Regimens (continued)

Acronym	Drug	Dosage	Indication
VBP	V—Vinblastine	0.2 mg/kg IV days 1 and 2 Repeat every 3 weeks for 5 courses	Testicular carcinoma
	B—Bleomycin	30 U/wk IV 6 hours after vinblastine on the second day of each week for 12 weeks until total dose of 360 U	
	P—Cisplatin	20 mg/m^2 IV days 1 to 5, 6 hours after vinblastine Repeat every 3 weeks for 3 courses	
VCAP	V—Vincristine	1 mg IV day 1	Multiple myeloma
	C—Cyclophosphamide	100 mg/m^2 PO days 1 to 4	
	A—Doxorubicin	25 mg/m^2 IV day 2	
	P—Prednisone	60 mg/m^2 PO days 1 to 4 Repeat every 4 weeks	
VCR–MTX–CF	VCR—Vincristine	2 mg/m^2 IV for 1 dose (maximum 2 mg)	Osteogenic sarcoma
	MTX—Methotrexate	3000 mg to 7500 mg/m^2 IV 6-hour infusion starting 30 minutes after vincristine	
	CF—Citrovorum factor (calcium leucovorin)	15 mg IV every 3 hours for 8 doses, then 15 mg PO every 3 hours for 8 doses	
VM	V—Vinblastine	5 mg/m^2 IV	Adenocarcinoma of lung
	M—Mitomycin	6 mg/m^2 IV Repeat every 2 weeks	
VMCP	V—Vincristine	1 mg IV day 1	Multiple myeloma
	M—Melphalan	5 mg/m^2 PO days 1 to 4	
	C—Cyclophosphamide	100 mg/m^2 PO days 1 to 4	
	P—Prednisone	60 mg/m^2 PO days 1 to 4 Repeat every 3 weeks	
VP	V—Vincristine	2 mg/m^2 IV every week for 4 weeks to 6 weeks (maximum 2 mg)	Acute lymphocytic leukemia
	P—Prednisone	60 mg/m^2 PO daily for 4 weeks, then taper weeks 5 to 7	
VP–L–Asparaginase	V—Vincristine	2 mg/m^2 IV every week for 4 weeks to 6 weeks (maximum 2 mg)	Acute lymphocytic leukemia
	P—Prednisone	60 mg/m^2 PO daily for 4 weeks to 6 weeks, then taper	
	L—Asparaginase	10,000 U/m^2 IV days 1 to 14	

Nutrients, Fluids, and Electrolytes

IX

Vitamins are commonly classified as either water soluble (B-complex, C) or fat soluble (A, D, E, K). The water-soluble vitamins are reviewed in this chapter and the fat-soluble vitamins are discussed in Chapter 76.

Vitamins—General Considerations

Vitamins are organic substances required by the body for synthesis of essential cofactors that catalyze metabolic reactions. The body does not have the capacity to provide enough of all the essential vitamins, hence dietary sources are necessary. Since the average diet is usually more than adequate in supplying most required vitamins, there is rarely a need for additional vitamins in the majority of persons, and indiscriminate use of single- or multiple-vitamin preparations should be discouraged.

There are, however, certain situations in which vitamin supplementation can be justified. Vitamin deficiency states can result from inadequate nutritional intake; impaired absorption; increased requirements; malnutrition (*e.g.,* from starvation, anorexia, extreme diets, food faddism); pathologic conditions (GI disorders, hyperthyroidism, intestinal surgery, carcinomas); alcoholism; prolonged stress; dialysis; and a variety of other conditions. Provided that a definite vitamin deficiency can be demonstrated based upon clinical symptoms, *selective* replacement of those vitamins that are lacking is indicated. Use of multivitamin formulations for replacement therapy, however, is usually unnecessary and can become a significant expense as well. A much more reasonable approach is to supply the deficient vitamins in the amounts required to eliminate the symptoms of the vitamin deficiency state. For example, thiamine is indicated for beriberi, niacin for pellagra, ascorbic acid for scurvy, and cyanocobalamin for pernicious anemia. It is important, however, to regard vitamins as *drugs* and as such, they should only be used where there is valid indication. Injudicious or excessive intake of vitamins is at best wasteful and can lead to untoward reactions, especially in the case of the fat-soluble vitamins (A, D, E, K). Moreover, continued self-medication with vitamin preparations may delay recognition or mask the symptoms of a more serious underlying disease. Vitamin supplementation should only be undertaken following consultation with a health-care professional, and the type and amount of individual vitamins prescribed should be based upon thorough clinical assessment of the patient's diet, health status, and presenting symptoms.

In the past, vitamin preparations were labeled with the minimum daily requirements (MDR) for each component, and these values represented the amounts necessary to prevent development of deficiency symptoms. Today, however, the standard by which vitamins are labeled is the recommended dietary allowance (RDA). RDAs are *not* requirements, but simply recommended daily intake levels believed to be adequate for the nutritional needs of most healthy persons subject to normal degrees of stress. RDA values vary according to the age and sex of the person, and are not intended to cover nutritional needs during disease or other

Water-Soluble Vitamins— Vitamins B and C

75

abnormal conditions (*e.g.,* anemia, alcoholism, malnutrition), in which certain vitamin requirements can be significantly elevated. The current RDAs for the B-complex and C vitamins are listed in Table 75-1 and for the fat-soluble vitamins (A, D, E, K) in Table 76-1 in Chapter 76.

There is no convincing evidence that use of excessive amounts (*i.e.,* megadoses) of certain vitamins can cure or prevent nonnutritional diseases. Despite the many, usually anecdotal, claims made by proponents of megadose vitamin therapy for beneficial effects in diseases ranging from alopecia to warts, use of quantities of vitamins beyond those needed for normal body functioning is at the very least wasteful and can be potentially quite hazardous.

Certain vitamins are readily soluble in water and are found together in many of the same foods. They are therefore usually grouped together as the water-soluble vitamins. They include the B-complex group and ascorbic acid (vitamin C). These substances are readily excreted in the urine and thus are potentially much less toxic following large doses than are the fat-soluble vitamins, which are metabolized slowly and can be stored in significant amounts in the body. Table 75-1 lists the water-soluble vitamins together with their RDAs, dietary sources, and other pertinent information.

B-Complex Vitamins

The vitamin B-complex group is composed of a number of compounds that differ in structure and biological activity,

but are obtained from many of the same sources, most notably liver and yeast. Of the 11 members of the B-complex family, the need for four—biotin, choline, inositol, and p-aminobenzoic acid (PABA)—in human nutrition has not been established. These substances are not considered here; they are discussed briefly in Chapter 77. Two others, cyanocobalamin (vitamin B_{12}) and folic acid (vitamin B_9) have been reviewed in Chapter 34, because they are primarily indicated in the treatment of pernicious anemia; cyanocobalamin is discussed here only as a nutritional supplement. The remaining five B-complex vitamins are examined individually in this chapter.

▶ **vitamin B_1 (thiamine)**

Betalin S, Biamine

Thiamine, or vitamin B_1, is an organic molecule that combines with ATP to form thiamine pyrophosphate, a coenzyme essential for carbohydrate metabolism. Thiamine requirements are closely linked to caloric intake and clinical manifestations of thiamine deficiency can range from mild (anorexia, weakness, paresthesias, hypothermia, hypotension) to moderate (polyneuritis, sensory and motor defects, cardiovascular disease) to severe (Wernicke's encephalopathy, Korsakoff's psychosis). Beriberi, a thiamine deficiency characterized by GI disturbances, peripheral neurologic complications ("dry beriberi"), and cardiovascular disease ("wet beriberi"), is frequently observed in far eastern countries where the diet consists largely of polished rice, which is very low in thiamine. Alcoholism, on the other hand, is

Table 75-1. Water-Soluble Vitamins

Vitamin	Major Dietary Sources	Recommended Dietary Allowances			Principal Symptoms of Deficiency States
		Infants	*Children*	*Adults*	
B-Complex					
Thiamine (B₁)	Liver, whole grain, enriched bread and cereals, pork	0.3 mg to 0.5 mg	0.7 mg to 1.2 mg	1.0 mg to 1.5 mg	Anorexia, constipation, beriberi (cardiac complications, peripheral neuritis)
Riboflavin (B₂)	Organ meats, milk, eggs, green vegetables, enriched bread and flour	0.4 mg to 0.6 mg	0.8 mg to 1.4 mg	1.2 mg to 1.7 mg	Stomatitis, glossitis, ocular itching or burning, photophobia, facial dermatitis, cheilosis, corneal vascularization
Nicotinic acid (Niacin, B₃)	Liver, fish, poultry, red meat, enriched bread and cereals	6 mg to 8 mg	9 mg to 16 mg	13 mg to 18 mg	Pellagra (nervousness, insomnia, dermatitis, diarrhea, confusion, delusions)
Pantothenic acid (B₅)	Organ meats, egg yolks, beef, peanuts, whole grains, cauliflower	*	*	*	Weakness, fatigue, mood changes, dizziness, "burning-foot" syndrome
Pyridoxine (B₆)	Red meat, liver, yeast, whole grains, soy beans, green vegetables	0.3 mg to 0.6 mg	0.9 mg to 1.6 mg	1.8 mg to 2.2 mg	Anemia, CNS lesions, epileptic convulsions in children
Cyanocobalamin (B₁₂)	Red meat, milk, liver, egg yolk, oysters, clams	0.5 mcg to 1.5 mcg	2 mcg to 3 mcg	3 mcg	Pernicious anemia, glossitis, paresthesias, muscle incoordination, confusion
Vitamin C (Ascorbic acid)	Citrus fruits, tomatoes, green vegetables, potatoes, strawberries, green peppers	35 mg	45 mg	50 mg to 60 mg	Scurvy (petechiae, bleeding gums, bruising, impaired wound healing, loosened teeth)

*RDA is not established

the most common cause of thiamine deficiency in the United States.

Mechanism

Interacts with ATP to form thiamine pyrophosphate, a coenzyme that functions in the decarboxylation of alpha-keto and pyruvic acids and in the utilization of pentose by the hexose-monophosphate shunt

Uses

1 Prevention and treatment of thiamine deficiency states (*e.g.,* beriberi, alcoholism)—see Table 75-1

Dosage

Oral: 5 mg to 30 mg/day
IM (Beriberi): 10 mg to 20 mg three times/day for 2 weeks, supplemented with a daily oral multivitamin containing 5 mg to 10 mg thiamine
IV (Beriberi with myocardial failure; Wernicke–Korsakoff syndrome): up to 30 mg three times/day

Fate

Oral absorption is limited to 8 mg to 15 mg/day. As intake exceeds the minimal requirement (1 mg–2 mg), tissue stores become saturated, and the excess appears in the urine, either as unchanged thiamine or as a pyrimidine metabolite.

Significant Adverse Reactions

(Usually with large doses) Feeling of warmth, pruritus, urticaria, sweating, nausea, restlessness, weakness, cyanosis, dyspnea, tightness of the throat, angioedema, pulmonary edema, and GI hemorrhage

Interactions

1 Thiamine can enhance the response to peripherally acting muscle relaxants.
2 Thiamine is unstable in alkaline solutions, for example, with carbonates, citrates or barbiturates.

▶ NURSING ALERTS

▷ 1 When thiamine is to be administered IV, perform an intradermal sensitivity test before injection, because deaths have resulted from thiamine hypersensitivity following IV use.
▷ 2 Be aware that thiamine-deficient patients may experience a sudden worsening of the symptoms of Wernicke's encephalopathy (*e.g.,* ataxia, diplopia, tremor, agitation) following IV glucose administration. Administer thiamine before a glucose load.

▶ NURSING CONSIDERATIONS

▷ 1 Do not use thiamine in combination with alkaline solutions (*e.g.,* citrates, carbonates, bicarbonates, barbiturates), because drug is unstable in alkaline or neutral solutions.
▷ 2 Rotate IM injection sites to minimize discomfort.
▷ 3 Recognize that simple thiamine deficiency is unusual and is most often accompanied by multiple vitamin deficiencies. Apropriate supplementary therapy should be instituted.
▷ 4 Be aware that clinically significant thiamine depletion

can occur within 3 weeks in the total absence of dietary thiamine.

▶ vitamin B₂ (riboflavin)
Riobin-50

Riboflavin, or vitamin B$_2$, derives its name from the presence of the sugar ribose as a component of the molecule and from the fact that the remainder of the structure is a yellow pigmented compound termed a *flavin*. Riboflavin functions as a coenzyme that plays an essential role in the metabolism of a variety of cellular respiratory proteins.

Mechanism

Converted to one of two riboflavin-containing biologically active coenzymes, flavin mononucleotide (FMN) and flavin adenine dinucleotide (FAD), which play a vital metabolic role in the action of tissue respiratory flavoproteins

Uses

1 Prevention and treatment of riboflavin deficiency (ariboflavinosis)—see Table 75-1

Dosage

Oral: 5 mg to 10 mg/day
IM: 50 mg

Fate

Well absorbed orally; widely distributed in the body but very little is stored; in small amounts, approximately 10% is excreted in the urine; larger doses are eliminated in increasing proportion in the urine; drug is present in the feces, but probably represents vitamin synthesized by intestinal microorganisms

Interactions

1 Riboflavin may inhibit the activity of tetracyclines when mixed together in solution.
2 Riboflavin can reduce chloramphenicol-induced bone marrow depression and optic neuritis.

▶ NURSING CONSIDERATIONS

▷ 1 Recognize that the symptoms of riboflavin deficiency (sore throat, stomatitis, glossitis, corneal vascularization, cheilosis, seborrheic dermatitis, blepharospasm, photophobia) will usually disappear shortly after beginning riboflavin replacement therapy.
▷ 2 Inform patients that riboflavin will impart a harmless yellowish color to the urine. Note, however, that this color may interfere with urinary catecholamine determinations.
▷ 3 Note that dietary riboflavin deficiency seldom occurs as a discrete entity, but is usually accompanied by a lack of other vitamins and nutrients as well. Multivitamin replacement therapy is usually indicated.

▶ vitamin B₃ (nicotinic acid, niacin)

Nicotinic acid or niacin (vitamin B$_3$) is a B-complex vitamin that serves as a constituent of two important coenzymes, NAD (coenzyme I) and NADP (coenzyme II). These coenzymes function in various oxidation-reduction reactions required for cellular and tissue respiration. Niacin is an essential dietary constituent, the lack of which results in pellagra, a condition that primarily affects the skin, GI tract, and CNS, and is often characterized by the three "D's," that is, dermatitis, diarrhea, and dementia. In addition to its value in treating pellagra and other nicotinic acid deficiency states, niacin is also employed in large doses as adjunctive therapy in various forms of hyperlipidemia and hypercholesterolemia. These latter indications are reviewed in detail in Chapter 33. Finally, its vasodilatory action has led to its use as a circulatory aid in peripheral vascular diseases (primarily as nicotinyl alcohol, see Chap. 32), but there is no conclusive evidence that the drug has a clinically beneficial effect in patients with circulatory impairment.

Large doses of nicotinic acid have been employed in treating schizophrenia, as part of what has been termed *orthomolecular psychiatry*. There is no convincing evidence that such treatment is effective, and use of high doses of nicotinic acid may be associated with significant toxicity, including liver damage, arrhythmias, peptic ulceration, sensory neuropathy, hyperglycemia, dermatoses, and GI distress.

Mechanism

Niacin is converted to either NAD or NADP, enzymes that play a vital role in cellular metabolism. Large doses exert a hypolipemic effect, presumably by reducing triglyceride synthesis and blocking the release of very low-density lipoproteins (VLDL) from the liver; may also increase cholesterol oxidation and inhibit mobilization of free fatty acids; exerts a direct, although relatively weak relaxing effect on peripheral vascular smooth muscle

Uses

1 Prevention and treatment of pellagra and other niacin deficiency states
2 Adjunctive therapy of hypercholesterolemia and hyperbetalipoproteinemia (Types IIb, III, IV, and V); see Chapter 33
3 Symptomatic treatment of peripheral vascular disorders; see Chapter 32

Dosage
Oral:
Niacin deficiency—50 mg to 100 mg/day
Pellagra—up to 500 mg/day, depending on severity of symptoms
Hyperlipidemias—1 g to 2 g three times a day (maximum 6 g/day)
IV (vitamin deficiencies only): 300 mg to 500 mg/day in divided doses every 2 hours to 3 hours by slow IV injection

Fate
Readily absorbed orally and widely distributed; peak serum concentrations occur in 45 minutes; approximately one third of a normal oral dose is excreted unchanged in the urine; with very large doses, the princial urinary excretary product is the unchanged drug.

Common Side-Effects
Cutaneous flushing and sensation of warmth, especially in the face or neck area; GI distress

Significant Adverse Reactions
(Especially with large doses) Headache, tingling, skin rash, pruritus, increased sebaceous gland activity, dryness of the skin, jaundice, allergic reactions, keratosis nigricans, activation of peptic ulcer, abdominal pain, vomiting, diarrhea, hypotension (orthostatic), dizziness, hyperuricemia, toxic amblyopia, and decreased glucose tolerance

Contraindications
Active peptic ulcer, hepatic dysfunction, severe hypotension, hemorrhaging or arterial bleeding

Interactions
1 Niacin may have additive blood pressure-lowering effects with antihypertensive drugs.
2 Niacin can reduce the effectiveness of oral antidiabetic agents by elevating blood glucose levels.

▶ NURSING ALERTS
▷ 1 Use cautiously in patients with glaucoma, jaundice, liver disease, peptic ulcer, gallbladder disease, diabetes, gout, or angina, in children and in pregnant or lactating women.
▷ 2 Caution patients against engaging in hazardous activities, because dizziness or weakness can occur, especially in the early stages of therapy.

▶ NURSING CONSIDERATIONS
▷ 1 Inform patients that tingling, itching, headache, or a sensation of warmth, esecially in the area of the head, neck, and ears can occur shortly after administration, but that these effects usually subside with continued therapy.
▷ 2 Administer drug with meals to minimize GI upset, and accompany with cold water. Avoid hot beverages because vasodilation may be intensified.
▷ 3 Begin therapy with small doses to minimize untoward reactions, and increase gradually to optimal level; initial therapeutic response usually occurs within 24 hours to 48 hours.
▷ 4 Be aware that parenteral therapy is only indicated for severe niacin deficiency, not for hyperlipidemia, and drug should be administered by slow IV injection if possible.
▷ 5 Caution patients against prolonged exposure to bright sunlight.
▷ 6 Consider use of niacinamide instead of niacin for vitamin replacement therapy if flushing is severe or bothersome. See next discussion.

▶ nicotinamide
Niacinamide

An amide of nicotinic acid, nicotinamide provides a source of niacin that can be utilized by the body, but that is devoid of hypolipidemic and vasodilatory effects. Thus, it is only indicated for treatment of niacin deficiency states, where it is preferred by many patients who find the flushing and paresthesias resulting from niacin itself unpleasant. Nicotinamide is available for oral or parenteral administration, and the dose is highly individualized based upon symptoms and response. The usual oral dosage range is 50 mg three to ten times a day. Parenteral dosage is 100 mg to 200 mg one to five times/day. Other than a reduced incidence of circulatory side-effects, the pharmacology of nicotinamide is essentially similar to that of nicotinic acid.

▶ **vitamin B₅ (pantothenic acid)**
▶ **calcium pantothenate**

Pantholin

Pantothenic acid, occasionally referred to as vitamin B₅, is incorporated into coenzyme A, which catalyzes a variety of metabolic reactions such as oxidative metabolism of carbohydrates, gluconeogenesis, synthesis and degradation of fatty acids, and synthesis of sterols and steroid hormones. Because pantothenic acid is found abundantly in the normal diet, deficiency states are quite rare. Although it is a necessary nutrient, the daily requirement is not precisely known and no RDAs are available. Pantothenic acid in the form of its calcium salt is commonly found in multivitamin preparations, but its presence is probably unnecessary.

Mechanism
Incorporated in coenzyme A, which functions as a cofactor for a variety of essential metabolic activities

Uses
1 Treatment of pantothenic acid deficiency, although this condition has *not* been recognized in humans with an ordinary diet

Dosage
10 mg to 20 mg/day, up to 100 mg/day

Fate
Readily absorbed orally; widely distributed in the body; not metabolized to any extent, but excreted largely unchanged in the urine

▶ NURSING CONSIDERATIONS
▷ 1 Note that while weakness, vomiting, abdominal cramps, dizziness, mood changes, altered gait, neurologic disturbances, and psychotic episodes have occurred in persons maintained on a low-pantothenic acid diet in conjunction with a pantothenic acid antagonist, no spontaneously occurring deficiency state has been reported in humans.
▷ 2 Be aware that calcium pantothenate is available with aluminum hydroxide and magnesium trisilicate as Durasil, but because the vitamin is essentially nontoxic, even in very large doses, the inclusion of antacids is probably unnecessary.

▶ **vitamin B₆ (pyridoxine)**

Beesix, Hexa-Betalin, Pyroxine, TexSix T.R.

Pyridoxine (vitamin B₆) is a naturally occurring substance that can be converted to pyridoxal and pyridoxamine. All three compounds possess similar biological activity, and thus should be regarded as different forms of vitamin B₆, although pyridoxine is the most commonly used term. Pyridoxine functions as a coenzyme at various stages in the metabolism of carbohydrates, fats, and proteins. The need for pyridoxine increases with the amount of protein in the diet, and RDAs are listed in Table 75-1.

Mechanism
All three forms of vitamin B₆ are converted *in vivo* to pyridoxal phosphate, the physiologically active form. Pyridoxal phosphate serves as a coenzyme for a number of essential metabolic reactions, including decarboxylation, transamination, and transulfuration of amino acids, conversion of tryptophan to serotonin or niacin, and glycogenolysis.

Uses
1 Treatment of pyridoxine deficiency, as seen, for example, with inadequate dietary intake, inborn errors of metabolism (*e.g.,* pyridoxine-dependent convulsions, pyridoxine-responsive anemia) or drug-induced deletion (*e.g.,* from isoniazid, alcohol, oral contraceptives)
2 Control of nausea and vomiting in pregnancy or that resulting from radiation (effectiveness not conclusively demonstrated)
3 Reversal of neurologic symptoms in hydrazine poisoning (investigational use only)

Dosage
Dietary deficiency: 10 mg to 20 mg/day orally for 3 weeks, followed by an oral multivitamin containing 2 mg to 5 mg pyridoxine (see Nursing Considerations)
Pyridoxine dependency syndrome: up to 600 mg/day initially, reduced to 50 mg/day for life
Isoniazid-induced deficiency: 100 mg/day for 3 weeks, followed by 50 mg/day
Isoniazid overdosage (10 g or more): give an equal amount of pyridoxine (4 g IV, followed by 1 g IM every 30 min)

Fate
Well absorbed orally; converted to pyridoxal phosphate; half-life is 15 days to 20 days; metabolized to 4-pyridoxic acid in the liver, which is excreted in the urine

Significant Adverse Reactions
(Usually only with large doses) Paresthesias, somnolence, flushing, reduced serum folic acid levels, and pain at injection site

Interactions
1 Pyridoxine can reduce the effectiveness of levodopa by accelerating its peripheral metabolism.
2 Pyridoxine requirement may be increased in patients

taking isoniazid, cycloserine, oral contraceptives, hydralazine, or penicillamine.

3 Chloramphenicol-induced optic neuritis can be prevented by pyridoxine.

▶ NURSING ALERTS

▷ 1 Use cautiously in nursing mothers, because pyridoxine can impair lactation by interfering with prolactin.

▷ 2 Be aware that a substantial number of alcoholics have a significant pyridoxine deficiency and should be given supplemental pyridoxine to prevent neurologic complications. Pyridoxine deficiency is also common in patients taking isoniazid and may also occur with use of oral contraceptives and certain other drugs. See Interactions.

▶ NURSING CONSIDERATION

▷ 1 Recognize that selective pyridoxine dietary deficiency is rare, and symptoms are usually best controlled with a multivitamin preparation once the pyridoxine levels are restored.

▶ vitamin B₁₂ (cyanocobalamin)

Kaybovite, Redisol

Cyanocobalamin, or vitamin B_{12}, is essential for normal growth and development, cell reproduction, hematopoiesis, and nucleoprotein and myelin synthesis. Insufficient GI absorption of cyanocobalamin, due primarily to decreased availability of the intrinsic factor, leads to pernicious anemia and is treated with large oral or parenteral doses (see Chap. 34). Oral preparations containing less than 500 mcg cyanocobalamin are *not* indicated for pernicious anemia, but are employed solely as a nutritional supplement, especially in persons on strict vegetarian diets. The recommended dosage range is 25 mcg to 250 mcg/day, although it should be remembered that the RDA for cyanocobalamin is only 3 mcg in adults.

Vitamin C

▶ ascorbic acid

various manufacturers

▶ calcium ascorbate

Calscorbate

▶ sodium ascorbate

Cenolate, Cevita

Vitamin C, or ascorbic acid, is an essential dietary substance that plays a major role in many metabolic reactions as well as the formation and maintenance of collagen and intracellular ground substance. The name *ascorbic acid* is a condensation of the term *antiscorbutic vitamin,* and is derived from the compound's ability to prevent scurvy, the principal ascorbic acid deficiency state. In normal therapeutic doses, ascorbic acid elicits few demonstrable pharmacologic effects except in the scorbutic person (*i.e.,* the patient with symptoms of scurvy). This disease is occasionally observed in elderly or debilitated persons, drug addicts, alcoholics, and others with poor diets. It is characterized by degenerative changes in connective tissue, bones, and capillaries. The symptoms of ascorbic acid deficiency (swollen and bleeding gums, petechiae, easy bruising, delayed wound healing, loosened teeth, joint pain, and bloody stools) are usually readily relieved by 200 mg to 400 mg ascorbic acid daily for several days; they can be prevented from recurring by small (50 mg–100 mg) daily supplemental doses of the vitamin. Although very large amounts (megadoses) of ascorbic acid have been advocated for a wide variety of disease states, ranging from prophylaxis of the common cold to treatment of carcinomas, *conclusive evidence* for the vitamin's effectiveness in megadose quantities for any of the proposed indications is lacking.

Mechanism

Participates in a number of essential biological functions, for example, formation of collagen and intracellular ground substance, cellular respiration, microsomal drug metabolism, steroid synthesis, tyrosine metabolism, and conversion of folic acid to folinic acid; important for the maintenance of tooth and bone matrix and capillary integrity, and may aid wound healing; reduces pH of the urine

Uses

1 Prevention and treatment of scurvy and other ascorbic acid deficiency states

2 Adjunctive therapy in extensive or deep burns, delayed wound healing, chronic or severe illnesses, and a variety of other disease states and stressful situations (effectiveness has not been conclusively demonstrated)

3 Acidification of the urine, usually in conjunction with a urinary anti-infective

Dosage

Oral:

Treatment of deficiency states—100 mg to 500 mg/day as needed

Prophylaxis—50 mg to 100 mg/day

Urinary acidification—4 g to 12 g/day of ascorbic acid in divided doses every 4 hours

IM, SC, IV:

Up to 2 g/day as needed for severe deficiency states; maintenance dose is 100 mg to 250 mg once or twice a day

Fate

Readily absorbed orally or parenterally and widely distributed; partly metabolized and excreted in the urine both as metabolites and unchanged drug; renal threshold is 1.5 mg/dl plasma, and the amount excreted markedly increases with large doses.

Significant Adverse Reactions

(Usually with large doses) Diarrhea, precipitation of oxalate or urate renal stones, soreness at IM or SC injection sites, and dizziness or faintness with too rapid IV injection

Contraindications

Use of sodium ascorbate injection in patients on sodium-restricted diets, or calcium ascorbate in patients receiving digitalis drugs

Interactions

1 Large doses of ascorbic acid lower urinary pH and thus may reduce excretion of acidic drugs (*e.g.*, salicylates, barbiturates) and increase excretion of basic drugs (*e.g.*, quinidine, atropine, amphetamines, tricyclic antidepressants, phenothiazines).
2 Ascorbic acid increases the possibility of crystalluria with the sulfonamides.
3 Large doses of ascorbic acid may shorten the prothrombin time in patients receiving oral anticoagulants.
4 Ascorbic acid can interfere with the effectiveness of disulfiram when it is used in the alcoholic patient (see Chap. 80).
5 Ascorbic acid in large doses may enhance the absorption of oral iron.
6 Mineral oil can retard absorption of ascorbic acid.
7 Ascorbic acid is chemically incompatible with penicillin G potassium and should not be mixed in the same syringe.
8 Intermittent administration of ascorbic acid may increase the risk of oral contraceptive failure.
9 Smoking may slightly reduce ascorbic acid serum levels; conversely, ascorbic acid can enhance excretion of nicotine, perhaps resulting in an increased desire to smoke.

▶ NURSING ALERT

▷ 1 Use cautiously in patients with glucose 6-phosphate dehydrogenase deficiency, hyperuricemia, or renal impairment, and in pregnant women.

▶ NURSING CONSIDERATIONS

▷ 1 Be aware that large doses may result in false readings in certain laboratory tests, for example, urine glucose, serum uric acid, and urinary steroids determinations.
▷ 2 Inject slowly IV to avoid dizziness and possibly fainting.
▷ 3 Do not inject calcium ascorbate SC and avoid IM injections in infants, as tissue necrosis can occur.

Summary. Water-Soluble Vitamins

Drug	Preparations	Usual Dosage Range
B-Complex Vitamins		
B$_1$ Thiamine (Betalin S, Biamine)	Tablets—5 mg, 10 mg, 25 mg, 50 mg, 100 mg, 250 mg, 500 mg Elixir—0.25 mg/5 ml, 1 mg/5 ml, 2.25 mg/5 ml Injection—100 mg/ml	Oral—5 mg to 30 mg/day IM—10 mg to 20 mg 3 times a day for 2 weeks, supplemented with 5 mg to 10 mg orally/day IV—up to 30 mg 3 times/day
B$_2$ Riboflavin (Riobin-50)	Tablets—5 mg, 10 mg, 25 mg, 50 mg, 100 mg Injection—50 mg/ml	Oral—5 mg to 10 mg/day IM—50 mg
B$_3$ Nicotinic acid (Niacin)	Tablets—50 mg, 100 mg, 500 mg Tablets (timed release)—150 mg Capsules (timed release)—125 mg, 200 mg, 250 mg, 300 mg, 400 mg, 500 mg Elixir—50 mg/5 ml Injection—50 mg/ml, 100 mg/ml	Oral: Niacin deficiency—50 mg to 100 mg/day Pellagra—up to 500 mg/day Hyperlipidemia—1 g to 2 g 3 times/day (maximum 6 g/day) IV: 300 mg to 500 mg/day in divided doses every 2 hours to 3 hours by slow infusion
Nicotinamide (Niacinamide)	Tablets—50 mg, 100 mg, 500 mg Capsules—500 mg Injection—100 mg/ml	Oral or parenteral—50 mg 3 to 10 times/day depending on severity of deficiency and clinical response
B$_5$ Calcium pantothenate (Pantholin)	Tablets—10 mg, 30 mg, 100 mg, 218 mg	10 mg to 20 mg/day, up to 100 mg/day

(continued)

Summary. Water-Soluble Vitamins (continued)

Drug	Preparations	Usual Dosage Range
B₆ Pyridoxine (Beesix, Hexa-Betalin, Pyroxine, TexSix T.R.)	Tablets—5 mg, 10 mg, 25 mg, 50 mg, 100 mg, 200 mg, 250 mg, 500 mg Capsules (timed release)—100 mg Injection—100 mg/ml	Dietary deficiency—10 mg to 20 mg/day for 3 weeks then 2 mg to 5 mg/day Pyridoxine dependency syndrome—up to 600 mg/day initially, then 50 mg/day Isoniazid-induced deficiency—100 mg/day for 3 weeks, then 50 mg/day Isoniazid overdosage—4 g IV, then 1 g IM every 30 minutes until an equal amount of pyridoxine is given
B₁₂ Cyanocobalamin (Kaybovite, Redisol)	Tablets—10 mcg, 25 mcg, 50 mcg, 100 mcg, 250 mcg Tablets (soluble)—25 mcg, 50 mcg, 100 mcg, 200 mcg Capsules—25 mcg	10 mcg to 250 mcg/day
Vitamin C		
Ascorbic acid (various manufacturers) Calcium ascorbate (Calscorbate) Sodium ascorbate (Cenolate, Cevita)	Tablets—25 mg, 50 mg, 100 mg, 250 mg, 500 mg, 1000 mg Chewable tablets—100 mg, 250 mg, 500 mg, 1000 mg Tablets (sustained release)—250 mg, 500 mg, 750 mg Capsules (timed release)—500 mg Syrup—100 mg/5 ml Drops—35 mg/0.6 ml, 60 mg/0.6 ml Injection (ascorbic acid)—50 mg/ml, 100 mg/ml, 200 mg/ml, 250 mg/ml, 500 mg/ml Injection (sodium ascorbate)—250 mg/ml, 500 mg/ml Injection (calcium ascorbate)—100 mg/ml	Oral: Deficiency states—100 mg to 500 mg/day as required Prophylaxis—50 mg to 100 mg/day Urinary acidification—(ascorbic acid only) 4 g to 12 g/day in divided doses every 4 hours IM, SC IV—up to 2 g/day as needed; maintenance dose is 100 mg to 250 mg once or twice a day

Unlike the B-complex and C vitamins discussed in Chapter 75, vitamins A, D, E, and K are poorly soluble in water but dissolve readily in fats. This property is responsible for certain characteristics that distinguish the fat-soluble vitamins from their water-soluble counterparts. While the B and C vitamins are readily absorbed orally, the fat-soluble vitamins require the presence of sufficient amounts of bile salts in the GI tract for adequate absorption. However, their absorption may be impaired by the presence of mineral oil or other fatty vehicles that can sequester the vitamins in the lumen of the intestine. Compared to the water-soluble vitamins, vitamins A, D, E, and K are stored in much larger amounts in various body tissues, such as adipose tissue, liver, and muscles. From these storage depots, small amounts are released over extended periods of time to meet nutritional needs; hence symptoms of a fat-soluble vitamin deficiency usually develop only after long periods of inadequate intake, that is, until body stores are depleted. Loss of fat-soluble vitamins in the urine is minimal and excretion proceeds at a very slow rate. The inefficient excretion of most fat-soluble vitamins can result in accumulation to toxic levels if excessive quantities of the vitamins are ingested to supplement the diet, and such a practice should be discouraged.

Characteristics of the fat-soluble vitamins are listed in Table 76-1, along with their recommended dietary allowances where available. The four vitamins making up the fat-soluble group are reviewed individually below.

In addition, two vitamin D metabolites, calcifediol and calcitriol, as well as a synthetic sterol, dihydrotachysterol, which is structurally and functionally related to ergocalciferol, are considered in this chapter. Finally, two vitamin A analogs, isotretinoin (a retinoic acid isomer) and tretinoin (retinoic acid itself), are discussed below with regard to their usefulness in treating acne vulgaris.

Fat-Soluble Vitamins— Vitamins A, D, E, and K

76

Vitamin A (Alphalin, Aquasol A)

The term *vitamin A* is commonly used to refer to a group of several biologically active compounds. Vitamin A_1 (retinol) is the principal naturally occurring substance and is formed from precursors termed *carotenes,* the most important of which is beta-carotene (provitamin A). The average adult receives about one-half of his daily dietary intake of vitamin A as preformed retinol and the remainder as carotene precursors. Vitamin A_2 (3-dehydroretinol) occurs mixed with retinol in many dietary sources. Most currently used preparations are synthetic retinol esters, which have largely replaced the natural vitamin A products previously extracted from fish liver oils, inasmuch as they are generally better absorbed and provide more consistent blood levels of the vitamin.

The potency of vitamin A preparations is expressed as international units (IU), one IU being equal to 0.3 mcg retinol or 0.6 mcg beta-carotene. Vitamin A is required for growth of bones and teeth, integrity of epithelial tissue, normal functioning of the retina (especially visual adaptation to darkness), reproduction, and embryonic development. In addition, vitamin-A deficiency can lower resistance to

Table 76-1. Fat-Soluble Vitamins

Vitamin	Major Dietary Sources	Recommended Dietary Allowances			Principal Symptoms of Deficiency States
		Infants	Children	Adults	
Vitamin A	Fish liver oils, eggs, milk, butter, green and yellow vegetables, tomatoes, squash	2000 IU to 2100 IU	2500 IU to 3500 IU	4000 IU to 5000 IU	Night blindness, xerophthalmia, keratinization of epithelial tissues, increased susceptibility to infection, retarded growth and development
Vitamin D (ergocalciferol, cholecalciferol)	Fish liver oils, egg yolk, milk, butter, margarine, salmon, sardines	400 IU	400 IU	200 IU to 400 IU	Rickets, osteomalacia
Vitamin E	Wheat germ, vegetable oils, green leafy vegetables, nuts, cereals, eggs, dairy products, meats	4 IU to 6 IU	7 IU to 10 IU	12 IU to 15 IU	Not established in humans; *possibly* hemolytic anemia, muscular lesions and necrosis, creatinuria
Vitamin K	Green leafy vegetables, liver, cheese, egg yolks, tomatoes, meats, cereals	*	*	*	Hypoprothrombinemia, hemorrhage

* RDAs are not established.

infection and reduce adrenal cortical steroid production. Deficiencies are rarely observed when reasonable dietary practices are followed, and liver stores of vitamin A are usually sufficient to satisfy up to 2-year requirement of the vitamin.

Mechanism

Complex and incompletely understood; among the actions ascribed to vitamin A are increased synthesis of RNA, proteins, steroids, mucopolysaccharides, and cholesterol; prevents growth retardation and preserves the integrity of epithelial cells; also necessary for formation of rhodopsin, a photosensitive pigment important for vision in dim light; may enhance healing of wounds

Uses

1 Treatment of vitamin-A deficiency states (*e.g.,* biliary or pancreatic disease, colitis, hepatic cirrhosis, celiac disease, regional enteritis)
2 Prophylaxis of vitamin-A deficiency during periods of increased requirements, for example, infancy, pregnancy, lactation, severe illness

Dosage

Adults:
Oral—100,000 IU to 500,000 IU/day for 3 days, then 50,000 IU/day for 2 weeks, then 10,000 IU to 20,000 IU/day for 2 months
IM—100,000 IU/day for 3 days, then 50,000 IU/day for 2 weeks
Children:
Oral—10,000 IU to 15,000 IU/day as a dietary supplement
IM (1 yr–8 yr)—17,500 IU to 35,000 IU/day for 10 days
Infants:
IM—7500 IU to 15,000 IU/day for 10 days

Fate

GI absorption of fat-soluble preparations is good in the presence of bile acids, pancreatic lipase, and dietary fat. Aqueous dispersions of the synthetic vitamin are more rapidly absorbed than oil solutions. Peak plasma concentrations occur in about 3 hours to 4 hours. Most of a dose is stored in the liver, with smaller amounts in many other body tissues. Vitamin E increases tissue storage of vitamin A. Plasma levels increase substantially when hepatic storage sites are saturated. It is slowly released from liver, and serum concentrations of vitamin A can be maintained for months by hepatic stores. Vitamin A is metabolized to water-soluble derivatives, and excreted largely in the urine. Little unchanged vitamin is excreted intact.

Significant Adverse Reactions

(Due to overdosage—hypervitaminosis A syndrome)
CNS—fatigue, irritability, malaise, lethargy, night sweats, vertigo, headache, increased intracranial pressure (may be manifest as papilledema)
Dermatologic—drying and fissuring of skin and lips, alopecia, gingivitis, pruritus, desquamation, increased pigmentation, tender swellings on the extremities
Musculoskeletal—retarded growth, arthralgia, premature closure of the epiphyses, bone pain
GI—abdominal pain, vomiting, anorexia
Other—liver and spleen enlargement, jaundice, leukopenia, hypomenorrhea, polydipsia, polyuria, hypercalcemia

Contraindications

Oral administration in patients with malabsorption syndrome, hypervitaminosis A, administration by the IV route

Interactions

1 Mineral oil, cholestyramine resin, and colestipol may impair absorption of vitamin A.

2 Increased plasma vitamin A levels have occurred in women taking oral contraceptives.

▶ NURSING ALERTS
▷ 1 Avoid use of vitamin A in excess of the RDA (*i.e.*, 6000 IU) during pregnancy, because fetal abnormalities have been produced by large doses in laboratory animals.
▷ 2 If signs of hypervitaminosis A are observed (see Significant Adverse Reactions), discontinue drug and advise physician. Symptoms usually subside quickly, but some may remain for months; for example, the tender swellings in the extremities.

▶ NURSING CONSIDERATIONS
▷ 1 Do not administer large doses over prolonged periods of time, because tissue accumulation can occur. Blood levels do not necessarily reflect total body concentration, because liver storage usually is extensive.
▷ 2 Be aware that preparations containing up to 25,000 IU can be sold over the counter, whereas higher strength preparations require a prescription.
▷ 3 Administer IM only when oral administration is unfeasible: for example, in presence of vomiting, unconsciousness, steatorrhea, or other malabsorption states.
▷ 4 Avoid use of mineral oil while taking vitamin A.

▶ isotretinoin
Accutane

Isotretinoin is an isomer of retinoic acid, a metabolite of retinol. It is used orally for treatment of *severe* acne and other cutaneous disorders of keratinization, such as ichthyosis, pityriasis, and other hyperkeratotic skin conditions. Due to its potential for eliciting serious untoward reactions, isotretinoin should be used with utmost caution and only under close supervision.

Mechanism
Not completely established; reduces sebum secretion and inhibits sebaceous gland differentiation; keratinization is also inhibited; elevates plasma triglycerides and cholesterol

Uses
1 Treatment of severe, recalcitrant cystic acne in patients unresponsive to conventional therapy, including antibiotics (*e.g.*, tetracyclines)
2 Treatment of disorders of excessive keratinization (*e.g.*, ichthyosis, pityriasis, hyperkeratosis plantaris, rubra pilaris)
3 Treatment of cutaneous T-cell lymphoma (mycosis fungoides)

Dosage
Usually, 1 mg/kg to 2 mg/kg/day in two divided doses for 15 weeks to 20 weeks; a second course of therapy may be initiated after a 2-month drug holiday. Doses of 0.05 mg/

kg to 0.5 mg/kg/day have been effective in some patients, but relapses are more common.

Fate
Oral bioavailability of the capsule dosage form is approximately 25%; peak plasma levels occur in about 3 hours; the drug is almost completely protein-bound; elimination half-life averages 10 hours (range 7 hr–35 hr); excreted in the urine and feces in approximately equal amounts

Common Side-Effects
Cheilitis, eye irritation, conjunctivitis, dry skin, skin fragility, pruritus, nosebleed, dryness of the nose and mouth, nausea, vomiting, abdominal pain, lethargy, white cells in urine, triglyceride elevation, and elevated sedimentation rate

Significant Adverse Reactions
Dermatologic—facial skin desquamation, nail brittleness, rash, alopecia, photosensitivity, skin infections, erythema nodosum, pigmentary changes, urticaria
GI—anorexia, regional ileitis, mild GI bleeding, inflammatory bowel disease, weight loss
CNS—insomnia, fatigue, paresthesias, headache, dizziness, visual disturbances, papilledema, corneal opacities
Musculoskeletal—arthralgia, joint and muscle pain and stiffness
Urinary—proteinuria, hematuria
Other—bruising, edema, respiratory infections, abnormal menses, herpes simplex infections, increased SGOT, SGPT, alkaline phosphatase and fasting serum glucose, elevated platelet counts, hyperuricemia, elevated cholesterol, decreased high-density lipoproteins

Contraindications
Pregnancy (drug causes fetal abnormalities), patients sensitive to parabens (preservatives in the formulation)

Interactions
1 Vitamin A supplements together with isotretinoin may result in increased toxicity.
2 Tetracyclines and isotretinoin can lead to pseudotumor cerebri or papilledema.
3 Concomitant ingestion of alcohol may further increase serum triglyceride levels.

▶ NURSING ALERTS
▷ 1 Do not use in women of childbearing potential unless contraceptive methods are employed, because drug has a significant teratogenic potential.
▷ 2 Perform baseline serum lipid determinations and repeat at weekly or biweekly intervals during therapy. Increased triglyceride and cholesterol and decreased high-density lipoprotein levels occur in up to 25% of patients but are reversible upon cessation of therapy.
▷ 3 Use cautiously in obese, alcoholic, or diabetic patients, because elevated serum triglycerides occur more frequently and levels are generally higher.
▷ 4 Note that musculoskeletal disorders occur in 15% to

20% of patients receiving isotretinoin, but symptoms are usually mild, seldom require discontinuation of therapy, and disappear upon cessation of the drug.

▷ 5 Perform periodic ophthalmic examinations during treatment and urge patients to report any changes in visual function.

▷ 6 Instruct patients to avoid prolonged exposure to sunlight, because photosensitivity reactions can occur.

▶ **NURSING CONSIDERATIONS**

▷ 1 Advise patients that a transient worsening of acne may occur during the initial stages of drug therapy.

▷ 2 Urge patients to reduce caloric intake, dietary fat, and alcohol consumption to minimize elevations in serum triglyceride levels.

▷ 3 Provide emotional support, as necessary, during drug treatment of severe acne.

▷ 4 If a second course of therapy is required, do not begin until at least 8 weeks after termination of the first course of therapy. Clinical improvement may continue during drug-free periods, however.

▶ **tretinoin**

Retin-A

Tretinoin (retinoic acid) is available for topical application in the treatment of acne vulgaris. Its effectiveness approaches that of steroid–antibiotic combinations and generally surpasses that of most other currently available topical acne preparations. Its use is frequently associated with erythema and desquamation, however, and some patients do not tolerate the drug. Tretinoin is available as a gel, cream, or liquid.

Mechanism
Promotes epidermal cell turnover and facilitates desquamation; suppresses keratin synthesis and prevents formation of comedones

Uses
1 Treatment of acne vulgaris, especially grades I, II, and III; not effective against acne conglobata (*i.e.,* deep cystic nodules and extensive pustules)
2 Treatment of several forms of skin cancer (investigational use)

Dosage
Apply once a day for at least 4 weeks to 6 weeks, at bedtime, and cover entire area lightly; reduce frequency of application as lesions respond.

Common Side-Effects
Stinging, feeling of warmth, dryness, peeling, and erythema

Significant Adverse Reactions
Edema, blistering, pigmentary changes, photosensitivity, and contact dermatitis (rare)

Interactions
1 Increased skin peeling can occur if tretinoin is used with sulfur, resorcinol, benzoyl peroxide, or salicylic acid.
2 Excessive skin drying can result from concomitant use of tretinoin and products containing high concentrations of alcohol, astringents, or lime.

▶ **NURSING ALERTS**

▷ 1 Caution patients to minimize exposure to sunlight or sunlamps, because photosensitivity reactions can occur. Experimental animal studies have indicated a tumorigenic potential for tretinoin upon exposure to UV light, although the significance of this effect in man is not clear.

▷ 2 Use with caution in patients with eczema, because severe irritation has occurred.

▶ **NURSING CONSIDERATIONS**

▷ 1 Keep away from the eyes, mouth, and other mucous membranes, because irritation can occur.

▷ 2 If significant erythema or irritation is noted, reduce frequency of application or temporarily discontinue medication.

▷ 3 Advise patients that slight stinging and feelings of warmth frequently occur and dryness and peeling of skin are to be expected.

▷ 4 Caution patients against use of topical preparations that have a drying effect (*e.g.,* alcohol, astringents, abrasive soaps or cleansers, cosmetics) with tretinoin, because *excessive* drying can result.

▷ 5 Inform users that a *temporary* worsening of the condition can occur in the early stages of therapy, due to the action of the drug on deeper, previously invisible lesions.

Vitamin D

Vitamin D is a term commonly applied to two related fat-soluble substances, ergocalciferol (D_2) and cholecalciferol (D_3), which are formed from the provitamins ergosterol and 7-dehydrocholesterol, respectively, by UV irradiation. The principal source of endogenous vitamin D in man is the synthesis of D_3 from 7-dehydrocholesterol upon exposure to the UV rays of the sun. Vitamin D_3 is then converted by hepatic microsomal enzymes to calcifediol (25-hydroxycholecalciferol), the principal transport form of vitamin D_3. Calcifediol possesses minor intrinsic vitamin D activity, and is further metabolized in the kidney to calcitriol (1,25 dihydroxycholecalciferol), the most active form of vitamin D_3. Both calcifediol and calcitriol are now available for clinical use, and are reviewed separately in this chapter. Vitamin D_2 is the form usually found in commercial vitamin preparations and in fortified milk, bread, and cereals. Because in humans there is no difference in activity between vitamin D_2 and D_3, *vitamin D* will be used as the collective term for all substances, natural and synthetic, having similar activity.

Vitamin D plays a major role in the regulation of plasma calcium levels and functions in much the same manner as the parathyroid hormone (see Chap. 41). Dihydrotachysterol is an analog of vitamin D_2 that is activated by the liver, resulting in formation of 25-hydroxy-dihydrotachysterol, a compound that elevates serum calcium levels. Dihydrotachysterol is also considered later in the chapter. In addition to calcium metabolism, phosphate and magnesium metabolism are also controlled by vitamin D. Dosage of the vitamin is measured in international units (IU), one IU of vitamin D activity being equal to 0.025 mcg ergocalciferol.

▶ ergocalciferol

Calciferol, Deltalin, Drisdol

Mechanism

Enhances the active absorption of calcium and phosphorus from the small intestine, facilitates their resorption from bone and promotes their reabsorption by the renal tubules; plasma levels of calcium and phosphorus are therefore maintained at levels adequate for neuromuscular activity, mineralization of bone, and other calcium-dependent functions.

Uses

1 Treatment of refractory (vitamin D-resistant) rickets and nutritional rickets
2 Treatment of hypoparathyroidism
3 Adjunctive treatment of infantile rickets and osteomalacia in adults
4 Treatment of hypophosphatemia associated with Fanconi's syndrome

Dosage

Vitamin D-resistant rickets
50,000 IU to 500,000 IU/day, depending on age and severity of disease

Nutritional rickets
Treatment: 1000 IU to 4000 IU/day
Prophylaxis: 400 IU/day

Hypoparathyroidism
50,000 IU to 400,000 IU/day plus 4 g calcium lactate six times a day

Fate

Well absorbed from the intestine, D_3 more completely and more rapidly than D_2; bile is essential for absorption; stored primarily in the liver, with small amounts in skin, bones, and CNS; in the plasma, vitamin D is bound to albumin and alpha globulins; plasma half-life of ergocalciferol is 20 hours to 24 hours, but drug may be stored in tissues for up to 6 months; converted in the liver to an active 25-hydroxy derivative (calcifediol), which has a plasma half-life of approximately 12 days to 22 days and is the principal circulating form of vitamin D; subsequently metabolized in the kidney to calcitriol (1,25 dihydroxycholecalciferol), the most active form of vitamin D, which has a half-life of 7 hours to 12 hours; about one half of an oral dose is excreted *via* the bile into the feces; only minimal amounts are eliminated in the urine

Significant Adverse Reactions

(Usually due to overdosage—Hypervitaminosis D syndrome)
Renal—polyuria, nocturia, elevated BUN, hypercalciuria, azotemia, nephrocalcinosis, proteinuria, urinary casts, renal insufficiency
GI—anorexia, nausea, vomiting, constipation or diarrhea, metallic taste, dry mouth
Other—acidosis, anemia, weakness, headache, irritability, photophobia, conjunctivitis, pancreatitis, hypertension, arrhythmias, vascular and soft-tissue calcification, muscle stiffness and pain, bone demineralization, mental retardation in children, dwarfism, hyperthermia, elevated SGOT and SGPT

Contraindications

Hypercalcemia, hyperphosphatemia, malabsorption syndrome, hypervitaminosis D, and renal osteodystrophy with hyperphosphatemia

Interactions

1 Mineral oil and cholestyramine resin can impair vitamin D absorption.
2 Phenytoin, primidone, and barbiturates may reduce the effectiveness of vitamin D by increasing its metabolic inactivation.
3 Thiazide diuretics may potentiate vitamin D-induced hypercalcemia in hypoparathyroid patients.
4 Vitamin D may increase the likelihood of cardiac arrhythmias with digitalis drugs.
5 The effects of verapamil and other calcium channel blockers may be reduced by vitamin D-induced hypercalcemia.

▶ NURSING ALERTS

▷ 1 Do not exceed RDA in pregnant women (400 IU/day), because animal studies have shown fetal abnormalities with high doses of vitamin D.
▷ 2 Avoid excessive or indiscriminate use of vitamin D, because cumulative toxicity can occur. Be alert for signs of hypervitaminosis D (see Significant Adverse Reactions), and promptly discontinue drug. Provide necessary supportive treatment (*e.g.,* increased fluid intake, acidification of urine, calcium restriction).
▷ 3 During high-dose therapy, perform frequent serum and urinary calcium, phosphate, potassium, and urea determinations. Blood calcium levels should be maintained between 9 mg to 10 mg/dl, because the range between therapeutic and toxic doses of vitamin D is often quite small.
▷ 4 Use cautiously in patients with impaired renal function or kidney stones.

▶ **NURSING CONSIDERATIONS**

▷ 1 Individualize dosage levels carefully and closely observe patients for signs of toxicity. Adjust doses as condition improves to minimize danger of hypervitaminosis D.

▷ 2 Recognize that persons with GI, biliary, or liver disease associated with malabsorption of vitamin D may require IM administration.

▷ 3 Ensure that dietary intake of calcium is adequate during vitamin D treatment.

▷ 4 Initiate vitamin D supplementation only after critical evaluation of the diet, because serious toxicity can result from excessive intake of vitamin D. Supplementation is usually not necessary in persons having a fortified diet and normal exposure to sunlight.

▶ **calcitriol**
Rocaltrol

The most active metabolite of vitamin D, calcitriol is a potent hypercalcemic agent that is primarily indicated for the treatment of hypocalcemia in patients undergoing renal dialysis. Its extreme potency and rather high cost limit its usefulness as a vitamin D substitute for vitamin D deficiency states.

Mechanism
See Vitamin D.

Uses

1 Management of hypocalcemia in patients on chronic renal dialysis

2 Treatment of metabolic bone disease

Dosage
0.25 mcg/day initially; may increase by 0.25-mcg/day increments every 2 weeks to 4 weeks until satisfactory response is obtained; usual maintenance range is 0.5 mcg to 1 mcg/day

Fate
Rapidly absorbed orally; peak serum levels occur within 4 hours; circulates largely bound to plasma proteins; metabolized by a renal enzyme and excreted both in the bile and urine

Significant Adverse Reactions
See Vitamin D.

Contraindications
Hypercalcemia, hypervitaminosis D

Interactions

1 Cholestyramine resin or colestipol may impair intestinal absorption of calcitriol.

2 Magnesium-containing antacids may result in hypermagnesemia if given concomitantly with calcitriol.

3 Calcitriol-induced hypercalcemia may increase the likelihood of digitalis toxicity.

4 Effects of calcium channel blockers may be antagonized by calcitriol.

▶ **NURSING ALERTS**

▷ 1 Determine serum calcium, phosphorus, magnesium, and alkaline phosphatase and 24-hour urinary calcium and phosphorus periodically during treatment (serum calcium twice weekly during early therapy). Discontinue drug immediately should hypercalcemia develop.

▷ 2 Use with extreme caution during pregnancy. Safety and efficacy have not yet been established in children.

▶ **NURSING CONSIDERATIONS**

▷ 1 Withhold all other vitamin-D supplementation during treatment to minimize risk of hypercalcemia.

▷ 2 Use aluminum carbonate or hydroxide gel in patients undergoing dialysis to control serum phosphate levels. Avoid magnesium-containing antacids or laxatives, because hypermagnesemia can occur.

▷ 3 Provide adequate calcium supplementation during therapy, because effectiveness of calcitriol depends on sufficient intake of calcium. Adult RDA for calcium is 1000 mg.

▷ 4 Be alert for the development of vomiting, weakness, or muscle or bone pain, because these symptoms may indicate hypercalcemia.

▷ 5 Urge strict compliance with dosage instructions, dietary recommendations, and calcium supplementation (if necessary) to minimize danger of untoward reactions.

▶ **calcifediol**
Calderol

Calcifediol, the hydroxylated metabolite of cholecalciferol, is the principal serum transport form of vitamin D_3. Its pharmacology is essentially similar to that of vitamin D_3 as well as calcitriol, the compound to which calcifediol is converted in the kidney, although its intrinsic activity is less than either D_3 or calcitriol.

Mechanism
See Vitamin D.

Uses

1 Treatment of metabolic bone disease and hypocalcemia associated with chronic renal failure

Dosage
Initially, 300 mcg to 350 mcg/week, on a daily or alternate day schedule; increase at 4-week intervals as necessary; usual maintenance range 50 mcg to 100 mcg/day

Fate
Rapidly absorbed from the GI tract; peak serum levels occur within 4 hours; transported bound to plasma proteins; serum half-life is approximately 2 weeks; converted in the kidney to calcitriol (1,25 dihydroxycholecalciferol)

Significant Adverse Reactions
See Vitamin D.

Contraindications
Hypercalcemia, hypervitaminosis D

Interactions
See Vitamin D.

▶ NURSING ALERTS
See Calcitriol.

▶ NURSING CONSIDERATIONS
See Calcitriol.

▶ dihydrotachysterol
DHT, Hytakerol

A reduction product of ergocalciferol, dihydrotachysterol is more effective than ergocalciferol in mobilizing calcium from bone. It is effective orally, but exhibits a shorter duration of action than ergocalciferol, thereby reducing the danger of severe hypercalcemia. Dihydrotachysterol is a potent vitamin D-like preparation (1 mg is equivalent to 120,000 U of vitamin D_2).

Mechanism
Similar to parathyroid hormone and vitamin D_2; increases intestinal absorption of calcium, mobilizes calcium from bone, and enhances urinary excretion of phosphate; may also increase intestinal absorption of sodium, potassium, and magnesium

Uses
1 Treatment of hypocalcemia associated with all forms of hypoparathyroidism
2 Suppression of hyperparathyroidism in chronic renal failure
3 Treatment of acute, chronic, or latent forms of postoperative or idiopathic tetany
4 Adjunctive treatment of vitamin D-resistant rickets, frequently with oral phosphate salts

Dosage
Initially, 0.8 mg to 2.4 mg/day for several days; maintenance 0.2 mg to 1 mg/day depending on serum calcium levels (may be supplemented with 10 g–15 g/day orally of calcium lactate or gluconate)

Fate
Onset of action occurs within several hours after administration but maximal hypercalcemic effects require 1 week to 2 weeks to develop; hypercalcemia may persist for up to 30 days following withdrawal; metabolized by the liver, partially to active metabolites, and excreted largely in the feces

Significant Adverse Reactions
(Usually result of drug-induced hypercalcemia) Constipation, nausea, vomiting, diarrhea, headache, dry mouth, thirst, polyuria, anorexia, metallic taste, abdominal pain, vertigo, tinnitus, ataxia, osteoporosis, neuromuscular disturbances, hypertension, irregular heart beat, mood changes, photosensitivity, convulsions, anemia, renal damage, albuminuria, and calcification of soft tissues (*e.g.,* heart, kidney, lungs)

Contraindications
Hypercalcemia, hypocalcemia associated with renal insufficiency and hyperphosphatemia, hypervitaminosis D, pregnancy, and renal stones

Interactions
See Vitamin D.

▶ NURSING ALERTS
▷ 1 Closely monitor serum calcium levels during treatment (normal range 9 mg–11 mg/100 ml). Safety margin with the drug is very small. Be alert for symptoms of hypercalcemia (see Significant Adverse Reactions).
▷ 2 If signs of hypercalcemia occur (see Significant Adverse Reactions), stop drug, give liberal amount of fluid, restrict dietary calcium, and provide other adjunctive measures as necessary (*e.g.,* laxatives, diuretics).
▷ 3 In cases of severe overdosage, be prepared to administer IV diuretics, corticosteroids (150 mg/day cortisone or equivalent), and sodium citrate (2.5% IV infusion).

▶ NURSING CONSIDERATIONS
▷ 1 Consult physician about allowable dietary calcium intake. Drug is often given with supplemental calcium salts and/or foods high in calcium because therapeutic response is enhanced by proper amount of additional calcium.
▷ 2 Note that clinical response is slow in developing (7 days–10 days) and that effects may persist for up to 30 days after cessation of therapy.
▷ 3 Do not store capsules in a cold place, because they may crack.

Vitamin E (Tocopherol)

Vitamin E is commonly used as a generic term to describe eight naturally occurring tocopherols possessing vitamin E activity. Alpha-tocopherol comprises about 90% of the tocopherols found in animal tissues, is the most biologically active of the eight, and is available both naturally in vegetable oils and other foods as well as synthetically. Because the potencies of the various forms of vitamin E vary somewhat, dosage is standardized in international units (IUs) based upon activity. The following list indicates relative potencies of *1 mg* of the various clinically available tocopherols:

d-alpha tocopherol = 1.49 IU
dl-alpha tocopherol = 1.1 IU
d-alpha tocopheryl acetate = 1.36 IU
dl-alpha tocopheryl acetate = 1.0 IU

d-alpha tocopheryl acid succinate = 1.21 IU
dl-alpha tocopheryl acid succinate = 0.89 IU
Although RDAs have been published for vitamin E, there is little conclusive evidence that it is of significant nutritional or therapeutic value. Deficiencies of vitamin E in humans are rare, inasmuch as adequate amounts are supplied in the ordinary diet. Low levels have occasionally been noted in severely malnourished infants and in patients with prolonged fat malabsorption or acanthocytosis. Based upon occasional relief of experimentally produced deficiency symptoms in laboratory animals, vitamin E has been advocated by some for treatment of an imposing array of human ills, including sterility, habitual abortion, muscular dystrophy, cardiovascular and peripheral vascular disorders, fever blisters, and schizophrenia. These claims have not been substantiated and use of vitamin-E supplementation, other than in clearly established deficiency states, cannot be justified.

Mechanism
Incompletely understood; action appears to be due to its antioxidant properties; prevents oxidation of essential cellular constituents and products; may serve as a cofactor in enzyme reactions, play a role in hematopoiesis and hemoglobin formation, protect red blood cells from hemolysis, interfere with platelet aggregation, and enhance utilization of vitamin A

Uses
1 Treatment of vitamin-E deficiency states
2 Treatment of anemia associated with extreme malnutrition, prematurity, or acanthocytosis
3 Reduce bronchopulmonary dysplasia and retrolental fibroplasia due to oxygen therapy in premature infants (investigational use only)
4 Control of dry or chapped skin and temporary relief of minor skin disorders, for example, itching, sunburn, abrasions (topical use only)

Dosage
Oral (deficiency states): 50 IU to 1000 IU/day, depending on severity (RDA is approximately 15 IU)
Topical: apply as needed

Fate
Readily absorbed from GI tract if fat absorption is adequate; widely distributed in the body and stored in tissues for extended periods of time, providing a continual source of the vitamin; placental transfer is poor; largely excreted in the feces by way of the bile, smaller amounts appearing as metabolites in the urine

Significant Adverse Reactions
Minimal, even at very large doses; occasionally GI distress, muscle weakness

Interactions
1 Vitamin E may enhance the action of oral anticoagulants by reducing levels of vitamin K-dependent clotting factors
2 Vitamin E can reduce the efficacy of oral iron preparations

▶ **NURSING CONSIDERATION**
▷ 1 Be aware that there is *no* conclusive evidence that vitamin E is beneficial for any condition other than those listed under Uses.

Vitamin K

Menadiol Sodium Diphosphate (K$_4$)	Menadione (K$_3$)
	Phytonadione (K$_1$)

Vitamin K refers to several structurally similar compounds that all possess the ability to promote hepatic synthesis of certain blood clotting factors. The primary source of vitamin K in humans is *via* absorption of phytonadione (vitamin K$_1$) synthesized in the gut by intestinal bacteria. In addition, vitamin K is found in many foods (see Table 76-1), although in most cases these represent a minor source of utilizable vitamin. Vitamin K$_1$ (phytonadione) is the only naturally occurring vitamin K used clinically; however, this lipid-soluble derivative is also prepared synthetically. Other synthetic vitamin K compounds employed therapeutically are menadione (vitamin K$_3$), a lipid-soluble derivative used orally, and menadiol sodium diphosphate (vitamin K$_4$), a water-soluble analog converted to menadione *in vivo*. Phytonadione is the preferred drug for treating hypoprothrombinemia, because it is the most potent of the derivatives, and exhibits the fastest onset and longest duration of action. However, adequate absorption of phytonadione occurs only in the presence of bile salts, whereas K$_3$ and K$_4$ can be adequately absorbed without bile salts.

The three available vitamin-K derivatives are discussed as a group, then listed individually in Table 76-2. Phytonadione has been reviewed previously in Chapter 35 as an antidote to overdosage with oral anticoagulants, and is considered only briefly here.

Mechanism
Promote hepatic synthesis of blood clotting factors II, VII, IX, and X, probably by functioning as an essential cofactor for microsomal enzyme systems that activate the precursors of these clotting factors

Uses
1 Treatment of vitamin-K deficiency due to anti-bacterial therapy
2 Treatment of hypoprothrombinemia secondary to impaired absorption or synthesis of vitamin K, for example, obstructive jaundice, biliary fistulas, ulcerative colitis, sprue, celiac disease, regional enteritis, intestinal resection, cystic fibrosis, salicylate therapy
3 Treatment of oral anticoagulant-induced prothrombin deficiency (phytonadione *only*)
4 Prophylaxis and treatment of hemorrhagic disease of the newborn (phytonadione *only*)

Dosage
See Table 76-2.

Table 76-2. Vitamin-K Preparations

Drug	Preparations	Usual Dosage Range	Remarks
K₁			
Phytonadione (AquaMEPHYTON, Konakion, Mephyton)	Tablets—5 mg Injection—2 mg/ml, 10 mg/ml	Hypoprothrombinemia and anticoagulant-induced prothrombin deficiency: 2.5 mg to 25 mg initially; repeat in 6 hours to 8 hours after parenteral injection or 12 hours to 48 hours after oral administration until prothrombin time is in desired range Hemorrhagic disease of newborn: Prophylaxis—0.5 mg to 2 mg IM or (less desirable) 1 mg to 5 mg to the mother 12 hours to 24 hours before delivery Treatment—1 mg to 2 mg SC or IM daily	Fat-soluble derivative that is the preferred antidote to oral anticoagulant overdose; only vitamin-K preparation indicated for hemorrhagic disease of the newborn; requires bile salts for oral absorption; injection is available as an aqueous colloidal solution (AquaMEPHYTON) for IV, SC, or IM use and as an aqueous dispersion (Konakion) for IM use only; do not exceed 1 mg/minute when injecting IV; use smaller doses for antidoting short-acting anticoagulants and larger doses for longer-acting anticoagulants; protect solutions from light
K₃			
Menadione (Menadione)	Tablets—5 mg	5 mg to 10 mg/day	Fat-soluble derivative with a slower onset and shorter duration of action than phytonadione; absorbed directly into the bloodstream, and does not require bile salts for adequate absorption; not used in newborn infants or pregnant women, because drug is not as safe as phytonadione; may induce erythrocyte hemolysis in patients having a glucose 6-phosphate dehydrogenase deficiency
K₄			
Menadiol sodium diphosphate (Synkayvite)	Tablets—5 mg Injections—5 mg/ml, 10 mg/ml, 37.5 mg/ml	Oral: 5 mg to 10 mg/day Parenteral (SC, IM, IV): Adults—5 mg to 15 mg 1 to 2 times a day Children—5 mg to 10 mg 1 to 2 times a day	Water-soluble derivative of vitamin K that is converted to menadione *in vivo;* approximately one half as potent as menadione; well absorbed orally, and does not require presence of bile salts; primarily used for hypoprothrombinemia due to obstructive jaundice, biliary fistulas, or administration of salicylates or antibiotics; single dose usually restores prothrombin time within 8 hours to 24 hours; may induce hemolysis of erythrocytes in glucose 6-phosphate dehydrogenase-deficient patients

Fate

Phytonadione is absorbed from the GI tract by way of the lymph and only in the presence of bile salts. Menadione and menadiol are absorbed directly into the blood stream even in the absence of bile. Bleeding is controlled within 6 hours to 12 hours following oral administration and within 1 hour to 2 hours following parenteral injection. It is initially concentrated in the liver but levels decline very rapidly. There is little accumulation in other tissues and drug is rapidly metabolized. It is excreted both in the bile and urine.

Common Side-Effects

Flushing sensation with IV injection

Significant Adverse Reactions

Oral—GI upset, vomiting, headache

Parenteral—dizziness, tachycardia, weak pulse, chills, fever, sweating, hypotension, dyspnea, cyanosis, hypersensitivity reactions, anaphylaxis, pain and swelling at injection site, and erythematous skin reactions; in newborns, hyperbilirubinemia, kernicterus, and hemolytic anemia

Contraindications

Menadione and menadiol are contraindicated in infants and in women during the last few weeks of pregnancy and during labor.

Interactions

1 Vitamin K antagonizes the anticoagulant action of coumarins and indandiones, but not heparin.
2 Mineral oil or cholestyramine may impair GI absorption of K_1 and K_3, but not K_4.
3 Antibiotics may reduce endogenous vitamin-K activity by decreasing its synthesis by intestinal flora. Increased bleeding can result.

▶ NURSING ALERTS

▷ 1 Use cautiously in patients with hepatic disease. Do not administer repeated large doses when the initial response is poor, because excessive doses can further depress hepatic function.
▷ 2 Be aware that a minimum of 1 hour to 2 hours is required to obtain a measurable increase in prothrombin time, even following parenteral administration. When a more immediate response is desired, or in the presence of severe blood loss, fresh whole blood or plasma is indicated.
▷ 3 Administer IV only when other routes of administration are not appropriate, because severe hypersensitivity reactions, some fatal, have occurred following IV injection of phytonadione. Use only normal saline or 5% Dextrose Solutions as diluent. If drug is given IV,

inject very slowly and closely monitor patient during administration.
▷ 4 Use the smallest dose that is effective in restoring normal prothrombin time (*i.e.,* 12 sec–14 sec), because large doses can provide the same conditions that previously increased the risk of clotting. Monitor prothrombin time frequently.
▷ 5 Use with extreme caution in infants (especially premature infants) in treating hemorrhagic disease of the newborn, because increased bilirubinemia, severe hemolytic anemia and kernicterus, possibly resulting in brain damage or death, can occur. Note that phytonadione is the only vitamin K analog indicated for this condition.

▶ NURSING CONSIDERATIONS

(See Table 76-2 for specific information on each derivative)

▷ 1 Be alert for development of allergic reactions and advise physician.
▷ 2 Advise patients stabilized on a vitamin-K regimen to avoid excessive intake of vitamin K-rich foods (see Table 76-1).
▷ 3 Note that patients receiving vitamin K may become temporarily unresponsive to oral anticoagulants. If an anticoagulant action is desired during this period of insensitivity, only heparin is effective.
▷ 4 Inform patient that temporary pain and swelling may occur with SC or IM injection. Administer IM by deep injection.
▷ 5 During vitamin-K therapy, reduce dose or discontinue use of other drugs that can interfere with coagulation mechanisms (*e.g.,* salicylates, antibiotics, quinidine).

Summary. Fat-Soluble Vitamins

Drug	Preparations	Usual Dosage Range
Vitamin A (Alphalin, Aquasol)	Tablets—5000 IU, 10,000 IU, 50,000 IU Capsules—5000 IU, 10,000 IU, 25,000 IU, 50,000 IU Drops—5000 IU/0.1 ml Injection—50,000 IU/ml	Oral: Adults—100,000 IU to 500,000 IU/day for 3 days, then 50,000 IU/day for 2 weeks, then 10,000 IU to 20,000 IU/day for 2 months Children—10,000 IU to 15,000 IU/day IM: Adults—100,000 IU/day for 3 days, then 50,000 IU/day for 2 weeks Children (1 yr–8 yr)—17,500 IU to 35,000 IU/day for 10 days Infants—7500 to 15,000 IU/day for 10 days
Isotretinoin (Accutane)	Capsules—10 mg, 20 mg, 40 mg	1 mg/kg to 2 mg/kg/day in 2 divided doses for 15 weeks to 20 weeks; a second course of therapy may be given following an 8-week drug-free period

Summary. Fat-Soluble Vitamins *(continued)*

Drug	Preparations	Usual Dosage Range
Tretinoin (Retin-A)	Cream—0.05%, 0.1% Gel—0.025%, 0.1% Liquid—0.05%	Apply daily at bedtime and cover lightly; continue until lesions have responded (4 wk–6 wk), then reduce frequency of application
Vitamin D Ergocalciferol (D_2) Cholecalciferol (D_3) (Calciferol, Deltalin, Drisdol)	Capsules—25,000 IU, 50,000 IU Tablets—50,000 IU Liquid—8,000 IU/ml Drops—200 IU/drop Injection—500,000 IU/ml	Vitamin D-resistant rickets: 50,000 IU to 500,000 IU/day Nutritional rickets: Treatment—1000 IU to 4000 IU/day Prophylaxis—400 IU/day Hypoparathyroidism: 50,000 IU to 400,000 IU/day together with 4 g calcium lactate 6 times a day
Calcitriol (Rocaltrol)	Capsules—0.25 mcg, 0.5 mcg	Initially 0.25 mcg/day; increase as needed by 0.25-mcg/day increments every 2 weeks to 4 weeks; maintenance range is usually 0.5 mcg to 1 mcg/day
Calcifediol (Calderol)	Capsules—20 mcg, 50 mcg	Initially 300 mcg to 350 mcg/week, on a daily or alternate-day schedule; may increase at 4-week intervals as needed; usual dosage range is 50 mcg to 100 mcg/day
Dihydrotachysterol (DHT, Hytakerol)	Tablets—0.125 mg, 0.25 mg, 0.4 mg Capsules—0.125 mg Solution—0.2 mg/ml, 0.25 mg/ml, 0.2 mg/5 ml	Initially 0.8 mg to 2.4 mg/day for several days; maintenance level 0.2 mg to 1 mg/day depending on serum calcium levels
Vitamin E (various manufacturers)	Capsules—50 IU, 100 IU, 200 IU, 400 IU, 600 IU, 800 IU, 1000 IU Tablets—100 IU, 200 IU, 400 IU, 1000 IU Chewable tablets—100 IU, 200 IU, 400 IU Drops—50 IU/ml Injection—200 IU/ml	Deficiency states: 50 IU to 1000 IU/day depending on severity Topical—apply several times a day as needed
Vitamin K	(See Table 76-2)	

The fluid composition of the body is normally maintained reasonably constant despite the many stresses placed upon it. Significant alterations in the volume and composition of the internal fluid environment can, however, result from disease, trauma, or drug therapy, as well as from a number of other external factors. Disturbances in fluid and electrolyte balance may involve changes in pH, volume, osmolarity, or concentrations of individual ions, and can seriously impair the normal metabolic activity of body organs. Thus, the various chemical constituents of the body (*i.e.,* electrolytes, minerals, amino acids, fluids, proteins, lipids) are often administered either individually or in combination to correct acute or chronic deficiency states, and such a procedure is termed *nutritional replacement therapy.*

This chapter considers those nutrients, fluids, and electrolytes, both oral and parenteral, that are commonly used to supply the nutritional needs of patients suffering from a deficiency state of one or more of these substances. The oral nutritional supplements are reviewed first, followed by a discussion of parenteral nutrients, including the hyperalimentation procedure. Not all of the substances used as nutritional supplements are considered here, inasmuch as several have been mentioned in other chapters dealing with drugs affecting specific organs with which a particular mineral or electrolyte is intimately associated. Thus, calcium is discussed with parathyroid hormone and calcitonin in Chapter 41, iron is reviewed along with other drugs used to treat anemia in Chapter 34, and iodine and iodide salts are considered in Chapter 40 with the thyroid hormones. The vitamins are discussed individually in Chapters 75 and 76.

Oral Nutritional Supplements

Bioflavonoids	Manganese
Calcium caseinate	Medium-chain triglycerides
Choline	Oral electrolyte mixture
Corn oil	Para-aminobenzoic acid
Fluoride	Phosphorus
Glucose polymers	Potassium
Inositol	Protein hydrolysates
Lactase	Safflower oil
Lecithin	Sodium chloride
L-Lysine	L-Tryptophan
Magnesium	Zinc

The substances used orally for correcting nutritional deficiency states include minerals, electrolytes, amino acids, proteins, and lipids, as well as a few other miscellaneous drugs. Perhaps the most widely used oral electrolytes are potassium and fluoride, and these preparations are considered individually in detail below. The remaining oral nutritional supplements are listed in Table 77-1.

▶ **potassium**

Potassium is the principal intracellular cation and is essential for many vital physiologic processes, including nerve

(Text continues on p. 734.)

Table 77-1. Oral Nutritional Supplements

Drug	Preparations	Usual Dosage Range	Remarks
Minerals and Electrolytes			
Magnesium (Almora, Magonate, Mg-PLUS)	Tablets—27 mg, 133 mg	27 mg to 133 mg 1 to 3 times a day	RDAs are 200 mg (children 4 yr–6 yr), 300 mg to 350 mg (adults), and 450 mg (pregnant or lactating women); excessive amounts may produce diarrhea; necessary in a number of enzyme systems and for nerve conduction and muscle contraction; deficiency is rare in well-nourished persons
Manganese (Mn-PLUS)	Tablets—5 mg	5 mg/day	Need in human nutrition is not established; functions as a cofactor in many enzyme systems; localized primarily in mitochondria
Oral electrolyte mixture (Infalyte, Lytren, Pedialyte)	Solution or powder (containing various electrolytes and dextrose or glucose)	Infants and young children—1500 ml to 2500 ml/m² Children (5 yr–10 yr)—1 qt to 2 qt/day Children (over 10 yr) and adults—2 qt to 3 qt/day (1 packet of powder is dissolved in 1 quart of water)	Used to replace water and electrolytes when food and fluid intake is sharply reduced (*e.g.,* postoperatively, starvation) or when fluid loss is excessive (*e.g.,* diarrhea, severe vomiting); severe, continual diarrhea requires parenteral replacement therapy; use only in recommended volumes to prevent electrolyte overload; reduce intake when other electrolytes are re-instituted; do not use in the presence of intestinal obstruction, intractable vomiting, adynamic ileus, perforated bowel, or impaired renal function; avoid mixing with other electrolyte-containing liquids (milk, fruit juice)
Phosphorus (K-Phos Neutral, Neutra-Phos, Neutra-Phos-K, Uro-KP-Neutral)	Tablets—173 mg, 250 mg (with sodium and potassium) Capsules—250 mg (with sodium and potassium) Powder for solution—250 mg/75 ml (reconstituted solution with sodium and potassium)	1 to 2 tablets 3 to 4 times a day *or* Contents of 1 capsule mixed with 75 ml water 4 times a day *or* 75 ml reconstituted solution 4 times a day	Used as dietary supplement where diet is deficient, needs are increased, or GI absorption is impaired; RDAs are 800 mg (adults and children 4 yr–6 yr) and 1200 mg (children 11 yr–18 yr and pregnant or lactating women); phosphate can lower urinary calcium levels; a laxative effect is common early in therapy; contraindicated in hyperkalemia and Addison's disease
Sodium chloride (Slo-Salt)	Tablets—650 mg, 1 g, 2.25 g Tablets (slow release)—600 mg Enteric-coated tablets—1 g	0.5 g to 1 g 5 to 10 times a day	Used to replace excessive loss of sodium and chloride (*e.g.,* resulting from perspiration or extreme diuresis) and to counteract excessive salt restriction; use cautiously in patients with congestive heart failure, renal disease, circulatory insufficiency, or electrolyte disturbances; also available with dextrose and vitamin B₁ (Sodium Chloride with Dextrose) and in fixed combination with potassium chloride, calcium carbonate, and dextrose (Thermotabs) or with potassium chloride, calcium phosphate, and magnesium carbonate (Heatrol)

(continued)

Table 77-1. Oral Nutritional Supplements *(continued)*

Drug	Preparations	Usual Dosage Range	Remarks
Zinc (Medizinc, Orazinc, Scrip Zinc, Verazinc, Zincate, Zinkaps)	Tablets—66 mg, 110 mg, 200 mg, 220 mg (equivalent to 15 mg, 25 mg, 45 mg, and 50 mg elemental zinc, respectively) Capsules—110 mg, 220 mg	15 mg to 55 mg elemental zinc a day	Important mineral for normal growth and repair of body tissues; symptoms of zinc deficiency include anorexia, loss of taste and olfactory sensation, mood changes, and growth retardation; used investigationally to treat delayed wound healing, acne, and rheumatoid arthritis, to improve the immune response in the elderly, and to delay onset of dementia in patients genetically at risk; RDAs are 10 mg (children 1 yr–10 yr), 15 mg (adults), 20 mg to 25 mg (pregnant or lactating women); excessive doses may produce severe vomiting, dehydration, and restlessness; GI upset can occur and can be minimized by taking drug with food or milk; zinc can impair absorption of tetracyclines

Miscellaneous Nutritional Factors

Drug	Preparations	Usual Dosage Range	Remarks
Bioflavonoids (C Speridin, C.V.P., duo-C.V.P., Hesper, Peridin, Span C	Tablets—100 mg, 150 mg, 200 mg, 300 mg Capsules—100 mg	100 mg to 500 mg/day	Derived from green citrus fruits; previously used to reduce capillary fragility and referred to as vitamin P ("permeability"); no evidence that they are effective and no established need in human nutrition
Calcium caseinate (Casec)	Powder—(containing 88% protein, 2% fat and 4.5% minerals)	Variable according to patient's requirements	Used as an infant formula modifier or as a diet supplement
Choline	Tablets—250 mg, 325 mg, 500 mg, 650 mg Powder	250 mg to 1 g/day	A component of lecithin that has a lipotropic action, and is essential for the formation of acetylcholine; average diet provides sufficient choline for body needs; has been used to treat fatty liver and cirrhosis, and relieve symptoms of CNS disorders such as Huntington's disease and tardive dyskinesias; can cause GI disturbances and imparts an odor of decaying fish to the feces and occasionally the breath; used as free choline as well as bitartrate, chloride, and dihydrogen citrate salts
Corn oil (Lipomul Oral)	Liquid—10 g/15 ml	Adults—45 ml 2 to 4 times a day Children—30 ml 1 to 4 times a day	Used to increase caloric intake in malnourished or debilitated patients; use cautiously in persons with diabetes and gallbladder dysfunction; each dose contains 270 cal and 30 g fat
Glucose polymers (Moducal, Polycose, Sumacal)	Liquid or powder—containing various amounts of carbohydrates, sodium, chloride, and potassium	Add to foods or beverages and give in small, frequent feedings	Derived from cornstarch; supplies calories in patients unable to meet caloric needs with usual food intake, or in patients on protein-, electrolyte-, and fat-restricted diets; *not* intended as the sole nutritional source; may be used for extended periods of time with diets containing all other essential nutrients

Table 77-1. Oral Nutritional Supplements (continued)

Drug	Preparations	Usual Dosage Range	Remarks
Inositol	Tablets—250 mg, 325 mg, 500 mg, 650 mg Powder	1 g to 3 g/day in divided doses	An isomer of glucose possessing lipotropic activity in animals; physiologic role in humans is obscure and there is no evidence that it is clinically effective, although it has been used to treat liver disorders and disordered fat metabolism; dietary sources include mainly vegetables
Lactase (Lact-Aid, Lactrase)	Liquid—1250 Neutral Lactase Units/4-drop dose Capsules—125 mg of standardized lactase enzyme	4 to 10 drops per quart of milk or 1 to 2 capsules either added to a quart of milk or taken along with milk or dairy products	Powdered enzyme preparation used to facilitate digestion of milk lactose in patients with lactose intolerance
Lecithin	Capsules—520 mg, 1.2 g Granules	1 to 4 capsules/day	A source of choline, inositol, phosphorus, and linoleic and linolenic acids employed as a dietary supplement (see Choline, above)
L-Lysine (Enisyl, L-Lysine)	Tablets—334 mg, 500 mg	334 mg to 1500 mg/day	An essential amino acid, used as a dietary supplement to increase utilization of vegetable proteins
Medium chain triglycerides (MCT)	Oil, consisting primarily of the triglycerides of C_8 and C_{10} saturated fatty acids	15 ml 3 to 4 times a day	A dietary supplement for persons who cannot efficiently digest and absorb conventional long-chain fatty acids; medium-chain triglycerides are more rapidly hydrolyzed than conventional food fat, and are not dependent on bile salts for emulsification; may be mixed with juices, poured on salads or other foods, incorporated into sauces, or used in cooking and baking; use with caution in persons with hepatic cirrhosis; one dose weighs approximately 14 g and contains 115 cal
Para-aminobenzoic acid (PABA, Potaba)	Tablets—30 mg, 100 mg, 250 mg, 500 mg Capsules—500 mg Powder	Adults—12 g/day in 4 to 6 divided doses Children—1 g/10 lb daily in divided doses	A substance found naturally associated with the B-complex vitamins and essential for the functioning of a number of important biologic processes; considered "possibly effective" for scleroderma, dermatomyositis, morphea, pemphigus, and Peyronie's disease; dissolve tablets in liquid to minimize GI upset; drug should be taken with food; adverse reactions include anorexia, nausea, fever, and rash; use cautiously in patients with kidney impairment; do not give concurrently with sulfonamides, because PABA interferes with the antibacterial action; has no known human nutritional value; acts as a sunscreen when applied topically
Protein hydrolysates (A/G Pro, PDP Liquid Protein, Pro-Mix, Propac, Protinex)	Tablets—542 mg (45% amino acids with minerals) Capsules—292 mg protein (with vitamins and minerals) Liquid—15 g protein/30 ml Powder	2 tablets 3 times a day or 1 capsule 3 times a day or 30 ml liquid/day or 1 tbsp to 2 tbsp powder in liquid/day	Preparations of amino acids and peptides obtained by hydrolysis of larger proteins; used as dietary supplement to correct or prevent protein deficiency; optimum daily intake of dietary protein is 1 g/kg

(continued)

Table 77-1. Oral Nutritional Supplements (continued)

Drug	Preparations	Usual Dosage Range	Remarks
Safflower oil (Microlipid)	Emulsion—50% fat	1 tbsp to 2 tbsp several times a day as necessary	A caloric and fatty-acid supplement used in malnourished patients and other persons with fatty-acid deficiencies; contains 4500 cal and 500 g fat per liter
L-Tryptophan (Trofan, Tryptacin)	Tablets—125 mg, 200 mg, 250 mg, 500 mg, 667 mg Capsules—200 mg, 250 mg	600 mg to 2 g/day in divided doses	An essential amino acid that serves as a precursor for serotonin; has been used experimentally as an antidepressant and hypnotic, although its clinical efficacy in this regard remains to be established

impulse transmission; skeletal, cardiac, and smooth muscle contraction; and maintenance of intracellular tonicity and renal function. Potassium depletion occurs most frequently as a result of diuretic therapy, but may also be due to hyperaldosteronism, severe diarrhea, or diabetic ketoacidosis. It is usually accompanied by chloride loss as well, and is therefore frequently associated with metabolic alkalosis. Symptoms of potassium depletion include muscle weakness, cramping, fatigue, disturbances in cardiac rhythm, and inability to concentrate urine. The salts of potassium available for oral use are the chloride, gluconate, acetate, citrate, and bicarbonate. When hypokalemia is associated with alkalosis, the chloride salt should be used. When acidosis is present, one of the other salts is indicated. When oral replacement therapy is not feasible (as with severe vomiting, prolonged diuresis, marked diabetic acidosis) parenteral (IV infusion) therapy is indicated (see Table 77-2).

The usual adult dietary intake of potassium ranges from 40 mEq to 150 mEq/day. Hypokalemia generally results from loss of 200 mEq or more of potassium from the total body store.

Mechanism
Essential ion for maintenance of excitability of nerves and muscles, as well as acid–base balance

Uses
1   Prevention and treatment of hypokalemia, for example, resulting from diuretic therapy, prolonged vomiting or diarrhea, diabetes, hepatic cirrhosis, inadequate dietary intake, malabsorption, hyperaldosteronism, or nephropathy

Dosage

10% solution = 20 mEq/15 ml

Prevention of hypokalemia: 16 mEq to 24 mEq/day
Treatment of deficiency states: 40 mEq to 100 mEq/day

Common Side-Effects
Nausea, abdominal discomfort, vomiting, and diarrhea

Significant Adverse Reactions
GI bleeding and perforation, hyperkalemia (paresthesias, flaccid paralysis, confusion, weakness, hypotension, respiratory distress, arrhythmias, cardiac depression, heart block)

Contraindications
Severe renal impairment with oliguria, anuria or azotemia, Addison's disease, acute dehydration, heat cramps, hyperkalemia in patients receiving potassium-sparing diuretics; in addition, solid dosage forms of potassium are contraindicated in patients in whom there is delayed passage of contents through the GI tract.

Interactions
1   Combinations of potassium salts with potassium-sparing diuretics can result in severe hyperkalemia.
2   Increased serum potassium decreases both toxicity and effectiveness of digitalis drugs.
3   Concurrent use of salt substitutes with potassium supplements can lead to hyperkalemia.

▶ NURSING ALERTS
▷ 1   Do not administer solid dosage forms (*i.e.*, tablets, powders) to any patient in whom there is reduced gastrointestinal (GI) passage, because gastric and intestinal ulceration can occur. Liquid dosage forms must be used.
▷ 2   Observe patients closely for development of severe vomiting, GI bleeding (*i.e.*, black stools), weakness, abdominal pain or distention, and discontinue drug immediately should these occur.
▷ 3   Use cautiously in patients with systemic acidosis, acute dehydration, chronic renal dysfunction, cardiac disease, adrenal insufficiency, or peptic ulcer.
▷ 4   Closely monitor acid–base balance, serum electrolytes, and ECG during treatment of hypokalemia with potassium salts to avoid potassium intoxication, which can result in arrhythmias and cardiac depression.
▷ 5   Never administer potassium chloride by IV push or in concentrated amounts by any route.

▶ NURSING CONSIDERATIONS
▷ 1   Be aware that *serum* potassium concentrations are not always an accurate indication of total *intracellular* potassium levels. Treatment of potassium depletion, therefore, requires careful assessment of clinical status as well as laboratory evaluations.
▷ 2   Monitor intake–output ratio and report immediately any significant change in renal function. Potassium intoxication with oral administration is rare in patients with normal kidney function.

▷ 3 Urge patients to avoid use of salt substitutes, many of which contain potassium. Caution against excessive use of laxatives, which can alter electrolyte balance.

▷ 4 Instruct patients to swallow coated tablets whole, because chewing will increase likelihood of GI irritation. Take with a full glass of water, preferably after meals or with food.

▷ 5 Dissolve powders or effervescent tablets in 4 oz to 8 oz cold water, juice, or other beverage, and sip slowly.

▶ fluoride

The fluoride ion, used either orally or topically, is employed as an aid in the prevention of dental caries. It is most commonly administered to young children combined with vitamins and minerals in the form of drops or tablets. Fluoride can also be used locally as a mouthwash by persons prone to develop frequent dental caries.

Mechanism
Incorporated into external layers of dental enamel, making it more resistant to erosion by acid; may also facilitate osteoblastic activity of bone

Uses
1 Aid in prevention of dental caries
2 Treatment of osteoporosis; doses up to 60 mg/day, in combination with calcium, vitamin D, and/or estrogen (investigational use only)

Dosage
(Prevention of dental caries)
Oral: 0.25 mg to 1 mg/day, depending on age
Topical: 5 ml to 10 ml once a day as a mouth rinse after brushing; rinse for 1 minute, then expectorate

Fate
Rapidly absorbed orally; widely distributed and quickly deposited in teeth and bone; quickly excreted by the kidney

Significant Adverse Reactions
Eczema, atopic dermatitis, urticaria, nausea, GI distress, headache, weakness, staining of the teeth (topical only)

Chronic overdosage can lead to mottling of the tooth enamel.

Contraindications
Intake of drinking water containing 0.7 ppm or more of fluoride, sodium-free diets

▶ NURSING CONSIDERATIONS
▷ 1 Administer tablets or drops after meals, but have patient avoid milk or dairy products with sodium fluoride tablets, because GI absorption is reduced.

▷ 2 Urge the use of rinses immediately after brushing and preferably just before retiring. Advise patients not to swallow while using the rinse and to avoid eating or drinking for at least 30 minutes afterward.

▷ 3 Use plastic containers for diluting rinses or drops.

▷ 4 Observe for staining or mottling of teeth with repeated use, and advise physician or dentist.

▷ 5 Note that acute fluoride overdosage can result in excessive salivation and GI disturbances. Emesis invariably occurs with ingestion of large amounts, and serves as a protective mechanism.

Parenteral Nutritional Supplements

Parenteral nutritional supplementation is provided for a number of reasons, ranging from correction of simple acute dehydration to chronic treatment of serious nutritional deficiencies resulting from such conditions as severe GI disorders, prolonged kidney failure, and extensive burns.

Substances provided in parenteral nutritional supplements include electrolytes, carbohydrates, fats, and proteins. Administration of nutritional solutions *via* peripheral veins (*i.e.,* peripheral parenteral nutrition) is generally adequate if caloric requirements are minimal and can be partially satisfied with oral supplements and if nutritional therapy will only be required for 1 week to 2 weeks. Conversely, in severely depleted patients or in patients who will require prolonged supplemental nutrition, central parenteral nutrition using a central venous catheter is usually indicated. This latter procedure, frequently termed *hyperalimentation,* is used to maintain an anabolic state when conventional oral or tube feeding is inappropriate and when peripheral IV therapy cannot meet the nutritional demands of the patient. Hyperalimentation is indicated following a major bowel resection, in the presence of obstructive or severe inflammatory conditions of the bowel, and in patients with prolonged paralytic ileus (such as following abdominal trauma or surgery). It is also employed to manage hypermetabolic states due to severe trauma such as extensive burns, infections, or multiple injuries, and to treat malabsorption states, as, for example those resulting from hepatic or pancreatic insufficiency.

Hyperalimentation solutions are hypertonic and contain a protein source (amino acids), together with varying amounts of dextrose, fat, vitamins, electrolytes, and trace minerals. Due to their hypertonicity, these solutions must be administered through a large vein having sufficient blood flow to provide adequate dilution. For this reason, the solution is given into the superior vena cava *via* the subclavian vein, and the procedure is carried out by surgically implanting a catheter into the appropriate vessel. Although the technical details of the hyperalimentation procedure are not reviewed here, this form of nutritional therapy is a potentially hazardous one, and requires personnel trained and experienced in the technique as well as in the care of patients undergoing the procedure.

The various types of substances used for parenteral nutrition are considered individually; however, as previously indicated, several different kinds of nutrients are usually administered together, depending on the clinical status and nutritional requirements of the patient.

Protein (Amino-Acid) Products

The protein products employed as parenteral nutrients include protein hydrolysates and mixtures of crystalline amino acids, with or without added electrolytes. Most products are used for central venous hyperalimentation, but some of the amino-acid preparations can be employed as dilute solutions for peripheral parenteral feeding. These products provide a concentrated form of utilizable amino acids for protein synthesis as well as varying amounts of electrolytes, but require addition of sufficient dextrose to provide for full caloric energy requirements when used for chronic hyperalimentation.

▶ crystalline amino-acid injection

Aminosyn, FreAmine III, Novamine, Procalamine, Travasol, Veinamine

Crystalline amino acids are hypertonic solutions of essential and nonessential l-amino acids or low-molecular-weight peptides with varying proportions of electrolytes that provide a substrate for protein synthesis and exert a protein-sparing effect. Preparations differ in degree of osmolarity, amino-acid ratios, and content of nitrogen. In addition to the general amino-acid formulations listed above, specialized formulations are available for use in patients with renal failure, hepatic failure/encephalopathy, or acute metabolic stress. These latter products are considered after the review of the general formulations.

Mechanism
Provide replacement of deficient amino acids and electrolytes; possess a nitrogen-sparing effect when used with a nonprotein caloric source; promote a positive nitrogen balance and increase protein synthesis

Uses
1 Prevention of nitrogen loss or treatment of negative nitrogen balance
2 Adjuncts in providing adequate total parenteral nutrition, as a component product of central parenteral nutrition (*i.e.*, hyperalimentation) in full strength or peripheral parenteral nutrition in diluted form

Dosage
Dosage is flexible and depends on daily protein requirements, patient's clinical response, and metabolic activity; see individual package instructions; average adult dose is 2 liters/day to provide 1 g to 2 g protein/kg

Common Side-Effects
Nausea, flushing, sensation of warmth (especially with rapid infusion)

Significant Adverse Reactions
Vomiting, chills, headache, abdominal pain, dizziness, allergic reactions, phlebitis, venous thrombosis, skin rash, papular eruptions; metabolic disturbances include acidosis, alkalosis, hypocalcemia, hypophosphatemia, hyperglycemia, glycosuria, hypovitaminosis, and other electrolyte imbalances.

Contraindications
Anuria, oliguria, severe liver or kidney impairment, metabolic disorders involving impaired nitrogen utilization, decreased circulating blood volume, inborn errors of amino-acid metabolism, hepatic coma or encephalopathy, and hyperammonemia

Interactions
1 Antianabolic drugs and tetracyclines may reduce the protein-sparing effects of amino acids
2 Addition of calcium to the infusion may precipitate the phosphate ion.

▶ NURSING ALERTS
▷ 1 Administer amino-acid injections only after a thorough assessment of the patient's fluid and electrolyte balance and nutritional status. Close monitoring of these parameters during therapy is essential for proper treatment.

▷ 2 Provide sufficient nonprotein calories in the form of concentrated dextrose solutions during infusions of amino-acid solutions over extended periods of time.

▷ 3 Do not premix amino-acid infusions with fat emulsions; rather, infuse simultaneously by means of a Y connector located near the infusion site.

▷ 4 Use amino-acid solutions cautiously in patients with reduced liver function and be alert for symptoms of hyperammonemia (reduced body temperature, weak pulse, GI distress). Discontinue administration and re-evaluate patient's status.

▷ 5 Do not administer simultaneously with blood through the same infusion site, because pseudoagglutination can occur.

▷ 6 Use aseptic technique in mixing solutions and in the insertion and maintenance of central venous catheters, because risk of sepsis is considerable. Use solution promptly after mixing and discard any unused portion. Do not mix antibiotics with protein–carbohydrate hyperalimentation solutions.

▷ 7 Discontinue infusion gradually (at least 24 hr) because sudden cessation of therapy may result in marked hypoglycemia.

▷ 8 Perform frequent blood and urine sugar determinations in diabetics and in patients with impaired glucose tolerance. Insulin dosage adjustments may be necessary.

▶ NURSING CONSIDERATIONS
▷ 1 Infuse slowly to minimize adverse effects. Too rapid infusion may result in hyperglycemia and glycosuria, which may require insulin administration to correct. Check for extravasation.

▷ 2 Monitor serum electrolytes during treatment, and supplement with appropriate electrolyte solutions as necessary.

▷ 3 Be alert for signs of fatty-acid deficiency (flaking skin, loss of hair) and assess plasma lipid level. IV fat emulsion will correct the deficiency.

▷ 4 Note that supplementary vitamins, minerals, electrolytes, heparin, or insulin may be given cautiously through the indwelling catheter, but administration of any *other* medications or withdrawal or transfusion of blood is not recommended by this route.

▷ 5 Use cautiously in patients with cardiac insufficiency to avoid circulatory overload.

▷ 6 Do *not* administer strongly hypertonic solutions (*e.g.,* stronger than 12.5% dextrose) by *peripheral* vein infusion. They should only be given through an indwelling central venous catheter with the tip located in the superior vena cava.

▷ 7 Relace all IV administration sets every 24 hours to 48 hours.

▷ 8 Recognize that most amino-acid infusions are indicated for hyperalimentation, except for Aminosyn 3.5%, FreAmine III 3% w/electrolytes, ProcalAmine, and Travasol 3.5% w/electrolyte 45.

▶ amino-acid formulation for renal failure
Aminosyn-RF, NephrAmine, RenAmin

Amino-acid formulation for renal failure is indicated to provide nutritional support for uremic patients where oral nutrition is impractical and dialysis is not feasible. The products are used in conjunction with dextrose, electrolytes, and vitamins, and are administered by central venous injection. Amino-acid formulation for renal failure supplies only essential amino acids, thus allowing urea nitrogen to be recycled to glutamate, which serves as a precursor for synthesis of nonessential amino acids. Therefore, use of these products in uremic patients results in utilization of retained urea and amelioration of azotemic symptoms. To promote urea reutilization, however, it is essential to provide adequate calories and to restrict intake of nonessential nitrogen.

▶ amino-acid formulation for high metabolic stress
FreAmine HBC

Amino-acid formulation for high metabolic stress is a mixture of essential and nonessential amino acids with high concentrations of the branched-chain amino acids isoleucine, leucine, and valine. Metabolic stress is often characterized by increased urinary excretion of nitrogen and by hyperglycemia, with decreased plasma levels of branched-chain amino acids. As a result, glucose utilization and fat mobilization are impaired. By supplying branched-chain amino acids, this formulation provides the substrates needed to meet the energy requirements of muscle and brain tissue.

▶ amino-acid formulation for hepatic failure or hepatic encephalopathy
HepatAmine

This formulation is very similar to the one above, being a mixture of essential and nonessential amino acids with high concentrations of branched-chain amino acids. It is used for treating hepatic encephalopathy in patients intolerant of general-purpose amino-acid injections. Replenishment of stores of branched-chain amino acids can reverse the abnormal plasma amino acid pattern seen in hepatic encephalopathy, with resultant improvement in mental status and EEG pattern. Nitrogen balance is also significantly improved.

Carbohydrates

Parenteral carbohydrate solutions are indicated primarily as a source of calories and fluid in patients with nutritional deficiencies who are unable to obtain the necessary nutrients orally. The available preparations include Dextrose in Water, Alcohol in Dextrose Infusion, Fructose in Water, and Invert Sugar (dextrose and fructose) in Water.

▶ dextrose in water injection
D-2½-W, D-5-W, D-10-W, D-20-W, D-25-W, D-30-W, D-38.5-W, D-40-W, D-50-W, D-60-W, D-70-W

Dextrose in Water Injection is available as solutions of varying concentrations of dextrose (D-glucose) in water for injection. Caloric content ranges from 85 cal/liter (2½%) to 2380 cal/liter (70%). The 5% solution is isotonic and along with the 2.5% and 10% solutions may be given by IV infusion into peripheral veins to provide calories where nonelectrolytic fluid is required. The 20% solution provides adequate calories in a minimal volume of water. The more concentrated solutions provide even greater caloric content with less fluid volume and may be irritating if given by peripheral infusion; they are usually administered by central venous catheters as a component of the hyperalimentation procedure. Dextrose is also available in several electrolyte solutions in various concentrations for IV infusion in patients having both a carbohydrate and an electrolyte deficit. Principal electrolytes used in fixed combination with dextrose are sodium, chloride, potassium, calcium, magnesium, phosphate, lactate, and acetate.

Mechanism
Provides a source of calories and fluid volume where nutritional or fluid deficiencies (or both) exist

Uses
1 Provide nonelectrolytic fluid and caloric replacement (usually 5% or 10% solution)
2 Component of total parenteral nutrition, in conjunction with other solutions of proteins, electrolytes, fats, vitamins (usually 40%, 50%, 60%, or 70% solution)
3 Treatment of insulin hypoglycemia to restore blood glucose levels (50% solution)
4 Treatment of acute symptomatic hypoglycemia in the neonate or older infant to restore depressed blood glucose levels (25% solution)

Dosage
Dependent on patient's status and nutritional state

Fate

Approximately 95% is retained if infusion rate is 800 mg/kg/hour; essentially 100% retention occurs at 400 mg to 500 mg/kg/hour

Significant Adverse Reactions

Thrombophlebitis (with prolonged infusion), irritation, tissue necrosis, infection at injection site, hypervolemia, mental confusion, hyperglycemia, glycosuria (especially with concentrated solutions or too-rapid administration), over-hydration, congestion, and pulmonary edema

Contraindications

Diabetic coma; use of concentrated solutions in patients with intracranial hemorrhage or delirium tremens

Interactions

1 Dextrose infusions may alter insulin or oral anti-diabetic drug requirements, and cause vitamin-B complex deficiency
2 Hyperglycemia and glycosuria may be intensified by diuretics that decrease glucose tolerance.

▶ **NURSING ALERTS**

▷ 1 Administer concentrated (hypertonic) solutions (25% or stronger) *slowly* by a central venous catheter. They are very irritating and may cause thrombosis if given into a peripheral vein.
▷ 2 Observe patients during administration for signs of hyperglycemia or hyperosmolarity (confusion, unconsciousness), and reduce or terminate infusion.
▷ 3 Be alert for development of fluid overload, leading to dilution of serum electrolytes, congestion, and possibly pulmonary edema.
▷ 4 If hypertonic dextrose infusion is abruptly terminated, administer 5% Dextrose to avoid a rebound hypoglycemic response.
▷ 5 Use carefully in patients with renal insufficiency, cardiac decompensation, hypervolemia, carbohydrate intolerance, or urinary tract obstruction.

▶ **NURSING CONSIDERATIONS**

▷ 1 Closely monitor blood and urine glucose during prolonged infusions, especially with concentrated solutions.
▷ 2 Add appropriate electrolytes to the infusion based on the electrolyte status of the patient.
▷ 3 Note that the maximum rate that dextrose can be infused without inducing glycosuria is 0.5 g/kg/hour.
▷ 4 Do not use unless solution is clear. Discard unused portion.

▶ **alcohol in dextrose infusion**

Alcohol in dextrose infusions are solutions of 5% Dextrose in Water containing 5% or 10% ethyl alcohol that provide a source of carbohydrate calories. They are not as commonly used as plain Dextrose in Water infusions due to the adverse effects of alcohol in many patients.

Mechanism

Supply a source of carbohydrate calories; may result in liver glycogen depletion and exert a protein-sparing action; alcohol can prevent premature labor, presumably by inhibiting release of oxytocin from the posterior pituitary.

Uses

1 Aid in increasing caloric intake in nutritional deficiencies
2 Prevent premature labor (10% solution)—investigational use only

Dosage

1 liter to 2 liters of a 5% solution in a 24-hour period by *slow* IV infusion
Children: 40 ml/kg/24 hours

Fate

Alcohol is metabolized at a rate of 10 ml to 20 ml/hour (200 ml–400 ml of a 5% solution)

Significant Adverse Reactions

(Usually with too-rapid infusion) Vertigo, flushing, sedation, confusion, alcoholic odor on breath, and pain and irritation at infusion site

Contraindications

Epilepsy, alcohol addiction, diabetic coma, urinary tract infections, severe kidney or liver impairment, shock, following cranial surgery

Interactions

1 Alcohol may shorten the effects of phenytoin, warfarin, and tolbutamide.
2 Alcohol can potentiate the postural hypotensive effects of antihypertensive drugs, vasodilators, and diuretics.
3 Additive CNS depressive effects can occur between alcohol and other CNS depressants, such as barbiturates, benzodiazepines, meprobamate, glutethimide, narcotics, phenothiazines, and so forth.
4 An acute alcohol intolerance syndrome (*e.g.,* flushing, sweating, tachycardia, nausea) has occurred with concurrent administration of disulfiram, metronidazole, moxalactam, cefamandole, cefoperazone, and sulfonylurea antidiabetic drugs.
5 Increased GI bleeding can occur with combined use of salicylates or other anti-inflammatory drugs.

▶ **NURSING ALERTS**

▷ 1 Use cautiously in diabetics, because the rate of metabolism of alcohol is slowed and blood sugar may decrease substantially.
▷ 2 Because alcohol readily crosses the placental barrier and passes into breast milk freely, use during pregnancy and nursing only when absolutely necessary.
▷ 3 Avoid extravasation during IV administration. Do not inject SC.
▷ 4 Use with caution in patients with liver or renal impairment, in the presence of shock, during postpartum hemorrhage, and following cranial surgery.

▶ **NURSING CONSIDERATIONS**

▷ 1 Use the largest available peripheral vein and a small-bore needle to minimize irritation. Infuse at a slow rate and observe for signs of alcohol intoxication (slurred speech, drowsiness, flushing, dizziness).

▷ 2 Be aware that 10% solutions of ethyl alcohol can be used by IV infusion to delay labor, presumably by decreasing release of oxytocin from the pituitary. Commercially available alcohol and dextrose infusions are not approved by the FDA for this particular indication.

▶ **fructose in water**

A 10% solution of Fructose (levulose) in Water provides approximately 375 cal/liter. Unlike dextrose, it does not require insulin for ultimate conversion to utilizable glucose, and produces lower serum and urinary glucose levels. In addition, it is more readiy converted to glycogen than dextrose. Thus, it may be preferred to dextrose in diabetic patients. However, it is of no value for treating hypoglycemia. It is principally an alternative source of calories and fluid, and the dosage must be adjusted to the caloric needs of the patient. Electrolyte and vitamin supplementation should be provided as needed.

Infusion rates should not exceed 1 g/kg/hour to minimize the danger of metabolic acidosis, especially in infants and small children. Fructose should not be given to patients with gout, because it may increase the serum uric acid level. Use with caution in patients with renal insufficiency, frank cardiac decompensation, hypervolemia, or urinary tract obstruction. The suitability of long-term fructose infusions is questionable, because significant depletion of liver ATP can occur.

▶ **invert sugar in water**

Travert

A solution comprising equal parts of dextrose and fructose, Invert Sugar in Water is available as a 10% concentration. The fructose reportedly enhances the utilization of dextrose and the combination represents an alternative to use of either agent alone. Refer to the respective monographs for each sugar for additional information.

Lipids

Fat emulsions designed for IV infusion are prepared from either soybean or safflower oil and contain a mixture of neutral triglycerides, which are largely polyunsaturated fatty acids. In addition, these products also contain 1.2% egg yolk phospholipids as an emulsifier and glycerin to adjust tonicity. Caloric content of the 10% IV fat emulsion is 1.1 cal/ml and that of the 20% emulsion is 2.0 cal/ml. These IV emulsions are isotonic, and may be given by either peripheral or central venous routes.

▶ **intravenous fat emulsion**

Intralipid 10%, 20%; Liposyn 10%, 20%; Soyacal 10%, 20%; Travamulsion 10%, 20%

Mechanism

Provide a source of calories and essential fatty acids in parenteral nutrition regimens

Uses

1 Supplemental source of calories and fatty acids for patients requiring total parenteral nutrition for extended periods of time whose caloric requirements cannot be met by glucose

2 Prevention and treatment of fatty-acid deficiency states

Dosage

(Note: Fat emulsion should comprise no more than 60% of the total caloric intake of the patient.)

Total parenteral nutrition
Adults:
10%—initially 1 ml/minute for 15 minutes to 30 minutes; gradually increase rate to 83 ml/hour to 125 ml/hour; infuse only 500 ml first day then gradually increase dose
20%—initially 0.5 ml/minute for 15 minutes to 30 minutes; gradually increase rate to 62 ml/hour; infuse only 250 ml first day
Do *not* exceed 3 g/kg/day
Children: (see Significant Adverse Reactions)
10%—initially 0.1 ml/minute for 10 minutes to 15 minutes
20%—initially 0.5 ml/minute for 10 minutes to 15 minutes; gradually increase rate of each to 1 g/kg/4 hour
Do *not* exceed 4 g/kg/day

Fatty-acid deficiency
Supply 8% to 10% of the caloric intake by IV fat emulsion.

Fate

Metabolized and utilized as a source of energy; cleared from the plasma in a manner similar to clearance of chylomicrons

Significant Adverse Reactions

Warning: Infusion of IV fat emulsion in premature infants has resulted in some fatalities, presumably due to fat accumulation in the lungs. Follow dosage guidelines strictly; infusion rate should be as slow as possible, not to exceed 1 g/kg in 4 hours. Carefully monitor the infant's ability to clear the fat from the circulation between infusions, for example, measurement of triglyceride or free fatty-acid levels. Lipemia *must* clear between daily infusions.

Dyspnea, cyanosis, allergic reactions, nausea, vomiting, flushing, headache, fever, sweating, insomnia, dizziness, chest or back pain, hyperlipemia, hypercoagulability, thrombophlebitis, irritation at injection site, transient increase in liver enzymes; with prolonged administration, hepatomegaly, jaundice, leukopenia, thrombocytopenia, splenomegaly, seizures, and shock

Contraindications

Disturbed fat metabolism, acute pancreatitis; in premature infants with bilirubin levels above 5 mg/dl, patients with severe egg allergies

▶ NURSING ALERTS

▷ 1 Use care when mixing with electrolyte nutrient solutions or other additive solutions (to avoid disturbing the emulsion) and do not use filters with this product. Observe emulsion for any separation and do not use if emulsion appears disturbed.

▷ 2 When administering together with carbohydrate or protein–amino-acid infusion solutions, either infuse into separate peripheral site or by means of a Y connector located near the infusion site. Keep lipid infusion line higher than dextrose–amino-acid infusion line to prevent backflow.

▷ 3 Use with caution in patients with liver damage, pulmonary disease, anemia, or coagulation disorders, or where there is danger of fat embolism.

▷ 4 Monitor liver function during extended administration and discontinue drug if liver dysfunction is noted. Monitor platelet count daily in neonates.

▷ 5 Assess patient's ability to clear the infused fat from the circulation during therapy. Lipemia must clear between daily infusions in order for therapy to proceed on a daily basis.

▷ 6 Closely monitor the hemogram, blood coagulation, plasma lipids, platelet count, and liver function. Discontinue drug if a significant abnormality occurs in any of the above parameters.

▶ NURSING CONSIDERATIONS

▷ 1 Recognize that IV fat emulsion should make up no more than 60% of patient's total caloric intake. Remainder should be supplied by carbohydrate and amino-acid sources.

▷ 2 Use only freshly opened solutions, and discard remainder of partially used dose.

▷ 3 Note that preparations should be stored at 25°C or below but not frozen.

▷ 4 Be aware that use of this product may result in deposition of a brown pigmentation in the reticuloendothelial system ("intravenous fat pigment"). The cause and significance are unknown.

Electrolytes

Ammonium	Phosphate
Bicarbonate	Potassium
Calcium	Sodium
Chloride	Tromethamine
Magnesium	

Parenteral electrolytes are sometimes supplied individually to correct a specific known deficiency (*e.g.,* hyponatremia, hypokalemia), but more commonly are used as combination electrolyte solutions for adjunctive treatment of nutritional disorders, dehydration, severe burns, trauma, and other emergency situations. Combined electrolyte solutions are also employed as part of the total parenteral nutrition (hyperalimentation) regimen. Serum electrolyte levels must be monitored closely during treatment, and the composition of the infusion solution as well as the rate of administration should be adjusted to provide as nearly optimal blood levels of each electrolyte as possible.

The various parenteral electrolytes are listed in Table 77-2, with available preparations, dosage, and pertinent remarks. Although the discussion afforded these preparations here is rather brief, anyone using these products routinely should become thoroughly familiar with their pharmacology and toxicology, because serious untoward reactions have occurred with improper selection or administration of parenteral electrolytes.

Table 77-2. Parenteral Electrolytes

Drug	Preparations	Usual Dosage Range	Remarks
Ammonium chloride	Injection—2.14% (0.4 mEq/ml), 26.75% (5 mEq/ml)	Dependent on patient's status; if edema or hyponatremia is not present, total dose is estimated as product of ECF volume (20% of body weight in kg) times serum chloride deficit in mEq/ml; initially, give one half calculated dose and check *p*H before giving remainder	Indicated for treatment of metabolic alkalosis or hypochloremic states sufficiently severe as to cause signs of impending tetany (severe or protracted vomiting, gastric suction); generally given with 20 mEq to 40 mEq potassium/liter to correct accompanying hypokalemia; contraindicated in severe hepatic impairment because danger of ammonia retention is present, and in patients with primary respiratory alkalosis and high CO_2; cautious use in renal dysfunction, cardiac edema, or pulmonary insufficiency; administer by *slow* IV infusion and

Table 77-2. Parenteral Electrolytes (continued)

Drug	Preparations	Usual Dosage Range	Remarks
			observe for signs of ammonia toxicity (sweating, irregular breathing, bradycardia, vomiting, twitching, arrhythmias); do not give SC, intraperitoneally, or rectally; low-strength solution may be given undiluted but higher strength solution should be diluted with normal saline; may increase excretion rate of basic drugs (*e.g.,* amphetamines, quinidine)
Calcium chloride	Injection—10% (1 g = 13.6 mEq)	Slow IV injection only: Hypocalcemia—500 mg to 1 g at 1-day to 3-day intervals Magnesium intoxication—500 mg at once; repeat as necessary Cardiac resuscitation—200 mg to 800 mg into the ventricular cavity or 500 mg to 1 g IV	Indicated for treatment of hypocalcemia requiring a prompt elevation in serum calcium levels (*e.g.,* neonatal tetany, parathyroid deficiency, alkalosis); also used to prevent hypocalcemia during exchange transfusions, as adjunctive therapy in treating serious insect bites, for managing lead colic and magnesium intoxication, and for cardiac resuscitation (calcium chloride only) when epinephrine therapy is ineffective; calcium chloride is highly irritating and severe necrosis and sloughing can occur; other calcium salts are preferred where possible; IM administration of calcium salts (except chloride—IV only) should be done only where IV administration is impractical or technically too difficult; do not mix calcium salts with sulfates, phosphates, carbonates, or tartrates in solution, because precipitation can occur; IV solutions should be warmed to body temperature and given slowly (0.5 ml–2 ml/min). Side-effects are infrequent at recommended doses; use with caution in digitalized patients and in patients with arrhythmias; calcium may antagonize the effects of verapamil
Calcium gluceptate	Injection—1.1 g/5 ml (1.1 g = 4.5 mEq)	Hypocalcemia: IM—2 ml to 5 ml IV—5 ml to 20 ml Exchange transfusions in newborn: 0.5 ml after each 100 ml of blood is exchanged	
Calcium gluconate (Kalcinate)	Injection—10% (1 g = 4.5 mEq)	Hypocalcemia: Adults—5 ml to 20 ml as needed by IV infusion Children—500 mg/kg/day in divided doses	
Magnesium sulfate	Injection—10% (0.8 mEq/ml), 12.5% (1 mEq/ml), 25% (2 mEq/ml), 50% (4 mEq/ml)	Mild magnesium deficiency: 1 g (2 ml 50% solution) IM every 6 hours for 4 doses Severe magnesium deficiency: IM—2 mEq/kg within 4 hours IV—5 g (40 mEq)/1000 ml infused over 3 hours Hyperalimentation: Adults—8 mEq to 24 mEq/day Infants—2 mEq to 10 mEq/day	Indicated for replacement therapy in magnesium-deficiency states, especially when accompanied by signs of tetany, and for treating hypomagnesemia resulting from hyperalimentation; may also be employed in certain acute convulsive states, e.g., toxemia, eclampsia, pre-eclampsia, epilepsy (1 g to 4 g 10%–20% solution IV) although other more effective and less toxic drugs are available (see Chap. 25); use with extreme caution in patients with renal impairment and observe closely for signs of overdosage (hypotension, respiratory depression, absence of patellar reflex); have respiratory assistance available; urine output

(continued)

Table 77-2. Parenteral Electrolytes (continued)

Drug	Preparations	Usual Dosage Range	Remarks
			should be maintained at a minimum of 100 ml/4 hours; do not exceed 1.5 ml/minute when infusing the 10% concentration (or equivalent volume of higher concentrations); dilute 50% solution to a concentration of 20% or less before infusing; however, the full-strength solution may be injected IM in adults; effects of CNS depressants can be potentiated by magnesium
Phosphate (Potassium phosphate, sodium phosphate)	Injection—3 mM phosphate/ ml and either 4 mEq sodium/ml or 4.4 mEq potassium/ml	Total parenteral nutrition (TPN): Adults—10 mM to 15 mM phosphorus (310 mg–465 mg elemental phosphorus) per liter of TPN solution Infants—1.5 mM to 2 mM/kg/ day	Primarily used to prevent or correct hypophosphatemia in patients undergoing hyperalimentation; contraindicated in diseases with high phosphate or low calcium levels; used IV only, diluted in a larger volume of fluid and slowly infused; monitor serum phosphorus, calcium, and sodium or potassium levels depending on which phosphate salt is used; be alert for symptoms of hypocalcemic tetany; use cautiously in patients with renal impairment, cardiac disease, arrhythmias, or adrenal insufficiency; symptoms of overdosage include weakness, confusion, paresthesias, hypotension, arrhythmias, flaccid paralysis, and ECG abnormalities
Potassium chloride	Injection—10 mEq, 20 mEq, 30 mEq, 40 mEq, 60 mEq, 90 mEq, in 5-ml, 10-ml, 20-ml, or 30-ml vials; 1,000 mEq/500 ml	Dependent on patient's status and governed by serum potassium level and ECG pattern; if serum potassium is less than 2 mEq/liter, maximum infusion rate is 40 mEq/hour to a total of 400 mEq/day; if serum potassium is greater than 2.5 mEq/liter, maximum infusion rate is 10 mEq/hr to a maximum of 200 mEq/day	Indicated for the prevention or treatment of moderate to severe potassium deficiency states and as adjunctive therapy in the management of cardiac arrhythmias, especially those due to digitalis overdosage; contraindicated in patients with anuria, oliguria, azotemia, adrenocortical insufficiency, acute dehydration, hyperkalemia, and severe hemolytic reactions; dilute injections with large volumes of parenteral solutions and administer slowly IV; direct injection of undiluted solution may be *fatal;* use cautiously in patients with cardiac disease, especially those taking digitalis drugs; monitor serum potassium levels, ECG, and urine flow frequently during therapy; be aware that toxic effects of potassium on the heart may be increased if serum sodium or calcium levels decrease or serum *p*H is reduced; most frequent adverse reactions are nausea, vomiting, diarrhea, and abdominal pain; avoid extravasation as irritation is often severe and tissue necrosis can occur
Potassium acetate	Injection—40 mEq/20 ml, 120 mEq/30 ml		

Table 77-2. Parenteral Electrolytes *(continued)*

Drug	Preparations	Usual Dosage Range	Remarks
Sodium acetate	Injection—2 mEq sodium and 2 mEq acetate/ml	Metabolic acidosis: Initially 2 mEq to 5 mEq/kg by IV infusion over 4 hours to 8 hours; adjust dose as necessary depending on clinical response	Indicated for acute treatment of metabolic acidosis, such as resulting from cardiac arrest, shock, or other circulatory insufficiency states, severe dehydration, or diabetic or lactic acidosis; also used to alkalinize the urine for treating certain drug intoxications and adjunctively in severe diarrhea to replace loss of bicarbonate; sodium lactate and sodium acetate are metabolized to bicarbonate, although conversion of lactate to bicarbonate is impaired in patients with hepatic disease; contraindicated in hypochloremia, metabolic or respiratory alkalosis, and hypocalcemia; use cautiously in patients with congestive heart failure, kidney impairment, edema, hypertension, or arrhythmias; do not exceed 8 mg/kg/day in small children, and infuse slowly because rapid injection or use of hypertonic solutions has resulted in decreased CSF pressure and intracranial hemorrhage; closely monitor *p*H and blood gases and electrolytes; avoid overdosage and subsequent production of alkalosis by giving repeated small doses; observe for signs of developing alkalosis (hyperirritability, restlessness, tetany) and discontinue drug; sodium bicarbonate is incompatible in solution with a wide variety of other drugs; administer alone to avoid undesirable interaction
Sodium bicarbonate (Neut)	Injection—4% (0.48 mEq/ml), 4.2% (0.5 mEq/ml), 5% (0.595 mEq/ml), 7.5% (0.892 mEq/ml), 8.4% (1.0 mEq/ml)	Cardiac arrest: Adults—initially 1 mEq/kg, followed by 0.5 mEq/kg every 10 minutes of arrest; use 7.5% or 8.4% solution	
Sodium lactate	Injection—0.167 mEq/ml, 5 mEq/ml	Children (under 2 yr)—initially 1 mEq to 2 mEq/kg over 1 minute to 2 minutes, followed by 1 mEq/kg every 10 minutes of arrest; use 4.2% solution	
Sodium chloride intravenous infusion	Infusion solution—0.45% (77 mEq/liter), 0.9% (154 mEq/liter), 3% (513 mEq/liter), 5% (855 mEq/liter)	(Dependent on patient's status and preparation being used) 0.9% solution—1.5 liters to 3 liters/24 hours	Used IV in various concentrations as a source of fluid and electrolytes; the 0.45% solution (hypotonic) is used when fluid loss exceeds electrolyte depletion; the 0.9% solution (isotonic) is most commonly used as replacement for fluid and sodium loss and as a diluent for many other drugs and nutrients; the 3% and 5% solutions (hypertonic) are indicated for hyponatremia and hypochloremia, extreme dilution of body fluids due to excessive water intake, and treatment of severe salt depletion; use with caution in patients with congestive heart failure, severe renal impairment, and edema with sodium retention; the 3% and 5% solutions should not be used when plasma sodium and chloride are elevated, normal, or even slightly decreased; monitor
Sodium chloride injection for admixtures	Injection—50 mEq/vial, 100 mEq/vial, 625 mEq/vial	0.45% solution—2 liters to 4 liters/24 hours	
Sodium chloride diluents	Injection—0.9% in various volumes	3% or 5% solution—maximum of 100 ml over 1 hour	

(continued)

Table 77-2. Parenteral Electrolytes *(continued)*

Drug	Preparations	Usual Dosage Range	Remarks
			intake–output ratio and serum electrolytes; also use cautiously in patients with decompensated cardiovascular or nephrotic diseases and in patients receiving corticosteroids; infuse higher strength solutions very slowly to avoid pulmonary edema
Tromethamine (Tham)	Infusion solution—18 g (150 mEq)/500 ml Powder for injection—36 g (300 mEq)/150 ml	Acidosis associated with cardiac arrest: 2 g to 6 g (62 ml–185 ml) injected into ventricular cavity *or* 3.6 to 10.8 g (111 to 333 ml) injected into a large peripheral vein; additional amounts as needed Acidosis during cardiac bypass surgery: 9.0 ml/kg (2.7 mEq/kg) to a maximum of 1000 ml in unusually severe cases Acidity of ACD priming blood: 0.5 to 2.5 g (15 ml–77 ml) added to each 500 ml blood (usually 2 g is adequate)	A highly alkaline, sodium-free organic amine that acts as a proton acceptor, combining with hydrogen ions to prevent or correct systemic acidosis associated with, for example, cardiac arrest or cardiac bypass surgery; also added to ACD priming blood to elevate pH; may function as an osmotic diuretic and increase urine flow and excretion of fixed acids, carbon dioxide, and electrolytes; contraindicated in anuria or uremia; should be administered slowly IV to avoid overdosage and alkalosis; may also be given by injection into ventricular cavity during cardiac arrest and by addition to pump oxygenator ACD blood or other priming fluid; treatment should not continue longer than a 24-hour period; determine blood values (pH, PCO_2, PO_2, glucose), electrolytes, and urinary output before treatment and frequently during drug administration to assess progress of treatment; adjust dose so that blood pH does not increase above normal (7.35–7.45); drug may depress respiration; have respiratory assistance available; avoid extravasation, because severe inflammation, vascular spasm, and tissue necrosis can result; transient hypoglycemia may occur, especially in infants; use cautiously in children, in patients with impaired renal function, and in pregnant women

Summary. Nutrients, Minerals, and Electrolytes

Drug	Preparations	Usual Dosage Range
Oral Nutritional Supplements		
Potassium (Various manufacturers)	Liquid—10 mEq/15 ml, 20 mEq/15 ml, 30 mEq/15 ml, 40 mEq/15 ml, 45 mEq/15 ml Powder—15 mEq/dose, 20 mEq/dose, 25 mEq/dose Effervescent tablets—20 mEq, 25 mEq, 50 mEq	Prevention—16 mEq to 24 mEq/day Replacement—40 mEq to 100 mEq/day

Summary. Nutrients, Minerals, and Electrolytes *(continued)*

Drug	Preparations	Usual Dosage Range
	Tablets—1 mEq, 2 mEq, 2.5 mEq, 4 mEq, 5 mEq, 6.7 mEq, 8 mEq, 10 mEq, 13.4 mEq	
Fluoride (Fluoritab, Luride, Phos-Flur, and various other manufacturers)	Tablets—0.25 mg, 0.5 mg, 1 mg Capsules (controlled release)—8 mEq Drops—0.125 mg/ml, 0.25 mg/ml, 0.5 mg/ml Rinse—0.02%, 0.09% Gel—0.1%, 0.5% Paste—2.3%	Oral—0.25 mg to 1 mg/day Topical—5 ml to 10 ml/day as a mouthwash; rinse for 1 minute, then expectorate

Other oral nutritional supplements—See Table 77-1

Parenteral Nutritional Supplements

Proteins/Amino Acids

Drug	Preparations	Usual Dosage Range
Crystalline amino-acid infusion (Aminosyn, FreAmine III, Novamine, Procalamine, Travasol, Veinamine)	Infusion solutions containing essential and nonessential amino acids with varying proportions of electrolytes	Dosage must be based on daily protein requirements, clinical response, and metabolic status; see individual package instructions
Amino-Acid Formulation for Renal Failure (Aminosyn-RF, NephrAmine, RenAmin)	Infusion solutions containing essential amino acids with varying proportion of electrolytes	Dosage must be based on daily protein requirements, clinical response, and metabolic status; see individual package instructions
Amino-Acid Formulation for High Metabolic Stress (FreAmine HBC)	Infusion solution containing essential and nonessential amino acids with high concentrations of branched-chain amino acids, and varying proportions of electrolytes	Dosage must be based on daily protein requirements, clinical response, and metabolic status; see individual package instructions
Amino-Acid Formulation for Hepatic Failure or Hepatic Encephalopathy (HepatAmine)	Infusion solution containing essential and nonessential amino acids with high concentrations of branched-chain amino acids, and varying proportions of electrolytes	Dosage must be based on daily protein requirements, clinical response, and metabolic status; see individual package instructions

Carbohydrates

Drug	Preparations	Usual Dosage Range
Dextrose in Water Injection (D-2½-W, D-5-W, D-10-W, D-20-W, D-25-W, D-30-W, D-38.5-W, D-40-W, D-50-W, D-60-W, D-70-W)	Infusion solutions containing 2½%, 5%, 10%, 20%, 25%, 30%, 38.5%, 40%, 50%, 60%, 70% Dextrose in Water for Injection	Individualized depending on patient's clinical status and nutritional state
Alcohol in Dextrose Infusion	Infusion solutions containing either 5% or 10% ethyl alcohol in 5% Dextrose in Water for Injection	Adults—1 liter to 2 liter 5% solution in a 24-hour period by *slow* IV infusion Children—40 ml/kg/24 hours
Fructose in Water	Infusion solution containing 10% Fructose in Water for Injection	Must be individualized depending on clinical status and nutritional state
Invert Sugar in Water (Travert)	Infusion solution containing either 5% or 10% Invert Sugar (dextrose and fructose) in Water for Injection	Must be individualized

(continued)

Summary. Nutrients, Minerals, and Electrolytes *(continued)*

Drug	Preparations	Usual Dosage Range
Lipids		
Intravenous fat emulsion (Intralipid, Liposyn, Soyacal, Travamulsion)	Emulsions for infusion containing 10% or 20% soybean oil (Intralipid, Soyacal, Travamulsion) or safflower oil (Liposyn) with 1.2% egg yolk phospholipids and 2.21% to 2.5% glycerin	Total Parenteral Nutrition Adults: 10%—initially 1 ml/minute for 15 minutes to 30 minutes; increase gradually to 83 ml to 125 ml/hour 20%—initially 0.5 ml/minute for 15 minutes to 30 minutes; increase gradually to 62 ml/ hour Do *not* exceed 3 g/kg/day Children: 10%—initially 0.1 ml/minute for 10 minutes to 15 minutes 20%—initially 0.05 ml/minute for 10 minutes to 15 minutes Gradually increase to 1 g/kg/4 hours; do *not* exceed 4 g/kg/ day Fatty acid deficiency: Adjust dose to supply 8% to 10% of caloric intake
Electrolytes		
See Table 77-2		

Miscellaneous Agents

X

Effective treatment of many disease states depends upon a critical assessment of the underlying pathology. To accomplish this, a number of diagnostic agents are available that assist the clinician in evaluating the clinical status of the patient as well as the functional capacity of many body organs. In most instances, proper use of diagnostic agents requires specially trained personnel and a thorough knowledge of the agent being employed. The extensive array of available diagnostic drugs precludes an in-depth discussion of each agent in a general pharmacology text of this type. Thus, this chapter presents a brief review of the principles of diagnostic drug usage, followed by tabular listings of the various categories of diagnostic agents. It is imperative, however, that health-care personnel using these drugs thoroughly familiarize themselves with the pharmacology and toxicology of the particular diagnostic agent being employed.

For purposes of discussion, the various diagnostic agents can be grouped into one of the four following categories:

I. *In vitro* diagnostic aids—agents usually employed at home or in the physician's office to monitor blood or urine levels of various substances such as glucose, proteins, or ketones as well as *p*H; also included in this category are the pregnancy screening tests, as well as tests for the presence of occult blood in the urine or feces

II. Intradermal diagnostic biologicals—agents used to skin test for sensitivity to certain diseases, notably tuberculosis, coccidioidomycosis, histoplasmosis, and mumps

III. *In vivo* diagnostic aids—agents usually employed to evaluate the functional status of various body organs, such as the liver, kidney, heart, pancreas, stomach, adrenal cortex, or pituitary; used in a hospital setting and require skilled personnel for administration and interpretation

IV. Radiographic diagnostic agents—opaque contrast substances, usually barium or iodinated compounds, that are impenetrable by x-rays; used to visualize internal structures such as the GI tract, kidneys, gallbladder, and bronchial tree

Diagnostic Agents

78

I   *In Vitro* Diagnostic Aids

A large number of preparations are used to rapidly screen the urine, feces, or blood for the presence of certain substances. These *in vitro* diagnostic aids commonly employ either (1) a reagent or tablet that is mixed in a test tube or on a slide with the sample to be analyzed or (2) a reagent-impregnated strip or tape that is dipped into the sample. Most are available over the counter and complete instructions for performing the test and analyzing the results are provided with the package. A few of these aids, however, such as tests for diagnosing mononucleosis, sickle cell anemia, and the presence of beta-hemolytic streptococci, are prescription-only items and require someone familiar with use of the product for proper interpretation. A fairly recent addition to the *in vitro* diagnostic aid group are the home pregnancy tests, which employ a reagent to be added to a urine sample. While certainly valuable as a preliminary screening method, confirmation of pregnancy should always be obtained professionally by use of one of the older, established pregnancy screening procedures.

Mention should also be made here of the currently approved method of reporting urine glucose concentrations using several of the *in vitro* diagnostic products. The previous system assigned a "plus value" ranging from one to four based upon the degree of color change either on the strip following immersion in urine or in the test tube following addition of a tablet to the urine sample. Confusion occasionally arose in the evaluation of the test due to nonuniformity among the different products with regard to assigning a particular number to a given urinary glucose concentration. The new method employs *percent* glucose relative to the color produced rather than a plus value, and is consistent among all the available *in vitro* diagnostic products (*e.g.,* 1% equals 1000 mg/dl). There is no consistent relationship among the available diagnostic products between the old "plus" system and the newer "percent" system. Thus, package literature must be consulted when comparing "plus" values obtained previously to "percent" values now being measured.

The various *in vitro* diagnostic aids are listed alphabetically by trade name in Table 78-1 with information regarding their dispensing status, type of preparation, and diagnostic uses.

II Intradermal Diagnostic Biologicals

The ability of selected biological products to elicit a local allergic reaction following intradermal injection is used to assess sensitivity to, but not necessarily the active presence of, certain diseases. The most commonly employed skin test is the tuberculin test, although sensitivity to mumps, histoplasmosis, and coccidioidomycosis can also be determined by intradermal testing. Interpretation of the tests is based upon the appearance of local hypersensitivity reaction at the site of intradermal injection, usually consisting of induration (tissue hardening) and, in some cases, erythema, in those patients previously exposed to the infecting organism.

Information relating to the available intradermal diagnostic drugs is presented in Table 78-2. Further information describing proper methods of administration and interpretation is provided with the individual drugs and should be consulted before performing the test.

III *In Vivo* Diagnostic Aids

The diagnostic agents used to assess the functional capacity of internal body organs are termed *in vivo* diagnostic aids

and are administered either orally or parenterally. Frequently, these compounds are designed to be concentrated in or excreted by the organ to be evaluated. Since they are administered systemically, a potential for untoward reactions does exist, and although these are generally mild and transient, patients should be observed carefully during, and for some time following, the testing procedure for development of more serious adverse reactions.

Several compounds that may be used for diagnostic purposes have been discussed in other chapters (*e.g.,* edrophonium for myasthenia gravis in Chap. 9; phentolamine for pheochromocytoma in Chap. 12; radioiodide 131 for thyroid function in Chap. 40), and are not considered here. Table 78-3 lists the important *in vivo* diagnostic drugs, together with their preparations, uses, and pertinent remarks. It should be recognized that the consideration given to the agents in this chapter is brief and is not intended to provide comprehensive information regarding their safe and effective use. Experienced personnel and proper facilities are necessary to derive maximum benefit from use of these diagnostic agents and to deal with any untoward reaction that may occur.

IV Radiographic Diagnostic Agents

With the exception of barium sulfate, the substances used for radiographic diagnostic procedures are all iodine-containing compounds. These agents are opaque chemicals that are employed as contrast media to enhance visualization of internal structures by x-ray examination. Localization of a substance to the particular area to be visualized is accomplished either through direct instillation into an organ (*e.g.,* uterus, colon, bronchioles, spinal column) or by incorporation of the radiopaque drug into an organic compound whose properties determine its distribution in the body (*e.g.,* excretion by way of the bile or urine or plasma protein binding).

Barium Sulfate

Barium sulfate is the most commonly used substance for visualization of the GI tract. It is a highly insoluble compound; thus, only minimal amounts are absorbed systemically and toxicity is quite low. Barium sulfate can be administered orally as a thick paste for examination of the esophagus or as a more dilute suspension for visualization of the stomach and upper intestinal tract. X-ray studies of the lower GI tract and colon may be performed following a cleansing enema and rectal instillation of barium sulfate suspension. Barium sulfate may be constipating and complete expulsion of the suspension from the GI tract following the examination usually requires use of a laxative or enema. The various barium-containing diagnostic agents are listed in Table 78-4.

(*Text continues on p. 760.*)

Table 78-1. *In Vitro* **Diagnostic Aids**

Trade Name	RX or OTC	Preparation	Diagnostic Uses
Acetest	OTC	Tablets	Serum/urinary ketones
Accusens T	OTC	Kit	Taste dysfunction
Acu-Test	OTC	Reagent	Pregnancy
Albustix	OTC	Strips	Urinary proteins
Answer	OTC	Reagent	Pregnancy
Azostix	OTC	Strips	Blood urea nitrogen
Beta-Neocept	Rx	Slide	Pregnancy
BetaPregnate	Rx	Slide	Pregnancy
Bili-Labstix	OTC	Strips	Urinary glucose, proteins, pH, blood, ketones, bilirubin
Bumintest	OTC	Tablets	Urinary protein
Chemstrip bG	OTC	Strips	Blood glucose
Chemstrip G	OTC	Strips	Urinary glucose
Chemstrip GP	OTC	Strips	Urinary glucose, protein
Chemstrip GK	OTC	Strips	Urinary glucose, ketones
Chemstrip K	OTC	Strips	Urinary ketones
Chemstrip LN	OTC	Strips	Urinary leukocytes, nitrite
Chemstrip 3	OTC	Strips	Urinary glucose, protein, pH
Chemstrip 4	OTC	Strips	Urinary glucose, protein, pH, blood
Chemstrip 5	OTC	Strips	Urinary glucose, protein, pH, blood, ketones
Chemstrip 6	OTC	Strips	Urinary glucose, protein, pH, blood, ketones, bilirubin
Chemstrip 7	OTC	Strips	Urinary glucose, protein, pH, blood, ketones, bilirubin, urobilinogen
Chemstrip 8	OTC	Strips	Urinary glucose, protein, pH, blood, ketones, bilirubin, urobilinogen, nitrite
Chemstrip 9	OTC	Strips	Urinary glucose, protein, pH, blood, ketones, bilirubin, urobilinogen, nitrite, leukocytes
Chemstrip 5L	OTC	Strips	Urinary glucose, protein, pH, blood, ketones, leukocytes
Chemstrip 6L	OTC	Strips	Urinary glucose, protein, pH, blood, ketones, bilirubin, leukocytes
Chemstrip 7L	OTC	Strips	Urinary glucose, protein, pH, blood, ketones, bilirubin, urobilinogen, leukocytes
Clinistix	OTC	Strips	Urinary glucose
Clinitest	OTC	Tablets	Urinary glucose
Clinitest 2-Drop	OTC	Reagent	Urinary glucose
Combistix	OTC	Strips	Urinary glucose, protein, pH
C-Stix	OTC	Strips	Urinary ascorbic acid
Daisy 2	OTC	Reagent	Pregnancy
Dextrostix	OTC	Strips	Blood glucose
Diastix	OTC	Strips	Urinary glucose
Entero-Test	OTC	Capsule	Upper intestinal bleeding, duodenal parasites
Entero-Test Pediatric	OTC	Capsule	Screening of gastroesophageal reflux
e.p.t.	OTC	Reagent	Pregnancy
Fact	OTC	Reagent	Pregnancy
Fleet Detecatest	OTC	Reagent	Fecal blood
Gastroccult	OTC	Reagent	Blood in gastric contents
Gastro-Test	OTC	Kit	Stomach pH
Gonodecten	Rx	Kit	Gonorrhea
Gravindex 90	Rx	Slide	Pregnancy
Hema-Chek	OTC	Slide	Fecal blood
Hema-Combistix	OTC	Strips	Urinary glucose, protein, pH, blood
Hemastix	OTC	Strips	Urinary blood
Hematest	OTC	Tablets	Fecal blood
Hemoccult	OTC	Slide	Fecal blood
Ictotest	OTC	Reagent	Urinary bilirubin
Keto-Diastix	OTC	Strips	Urinary glucose, ketones
Ketostix	OTC	Strips	Urinary/blood ketones
Labstix	OTC	Strips	Urinary glucose, protein, pH, blood, ketones
Microstix-3	OTC	Strips	Urinary nitrite, total bacteria, gram-negative bacteria
Microstix-Nitrite	OTC	Strips	Urinary nitrite
MicroTrax Chlamydia	Rx	Slide	*Chlamydia trachomatis* in tissue culture
Model Urine HCG Assay	Rx	Reagent	Pregnancy
Mono-Chek	Rx	Reagent	Mononucleosis
Mono-Diff Test	Rx	Reagent	Mononucleosis
Monospot	Rx	Reagent	Mononucleosis
Monosticon Dri-Dot	Rx	Reagent	Mononucleosis
Mono-Test	Rx	Reagent	Mononucleosis
MPS Papers	OTC	Strips	Urinary acid mucopolysaccharides

(continued)

Table 78-1. *In Vitro* Diagnostic Aids *(continued)*

Trade Name	RX or OTC	Preparation	Diagnostic Uses
Multistix	OTC	Strips	Urinary glucose, protein, *p*H, blood, ketones, bilirubin, urobilinogen
Nitrazine Paper	OTC	Strips	Urinary *p*H
N-Multistix	OTC	Strips	Urinary glucose, protein, *p*H, blood, ketones, bilirubin, urobilinogen, nitrite
N-Multistix-C	OTC	Strips	As above, plus ascorbic acid
N-Uristix	OTC	Strips	Urinary glucose, protein, nitrite
Phadebact Streptococcus Test	Rx	Reagent	Beta-hemolytic streptococci, groups A, B, C, and G
Phenistix	OTC	Strips	Phenylketonuria
Placentex	Rx	Reagent	Pregnancy
Predictor	OTC	Reagent	Pregnancy
Pregnate	Rx	Slide	Pregnancy
Pregnosis	Rx	Slide	Pregnancy
Pregnosticon Dri-Dot	Rx	Slide	Pregnancy
Rubacell II	Rx	Reagent	Serum rubella virus antibodies
Sensi-Tex	Rx	Reagent	Pregnancy
Sensi-Slide	Rx	Slide	Pregnancy
Serameba	Rx	Slide	Serum amebic antibodies
Sickledex Test	Rx	Strips	Hemoglobin S (sickle cells)
Streptonase-B	Rx	Reagent	Serum-B antibodies (streptococcal infection)
Strepto-Sec	Rx	Slide	Beta-hemolytic streptococci, groups A, B, C, and G
Tes-Tape	OTC	Strips	Urinary glucose
UCG-Slide Test	Rx	Slide	Pregnancy
Uristix	OTC	Strips	Urinary glucose, protein
Urobilistix	OTC	Strips	Urinary urobilinogen
Visidex	OTC	Strips	Blood glucose

Table 78-2. Intradermal Diagnostic Biologicals

Diagnostic Agent	Preparations	Uses	Remarks
Candida and *Trichophyton* (Dermatophytin, Dermatophytin "O")	Injection—filtrates of cultures of *Trichophyton mentagrophytes, T. rubrum, T. tonsurans,* and *Candida albicans*	Diagnosis of ringworm infections of the skin	Available as undiluted extract and diluted solution of *Trichophyton* (Dermatophytin) and *Candida* (Dermatophytin "O"); a positive *Trichophyton* reaction must occur at a concentration of 1:30 or weaker, intradermally, while a *Candida*-positive reaction must occur with a concentration no stronger than 1:100; a positive reaction consists of erythema and induration 5 mm or greater; refer to package literature for complete dilution instructions and for procedure to be followed for use of extracts for treatment if reaction is positive
Coccidioidin (Spherulin)	Injection—1:10, 1:100	Diagnosis of coccidioidomycosis. Differentiation of coccidioidomycosis from other diseases with similar clinical findings, *e.g.,* histoplasmosis, sarcoidosis	Diluted with Sodium Chloride Injection; 0.1 ml of 1:10,000 is injected intradermally; if negative, repeat with 1:1000 and finally 1:100; positive reaction is appearance of area of induration measuring 5 mm or greater; erythema without induration is considered negative; reaction is readable at 24 hours and maximal at 36 hours, and indicative that contact with the fungus has occurred in the past but patient does not necessarily have an active infection; false positive skin reactions do *not* occur; sensitive individuals may exhibit an intense local response

Table 78-2. Intradermal Diagnostic Biologicals *(continued)*

Diagnostic Agent	Preparations	Uses	Remarks
Diphtheria (Diphtheria Toxin for Schick Test)	Injection—1 vial of toxin and 1 vial of control	Diagnosis of serologic immunity to diphtheria	Injected intradermally on flexor surface or forearm, control solution on one arm and toxin on other arm; results are read on day 4 or 5; positive reaction is appearance of circumscribed area of redness and slight infiltration measuring 1 cm or more in diameter, and indicates person has little or no antitoxin to diphtheria and is susceptible to infection; aspirate prior to injection to ensure needle is not in blood vessel
Histoplasmin (Histoplasmin, Diluted; Histolyn-CYL)	Injection—1.0 ml/vial in 10 0.1-ml doses, 1.3-ml multidose vial	Diagnosis of histoplasmosis Differentiation of histoplasmosis from other mycotic or bacterial infections, *e.g.,* coccidioidomycosis, sarcoidosis	A sterile filtrate from cultures of *Histoplasma capsulatum;* 0.1 ml is injected *intradermally* into flexor surface of the forearm and reaction is read in 48 hours to 72 hours; induration of 5 mm or greater is considered positive and may indicate a previous mild, subacute, or chronic infection with *Histoplasma capsulatum* or immunologically related organisms; little value in diagnosing acute, fulminating infections because a negative reaction usually occurs; large doses can produce severe erythema and induration with ulceration and necrosis; systemic allergic reactions can occur; infrequently used test
Mumps skin test antigen	Injection—1 ml (10 tests)	Determination of sensitivity to mumps virus	Suspension of killed mumps virus used to determine skin sensitivity to mumps; effectiveness has not been conclusively established; may be useful in adolescence for identifying those who should be protected against the disease; however, most of the population have had contact with mumps virus and will demonstrate a delayed cutaneous hypersensitivity to the antigen; following injection of 0.1 ml intradermally on inner surface of forearm, reaction is read in 24 hours to 36 hours; erythema of 1.5 cm or more indicates sensitivity to virus and probable immunity; negative reaction suggests probable susceptibility; do not use in persons sensitive to chicken, eggs, or feathers because preparation is cultivated in chicken embryo
Tuberculin purified protein derivative—Tuberculin PPD (Aplisol, Tubersol-Connaught)	Injection—1 U/0.1 ml, 5 U/0.1 ml, 250 U/0.1 ml	Aid in diagnosis of tuberculosis	Aqueous solution of a purified protein fraction from filtrates of cultured human strains of *Mycobacterium tuberculosis;* use only *fresh* tuberculin preparations for testing; injected intradermally (5 U) on the flexor or dorsal surface of the forearm; reaction is

(continued)

Table 78-2. Intradermal Diagnostic Biologicals (continued)

Diagnostic Agent	Preparations	Uses	Remarks
			read in 48 hours to 72 hours; induration of 10 mm or more is a positive reaction, whereas induration of 5 mm or less is negative; erythema is not of diagnostic significance, but may indicate incorrect administration; retesting is indicated if induration measures 5 mm to 9 mm; positive reaction does not indicate an active infection, but suggests further evaluation is necessary; positive reaction may also indicate previous BCG vaccination; preferred over old tuberculin (OT) test due to greater purity; highly sensitive persons may experience vesiculation, ulceration, and necrosis, and persons suspected of being highly sensitive should receive an initial dose of only 1 U; the 250-U injection is *only* used for persons who do not react to 5 U, although individuals not reacting to 5 U may be considered tuberculin negative
Tuberculin PPD, multiple puncture device (Aplitest, Sclavo Test-PPD)	Cylindrical plastic units	See Tuberculin PPD	A single-use device consisting of 4 stainless steel tines coated with tuberculin PPD, standardized to give reactions equivalent to 5 U of intradermal tuberculin PPD
Old tuberculin, multiple puncture devices (Tuberculin Mono-Vacc Test, Tuberculin Old Tine Test)	Individual units	See Tuberculin PPD	Single-use, multiple puncture device standardized to give reactions equivalent to 5 U of standard solution of old tuberculin administered intradermally; test is read 48 hours to 96 hours after administration; positive reaction is vesiculation or induration of 1 mm or greater, but further diagnostic tests are necessary to establish presence of infection; infrequently used preparation

Table 78-3. *In Vivo* Diagnostic Aids

Diagnostic Agent	Preparations	Uses	Remarks
Aminohippurate sodium (PAH)	Aqueous solution—20%	Assessment of renal blood flow and tubular secretory mechanisms	Occasionally used to study certain aspects of kidney function; used by IV injection; not metabolized and excreted solely by the kidney; low plasma concentrations (1 mg–2 mg/dl) are used to measure renal blood flow; higher concentrations (40 mg to 60 mg/dl) are employed to determine maximal tubular secretory capacity; may elicit nausea, feelings of warmth, and urge to defecate
L-Arginine (R-Gene 10)	Solution—10% in Sterile Water for Injection for IV infusion	Determination of pituitary human growth hormone reserve; diagnosis of panhypopituitarism, pituitary	Stimulates pituitary to release growth hormone; dosage is 300 ml in adults and 5 ml/kg in children; rate of false positive

Table 78-3. *In Vivo* **Diagnostic Aids** *(continued)*

Diagnostic Agent	Preparations	Uses	Remarks
		dwarfism, pituitary trauma, and other hypopituitary conditions	reactions is 32% and false negative is 27%; do not use in patients with strong allergic tendencies; excessive infusion rates can result in irritation, nausea, vomiting, and flushing; have antihistamine available in case of allergic reactions; do not use if solution is not clean or if bottle lacks a vacuum; refer to package literature for interpretation of results
Bentiromide (Chymex)	Solution—500 mg/7.5 ml	Screening test for pancreatic exocrine insufficiency	A peptide containing 170 mg para-aminobenzoic acid (PABA) per 500 mg dose; following oral administration, bentiromide is hydrolyzed by pancreatic chymotrypsin, liberating PABA, which is excreted in the urine; if exocrine pancreatic function is normal, over 50% of the PABA contained in bentiromide appears in the urine within 6 hours and can be detected using the Smith modification of the Bratton–Marshall test for arylamines; patients should fast at least 8 hours before receiving a test dose; diarrhea, headache, nausea, flatulence, and weakness can occur; instruct patient to urinate immediately before receiving bentiromide; falsely elevated readings can occur if the patient is taking other drugs metabolized to arylamines, such as acetaminophen, chloramphenicol, lidocaine, procaine, procainamide, sulfonamides, or thiazide diuretics
Benzylpenicilloyl-polylysine (Pre-Pen)	Ampules	Skin test for penicillin hypersensitivity in patients who have previously received penicillin and demonstrated a clinical hypersensitivity reaction	May be applied either by scratching forearm (preferred method) or by intradermal injection on upper outer arm surface; positive reaction consists of whealing, erythema, and itching; occurs usually within 10 minutes, and is associated with an incidence of allergic reactions to systemic benzylpenicillin or penicillin G of greater than 20%; a negative skin test response predicts a less than 5% incidence of allergic complications; of doubtful value in assessing sensitivity to semisynthetic penicillins or cephalosporins; may produce an intense local inflammatory response and occasionally systemic allergic reactions
Betazole (Histalog)	Injection—50 mg/ml	Evaluation of gastric acid secretory capacity	Structural analog of histamine; stimulates gastric acid secretion with minimal effects on other organs; lower incidence of side-effects compared to histamine itself; administered IM or SC (50

(continued)

Table 78-3. *In Vivo* **Diagnostic Aids** *(continued)*

Diagnostic Agent	Preparations	Uses	Remarks
			mg); maximal secretory response occurs in 45 minutes to 60 minutes, and lasts 2 hours to 3 hours; flushing, headache, and urticaria can occur; overdosage results in weakness and syncope; use with caution in patients with a history of allergic reactions; not as commonly used as pentagastrin for assessing GI secretory capacity
Ceruletide diethylamine (Tymtran)	Injection—40 mcg/2 ml	Aid in oral cholecystography to facilitate contraction of the gallbladder; adjunctive use in small bowel radiologic examination	Effects are similar to those of cholecystokinin; contracts gallbladder, stimulates pancreatic and gastric secretion, delays gastric emptying, inhibits proximal duodenal motility, and increases motility of distal duodenum, jejunum, and ileum; administered IM (0.3 mcg/kg); films are taken 10 minutes and 30 minutes after injection; do not use in pregnant women near term, because premature labor can be induced; abdominal pain, cramping, and nausea are common (10%), and pain at injection site has been reported frequently; may be diluted with 0.5 ml normal saline to reduce pain on injection
Cholecystokinin (CCK)	Powder for injection—75 Ivy Dog Units/vial	Aid in cholecystography, cholangiography, x-ray studies of the small bowel; diagnosis of pancreatic insufficiency (with the secretin test—see Sincalide)	Natural hormone found in small intestine which stimulates flow of bile, gallbladder contraction, and secretion of pancreatic enzymes; also inhibits contraction of lower esophageal sphincter and enhances motility of the stomach and intestines; stomach pain and epigastric distress can occur; too-rapid injection may elicit flushing; powder is stable for 1 year at 0°C; discard any unused reconstituted solution; see package literature for dosage recommendations
Cosyntropin (Cortrosyn)	Vials with diluent—0.25 mg with 10 mg mannitol	Diagnosis of adrenal cortical insufficiency	Synthetic subunit of human ACTH used IM or by IV infusion to differentiate primary (adrenal) from secondary (pituitary) adrenocortical insufficiency; in primary Addison's disease, 24-hour urinary 17-hydroxycorticosteroid levels fail to rise following IV infusion and plasma cortisol levels do not increase significantly within 30 minutes following IM injection; secondary pituitary failure is characterized by a *slow increase* in urinary steroids following IV infusion; produces fewer allergic reactions than ACTH injection
Gonadorelin (Factrel)	Powder for injection—100 mcg/vial, 500 mcg/vial	Evaluation of hypothalamic–pituitary–gonadotropic function	Used SC or IV; in females, test should be performed in early follicular phase of the menstrual

Table 78-3. *In Vivo* Diagnostic Aids *(continued)*

Diagnostic Agent	Preparations	Uses	Remarks
		Evaluation of residual gonadotropic function following hypophysectomy Investigational uses include induction of ovulation and treatment of precocious puberty	cycle; do not give concurrently with gonadal hormones, glucocorticoids or spironolactone, because pituitary secretion of gonadotropins can be affected; SC injection can result in localized pain, swelling and itching; use during pregnancy only where clearly needed; refer to package prescribing information for testing methodology
Histamine phosphate	Injection: Gastric test—0.55 mg (0.2 mg base)/ml	Assessment of gastric acid secretory capacity	Basal acid secretion is measured, then 0.01 mg to 0.04 mg histamine base/kg is injected SC and gastric contents are collected in 4 15-minute specimens and analyzed for volume, *p*H, and acidity; an antihistamine should be administered IM before histamine; many side-effects noted and severe allergic reactions (*e.g.*, asthma) can occur; largely replaced by other, safer diagnostic measures (*e.g.*, pentagastrin)
	Pheochromocytoma—0.275 mg (0.1 mg base)/ml	Presumptive diagnosis of pheochromocytoma	Once used for diagnosis of pheochromocytoma (positive response was at least a 60 mm/40 mm rise in blood pressure above the base line or an increase of at least 20 mm/10 mm above that obtained in the cold pressor test); very hazardous procedure; phentolamine must be readily available to control excessive increases in blood pressure; rarely employed today with the availability of more accurate and less dangerous procedures
Hysteroscopy fluid (Hyskon)	Solution—32% w/v dextran 70 in 10% w/v dextrose	Aid in distending the uterine cavity and visualizing its surfaces	Introduced into uterine cavity *via* cannula under low pressure until uterus is sufficiently distended to permit adequate visualization; volume usually required is 50 ml to 100 ml; allergic reactions, including anaphylaxis, can result if drug is absorbed systemically; do not exceed 150 mm Hg infusion pressure
Indocyanine green (Cardio-Green)	Vials—25 mg, 50 mg Disposable units—10 mg, 40 mg	Determination of cardiac output, hepatic function, and liver blood flow Aid in ophthalmic angiography	A water-soluble dye that is injected IV, is quickly bound to plasma proteins, and is taken up almost exclusively by hepatic parenchymal cells; dilution of dye in blood samples obtained from different sites at various times following administration are an indication of blood flow in a particular area; adverse effects are minimal; drug contains a small amount of sodium iodide and may interfere with radioactive iodine-uptake studies
Inulin	Injection—100 mg/ml	Measurement of glomerular filtration rate	Polymer of fructose given by IV infusion; drug is rapidly filtered by

(continued)

Table 78-3. *In Vivo* **Diagnostic Aids** *(continued)*

Diagnostic Agent	Preparations	Uses	Remarks
			the kidney, and neither secreted nor reabsorbed; following a loading dose, samples of urine are collected at regular intervals and concentration of inulin in each sample is determined colorimetrically; normal adult inulin clearance is 100 ml to 160 ml/minute
Mannitol	Solution—5%, 10%, 15%, 20%, 25%	Measurement of glomerular filtration rate	An osmotic diuretic (see Chap. 37) that is also used to measure glomerular filtration rate (GFR); 100 ml of a 20% solution is diluted with 180 mg normal saline and infused at a rate of 20 ml/minute; urine is collected by a catheter for a specific time period and a blood sample is drawn at the beginning and end of the collection period; mannitol concentrations (mg/ml) are determined for each sample and the GFR is calculated as ml of plasma that must be filtered to yield the amount of mannitol excreted per minute in the urine
Metyrapone (Metopirone)	Tablets—250 mg	Diagnosis of hypothalamus–pituitary function	Used to test whether pituitary secretion of ACTH is adequate; ability of adrenals to respond to ACTH should be demonstrated by ACTH or cosyntropin test before giving metyrapone; following a 2-day rest period, 15 mg/kg is administered orally every 4 hours for 6 doses, then urinary 17-hydroxycorticosteroids (17-OHCS) are collected for 24 hours; normal pituitary function is indicated by a 2- to 4-fold increase in 17-OHCS over control levels obtained before drug administration; excessive excretion of 17-OHCS suggests Cushing's syndrome (adrenal hyperplasia), while subnormal excretion indicates hypopituitarism
Pentagastrin (Peptavlon)	Injection—0.25 mg/ml	Evaluation of gastric acid secretory capacity	Action resembles that of natural gastrin; following SC injection of 6 mcg/kg, acid secretion begins within 10 minutes peaks in 20 minutes to 30 minutes and lasts 60 minutes to 90 minutes; elicits fewer and less intense side-effects than either histamine or betazole, and is the preferred drug for measuring gastric acid secretion; children's doses have not been established; cautious use in patients with hepatic, biliary, or pancreatic disease
Phenolsulfonphthalein	Injection—6 mg/ml	Renal function testing	A relatively quick screening procedure for evaluating kidney function; after forcing fluids for 1 hour to 2 hours, the bladder is emptied completely and 1 ml (6 mg) of the dye is injected IV or IM; urine samples are collected at

Table 78-3. *In Vivo* Diagnostic Aids *(continued)*

Diagnostic Agent	Preparations	Uses	Remarks
			specified intervals and the amount of dye excreted at each time is measured spectrophotometrically and compared to normal ranges; allergic reactions have occurred on occasion
Protirelin (Relefact TRH, Thypinone)	Injection—0.5 mg/ml	Evaluation of thyroid function	Synthetic peptide similar in action to thyrotropin-releasing hormone (TRH); following IV injection (adults—500 mcg; children—7 mcg/kg), protirelin causes release of thyroid-stimulating hormone (TSH) from anterior pituitary; TSH blood levels are determined before injection and again 30 minutes after injection; thyroid function is characterized by comparing baseline TSH serum levels to those obtained following drug injection; if test is repeated, allow an interval of 7 days; discontinue thyroid drugs at least 7 days before performing test; most common side-effects are nausea, urinary urgency, flushing, lightheadedness, headache, dry mouth, and abdominal discomfort; patient should be supine during testing to minimize changes in blood pressure
Saralasin (Sarenin)	Injection—18 mg/30 ml	Detection of angiotensin II-dependent hypertension, when results are combined with those of other suitable tests	Binds to angiotensin II receptors, but exerts less vasoconstrictive activity then angiotensin II itself; thus, it acts as an *antagonist* in the presence of high levels of circulating angiotensin II, and lowers blood pressure; conversely, when circulating levels of angiotensin II are low, saralasin behaves as an *agonist,* and elevates blood pressure; fluid and electrolyte status can markedly affect results; thus the drug is intended to be used as one of several tests (*e.g.,* plasma renin activity, intravenous pyelogram, renal arteriogram) to detect cause of hypertension; monitor patients carefully due to danger of exaggerated pressor or depressor responses
Secretin (Secretin-Boots, Secretin-Kabi)	Injection—10 U/ml when reconstituted according to package instructions	Diagnosis of pancreatic exocrine disease or gastrinoma (Zollinger-Ellison syndrome)	Hormone obtained from porcine duodenal mucosa that increases volume and bicarbonate content of pancreatic secretions; powder is dissolved in 10 ml Sodium Chloride Injection and administered by slow IV injection (5 min) at a dose of 1 U to 2 U/kg; samples are collected with a gastric tube and analyzed for volume, enzyme and bicarbonate content, occult blood, biliary pigment; cautious use in acute pancreatitis; frequently given with sincalide (see below)

(continued)

Table 78-3. *In Vivo* Diagnostic Aids *(continued)*

Diagnostic Agent	Preparations	Uses	Remarks
Sincalide (Kinevac)	Injection—5 mcg/vial for reconstitution to 1 mcg/ml	Stimulate pancreatic or gallbladder secretions	Synthetic subunit of cholecystokinin that produces gallbladder contraction following IV injection; also enhances pancreatic secretions when given in combination with secretin; to contract gallbladder, 0.02 mcg/kg is given by rapid (30 sec–60 sec) IV injection, which may be repeated in 15 minutes at 0.04 mcg/kg; for secretin–sincalide test of pancreatic function, 0.02 mcg/kg is infused over a 30-minute period beginning 30 minutes after the secretion infusion; safety not established in children or pregnant women; abdominal discomfort and urge to defecate frequently occur
Tolbutamide sodium (Orinase Diagnostic)	Injection—1 g with diluent	Diagnosis of pancreatic islet cell adenoma or diabetes	Patients with pancreatic cell insulinomas show a *sharp, intense* drop in blood glucose following IV injection of 1 g tolbutamide sodium; hypoglycemia may persist for several hours, and may require treatment if symptoms are too intense; diabetic patients show a *gradual* decrease in blood glucose, whereas normal persons evidence a prompt reduction (15 min–20 min) associated with an elevation in serum insulin
D-Xylose (Xylo-Pfan)	Powder	Test for intestinal malabsorption states	Nonmetabolizable sugar given orally (25 g) to assess absorptive capacity of GI tract; normal values are 5 g to 8 g in urine within 5 hours and 40 mg/100 ml blood within 2 hours

Iodinated Radiopaque Agents

A variety of iodine-containing organic compounds can be used either orally or parenterally to visualize a number of different body organs. The opacity of these agents depends upon the percentage of iodine in the molecule and the amount of drug concentrated at a particular site. Patients should be questioned concerning iodine hyperesensitivity before administration of one of these compounds. Severe, *sometimes fatal*, allergic reactions have occurred with use of these agents, and patients with a history of bronchial asthma or other allergies must be closely monitored during and for at least 1 hour following administration. Appropriate antidotal measures, including respiratory aids, epinephrine, and corticosteroids should be available.

Adverse reactions are uncommon, but the possibility of their occurrence must not be overlooked. Among the untoward reactions reported with use of radiographic contrast media are urticaria, wheezing, dyspnea, angioneurotic edema, laryngeal spasm, anaphylaxis, hyperthermia, head-ache, chest tightness, and tremor. Reactions that are probably attributable to volume, speed, and site of injection are flushing, dizziness, nausea, generalized vasodilation, and hypotension. Pain and irritation at the injection site have been noted, as well as paresthesias, numbness, hematomas, ecchymoses, and thrombophlebitis.

The various iodinated radiographic contrast agents are listed in Table 78-5. Their dosage forms, iodine content, composition, and diagnostic use are given as well. Because their dose and route of administration depend on their diagnostic intent, the information included with each drug must be consulted before administration.

An adjunctive drug that is sometimes used in lymphography to facilitate visualization of the lymphatic system is isosulfan blue (Lymphazurin 1%). Following SC injection of 0.5 ml into three interdigital spaces of each extremity per study, isosulfan is selectively concentrated in the lymphatic vessels, which are colored a bright blue. Adverse reactions are relatively infrequent (1%–2%), and are largely of an allergic nature, ranging from itching and swelling of the hands to generalized edema and respiratory distress in rare instances.

Table 78-4. Barium-containing Diagnostic Agents

Trade Name	Preparations	Uses	Dosage
Barodense	Powder for suspension—97% micronized barium sulfate with suspending agents	Esophageal, upper and lower GI, and colon studies Air-contrast studies	Esophageal—5 oz to 6 oz in 240 ml water Upper/lower GI—4 oz in 240 ml water Colon—16 oz to 18 oz in 2 qt water Air contrast—20 oz to 22 oz in 2 qt water
Baroflave	Powder—100% barium sulfate	Upper and lower GI studies	50 g to 500 g suspended in water
Baroloid	Powder for suspension—97% barium sulfate with flavoring and suspending agents	Esophageal, upper and lower GI, and colon studies	Esophageal—add powder to desired consistency Upper GI/small bowel—90 g to 120 g in 240 ml water Colon—360 g in 1,680 ml water by enema
Barosperse	Powder for suspension—95% barium sulfate in single-dose cups, disposable enemas, and air-contrast units	Esophageal, upper and lower GI, and colon studies Air-contrast studies	Esophageal—45 g in 15 ml water Upper/lower GI, air contrast—225 g in 150 ml to yield a 60% suspension Colon—dilute 500 ml 60% suspension with 1,500 ml to make 23% suspension; use by enema
Barosperse 110	Powder for suspension—95% barium sulfate	Upper and lower GI and colon studies	Upper GI/colon—add 600 ml water to make a 60% suspension Low-density upper GI—add 875 ml water to make a 50% suspension
Barotrast	Powder for suspension—92.5% barium sulfate with saccharin sodium and suspending agents	Esophageal, upper GI, small bowel, and colon studies	Oral—60 g to 450 g Rectal—150 g to 750 g in appropriate amounts of water
Esophotrast	Oral cream—56% barium sulfate with flavoring and suspending agents	Esophageal studies	Chew 1 tbsp thoroughly, then swallow; repeat with a second tablespoonful
Fleet Barobag	Powder for suspension—98% barium sulfate with suspending agents in disposable enema	Lower GI studies	Add 1000 ml to 3000 ml water to desired concentration; use as enema
Fleet Oral Barium	Powder for suspension—96% barium sulfate with flavoring and suspending agents in single-dose cup	Upper GI studies	Add water to cup to make either a 45%, 50%, or 60% suspension
Oratrast	Powder for suspension—92% barium sulfate with flavoring and suspending agents	Upper and lower GI studies	Add 150 g to 250 ml water to make a 35% solution
Ultrapaque C	Powder for suspension—96% barium sulfate with chocolate flavoring and suspending agents	Esophageal and upper GI studies	Esophageal—1 tbsp in 60 ml to 90 ml water Upper GI—3 tbsp in 300 ml water

Table 78-5. Iodinated Radiographic Diagnostic Agents

Trade Name	Dosage Form	Iodine Content	Composition	Diagnostic Uses
Amipaque	Injection	48.25%	13.5%, 18.75% Metrizamide	Myelography Computerized tomography of intracranial subarachnoid spaces Peripheral arteriography Pediatric angiocardiography
Angio-Conray	Injection	48%	80% Iothalamate	Angiocardiography Aortography
Angiovist 282	Injection	28%	60% Diatrizoate meglumine	Angiography Arthrography

(continued)

Table 78-5. Iodinated Radiographic Diagnostic Agents *(continued)*

Trade Name	Dosage Form	Iodine Content	Composition	Diagnostic Uses
				Cholangiography Discography Excretory urography Peripheral arteriography Pyelography Splenoportography Venography
Angiovist 292	Injection	29.2%	52% Diatrizoate meglumine and 8% diatrizoate sodium	See Angiovist 282
Angiovist 370	Injection	37%	66% Diatrizoate meglumine and 10% diatrizoate sodium	See Angiovist 282
Bilivist	Capsules	61.4%	500 mg Ipodate sodium	Cholangiography Cholecystrography
Bilopaque	Capsules	57.4%	750 mg Tyropanoate sodium	Cholecystography
Cardiografin	Injection	40%	85% Diatrizoate meglumine	Angiocardiography Thoracic aortography
Cholebrine	Tablets	62%	750 mg Iocetamic acid	Cholecystography
Cholografin	Injection	5.1%	10.3% Iodipamide meglumine	Cholecystography Cholangiography
Cholografin	Injection	26%	52% Iodipamide meglumine	Cholecystography Cholangiography
Conray	Injection	28.2%	60% Iothalamate meglumine	Cerebral angiography Drip infusion pyelography Peripheral arteriography Urography Venography
Conray-30	Injection	14.1%	30% Iothalamate meglumine	Infusion urography
Conray-43	Injection	20.2%	43% Iothalamate meglumine	Lower extremity venography
Conray-325	Injection	32.5%	54.3% Iothalamate sodium	Excretory urography
Conray-400	Injection	40%	66.8% Iothalamate sodium	Angiocardiography Aortography Excretory urography IV pyelography Renal arteriography
Cysto-Conray	Instillation solution	20.2%	43% Iothalamate meglumine	Cystography Cystourethrography Retrograde pyelography
Cysto-Conray II	Instillation solution	8.1%	17.2% Iothalamate meglumine	Cystography Cystourethrography Retrograde pyelography
Cystografin	Instillation solution	14.1%	30% Diatrizoate meglumine	Cystourethrography Retrograde pyelography
Diatrizoate meglumine 76%	Injection	35.8%	76% Diatrizoate meglumine	Aortography Excretory urography Pediatric angiocardiography Peripheral arteriography
Ethiodol	Injection	37%	Ethiodized oil	Hysterosalpingography Lymphography
Gastrografin	Oral/rectal solution	37%	66% Diatrizoate meglumine and 10% diatrizoate sodium	GI radiography
Gastrovist	Oral/rectal solution	37%	66% Diatrizoate meglumine and 10% diatrizoate sodium	GI radiography
Hypaque 20%	Instillation solution	12%	20% Diatrizoate sodium	Retrograde pyelography
Hypaque 25%	Injection	15%	25% Diatrizoate sodium	Drip infusion pyelography (excretory urography)

Table 78-5. Iodinated Radiographic Diagnostic Agents (continued)

Trade Name	Dosage Form	Iodine Content	Composition	Diagnostic Uses
Hypaque 50%	Injection	30%	50% Diatrizoate sodium	Angiography (cerebral and peripheral) Aortography Cholangiography Hysterosalpingography Intraosseous venography Splenoportography
Hypaque-M 75%	Injection	38.5%	50% Diatrizoate meglumine and 25% diatrizoate sodium	Abdominal aortography Angiocardiography Arteriography (coronary, peripheral and renal) Urography
Hypaque-M 90%	Injection	46.2%	60% Diatrizoate meglumine and 30% diatrizoate sodium	Abdominal aortography Angiocardiography Arteriography (coronary and peripheral) Hysterosalpingography Urography
Hypaque-Cysto	Instillation solution	14.1%	30% Diatrizoate meglumine	Retrograde cystourethrography
Hypaque meglumine 30%	Injection	14.1%	30% Diatrizoate meglumine	Infusion urography Computed tomography
Hypaque meglumine 60%	Injection	28.2%	60% Diatrizoate meglumine	Arthrography Cerebral angiography Cholangiography Diskography Excretory urography Peripheral arteriography and venography Splenoportography
Hypaque sodium	Liquid	24.9%	2.4 g Diatrizoate sodium/ml	GI radiography
Hypaque sodium	Powder for oral solution	59.8%	—	GI radiography
Hypaque 76	Injection	37%	66% Diatrizoate meglumine and 10% diatrizoate sodium	See Angiovist 282
MD-76	Injection	37%	66% Diatrizoate meglumine and 10% diatrizoate sodium	See Angiovist 282
Oragrafin calcium	Granules for oral suspension	61.7%	3 g Ipodate calcium/8-g packet	Cholangiography Cholecystography
Oragrafin sodium	Capsules	61.4%	500 mg Ipodate sodium	Cholecystography
Renografin-60	Injection	29%	52% Diatrizoate meglumine and 8% diatrizoate sodium	Arthrography Cerebral angiography Cholangiography Computerized tomography Diskography Excretory urography Peripheral arteriography Pyelography Splenoportography Venography
Renografin-76	Injection	37%	66% Diatrizoate meglumine and 10% diatrizoate sodium	See Renografin-60
Reno-M-30	Instillation solution	14%	30% Diatrizoate meglumine	Retrograde or ascending pyelography
Reno-M-60	Injection	28%	60% Diatrizoate meglumine	Arthrography Cerebral angiography Cholangiography Diskography

(continued)

Table 78-5. Iodinated Radiographic Diagnostic Agents *(continued)*

Trade Name	Dosage Form	Iodine Content	Composition	Diagnostic Uses
				Excretory urography Peripheral arteriography Pyelography Splenoportography Venography
Reno-M-Dip	Injection	14%	30% Diatrizoate meglumine	Computerized tomography Drip infusion pyelography
Renovist	Injection	37%	34.3% Diatrizoate meglumine and 35% diatrizoate sodium	Angiocardiography Aortography Excretory urography Peripheral arteriography and venography Venocavography
Renovist II	Injection	31%	28.5% Diatrizoate meglumine and 29.1% diatrizoate sodium	See Renovist
Renovue-65	Injection	30%	65% Iodamide meglumine	Excretory urography
Renovue-Dip	Injection	11.1%	24% Iodamide meglumine	Excretory urography
Sinografin	Injection	38%	52.7% Diatrizoate meglumine and 26.8% iodipamide meglumine	Hysterosalpinography
Telepaque	Tablets	66.7%	500 mg Iopanoic acid	Cholecystography
Urovist Cysto	Instillation solution	14.1%	30% Diatrizoate meglumine	Cystourethrography Retrograde pyelography
Urovist Meglumine DIV/CT	Injection	14.1%	30% Diatrizoate meglumine	Drip-infusion pyelography Computed tomography Venography
Urovist Sodium 300	Injection	30%	50% Diatrizoate sodium	See Hypaque 50%
Vascoray	Injection	40%	52% Iothalamate meglumine and 26% iothalamate sodium	Angiocardiography Aortography Arteriography (coronary and renal) Excretory urography

The ability of circulating antibodies to render a person resistant to a particular disease is known as *immunity*. Immunity may be of two types, natural or acquired. Persons born with resistance to a certain disease state are said to have *natural* immunity; however, this is a relatively rare occurrence. Most types of immunity are *acquired,* that is, attained during the person's lifetime, either by production of antibodies in response to an invasion by foreign microorganisms (*active* acquired immunity) or by utilization of antibodies obtained from an animal or another human immunized against a particular disease (*passive* acquired immunity). Active immunity, therefore, is acquired through contact with the antigen itself, which stimulates the body to produce its own specific antibodies to combat it. If the antibodies develop in response to exposure to an actual disease state, whether clinical symptoms are present or not, the active immunity is said to be *naturally* acquired. Conversely, if the antibodies form in response to inoculation into the body of killed or attenuated microorganisms or their toxic by-products, the active immunity is referred to as *artificially* acquired.

The various biological preparations used to confer immunity may be categorized in the following manner:

I. Agents for active immunity
   A. Toxoids (*e.g.,* diphtheria, tetanus)
   B. Vaccines
      1. Bacterial (*e.g.,* BCG, cholera, typhoid)
      2. Viral (*e.g.,* influenza, measles, poliovirus)
II. Agents for passive immunity
   A. Antitoxins/antivenins (*e.g.,* diphtheria, tetanus, black widow spider)
   B. Human immune serums (*e.g.,* immune globulins)
III. Rabies prophylaxis products (*e.g.,* antirabies serum, rabies immune globulin, rabies vaccine)

Serums and Vaccines

79

I Agents for Active Immunity

Agents used for active immunization contain specific antigens that induce the formation of antibodies when injected into the body. These antigenic substances are of two types, toxoids and vaccines. Toxoids are toxins derived from microorganisms that have been modified (*i.e.,* detoxified) usually with formaldehyde, so that they are no longer toxic but are still antigenic, and thus are capable of stimulating antibody production. Vaccines are suspensions of whole microorganisms, either killed or chemically attenuated to reduce their virulence, which are capable of inducing the formation of antibodies without causing an outbreak of the disease. Active immunity with toxoids or vaccines requires several days or even weeks to develop, because sufficient antibody levels need to be attained. In some cases, more than one dose may be required. Thus, toxoids and vaccines are of limited value in treating *active* infections. Once acquired, however, active immunity can usually be made to last a lifetime, especially if reinforced by periodic "booster" doses at appropriate intervals.

A   Toxoids

Diphtheria	Diphtheria and tetanus and
Diphtheria and tetanus	pertussis vaccine
	Tetanus

Toxoids are generally prepared by treating exotoxins with formaldehyde, which renders them nontoxic but still antigenic. Stimulation of antibody production by toxoids can be increased by precipitating the toxoid with alum or adsorbing it onto colloids such as aluminum hydroxide. The precipitated or adsorbed products are absorbed and excreted more slowly, and persist in tissues a longer period of time than do plain toxoids, resulting in higher antibody production. The principal disadvantage of these precipitated or adsorbed toxoids is that their use is frequently associated with pain, swelling, and tenderness at the injection site, especially in older children and adults. These reactions are sometimes quite severe. The most commonly employed toxoids are diphtheria and tetanus, which are frequently given in combination with pertussis vaccine as DTP for routine immunization in preschool children. Table 79-1 lists the various toxoids.

B   Vaccines

BCG	Plague
Cholera	Pneumococcal
Hepatitis B	Poliomyelitis
Influenza virus	Rubella
Measles	Rubella and mumps
Measles and rubella	Smallpox
Measles, rubella, and mumps	Typhoid
Meningitis	Yellow fever
Mixed respiratory	

Vaccines are suspensions of killed or attenuated microorganisms of bacteria or viruses that are capable of stimulating antibody production but that are in themselves nonpathogenic. The live, attenuated vaccines are claimed to provide longer lasting immunity in most cases than the killed or inactivated vaccines, although both types are quite effective in increasing antibody levels. Caution must be observed, however, in using a vaccine grown and cultivated in living tissues, for example, chick embryo, because allergic reactions can occur in patients hypersensitive to the specific foreign proteins. Since most vaccines can produce both local and systemic allergic reactions, epinephrine, corticosteroids, and other antidotal measures should be available. Patients receiving immunosuppressive drugs (such as corticosteroids or antineoplastics) should not receive vaccines concomitantly, because these persons may exhibit an impaired antibody response

In the case of certain viral vaccines, a subclinical disease state may be induced by the vaccine itself, accompanied by fever, myalgia, and other manifestations of the particular viral disease (*e.g.,* rash, urticaria, parotitis). These symptoms are generally mild and transient and usually require nothing more than symptomatic management with medications such as antipyretics or analgesics. Vaccines do not afford immediate protection, because several days or occasionally weeks are required to produce sufficient serum antibody levels. A second and, occasionally, third injection at 4- to 8-week intervals are frequently given with certain vaccines to ensure adequate antibody levels. Active or imminent infections, therefore, require administration of one of the immune serums or antitoxins.

The various bacterial and viral vaccines are listed in Table 79-2, along with dosage guidelines and pertinent remarks.

In addition to the commercially available vaccines listed in Table 79-2, several other vaccines are available from the Centers for Disease Control in Atlanta for nonemergency use in persons at high risk for exposure in the laboratory. These vaccines include Anthrax Vaccine (adsorbed), Botulinum Toxoid (pentavalent), Eastern Equine Encephalitis (EEE) Vaccine (live, attenuated), Tularemia Vaccine (live, attenuated), and Venezuelan Equine Encephalitis (VEE) Vaccine.

II   Agents for Passive Immunity

Substances used to confer passive immunity are termed *immune serums* and consist of preformed antibodies derived from either human or animal sources. Human immune serums contain globulins possessing antibodies against a number of bacterial and viral diseases and are derived from human serum or plasma. Conversely, immune serums obtained by actively immunizing an animal against a specific disease, then removing and purifying the serum, which contains antibodies against that disease, are generally termed *antitoxins* or *antivenins.* Although both types of immune serums are effective in protecting against certain diseases, the human immune serums are much less likely to elicit hypersensitivity reactions, inasmuch as they do not contain foreign (*i.e.,* animal-derived) proteins.

A   Antitoxins/Antivenins

Black widow spider antivenin	North American coral snake
Crotalidae antivenin	antivenin
Diphtheria antitoxin	Tetanus antitoxin

Antitoxins and antivenins are prepared by repeatedly inoculating an animal, usually a horse, with a toxoid (*e.g.,* diphtheria, tetanus) or a venom (*e.g.,* from a snake, black widow spider), then bleeding the animal, and concentrating the antibody-containing fraction of the plasma. The partially purified antibodies or antitoxins can then be administered

(Text continues on p. 772.)

Table 79-1. Toxoids

Preparations	Administration	Remarks
Diphtheria toxoid, adsorbed, pediatric	2 injections (0.5 ml) IM 6 weeks to 8 weeks apart, then a third dose 1 year later *Booster:* 5-year to 10-year intervals	Used in infants and children under 6 years; do not administer subcutaneously; avoid giving during active infections or in patients receiving corticosteroids, because antibody response is diminished; cautious use in children with neurologic or convulsive disorders
Diphtheria and tetanus toxoids, combined, pediatric	2 injections (15 U diphtheria/ 0.5 ml) IM 4 weeks to 8 weeks apart, then a third dose 1 year later *Booster:* at 5 years of age	Used only in children 6 years or under; indicated only where the triple antigen (DTP) is contraindicated; do not administer during acute infection or in patients receiving immunosuppressant drugs; note that *pediatric* preparation is 7½ times as potent as adult preparation with respect to diphtheria toxoid
Diphtheria and tetanus toxoids, combined, adult	2 injections (2 U diphtheria/ 0.5 ml) IM 4 weeks to 8 weeks apart, then a third dose 6 months to 12 months later *Booster:* 10-year intervals	Reduced amount of diphtheria toxoid provides adequate immunization in adults with minimal risk of hypersensitivity reactions; tetanus toxoid content is identical in pediatric and adult preparations; cautious use during pregnancy and in debilitated individuals
Diphtheria and tetanus toxoids and pertussis vaccine, adsorbed–DTP (Tri-Immunol)	3 injections (0.5 ml) IM at 4-week to 8-week intervals, beginning at 2 months then a fourth dose 1 year thereafter *Booster:* at 4 years to 6 years of age	Most commonly used preparation for routine immunization of young children; not recommended in adults or children over 7 years; do not use in children with history of CNS disease or convulsions; defer administration during an acute febrile illness, shock, alterations in consciousness, extremely agitated behavior, or if patient is receiving immunosuppressive therapy; slight fever and malaise frequently occur following injection
Tetanus toxoid, fluid or adsorbed	Fluid—0.5 ml at 3-week to 4-week intervals for 3 doses, then a fourth dose 6 months to 12 months later Adsorbed—0.5 ml at 4-week to 6-week intervals for 2 doses, then a third dose 1 year later *Booster:* Every 10 years for each	Adsorbed toxoid gives higher antibody levels and longer protection than fluid toxoid, and is the preferred agent; adsorbed preparation is given IM only, but fluid preparation can be administered IM or SC; do not use in patients with acute respiratory infection, active tetanus infection, or convulsive disorders, or in persons receiving immunosuppressive therapy; local irritation and erythema are *common,* especially in adults

Table 79-2. Vaccines

Vaccine	Preparations	Administration	Remarks
Bacterial			
BCG vaccine (BCG)	Injection—8 million U to 26 million U/ml of standardized BCG bacillus prepared from culture	0.1 ml intradermally (0.05 ml in newborns)	Live, attenuated vaccine used in tuberculin-negative patients exposed to persons with active tuberculosis; contraindicated in tuberculin-positive patients, burn patients, and persons receiving chronic corticosteroid therapy; low incidence of untoward reactions, but can produce skin ulceration and abscesses; sterilize unused portion before disposal
Cholera vaccine	Injection—suspension of killed *Vibrio cholerae* organisms	Adults—0.5 ml SC or IM followed in 1 week to 4 weeks by a second 0.5-ml dose Children—0.2 ml to 0.3 ml SC or IM; repeat in 1 week to 4 weeks *Booster*—0.2 ml to 0.5 ml (depending on age) given every 6 months as long as protection is desired	Immunity is short-lived (3 mo–6 mo); therefore repeated doses are necessary to confer long-lasting protection; protection is not absolute, and disease can still be contacted if exposure occurs; injections *often* cause local pain, erythema, swelling, and a febrile reaction; for mass immunization during epidemics, a *single* dose of 1.0 ml can be used
Meningitis vaccines (Menomune-A, Menomune-C, Menomune-A/C, Menomune-A/C/Y/W-135)	Injection—suspensions of polysaccharides from *meningococcus*, groups A, C, Y, and W-135 as indicated	0.5 ml (50 mcg meningococcal isolated product) SC as a single injection (children under 2 yr—0.5 ml SC injections of group A vaccine 1 month apart)	Stimulates antibody production against *Neisseria meningitidis* groups A, C, Y, and W-135 depending upon vaccine content; used in persons at risk in epidemic or endemic areas; infants and children under 2 years should receive group A only and persons under 18 years should receive groups A and C only, because efficacy of other groups in these populations has not been established; do not give intradermally or IV; adverse reactions include chills, fever, malaise, local soreness; contraindicated in presence of active infections in persons taking corticosteroids and in pregnant women
Mixed respiratory vaccine (MRV)	Injection—suspensions of several strains of bacterial organisms present in common respiratory infections, *e.g.*, *Staphylococcus aureus*, *Streptococcus pneumoniae*, *Klebsiella pneumoniae*, *Hemophilus influenzae*	Initially, 0.05 ml SC; increase by 0.05 ml to 0.1 ml at 4-day to 7-day intervals until a maximum of 1 ml is given; maintenance dose 0.5 ml every 1 week to 2 weeks	Used to prevent bacterial hypersensitization in respiratory infections that can lead to asthma, urticaria, rhinitis; effectiveness has *not* been conclusively demonstrated; repeat doses should not be given until all local reactions from previous dose have disappeared; frequency of administration is highly individualized; children's dose is the same as adults; observe for symptoms of allergic reaction and, if severe, administer epinephrine, corticosteroids, or antihistamines; local hypersensitivity reactions are common and are not a cause for alarm
Plague vaccine	Injection—2 billion killed plague bacilli/ml	Adults—1.0 ml IM, followed in 1 month to 3 months by 0.2 ml IM; third injection of 0.2 ml IM after 3 months to 6 months is recommended	Suspension of inactivated *Yersinia pestis* organisms grown in artificial media; repeated injections increase the likelihood of adverse reactions, especially local allergic

Table 79-2. Vaccines (continued)

Vaccine	Preparations	Administration	Remarks
		Booster: 0.1 ml to 0.2 ml at 6-month intervals during active exposure Children— (Under 1 yr) $^1/_5$ adult dose (1 yr–4 yr) $^2/_5$ adult dose (5 yr–10 yr) $^3/_5$ adult dose	effects; *common* initial side-effects are malaise, headache, fever, local erythema, and mild lymphadenopathy; vaccine is recommended for those persons who must be in known plague areas, *e.g.,* Far East, South America, China, Saudi Arabia, and parts of Western U.S.
Pneumococcal vaccine, polyvalent (Pneumovax, Pnu-Immune)	Injection—25 mcg each of 23 polysaccharide isolates derived from pneumonococci/0.5 ml	0.5 ml SC or IM; revaccination at not less than 5-year intervals	Used for protection against pneumococcal pneumonia and bacteremia resulting from any of the 23 most prevalent capsular types of *pneumococci,* accounting for approximately 90% of all cases; indicated in persons over 2 years of age with increased risk of morbidity or mortality (*e.g.,* chronic debilitating disease or metabolic disorders, persons over 50, patients in chronic care facilities); also used to prevent pneumococcal otitis media in children under 2 years who are at high risk; protection is conferred for extended periods of time, and too frequent revaccination results in increasingly severe local reactions; do not inject IV or intradermally; local soreness and induration are very common within 2 days but quickly disappear
Typhoid vaccine	Injection—8 protective U/ml of a suspension of killed Ty-2 strain of *Salmonella typhosa* organisms	Adults—2 0.5-ml doses SC at 4-week intervals *Booster:* 0.5 ml SC or 0.1 ml intradermally every 3 years Children (under 10 yr)—2 0.25-ml doses, SC, at least 4 weeks apart *Booster:* 0.25 ml SC or 0.1 ml intradermally every 3 years	Used for immunization against typhoid fever in persons exposed to a known typhoid carrier or travelling to areas where the disease is endemic; commonly causes local erythema, tenderness, and induration as well as malaise, headache, fever, and myalgia; do *not* administer during other active infections

Viral

Vaccine	Preparations	Administration	Remarks
Hepatitis B vaccine (Heptavax-B)	Injection—20 mcg hepatitis B antigen per ml	Adults—1.0 ml initially, 1.0 ml at 1 month, and 1.0 ml at 6 months Children (under 10 yr)—0.5 ml initially, 0.5 ml at 1 month, and 0.5 ml at 6 months *Booster:* at 5 years to maintain immunity	Vaccine containing highly purified, formalin-inactivated hepatitis B surface antigen derived from plasma of chronic carriers of the antigen; affords a high degree of protection (90%–95%) against hepatitis B virus, a significant health risk for health-care professionals, drug abusers, homosexuals, patients undergoing hemodialysis or renal transplantation, cancer patients, and patients receiving multiple blood transfusions; hepatitis B infections have also been linked to hepatocellular carcinoma; effectiveness of vaccine in preventing hepatitis B when given after exposure to virus is not conclusively established, but vaccine has been given with Hepatitis B Immune Globulin with no deleterious effects

(continued)

Table 79-2. Vaccines (continued)

Vaccine	Preparations	Administration	Remarks
Influenza virus vaccines (Fluogen, Fluzone-Connaught)	Injection—suspension of inactivated influenza virus particles of the currently prevailing types	Over 13 years—0.5 ml IM in a single dose 3 years to 12 years—2 doses of 0.5 ml IM at least 4 weeks apart Under 3 years—2 doses of 0.25 ml IM at least 4 weeks apart	Composition of vaccine changes yearly depending on prevalent virus strains; recommended in persons at high risk for adverse reactions from lower respiratory infections, such as those with heart disease, chronic pulmonary disease, renal dysfunction, diabetes, or debilitation, contraindicated during first trimester of pregnancy, in persons with severe neurologic disorders, and in patients with a history of Guillain–Barré syndrome; use with caution in hypersensitive persons, because vaccine is egg-grown; defer immunization in patients with acute respiratory disease or other active infection; not effective against *all* influenza viruses; available as "whole-virus" or "split-virus" preparations; split virus associated with fewer adverse effects in children and is preferred in patients under 12 years; a single dose is sufficient for persons inoculated within the previous 2 years; vaccine may reduce elimination of drugs metabolized by cytochrome P-450 system in the liver (*e.g.,* theophylline, warfarin)
Measles vaccine—Rubeola (Attenuvax)	Injection—Suspension of Edmonston strain of measles virus in single-dose vials with diluent	Administer total volume of reconstituted vaccine SC *Booster:* not necessary	Live, attenuated strain of measles virus grown in chick embryo tissue culture; most often given together with mumps and rubella vaccines as a single preparation (see below); produces a mild measles infection (*e.g.,* fever, rash), which induces immunity in 97% of susceptible individuals; immune serum globulin (human) is frequently given IM (0.02 ml/kg) concomitantly with measles vaccine to lessen the severity of response to the live vaccine; recommended in children 15 months or older; revaccination is *not* required if child was over 12 months when initially vaccinated; contraindicated in pregnancy; use cautiously in children with a history of febrile convulsions or cerebral injury; discard if not used within 8 hours
Measles and rubella vaccine (M-R-Vax II)	Injection—single-dose vials with diluent containing a combination of live, attenuated strains of measles and rubella viruses	Administer total volume of reconstituted vaccine SC *Booster:* not necessary	Indicated for simultaneous immunization against measles and rubella (German measles) in children over 15 months; see measles vaccine and rubella vaccine for additional information; most frequently given together with mumps vaccine as a single preparation (see below)
Measles, mumps, and rubella vaccine (M-M-R II)	Injection—single-dose vials, with diluent containing live, attenuated strains of measles, mumps, and rubella viruses	Administer total volume of reconstituted vaccine SC *Booster:* not necessary	Indicated in children over 15 months for simultaneous immunization against measles, mumps, and rubella; highly effective (95%–98% of children develop effective

Table 79-2. Vaccines (continued)

Vaccine	Preparations	Administration	Remarks
			antibody levels to all three viruses) and generally well tolerated; widely used preparation; immunity persists for at least 8 years to 10 years; thus revaccination is not required; see Remarks for measles, mumps, and rubella vaccines
Mumps vaccine (Mumps vax)	Injection—single-dose vials with diluent containing live, attenuated Jeryl Lynn (B) mumps virus grown in chick embryo cell cultures	Administer total volume of reconstituted vaccine SC *Booster:* not necessary	Used for immunization of children over 15 months and adults; immunity is produced in 97% of children and 93% of adults with a single dose, and persists for at least 10 years; do *not* use in pregnant women; allergic reactions can occur (vaccine is derived from chick embryo); be prepared with epinephrine, antihistamines; fever and parotitis have occurred but are generally mild
Poliomyelitis vaccine, inactivated—IPV (Poliomyelitis Vaccine-Connaught)	Injection—suspension of 3 types of poliovirus (types 1, 2, 3) grown in monkey kidney cell cultures	3 doses (1.0 ml each) given SC at 4-week to 6 week intervals, followed by a fourth dose (1.0 ml) 6 months to 12 months after the third dose *Booster:* every 2 to 3 years	Indicated for polio immunization in persons with compromised immune systems; oral polio vaccine (Sabin) is vaccine of choice in other persons; dosage schedule is often integrated with that of DTP immunization and begun at 6 weeks to 12 weeks of age; vaccine should be clear red; do not use if cloudy, discolored, or precipitated; defer injections during periods of other active infections; hypersensitivity reactions can occur; have epinephrine injection available
Poliovirus vaccine, live oral trivalent—TOPV, Sabin (Orimune)	Dispettes—single-dose (0.5 ml) containing types 1, 2, and 3 poliovirus grown in monkey kidney cell cultures Vial with dropper—As above	3 doses (0.5 ml each) given orally at 6 weeks to 12 weeks of age, 8 weeks later, and 8 months to 12 months after the second dose *Booster:* 5 years of age	Vaccine of choice for primary immunization against poliovirus; advantages over Salk vaccine are ease of administration, longer lasting immunity, protection against infection by wild polioviruses, and lack of need for periodic booster doses; do *not* administer if persistent vomiting or diarrhea is present; store in a freezer, thaw before use, refrigerate vial after opening, and use contents within 7 days
Rubella vaccine (Meruvax II)	Injection—single-dose vials with diluent, containing Wistar RA 27/3 strain of rubella virus propagated in human diploid cell culture	Administer total volume of reconstituted vaccine SC	Live, attenuated rubella virus strains used to immunize against rubella in children from 15 months to puberty; antibody levels persist for at least 6 years; useful in adolescents and adults to prevent outbreaks in high-risk situations; do *not* administer to pregnant women and use cautiously in women of childbearing age, because congenital abnormalities can occur; usually given combined with measles and mumps vaccines (see MMR); side-effects are uncommon, but can include symptoms of the disease (rash, urticaria, sore throat, malaise, fever, headache,

(continued)

Table 79-2. Vaccines (continued)

Vaccine	Preparations	Administration	Remarks
			lymphadenopathy); arthralgia is fairly common in women (12%–20%)
Rubella and mumps vaccine (Biavax II)	Injection—single-dose vials with diluents, containing a mixture of mumps and rubella virus strains	Administer total volume of reconstituted vaccine SC	Combination vaccine yielding effective antibody levels in 97% to 100% of susceptible children; may be given as early as 1 year of age; not as frequently used as measles, mumps, and rubella vaccine (MMR); see Remarks for rubella and mumps vaccines
Smallpox vaccine (Dryvax)	Vials with diluent	Administer vaccine with puncture needles according to package instructions	Suspension of vaccinia viruses isolated from calf lymph; routine vaccination is no longer indicated but is recommended in individuals at high risk, such as laboratory workers directly involved with smallpox or related (variola, monkeypox) viruses; revaccination is recommended approximately every 3 years in these special risk groups; positive vaccination is indicated by appearance of vesicle at injection site 6 days to 8 days after inoculation; *contraindicated* in persons with eczema or other skin disease, malignancies, or those receiving x-ray or other forms of immunosuppressive therapy, and during pregnancy
Yellow fever vaccine (YF-Vax)	Injection—vials with diluent, for needle injection or jet-injector use, containing a live, attenuated 17D strain virus cultured in chick embryo	0.5 ml SC	Indicated for immunization of persons traveling to countries requiring vaccination against yellow fever; immunity develops within 7 days and can last for up to 10 years; administer at least 1 month apart from other live viruses; fever and malaise occur in about 10% of patients; keep frozen until reconstituted and then use within 1 hour; do not use if vaccine has been exposed to temperatures above 5°C

to humans to neutralize toxins produced by invading microorganisms or introduced by a bite.

It is imperative that a skin or conjunctival hypersensitivity test be performed before administering any of the horse serum antitoxins to determine if the patient might exhibit an allergic reaction to the foreign serum. Package literature describing the appropriate hypersensitivity testing procedure should always be consulted before utilizing one of these products. Even a negative sensitivity test result, however, does not completely rule out the possibility of an allergic reaction and epinephrine injection should always be available when an antitoxin is administered. Adverse reactions to antitoxins range from local pain and erythema at the injection site, to serum sickness and anaphylaxis, the incidence of the more serious allergic reactions being approximately 5% to 10%.

Information pertaining to the commercially available antitoxins and antivenins is presented in Table 79-3. In addition,

Botulism Equine Antitoxin (ABE) is available by request to the Centers for Disease Control in Atlanta.

B Human Immune Serums

Hepatitis B immune globulin
Immune globulin, human
Lymphocyte immune globulin
Pertussis immune globulin

Tetanus immune globulin
Rh₀(D) immune globulin
Varicella zoster immune globulin

Immune globulins containing antibodies against certain diseases can be obtained from human serum, and these products are generally preferred over animal-derived globulins because of the lower incidence of hypersensitivity reactions. Human immune globulins may be obtained from pooled plasma of human donors, in which case the preparation

(Text continues on p. 776.)

Table 79-3. Antitoxins/Antivenins

Antitoxin/Antivenin	Preparations	Administration	Remarks
Antivenins			
Black widow spider antivenin (Antivenin *Latrodectus mactans*)	Injection—6000 U/vial with diluent plus vial of normal horse serum for sensitivity testing	2.5 ml reconstituted antivenin IM *or* 2.5 ml in 10 ml to 50 ml saline by IV infusion	Used to treat persons bitten by black widow spider; prompt administration yields most effective results; use of muscle relaxants appears to be most important during early reaction phase
Crotalidae antivenin, polyvalent	Injection—vial of lyophilized serum with diluent plus vial of normal horse serum for sensitivity testing	Dosage depends on severity of bite; *Mild*—2 to 4 vials IV *Moderate*—5 to 9 vials IV *Severe*—10 to 20 vials IV	Preparation of serum globulins containing protective antibodies against a number of crotalids, including pit vipers, rattlesnakes, cottonmouths, copperheads, bushmasters (see package instructions); administer as soon as possible after bite and immobilize patient to minimize spread of venom; do *not* administer at or around the site of the bite; children have less resistance and require proportionately larger doses than adults; subsequent injections depend on clinical response; use barbiturates and narcotics with caution, because increased respiratory depression can result
North American coral snake antivenin (Antivenin *Micrurus fulvius*)	Injection—vial with diluent	3 to 5 vials (30 ml–50 ml) slowly injected directly into IV infusion tubing or added to reservoir bottle of IV drip	Concentrated solution of serum globulins obtained from horses immunized against eastern coral snake venom; bitten area should be completely immobilized; first several milliliters of antivenin should be administered over a 5-minute period and patient carefully observed for evidence of allergic reaction; up to 10 vials have been required in some persons with severe or multiple bites; drugs that depress respiration should be used cautiously; because snake venom itself produces respiratory depression and paralysis
Antitoxins			
Diphtheria antitoxin	Injection—10,000 or 20,000 U/vial	Adults and children—20,000 U to 120,000 U IM or IV depending on severity and duration of infection; repeat in 24 hours if clinical improvement is not apparent Prophylaxis—5000 U to 10,000 U IM	Concentrated solution of purified globulins obtained from the serum of horses immunized against diphtheria toxin; delay in beginning therapy increases dosage requirements and reduces beneficial effects; continue treatment until all symptoms are controlled; appropriate antimicrobial agents should be used concurrently; nonimmunized patients exposed to diphtheria should receive a low dose (see Administration) to produce a temporary passive immunity; sensitivity testing is necessary before administration
Tetanus antitoxin	Injection—1500 or 20,000 U/vial	Treatment—50,000 U to 100,000 U IV	Concentrated solution of serum globulins from horses immunized

(continued)

Table 79-3. Antitoxins/Antivenins *(continued)*

Antitoxin/Antivenin	Preparations	Administration	Remarks
		Prophylaxis—1500 U to 5000 U IM or SC depending on body weight	against tetanus toxin; indicated *only* when tetanus immune globulin is not available; protection lasts about 2 weeks with a single prophylactic dose; tetanus toxoid, adsorbed, is usually given with the antitoxin to initiate active immunization; most children are routinely immunized against tetanus and the need for the antitoxin seldom occurs

Table 79-4. Human Immune Serums

Immune Serum	Preparations	Administration	Remarks
Hepatitis B immune globulin (H-BIG, Hep-B-Gammagee, HyperHep)	Injection—1-ml, 5-ml vials	0.06 ml/kg IM as soon after exposure as possible; repeat in 1 month	Solution of immunoglobulins containing a high titer of antibodies to hepatitis B surface antigen; indicated for prophylaxis following accidental oral, parenteral, or direct mucous membrane exposure to antigen-containing materials such as blood or serum
Immune globulin—Intramuscular (ISG) (Gamma Globulin, Gamastan, Gammar, Immuglobin)	Injection—2-ml, 10-ml vials	IM injection only: Bacterial infections—0.5 ml to 3.5 ml/kg Hepatitis A—0.02 ml/kg Hepatitis B—0.06 ml/kg; repeat in 1 month Immunoglobulin deficiency—1.2 ml/kg initially, then 0.6 ml/kg every 3 weeks to 4 weeks Measles—0.2 ml/kg Rubella—20 ml (pregnant women *only*) Varicella—0.6 ml to 1.2 ml/kg	Solution of globulins obtained from pooled human serum, containing antibodies to a number of organisms; used to decrease the severity of certain diseases (hepatitis, measles, varicella) in persons exposed to an active infection; also indicated as replacement therapy for immunoglobulin deficiency states and as adjunctive treatment to antibiotics in severe bacterial infections or burns; may be of benefit in pregnant women exposed to rubella virus to lessen possibility of fetal damage, but routine use in early pregnancy cannot be justified; injections can be very painful
Immune globulin, intravenous (Gamimune)	Injection—5% (in 10% maltose)	IV infusion only: 100 mg/kg (2 ml/kg) once a month by IV infusion (0.01 ml/kg–0.04 ml/kg/min for 30 min)	Provides *immediate* antibody levels; half-life is approximately 3 weeks; preferred to immune globulin, IM, in patients requiring rapid increase in IgG antibodies, in patients with a small muscle mass, and in patients with bleeding tendencies; maltose is added to stabilize the protein, reducing the incidence of adverse effects; may cause a precipitous drop in blood pressure, especially at rapid infusion rates; monitor vital signs carefully during infusion; have epinephrine available for allergic reactions
Lymphocyte immune globulin—anti-thymocyte globulin (Atgam)	Injection—50 mg/ml	IV infusion only: Adults—10 mg/kg to 30 mg/kg/day Children—5 mg/kg to 25 mg/kg/day	A lymphocyte-selective immunosuppressant that reduces the number of circulating, thymus-dependent lymphocytes; used by *experienced personnel only* for management of allograft rejection in renal transplant patients and as an adjunct to other immunosuppressive therapy to delay onset of first

Table 79-4. Human Immune Serums *(continued)*

Immune Serum	Preparations	Administration	Remarks
			rejection; discontinue if anaphylaxis or *severe* thrombocytopenia or leukopenia occurs; frequently encountered adverse reactions are fever, chills, rash, pruritus, urticaria, leukopenia, and thrombocytopenia; drug must be diluted in saline before infusion; do not dilute with dextrose solutions or highly acidic solutions, because precipitation can occur; a dose should not be infused in less than 4 hours; have resuscitative materials available (*e.g.,* epinephrine, antihistamines, steroids, *etc.*)
Pertussis immune globulin (Hypertussis)	Injection—1.25-ml vials	Treatment: 1.25 ml to 2.5 ml IM, repeated at 24-hour to 48-hour intervals Prophylaxis: 1.25 ml to 2.5 ml IM followed by a second dose 1 week to 2 weeks later	Used for prophylaxis and adjunctive treatment of pertussis (whooping cough) in young children who have not been immunized previously; clinical efficacy has not been completely established
Tetanus immune globulin (Homo-Tet, Hu-Tet, Hyper-Tet)	Injection—250 U/vial or disposable syringe	Treatment: 3000 U to 6000 U IM Prophylaxis: 250 U IM	Indicated for passive tetanus prophylaxis in persons not actively immunized or whose immunization status is uncertain; not generally necessary if person has had at least 2 doses of tetanus toxoid; produces effective levels of circulating antibodies for much longer periods of time than tetanus antitoxin; does not interfere with immune response to tetanus toxoid given at the same time; thorough cleansing of wounds and removal of all foreign particles is important to prevent infection
Rho(D) immune globulin (Gamulin Rh, HypRho-D, RhoGAM)	Injection—vial with diluent	Inject contents of 1 vial IM for every 15 ml fetal packed red cell volume within 72 hours following delivery, miscarriage, abortion, or transfusion (See package instructions for mixing and injecting directions)	Used to prevent sensitization in a subsequent pregnancy to the Rho(D) factor in an Rh-negative mother who has given birth to an Rh-positive infant by an Rh-positive father; also may be employed to prevent Rho(D) sensitization in Rh-negative patients accidentally transfused with Rh-positive blood; consult product information for blood typing and drug administration procedures; do not give IV; also available in microdose form (MICRhoGAM) to prevent maternal Rh-immunization following miscarriage or abortion up to 12-weeks gestation
Varicella-Zoster immune globulin (human)—VZIG	Injection—10% to 18% solution of the globulin fraction of human plasma containing 125 U of antibody to varicella-zoster virus in a single-dose vial	IM injection only: 125 U to 625 U (1 to 5 vials) depending on patient's weight	Globulin fraction of adult human plasma (primarily immunoglobulin G) with high titer of varicella-zoster antibodies; used for passive immunization of *immunodeficient* children following exposure to varicella; most effective if given within 96 hours after exposure; not indicated prophylactically; do *not* administer IV; no more than 2.5 ml should be injected at a single IM site (1.25 ml maximum if patient weighs less than 10 kg); VZIG must be requested from regional distribution centers of American Red Cross Blood Services

contains antibodies against a number of diseases (*e.g.*, hepatitis, rubella, varicella) or from the blood of persons recently recovered from or hyperimmunized against a *particular* disease, in which case the globulins contain high antibody titers against that particular disease. These human immune serums should be used cautiously in individuals with immunoglobulin A deficiency, thrombocytopenia, or coagulation disorders, and in pregnant women. Skin testing for hypersensitivity is meaningless with human immune serums, because intradermal injections frequently give rise to a local inflammatory response that can be misinterpreted as an allergic reaction. True hypersensitivity reactions to human immune globulins are extremely rare.

The human immune serums are listed in Table 79-4 along with dosages and other pertinent information.

III   Rabies Prophylaxis Products

Antirabies serum, equine   Rabies vaccine, human diploid
Rabies immune globulin   cell culture

Rabies is an acute viral disease of animals that can be transmitted to other animals and humans by the bite of an infected animal. Although many animals are susceptible to rabies, it occurs most commonly in dogs, cats, raccoons, skunks, coyotes, and wolves. The virus has a high affinity for the nervous system, and is inevitably fatal unless appropriate immunologic therapy is instituted quickly.

Products used for rabies prophylaxis include the following:

Table 79-5. Rabies Prophylaxis Products

Immune Serum	Preparations	Administration	Remarks
Antirabies serum, equine	Injection—1000 U/vial	55 U/kg (1000 U/40 lb) IM in a single dose	Used to promote passive immunity to rabies when rabies immune globulin is unavailable; delays propagation of virus, thus allowing time for rabies vaccine to induce sufficient antibodies; give as soon as possible after exposure; sensitivity testing (intradermal or conjunctival) should be done before administration; part of the serum should be infiltrated into the tissue around the wound; usually given in conjunction with rabies vaccine, although not in the same syringe
Rabies immune globulin, human (Hyperab, Imogam)	Injection—150 U/ml	20 U/kg (9.1 U/lb); ½ the dose IM and ½ the dose to infiltrate the wound	Used to provide rabies antibodies immediately; given in conjunction with rabies vaccine; reduces risk of serum sickness to equine vaccine; should be given as soon as possible following exposure, but regardless of interval, immune globulin is still recommended; do not give repeated doses once vaccine has been administered
Rabies vaccine, human diploid cell cultures—HDVC (Imovax, WYVAC)	Injection—single-dose lyophilized preparation with diluent	Preexposure—3 injections, IM, of 1.0 ml each on days 0, 7, and 28 *Boosters:* every 2 years in high-risk individuals Postexposure—5 injections, IM, of 1.0 ml each on days 0, 3, 7, 14, and 28 with a dose of rabies immune globulin on day 0	Preferred rabies vaccine due to greater efficacy and safety compared to duck embryo vaccine; antibody response is virtually 100% with recommended 5 doses; pre-exposure vaccination is indicated for persons in contact with rabid animals or patients or those handling rabies virus or contaminated articles; postexposure treatment should also include rabies immune globulin; adverse reactions to vaccine are infrequent; local swelling and erythema have occurred; corticosteroids and other immunosuppressive agents can interfere with development of active immunity to vaccine; do not administer together

A. *Human diploid cell vaccine* (HDCV)—suspension of Wistar rabies virus strain grown in human diploid cell cultures

B. *Rabies immune globulin* (RIG)—human immune globulin obtained from plasma of hyperimmunized donors

C. *Antirabies serum, equine origin* (ARS)—concentrated serum obtained from hyperimmunized horses

Postexposure treatment is best accomplished by a combination of active and passive immunization, that is, vaccine and immune globulin. For passive immunization, rabies immune globulin is the drug of choice, and the equine antirabies serum should only be used when the immune globulin is unavailable. For active immunization, HDCV is utilized.

The various rabies prophylaxis products are briefly reviewed in Table 79-5. It is important, however, that anyone using any of the products become thoroughly familiar with the indications, precautions, and general handling procedures of each particular preparation by consulting the product literature.

80 Miscellaneous Drug Products

There are several pharmacologic agents that do not fall into one of the previously discussed categories of drugs and thus will be reviewed here under a miscellaneous heading.

▶ alprostadil
Prostin VR Pediatric

Alprostadil (prostaglandin E_1) is a solution for IV infusion that is used in neonates with congenital heart defects to temporarily maintain the patency of the ductus arteriosus until corrective surgery can be performed.

Mechanism
Relaxes smooth muscle of the ductus arteriosus, thereby providing for adequate blood oxygenation. Other actions of PGE_1 include vasodilation, increased tone of intestinal and uterine smooth muscle, and inhibition of platelet aggregation.

Uses
1 Palliative therapy of neonates with congenital heart defects (*e.g.,* pulmonary stenosis, tricuspid atresia, tetralogy of Fallot, aortic coarctation) to maintain patency until corrective surgery can be performed

Dosage
Initially, 0.1 mcg/kg/minute until improvement is noted; reduce infusion rate to lowest dose that maintains the response (0.01–0.05 mcg/kg/min); maximum dose—0.4 mcg/kg/minute

Fate
Rapidly metabolized upon first pass through the lungs; metabolites are excreted primarily by the kidney; does not appear to be retained in body tissue

Common Side-Effects
Fever, apnea (see Nursing Alerts), flushing, bradycardia, and hypotension

Significant Adverse Reactions
Cardiovascular—tachycardia, edema, second-degree heart block, hyperemia, shock, congestive heart failure, ventricular fibrillation, cardiac arrest
CNS—seizures, hyperirritability, lethargy, hypothermia, cerebral bleeding, hyperextension of the neck
Hematologic—disseminated intravascular coagulation, anemia, thrombocytopenia, bleeding
GI—diarrhea, regurgitation, hyperbilirubinemia
Respiratory—wheezing, hypercapnia, respiratory depression
Other—anuria, hematuria, sepsis, peritonitis, hypokalemia, hypoglycemia, cortical proliferation of long bones

Contraindication
Respiratory distress syndrome (hyaline membrane disease)

▶ **NURSING ALERTS**

▷ 1 Be aware that apnea occurs in 10% to 12% of neonates treated with alprostadil, most often in those weighing less than 2 kg at birth. Monitor respiratory status closely during infusion, and always have respiratory assistance immediately available.

▷ 2 Use with caution in neonates with bleeding tendencies, because drug inhibits platelet aggregation.

▷ 3 Be alert for symptoms of overdosage (*e.g.,* bradycardia, apnea, flushing, pyrexia) and discontinue infusion. Reinitiate infusion cautiously when symptoms subside and closely observe patient.

▶ **NURSING CONSIDERATIONS**

▷ 1 Infuse drug at the lowest dose and for the shortest time to produce the desired effect.

▷ 2 Monitor arterial pressure during drug administration, and reduce perfusion rate should pressure fall significantly.

▷ 3 Assess efficacy of treatment by monitoring blood oxygenation in infants with decreased pulmonary flow and by monitoring systemic blood pressure and blood *p*H in infants with compromised systemic blood flow.

▶ **antidotes**

Deferoxamine mesylate	Edetate calcium disodium
Dimercaprol-BAL	

Most drugs employed as specific antidotes (*e.g.,* narcotic antagonists, protamine sulfate, vitamin K, diazoxide, leucovorin) have been considered previously in the individual chapters dealing with the pharmacologic agents that they specifically antagonize. Certain other drugs have the ability to complex with various heavy metals (such as iron, lead, gold, mercury) and are employed to treat poisoning with these substances. Such poisoning can occur either from drug overdosage, for example, with use of gold salts for rheumatoid arthritis or iron for severe anemias, or accidental ingestion, such as lead-containing paints, insecticides, or pesticides. Heavy metal intoxication often results in impaired enzymatic functions, which, if severe, can lead to cellular anoxia and possibly death.

Table 80-1 lists the various heavy metal antidotes, together with their indications, dosage, and pertinent remarks.

▶ **azathioprine**

Imuran

Azathioprine is an immunosuppressive agent used to prevent rejection in renal transplantations. It is a potent bone marrow depressant, and frequent blood counts are necessary during therapy. Azathioprine has been used experimentally in treating other disorders beieved to be the result of altered immunologic function, such as severe rheumatoid arthritis, systemic lupus erythematosus, and idiopathic thrombocytopenic purpura.

Mechanism

Not completely established; converted to 6-mercaptopurine, which appears to interfere with nucleic acid and protein synthesis and coenzyme function (see Mercaptopurine, Chap. 74); may also alter cellular metabolism

Uses

1 Adjunct for prevention of rejection in renal homotransplantation

2 Treatment of severe, active rheumatoid arthritis in patients not responsive to conventional therapy (*i.e.,* aspirin, nonsteroidal anti-inflammatory drugs, corticosteroids, gold)

Dosage

Prevention of rejection: initially 3 mg/kg to 5 mg/kg/day IV beginning at the time of transplant; switch to oral therapy as soon as feasible; usual maintenance range is 1 mg/kg to 2 mg/kg/day

Rheumatoid arthritis: initially 1 mg/kg as a single dose or two divided doses; increase stepwise at 4-week to 6-week intervals if response is not satisfactory and no serious toxicity is noted; maximum dose is 2.5 mg/kg/day

Fate

Largely converted to 6-mercaptopurine following administration; most is metabolized in the liver and excreted by the kidneys; partially (30%) bound to plasma proteins

Common Side-Effects

Leukopenia, infections (fever, chills, sore throat, cold sores), nausea, and vomiting

Significant Adverse Reactions

Anemia, thrombocytopenia, bleeding, jaundice, diarrhea, alopecia, oral mucosal lesions, pancreatitis, arthralgia, steatorrhea, severe secondary infections, toxic hepatitis, and biliary stasis

Contraindications

Treatment of rheumatoid arthritis in pregnant women or in patients previously treated with alkylating agents

Interactions

1 Allopurinol inhibits azathioprine and mercaptopurine metabolism and can increase the toxic effects of these drugs.

▶ **NURSING ALERTS**

▷ 1 Perform complete blood counts and liver and kidney function tests at least weekly during initial therapy, and every 2 weeks to 3 weeks during prolonged treatment. Rapid fall or persistent decrease in leukocyte count mandates a dosage reduction or drug withdrawal.

▷ 2 Observe closely for indications of thrombocytopenia (abnormal bleeding or bruising, mucosal ulceration) or other blood dyscrasias, and advise physician.

▷ 3 Be alert for occurrence of hepatic dysfunction (pru-

Table 80-1. Heavy Metal Antidotes

Drug	Preparations	Indications	Usual Dosage Range	Remarks
Deferoxamine mesylate (Desferal Mesylate)	Powder for injection—500 mg/vial	Acute iron intoxication Chronic iron overload (*e.g.*, multiple transfusions)	Acute intoxication: 1 g IM, followed by 0.5 g every 4 hours for 2 doses, then every 4 hours to 12 hours as needed IV infusion—same as IM dose at rate of 15 mg/kg/hour Chronic overload: IM—0.5 g to 1 g/day IV—2 g at a rate of 15 mg/kg/hour SC—1 g to 2 g/day over 8 hours to 24 hours with a mini-infusion pump Children—50 mg/kg IM or IV every 6 hours or up to 15 mg/kg/hour by IV infusion	Chelates iron in the ferric state, forming a stable, water-soluble, readily excretable complex; no effect on electrolyte or trace metal excretion; contraindicated in severe renal disease; should be used in conjunction with other appropriate antidotal measures (emesis, lavage, correction of acidosis, control of shock, respiratory assistance); pain on injection, allergic reactions, blurred vision, diarrhea, abdominal pain, tachycardias, and fever have been reported; Urine may be colored red
Dimercaprol-BAL (Bal In Oil)	Injection—100 mg/ml	Arsenic, gold and mercury poisoning Acute lead poisoning (in combination with calcium EDTA	IM only: Arsenic/gold poisoning—2.5 mg to 3 mg/kg 4 to 6 times a day for 2 days, then 2 to 4 times a day on the third day, then 1 to 2 times a day for 10 days Mercury poisoning—5 mg/kg initially, then 2.5 mg/kg 1 to 2 times a day for 10 days Lead poisoning—4 mg/kg at 4-hour intervals in combination with calcium sodium EDTA at a different site	Complexes with various heavy metals forming stable, water-soluble chelates that are readily excreted by the kidney; sulfhydryl enzymes are thus protected from the toxic action of the metals; do not use in iron, cadmium, or selenium poisoning, because resultant complexes are more toxic than the metals; most effective when given as soon as possible after metal ingestion; urine should be kept alkaline to minimize kidney damage as chelate is being excreted; local pain is frequent at site of injection; contraindicated in hepatic insufficiency; large doses may increase blood pressure and heart rate; other adverse effects include fever in children (30% frequency), nausea, vomiting, headache, burning in the mouth and throat, chest constriction, lacrimation, salivation, and paresthesias; other supportive measures are necessary (fluids, electrolytes, respiratory assistance)
Edetate calcium disodium (Calcium Disodium Versenate, Calcium EDTA)	Injection—200 mg/ml	Acute and chronic lead poisoning and lead encephalopathy	IV—1 g diluted to 250 ml to 500 ml and infused over 1 hour; administer twice a day for up to 5 days, stop 2 days, then resume for another 5 days if necessary IM (preferred in children)—50 mg to 75 mg/kg/day in 2 equally divided doses for 3 days to 5 days	Calcium in the compound is displaced by a heavy metal (*e.g.*, lead), resulting in formation of a stable metal–drug complex that is removed by the kidneys; potentially a very toxic compound; recommended dosage levels should not be exceeded; do not infuse rapidly in patients with lead encephalopathy; increased intracranial pressure can be fatal; IM is the preferred route of administration; closely monitor renal function; do not give to patients with impaired kidney function; refer to package instructions for mixing and administering directions

ritus, darkened urine, light colored stools, yellowing of skin or sclera), and alert physician.

▷ 4 Use with caution in patients with liver or kidney dysfunction, during a clinically active infection, in pregnant or nursing women, and in women of childbearing potential.

▷ 5 Recognize that azathioprine is carcinogenic in animals and may increase the risk of neoplasia, especially in transplant recipients. The benefit/risk ratio must be carefully assessed when using azathioprine; acute myelogenous leukemia and solid tumors have occurred in rheumatoid arthritis patients receiving the drug.

▶ NURSING CONSIDERATIONS

▷ 1 Observe patient closely during therapy, and adjust dosage to obtain the maximum therapeutic benefit with minimal toxicity.

▷ 2 Monitor intake–output ratio and renal clearance of azathioprine to prevent cumulation toxicity.

▷ 3 Reduce dosage if negative nitrogen balance occurs.

▷ 4 Stress good hygiene and urge avoidance of persons or situations that may result in development of colds or infections during azathioprine treatment. If infection develops, treat immediately with appropriate drugs; a dosage reduction for azathioprine may also be necessary.

▷ 5 Reduce dose of azathioprine to one third to one fourth normal dose if given concurrently with allopurinol.

▶ **bromocriptine**

Parlodel

An ergot derivative exhibiting dopamine agonist activity, bromocriptine markedly reduces secretion of prolactin with minimal effects on other pituitary hormones. It is used for treating amenorrhea and galactorrhea resulting from hyperprolactinemia, for suppressing postpartum lactation, and as adjunctive therapy in treating Parkinson's disease (see Chap. 26).

Mechanism

Activates postsynaptic dopamine receptors in the tuberoinfundibular dopaminergic neuronal system, resulting in secretion of prolactin inhibitory factor (PIF) from the hypothalamus; PIF blocks liberation of prolactin from the anterior pituitary in patients with hyperprolactinemia; also stimulates dopamine receptors in the corpus striatum, thus relieving some of the symptoms of parkinsonism

Uses

1 Short-term treatment of amenorrhea–galactorrhea associated with hyperprolactinemia, except where a demonstrable pituitary tumor is present (not indicated in patients with normal prolactin levels)

2 Prevention of postpartum lactation occurring after parturition, stillbirth, or abortion

3 Treatment of female infertility associated with hyperprolactinemia

4 Adjunctive treatment of parkinsonism (see Chap. 26)

5 Reduce plasma growth hormone levels in patients with acromegaly (investigational use only)

Dosage

Amenorrhea–galactorrhea: 2.5 mg two to three times a day; not to exceed 6 months

Prevention of lactation: 2.5 mg two to three times a day for 14 days to 21 days

Treatment of infertility: initially 2.5 mg once daily; increase to two to three times a day within the first week

Parkinsonism: initially 2.5 mg/day in two divided doses; increase every two weeks to four weeks by 2.5 mg/day as necessary

Fate

About one fourth of an oral dose is absorbed from the GI tract; metabolized completely and excreted largely in the feces, *via* the bile; less than 5% of the dose appears in the urine; highly (90%–95%) bound to plasma proteins

Common Side-Effects

Nausea, dizziness, headache, hypotension, fatigue, abdominal cramping, lightheadedness, and nasal congestion

Significant Adverse Reactions

Vomiting, diarrhea, syncope, altered behavior, dyskinesias, seizures, dyspnea, blurred vision, diplopia, GI bleeding, exacerbation of angina, bladder disturbances, Raynaud's phenomenon, alcohol intolerance, hypertension, and cerebrovascular accident

Contraindications

Ischemic heart disease, peripheral vascular disease, pregnancy, and lactation

Interactions

1 Bromocriptine may potentiate other drugs that can also lower blood pressure.

2 Phenothiazines and other antipsychotic drugs can reduce the effects of bromocriptine by blocking dopamine receptor sites.

3 Oral contraceptives may cause amenorrhea or galactorrhea and reduce the effectiveness of bromocriptine.

4 Methyldopa, metoclopramide, MAO inhibitors, and reserpine can increase serum prolactin levels, thus reducing the effectiveness of bromocriptine.

▶ NURSING ALERTS

▷ 1 Discontinue treatment immediately if pregnancy occurs during bromocriptine administration.

▷ 2 Do not begin therapy for postpartum lactation until patient's vital signs have stabilized and no sooner than 4 hours after delivery, because incidence of hypotension is quite high in early postpartum period.

▷ 3 Caution patients against operating machinery or engaging in other potentially hazardous activities during bromocriptine therapy, because dizziness and fainting have occurred.

▷ 4 Be aware that treatment of amenorrheic women with bromocriptine may result in restoration of fertility. Urge birth control measures (other than oral contraceptives; see Interactions) during treatment and perform periodic pregnancy tests.

▷ 5 Determine if pituitary tumor is present before beginning bromocriptine therapy for galactorrhea, because drug will lower serum prolactin levels even if a tumor is present, but will not obviate the need for surgery or radiotherapy.

▷ 6 Use with caution in patients with hepatic disease or hypertension, and in children under 15 years of age.

▷ 7 Monitor blood pressure frequently during administration of bromocriptine for suppression of lactation, because hypertension has occurred up to 9 days postpartum. Blood pressure returns to pretreatment levels upon cessation of therapy.

▶ NURSING CONSIDERATIONS

▷ 1 Inform postpartum patients that they may experience rebound breast engorgement and secretion once bromocriptine therapy is stopped.

▷ 2 Note that menses are usually re-established within 6 weeks to 8 weeks, but galactorrhea may take somewhat longer to control, for example, 8 weeks to 12 weeks.

▷ 3 Be aware that recurrence rates are quite high for amenorrhea–galactorrhea following termination of therapy, and safety of long-term or repeated therapy is not known.

▷ 4 Recognize that dose of bromocriptine effective in parkinsonism (25 mg–100 mg/day) is approximately 10 times higher than that used for galactorrhea and adverse effects are more frequent and often more severe.

▶ cyclosporine
Sandimmune

Cyclosporine (cyclosporin A) is an immunosuppressant that may be employed to prolong and assist survival of allogeneic transplants involving the heart, kidney, liver, and possibly also the bone marrow, pancreas, and lung.

Mechanism
Not completely established; appears to specifically and reversibly inhibit T-lymphocytes, including the T-helper cell and T-suppressor cell; lymphokine production is also impaired, and release of interleukin-2 or T-cell growth factor may be reduced

Uses
1 Prevention of organ rejection in kidney, liver, or heart transplants, in conjunction with adrenal corticosteroids
2 Treatment of chronic rejection in patients previously treated with other immunosuppressive drugs

Dosage
Oral: initially 15 mg/kg/day, 4 hours to 12 hours prior to transplantation; continue for 1 week to 2 weeks postoperatively, then taper by 5%/week to a maintenance level of 5 mg/kg to 10 mg/kg/day
IV (see Nursing Alerts): initially 5 mg/kg to 6 mg/kg/day 4 hours to 12 hours prior to transplantation, as a slow (2 hr–6 hr) infusion of dilute solution (50 mg per 20 to 100 ml of Sodium Chloride Injection or 5% Dextrose Injection)

Fate
Oral absorption is erratic and incomplete; peak serum levels are attained in 3 hours to 4 hours; distributes to erythrocytes, granulocytes, leukocytes, and plasma, where it is approximately 90% protein-bound; extensively metabolized and excreted primarily *via* the bile, with only about 60% of the dose eliminated in the urine

Common Side-Effects
Renal dysfunction, tremor, hirsutism, hypertension, gum hyperplasia, and secondary infections

Significant Adverse Reactions
CNS—headache, confusion, convulsions, flushing, paresthesias
GI—diarrhea, vomiting, abdominal pain, gastritis, peptic ulcer, anorexia, hepatotoxicity
Dermatologic—acne, brittle nails
Other—anxiety, depression, muscle weakness, joint pain, chest pain, visual disturbances, gynecomastia, difficulty in swallowing, upper GI bleeding, pancreatitis, mouth sores, constipation, night sweats, leukopenia, lymphoma, anemia, thrombocytopenia

Interactions
1 Cyclosporine can enhance the nephrotoxicity of aminoglycosides, loop diuretics, and other drugs that can damage the kidney.
2 Ketoconazole and amphotericin B can elevate the plasma levels of cyclosporine.
3 Concomitant use of cyclosporine with other immunosuppressive drugs can result in increased susceptibility to infection and possible development of lymphoma.

▶ NURSING ALERTS

▷ 1 Recognize that patients receiving cyclosporine should be managed by health-care personnel skilled in the administration and monitoring of the drug. Adequate laboratory and supportive resources must be readily available.

▷ 2 Be aware that drug is highly insoluble and that the IV form is prepared in a cremophor vehicle. This vehicle is allergenic, and its use can result in anaphylactic reactions. Be prepared to treat severe allergic reactions should they develop.

▷ 3 Do not use cyclosporine with any other immunosuppressive drugs (except adrenal steroids), because serious toxicity can result—see Interactions.

▷ 4 Closely monitor renal and hepatic function and perform frequent determinations of BUN, serum creatinine, serum bilirubin, and liver enzymes. Serum creatinine and BUN are commonly elevated during therapy but are usually responsive to dosage reduction. Persistent elevations unresponsive to a dosage alteration may necessitate switching to another immunosuppressant.

▷ 5 Notify physician immediately if fever, sore throat, abnormal bruising, or unusual tiredness occur, because they may be early indications of a developing blood dyscrasia.

▷ 6 Use cautiously in hypertensive patients (blood pressure elevations are common) and in pregnant or nursing mothers. Although safety and efficacy have not been established in children, cyclosporine has been used in patients as young as 6 months with no apparent deleterious effects.

▶ NURSING CONSIDERATIONS
▷ 1 Note that oral absorption of cyclosporine is erratic. Make frequent determinations of cyclosporine blood levels and adjust dosage as necessary to minimize toxicity due to excessive plasma levels.

▷ 2 Mix oral solution of drug with milk, chocolate milk, or orange juice at room temperature to improve palatability.

▷ 3 Advise patients receiving the drug of the potential risks of teratogenicity should pregnancy occur during therapy.

▷ 4 Switch patients from the IV solution to the oral solution as soon as possible following surgery.

▶ dexpanthenol
Ilopan, Panol

Dexpanthenol is used either by IM injection as a GI stimulant for treating adynamia or as a lotion or cream (Panthoderm) for use as an emollient to relieve skin itching and lesioning.

Mechanism
Not established; drug is a derivative of pantothenic acid, a precursor of coenzyme A, which serves as a cofactor in the synthesis of acetylcholine (ACh); ACh exerts a range of functions in the body, including maintenance of intestinal tone and peristalsis

Uses
1 Prevention of paralytic ileus and intestinal atony following abdominal surgery (IM)
2 Treatment of adynamic ileus (IM)
3 Relief of itching and to assist healing of skin lesions in minor skin conditions (topical)

Dosage
Prevention of paralytic ileus: 250 mg to 500 mg IM; repeat in 2 hours, then every 6 hours until danger of adynamic ileus has passed

Treatment of adynamic ileus: 500 mg IM; repeat in 2 hours and again every 6 hours as needed
Skin lesions: apply topically one to four times a day

Significant Adverse Reactions
Itching, erythema, dermatitis, urticaria, dyspnea, intestinal colic, hypotension, vomiting, and diarrhea

Contraindication
Hemophilia

Interactions
1 Concomitant use of antibiotics, barbiturates, or narcotics may increase the likelihood of allergic reactions.
2 Respiratory difficulty has occurred when dexpanthenol was administered following succinylcholine.

▶ NURSING ALERTS
▷ 1 Do not administer IV or give within one hour of succinylcholine (see Interactions).
▷ 2 Use with caution in pregnant or nursing mothers, in children, and in elderly persons.

▶ NURSING CONSIDERATIONS
▷ 1 Discontinue drug if signs of a hypersensitivity reaction are noted.

▶ dimethyl sulfoxide
Rimso-50

Dimethyl sulfoxide (DMSO) is a clear, colorless solvent possessing a wide range of pharmacologic actions, but only a very limited clinical applicability, because the compound has not been adequately tested and its potential toxicity is rather high. It is approved for use as a bladder irrigant for the treatment of interstitial cystitis, but has been used experimentally by topical application for treatment of various musculoskeletal disorders and collagen diseases. Dimethyl sulfoxide can also serve as a vehicle to enhance percutaneous absorption of other drugs and has been reported to possess diuretic, local anesthetic, vasodilatory, muscle relaxant, and bacteriostatic activity, although data to support these claims are insufficient. Principal adverse effects are a garlic-like odor on the breath and skin, topical irritation, and allergic reactions due to histamine release. Ocular disturbances have been noted in experimental animals. The following discussion is limited to the use of dimethyl sulfoxide as a bladder irrigant. Its topical application should be discouraged until the efficacy and safety of the drug have been conclusively established.

Mechanism
Not established; appears to exert anti-inflammatory, local anesthetic, diuretic, muscle relaxing, vasodilatory, and bacteriostatic activity

Uses
1 Symptomatic treatment of interstitial cystitis

Dosage

Instill 50 ml into the bladder and allow to remain at least 15 minutes; repeat every 2 weeks or more as needed

Common Side-Effects

Garlic-like taste, discomfort upon bladder instillation

Significant Adverse Reactions

Hypersensitivity reactions (nasal congestion, dyspnea, angioedema, pruritus, urticaria)

▶ NURSiNG ALERTS

▷ 1 Use cautiously in pregnant or nursing women, children, and in patients with liver or kidney disease.
▷ 2 Perform periodic ophthalmic examinations and kidney and liver function tests during therapy. Changes in refractive index and lens opacities have occurred in experimental animals, but not in patients receiving the drug by bladder instillation.

▶ NURSING CONSIDERATIONS

▷ 1 Advise patients that garlic-like odor and taste may appear within several minutes and persist for up to 72 hours.

▶ disulfiram

Antabuse

Disulfiram is an antoxidant that blocks the oxidative metabolism of alcohol at the acetaldehyde stage. Thus, ingestion of even small amounts of alcohol in the presence of disulfiram results in a 5- to 10-fold increase in blood acetaldehyde levels, which elicits a range of unpleasant symptoms known as the disulfiram reaction or *mal rouge.* Thus, disulfiram is employed for the management of properly motivated chronic alcoholics who *desire* to be placed in a situation of enforced sobriety. The threat of illness upon consumption of alcohol is the prime deterrent with this drug. The drug is slowly absorbed and excreted, and the effects persist for up to 2 weeks after the last dose has been taken. Users must be made aware of the consequences of ingesting even small amounts of alcohol in any form whatsoever (*e.g.,* cough syrups, mouthwashes, cold preparations, food sauces, vinegars). Also, application of alcohol-containing liniments or lotions (rubbing alcohol, colognes, toilet waters, aftershaves) should be avoided, because the alcohol may be absorbed systemically. The disulfiram–alcohol reaction consists of flushing, nausea, sweating, thirst, throbbing in the head, dyspnea, palpitations, chest pain, tachycardia, hypotension, weakness, vertigo, blurred vision, confusion, and syncope. With large amounts of alcohol, serious adverse reactions can occur, including arrhythmias, congestive heart failure, respiratory depression, convulsions, and even death. The intensity of the reaction is dependent on the amounts of disulfiram and alcohol ingested. Symptoms are usually fully developed at a blood alcohol level of 50 mg%, and unconsciousness occurs at 125 mg% to 150 mg%.

Mechanism

Blocks conversion of acetaldehyde to acetate during alcohol metabolism by inhibiting the enzyme aldehyde dehydrogenase, thereby elevating plasma levels of acetaldehyde, a toxic intermediate

Uses

1 Adjunctive treatment of chronic alcoholism, in conjunction with supportive therapy and proper motivation

Dosage

Initially 500 mg/day in a single dose for 1 week to 2 weeks; maintenance doses range from 125 mg to 500 mg once daily until patient is fully recovered

Fate

Rapidly and completely absorbed orally; highly lipid-soluble and localized initially in fatty tissue; slowly metabolized by the liver and excreted in the urine; effects persist for up to 2 weeks following withdrawal of medication

Common Side-Effects

Drowsiness

Significant Adverse Reactions

Impotence, headache, restlessness, fatigability, skin eruptions, metallic taste, optic or peripheral neuritis, polyneuritis, tremor, psychotic reactions, and arthropathy

See above introductory section for disulfiram–alcohol reaction syndrome.

Contraindications

Severe myocardial disease, coronary occlusion, psychoses, pregnancy, and in patients who have recently received alcohol or alcohol-containing products, metronidazole, or paraldehyde

Interactions

1 Disulfiram may potentiate the effects of diazepam, chlordiazepoxide, oral anticoagulants, and phenytoin.
2 Disulfiram plus isoniazid can result in coordination difficulties and behavioral changes.
3 Paraldehyde is partially metabolized to acetaldehyde and can produce toxic reactions in the presence of disulfiram.
4 Metronidazole given together with disulfiram can elicit psychotic reactions.

▶ NURSING ALERTS

▷ 1 Do not undertake treatment with disulfiram unless patient and family are *fully* informed of the rationale for therapy and the consequences of ingesting or absorbing alcohol in any form (see introductory paragraph). Never administer to an intoxicated patient.
▷ 2 Recognize that disulfiram is not a cure for alcoholism, but is merely an adjunct to other forms of therapy in managing the chronic alcoholic who *desires* to abstain.
▷ 3 Use with extreme caution in persons with epilepsy, diabetes, cerebral damage, hypothyroidism, hepatic cirrhosis, or nephritis.

▷ 4 Do not initiate therapy until patient has abstained from alcohol for at least 12 hours. Warn patients that *mal rouge* reactions can occur up to 2 weeks after the last dose of disulfiram if alcohol is ingested during that time.

▷ 5 Urge caution in driving and performing other hazardous tasks, because drowsiness can occur.

▷ 6 Institute appropriate measures (*e.g.,* oxygen, IV vitamin C, ephedrine, antihistamines) in case of severe disulfiram reactions.

▶ **NURSING CONSIDERATIONS**

▷ 1 Perform blood studies (CBC, SMA-12) and liver function tests at regular intervals during treatment.

▷ 2 Urge patients to always carry identification indicating drug being taken, physician's name and phone number, and other pertinent information in case of an unexpected reaction.

▷ 3 Inform patients that some side-effects may occur during first 2 weeks of therapy (metallic taste, drowsiness, headache, weakness, skin eruptions) but generally disappear with continued treatment.

▷ 4 Administer tablet in the morning unless sedation becomes a problem. Crush and mix tablet with a liquid if necessary.

▷ 5 Alert patients to the fact that tolerance does not develop with prolonged use; rather, sensitivity to alcohol increases the longer the drug is used.

▶ **enzyme preparations**

Carica papaya	Hyaluronidase
Chymotrypsin	Papain
Collagenase	Sutilains
Fibrinolysin and desoxyribonuclease	Trypsin

A number of enzymes are available for either topical or systemic use, most of which are employed to assist removal of excess fluids, tissue exudates, or clotted blood from ulcerated, inflamed, infected, or otherwise injured areas. Topical enzyme preparations may also be used for debriding surface ulcers, surgical or other types of wounds, and second- and third-degree burns. Since the various enzyme preparations differ with regard to route of administration, indications, and precautions to be observed with their use, they are considered individually in Table 80-2.

▶ **flavoxate**

Urispas

Mechanism

Exerts a direct relaxant effect on smooth muscle of the urinary tract; also possesses anticholinergic, local anesthetic, and possibly analgesic properties

Uses

1 Symptomatic relief of dysuria, urgency, nocturia, suprapubic pain, and incontinence resulting from cystitis, urethritis, prostatitis, and other genitourinary conditions

Dosage

100 mg to 200 mg orally three to four times/day

Significant Adverse Reactions

Drowsiness, dizziness, blurred vision, dry mouth, headache, nervousness, increased intraocular tension, confusion, urticaria, dermatoses, tachycardia, palpitation, hyperpyrexia, eosinophilia, and leukopenia

Contraindications

Pyloric or duodenal obstruction, obstructive intestinal lesions, achalasia, and GI hemorrhage

▶ **NURSING ALERTS**

▷ 1 Use with caution in patients with glaucoma and in pregnant women.

▷ 2 Urge caution in driving or performing tasks requiring alertness, because drug can cause drowsiness, dizziness, and blurred vision.

▶ **NURSING CONSIDERATIONS**

▷ 1 Suggest use of hard candy or gum to alleviate dry mouth.

▶ **metoclopramide**

Reglan

Metoclopramide is a smooth muscle stimulant that acts largely on the upper GI tract. It increases gastric contractions and peristalsis of the duodenum and jejunum but relaxes the pyloric sphincter and duodenal bulb, thus accelerating gastric emptying and upper intestinal transit. Metoclopramide has little if any effect on colonic or gallbladder motility or on intestinal, biliary, and pancreatic secretions. It is used IV to assist intubation of the small intestine *via* a pyloric entry, and to increase elimination of barium from the upper intestinal tract, and orally for relief of the nausea, vomiting, anorexia, and persistent feeling of fullness associated with acute and recurrent diabetic gastroparesis.

Mechanism

Stimulates upper GI motility and decreases normal inhibitory tone, probably by blocking dopamine receptors and sensitizing tissues to the action of acetylcholine; action is not dependent on intact vagal innervation and can be reversed by anticholinergic drugs

Uses

1 Facilitates small bowel intubation in patients in whom the tube does not pass the pylorus by conventional methods (IV use)

2 Stimulates gastric emptying and upper intestinal transit

Table 80-2. Enzyme Preparations

Drug	Preparations	Indications	Administration and Dosage	Remarks
Topical Only				
Collagenase (Biozyme-C, Santyl)	Ointment—250 U/g	Debridement of dermal ulcers and severe burns	Apply once daily or once every other day	Digests collagen and promotes formation of granulation tissue and epithelization of ulcers and burns; optimal pH range for enzymatic activity is 6 to 8; cleanse lesion before application and cover wound with sterile gauze after using ointment; remove excess ointment each time dressing is changed; a suitable antibacterial ointment is used when infection is present; avoid soaks or washing with solutions containing metal ions or acidic substances, because they reduce enzymatic activity
Fibrinolysin and Desoxyribonuclease (Elase)	Ointment—30 U fibrinolysin and 20,000 U DNAase per 30 g. Powder—25 U fibrinolysin and 15,000 U DNAase per 30-ml container	Topically—debridement of inflamed or infected lesions. Intravaginal—adjunctive treatment of vaginitis and cervicitis	Topically—apply as ointment or solution prepared from powder in the form of a spray or wet dressing. Change dressing 2 to 3 times a day, removing debris and exudates each time. Vaginally—instill 5 g of ointment or 10 ml of solution (1 vial/10 ml) deep into vagina at bedtime for 5 days	Combination of two enzymes that attack both DNA and fibrin, thus breaking down necrotic tissue and fibrinous exudates; do not use parenterally, because bovine fibrinolysin may be antigenic; solutions from dry powder must be used within 24 hours; following instillation of solution into vagina, wait 1 to 2 minutes, then insert a tampon for 12 hours to 24 hours; affected area must be cleaned, and dense, dry, escharotic tissue removed before application of drug, because enzymes must be in contact with the tissue to be removed to be effective; also available as ointment with 10 mg/g chloramphenicol as Elase-Chloromycetin
Papain (Panafil)	Ointment—10% with 10% urea	Debridement of surface lesions	Apply directly to lesion 1 to 2 times a day	Enzyme derived from *Carica papaya;* cover with gauze and remove accumulated necrotic tissue at each redressing; hydrogen peroxide may inactivate papain; itching or stinging can occur with topical application
Sutilains (Travase)	Ointment—82,000 casein U/g	Debridement of burned areas, decubitus ulcers, incisional or traumatic wounds and surface ulcers resulting from peripheral vascular diseases	Apply in a thin layer to moistened wound area 3 to 4 times a day	Proteolytic enzyme that digests necrotic tissue, thus facilitating formation of granulation tissue; avoid contact of ointment with eyes; a moist environment is essential for optimal enzymatic activity; action of enzyme is reduced by iodine, thimerosal, hexachlorophene, benzalkonium chloride, and nitrofurazone; side-effects include mild pain, paresthesias, dermatitis, and possibly bleeding
Trypsin (Granulex)	Aerosol—0.1 mg trypsin/0.82 ml with balsam of Peru and castor oil	Treatment of decubitus and varicose ulcers, wounds, and severe sunburn	Spray twice daily	Used as a spray for debriding necrotic areas

Table 80-2. Enzyme Preparations *(continued)*

Drug	Preparations	Indications	Administration and Dosage	Remarks
Systemic Only				
Carica papaya proteolytic enzymes (Papase)	Tablets—10,000 U	Relief of symptoms of episiotomy and other surgical lesions (possibly effective)	2 tablets 4 times a day for at least 5 days; Prophylactically—2 tablets 1 hour to 2 hours before episiotomy	Proteolytic enzymes derived from *Carica papaya;* tablets may be swallowed or chewed; contraindicated with oral anticoagulants; use cautiously in patients with systemic infections, clotting disorders, or renal or hepatic disease, and during pregnancy; effectiveness has not been conclusively demonstrated
Chymotrypsin (Avazyme)	Tablets—50,000 U, 100,000 U	Adjunctive treatment of traumatic or surgical wounds (possibly effective)	1 to 2 tablets 4 times a day	Crystalline chymotrypsin preparation; see Bromelains; also available in combination with trypsin (Chymoral, Orenzyme); no advantage over other systemic enzymes; effectiveness has not been conclusively demonstrated
Hyaluronidase (Wydase)	Injection—150 U/ml, 1500 U/10 ml	Aid to increasing absorption and dispersion of other injected drugs and diagnostic agents Adjunct in subcutaneous urography Aid in hypodermoclysis	Absorption of other drugs—150 U added to drug solution Hypodermoclysis—150 U injected SC before clysis or into rubber tubing during procedure Urography—75 U SC injected over each scapula	Mucolytic enzyme that hydrolyzes hyaluronic acid, thus aiding diffusion of fluids through tissues; extent of diffusion depends on amount of enzyme present and volume of solution; do not inject into acutely inflamed, infected, or cancerous areas; use caution when adding to clysis solution to prevent overhydration, because enzyme can facilitate excess water absorption; monitor infusion rate carefully; preliminary skin test (0.02 ml intradermally) is often used to detect sensitive individuals; whealing and itching are positive signs of hypersensitivity

of barium where delayed passage interferes with radiologic examination (IV use)

3 Prophylaxis of vomiting associated with cisplatin cancer chemotherapy (IV use)

4 Relieves symptoms (nausea, anorexia, vomiting, fullness) associated with acute or recurrent diabetic gastroparesis (oral use)

5 Investigational uses include aid to lactation, treatment of gastroesophageal reflux, prophylaxis of chemotherapy-induced vomiting due to drugs other than cisplatin, prevention of relapsing gastric ulcers, and treatment of anorexia nervosa

Dosage
Oral:

10 mg 30 minutes before each meal and at bedtime for 2 weeks to 8 weeks

IV:

Adults—10 mg by slow IV injection (1 min–2 min)

Children (6 yr–14 yr)—2.5 mg to 5 mg

Children (under 6 yr)—0.1 mg/kg

Prevention of cisplatin-induced vomiting:

Initially 2 mg/kg of a dilute solution infused over a 15-minute period 30 minutes before cisplatin and repeated every 2 hours for two doses, then every 3 hours for three doses

Fate
Onset of action is 1 minute to 3 minutes IV and 30 minutes to 60 minutes orally; duration 1 hour to 2 hours; excreted largely (80%–90%) in the urine as unchanged drug or metabolites; half-life is approximately 3 hours to 6 hours

Common Side-Effects
Drowsiness, fatigue, and restlessness

Significant Adverse Reactions
CNS—extrapyramidal reactions, akathisia, dizziness, dystonia, anxiety, insomnia, headache, depression

GI—nausea, diarrhea

Other—hypertension, tachycardia

Contraindications

GI obstruction, perforation or hemorrhage, pheochromocytoma, and epilepsy

Interactions

1 The action of metoclopramide can be antagonized by anticholinergics and narcotic analgesics.
2 Metoclopramide may impair absorption of drugs from the stomach (*e.g.,* digitalis glycosides, cimetidine) and increase absorption of drugs from the small intestine (*e.g.,* acetaminophen, ethanol, tetracyclines, levodopa).
3 Increased sedation may be observed when metoclopramide is given with alcohol, barbiturates, narcotics, or other sedatives and hypnotics.
4 Metoclopramide may alter insulin requirements by influencing the timing of food delivery to the intestines.

▶ NURSING ALERTS

▷ 1 Inject slowly IV (1 min–2 min) to minimize incidence of restlessness and anxiety, which are often intense if injection is rapid.
▷ 2 Be alert for development of extrapyramidal reactions (approximately 0.2%–1% of patients) and administer anticholinergics or antiparkinsonian drugs as necessary to control symptoms.
▷ 3 Use with caution in patients with diabetes, depression, and in pregnant or nursing women.

▶ NURSING CONSIDERATIONS

▷ 1 Urge patients to exhibit caution for several hours following administration, because drowsiness and dizziness can occur.
▷ 2 Note that drug is usually not given unless tube has not passed the pylorus within 10 minutes with conventional maneuvers.
▷ 3 Be aware that metoclopramide has been used experimentally to prevent relapsing gastric ulcers by suppressing bile reflux, but this is not an approved indication.

▶ plasma expanders

Dextran 40   Hetastarch
Dextran 70, 75

Dextran, a synthetic polysaccharide of varying molecular weights, and hetastarch, a chemically modified corn starch, are employed to expand reduced plasma volume, which can occur in hypovolemic shock resulting from hemorrhage, extensive burns, surgery, sepsis, or other forms of trauma. Their principal advantages over whole blood or plasma for volume replacement are their relatively low cost, wide availability, and lack of incompatibility problems, as well as the fact that they are not associated with the danger of transmitting diseases such as viral hepatitis or AIDS. However, these synthetic polysaccharides can produce allergic reactions, occasionally severe, and may also interfere with platelet function, resulting in increased bleeding tendencies. Of course, these plasma expanders are no substitute for whole blood where large quantities of red cells have been lost.

The agents used as plasma expanders are considered as a group, and then are listed individually in Table 80-3.

Mechanism

Plasma expanders elevate the osmotic pressure of the blood, thus drawing water from extravascular spaces into the bloodstream. Plasma volume expands slightly in excess of the volume of drug solution infused. The drugs also decrease blood viscosity and reduce erythrocyte aggregation and rouleau formation, thus improving microcirculation. They reduce platelet adhesiveness and can alter the structure of fibrin clots, thus reducing the likelihood of thrombus formation. Secondary cardiovascular effects include increased blood pressure, venous return, cardiac output, and urine flow, and decreased heart rate and peripheral resistance.

Uses

1 Adjunctive treatment of shock due to hemorrhage, burns, surgery, sepsis, or other trauma (*NOT* to be viewed as a substitute for blood or plasma)
2 Priming fluid in pump oxygenators during extracorporeal circulation (Dextran *40* only)
3 Prophylaxis against venous thrombosis and pulmonary embolism in patients undergoing high-risk procedures, for example, hip surgery (Dextran *40* only)
4 Adjunctive use in leukapheresis to increase granulocyte yield (Hetastarch only)

Dosage

See Table 80-3.

Fate

Onset of volume-expanding action varies from several minutes (Dextran 40) to about 1 hour (Dextran 75); hemodynamic status is improved for at least 12 hours (Dextran 40) to over 24 hours (Dextran 75, Hetastarch) with a single infusion; molecules less than 50,000 molecular weight are eliminated by the kidneys, 40% to 75% within 24 hours; larger-molecular-weight molecules are slowly metabolized to smaller sugars and either excreted in the urine or eliminated as breakdown products (*e.g.,* carbon dioxide and water); small amounts of drugs are excreted in the feces

Significant Adverse Reactions

Allergic reactions (nasal congestion, urticaria, wheezing, dyspnea, hypotension), anaphylactic reactions (rare), nausea, vomiting, headache, fever, joint pain, infection at injection site, phlebitis, hypervolemia, pulmonary edema, osmotic nephrosis, renal failure (rare), prolongation of bleeding time; *also with Hetastarch*—submaxillary and parotid gland enlargement, flu-like symptoms, and edema of the lower extremities

Contraindications

Severe cardiac decompensation, renal failure, and marked

Table 80-3. Plasma Expanders

Drug	Preparations	Usual Dosage Range	Remarks
Dextran 40—low molecular weight (Gentran 40, 10% LMD, Rheomacrodex)	Injection—10% in either sodium chloride or 5% dextrose	Shock—20 ml/kg/24 hours by IV infusion the first day; thereafter, 10 ml/kg/day for a maximum of 5 days Extracorporeal circulation—10 ml/kg to 20 ml/kg added to perfusion circuit Prophylaxis of venous thromboses—10 ml/kg on day of surgery, then 500 ml/day for 2 days to 3 days, then 500 ml every 2 days to 3 days for 2 weeks	Low-molecular-weight dextran is effective in reducing erythrocyte clumping and sludging and is reported to be able to disrupt thrombi; bleeding time can be prolonged and platelet function may be depressed by large doses; monitor coagulation time closely during therapy and observe for early signs of bleeding (epistaxis, petechiae)
Dextran 70, 75—high molecular weight (Gentran 75, Macrodex)	Injection—6% in either sodium chloride or dextrose	Shock: Adults—10 ml/kg to 20 ml/kg/24 hours by IV infusion; usually, 500 ml is given at a rate of 20 ml to 40 ml/minute for emergency treatment Children—Maximum dose 20 ml/kg	High-molecular-weight dextran is slower in onset, but more prolonged acting than low-molecular-weight dextran; be alert for allergic reactions, which most often develop in first few minutes of infusion; may adversely affect capillary flow by increasing blood viscosity; can interfere with platelet aggregation, and transiently prolong bleeding time
Hetastarch (Hespan)	Injection—6% in sodium chloride	Volume expansion—500 ml to 1000 ml/day (maximum 1500 ml/day); in acute situations, infusion rate is 20 ml/kg/hour Leukapheresis—250 ml to 700 ml infused at a fixed ratio (*e.g.*, 1:8) to venous whole blood	Synthetic polymer prepared from amylopectin; similar to dextran in action and can also increase erythrocyte sedimentation rate; thus is used to improve efficiency of granulocyte collection by centrifugation; may elevate bilirubin levels; use with caution in patients with liver disease; during leukapheresis, hemoglobin and platelet counts may be temporarily reduced due to volume expanding effects of hetastarch; blood counts, hemoglobin determinations, and prothrombin times should be performed during therapy

hemostatic defects (hyperfibrinogenemia, thrombocytopenia)

Interactions
1 Effects of anticoagulants can be potentiated by plasma expanders.

▶ NURSING ALERTS
▷ 1 Observe patients closely during infusion and discontinue drug at first sign of allergic reaction. Have resuscitative measures available (*e.g.*, epinephrine, antihistamines, and corticosteroids).

▷ 2 Monitor central venous pressure during drug administration and observe for indications of circulatory overload (dyspnea, wheezing, coughing, increased pulse and respiratory rate). Discontinue drug and advise physician.

▷ 3 Determine urine output and specific gravity at regular intervals. Be alert for oliguria, anuria, or altered specific gravity, and report immediately. Marked elevations in specific gravity can indicate reduced urine flow.

▷ 4 Use with caution in patients with active hemorrhaging, liver or kidney impairment, severe dehydration, or history of allergic reactions, and in pregnant women.

▷ 5 Do not administer solutions containing sodium chloride to patients with congestive heart failure or renal insufficiency or to persons receiving corticosteroids.

▶ NURSING CONSIDERATIONS
▷ 1 Determine hematocrit following drug administration and advise physician if value falls below 30 mg/dl.

▷ 2 Do not exceed recommended dose or flow rate, because excessive doses can precipitate renal failure.

▷ 3 Note that dextran may cause false elevations in blood glucose, urinary proteins, bilirubin, and total protein assays, and can give unreliable readings in blood typing and cross-matching procedures.

▷ 4 Do not confuse low-molecular-weight dextran (40) with high-molecular-weight dextran (70, 75). High-molecular-weight dextran is reported to have fewer adverse reactions (except allergic), but is slower in onset, not cleared as rapidly, more viscous, and exhibits much less of an effect in retarding rouleau formation and erythrocyte clumping.

▷ 5 Discard partially used containers, because solution contains no bacteriostatic agent. Store at room temperature to prevent crystallization. Do not use if solution is not clear or under vacuum.

▶ plasma protein fractions

Albumin, human   Plasma protein fraction

The plasma protein fractions are obtained by fractionating human plasma, and include normal serum albumin and plasma protein fraction. These products are primarily employed to expand plasma volume, as they raise the osmotic pressure of the blood. Since they both are heat treated to destroy hepatitis B virus, they are considered somewhat safer than whole blood or plasma as volume expanders.

Normal serum albumin is available in two concentrations, a 5% solution, which is approximately osmotically and isotonically equivalent to human plasma, and a 25% solution, osmotically equivalent to five times the volume of plasma. Plasma protein fraction is a 5% solution of human plasma proteins (83%–90% albumin with small amounts of alpha and beta globulins) that is osmotically equivalent to human plasma. These albumin preparations do not appear to interfere with normal coagulation mechanisms, and do not require cross-matching. The absence of cellular elements, moreover, greatly reduces the risk of sensitization with repeated administration.

The plasma protein fractions will be discussed together, then listed individually in Table 80-4.

Mechanism
Increase intravascular osmotic pressure, thereby drawing extracellular fluid into the bloodstream, expanding plasma volume; bind bilirubin in the plasma

Uses
1 Adjunctive emergency treatment of hypovolemic shock
2 Temporary replacement of blood loss to prevent hemoconcentration following severe burns

Table 80-4. Plasma Protein Fractions

Drug	Preparations	Usual Dosage Range	Remarks
Albumin, human (Albuminar, Albutein, Buminate, Plasbumin)	Injection—5%, 25%	Variable, depending upon diagnosis, severity of condition, patient's age and concentration of solution; usually, the equivalent of 25 g to 100 g albumin per day is given by slow IV infusion (1 ml–4 ml/min depending on concentration); maximum recommended dose is 250 g/48 hours	Available in two strengths, 5% and 25%, both containing 130 mEq to 160 mEq/liter; the 25% solution allows administration of large amounts of albumin quickly, and 100 ml provides as much plasma protein as 500 ml plasma or 2 pints whole blood; concentrated solution usually requires supplemental fluids in dehydrated patients; thus 5% solution may be preferred for routine use, because maximum osmotic effect is attained without additional fluids; preparations may cause an elevation of alkaline phosphatase levels; the 25% solution is preferred in most patients requiring sodium restriction
Plasma protein fraction (Plasmanate, Plasma-Plex, Plasmatein, Protenate)	Injection—5%	Hypovolemic shock: Adults—250 ml to 500 ml by IV infusion Children—20 ml/kg to 30 ml/kg Hypoproteinemia—1000 ml to 1500 ml/day	Rate of infusion is determined by condition and patient's age and body weight; maximum infusion rate is 10 ml/minute in shock and 5 ml to 8 ml/minute in hypoproteinemia; do not give more than 250 g in 48 hours; monitor patients carefully for signs of volume overload; slow infusion if blood pressure declines; use cautiously in sodium-restricted patients; solution contains 130 mEq to 160 mEq/liter; if edema is present, or if large amounts of protein are lost, use 25% albumin solution

3 Treatment of hypoproteinemia due to nephrotic syndrome, hepatic cirrhosis, toxemia of pregnancy, and tuberculosis, and in postoperative patients and premature infants

4 Adjunctive therapy during exchange transfusions in hyperbilirubinemia and erythroblastosis fetalis

5 Adjunctive treatment of acute liver failure, adult respiratory distress syndrome, acute peritonitis, pancreatitis, or mediastinitis and during cardiopulmonary bypass or renal dialysis

Dosage
See Table 80-4.

Significant Adverse Reactions
Hypotension, allergic reactions (fever, chills, flushing, urticaria, rash), headache, nausea, vomiting, tachycardia, salivation, back pain, and respiratory irregularities

Vascular overload and pulmonary edema can occur with too-rapid infusion.

Contraindications
Cardiac failure, severe anemia, and normal or increased intravascular volume

In addition, plasma protein fraction is contraindicated in patients on cardiopulmonary bypass.

▶ NURSING ALERTS
▷ 1 Maintain a slow infusion rate (see Table 80-4; rapid infusion may produce hypotension) and observe patients for signs of vascular overload (coughing, dyspnea, tachycardia, distended neck veins).

▷ 2 Recognize that albumin preparations are not a substitute for whole blood, and large volume requirements should be satisfied with supplemental whole blood or plasma.

▷ 3 Use cautiously in patients with mild anemia, low cardiac reserve, hepatic or renal failure, or congestive heart failure.

▶ NURSING CONSIDERATIONS
▷ 1 Do not use solutions that appear turbid or show evidence of sedimentation.

▷ 2 Use promptly after opening (*i.e.,* within 4 hr), and discard unused portions because solution contains no preservatives or bacteriostatic substances.

▷ 3 Monitor blood pressure and pulse and respiratory pattern during infusion, and report any significant changes in any parameter.

▷ 4 Administer additional fluids to patients with marked dehydration to minimize excessive depletion of tissue fluid.

▷ 5 Observe patients for signs of external bleeding, because blood pressure may be elevated following too-rapid administration. If bleeding is noted, be prepared to deal with new hemorrhaging or possibly shock.

▷ 6 While drug solution can be added to usual IV infusion solutions, do not infuse together with solutions containing alcohol or protein hydrolysates, because albumin may precipitate.

▶ psoralens

Methoxsalen	Trioxsalen

Two psoralen compounds, methoxsalen and trioxsalen, have the ability to increase the deposition of the pigment melanin in the skin in response to ultraviolet (UV) radiation. They may be employed either orally or topically to facilitate repigmentation in patients with vitiligo, a disorder characterized by patchy areas of nonpigmented skin. The oral dosage form of these two drugs can also be used to increase tolerance to sunlight in persons with fair complexions who suffer severe reactions upon exposure. Finally, much interest is centered around the possible beneficial effects of these drugs in treating severe psoriasis, when followed by controlled exposure to long-wave-length UV light (320 nm–400 nm). Such treatment, known as PUVA therapy, shows promise of being a very effective, albeit potentially toxic, form of therapy.

In vitiligo, repigmentation varies in time of onset, degree of completeness, and duration. Although some effect may be evident within several weeks after beginning therapy, significant repigmentation may take 6 months to 12 months. The psoralens are only effective in enhancing pigmentation when followed by exposure of affected skin areas to UV light, either artificial or natural (sunlight).

Mechanism
Not established; may increase the number of functional melanocytes and activate resting or dormant cells; also initiate a local inflammatory response; can increase synthesis of melanosome and activity of tyrosinase, an enzyme involved in conversion of tyrosine to dihydroxyphenylalanine, a precursor of melanin; activity is dependent on the presence of functional melanocytes and activation of the psoralen agent by UV radiation, either artificial or sunlight

Uses
1 Repigmentation of idiopathic vitiligo
2 Aid to increasing tolerance to sunlight (trioxsalen only)
3 Treatment of severe recalcitrant, disabling psoriasis not responsive to other forms of therapy—given *only* in conjunction with controlled doses of long-wave UV radiation

Dosage
See Table 80-5.

Fate
Oral absorption is 95% complete. Food appears to increase serum concentrations. Following oral ingestion, skin sensitivity to UV radiation is maximal in 2 hours and disappears within 8 hours. Psoralens are metabolized in the liver and excreted primarily (90%) in the urine. Topical application produces a rapid sensitivity.

Common Side-Effects
Nausea, pruritus, and erythema

Table 80-5. Psoralens

Drug	Preparations	Usual Dosage Range	Remarks
Methoxsalen (Oxsoralen)	Lotion—1% Capsules—10 mg	Topical—apply once weekly to small, well-defined lesions, then expose area to UV light for 1 minute; subsequent exposure times should be increased with caution Oral—2 capsules/day in a single dose, followed in 2 hours to 4 hours by a 5-minute exposure to UV light; gradually increase exposure time to 30 minutes to 35 minutes	Pigmentation may begin within several weeks, but significant repigmentation may require treatment for 6 months to 9 months; do not increase dosage of oral preparation; perform liver function tests periodically during therapy, and stop drug if liver impairment occurs; topical preparation is only used on small, well-defined vitiliginous lesions that can be protected from excessive exposure; use of bandages or sunscreens or both may be necessary
Trioxsalen (Trisoralen)	Tablets—5 mg	Vitiligo—10 mg/day, followed by 2 hours to 4 hours by UV exposure ranging from 15 minutes to 30 minutes Sunlight tolerance—10 mg/day, 2 hours before exposure to sun, for a maximum of 14 days	More active than methoxsalen, yet its median lethal dose is 6 times higher; do not increase dosage and only lengthen exposure times in gradual increments; discontinue drug if repigmentation is not evident within 3 months to 4 months

Significant Adverse Reactions

Warning: Use of psoralens together with UV radiation must be undertaken only by health-care personnel experienced in photochemical treatment of psoriasis and vitiligo. Severe adverse reactions can occur (burns, ocular damage, skin aging, skin cancer) and patients must be informed of the risks inherent in such treatment.

Topical—skin irritation, erythema, blistering
Oral—GI upset, nervousness, insomnia, depression, edema, dizziness, headache, hypopigmentation, vesiculation, nonspecific rash, urticaria, folliculitis, leg cramps, hypotension, severe burns from UV light, cataracts from UV exposure

Contraindications

Melanoma, invasive squamous cell carcinoma, aphakia, albinism, porphyria, acute lupus erythematosus, leukoderma of infectious origin; in children under 12 years of age (trioxsalen only); and concurrent use of a photosensitizing drug

▶ NURSING ALERTS

▷ 1 Be aware that overdosage or overexposure can result in severe blistering and burning. Do not exceed prescribed dose or exposure time, and keep patients under *constant* supervision during therapy.

▷ 2 Do not dispense topical preparations for home use; they should be applied and monitored only by trained personnel under strictly controlled light conditions.

▷ 3 Instruct patients receiving topical preparations to keep treated area protected from sunlight, except for desired exposure periods, because severe burns can occur if treated area is exposed to additional UV light.

▷ 4 Use products cautiously in patients with impaired liver function and in pregnant or nursing women.

▶ NURSING CONSIDERATIONS

▷ 1 Administer oral preparations with food or milk to minimize GI distress, or divide oral dose into two portions taken one half hour apart.

▷ 2 Advise patients to protect lips and eyes during UV exposure periods.

▷ 3 Be aware that sensitivity to light is greatest during the first few days of therapy. Observe patients for signs of irritation or blistering.

▷ 4 Perform a CBC, antinuclear antibody test, liver and kidney function tests, and an ophthalmologic examination prior to therapy and at 6-month to 12-month intervals during prolonged therapy.

▶ sclerosing agents

Morrhuate sodium	Sodium tetradecyl sulfate

Sclerosing agents are primarily used to obliterate varicose veins. They produce their effects by irritating the vessel lining, producing a thrombus that occludes the damaged vessel.

Mechanism

Directly irritate the venous intimal endothelium following injection, resulting in development of a blood clot that occludes the vein and leads to formation of fibrous tissue

Uses

1 Treatment of small, uncomplicated varicose veins of the lower extremities

2 Supplement to venous ligation to obliterate residual varicosed veins or reduce risk of surgery

Table 80-6. Sclerosing Agents

Drug	Preparations	Usual Dosage Range	Remarks
Morrhuate sodium (CMC)	Injection—50 mg/ml	50 to 250 mg IV (1 ml–5 ml) depending on size of vein, given as multiple injections at the same time, or a single dose; repeat at 5-day to 7-day intervals as needed	To determine patient sensitivity, 0.25 ml to 1 ml is given into a varicosity 24 hours before administration of a large dose; vial should be warmed before injecting; use a large-bore needle to fill syringe, because solution froths easily; however, a small-bore needle is used for injection; pulmonary embolism has occurred
Sodium tetradecyl sulfate (Sotradecol)	Injection—10 mg/ml, 50 mg/ml	0.5 ml to 2 ml of either strength solution depending on size of varicosity	Initially 0.5 ml of 1% solution should be given to determine patient sensitivity; observe for several hours before giving a larger amount; may *permanently* discolor vein at injection site; do *not* use for injecting veins for cosmetic purposes; caution in patients taking oral anticoagulants

3 Treatment of internal hemorrhoids (effectiveness is not conclusively established)
4 Treatment of esophageal varices (investigational use)

Dosage
See Table 80-6.

Fate
Injected directly into the varicosed vein

Common Side-Effects
Burning and cramping at injection site

Significant Adverse Reactions
Urticaria, tissue sloughing and necrosis; rarely, drowsiness, headache, hypersensitivity reactions (dizziness, weakness, respiratory difficulty, GI upset, vascular collapse, anaphylaxis)

Contraindications
Acute thrombophlebitis, uncontrolled diabetes, sepsis, blood dyscrasia, thyrotoxicosis, tuberculosis, neoplasms, asthma, acute respiratory or skin disease, varicosities due to abdominal or pelvic tumors, bedridden patients, and persistent occlusion of deep veins

▶ **NURSING ALERTS**
▷ 1 Do not use unless deep vein patency is established. Perform a preinjection evaluation for valvular competence and slowly inject a small amount (2 ml) of drug solution into the varicosity.
▷ 2 Avoid intra-arterial injection, because severe ischemia can result.

▶ **NURSING CONSIDERATIONS**
▷ 1 Have emergency measures (*e.g.,* antihistamines, epinephrine, corticosteroids) readily available should an allergic reaction develop.
▷ 2 Use only clear solutions. Avoid extravasation.
▷ 3 Advise patients that following injection the vein will become hard and swollen, and will be tender to the touch. Aching and a feeling of stiffness will usually occur and may persist for 48 hours.

Summary. Miscellaneous Drug Products

Drug	Preparations	Usual Dosage Range
Alprostadil (Prostin VP Pediatric)	Injection—500 mcg/ml	Initially 0.1 mcg/kg/minute until improvement is noted; reduce infusion rate to 0.01 mcg/kg to 0.05 mcg/kg/minute; maximum dose 0.4 mcg/kg/minute
Antidotes	See Table 80-1	
Azathioprine (Imuran)	Tablets—50 mg Injection—100 mg/20 ml	Initially 3 mg to 5 mg/kg/day IV Switch to oral as soon as possible

(continued)

Summary. Miscellaneous Drug Products (continued)

Drug	Preparations	Usual Dosage Range
Bromocriptine (Parlodel)	Tablets—2.5 mg	Usual maintenance dose 1 mg/kg to 2 mg/kg/day Amenorrhea–galactorrhea—2.5 mg 2 to 3 times a day for up to 6 months Postpartum lactation—2.5 mg 2 to 3 times a day for 14 days to 21 days Infertility—initially 2.5 mg once daily; increase to 2 to 3 times/day within the first week Parkinsonism—initially 2.5 mg/day in 2 divided doses; increase every 2 weeks to 4 weeks by 2.5 mg/day
Cyclosporine (Sandimmune)	Oral solution—100 mg/ml IV solution—50 mg/ml	Oral—initially 15 mg/kg/day, 4 hours to 12 hours prior to transplantation; continue for 1 week to 2 weeks postoperatively, then taper by 50%/week to a level of 5 mg/kg to 10 mg/kg/day IV—initially 5 mg/kg to 6 mg/kg/day 4 hours to 12 hours prior to transplantation as a slow IV infusion
Dexpanthenol (Ilopan, Panol, Panthoderm)	Injection—250 mg/ml Tablets—50 mg, with 25 mg choline bitartrate Cream—2% Lotion—2%	IM—250 mg to 500 mg; repeat in 2 hours, then every 6 hours as needed Oral—2 to 3 tablets, 3 times/day Topical—apply 1 to 4 times/day
Dimethyl sulfoxide (Rimso-50)	Solution—50%	Instill 50 ml into the bladder and retain for at least 15 minutes; repeat every 2 weeks or more as needed
Disulfiram (Antabuse)	Tablets—250 mg, 500 mg	Initially 500 mg/day in a single dose for 2 weeks; maintenance range 125 mg to 500 mg/day
Enzyme preparations	See Table 80-2	
Flavoxate (Urispas)	Tablets—100 mg	100 mg to 200 mg 3 to 4 times/day
Metoclopramide (Reglan)	Tablets—10 mg Injection—10 mg/2 ml	Oral: 10 mg 30 minutes before each meal and at bedtime for 2 weeks to 8 weeks IV: Adults—10 mg by slow injection (1 min–2 min) Children (6 yr–14 yr)—2.5 mg to 5 mg Children (under 6 yr)—0.1 mg/kg Prevention of cisplatin-induced vomiting: Initially 2 mg/kg IV infusion over a 15-minute period 30 minutes before cisplatin; repeat every 2 hours for 2 doses, then every 3 hours for 3 doses
Plasma expanders	See Table 80-3	
Plasma protein fractions	See Table 80-4	
Psoralens	See Table 80-5	
Sclerosing agents	See Table 80-6	

Drug Dependence and Addiction

XI

The misuse and abuse of drugs, a part of cultures from the beginnings of recorded medical history, have in recent years reached near epidemic proportions in certain segments of the population and show no signs of abating. Rather, improper use of mind-altering substances, whether legally prescribed or illegally obtained, has risen significantly in the last decade, and it is likely that the incidence of drug abuse will continue to increase in the foreseeable future in spite of the many legal and educational efforts being made to reverse the trend.

Drug abuse is a nebulous term, broadly applied to the use of any drug in a manner that deviates from the generally accepted medicosociological norm. The precise interpretation of this definition, however, is dependent on the variability from culture to culture regarding acceptable behavioral patterns in drug-taking individuals. For example, chronic cigarette smokers are not usually viewed in the same light as chronic narcotic users in terms of drug abuse, yet both forms of behavior may be considered a misuse of a drug substance. Thus, the term *drug abuse* does not necessarily connote legally or socially unacceptable behavior, and therein frequently lies a significant deterrent to its eradication.

Drug abuse has many origins and an equal number of perpetuating factors. Precipitating circumstances include indiscriminate prescribing and inadequate monitoring of psychoactive drugs, emotional instability, peer pressure, and an environment that permits or encourages drug usage. The compulsion to continue one's drug-taking habit may be reinforced by a number of factors, including availability, parental behavior patterns, stressful demands of everyday life, and desire for social acceptance. Drug abuse, therefore, is an extremely complex phenomenon involving environmental, sociological, and psychological aspects.

The discussion that follows focuses primarily on the pharmacology of the various drugs of abuse, and reviews methods for proper recognition and treatment of the drug-intoxicated state. An extensive listing of "street" names of abused drugs is provided at the end of the chapter to acquaint the reader with some of the terminology used by many drug abusers.

A useful, but by no means complete, classification of drugs subject to abuse is as follows:

I. CNS depressants
   A. Alcohol
   B. Barbiturates
   C. Nonbarbiturate sedatives and antianxiety agents
II. CNS stimulants
   A. Amphetamines
   B. Anorectics
   C. Cocaine
III. Narcotics
IV. Psychotomimetics, for example, LSD, DOM, STP, psilocybin, DMT, mescaline
V. Phencyclidine (PCP)
VI. Volatile inhalants, for example, acetone, benzene, trichloroethylene, toluene
VII. Marijuana
VIII. Nicotine

Drugs of Abuse— A Review

81

In discussing the drugs of abuse, frequent reference is made to the various *schedules* in which controlled drugs are categorized. These schedules reflect the different regulations governing the prescribing and dispensing of each agent and the penalties for illegal possession. Descriptions of the various schedules for controlled substances and a listing of drugs in each schedule are found in the appendix.

Before reviewing the pharmacology of abused drugs, it is necessary to briefly describe a few terms that appear throughout the discussion, recognizing, of course, that the following descriptions are by no means complete or universally accepted:

Habituation—a pattern of repeated drug usage, although the actual physical need for the drug is minimal. There is no desire to increase the amount taken and removal of the drug is usually *not* accompanied by withdrawal symptoms, nor by a compulsive need to obtain the drug at any cost.

Tolerance—a reduced effect of a drug resulting from repeated exposure to that particular drug or to a similar drug. The latter condition is also known as cross-tolerance.

Drug dependence—a state of reliance on a drug's effects to such an extent that absence of the drug impairs the ability to function continually in a socially acceptable manner; often interchanged with habituation; two distinct types are recognized:

1 *Psychological dependence*—a compulsive need to experience a pleasurable drug reaction, ranging from a mild desire for the drug on a routine basis to an overwhelming need to have the drug at any cost; very similar to habituation and often used interchangeably; with many drugs, can lead to a more severe type of dependence, namely:

2 *Physical dependence*—an altered physiologic state resulting from prolonged use of a drug; regular drug usage is *necessary* to avoid precipitation of withdrawal reactions that are often severe depending on the drug and duration of use.

Addiction—a vague term that can refer to compulsive drug usage, the necessity of obtaining the drug at any cost, and the appearance of withdrawal symptoms if the drug is unavailable; a *quantitative* term that is usually applied to *severe* habituation or physical dependence.

I CNS Depressants

A Alcohol

Alcohol abuse is the major drug problem in the United States in terms of damaged health, accidents, family strife, business interruptions, and socially unacceptable behavior. The characteristics of acute alcohol intoxication depend largely on the blood level, and range from euphoria and altered judgment (50 mg/dl), to impaired motor coordination, concentration, and memory (100 mg–150 mg/dl), to profound respiratory and cardiovascular depression and coma (300 mg–

400 mg/dl). More insidious and dangerous, however, are the consequences of prolonged alcohol consumption. Chronic alcohol abuse is associated with GI disturbances, liver damage, pancreatitis, neuronal damage, cardiac impairment, malnutrition, and psychotic disturbances. In addition, alcohol in combination with other CNS depressants creates the most frequently observed drug-related hospital emergency and is responsible for more fatalities than any other drug or combination of drugs.

Chronic alcohol ingestion results in development of tolerance and ultimately physical dependence similar to that seen with barbiturates and narcotics. Cessation of alcohol after several weeks of steady consumption may result in tremors, GI disturbances, anxiety, confusion, weakness, insomnia, and possibly delusions. Longer periods of alcohol abuse can, upon abrupt termination, lead to delirium tremens (fever, tachycardia, tremors, profuse sweating), agitation, disorientation, intense hallucinations, and convulsions.

Treatment of acute alcohol withdrawal is largely symptomatic and usually involves use of sedatives or anticonvulsants (*e.g.*, diazepam, barbiturates) or both, along with necessary supportive therapy. Effective management of chronic alcoholism, on the other hand, often requires a combination of supportive social interaction (*e.g.*, Alcoholics Anonymous), psychiatric counseling, and appropriate pharmacotherapy, such as anti-anxiety agents or disulfiram (see Chap. 80).

B Barbiturates

The barbiturates are valuable therapeutic agents for certain indications, for example, induction anesthesia, insomnia, epilepsy, and other acute convulsive states. Members of the drug subculture, however, frequently employ these agents for their anxiety-reducing effects, often to quell the central excitatory action resulting from excessive stimulant abuse. The various barbiturates are classified into either Schedule II, III, or IV, depending on their potency, duration of action, and tendency to produce dependence. The shorter acting drugs (amobarbital, pentobarbital, secobarbital, and combinations thereof) are most sought by abusers, because they produce a degree of euphoria following ingestion. These agents are all Schedule II drugs.

Symptoms of barbiturate intoxication closely resemble those of alcohol intoxication, and depend primarily on the blood level of the drug. Slurred speech, disorientation, impaired motor coordination, poor judgment, confusion, and emotional instability are frequent occurrences with excessive barbiturate usage. Serious overdosage may be associated with decreased respiration, rapid and weak pulse, cyanosis, mydriasis, and ultimately coma and respiratory paralysis. The CNS effects of barbiturates are additive to those of other CNS depressants, and combinations with alcohol or narcotics often prove fatal. Regular barbiturate use reduces the amount of time spent in rapid eye movement (REM) sleep and can lead to irritability and possibly to personality and behavioral changes.

Withdrawal reactions occur upon abrupt termination of excessive barbiturate use, and range from anxiety, weakness, confusion, anorexia, and mild tremors, to delirium, disorientation, hallucinations, and convulsions. Symptoms are generally more severe with the shorter acting derivatives. Management of the withdrawal state is symptomatic. Treatment of chronic barbiturate dependence may be accomplished by substituting phenobarbital for the barbiturate being abused at a dose that initially provides a similar effect, then gradually reducing the phenobarbital dose over a period of weeks.

C   Nonbarbiturate Sedatives and

Antianxiety Agents

Chronic use of a number of other hypnotic, sedative, and antianxiety drugs can result in dependence and an abstinence syndrome resembling that of the barbiturates. Glutethimide, methyprylon, and ethchlorvynol are among the hypnotic drugs employed as barbiturate alternatives, but they offer no significant advantages. Habituation commonly results from their prolonged use. Glutethimide, in particular, is an undesirable agent, inasmuch as convulsions and toxic psychoses have occurred *during* its continued administration; and its long duration of action makes reversal of acute overdosage extremely difficult.

Methaqualone, a Schedule II drug, has been withdrawn from the market but nevertheless remains one of the "street drugs of choice" and is widely abused by a large number of persons. The number of medical emergencies resulting from methaqualone has risen dramatically. Methaqualone is used orally and produces effects resembling those of the barbiturates; in addition, paresthesias are experienced by many persons before the onset of the hypnotic effect. Although acute toxicity is usually not accompanied by severe respiratory and cardiovascular depression, other effects such as convulsions, rigidity, and coma can occur. Prolonged use invariably leads to dependence. A combination of methaqualone and the antihistamine diphenhydramine is marketed in Great Britain as Mandrax, and is a more dangerous preparation than methaqualone alone, because the antihistamine can produce excitation, ataxia, and psychotic behavior in large doses. Withdrawal symptoms noted following cessation of methaqualone use include nausea, headache, cramping, insomnia, and occasionally toxic psychoses and severe convulsions.

Meprobamate is viewed as a minor tranquilizer, and is used mainly for relief of anxiety, tension, and accompanying muscle spasms. It is somewhat less potent than the barbiturates and correspondingly less toxic, although tolerance occurs rather easily and physical dependence has been reported with as little as 3 g/day for several weeks. Meprobamate withdrawal is usually characterized by insomnia, anxiety, and tremors, but can include hallucinations, convulsions, and coma. Fatalities have occurred with meprobamate overdosage.

The benzodiazepines are the most widely used antianxiety drugs, primarily because their margin of safety is greater than with other sedatives or hypnotics. Diazepam is the most frequently prescribed benzodiazepine and is involved in more reported emergency room cases than any other drug, with the exception of alcohol. Although not preferred as "street" drugs, benzodiazepines are frequently misused by patients being treated for anxiety neuroses or other psychosomatic disorders. A principal hazard with these drugs is the possibility of serious intoxication when they are combined with other depressants, most notably alcohol; deaths have resulted from this combination. Prolonged use of the benzodiazepines has resulted in both psychological and physical dependence; abrupt discontinuation of treatment (60 mg–120 mg/day) after 2 months has resulted in the appearance of cramping, sweating, agitation, disorientation, confusion, tremors, depression, auditory and visual hallucinations, and paranoia.

Flurazepam, temazepam, and triazolam are benzodiazepine analogs used for short-term treatment of insomnia, and are claimed to have several advantages over the barbiturates (no hangover, no depression of REM sleep, greater safety margin). They are habituating drugs, nevertheless, and therefore should be accorded the same respect as any other hypnotic agent.

II   CNS Stimulants

A   Amphetamines

The three amphetamines (DL-amphetamine, dextroamphetamine, methamphetamine), as well as the structural analogs phenmetrazine and methylphenidate, are classed as Schedule II drugs. Their approved clinical indications are limited, and currently include *only* treatment of the minimal brain dysfunction syndrome in children, short-term treatment of obesity, and symptomatic control of narcolepsy. They are, however, a widely abused group of drugs, and together with the anorectics (see next discussion) are misused for their CNS-stimulating effects. Students, truck drivers, housewives, executives, athletes, and health professionals (e.g., doctors, nurses, pharmacists) have all employed amphetamines in therapeutic doses to suppress fatigue, increase alertness, enhance psychomotor performance, and generally induce a temporary state of well-being. While potentially hazardous, and in some instances illegal, this type of amphetamine use is usually not labeled abuse. Amphetamine abuse refers to the parenteral or oral administration of large doses of the drugs to attain the intense "rush" or rapid "high" characteristic of these agents. Methamphetamine or "speed" is a favorite among drug abusers, because an IV injection elicits an almost instantaneous euphoria or orgasmic-like reaction. However, tolerance to this effect develops rapidly, so that increasingly larger doses must be administered to experience the same sensation. Whereas normal therapeutic doses are in the 5 mg to 15 mg/day range, "speed freaks" have been known to use as much as 5000 mg/day. Obviously this behavior cannot continue for long, and after a period of several days to, occasionally, weeks, the person becomes exhausted to the point of lapsing into long periods of sleep and depression, the so-called crash.

Symptoms of mild amphetamine intoxication include insomnia, increased blood pressure and pulse rate, excitation, hyperactive reflexes, mydriasis, anorexia, and palpitations. More severe overdosage is reflected by extreme agitation, hostility, impulsiveness, hallucinations, confusion, bizarre behavior, aggressiveness, paranoid ideation, convulsions, and possibly death. The social implications of amphetamine abuse are obvious. Methamphetamine abuse, moreover, can result in cerebral vascular spasm, systemic necrotizing angiitis, cerebral hemorrhaging, arrhythmias, and severe abdominal pain. Effects of acute amphetamine intoxication have been treated with haloperidol, a dopamine antagonist with minimal anticholinergic effects.

Although amphetamines are not believed to induce a true physical dependence, abrupt withdrawal does result in the appearance of fatigue, muscle pain, lethargy, and depression. Withdrawal should be accomplished by allowing the patient to remain in a quiet environment and providing support of vital functions where necessary. Diazepam may be employed if sedation is needed; however, caution must be exercised to avoid adding to the subsequent depression. Acidification of the urine (e.g., with ammonium chloride) markedly increases the excretion of amphetamines, and is frequently used to facilitate their removal. Conversely, the amphetamine "high" can be prolonged by concurrent use of antacids, sodium bicarbonate, or other urinary alkalinizers that slow renal excretion of the drug, and this is a technique commonly used by abusers.

Although the legal production of amphetamines has been sharply curtailed, clandestine laboratories are currently providing vast amounts of these drugs, especially methamphetamine, for the street market. Amphetamine abuse remains a serious sociological and medical problem.

Phenmetrazine, an anorectic, and methylphenidate, a drug principally used in minimal brain dysfunction, are two structurally related compounds classified as Schedule II drugs that possess pharmacologic and toxicologic actions similar to the amphetamines. Although administered orally for their clinical indications, the tablets are frequently dissolved in water by abusers and injected IV. A major danger associated with parenteral use of these drugs is the presence of insoluble particles in the injected solution, which can result in circulatory impairment and talc deposits in the lungs and eye.

B Anorectics

A number of other amphetamine-related drugs termed *anorectics* are employed as adjuncts in the treatment of obesity and are discussed in Chapter 27. Their pharmacology in most cases is similar to that of the amphetamines, but they are less potent CNS stimulants and generally not as desirable as street drugs. They are, however, frequently misused as appetite suppressants, and chronic ingestion of these agents

produces many of the symptoms of prolonged amphetamine use, namely insomnia, elevated blood pressure, tachycardia, and anxiety. Severe overdosage can result in a syndrome resembling amphetamine intoxication; these drugs should never be used continuously for longer than several weeks at a time. Most of these drugs are found in Schedule III, while phentermine and fenfluramine are listed in Schedule IV.

C Cocaine

Cocaine is a natural product extracted from the leaves of the coca plant and has been employed clinically as a local anesthetic, especially for the nose and oral cavity. It is currently a very popular drug of abuse; its systemic effects resemble those of amphetamine, but are of much shorter duration. The powdered drug is most commonly administered by inhalation or "snorting" through the nasal passages, although it has been injected IV as well. Irrespective of its mode of administration, it quickly elicits a pleasurable high that may be accompanied by tachycardia, elevated blood pressure, restlessness, and mydriasis. Cocaine, a Schedule II drug, induces neither tolerance nor classic physical dependence, and there is no characteristic abstinence syndrome upon abrupt withdrawal. However, repeated use can lead to an overwhelming psychological dependence, characterized by an extreme involvement in procuring and using the drug on a daily basis. Because the cost of the illicit drug is quite high, a chronic cocaine habit is a very expensive type of drug abuse. Moreover, the cocaine powder is commonly adulterated with various sugars as well as with local anesthetics at every level of distribution to increase pushers' profits.

Prolonged use of cocaine may result in ulceration and necrosis of the nasal membranes, insomnia, weight loss, nausea, anxiety, irritability, "tactile" hallucinations (i.e., imaginary skin insects or "cocaine bugs"), and visual disturbances (flashing lights, "snow effect").

Overdosage with cocaine can lead to arrhythmias, tremors, convulsions, delirium, paranoia, respiratory complications, and, occasionally, death. Treatment of acute intoxication requires use of sedatives along with appropriate supportive therapy, and must include careful monitoring of cardiovascular and respiratory function.

III Narcotics

The narcotic drugs, both the natural alkaloids of the opium plant (morphine and codeine) as well as the many semisynthetic and synthetic derivatives (see Chap. 18), are widely used for their potent analgesic, antitussive, and antidiarrheal actions. The alleviation of pain induced by these drugs frequently results in a temporary state of euphoria and relief from the accompanying anxiety and is a very pleasurable sensation. However, despite the fact that healthy, well-adjusted persons do not always experience the euphoric effects of opiates, it is precisely the desire to repeat this effect when it occurs that leads to opiate abuse.

Heroin, a Schedule I narcotic, is the most widely abused street opiate, because it is the most potent of the available narcotics. Pure heroin is rarely obtainable, and most illicit heroin usually contains only 1% to 10% active drug, the remainder consisting of fillers such as sugars, starches, or quinine. This variable composition is a major cause of overdosage (*i.e.,* when the percentage of opiate is significantly larger than expected). Most other narcotics are qualitatively if not quantitatively similar in their effects, and are variously classified in Schedule II, III, IV, or V. Other favorite narcotics of abuse are hydromorphone (Dilaudid), a potent, short-acting opiate used either orally or parenterally, and oxycodone, available for oral administration in combination with either aspirin as Percodan or acetaminophen as Percocet.

IV injection of heroin and other potent narcotics results in a sensation of exquisite pleasure, the so-called orgasmic effect or rush, and a feeling of extreme contentment. Oral use of narcotics does not produce the rush, but usually leads to relaxation, euphoria, and a feeling of detachment or indifference to anxiety or pain. Other effects of narcotic drugs unrelated to their abuse potential are miosis, drowsiness, constipation, nausea, vomiting, and depression of vital functions.

Repeated use of narcotics invariably results in tolerance to the pleasurable effects of the drugs, resulting in the compulsion to continually increase the dose. Eventually, a state of physical dependence ensues and the abuser soon *requires* the drug, not to provide the euphoric effect, but to prevent development of withdrawal symptoms. Overdosage leading to respiratory paralysis is a common cause of opiate fatalities, because the dose is pushed to extreme limits in the desire to continue to experience the rush. Other related hazards of narcotic addictions are malnutrition, infections due to unsterile injection equipment and poor hygiene, toxic reactions to contaminants injected along with the narcotic, hepatitis, vasculitis, and thromboembolic complications.

Acute opiate overdosage is marked by stupor, slow and shallow respiration, pinpoint pupils, cold and clammy skin, hypotension, bradycardia, and possibly coma. Treatment involves a narcotic antagonist (naloxone) along with necessary supportive treatment (respiratory assistance, vasopressors). Dosage of the narcotic antagonist must be carefully controlled to avoid precipitation of acute withdrawal symptoms.

When narcotics are unavailable to a physically dependent individual, withdrawal symptoms usually begin within 8 hours to 12 hours, reach a maximum intensity in 36 hours to 72 hours, and can persist for up to 7 days to 10 days. The severity of these symptoms depends on the degree of dependence, a function of the length of time the drugs have been used, and the average amount administered. Initial signs of withdrawal include yawning, perspiration, lacrimation, sneezing, and restlessness. Progressively severe symptoms encompass anorexia, irritability, insomnia, anxiety, vomiting, generalized body aches, stomach cramping, diarrhea, fever, chills, tremors, jerking movements, muscle spasms, tachycardia, and elevated blood pressure. Although frightening to the patient, symptoms experienced during narcotic withdrawal are not usually life-threatening, in contrast to those associated with barbiturate withdrawal, which have resulted in fatalities.

Withdrawal symptoms can be suppressed by administration of another narcotic, frequently oral methadone, in an initial stabilizing amount, 20 mg once or twice a day, then a gradual reduction of the dose. Methadone's long duration of action (up to 24 hr) also permits *single* daily dosing. However, it should be recognized that methadone is also a potent narcotic, and methadone abuse has now become a significant problem as well. Withdrawal from methadone is more prolonged than from opiates, but symptoms are often less severe. Methadone and a newer chemically related compound, levo-alpha-acetylmethadol (LAAM), an even longer acting drug (48 hr–72 hr), are being used for management of narcotic addiction. This procedure involves stabilizing a patient on a regular oral dose of one of the compounds, resulting in development of cross-tolerance to the abused opiate, for example, heroin. Thus, the addict no longer experiences the rush or euphoria characteristic of heroin, and theoretically at least, can now slowly be withdrawn from methadone or LAAM. In reality, however, only a small percentage of narcotic abusers completely overcome their habit, and most either resume their addictive behavior toward heroin or require continual methadone or LAAM administration.

This type of detoxification program works best in conjunction with psychiatric and social counseling. Because the addict's daily behavior is usually structured completely around obtaining and using narcotic drugs, withdrawal alone is rarely entirely successful in overcoming narcotic dependence.

IV Psychotomimetics

Psychotomimetic drugs, often termed *hallucinogens,* are a group of both naturally occurring compounds (such as psilocybin, mescaline) and synthetic compounds (*e.g.,* LSD, DOM) capable of producing profound distortion of reality. Their clinical applications are currently experimental (*e.g.,* as psychiatric aids), and the principal interest in these substances is as drugs of abuse. Psychotomimetics are Schedule I drugs that can cause serious psychological harm to the occasional, as well as the habitual, user. They have the capacity to distort mental function, often resulting in confusion, delirium, amnesia, and a distorted sense of direction, time, and distance. In large doses, delusions and hallucinations are common and seriously impaired judgment and severe depression have frequently resulted from ingestion of these drugs. While the drugs are usually employed in a desire to experience the "pleasant" psychic alterations such as euphoria, elation, vivid color imagery, and synesthesias ("hearing" colors, "seeing" sounds), the psychological state induced by these agents depends on many variables, most importantly the personality and expectations of the user and the environmental situation. Some persons experience the opposite type of effects, such as anxiety, dysphoria, panic, severe depression, despair, and suicidal tendencies, the so-called bad trip. These latter effects tend to occur following ingestion of large doses by inexperienced, nontolerant persons, especially those persons with preexisting psychological disturbances. Unpleasant reactions are also observed more commonly in threatening, hostile, or disturbing surroundings. Treatment of such bad trips may be accomplished by placing the patient in a nonthreatening, supportive environment, and maintaining reassuring verbal contact ("talking down"). Mild sedatives (such as benzodiazepines) are recommended, but use of phenothiazines should be avoided.

Recurrences of the various perceptual distortions are experienced in a large number of psychotomimetic drug users, especially with LSD, and can occur up to a year after the initial usage. These "flashbacks" vary in duration from seconds to minutes, and although occasionally spontaneous, are most frequently triggered by periods of stress or anxiety or by use of other psychotropic drugs, such as marijuana. These flashback episodes may be potentially harmful to the person depending on their severity and place of occurrence.

While a significant degree of tolerance to the behavioral and psychological effects of LSD develops within a short period of time, marked psychological dependence is rare and physical dependence does not occur. There are no characteristic symptoms following abrupt discontinuation of drug usage.

Chronic episodes of psychotic behavior are not uncommon following use of psychotomimetic drugs. Most occur in persons who exhibit underlying emotional instability. The extent to which use of hallucinogens contributes to the protracted disturbed behavior of these people is difficult to assess accurately. Unfortunately, it is just such unstable persons who frequently become involved with use of psychotomimetic agents.

The most commonly used hallucinogens are the following:

▶ LSD

The most potent hallucinogen currently available; effects usually last 8 hours to 12 hours; tolerance develops quickly and effects usually cannot be duplicated for several days; sold as tablets, thin squares of gelatin ("window panes"), or impregnated paper ("blotter acid"); average effective oral dose is 25 mcg to 50 mcg

▶ mescaline

Active ingredient of the flowering heads of the peyote cactus; oral doses of 250 mg–500 mg produce hallucinations lasting 6 hours to 12 hours

▶ DOM

Structural analog of mescaline, also known as STP, an acronym for "serenity, tranquility, and peace;" a potent, synthetic psychotomimetic producing intense, prolonged psychic alterations at a dose of 5 mg, occasionally lasting for several days following a single oral dose; frequently sold on the illicit market as mescaline

▶ DMT

A naturally occurring hallucinogen, N,N-dimethyltryptamine is not effective orally, and must be inhaled or smoked; produces a rapid, brief alteration in perception and mood

▶ psilocybin and psilocyn

Active ingredients of Psilocybe mushrooms, chemically related to LSD, although much less potent and shorter acting; usually administered orally

There are many other substances used for their hallucinogenic effects, many being amphetamine derivatives or centrally acting anticholinergics. One compound in particular, phencyclidine, is chemically related to the dissociative anesthetic ketamine and has become a very dangerous, widely misused drug in the United States. It is discussed separately below.

V   Phencyclidine (PCP)

A Schedule II drug, phencyclidine (PCP, "angel dust") is a potent psychotomimetic that may be the most dangerous of all currently used drugs of abuse. Related to ketamine, PCP has been used as a veterinary anesthetic, but production of the drug was stopped in 1978. Thus, the PCP available on the street is a product of clandestine laboratories, often highly contaminated, and frequently misrepresented as LSD, THC, cocaine, or mescaline. Although occasionally administered orally or IV, it is most often used by smoking or nasal inhalation (snorting), thus allowing the user to regulate more carefully the amount consumed and to reduce the danger of overdosage.

Effects of PCP are dependent on the dose and route of administration. Small amounts elicit euphoria, numbness of the extremities, and a sense of detachment. Larger amounts can result in analgesia, impaired speech, loss of coordination, agitation, muscle rigidity, tachycardia, elevated blood pressure, exaggerated gait, auditory hallucinations, acute anxiety, self-destructive behavior, and severe mood disorders, including paranoia, violent hostility, and feelings of depersonalization or doom. A psychotic state indistinguishable from paranoid schizophrenia is often a result of prolonged use of the drug, but has occurred in some cases after only a single dose. Delayed psychological reactions have been observed for up to several weeks following administration.

Undesirable reactions ("bad trips") have become a significant problem with PCP, and the drug is capable of producing severe behavioral disturbances, frequently prolonged. Treatment of overdosage is best carried out by use of sedatives to control agitation and urinary acidifiers to facilitate excretion, and by isolation of the patient. Verbal contact should be kept to a minimum during the acute recovery stage, which is frequently accompanied by involuntary movements, facial grimacing, torticollis, and catatonic-like posturing. Although usually rapid, recovery can take several days or even weeks, and patients should be kept under close observation during this time.

VI Volatile Inhalants

Volatile hydrocarbons such as acetone, benzene, carbon tetrachloride, trichloroethane, trichloroethylene, and toluene are present in many household products, including glue, paint, lighter fluid, nail polish remover, and varnish thinner, and are frequently abused by young persons. These volatile liquids are commonly placed on a rag or handkerchief or in a bag, and inhaled. The initial effects are CNS excitation, characterized by a sense of exhilaration, dizziness, and occasionally auditory or visual hallucinations, accompanied by tinnitus, blurred vision, slurred speech, and a staggering gait. These effects generally last 30 minutes to 60 minutes. Larger amounts of inhaled vapors can lead to drowsiness, hypotension, delirium, stupor, unconsciousness, and possibly coma. Amnesia frequently follows recovery. Fatalities have resulted, either from drug-induced respiratory failure or due to suffocation from the plastic bags placed over the face. Cardiac arrest has also been reported.

Psychological dependence can develop, but physical dependence is rare, primarily due to the rather brief duration of action. Chronic misuse of volatile hydrocarbons can result in significant organ damage, especially to the liver, kidneys, heart, and CNS, and it is this dangerous aspect of volatile inhalant abuse that is frequently overlooked by youthful users.

Treatment of acute intoxication resembles that of barbiturate overdosage, and employs oxygen and respiratory assistance along with other supportive care as needed. Injections of vasopressors (such as epinephrine) should be avoided, however, due to the danger of myocardial sensitization by the volatile hydrocarbon, resulting in precipitation of arrhythmias in the presence of adrenergic amines.

VII Marijuana

Marijuana is obtained from the hemp plant, *Cannabis sativa,* and constitutes a mixture of dried leaves, flowering tops, and other parts of the plant. The biologically active constituents of marijuana are termed *cannabinoids* and among the more than 60 known compounds, delta-9-tetrahydrocannabinol (THC) appears to be the major psychoactive derivative. Marijuana may be administered orally, but it is several times more potent when the powder is rolled loosely

into cigarettes ("joints") and smoked. Depending on the potency, peak psychopharmacologic effects occur within 10 minutes to 20 minutes of inhalation and persist for 1 hour to 4 hours. The average "joint" contains between 2% and 4% THC (approximately 10 mg–20 mg), of which approximately one half is usually absorbed.

The psychic and perceptual effects of marijuana vary widely among individuals, and depend on the mental status, mood, previous experience, and expectations of the users, as well as the environment and circumstances surrounding its use. Typical psychic reactions include a sense of relaxation and well-being, perhaps even euphoria, impaired time and space orientation, altered sensory perception (especially sound and color), and spontaneous, often uncontrolled laughter. Short-term memory may be affected, psychomotor performance may be somewhat impaired, and attention span can be reduced. Although reflexive driving ability does not appear to be markedly compromised, perceptual difficulties can prove hazardous to a person behind the wheel. Large doses may result in image distortion, depersonalization, disorganized thought and speech, fantasies, and, rarely, hallucinations.

Physiologic changes accompanying marijuana usage can include elevated pulse rate and conjunctival congestion, which occur routinely, and erythema, enhanced appetite, disturbed equilibrium, xerostomia, oropharyngeal irritation, tinnitus, paresthesias, and vomiting, all of which may or may not be present.

Adverse reactions may appear to be minimal with occasional use in emotionally stable persons. Reported untoward reactions to marijuana comprise mild depression, anxiety, agitation, and a "panic" state, most frequently observed in first-time users. Acute intoxication from high doses (toxic psychosis) is manifested by hallucinations, severe agitation, and paranoia, and usually resolves within 24 hours. It is seen most frequently in patients prone to schizophrenia. THC can disrupt pituitary production of gonadotropic hormones, crosses the placental barrier, and is excreted in breast milk; these actions strongly suggest that pregnant and lactating women should refrain from marijuana use.

Prolonged usage of marijuana has been implicated in pulmonary toxicity (precancerous cellular changes), suppression of cellular-mediated immune responsiveness, and personality and behavioral changes. Severe psychic disturbances, however, occur primarily in persons with preexisting emotional disorders.

Chronic use of marijuana may result in psychological dependence, but physical dependence is rare. A phenomenon of "reverse" tolerance has been reported in some marijuana users, whereby smaller amounts of the drug are able to elicit the desired psychic effects with repeated administration. This may be due in part to cumulation effects of the drug with frequent usage.

Although acute overdosage with marijuana is rare, episodes can be managed by appropriate support of respiration, blood pressure, and other vital functions as required. A quiet environment and reassuring attitude is quite helpful during the acute psychotic phase, and extreme agitation is best treated with benzodiazepines such as diazepam.

Although marijuana and its active constituents are Schedule I drugs, their potential clinical applications are receiving much attention. Two areas of potential therapeutic benefit for the cannabinoids, especially THC, are the control of nausea and vomiting produced by chemotherapeutic agents and reduction of elevated intraocular pressure in glaucoma. Other properties of THC currently being investigated for possible clinical use are its analgesic, anti-inflammatory, tranquilizing, bronchodilatory, and anticonvulsant actions.

The resinous secretions from the flowering tops of the cannabis plant are also available as hashish. These secretions are usually dried and then either smoked or compressed into a variety of other dosage forms, such as cookies, cakes, or candies. While hashish ranges in potency depending upon the source, it is generally between 5 and 10 times more potent than marijuana itself. Hashish oil, a concentrated liquid extract of Cannabis plant materials, contains a high percentage of THC (10%–50%) and several drops are equivalent to a single "joint" of marijuana. Hashish oil has also been administered IV, but this procedure is associated with a significant mortality rate.

VIII Nicotine

Nicotine is an alkaloid found in tobacco in a concentration usually between 1% and 2%. It is rapidly absorbed by the lungs and has a mild central stimulatory effect. At the same time, there is decreased skeletal muscle tone, reduced appetite, and, in naive users, occasionally nausea, vomiting, dizziness, and irritability. Tolerance usually develops to these latter effects, but is of a very variable nature and duration. Withdrawal is not a clearly established phenomenon, but cessation of nicotine usage can result in nausea, diarrhea, increased appetite, headache, drowsiness, insomnia, irritability, and poor concentration. Following extended abstinence, blood pressure and heart rate decrease, peripheral blood flow increases, and respiratory difficulties are reduced, but weight gain is common, because food is often used as a substitute form of oral gratification. Gradual reduction in nicotine consumption is usually less effective over the long term than abrupt cessation.

The other major risk factors associated with cigarette smoking (bronchogenic carcinoma, coronary artery disease, emphysema, and other chronic pulmonary disorders) cannot be exclusively linked to the nicotine content of the tobacco, but probably result from constant exposure to the many other products of combustion inhaled as well in cigarette smoke.

Glossary of "Street Names" for Drugs of Abuse

Acapulco Gold	Marijuana
Acid	LSD
Angel Dust	Phencyclidine
Beans	Amphetamines
Bennies	Amphetamines
Big H	Heroin
Black Beauties	Amphetamines
Black Mollies	Amphetamines

Glossary of "Street Names" for Drugs of Abuse (continued)

Blockbusters	Barbiturates
Blotter Acid	LSD
Blow	Cocaine
Bluebirds	Barbiturates
Blue Devils	Barbiturates
Blues	Barbiturates
Boy	Heroin
Brown	Heroin
Brownies	Amphetamines
Brown Sugar	Heroin
Buttons	Peyote
C	Cocaine
Caballo	Heroin
Cactus	Peyote
California Sunshine	LSD
Cannabis	Marijuana
Charley	Cocaine
Christmas Tree	Barbiturates
Chiva	Heroin
Coca	Cocaine
Coke	Cocaine
Colombian	Marijuana
Copilots	Amphetamines
Crank	Methamphetamine
Crap	Heroin
Crossroads	Amphetamines
Crystal	Methamphetamine, phencyclidine
Cube	Morphine, LSD
Cubes	LSD
Cyclone	Phencyclidine
Dexies	Dextroamphetamine
Dillies	Dilaudid
Dollies	Methadone
Double Cross	Amphetamines
Downers	Barbiturates
Estuffa	Heroin
First Line	Morphine
Flake	Cocaine
Footballs	Amphetamines
Ganga	Marijuana
Girl	Cocaine
Goma	Morphine
Grass	Marijuana
Green Dragons	Barbiturates
Griffa	Marijuana
H	Heroin
Hash	Hashish
Haze	LSD
Hazel	Heroin
Hearts	Dextroamphetamine
Heaven Dust	Cocaine
Hemp	Marijuana
Herb	Marijuana
Hero	Heroin
Hog	Phencyclidine, chloral hydrate
Hombre	Heroin
J	Marijuana
Jay	Marijuana
Joint	Marijuana
Junk	Heroin
Lady	Cocaine
Log	Marijuana
Mary Jane	Marijuana
Mesc	Peyote, mescaline
Mescal	Peyote
Meth	Methamphetamine
Mexican Mud	Heroin
Mexican Reds	Barbiturates, secobarbital
Microdots	LSD

Glossary of "Street Names" for Drugs of Abuse
(continued)

Minibennies	Amphetamines
Morf	Morphine
Morpho	Morphine
Morphy	Morphine
Mota	Marijuana
Mud	Morphine
Mujer	Cocaine
Mutah	Marijuana
Nebbies	Barbiturates, pentobarbital
Nimbies	Barbiturates, pentobarbital
Nose Candy	Cocaine
Oranges	Amphetamines
Panama Red	Marijuana
Paper Acid	LSD
Paradise	Cocaine
PCP	Phencyclidine
Peace Pill	Phencyclidine
Pep Pills	Amphetamines
Perico	Cocaine
Pink Ladies	Barbiturates
Pinks	Barbiturates, secobarbital
Polvo	Heroin
Polvo Blanco	Cocaine
Pot	Marijuana
Purple Haze	LSD
Quacks	Methaqualone
Quads	Methaqualone
Rainbows	Barbiturates, Tuinal
Red and Blues	Barbiturates, Tuinal
Redbirds	Barbiturates, secobarbital
Red Devils	Barbiturates, secobarbital
Reds	Barbiturates, Tuinal
Reefer	Marijuana
Roach	Marijuana

Glossary of "Street Names" for Drugs of Abuse
(continued)

Rock	Cocaine
Rocket Fuel	Phencyclidine
Roses	Amphetamines
Sativa	Marijuana
Scag	Heroin
Sleeping Pills	Barbiturates
Smack	Heroin
Smoke	Marijuana
Snow	Cocaine
Soapers	Methaqualone
Soles	Hashish
Sopes	Methaqualone
Sparklers	Amphetamines
Speed	Methamphetamine
Stick	Marijuana
Stumblers	Barbiturates
Stuff	Heroin
Sunshine	LSD
Supergrass	Phencyclidine
T's and Blues	Pentazocine and tripelennamine
Tea	Marijuana
THC	Tetrahydrocannabinol
Thing	Heroin
Thrusters	Amphetamines
Tic Tac	Phencyclidine
Truck Drivers	Amphetamines
Uppers	Amphetamines
Wake-ups	Amphetamines
Wedges	LSD
Weed	Marijuana
Whites	Amphetamines
Window Panes	LSD
Yellow Jackets	Barbiturates, pentobarbital
Yellows	Barbiturates, pentobarbital

Appendix

XII

Since the enactment of the first federal drug law in 1906, the Pure Food and Drug Act, Congress has passed more than 50 pieces of legislation pertaining to the control and distribution of drugs. Except for the Durham–Humphrey amendment to the Federal Food, Drug, and Cosmetic Act of 1938, which restricted certain drugs to a "prescription only" status, the previous drug laws were all repealed by the passage on May 1, 1971, of the Comprehensive Drug Abuse Prevention and Control Act of 1970. This piece of legislation, commonly referred to as the Controlled Substances Act, was designed to control the manufacturing, distribution, administration, and disposition of narcotics, depressants, stimulants, and other drugs with an abuse potential as designated by the Drug Enforcement Administration (DEA).

Among its many provisions, the Controlled Substances Act classified the various drugs subject to abuse into one of five *Schedules* according to their medical usefulness and potential for abuse. The drugs comprising the various schedules are given in the accompanying list. Regulations governing each group of drugs are as follows:

Schedule I

Drugs in Schedule I have a *high* abuse potential and *no accepted* medical use in the United States. They are not available for routine prescription use, but may be obtained for investigational studies by proper application to the Drug Enforcement Administration.

Schedule II

Drugs in Schedule II have valid medical indications, but exhibit a *high* abuse potential. Misuse of these substances can lead to profound psychological and physical dependence.

Schedule III

Drugs in Schedule III have a potential for abuse less than those in Schedule I or II; however, misuse can still lead to moderate to low physical dependence and rather high psychological dependence.

Schedule IV

Drugs in Schedule IV have a lower abuse potential than Schedule III drugs. Misuse most often results in varying degrees of psychological dependence, with occasional reports of limited physical dependence.

Schedule V

Schedule V drugs consist mainly of preparations containing moderate amounts of opioid drugs, generally for antitussive or antidiarrheal use. Their abuse potential is less than Schedule IV drugs.

Each commercial container of a controlled substance bears on its label a symbol designating the schedule to which it belongs. Symbols are a large red "C," either enclosing or followed by the Roman numeral I through V referring to the schedule to which the drug belongs.

Drug Legislation and Regulations

Dispensing Controlled Substances

The requirements for dispensing a controlled drug outlined below are the currently mandated federal regulations. However, it should be stressed that in many instances, individual *state* laws are more stringent than the *federal* law, and must be observed by all practitioners within a particular state. Persons handling controlled substances must therefore acquaint themselves with those specific state regulations, if any, that supersede the federal law.

All prescription orders for Schedule II drugs must be either typewritten or written in ink or indelible pencil and signed by the physician. No prescriptions for Schedule II drugs may be refilled and all records and inventory information must be maintained separately from the other pharmacy records. A triplicate order form is necessary for ordering Schedule II drugs. Under certain emergency situations outlined below, a Schedule II drug may be dispensed upon oral authorization.

Orders for Schedule III, IV, and those Schedule V drugs requiring a prescription (see below) may be issued either orally or in writing and may be refilled up to five times within 6 months of the original prescription date if so authorized by the physician. Oral prescription orders must be immediately committed to writing. Prescriptions for drugs in Schedule III, IV, or V must be readily retrievable from the files, and if these controlled substances prescriptions are filed with the remainder of the prescription orders (except Schedule II drugs), each prescription for a Schedule III, IV, or V drug must be marked with the letter "C" in red ink to facilitate retrieval. Records must be maintained for at least 2 years.

Each time a prescription for a Schedule III, IV, or V drug is refilled, the date and amount of drug dispensed must be noted on the back of the order blank and initialed by the dispenser. The label of any controlled drug in Schedule II, III, or IV must contain the following statement: "Caution: Federal law prohibits the transfer of this drug to any person other than the patient for whom it was prescribed."

Nonprescription Dispensing

of Schedule V Drugs

Certain Schedule V preparations may be dispensed without a prescription providing the following conditions are met:

1 The dispensing is made only by a pharmacist or pharmacist–intern.

2 The purchaser is at least 18 years of age (proof of age is necessary if the purchaser is unknown to the dispenser)

3 Not more than 240 ml or not more than 48 solid dosage units of any substance containing opium, nor more than 120 ml or not more than 24 solid dosage units of any other controlled substance may be distributed to the same purchaser within 48 hours.

4 The name and address of the purchaser, kind and quantity of substance purchased, date of sale, and pharmacist's initials must be recorded for each sale in a Schedule V record book and records maintained for 2 years.

State and local laws often are more stringent with respect to retail distribution of Schedule V substances, and must be observed in lieu of the federal law.

Partial Distribution of Controlled Substances

If the full quantity of a Schedule II drug cannot be supplied with the original prescription order, the remaining portion may be dispensed within 72 hours provided the quantity dispensed with the initial order is noted on the face of the written prescription. Additional partial quantities may not be supplied beyond the 72-hour time limit except on a new prescription order.

Partial dispensing of Schedule III and IV drugs is allowed provided the quantity dispensed is noted on the back of the prescription order. The balance of the partial quantities dispensed may not exceed the total amount authorized (*i.e.*, original quantity plus allowable refills), nor extend past the 6-month time limit.

Emergency Dispensing of Schedule II Drugs

In the event of an emergency situation, a Schedule II controlled substance can be dispensed upon oral authorization provided certain conditions are satisfied. An emergency situation is defined as one in which:

1 *Immediate* administration of the drug is necessary for proper treatment.

2 No appropriate alternative treatment is available.

3 A written prescription cannot reasonably be provided by the prescribing physician before the drug is required.

The provisions for dispensing a Schedule II drug under an emergency situation are as follows:

1 Quantity dispensed must be limited to the amount necessary to treat the patient during the emergency period.

2 Prescription order must be reduced to writing immediately.

3 All efforts to verify the identity of the prescriber should be made, in the event that he is not known to the dispenser.

4 A written prescription with the notation "Authorization for Emergency Dispensing" must be delivered to the dispenser within 72 hours of the oral authorization, or, if mailed, postmarked within 72 hours.

A practitioner (physician, dentist, veterinarian) must apply for permission to dispense controlled drugs by registering with the Drug Enforcement Administration and, upon approval, receives a 7-digit registration number (DEA number) that must appear on every order for controlled substances. This registration must be renewed annually. Likewise, every pharmacy that dispenses controlled drugs must register annually with the Drug Enforcement Administration, and their DEA number must be available for inspection at the location of business.

Schedules of Controlled Drugs

Schedule I

Benzylmorphine
Cannabinols, *e.g.,* hashish, marijuana, tetrahydrocannabinol
Dihydromorphine
Hallucinogens, *e.g.,* bufotenin, DET, DMT, DOB, DOM, ibogaine, LSD, MDA, mescaline, peyote, PMA, psilocybin, psilocyn
Ketobemidone
Levomoramide
Nicocodeine
Nicomorphine
Racemoramide

Schedule II

Depressants

Amobarbital
Methaqualone
Pentobarbital
Phencyclidine
Secobarbital

Narcotics

Alphaprodine
Codeine
Etorphine
Fentanyl
Hydromorphone
Levorphanol
Meperidine
Methadone
Opium and opium alkaloids *e.g.,* morphine and codeine
Oxycodone
Oxymorphone
Phenazocine

Stimulants

Amphetamine
Coca leaves
Cocaine
Dextroamphetamine
Methamphetamine
Methylphenidate
Phenmetrazine

Schedule III

Depressants

Aprobarbital
Butabarbital
Chlorhexadol
Glutethimide
Hexobarbital

Schedule III (*continued*)

Metharbital
Methyprylon
Talbutal
Thiamylal
Thiopental

Narcotics

Opiates in combination with other non-narcotic drugs, *e.g.,* Empirin with Codeine, Tylenol with Codeine, Hycodan
Paregoric
Nalorphine (narcotic antagonist)

Stimulants

Benzphetamine
Chlorphentermine
Chlortermine
Mazindol
Phendimetrazine

Schedule IV

Depressants

Barbital
Benzodiazepines (alprazolam, chlordiazepoxide, clonazepam, clorazepate, diazepam, flurazepam, halazepam, lorazepam, oxazepam, prazepam, temazepam, triazolam)
Chloral hydrate
Ethchlorvynol
Ethinamate
Meprobamate
Mephobarbital
Methohexital
Paraldehyde
Phenobarbital

Narcotics

Pentazocine
Propoxyphene

Stimulants

Diethylpropion
Fenfluramine
Pemoline
Phentermine

Schedule V

Diphenoxylate and atropine (*e.g.,* Lomotil)
Loperamide
Narcotic drugs in combination with other non-narcotic agents, generally used as antitussives, where the amount of narcotic (*e.g.,* codeine, dihydrocodeine) is limited. See above discussion.

Abbreviations

aa	of each (equal parts)	mg	milligram
ac	before meals	ml	milliliter
ad	up to	no	number
ad lib	as desired	non rep (NR)	no refill
aq (dest)	water (distilled)	noct	night
aur (a)	ear	O	pint
au	each (both) ear (s)	od	right eye *or* every day
ad	right ear	oh	every hour
as	left ear	os	mouth
bid	twice a day	os	left eye
c̄	with	ou	each eye
caps	capsule	oz	ounce
comp	compound	pc	after meals
d	day *or* right	po	by mouth
dil	dilute	prn	as needed
disp	dispense	pulv	powder
dr	dram	q	every
dtd	dispense such doses	qid	4 times a day
		qod	every other day
elix	elixir	qs	a sufficient quantity
et	and	R$_x$	recipe (take)
ext	extract	rep	repeat
F (ft)	make	s̄	without
fl	fluid	s̄s̄	half
g (gm)	gram	Sig (S)	(write on) label
gr	grain	sol	solution
gtt (s)	drop (s)	stat	immediately
h	hour	supp	suppository
hs	bedtime (hour of sleep)	syr	syrup
		tab	tablet
IM	intramuscular	tid	3 times a day
IV	intravenous	tinct (tr)	tincture
L	liter	ung	ointment
M	mix	ut dict (UD)	as directed
m$_x$	minim		

References

Pharmacology

Abrams AC: Clinical Drug Therapy—Rationales for Nursing Practice. Philadelphia, JB Lippincott, 1983

Albanese JA: Nurses' Drug Reference, 2nd ed. New York, McGraw-Hill, 1982

Albanese JA, Bond T: Drug Interactions: Basic Principles and Clinical Problems. New York, McGraw-Hill, 1978

Annual Review of Pharmacology. Palo Alto, CA, Annual Reviews, Inc.

Asperheim MK, Eisenhauer LA: The Pharmacologic Basis of Patient Care. Philadelphia, WB Saunders, 1981

Avery GS (ed): Drug Treatment, 2nd ed. Littleton, MA, Publishing Sciences Group, 1980

Barber JM: Handbook of Emergency Pharmacology. St Louis, CV Mosby, 1978

Beeson PB, McDermott W, Wyngaarden J (eds): Cecil-Loeb Textbook of Medicine, 15th ed. Philadelphia, WB Saunders, 1979

Bevan JA, Thompson JH (eds): Essentials of Pharmacology, 3rd ed. Philadelphia, Harper & Row, 1983

Bowman WC, Rand MJ: Textbook of Pharmacology, 2nd ed. Oxford, England, Blackwell Scientific Publications, 1980

Brunner LS, Suddarth DS: Textbook of Medical-Surgical Nursing, 5th ed. Philadelphia, JB Lippincott, 1984

Clark JB, Queener SF, Karb VB: Pharmacological Basis of Nursing Practice. St Louis, CV Mosby, 1982

Cooper JR, Bloom FE, Roth RH: The Biochemical Basis of Neuropharmacology, 4th ed. New York, Oxford University Press, 1982

DiPalma JR (ed): Drill's Pharmacology in Medicine, 4th ed. New York, McGraw-Hill, 1971

Eisenhauer LA, Gerald MC: The Nurse's Guide to Drug Therapy. Englewood Cliffs, NJ, Prentice-Hall, 1984

Facts and Comparisons. Philadelphia, JB Lippincott (updated monthly)

Feldman RS, Quenzer LF: Fundamentals of Neuropsychopharmacology. Sunderland, MA, Sinauer Associates, 1984

Gahart BL: Intravenous Medications, 3rd ed. St Louis, CV Mosby, 1981

Gilman AG, Goodman LS, Gilman A (eds): The Pharmacological Basis of Therapeutics, 6th ed. New York, Macmillan, 1980

Goth A: Medical Pharmacology, 10th ed. St Louis, CV Mosby, 1981

Govoni LE, Hayes JE: Drugs and Nursing Implications, 4th ed. New York, Appleton-Century-Crofts, 1982

Hahn AB, Barkin RL, Oestreich SJ: Pharmacology in Nursing, 15th ed. St Louis, CV Mosby, 1982

Handbook of Nonprescription Drugs, 7th ed. Washington, DC, American Pharmaceutical Association, 1982

Howry LB, Bindler RM, Tso Y: Pediatric Medications. Philadelphia, JB Lippincott, 1981

Irons PD: Psychotropic Drugs and Nursing Intervention. New York, McGraw-Hill, 1978

Iversen SD, Iversen LL: Behavioral Pharmacology, 2nd ed. New York, Oxford University Press, 1981

Johns MP: Drug Therapy and Nursing Care. New York, Macmillan, 1979

Katzung BC (ed): Basic and Clinical Pharmacology 2nd ed. Los Altos, CA, Lange Medical Publications, 1984

Long JW: The Essential Guide to Prescription Drugs, 3rd ed. New York, Harper & Row, 1982

Martin EW: Hazards of Medication, 2nd ed. Philadelphia, JB Lippincott, 1978

The Medical Letter on Drugs and Therapeutics. New Rochelle, NY, Medical Letter, Inc. (biweeky)

Melmon KL, Morrelli HF (eds): Clinical Pharmacology, 2nd ed. New York, Macmillan, 1978

Modell W, Schild HO, Wilson A: Applied Pharmacology. Philadelphia, WB Saunders, 1976

Physicians' Desk Reference, 38th ed. Oradell, NJ, Medical Economics, 1984

Poe WD, Holloway DA: Drugs and the Aged. New York, McGraw-Hill, 1980

Rodman MJ, Karch AM, Boyd EH: Pharmacology and Drug Therapy in Nursing, 3rd ed. Philadelphia, JB Lippincott, 1985

Russell H: Pediatric Drugs and Nursing Intervention. New York, McGraw-Hill, 1980

Sager DP, Bomar SK: Intravenous Medications. Philadelphia, JB Lippincott, 1980

Schmidt RM, Margolin S: Harper's Handbook of Therapeutic Pharmacology. Philadelphia, Harper & Row, 1981

Spencer RT, Nichols LW, Waterhouse HP et al: Clinical Pharmacology and Nursing Management. Philadelphia, JB Lippincott, 1983

United States Pharmacopeia Dispensing Information. St Louis, CV Mosby, 1984

Wiener MB, Pepper GA, Kuhn-Weisman G et al: Clinical Pharmacology and Therapeutics in Nursing. New York, McGraw-Hill, 1979

Physiology

Annual Review of Physiology. Palo Alto, CA, Annual Reviews, Inc.

Chaffee EE, Lytle IM: Basic Physiology and Anatomy, 4th ed. Philadelphia, JB Lippincott, 1980

Ganong WF: Review of Medical Physiology, 10th ed. Los Altos, CA, Lange Medical Publications, 1981

Guyton AC: Human Physiology and Mechanisms of Disease, 3rd ed. Philadelphia, WB Saunders, 1982

Guyton AC: Textbook of Medical Physiology, 6th ed. Philadelphia, WB Saunders, 1981

Hole JW: Human Anatomy and Physiology, 3rd ed. Dubuque, IA, WC Brown, 1984

Jensen D: The Principles of Physiology, 2nd ed. New York, Appleton-Century-Crofts, 1980

Selkurt EE: Basic Physiology for the Health Sciences, 2nd ed. Boston, Little, Brown & Co, 1982

Spence AP, Mason EB: Human Anatomy and Physiology, 2nd ed. Menlo Park, CA, Benjamin/Cummings, 1983

Tortora GJ: Principles of Human Anatomy, 3rd ed. New York, Harper & Row, 1983

Tortora GJ, Evans RL, Anagnostakos NP: Principles of Human Physiology. New York, Harper & Row, 1982

Vander AJ, Sherman JH, Luciano DS: Human Physiology: The Mechanisms of Body Function, 3rd ed. New York, McGraw-Hill, 1980

Index

Drugs are listed by both generic and proprietary names in the following manner: generic (proprietary) and proprietary (generic). Names within parentheses are generic if not capitalized and proprietary if capitalized. Numbers followed by *t* indicate tables; numbers followed by *f* indicate figures.